DERMATOTOXICOLOGY

[6TH EDITION]

DERMATOTOXICOLOGY

[6TH EDITION]

EDITED BY

HONGBO ZHAI AND HOWARD I. MAIBACH

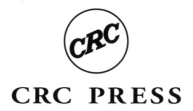

CRC PRESS

Boca Raton   London   New York   Washington, D.C.

Library of Congress Cataloging-in-Publication Data

Catalog record is available from the Library of Congress

Visit the CRC Press Web site at www.crcpress.com

Dermatotoxicology
Sixth Edition

CONTRIBUTORS xiii
FOREWORD FROM THE FIFTH EDITION xxi
PREFACE TO THE SIXTH EDITION xxv

PART I
Concepts

CHAPTER 1

Skin Permeability 3
Ronald C. Wester and Howard I. Maibach

CHAPTER 2

Occlusion and Barrier Function 13
Hongbo Zhai and Howard I. Maibach

CHAPTER 3

Percutaneous Absorption of Complex Chemical Mixtures 29
Jim E. Riviere

CHAPTER 4

Anatomical Factors Affecting Barrier Function 43
Nancy A. Monteiro-Riviere

CHAPTER 5

Percutaneous Absorption: Role of Lipids 71
Philip W. Wertz

CHAPTER 6

Percutaneous Absorption: Short-Term Exposure, Lag Time,
Multiple Exposures, Model Variations, and Absorption
from Clothing 83
Ronald C. Wester and Howard I. Maibach

CHAPTER 7

Chemical Partitioning into Powdered Human Stratum
Corneum: A Useful *In Vitro* Model for Studying Interaction
of Chemical and Human Skin 105
*Xiaoying Hui, Ronald C. Wester, Hongbo Zhai
and Howard I. Maibach*

CHAPTER 8

Sensitive Skin 123
Harald Löffler, Jún Aramaki, Isaak Effendy and Howard I. Maibach

CHAPTER 9

Transdermal Drug Delivery System — An Overview 137
Cheryl Levin and Howard I. Maibach

CHAPTER 10

Iontophoresis 151
Angela N. Anigbogu and Howard I. Maibach

CHAPTER 11

Irritant Dermatitis (Irritation) 181
Sara Weltfriend, Michal Ramon and Howard I. Maibach

CHAPTER 12

Allergic Contact Dermatitis 229
Francis N. Marzulli and Howard I. Maibach

CHAPTER 13

Irritant Contact Dermatitis versus Allergic Contact
Dermatitis 237
Iris S. Ale and Howard I. Maibach

CHAPTER 14

Molecular Basis of Allergic Contact Dermatitis 265
Jean-Pierre Lepoittevin and Valérie Berl

CHAPTER 15

Systemic Contact Dermatitis 285
Niels K. Veien, Torkil Menné and Howard I. Maibach

CHAPTER 16

Permeability of Human Skin to Metals and Paths
for Their Diffusion 321
Jurij J. Hostýnek

CHAPTER 17

Photoirritation (Phototoxicity, Phototoxic Dermatitis) 341
Francis N. Marzulli and Howard I. Maibach

CHAPTER 18

Chemically Induced Scleroderma 353
Glenn G. Russo

CHAPTER 19

Chemical Agents that Cause Depigmentation 375
Leslie P. McCarty and Howard I. Maibach

CHAPTER 20

Sulfur Mustard: A Chemical Vesicant Model 389
*Frederick R. Sidell, William J. Smith, John P. Petrali
and Charles G. Hurst*

CHAPTER 21

Carcinogenesis: Current Trends in Skin Cancer Research 409
Karen J. Auborn

CHAPTER 22

Retinoids and Their Mechanisms of Toxicity 419
William J. Cunningham and Graeme F. Bryce

CHAPTER 23

Skin Disorders Caused by Cosmetics in China 441
Shaoxi Wu, Ningru Guo, Weili Pan and Zheng Min

CHAPTER 24

Drug Induced Ocular Phototoxicity 449
Joan E. Roberts

CHAPTER 25

Water: Is It an Irritant? 471
Tsen-fang Tsai and Howard I. Maibach

CHAPTER 26

Sodium Lauryl Sulfate in Dermatotoxicology 479
Cheol Heon Lee and Howard I. Maibach

CHAPTER 27

Barrier Creams 507
Hongbo Zhai and Howard I. Maibach

PART II

Methods

CHAPTER 28

Methods for *In Vitro* Percutaneous Absorption 519
Robert L. Bronaugh

CHAPTER 29

Tape Stripping Method and Stratum Corneum 531
Myeong Jun Choi, Hongbo Zhai and Howard I. Maibach

CHAPTER 30

Percutaneous Absorption of Hazardous Substances
from Soil and Water 549
Ronald C. Wester and Howard I. Maibach

CHAPTER 31

Isolated Perfused Porcine Skin Flap 563
Jim E. Riviere

CHAPTER 32

Physiologically Based Pharmacokinetic Modeling 589
James N. McDougal

CHAPTER 33

Methods for *In Vitro* Skin Metabolism Studies 621
Robert L. Bronaugh

CHAPTER 34

Transdermal Drug Delivery Systems: Dermatologic
and Other Adverse Reactions 631
Cheryl Levin and Howard I. Maibach

CHAPTER 35

Predictive Toxicology Methods for Transdermal
Delivery Systems 653
*Anne Chester, Wei-Qi Lin, Mary Prevo, Michel Cormier
and James Matriano*

CHAPTER 36

Animal, Human, and *In Vitro* Test Methods for
Predicting Skin Irritation 677
Cheryl Levin and Howard I. Maibach

CHAPTER 37

Analysis of Structural Change in Intercellular Lipids
of Human Stratum Corneum Induced by Surfactants:
Electron Paramagnetic Resonance (EPR) Study 695
*Yoshiaki Kawasaki, Jun-ichi Mizushima
and Howard I. Maibach*

CHAPTER 38

Test Methods for Allergic Contact Dermatitis in Animals 725
Georg Klecak

CHAPTER 39

Test Methods for Allergic Contact Dermatitis in Humans 763
Francis N. Marzulli and Howard I. Maibach

CHAPTER 40

Immunoadjuvants in Prospective Testing for Contact
Allergens 775
Henry C. Maguire, Jr.

CHAPTER 41

The Local Lymph Node Assay 793
*Ian Kimber, David A. Basketter, G. Frank Gerberick
and Rebecca J. Dearman*

CHAPTER 42

Contact Urticaria and the Contact Urticaria Syndrome
(Immediate Contact Reactions) 817
Smita Amin, Arto Lahti and Howard I. Maibach

CHAPTER 43

An Optimized *In Vitro* Approach to Assess Skin Irritation
and Phototoxicity of Topical Vehicles 849
Bart De Wever, Martin Rosdy and Alan M. Goldberg

CHAPTER 44

Photoirritation (Phototoxicity) Testing in Humans 871
Francis N. Marzulli and Howard I. Maibach

CHAPTER 45

Measuring and Quantifying Ultraviolet Radiation Exposure 879
David H. Sliney

CHAPTER 46

Use of Pig Skin Preparations in Novel Diffusion Cell Arrays
to Measure Skin Absorption and to Evaluate Potential
Chemical Toxicity 901
William G. Reifenrath, Victoria L. Garzouzi and Harold O. Kammen

CHAPTER 47

Determination of Subclinical Changes of Barrier Function 937
Véranne Charbonnier, Marc Paye and Howard I. Maibach

CHAPTER 48

Assessing the Validity of Alternative Methods for
Toxicity Testing 957
Leon H. Bruner, G.J. Carr, M. Chamberlain and R.D. Curren

CHAPTER 49

Animal Models for Immunologic and Nonimmunologic
Contact Urticaria 999
Antti Lauerma and Howard I. Maibach

CHAPTER 50

Diagnostic Tests in Dermatology: Patch and Photopatch
Testing and Contact Urticaria 1007
Smita Amin, Antti Lauerma and Howard I. Maibach

CHAPTER 51

Cosmetic Reactions 1021
*Sara P. Modjtahedi, Jorge R. Toro, Patricia Engasser
and Howard I. Maibach*

CHAPTER 52

Evaluating Efficacy of Barrier Creams: *In Vitro* and
In Vivo Models 1087
Hongbo Zhai and Howard I. Maibach

CHAPTER 53

Light-Induced Dermal Toxicity: Effects on the Cellular
and Molecular Levels 1105
Andrija Kornhauser, Wayne G. Wamer and Lark A. Lambert

INDEX 1179

Contributors

Iris S. Ale, M.D.
Arazati 1194
11300 Montevideo, Uruguay
Tel/fax: 598 2 6220882
Email: *irisale@apolo.hc.edu.uy*
Email: *iris.a@medscape.com*

Smita Amin, M.D.
250 Harding Boulevard West
Suite 210
Richmond Hill
Ontario L4C 9M7, Canada
Tel: (905) 737-1245
Fax: (905) 737-1246
Email: *smita.amin@utoronto.ca*

Angela N. Anigbogu, Ph.D.
Watson Labs-Transdermal Research
577 Chipeta Way
Salt Lake City, UT 84108
Tel: (801) 588-6619
Fax: (801) 588-6620
Email: *aanigbogu@watsonpharm.com*

Jún Aramaki (Imura)
Shinjuku-ku
Ichigayasanae-cyo
21 Arisukan 302
Tokyo 162-0846, Japan

Karen Auborn, Ph.D.
North Shore-Long Island Jewish
  Research Institute
Boas-Marks Biomedical Science
  Research Center
350 Community Drive
Manhasset, NY 11030
Tel: (516) 562-1184
Fax: (516) 562-1022
Email: *kauborn@nshs.edu*

David A. Basketter, Ph.D.
Safety and Environmental Assurance
  Centre
Unilever Colworth Laboratory
Sharnbrook
Bedford MK44 1LQ, United Kingdom

Valérie Berl
Laboratoire de Dermato-Chimie
Clinique Dermatologique
Universite Louis Pasteur, CHU
F-67091 Strasbourg Cédex, France

Robert L. Bronaugh, Ph.D.
Skin Absorption and Metabolism
  Section
HFS-128, Food and Drug
  Administration
8301 Muirkirk Road
Laurel, MD 20708
Tel: (301) 210-2168
Fax: (301) 210-0220
Email: *robert.bronaugh@cfsan.fda.gov*

Leon H. Bruner, D.V.M., Ph.D.
The Gillette Company
Gillette Medical Evaluation
  Laboratory
37 A Street
Needham, MA 02492-9120
Tel: (781) 292-8101
Fax: (781) 292-8115
Email: *leon_bruner@gillette.com*

Graeme F. Bryce, Ph.D.
GFB Associates, Inc.
245 N. Mountain Avenue
Montclair, NJ 07043
Tel: (973) 746-9568
Fax: (973) 746-1723
Email: *gfbryce@comcast.net*

Gregory J. Carr
The Gillette Company
Gillette Medical Evaluation
  Laboratory
37 A Street
Needham, MA 02492-9120
Tel: (781) 292-8101
Fax: (781) 292-8115

M. Chamberlain
The Gillette Company
Gillette Medical Evaluation
  Laboratory
37 A Street
Needham, MA 02492-9120
Tel: (781) 292-8101
Fax: (781) 292-8115

Véranne Charbonnier, Ph.D.
65, Chemin Collet de Rafféo
06670 Colomars, France
Tel/fax: 33 (0)4 93 37 84 65
Email: *veranne-charbonnier@club-internet.fr*

Anne Chester
ALZA Corporation
1900 Charleston Road
P.O. Box 7210
Mountain View, CA 94039-7210
Tel: (650) 564-2753
Fax: (650) 564-2770
Email: *achester@alzus.jnj.com*

Myeong Jun Choi, Ph.D.
Department of Dermatology
University of California
School of Medicine
Box 0989, Surge 110
90 Medical Center Way
San Francisco, CA 94143-0989
Tel: (415) 476-4997
Fax: (415) 753-5304
Email: *mjchoi@itsa.ucsf.edu*

Michel Cormier
ALZA Corporation
1900 Charleston Road
P.O. Box 7210
Mountain View, CA 94039-7210
Tel: (650) 564-2708
Fax: (650) 564-2770

William J. Cunningham, M.D.
Cu-Tech, LLC
36 Midvale Road
Mountain Lakes, NJ 07046
Tel: (973) 331-1620
Fax: (973) 331-1622
Email: *studyskin@cu-tech.com*

R.D. Curren
The Gillette Company
Gillette Medical Evaluation
  Laboratory
37 A Street
Needham, MA 02492-9120
Tel: (781) 292-8101
Fax: (781) 292-8115

Bart De Wever
SkinEthic Laboratories
45, Rue St. Philippe
06000 Nice, France
Tel: 33 493 97 77 27
Fax: 33 493 97 77 28
E-mail: *bdewever@skinethic.com*

Rebecca J. Dearman, Ph.D.
Syngenta Central Toxicology
  Laboratory
Alderley Park, Macclesfield
Cheshire SK10 4TJ, United Kingdom

Isaak Effendy, M.D.
Department of Dermatology of
  Bielefeld
Academic Teaching Hospital of the
  University of Muenster
Teutoburger Str. 50
D-33604 Bielefeld, Germany
Tel: 49 521 581 3600
Fax: 49 521 581 3699
Email: *isaak.effendy@sk-bielefeld.de*

Patricia Engasser, M.D.
34 Ashfield Road
Atherton, CA 94027
Tel: (650) 322-6498
Fax: (650) 322-6494
Email: *engasser@yahoo.com*

Victoria L. Garzouzi
Stratacor, Inc.
1315 South 46th Street
Building 154
Richmond, CA 94804
Tel: (510) 231-9463
Fax: (510) 231-9464

G. Frank Gerberick, M.D.
Procter and Gamble Company
Miami Valley Laboratories
Cincinnati, OH 45253-8707

Alan M. Goldberg, Ph.D.
Center for Alternatives to Animal
 Testing
Johns Hopkins University
Bloomberg School of Public Health
Department of Environmental Health
 Sciences
111 Market Place, Suite 840
Baltimore, MD 21202-6709
Tel: (410) 223-1692
Fax: (410) 223-1603
Email: *goldberg@jhsph.edu*

Ningru Guo, M.D.
Institute of Dermatology
Chinese Academy of Sciences
Jiangwangmiao
Nanjing, 210042, Jiangsu, People's
 Republic of China
Tel: 86 25 5420814
Fax: 86 25 5414477
Email: *nanadamwu@yahoo.com*

Jurij J. Hostýnek, Ph.D.
ETRI
3644 Happy Valley Road
Lafayette, CA 94549
Tel: (925) 283-5939
Fax: (925) 284-1157
Email:*jurijj@hotmail.com*

Xiaoying Hui, M.D.
Department of Dermatology
University of California
School of Medicine
Box 0989, Surge 110
90 Medical Center Way
San Francisco, CA 94143-0989
Tel: (415) 502-7761
Fax: (415) 753-5304
Email: *xhui@itsa.ucsf.edu*

Charles G. Hurst
Chemical Casualty Care Division
U.S. Army Medical Research Institute
 of Chemical Defense
Aberdeen Proving Ground
Edgewood, MD 21010

Harold O. Kammen
Stratacor, Inc.
1315 South 46th Street
Building 154
Richmond, CA 94804
Tel: (510) 231-9463
Fax: (510) 231-9464

Yoshiaki Kawasaki, Ph.D.
U.S. Cosmetics Corporation
110 Louisa Viens Drive
P.O. Box 859
Dayville, CT 06241
Tel: (860) 779-3990
Fax: (860) 779-3994
Email: *yoshiakik@us-cosm.com*

Ian Kimber, Ph.D.
Syngenta Central Toxicology
 Laboratory
Alderly Park, Macclesfield
Cheshire SK10 4TJ, United Kingdom
Tel: 44 1625 515408
Fax: 44 1625 590996
Email: *ian.kimber@syngenta.com*

Georg Klecak, M.D.
Muhlezelgstrasse 15
8047 Zurich, Switzerland

Andrija Kornhauser, Ph.D.
Office of Cosmetics and Colors
Food and Drug Administration
HFS-128, 200 C Street S.W.
Washington, DC 20204
Email:
Andrija.Kornhauser@cfsan.fda.gov

Arto Lahti, M.D.
Department of Dermatology
University of Oulu
SF 902 20, Oulu, Finland

Lark A. Lambert, B.S.
Office of Cosmetics and Colors
Food and Drug Administration
HFS-128, 200 C Street S.W.
Washington, DC 20204

Antti Lauerma, M.D., Ph.D.
Skin and Allergy Hospital
Helsinki University Central Hospital
Meilahdentie 2
FIN-00250 Helsinki, Finland
Tel: 358 9 471 961 86347
Fax: 358 9 471 961 86561
Email: *antti.lauerma@helsinki.fi*
Email: *antti.lauerma@hus.fi*

Cheol Heon Lee, M.D.
Department of Dermatology
Kangnam Sacred Heart Hospital
College of Medicine
Hallym University
948-1 Daerim-1-Dong
Youngdeungpo-ku
Seoul 150-950, Korea
Fax: 82 2 832 3237
Email: *dermlee@yahoo.co.kr*

Jean-Pierre Lepoittevin, D.Sc.
Laboratoire de Dermato-Chimie
Clinique Dermatologique
Universite Louis Pasteur, CHU
F-67091 Strasbourg Cédex, France
Tel: 33 3 8835 0664
Fax: 33 3 8814 0447
Email: *jplepoit@chimie.u-strasbg.fr*

Cheryl Levin, MSIII
Stanford University School of Medicine
Stanford, CA 94305
Tel: (650) 326-3663
Email: *clevin@stanford.edu*

Wei-qi Lin, M.D.
ALZA Corporation
1900 Charleston Road
P.O. Box 7210
Mountain View, CA 94039-7210
Tel: (650) 564-2721
Fax: (650) 564-2770
Email: *wlin3@alzus.jnj.com*

Priv.-Doz. Dr. med. Harald Löffler
Klinik für Dermatologie und
Allergologie
Philipps-Universität Marburg
Deutschhausstr. 9
35033 Marburg, Germany
Tel: 49 6421 286 2321
Fax: 49 6421 286 2324
Email:
Harald.Loeffler@mailer.uni-marburg.de

Howard I. Maibach, M.D.
Department of Dermatology
University of California
School of Medicine
Box 0989, Surge 110
90 Medical Center Way
San Francisco, CA 94143-0989
Tel: (415) 476-2468
Fax: (415) 753-5304
Email: *himjlm@itsa.ucsf.edu*

Henry C. Maguire, Jr.
University of Pennsylvania
School of Medicine
Pathology & Laboratory Medicine
  Department
422 Curie Building
Philadelphia, PA 19104-6160
Tel: (215) 662-2352
Fax: (215) 573-9436
Email: *hmaguire@mail.med.upenn.edu*

Francis N. Marzulli, Ph.D.
8044 Park Overlook Drive
Bethesda, MD 20817
Tel/fax: (301) 469-7513

James Matriano
ALZA Corporation
1900 Charleston Road
P.O. Box 7210
Mountain View, CA 94039-7210
Tel: (650) 564-2722
Fax: (650) 564-2770

Leslie P. McCarty, Ph.D. (deceased)
111 East Chapel Lane
Midland, MI 48642

James N. McDougal, Ph.D.
Department of Pharmacology and
  Toxicology
Wright State University
School of Medicine
3640 Colonel Glenn Highway
Dayton, OH 45435-0001
Tel: (937) 775-3697
Fax: (937) 775-7221
Email: *james.mcdougal@wright.edu*

Torkil Menné, Ph.D.
Department of Dermatology
Niels Andersens Vej 65
University of Copenhagen
Hellerup, 2900, Denmark
Tel: 45 39773206
Fax: 45 39657137
Email: *tomen@gentoftehosp.kbhamt.dk*

Zheng Min, M.D.
Department of Dermatology
Second Affiliated Hospital
Zhejiang University
88 Jie-fang Road
Hangzhou, 310009, People's Republic
  of China
Tel: 86 57 187783791
Fax: 86 57 187215882
Email: *minz@mail.hz.zj.cn*

Jun-ichi Mizushima
Department of Dermatology
Tokyo Women's Medical University
8-1 Kawada-cho
Shinjuku, Tokyo 162-8666, Japan

Sara P. Modjtahedi
Department of Dermatology
University of California
School of Medicine
Box 0989, Surge 110
90 Medical Center Way
San Francisco, CA 94143-0989
Tel: (415) 476-4997
Fax: (415) 753-5304
Email: *spmodjta@ucla.edu*

Nancy A. Monteiro-Riviere, Ph.D.
Center for Chemical Toxicology
Research and Pharmacokinetics
North Carolina State University
College of Veterinary Medicine
Department of Clinical Sciences
4700 Hillsborough Street
Raleigh, NC 27606
Tel: (919) 513-6426
Fax: (919) 513-6358
Email: *nancy_monteiro@ncsu.edu*

Weili Pan, M.D.
Department of Dermatology
People's Hospital of Zhejiang Province
4 Zhaohui District
Hangzhou, 310014 People's Republic
  of China
Tel: 86 57 185239988-3309
Fax: 86 57 185131448
Email: *pwlhz@163.net*

Marc Paye
Colgate-Palmolive Research and
  Development
Milmort, Belgium

John P. Petrali
Comparative Pathology Branch
Comparative Medicine Division
U.S. Army Medical Research Institute
  of Chemical Defense
Aberdeen Proving Ground
Edgewood, MD 21010

Mary Prevo, M.A.
ALZA Corporation
1900 Charleston Road
P.O. Box 7210
Mountain View, CA 94039-7210
Tel: (650) 564-2780
Fax: (650) 564-2882

Michal Ramon, M.D.
Department of Dermatology
Rambam Medical Center
University of Haifa
Haifa 31096, Israel

William G. Reifenrath
Stratacor, Inc.
1315 South 46th Street
Building 154
Richmond, CA 94804
Tel: (510) 231-9463
Fax: (510) 231-9464
Email: *WmReifenrath@cs.com*

Jim E. Riviere, D.V.M., Ph.D., FATS
Center for Chemical Toxicology
Research and Pharmacokinetics
College of Veterinary Medicine
North Carolina State University
Raleigh, NC 27606
Phone: (919) 513-6305
Fax: (919) 513-6358
Email: *jim_riviere@ncsu.edu*

Joan E. Roberts, Ph.D.
Department of Natural Sciences
Fordham University at Lincoln Center
113 West 60th Street
New York, NY 10023-7404
Tel: (212) 636-6323
Fax: (212) 636-7217
Email: *jroberts@fordham.edu*

Martin Rosdy
SkinEthic Laboratories
45, Rue St. Philippe
06000 Nice, France
Tel: 33 493 97 77 27
Fax: 33 493 97 77 28

Glenn G. Russo, M.D.
Department of Dermatology TB36
School of Medicine
Tulane University Health Sciences
 Center
1430 Tulane Avenue
New Orleans, LA 70112-2699
Tel: (504) 588-5114
Fax: (504) 587-7382
Email: *grusso@tulane.edu*

Frederick R. Sidell, M.D.
Chemical Casualty Care Division
U.S. Army Medical Research Institute
 of Chemical Defense
Aberdeen Proving Ground
Edgewood, MD 21010
Email: *hbpub@aol.com*

David H. Sliney, Ph.D.
Laser/Optical Radiation Program
U.S. Army Center for Health
Promotion and Preventive Medicine
Attn: MCHB-TS-OLO (Bldg. E-1950)
Aberdeen Proving Ground
Edgewood, MD 21010-5422
Tel: (410) 436-3002
Fax: (410) 436-5054
Email: *david.sliney@apg.amedd.army.mil*

William J. Smith
Biochemical Pharmacy Branch
U.S. Army Institute of Chemical
 Defense
Aberdeen Proving Ground
Edgewood, MD 21010

Jorge R. Toro, M.D.
Dermatology Branch
Building 10, Room 12N238
National Cancer Institute
10 Center Drive, MSC 1908
Bethesda, MD 20892-1908
Tel: (301) 451-4562
Fax: (301) 402-4489
Email: *torojo@exchange.nih.gov*
Email: *toroj@mail.nih.gov*

Tsen-Fang Tsai, M.D.
Department of Dermatology
National Taiwan University Hospital
7 Chung-Shan South Road
Taipei, Taiwan, Republic of China
Email: *tftsai@yahoo.com*

Niels K. Veien, M.D., Ph.D.
Vesterbro 99
DK-9000 Aalborg, Denmark
Tel: 45 9812 5259
Fax: 45 9816 8173
Email: *veien@dadlnet.dk*

Wayne G. Wamer
Office of Cosmetics and Colors
Food and Drug Administration
HFS-128, 200 C Street S.W.
Washington, DC 20204

Sara Weltfriend, M.D.
Department of Dermatology
Rambam Medical Center
University of Haifa
Haifa 31096, Israel
Tel: 972 4 8542610
Fax: 972 4 8542951
Email: *dermatology@rambam.health.gov.il*
Email: *s_weissman@rambam.health.gov.il*

Philip W. Wertz, Ph.D.
N450 DSB
University of Iowa
Iowa City, IA 52242
Tel: (319) 335-7409
Fax: (319) 335-8895
Email: *philip-wertz@uiowa.edu*

Ronald C. Wester, Ph.D.
Department of Dermatology
University of California
School of Medicine
Box 0989, Surge 110
90 Medical Center Way
San Francisco, CA 94143-0989
Tel: (415) 476-2468
Fax: (415) 753-5304
Email: *rcwgx@itsa.ucsf.edu*

Shaoxi Wu, M.D.
Institute of Dermatology
Chinese Academy of Sciences
Jiangwangmiao
Nanjing, 210042, Jiangsu, People's
  Republic of China
Tel: 86 25 5420814
Fax: 86 25 5414477
Email: *nanadamwu@yahoo.com*

Hongbo Zhai, M.D.
Department of Dermatology
University of California
School of Medicine
Box 0989, Surge 110
90 Medical Center Way
San Francisco, CA 94143-0989
Tel: (415) 514-1537
Fax: (415) 753-5304
Email: *hongbo@itsa.ucsf.edu*

Foreword from the Fifth Edition

The field of toxicology is at an exciting juncture as we approach the turn of the century. It is an appropriate time to look at the past, consider the present, and anticipate the future for toxicology. Publication of the fifth edition of *Dermatotoxicology* provides an excellent opportunity for such reflection.

The roots of toxicology are ancient and undoubtedly predate recorded history. The earliest references to toxicology most often deal with poisons or potions. Other references call attention to the close relationship between poisons and remedies, as in this succinct and often quoted statement of Paracelsus: "All substances are poisons; there is none which is not a poison. The right dose differentiates a poison and a remedy." And some other references note poisonings related to occupation, such as the mad hatter syndrome from intake of mercury. The roots of toxicology, whether related to poisons, drugs, or agents encountered in the workplace or environment, usually had a strong orientation and most often concerned individuals rather than populations. An exposure to or intake of toxicants occurred and an effect was observed, usually of an obvious nature and within a short period of time. This kind of knowledge was readily applied to similar situations to avoid further poisonings or in some cases to assure that intended poisoning was carried out in an even more crafty way.

In this century and especially after World War II, the field of toxicology has changed markedly. Descriptive toxicology and direct application to similar situations have been supplanted by the need to predict or estimate toxicity for exposure situations that differ from those for which actual observations exist. Increasingly, toxicologists have been called on to predict the potential nature and magnitude of adverse health effects at exposure levels much lower than those for which human observations are available and in some cases for materials for which human data do not exist. The earlier concern for acute effects is now overridden by concern for diseases such as cancer that occur years after initial intake of a suspected toxicant. Cancer, for example, may be expected to occur at very low incidence in excess of the disease incidence occurring spontaneously; in other words, one cancer added to the base incidence of more than 200,000 cancer cases may be expected to occur from all causes in a population of a million individuals. Without question, emphasis has shifted from poisoning of individuals to individuals within a population. The exposure levels of concern are frequently orders of magnitude lower than those for which any human data exist, giving rise to the need for extrapolation. Furthermore, human data in many cases are unavailable or insufficient, making it necessary to obtain information from studies using laboratory animals, tissues, and macromolecules and conducted with exposure levels much higher than the exposure levels likely to be of concern for people. Thus, multiple extrapolations may be required—across species, downward in exposure level, from subanimal systems to the intact mammal, and from a few individuals to large populations.

The earliest extrapolations were usually quite simplistic, involving the use of no-observed-effect levels and safety factors. Such approaches are most readily justified when dealing with health endpoints for which thresholds may exist. Even when thresholds exist, the situation becomes complicated when dealing with large populations containing individuals of varying sensitivity. When dealing with induction of cancers, some types of which may not exhibit a demonstrable threshold between exposure and incidence, the extrapolation may be accomplished using mathematical models. The validity of the biological assumptions underlying some models has been challenged. Unfortunately, economic and logistical limitations on the size of populations that can be studied will probably preclude validation of most of the models by direct observations.

During the past two decades, it has become a tenet of faith of most toxicologists that increased confidence can be developed in the extrapolations noted above as we develop an improved understanding of the mechanisms of action of toxic agents. Some progress has been made in improving our knowledge of the mechanisms of action of toxicants. To date, however, such information has not been used in regulatory decisions as often as one would like.

As we look to the future of toxicology, one of the critical issues is how to incorporate a better understanding of mechanisms of action of toxicants, as some might say—the relevant biology—into the various extrapolations that must be made as part of the process of controlling exposures to toxicants, thereby limiting the occurrence of adverse health outcomes. I submit that progress will be most notable when the experimentalist and regulator, after compiling and integrating the available data, identify the gaps in our knowledge that, if filled, will have the greatest impact on reducing the uncertainty in estimating health risks at relevant levels of human exposure. Meeting these data needs will be a formidable challenge because it will focus attention on the need to understand mechanisms of action at exposure levels that are difficult and perhaps not even possible to study with traditional experimental approaches.

Success with this new toxicology, with an emphasis on reducing the uncertainty in our assessment of toxicant risks through an understanding of mechanisms of action at relevant exposure levels, will depend greatly on developing an improved capability for integrating data obtained from studies at various levels of biological organization ranging from macromolecules to cells to tissues and organs to intact mammals to populations of laboratory animals and, ultimately, to people. The explosion in our knowledge and capability at the molecular and cellular levels provides us with both opportunity and challenge. The opportunity relates to the immenseness of the knowledge and the power of the techniques. The challenge for toxicology is to integrate the information with a view to better understanding diseases that occur in intact individuals with complex modulating systems as members of large populations that may vary greatly in individual susceptibility to specific toxicants.

Of the various subspecialties of toxicology, none has received more pressure than dermatotoxicology for using approaches other than the study of whole animals as alternatives for assessing the toxic effect of materials applied to the skin. I hope that past emphasis on alternatives will shift to concern for integrating data obtained from complementary systems and a reduction in rather than elimination of the use of laboratory animals. If data from laboratory animals are not available, human populations may serve as the test system for validation of our estimates of toxicity derived from using cells, tissues, and computer models. This could have unfortunate consequences.

The fifth edition of *Dermatotoxicology* illustrates well the extent to which the field is at a juncture. The revisions of old chapters and the many new chapters clearly describe the current state of our knowledge of dermatotoxicology. The book is a careful blending of fundamental information on the mechanisms of action of toxicants on skin, practical information on the varied responses of skin to specific toxicants, and approaches to evaluating dermal toxicity. Equally as important, many of the chapters convey a sense of where the field is going. I am confident that the book will be useful to a broad spectrum of readers: dermatotoxicologists, general toxicologists, occupational physicians, and regulatory authorities, all of whom are concerned with minimizing the occurrence of toxicant-induced skin disease.

Roger O. McClellan
Chemical Industry Institute of Toxicology
(Past President, Society of Toxicology, 1989–1990)

Preface to the Sixth Edition

The Sixth Edition of Dermatotoxicology has the benefit of decades of practical experience in classrooms, government laboratories, regulatory environments, and in industry. We are indebted to our contributors for their diligence and thoughtfulness; we are equally appreciative of the editorial team at Taylor and Francis, including Catherine Russell and Dilys Alam, for their painstaking handling of our complex scientific language.

Although we would have liked to include every important contribution from each of the five editions in this one volume, very few of us would be able to lift the result. For this reason, we strongly suggest that Editions 1 through 5 be reviewed for chapters that were not repeated in this edition.

Howard I. Maibach, M.D.

Hongbo Zhai, M.D.

PART I

Concepts

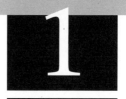

Skin Permeability

RONALD C WESTER AND HOWARD I MAIBACH

Contents

1.1   Introduction

1.2   Method analyses: Atrazine

1.3   Method analyses: Borates

1.4   Limitations

1.5   Discussion

1.1 INTRODUCTION

The rate determining step for human risk assessment is bioavailability, that amount of chemical in the environment which gets into the human body. If the exposure includes skin, then skin permeability becomes a rate determining step.

Various methods are available to assess skin permeability. These include *in vivo*, *in vitro* and computer model methods. Cost/benefit would favor the *in vitro* system (this is assumed) and certainly the computer calculated permeability is cost friendly (not to mention manpower friendly). The down side is that errors can cost money and human suffering. This chapter gives examples of the different methodologies, showing when they work and where validation points out method shortcomings.

1.2 METHOD ANALYSES: ATRAZINE

Table 1.1 gives the *in vivo* human percutaneous absorption of [^{14}C] atrazine. Two dose levels, 6.7 and 79 µg/cm^2, were applied to the ventral forearm of volunteers (from whom consent had been obtained) and total urinary and fecal radioactivity determined. A previous *in vivo* intravenous study in the rhesus monkey showed that all of the iv dose was excreted within 7 days, and this was the case with the human volunteers with topical dose application. Total percent dose absorbed was 5.6 ± 3.0 and total dose accountability (absorbed plus washes) was 101.2 ± 3.4 percent for the 6.7 µg/cm^2 dose. Similar results were obtained

TABLE 1.1:

Atrazine human *in vivo* percutaneous absorption

		Dose A[a] (n = 4)			Dose B[a] (n = 6)		
Dose		6.7 µg/cm^2			79 µg/cm^2		
Excretron:	Urinary (%)	5.0	±	2.9	1.1	±	0.9
	Fecal (%)	0.6	±	0.3	0.1	±	0.1
	Total (%)	5.6	±	3.0	1.2	±	1.0
Dose absorbed (%)		5.6	±	3.0	1.2	±	10
Total dose accountability (%)		101.2	±	3.4	92.3	±	2.8
Flux (µg/cm^2/hr)		0.0156	±	0.0084	0.0379	±	0.0332
Half-life (hr) ^{14}C		17.5	±	5.4	24.5	±	9.0

Dose applied to ventral forearm, covered with non-occlusive raised patch for 24 hours, then dose side washed with soap and water.

[a]Mean ± SD

for the higher dose. This is considered the gold standard for skin permeability. Definitive percent dose absorbed and flux are obtained and all of the applied dose is accounted for.

The *in vivo* urine samples were further validated. Split urine aliquots were analyzed by accelerator mass spectrometry (Gilman *et al.*, 1998). Data from these two methods (scintillation counting and accelerator MS) have a correlation coefficient of 0.998 for a linear plot of the entire sample set. Urinary metabolites were also determined using HPLC—accelerator mass spectrometry (Buchholz *et al.*, 1999).

Table 1.2 gives atrazine *in vitro* percutaneous absorption through human skin (Ademola *et al.*, 1993). The human skin was used under conditions which ensure skin viability (Wester *et al.*, 1998a) and atrazine metabolites were determined. In this *in vitro* study receptor fluid accumulation and skin content (at end of study) were determined for skin permeability. A basic question with *in vitro* methodology is: does one use only receptor fluid content or both receptor fluid and skin content to determine skin permeability. Without knowledge of *in vivo* human absorption (Table 4.1) which is the proper choice?

Table 1.3 summarizes atrazine flux in humans using the *in vivo* data (0.0156 μg/cm^2/hr) and *in vitro* data (0.0081 μg/cm^2/hr for receptor fluid only and 0.038 μg/cm^2/hr using combined receptor fluid and skin content). For comparison purposes the flux was calculated using Guy and Potts (1992) as 0.044 μg/cm^2/hr. All three flux calculations are relatively in agreement.

Atrazine is a "friendly" chemical for these types of analysis because the molecular weight (215.69), water solubility (34.7 mg/L) and Log P (octanol-water) of 2.61 are amendable to all systems. However, there are exceptions to the rule.

TABLE 1.2:

Atrazine *in vitro* percutaneous absorption human skin

Distribution	Percent Dose Absorbed		
Receptor fluid	3.5	±	0.3
Skin	12.8	±	1.2
Surface wash	66.8	±	6.9
Total recovery	83.0	±	7.3

Dose is 4.6 μg/cm^2
Each value: mean ± SEM (n = 14) for 20 hours

Source: Ademola *et al.* (1993)

TABLE 1.3:

Atrazine Flux In Humans

Method	Flux ($\mu g/cm^2/hr$)
In vivo human	0.016
In vitro	
Receptor fluid	0.008
Receptor fluid and skin	0.038
Calculated[b]	0.044

[a] Based upon 6.7 $\mu g/cm^2$ dose
Source: Guy and Potts (1992)

1.3 METHOD ANALYSES: BORATES

Boron is an ubiquitous element in rocks; soil and water. A small amount of boron is essential to life. Borates come in contact with human skin in many ways (mining, detergent, fertilizer, wood treatment, organic insecticide).

Table 1.4 gives the *in vivo* percutaneous absorption in human volunteers (from whom informed consent was obtained) for the borates 5 percent boric acid, 5 percent borax and 10 percent disodium octaborate tetrahydrate (DOT). These dose concentration are near water solubility limitation (Wester *et al.,*

TABLE 1.4:

In vivo absorption, flux and permeability content for [10]boron as 5% boric acid, 5% borax, and 10% disodium octaborate tetrahydrate (dot) in normal human volunteers

Dose	Dose ^{10}B (μg)	Percentage of dose	Flux ($\mu g/cm^2/h$)	Permeability constant (K_p) (cm/h)		
5% boric acid						
No treatment	14,200	0.226	0.00912	1.9	$\times$	10^{-7}
SLS treatment[a]	14,200	0.239	0.00966	2.0	$\times$	10^{-7}
5% borax						
No treatment	9270	0.210	0.00855	1.8	$\times$	10^{-7}
SLS treatment[a]	9220	0.185	0.00746	1.5	$\times$	10^{-7}
10% DOT						
No treatment	34,700	0.122	0.00975	1.0	$\times$	10^{-7}
SLS treatment[a]	34,800	0.107	0.00878	0.9	$\times$	10^{-7}

[a]SLS = sodium lauryl sulfate
Dose was spread over 900 cm^2 area of the back

Source: Wester *et al.,* 1998b

CHAPTER 1

TABLE 1.5:

In vitro percutaneous absorption of boron administrated as boric acid, borax, and disodium octaborate tetrahydrate (DOT) in normal human skin

Dosing solution	Percentage of dose absorbed geometric mean (95% CI)	Flux (μg/cm^2/h)	Kp (cm/h)
Boric acid (w/v)			
5% at 2μl/cm^2	1.75 (0.18—17)	0.07	1.4 $\times$ 10^{-6}
5% at 1000μl/cm^2	0.70 (0.072—6.81)	14.58	2.9 $\times$ 10^{-4}
0.5 at 1000μl/cm^2	0.28 (0.029—2.72)	0.58	1.2 $\times$ 10^{-4}
0.05% at 1000μl/cm^2	1.20 (0.012—11.7)	0.25	5.0 $\times$ 10^{-4}
Borax			
5% at 1000μl/cm^2	0.41 (0.042—3.99)	8.5	1.7 $\times$ 10^{-4}
DOT			
10% at 1000μl/cm^2	0.19 (0.018—1.81)	7.9	0.8 $\times$ 10^{-4}

Source: Wester *et al.* (1998b)

1998b): the *in vivo* permeability contants (K_p) range from $1 - 2 \times 10^{-7}$ for these borates. The human skin *in vitro* percutaneous absorption is in Table 1.5. Comparison of Tables 1.4 and 1.5 yield some interesting data relative to *in vivo* and *in vitro* methodology.

The *in vitro* permeability coefficient (K_p) for the 5 percent boric acid, 5 percent borax and 10 percent DOT range from $0.8 - 2.9 \times 10^{-4}$. This is a 1000-fold increase over *in vivo* K_ps.

The *in vivo* studies were done with a dose of 2μl/cm^2 (any more would run off the skin). The *in vitro* doses were at 1000 μl/cm^2. However one *in vitro* 5 percent boric acid was dosed at 2 μl/cm^2. Interestingly, the 5 percent boxic acid K_p at 1000 μl/cm^2 was 2.9×10^{-4} while the 5 percent boric acid K_p at 2 μl/cm^2 was 1.4×10^{-6}, a 200-fold difference. The amount of vehicle (water) was the determining factor in boric acid *in vitro* human percutaneous absorption.

The relationship between flux and permeability coefficient (flux is concentration dependent while K_p is independent) was true for this *in vitro* study (Figure 1.1).

1.4 LIMITATIONS

Regulatory agencies have developed an affinity for a calculated permeability coefficient (K_p) for risk assessment. Permeability coefficients are easiest determined from the time course of chemical diffusion from a vehicle across the skin

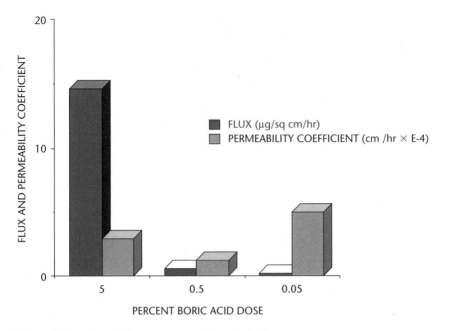

Figure 1.1: Boric acid dose response at 1000 μl/cm².

barrier into a receptor fluid. Table 1.6 compares *in vitro* diffusion receptor fluid absorption with *in vivo* percutaneous absorption. Receptor fluid accumulation for the higher logP chemicals (Table 1.7) is negligible. This is due to basic chemistry—the compounds are not soluble in the water based receptor fluid. Based on these receptor fluid accumulations these chemicals are not absorbed skin. Risk assessment would contain an extreme false negative component. That point where the diffusion system and receptor fluid accumulation gives a true K_p or manufactures a false K_p has not been determined. Regulatory agents should have some *in vivo* validation before blindly accepting an *in vitro* K_p. Also, computer models based on *in vitro* data have the same risk.

1.5 DISCUSSION

Human skin was developed during evolutionary history, basically designed as a physical barrier to the environment and to contain our water based body chemistry. The industrial revolution introduced a new wave of chemicals for the skin to deal with. Considering skin's barrier properties, a lot of protection is provided. However, chemicals do permeate the skin barrier and human health

TABLE 1.6:

In vitro receptor fluid versus *in vivo* percutaneous absorption

Compound	Vehicle	*In vitro* Receptor fluid			*In vivo*		
DDT	Acetone	0.08	±	0.02	18.9	±	9.4
	Soil	0.04	±	0.01	3.3	±	0.5
Benzo[a]pyrene	Acetone	0.09	±	0.06	51.0	±	22.0
	Soil	0.01	±	0.06	13.2	±	3.4
Chlordane	Acetone	0.07	±	0.06	6.0	±	2.8
	Soil	0.04	±	0.05	4.2	±	1.8
Pentachlorophenol	Acetone	0.6	±	0.09	29.2	±	5.8
	Soil	0.01	±	0.00	24.4	±	6.4
PCBs (1242)	Acetone	—			21.4	±	8.5
	TCB	—			18.0	±	8.3
	Mineral oil	0.3	±	0.6	20.8	±	8.3
	Soil	0.04	±	0.05	14.1	±	1.0
PCBs (1254)	Acetone	—			14.6	±	3.6
	TCB	—			20.8	±	8.3
	Mineral oil	0.1	±	0.07	20.4	±	8.5
	Soil	0.04	±	0.05	13.8	±	2.7
2,4-D	Acetone	—			2.6	±	2.1
	Soil	0.02	±	0.01	15.9	±	4.7
Arsenic	Water	0.9	±	1.1	2.0	±	1.2
	Soil	0.03	±	0.5	3.2	±	1.9
Cadmium	Water	0.4	±	0.2	—		
	Soil	0.03	±	0.02	—		
Mercury	Water	0.07	±	0.01	—		
	Soil	0.06	±	0.01	—		

TABLE 1.7:

Octanol / water partition coefficients of compounds

Compounds	LogP
DDT	6.91
Benzo[a]pyrene	5.97
Chlordane	5.58
Pentachlorophenol	5.12
2,4-D	2.81
PCBs	mixture
Aroclor 1242	(high logP)
Aroclor 1254	(high logP)

requires knowledge and regulation to maintain safety. Skin permeability can best be determined *in vivo* in human volunteers (gold standard). *in vitro* diffusion methodology and predictive models can aid in predicting skin permeability, but they do have limitation. If these limitations are not vigorously defined and validated, the consequences can be severe. False positive errors can be financially costly and false negative errors can be deadly.

REFERENCES

ADEMOLA, J.I., SEDIK, L.E., WESTER, R.C. and MAIBACH, H.I. (1993) *In vitro* percutaneous absorption and metabolism in man of 2-chloro-4-ethylamino-6-isopropylamine-5-triazine (Atrazine). *Arch. Toxicol.* **67**, 85–91.

BUCHHOLZ, B.A., FULTZ, E., HAACK, K.W., VOGEL, S., GILMAN, S.D., GEE, S.J., HAMMOCK, B.D., HUI, X., WESTER, R.C., MAIBACH, H.I. (1999) APLC-accelerator MS measurement of atrazine metabolites in human urine after dermal exposure. *Anal. Chem.* **71**, 3519–3525.

GILMAN, S.D., GEE, S.J., HAMMOCK, B.D., VOGEL, J.S., HAACK, K.W., BUCHHOLZ, B.A., FREEMAN, S.P.H.T., WESTER, R.C., HUI, X., MAIBACH, H.I. (1998) Analytical performance of accelerator mass spectrometry and liquid scintillation counting for detection of ^{14}C-labeled atrazine metabolites in human urine. *Anal. Chem.* **70**, 3463–3469.

GUY, R.H. and POTTS, R.O. (1992) Structure-permeability relationship in percutaneous penetration. *J. Pharm. Sci.* **81**, 603–604.

WESTER, R.C., CHRISTOPHER, J., HARTWAY, T., POBLETE, N., MAIBACH, H.I. and FORSELL, J., (1998a) Human cadaver skin viability for *in vitro* percutaneous absorption: storage and detrimental effects of heat-separation and freezing. *Pharm. Res.* **15**, 82–84.

WESTER, R.C., HUI, X., HAACK, K.W., POBLETE, N., MAIBACH, H.I., BELL, K., SCHELL, M.J., NORTINGTON, D.J., STRONG, P. and CULVER, B.D. (1998b) *In vivo* percutaneous absorption of boric acid, borax, and disodium octaborate tetrahydrate in humans compared to *in vitro* absorption in human skin from infinite and finite doses. *Toxicol. Sci.* **45**, 42–51.

Occlusion and Barrier Function

HONGBO ZHAI AND HOWARD I MAIBACH

Contents

2.1   Introduction

2.2   Occlusion and its application

2.3   Skin barrier function

2.4   Effects of occlusion on barrier function

2.5   Quantification with bioengineering techniques

2.6   Conclusions

2.1 INTRODUCTION

Occlusion has been used in dermatology to increase topical corticosteroids efficacy (Scholtz, 1961; Sulzberger and Witten, 1961). It may increase percutaneous absorption of applied compounds but with important exception (Bucks et al., 1988; Bucks et al., 1991; Bucks and Maibach, 1999). In turn, it obstructs normal ventilation of the skin surface; increases stratum corneum hydration and hence may compromise skin barrier function (Kligman, 1996; Warner et al., 1999; Kligman, 2000). Evaluation and investigation of the impact of occlusion on barrier function are important in many fields: skin physiology, pathology, pharmacology, and dermatology. Zhai and Maibach (2002) recently reviewed this topic. This chapter emphasizes the effects of occlusion on skin barrier function, in particularly, as defined with objective skin bioengineering technology.

2.2 OCCLUSION AND ITS APPLICATION

With occlusion, the skin is covered directly or indirectly by impermeable films or substances such as diapers, tape, chambers, gloves, textiles garments, wound dressings, transdermal devices, etc. (Kligman, 1996). In addition, certain topical vehicles that contain fats and/or polymers oils (petrolatum, paraffin, etc.) may also generate occlusive effects (Berardesca and Maibach, 1988).

Due to its simplicity, occlusion is widely utilized to enhance the penetration of applied drugs in clinical practice. However, occlusion does not increase percutaneous absorption to all chemicals (Bucks et al., 1988; Bucks et al., 1991; Bucks and Maibach, 1999). It may increase penetration of lipid-soluble, nonpolar molecules but has less effect on polar molecules: a trend of occlusion-induced absorption enhancement with increasing penetrant lipophilicity is apparent (Bucks et al., 1988; Treffel et al., 1992; Cross and Roberts, 2000). In practice, increasing skin penetration rates of applied drug is far from simple. Skin barrier function can be ascribed to the macroscopic structure of the stratum corneum, consisting of alternating lipoidal and hydrophylic regions. For this reason, physico-chemical characteristics of the chemical, such as partition coefficient, structure, and molecular weight, play an important role in determining the facility of absorption (Wiechers, 1989; Hostynek et al., 1996). Another factor to consider in drug percutaneous absorption, is the vehicle, in which the drug is formulated, acts on drug release from the formulation (Hotchkiss et al., 1992; Cross and Roberts, 2000). In addition, the anatomical site may also influence the effects of occlusion on percutaneous absorption (Qiao et al., 1993).

■ CHAPTER 2 ■

In many industrial and food fields, protective gloves or clothing are required to protect the workers from hazardous materials or for hygiene. On other hand, these protective measures may also produce negative events because of the nature of occlusion, which often causes stratum corneum hyper-hydration and reduces the protective barrier properties of the skin (Graves *et al.*, 1995). Many gloves do not resist the penetration of low molecular weight chemicals. As results, those chemicals may enter the glove and become trapped on the skin under occlusion for many hours, possibly leading to irritation, and more seriously to dermatitis or eczematous changes (Van der Valk and Maibach, 1989; Mathias, 1990; Estlander *et al.*, 1996).

Wound dressings have been employed to speed the healing processes in acute and chronic wounds. They keep healing tissues moist and increase superficial wound epithelialization (Winter, 1962; Winter and Scales, 1963; Hinman and Maibach, 1963; Alvarez *et al.*, 1983; Eaglstein, 1984; Berardesca and Maibach, 1988). However, occlusive or semiocclusive dressings can increase micro-organisms and hence induce wound infections (Aly *et al.*, 1978; Rajka *et al.*, 1981; Faergemann *et al.*, 1983; Mertz and Eaglstein, 1984; Berardesca and Maibach, 1988). A significant increase in the density of *Staphylococcus aureus* and lipophilic diphtheroids were observed after 24 h occlusion in eczematous and psoriatic skin (Rajka *et al.*, 1981).

Thus, the effects of occlusion on skin are complex and may produce profound changes that include altering epidermal lipids, DNA synthesis, epidermal turnover, pH, epidermal morphology, sweat glands, Langerhans cells stresses, etc. (Faergemann *et al.*, 1983; Berardesca and Maibach, 1988; Bucks *et al.*, 1991; Matsumura *et al.*, 1995; Kligman, 1996; Berardesca and Maibach, 1996; Leow and Maibach, 1997; Denda *et al.*, 1998; Bucks and Maibach, 1999; Warner *et al.*, 1999; Kömüves *et al.*, 1999; Fluhr *et al.*, 1999; Kligman, 2000).

2.3 SKIN BARRIER FUNCTION

Skin has numerous functions, one of which is to serve as a water permeability barrier to keep body fluids in and minimize dehydration. This function takes place largely in the stratum corneum (SC) or horny layer (Baker, 1972). SC has been referred to as a brick and mortar structure. The bricks are protein rich corneocytes separated by lipid rich intercellular domains consisting of stacks of bilaminar membrane (Kligman, 2000). Normally, the passage of water through the skin is closely controlled—allowing 0.5 cm^2/hour to evaporate. When water content falls too low, water barrier function is impaired and the skin becomes more sensitive to repeated use of water, detergents and other irritants. Barrier function may be disturbed by physical, chemical, pathological factors, and environmental changes (Denda *et al.*, 1998).

Maintenance of the SC structural integrity is critical to barrier function. Increasing SC hydration can progressively reduce barrier efficiency (Bucks *et al.*, 1991; Matsumura *et al.*, 1995; Berardesca and Maibach, 1996; Kligman, 1996; Leow and Maibach, 1997; Bucks *et al.*, 1988; Haftek *et al.*, 1998; Warner *et al.*, 1999; Bucks and Maibach, 1999; Fluhr *et al.*, 1999; Tsai and Maibach, 1999; Kligman, 2000). SC is extremely hygroscopic: it can pick up 500 percent of its dry weight in less than 1 h following immersing in water, swelling vertically to 4–5 times its original width (Kligman, 2000).

2.4 EFFECTS OF OCCLUSION ON BARRIER FUNCTION

Healthy stratum corneum typically has a water content of 10–20 percent (Baker, 1972). Occlusion can block diffusional water loss from skin surface, increasing stratum corneum hydration, thereby swelling the corneocytes, and promoting water uptake into intercellular lipid domains (Bucks *et al.*, 1991; Bucks and Maibach, 1999). Water content can be increased up to 50 percent with occlusion (Bucks *et al.*, 1991; Bucks and Maibach, 1999): even short time (30 min) exposure can result in significantly increased stratum corneum hydration (Ryatt *et al.*, 1988). With 24 h occlusion, the relative water content in stratum corneum can be increased significantly from 53 percent before occlusion to 59 percent (Faergemann *et al.*, 1983). Morphological changes on the surface can be induced by 24 h occlusion, deepening skin furrows (Matsumura *et al.*, 1995). Zhai *et al.* (2002) determined the level of skin hydration and skin permeability to nicotinates following occlusive patches and diapers at different exposure times. They found that permeation of nicotinates was increased for hydrated skin versus control even after only 10 minutes of patch exposure. No evidence of increased permeation rates with increased hyperhydration once a relatively low threshold of hyperhydration was achieved (e.g., which reached after a 10 min wet patch). Water under occlusion may disrupt barrier lipids and damage stratum corneum similar to surfactants (Warner *et al.*, 1999). Kligman (1996) studied hydration dermatitis in man: one week of an impermeable plastic film did not injure skin: 2 weeks was moderately harmful to some but not all subjects: 3 weeks regularly induced dermatitis. Hydration dermatitis was independent of race, sex, and age. They examined the potential role of microorganisms in developing hydration

CHAPTER 2

dermatitis by using antibiotic solutions immediately following occlusion with plastic wrapping: microorganisms had no impact. In addition, hydrogels did not appreciably hydrate or macerate the surface by visual inspection when left in place for 1 week.

Some transdermal drug delivery systems (TDDS) may indeed provoke a dermatitis when applied twice weekly to the same site. These occlusive devices demonstrated marked cytotoxicity to Langerhans cells, melanocytes and keratinocytes (Kligman, 1996). However, Nieboer *et al.* (1987) evaluated the effects of occlusion with transdermal therapeutic systems (TTS) on Langerhans cell and skin irritation at different times ranging (6 hours, 1, 2, 4 and 7 days). Irritation was judged on morphology, histopathologic and immunofluorescence findings, and changes in the Langerhans cell systems. Occlusion provoked only slight or no skin irritation. Fluhr *et al.* (1999) evaluated the barrier damage by prolonged occlusion on the forearm for 24 to 96 h and did not find significant changes in hydration and water holding capacity. But, transepidermal water loss (TEWL) increased reaching a plateau on day 2, concluding that occlusion induced barrier damage without skin dryness.

2.5 QUANTIFICATION WITH BIOENGINEERING TECHNIQUES

Recently, noninvasive bioengineering techniques have been utilized to better quantify skin barrier function. Modern noninvasive techniques can assess the mechanical and physiological properties of skin in health and disease. Their great value becomes apparent in providing accurate, reproducible, and objective measurements that can determine subtle differences before visual clinical signs. The unaided eye is not reliable for determining subclinical changes.

We briefly introduce some common useful noninvasive bioengineering techniques below. Background, principles, extensive details, and validations of these techniques can be found in textbooks (Frosch and Kligman, 1993; Elsner *et al.*, 1994; Serup and Jemec, 1995; Berardesca *et al.*, 1995a; Berardesca *et al.*, 1995b; Wilhelm *et al.*, 1997).

A. TEWL, as a marker of barrier function and structure changes can be monitored by an evaporimeter (Tewameter) (Courage & Khazaka, Cologne, Germany, and Acaderm Inc., Menlo Park, CA, USA). It may also act as an indicator for the recovery of barrier function (Grubauer *et al.*, 1989). Standard guidelines are utilized (Pinnagoda *et al.*, 1990).

B. Cutaneous blood flux of test sites can be observed with a Laser Doppler Flowmeter (LDF) (Moor Instruments, Axminster, England) or Laser Doppler Velocimeter (LDV) (Acaderm Inc., Menlo Park, CA, USA). Methods and standard guidelines are described elsewhere (Bircher *et al.*, 1994).

C. Skin color can be measured by a reflectance meter (such as a colorimeter) (Minolta, Osaka, Japan, and Acaderm Inc., Menlo Park, CA, USA), and the a* value (red-green axis) is considered a reliable quantification of erythema (Wilhelm *et al.*, 1989; Wilhelm and Maibach, 1989). Standard guidelines and measuring principle have been described in detail (Fullerton *et al.*, 1996).

D. Capacitance as a parameter of stratum corneum hydration (or water content) can be determined with a capacitance meter (such as a Corneo-meter) (Courage & Khazaka, Cologne, Germany, and Acaderm Inc., Menlo Park, CA, USA). The measuring principle and methods are elsewhere (Triebskorn and Gloor, 1993).

Brief quantification data of bioengineering measurements on occlusive skin conditions are summarized in Table 2.1.

2.6 CONCLUSIONS

The effects of occlusion on skin barrier function have been defined with various techniques. Obviously, occlusion alone may damage skin barrier function. With application of chemicals/drugs under occlusion conditions, it can increase penetration of chemicals and antigens into the skin and therefore also increases dermatitis (Berardesca and Maibach, 1988; Kligman, 1996). Local reactions (i.e., irritation and/or sensitization) of TDDS which are typically occlusive patches placed on the skin surface for 1–7 days to deliver the drugs into the systemic circulation have been widely reported (Boddé *et al.*, 1989; Hogan and Maibach, 1990; Hogan and Maibach, 1991; Patil *et al.*, 1996; Murphy and Carmichael, 2000). However, reactions can be minimized with immunosuppressive agents, antioxidants, local anesthetics, and other anti-irritant technologies (Kydonieus and Wille, 2000). Topical corticoids are another alternative but their role in the suppression of TDDS induced dermatitis needs better definition, especially for patients who require continued treatment with long-term application of such devices (Hogan and Maibach, 1990). Advancements in design and construction of protective garments and wound dressings may reduce the level of skin hydration and dermatitis. Application of optimal hydrocolloid patches that

CHAPTER 2

TABLE 2.1:

Brief results of bioengineering measurements on occlusive skin condition.

Occlusive manner and time	Bioengineering techniques	Results	Authors and References
Plastic film for 5 days	TEWL	TEWL increased from 0.56 mg/cm2/h (baseline) to 1.87 mg/cm2/h (occlusion) and showed essentially saturated after 2 days.	Aly et al., (1978)
Plastic film for 1 h	TEWL and capacitance	Post-occlusion TEWL were significantly greater than the normal sites.	Orsmark et al. (1980)
Plastic film for 1, 3, and 8 days	TEWL and electromagnetic wave	Occlusion significantly increased TEWL and water content within 24 h.	Faergemann et al. (1983)
Occlusion with polypropylene chamber or vehicles for 30 min; hexyl nicotinate (HN) as an indicator	LDV	The onset of action and time to peak were significantly shortened, and the peak height and AUC significantly increased under occlusion conditions.	Ryatt et al. (1986)
Polypropylene chambers for 30 min; HN as an indicator	LDV	Occlusion significantly shortened both the time of onset of the LDV-detected response to HN and the time to peak response. In addition, the magnitude of the peak LDV response to HN and the area under curve (AUC) were significantly increased. Occlusion was also significantly elevated the stratum corneum water content. There was a significant correlation between stratum corneum water content and area under the LDV response-time curve after 30 min occlusion.	Ryatt et al. (1988)
Post-application occlusion after short-term SLS exposure for 5 consecutive days	TEWL	Occluded skin sites had a significant increase TEWL values (every-day and alternate-day schedule) when compared to unoccluded sites. Results indicated that post-exposure occlusive treatment markedly enhanced irritant response.	Van der Valk and Maibach (1989)
Chambers with 0.5% SLS, water, and empty chambers only for 3 h	TEWL	All values from SLS, water, and empty chambers were significantly increased as compared to normal skin.	Pinnagoda et al. (1990)
Aluminum chambers and chambers with water, physiological saline, a paper disc or 0.002% of SLS for 24 h	Electrical impedance	Occlusion did not affect readings of electrical skin impedance taken 24 h or later after removal, but increased variance for readings taken 1 h after removal.	Emtestam and Ollmar (1993)

Method	Parameters	Results	Reference
Glove patch for 4 h and 8, and empty dressing; HN as an indicator	LDV, TEWL, and skin surface roughness	Percorneal permeability, TEWL, compliance parameter were significantly increased after occlusion 4 and 8 h, and skin surface roughness was significantly reduced in terms of roughness parameters Ra and Rz by 4 and 8 h occlusion.	Graves et al. (1995)
Plastic chambers with a series of sodium alkyl sulfates for 24 h.	TEWL, capacitance, and a* values	All alkyl sulfates with the exception of sodium lauryl sulfate resulted in a temporary decrease of SC hydration 1 h after patch removal. At day 2, SC hydration levels of surfactant treated skin were not significantly different from controls. Thereafter, a second decrease in capacitance value was observed with lowest hydration at day 7.	Wilhelm (1995)
Different occlusive and semipermeable dressings for 23 and 46 h on irritation and tape stripping skins	TEWL and capacitance	Occlusion did not significantly delay barrier repair.	Welzel et al. (1995; 1996)
Short-term (6 h/day for 3 days) gloves on normal skin and gloves on SLS-compromised skin	TEWL, capacitance, and erythema index	Glove occlusion on normal skin for short-term exposure did not significantly change the water barrier function but caused a significantly negative effect on SLS-compromised skin for the same period.	Ramsing and Agner (1996a)
Long-term (6 h/day for 14 days) gloves on normal skin and a cotton glove worn under the occlusive glove	TEWL, capacitance, and erythema index	This long-term using glove occlusion on normal skin caused a significant negative effect on skin barrier function, as measured by TEWL, which was prevented by the cotton glove.	Ramsing and Agner (1996b)
Plastic chambers at 24, 48, 72 and 96 h	TEWL and capacitance	A significantly progressive increase under occlusion and reaching a plateau on day 2. Hydration and water holding capacity did not show significant changes.	Fluhr et al. (1999)
Occlusion with patches and diapers at different exposure times. Nicotinates as markers to evaluate skin permeability	Water evaporation rate (WER), skin blood flow volume (BFV), capacitance, and redness (a*)	Permeation of nicotinates was increased for hydrated skin versus control even after only 10 minutes of patch exposure. No evidence of increased permeation rates with increased hyperhydration once a relatively low threshold of hyperhydration was achieved (e.g., which reached after a 10 min wet patch).	Zhai et al. (2002)

absorb water in both liquid and vapor form can also decrease irritant reactions (Hurkmans *et al.*, 1985; Fairbrother *et al.*, 1992; Hollingsbee *et al.*, 1995). A natural, pure, and non-woven dressing has been made from calcium alginate fibers (Williams, 1999). It can rapidly absorb and retain wound fluid to form an integral gellified structure, thereby maintaining an ideal moist wound healing environment. It can also trap and immobilize pathogenic bacteria in the network of gellified fibers, stimulates macrophage activity and activate platelets, resulting in hemostasis and accelerated wound healing.

Today, with the rapid development of the new technologies in the bioscience, we expect greater efficacy and optimal dressings or materials that can absorb excess water and reduce the unfavorable effects of occlusion.

REFERENCES

AGNER, T. and SERUP, J. (1993) Time course of occlusive effects on skin evaluated by measurement of transepidermal water loss (TEWL). Including patch tests with sodium lauryl sulfate and water. *Contact Dermatitis* **28**, 6–9.

ALVAREZ, O.M., MERTZ, P.M. and EAGLSTEIN, W.H. (1983) The effect of occlusive dressings on collagen synthesis and re-epithelialization in superficial wounds. *Journal of Surgical Research* **35**, 142–148.

ALY, R., SHIRLEY, C., CUNICO, B. and MAIBACH, H.I. (1978) Effect of prolonged occlusion on the microbial flora, pH, carbon dioxide and transepidermal water loss on human skin. *Journal of Investigative Dermatology* **71**, 378–381.

BAKER, H. (1972) The skin as a barrier. In: ROOK, A. ,WILKINSON, D.S. and EBLING, F.J.G. (eds) *Textbook of Dermatology,* 2nd ed. Oxford: Blackwell Scientific Publications, 249–255.

BERARDESCA, E. and MAIBACH, H.I. (1988) Skin occlusion: treatment or drug-like device? *Skin Pharmacology* **1**, 207–215.

BERARDESCA, E. and MAIBACH, H.I. (1996) The plastic occlusion stress test (POST) as a model to investigate skin barrier function. In: Maibach, H.I. (ed.) *Dermatologic Research Techniques,* Boca Raton: CRC Press, 179–186.

BERARDESCA, E., ELSNER, P. and MAIBACH, H.I. (1995a) *Bioengineering of the Skin: Cutaneous blood flow and erythema.* Boca Raton: CRC Press.

BERARDESCA, E., ELSNER, P., WILHELM, K-P. and MAIBACH, H.I. (1995b) *Bioengineering of the Skin: Methods and instrumentation.* Boca Raton: CRC Press.

BIRCHER, A., DE BOER, E.M., AGNER, T., WAHLBERG, J.E. and SERUP, J. (1994)

Guidelines for measurement of cutaneous blood flow by laser Doppler flowmetry. *Contact Dermatitis* **30**, 65–72.

BODDÉ, H.E., VERHOEVEN, J., VAN DRIEL, L.M.J. (1989) The skin compliance of transdermal drug delivery systems. *Critical Reviews in Therapeutics Drug Carrier Systems* **6**, 87–115.

BUCKS, D.A., McMASTER, J.R., MAIBACH, H.I. and GUY, R.H. (1988) Bioavailability of topically administered steroids: a "mass balance" technique. *Journal of Investigative Dermatology* **91**, 29–33.

BUCKS, D. and MAIBACH, H.I. (1999) Occlusion does not uniformly enhance penetration *in vivo*. In: BRONAUGH, R.L. and MAIBACH, H.I., eds. *Percutaneous Absorption: Drug-cosmetics-mechanisms-methodology*, 3rd ed. New York: Marcel Dekker, 81–105.

BUCKS, D., GUY, R. and MAIBACH, H.I. (1991) Effects of occlusion. In: BRONAUGH, R.L. and MAIBACH, H.I. eds. *In Vitro Percutaneous Absorption: Principles, fundamentals, and applications*, Boca Raton: CRC Press, 85–114.

CROSS, S.E. and ROBERTS, M.S. (2000) The effect of occlusion on epidermal penetration of parabens from a commercial allergy test ointment, acetone and ethanol vehicles. *Journal of Investigative Dermatology* **115**, 914–918.

DENDA, M., SATO, J., TSUCHIYA, T., ELIAS, P.M. and FEINGOLD, K.R. (1998) Low humidity stimulates epidermal DNA synthesis and amplifies the hyper-proliferative response to barrier disruption: implication for seasonal exacerbations of inflammatory dermatoses. *Journal of Investigative Dermatology* **111**, 873–878.

EAGLSTEIN, W.H. (1984) Effect of occlusive dressings on wound healing. *Clinics in Dermatology* **2**, 107–111.

ELSNER, P., BERARDESCA, E. and MAIBACH, H.I. (1994) *Bioengineering of the Skin: Water and the stratum corneum*. Boca Raton: CRC Press.

EMTESTAM, L. and OLLMAR, S. (1993) Electrical impedance index in human skin: measurements after occlusion, in 5 anatomical regions and in mild irritant contact dermatitis. *Contact Dermatitis* **28**, 104–108.

ESTLANDER, T., JOLANKI, R. and KANERVA, L. (1996) Rubber glove dermatitis: A significant occupational hazard-prevention. In: ELSNER, P., LACHAPELLE, J.M., WAHLBERG, J.E. and MAIBACH, H.I., eds. *Prevention of Contact Dermatitis. Current problem in dermatology*, Basel: Karger, 170–176.

FAERGEMANN, J., ALY, R., WILSON, D.R. and MAIBACH, H.I. (1983) Skin Occlusion: effect on pityrosporum orbiculare, skin P CO2, pH, transepidermal water loss, and water content. *Archives of Dermatological Research* **275**, 383–387.

CHAPTER 2

FAIRBROTHER, J.E., HOLLINGSBEE, D.A. and WHITE, R.J. (1992) Hydrocolloid dermatological patches–corticosteroid combinations. In: MAIBACH, H.I. and SURBER, C., eds. *Topical Corticosteroids*, Basel: Karger, 503–511.

FLUHR, J.W., LAZZERINI, S., DISTANTE, F., GLOOR, M. and BERARDESCA, E. (1999) Effects of prolonged occlusion on stratum corneum barrier function and water holding capacity. *Skin Pharmacology and Applied Skin Physiology* **12**, 193–198.

FROSCH, P.J. and KLIGMAN, A.M. (1993) *Noninvasive Methods for the Quantification of Skin Functions*. Basel: Karger.

FULLERTON, A., FISCHER, T., LAHTI, A., WILHELM, K.P., TAKIWAKI, H. and SERUP, J. (1996) Guidelines for measurement of skin colour and erythema. *Contact Dermatitis* **35**, 1–10.

GRAVES, C.J., EDWARDS, C. and MARKS, R. (1995) The occlusive effects of protective gloves on the barrier properties of the stratum corenum. In: ELSNER, P. and MAIBACH, H.I. (eds) *Irritant Dermatitis. New clinical and experimental aspects. Current problem in dermatology*, Basel: Karger, 87–94.

GRUBAUER, G., ELIAS, P.M. and FEINGOLD, K.R. (1989) Transepidermal water loss: the signal for the recovery of barrier structure and function. *Journal of Lipid Research* **30**, 323–333.

HAFTEK, M., TEILLON, M.H. and SCHMITT, D. (1998) Stratum corneum, corneodesmosomes and ex vivo percutaneous penetration. *Microscopy Research and Technique* **43**, 242–249.

HINMAN, C.D. and MAIBACH, H.I. (1963) Effect of air exposure and occlusion on experimental human skin wounds. *Nature* **200**, 377–378.

HOGAN, D.J. and MAIBACH, H.I. (1990) Adverse dermatologic reactions to transdermal drug delivery systems. *Journal of the American Academy of Dermatology* **22**, 811–814.

HOGAN, D.J. and MAIBACH, H.I. (1991) Transdermal drug delivery systems: adverse reaction—dermatologic overview. In: MENNE, T. and MAIBACH, H.I., eds. *Exogenous Dermatoses: Environmental dermatitis*, Boca Raton: CRC Press, 227–234.

HOLLINGSBEE, D.A., WHITE, R.J. and EDWARDSON, P.A.D. (1995) Use of occluding hydrocolloid patches. In: SMITH, E.W. and MAIBACH, H.I. (eds) *Percutaneous Penetration Enhancers*, Boca Raton: CRC Press, 35–43.

HOSTYNEK, J.J., MAGEE, P.S. and MAIBACH, H.I. (1996) QSAR predictive of contact allergy: scope and limitations. In: ELSNER, P., LACHAPELLE, J.M. WAHLBERG,

J.E. and MAIBACH, H.I. (eds) *Prevention of Contact Dermatitis. Current problem in dermatology,* Basel: Karger, 18–27.

HOTCHKISS, S.A., MILLER, J.M. and CALDWELL, J. (1992) Percutaneous absorption of benzyl acetate through rat skin *in vitro.* 2. Effect of vehicle and occlusion. *Food and Chemical Toxicology* **30**, 145–153.

HURKMANS, J.F., BODDÉ, H.E., VAN DRIEL, L.M., VAN DOORNE, H. and JUNGINGER, H.E. (1985) Skin irritation caused by transdermal drug delivery systems during long-term (5 days) application. *British Journal of Dermatology* **112**, 461–467.

KLIGMAN, A.M. (1996) Hydration injury to human skin. In: VAN DER VALK, P.G.M. and MAIBACH, H.I., eds. *The Irritant Contact Dermatitis Syndrome,* Boca Raton: CRC Press, 187–194.

KLIGMAN, A.M. (2000) Hydration injury to human skin: A view from the horny layer. In: KANERVA, L., ELSNER, P., WAHLBERG, J.E. and MAIBACH, H.I., eds. *Handbook of Occupational Dermatology,* Berlin: Springer, 76–80.

KÖMÜVES, L.G., HANLEY, K., JIANG, Y., KATAGIRI, C., ELIAS, P.M., WILLIAMS, M.L. and FEINGOLD, K.R. (1999) Induction of selected lipid metabolic enzymes and differentiation-linked structural proteins by air exposure in fetal rat skin explants. *Journal of Investigative Dermatology* **112**, 303–309.

KYDONIEUS, A.F. and WILLE, J.J. (2000) Modulation of skin reactions: a general overview. In: KYDONIEUS, A.F. and WILLE, J.J. (eds) *Biochemical Modulation of Skin Reactions. Transdermals, topicals, cosmetics,* Boca Raton: CRC Press, 205–221.

LEOW, Y.H. and MAIBACH, H.I. (1997) Effect of occlusion on skin. *Journal of Dermatological Treatment* **8**, 139–142.

MATHIAS, C.G.T. (1990) Prevention of occupational contact dermatitis. *Journal of the American Academy of Dermatology* **23**, 742–748.

MATSUMURA, H., OKA, K., UMEKAGE, K., AKITA, H., KAWAI, J., KITAZAWA, Y., SUDA, S., TSUBOTA, K., NINOMIYA, Y., HIRAI, H., MIYATA, K., MORIKUBO, K., NAKAGAWA, M., OKADA, T. and KAWAI, K. (1995) Effect of occlusion on human skin. *Contact Dermatitis* **33**, 231–235.

MERTZ, P.M. and EAGLSTEIN, W.H. (1984) The effect of a semiocclusive dressing on the microbial population in superficial wounds. *Archives of Surgery* **119**, 287–289.

MURPHY, M. and CARMICHAEL, A.J. (2000) Transdermal drug delivery systems and skin sensitivity reactions. Incidence and management. *American Journal of Clinical Dermatology* **1**, 361–368.

■ CHAPTER 2 ■

NIEBOER, C., BRUYNZEEL, D.P. and BOORSMA, D.M. (1987) The effect of occlusion of the skin with transdermal therapeutic system on Langerhans cells and the induction of skin irritation. *Archives of Dermatology* **123**, 1499–1502.

ORSMARK, K., WILSON, D. and MAIBACH, H.I. (1980) *In vivo* transepidermal water loss and epidermal occlusive hydration in newborn infants: anatomical region variation. *Acta Dermato-Venereologica* **60**, 403–407.

PATIL, S., HOGAN, D.J. and MAIBACH, H.I. (1996) Transdermal drug delivery systems: Adverse dermatologic reactions. In: MARZULLI, F.N. and MAIBACH, H.I. (eds) *Dermatotoxicology*, 5th edn. Washington DC: Taylor & Francis, 389–396.

PINNAGODA, J., TUPKER, R.A., AGNER, T. and SERUP, J. (1990) Guidelines for transepidermal water loss (TEWL) measurement. *Contact Dermatitis* **22**, 164–178.

QIAO, G.L., CHANG, S.K. and RIVIERE, J.E. (1993) Effects of anatomical site and occlusion on the percutaneous absorption and residue pattern of 2,6-[ring-14C] parathion *in vivo* in pigs. *Toxicology and Applied Pharmacology* **122**, 131–138.

RAJKA, G, ALY, R., BAYLES, C., TANG, Y. and MAIBACH, H.I. (1981) The effect of short-term occlusion on the cutaneous flora in atopic dermatitis and psoriasis. *Acta Dermato-Venereologica* **61**, 150–153.

RAMSING, D.W. and AGNER, T. (1996a) Effect of glove occlusion on human skin. (I). short-term experimental exposure. *Contact Dermatitis* **34**, 1–5.

RAMSING, D.W. and AGNER, T. (1996b) Effect of glove occlusion on human skin (II). Long-term experimental exposure. *Contact Dermatitis* **34**, 258–262.

RYATT, K.S., MOBAYEN, M., STEVENSON, J.M., MAIBACH, H.I. and GUY, R.H. (1988) Methodology to measure the transient effect of occlusion on skin penetration and stratum corneum hydration *in vivo*. *British Journal of Dermatology* **119**, 307–312.

RYATT, K.S., STEVENSON, J.M., MAIBACH, H.I. and GUY, R.H. (1986) Pharmacodynamic measurement of percutaneous penetration enhancement *in vivo*. *Journal of Pharmaceutical Science* **75**, 374–377.

SCHOLTZ, J.R. (1961) Topical therapy of psoriasis with fluocinolone acetonide. *Archives of Dermatology* **84**, 1029–1030.

SERUP, J. and JEMEC, G.B.E. (1995) *Handbook of Non-invasive Methods and the Skin*. Boca Raton: CRC Press.

SULZBERGER, M.B. and WITTEN, V.H. (1961) Thin pliable plastic films in topical dermatologic therapy. *Archives of Dermatology* **84**, 1027–1028.

TREFFEL, P., MURET, P., MURET-D'ANIELLO, P., COUMES-MARQUET, S. and AGACHE, P. (1992) Effect of occlusion on *in vitro* percutaneous absorption of two compounds with different physicochemical properties. *Skin Pharmacology* **5**, 108–113.

TRIEBSKORN, A. and GLOOR, M. (1993) Noninvasive methods for the determination of skin hydration. In: FROSCH, P.J. and KLIGMAN, A.M., eds. *Noninvasive Methods for the Quantification of Skin Functions,* Basel: Karger, 42–55.

TSAI, T-F. and MAIBACH, H.I. (1999) How irritant is water? An overview. *Contact Dermatitis* **41**, 311–314.

VAN DER VALK, P.G.M. and MAIBACH, H.I. (1989) Post-application occlusion substantially increases the irritant response of the skin to repeated short-term sodium lauryl sulfate (SLS) exposure. *Contact Dermatitis* **21**, 335–338.

WARNER, R.R., BOISSY, Y.L., LILLY, N.A., SPEARS, M.J., MCKILLOP, K., MARSHALL, J.L. and STONE, K.J. (1999) Water disrupts stratum corneum lipid lamellae: damage is similar to surfactants. *Journal of Investigative Dermatology* **113**, 960–966.

WELZEL, J., WILHELM, K.P. and WOLFF, H.H. (1995) Occlusion does not influence the repair of the permeability barrier in human skin. In: ELSNER, P. and MAIBACH, H.I., eds. *Irritant Dermatitis. New clinical and experiemntal aspects. Current problem in dermatology*, Basel: Karger, 180–186.

WELZEL, J., WILHELM, K.P. and WOLFF, H.H. (1996) Skin permeability barrier and occlusion: no delay of repair in irritated human skin. *Contact Dermatitis* **35**, 163–168.

WIECHERS, J.W. (1989) The barrier function of the skin in relation to percutaneous absorption of drugs. *Pharmaceutisch Weekblad* **11**, 185–198.

WILHELM, K.P. (1995) Effects of surfactants on skin hydration. In: SURBER, C. ELSNER, P. and BIRCHER, A.J. (eds) *Exogenous Dermatology. Current problem in dermatology*, Basel: Karger, 72–79.

WILHELM, K.P. and MAIBACH, H.I. (1989) Skin color reflectance measurement for objective quantification of erythema in human beings. *Journal of the American Academy of Dermatology* **21**, 1306–1308.

WILHELM, K.P., SURBER, C. and MAIBACH, H.I. (1989) Quantification of sodium lauryl sulfate dermatitis in man: comparison of four techniques: skin color

CHAPTER 2

reflectance, transepidermal water loss, laser Doppler flow measurement and visual scores. *Archives of Dermatological Research* **281**, 293–295.

WILHELM, K-P., ELSNER, P., BERARDESCA, E. and MAIBACH, H.I. (1997) *Bioengineering of the Skin: Skin surface imaging and analysis.* Boca Raton: CRC Press.

WILLIAMS, C. (1999) Algosteril calcium alginate dressing for moderate/high exudate. *British Journal of Nursing* **8**, 313–317.

WINTER, G.D. (1962) Formation of the scab and the rate of epithelization of superficial wounds in the skin of the young domestic pig. *Nature* **193**, 293–294.

WINTER, G.D. and SCALES, J.T. (1963) Effect of air drying and dressings on the surface of a wound. *Nature* **197**, 91–92.

ZHAI, H. and MAIBACH, H.I. (2002) Occlusion versus skin barrier function. *Skin Research and Technology* **8**, 1–6.

ZHAI, H., EBEL, J.P., CHATTERJEE, R., STONE, K.J., GARTSTEIN, V., JUHLIN, K.D., PELOSI, A. and MAIBACH, H.I. (2002) Hydration versus skin permeability to nicotinates in man. *Skin Research and Technology* **8**, 13–18.

Percutaneous Absorption of Complex Chemical Mixtures

JIM E RIVIERE

Contents

3.1   Introduction

3.2   Levels of interaction

3.3   Examples of mixture interactions

3.4   Conclusions

3.1 INTRODUCTION

The percutaneous absorption of chemicals is most often studied using single chemicals applied to the surface of skin, often in a vehicle if solubilization is necessary. Exposure in most environmental and occupational scenarios occurs to combinations of chemicals. Similarly, most dermatological drugs are dosed in formulations composed of multiple additives. The difference is that in the pharmaceutical sector, components of a formulation are usually added for a specific purpose and their effects on drug absorption have been studied. In environmental and occupational scenarios, the chemicals to which an individual is exposed are a function of their occurrence in the environment. The effect of one chemical modulating absorption of a second mixture component is not known. Risk assessments on topical exposure to chemical mixtures are presently an area of intense interest.

The potential for chemical mixture interactions affecting systemic drug and chemical disposition and toxicity has been well recognized for many years and has been comprehensively reviewed elsewhere (Bliss, 1939; Yang, 1994; Pohl *et al.*, 1997; Haddad *et al.*, 2000, 2001; Borgert *et al.*, 2001; Groten *et al.*, 2001). Similarly, the potential for drug–drug pharmacokinetic interactions has been recognized and debated in the context of the development of cassette dosing in drug discovery screening (White and Manitpisitkul, 2001; Christ, 2001). Despite this widespread acknowledgment of the importance of chemical interactions in systemic pharmacology and toxicology, little attention outside of the dermatological formulation arena has been paid to interactions that may occur after topical exposure to complex mixtures. The focus of this chapter is to provide a brief review into factors that should be considered when chemical mixtures are topically applied to skin.

3.2 LEVELS OF INTERACTION

The focus on any interaction is usually related to a compound of pharmacological or toxicological interest. The concern is then on how other chemicals in the mixture modulate the percutaneous absorption or dermatotoxicity of this chemical of interest. To clarify this discussion, we will refer to the compound of pharmacological or toxicological interest as the "marker" compound and all other substances present in the mixture as "components." In a simple binary mixture, the component would be the vehicle. It must be stressed that the purpose of selecting a component of a mixture as a "marker" compound does not confer special importance to this chemical relative to the other "components" present. It is purely an artificial construct to provide a frame of reference on which chemical interactions can be discussed. In many cases, multiple components may in fact be toxic or cause irritation.

Previously, we have presented a conceptual framework upon which the study of chemical interactions involved in compound percutaneous absorption can be based, termed Mechanistically-Defined Chemical Mixtures (MDCM) (Baynes *et al.*, 1996; Qiao *et al.*, 1996; Williams *et al.*, 1996). This approach assumes that components that are capable of modulating a marker's absorption or cutaneous disposition would result in an altered pharmacological or toxicological effect. Table 3.1 lists a series of levels in which chemical and biological interactions could occur.

The first potential for chemical–chemical interactions is on the surface of the skin. The types of phenomena that could occur are governed by the laws of solution chemistry, and include factors such as altered solubility, precipitation, super-saturation, solvation or volatility; as well as physical chemical effects such as altered surface tension from the presence of surfactants, changed solution viscosity and micelle formation (Idson, 1983; Williams and Barry, 1998; Barry, 2001; Moser *et al.*, 2001). For some of these effects, chemicals act independent of one another. However, for many the presence of other component chemicals may modulate the effect seen. Chemical interactions may further be modulated by interaction with adnexial structures or their products such as hair, sebum or sweat secretions. The result is that when a marker chemical is dosed on the

TABLE 3.1:

Levels of potential interactions after topical exposure to chemical mixtures

Surface	Chemical–chemical (binding, ion-pair formation, etc.)
	Altered physical-chemical properties
	(e.g. solubility, volatility, critical micelle concentration)
	Altered rates of surface evaporation
	Occlusive behavior
	Binding or interaction with adnexial structures or their
	products (e.g. hair, sweat, sebum).
Stratum corneum	Altered permeability through lipid pathway (e.g. enhancer)
	Altered partitioning into stratum corneum
	Extraction of intercellular lipids
Epidermis	Altered biotransformation
	Induction of and/or modulation of inflammatory mediators
Dermis	Altered vascular function
	(direct or secondary to mediator release)

skin as a component of a chemical mixture, the amount freely available for subsequent absorption may be significantly affected. The primary driving force for chemical absorption in skin is passive diffusion that requires a concentration gradient of thermodynamically active (free) chemical.

The next level of potential interaction are those involving the marker and/or component chemicals with the constituents of the stratum corneum. These include the classic enhancers such as oleic acid, Azone®, or ethanol, widely reviewed elsewhere (Williams and Barry, 1998). These chemicals alter a compound's permeability within the intercellular lipids of the stratum corneum. Similarly, the partition coefficient between the drug in the surface dosing vehicle and stratum corneum lipids may be altered if chemical components of the mixture also partition and diffuse into the lipids and thus alter their composition. Organic vehicles on the surface of the skin may extract stratum corneum lipids that would alter permeability to the marker chemical (Monteiro-Riviere *et al.*, 2001; Rastogi and Singh, 2001). Compounds may also bind to stratum corneum constituents forming a depot.

The next level of interaction would be with the viable epidermis. The most obvious point of potential interaction would be with a compound that undergoes biotransformation (Bronaugh *et al.*, 1989; Mukhtar, 1992). A marker and component could interact in a number of ways, including competitive or non-competitive inhibition for occupancy at the enzyme's active site, or induction or inhibition of drug metabolizing enzymes. Other structural and functional enzymes could also be affected (e.g. lipid synthesis enzymes) which would modify barrier function (Elias and Feingold, 1992). A penetrating marker or component could also induce keratinocytes to release cytokines or other inflammatory mediators (Luger and Schwarz, 1990; Allen *et al.*, 2000). Monteiro-Riviere *et al.* (2003) which could ultimately alter barrier function in the stratum corneum or vascular function in the dermis. Alternatively, cytokines may modulate biotransformation enzyme activities (Morgan, 2001). A dermato-pharmacokinetic scheme taking into account marker and a single component (vehicle) compound penetration and potential interaction is depicted in Figure 31.6 of the present text.

The final level of potential interaction is in the dermis where a component chemical may directly or indirectly (e.g. via cytokine release in the epidermis) modulate vascular uptake of the penetrated marker (Riviere and Williams, 1992; Williams and Riviere, 1993). In addition to modulating transdermal flux of chemical, such vascular modulation could also affect the depth and extent of marker penetration into underlying tissues.

■ CHAPTER 3 ■

TABLE 3.2:

Experimental model systems used to assess levels of interactions.

In vitro physical-chemical determinations	Solubility Viscosity Critical Micelle Concentration Partition coefficients
In vitro silicone membrane diffusion cells	*Above effects* Assess partitioning and diffusion through defined membrane.
In vitro dermatomed skin diffusion cells[a]	*Above effects* Partitioning and diffusion parameters through stratum corneum and viable epidermis Epidermal biotransformation
Ex vivo isolated perfused porcine skin flaps (IPPSF)	*Above effects* Vascular modulation Inflammatory mediators Dermal binding and metabolism
In vivo whole animals or humans	*All above effects* Systemic feedback operative

[a] Human and porcine skin (correlated to IPPSF and *in vivo*)

It must be stressed that interactions at all of these levels could occur simultaneously, and multiple components could be affecting marker penetration, as well as other component disposition in skin. These can optimally be teased apart using a hierarchy of experimental model systems which are only responsive to specific levels of interactions. A scheme used in our laboratory to study these effects is depicted in Table 3.2. The important point to stress about this scheme is that when a chemical mixture absorption is being assessed, the biological complexity of the experimental model system must be sufficient to detect the interaction. It is the sum of all interactions that ultimately determines the mixture's effect on marker absorption or skin disposition.

3.3   EXAMPLES OF MIXTURE INTERACTIONS

The above conceptual framework for assessing the importance of chemical mixture interactions on a marker chemical absorption or cutaneous disposition is by no way unique. As mentioned earlier, many of these interactions have been defined in binary mixtures consisting of marker chemical and vehicle, and thus are often categorized as vehicle effects. The problems occur when the absorption of complex mixtures, such as environmental contaminants at waste sites ($\approx$ 50) or hydrocarbon fuels (> 200) are considered. Many "simple" occupational mixtures may contain upwards of 5–10 compounds. Some interactions may be synergistic, others antagonistic. The result observed is a vectorial sum of all interactions. The principles of complexity and chaotic systems teach us that when simple systems are added together, emergent behavior may occur which is not predictable from examining simpler systems with fewer components (Bar-Yum, 1997). We have demonstrated this lack of predictability when the behavior of single and 2×2 combinations of jet fuel additives did not predict the behavior of hydrocarbon marker absorption when all three additives were present (Baynes *et al.*, 2001).

A number of investigators have probed non-vehicle type mixture effects on topical absorption. Reifenrath and co-workers (1996) demonstrated that exposure of skin to a complex chemical irritant (hydroxylammonium nitrate, triethanolammonium nitrate, water) resulted in enhanced skin permeability of subsequently applied benzoic acid using *in vitro* and *in vivo* models. Based on their own data and an interpretation of other irritant studies (Bronaugh and Stewart, 1985; Wilhelm *et al.*, 1991), they concluded that *in vitro* and *in vivo* studies agree when alterations occur to the stratum corneum barrier. However, when irritants influence other aspects of cutaneous physiology (e.g. vesication, erythema), then the *in vivo* response may be exaggerated. A role of estradiol in modulating phenol absorption has been reported (Abou-Hadeed *et al.*, 1998).

Our laboratory initially implemented the MDCM approach studying the effects of sodium lauryl sulfate (surfactant), methyl nicotinate (rubefacient) and stannous chloride (reducing agent) in aqueous mixtures containing either acetone or DMSO on the percutaneous absorption of parathion (Qiao *et al.*, 1996) and benzidine (Baynes *et al.*, 1996). These studies in parathion mixtures containing up to six components demonstrated significant modulation (eleven-fold) of marker compound absorption and skin penetration depending on the composition of the dosed mixture. Higher level statistical interactions between mixture components were detected. Benzidine absorptions were modulated ten-fold. In both studies, some compounds tended to enhance absorption (sodium lauryl sulfate, DMSO) while others (stannous chloride) tended to retard absorption when present in a mixture. Methyl nicotinate blunted parathion absorptive flux and changed the shape of the absorption profile. The effects of some mixture components were most dramatically evidenced by changes in the absorption/skin deposition ratios. Stratum corneum barrier function as measured by transepidermal water loss in the benzidine study changed as a function of mixture composition (Baynes *et al.*, 1997). These studies concluded

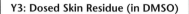

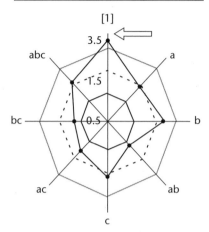

Figure 3.1: Compass plot illustrating a three component chemical interaction. Mean (---) and confidence intervals (——) are depicted for all combinations of treatments a, b, and c. Points outside of this polygon (⇒) are significantly different.

that the percutaneous absorption and skin deposition of the marker compounds benzidine and parathion were significantly dependent upon the composition of the chemical mixture in which they were dosed. Compass plots (Figure 3.1), a novel graphical tool was developed to statistically evaluate and illustrate the interactions present in such complex mixtures (Budsaba *et al.*, 2000).

Similar mixture interactions were detected in a study of pentachlorophenol (PCP) percutaneous absorption (Riviere *et al.*, 2001), where PCP flux varied twelve-fold depending on the mixture applied. These data are illustrated in Figure 3.2. In contrast, absorption of 3,3′,4,4′ tetrachlorobiphenyl (TCB) and 3,3′,4,4′,5-pentachlorobiphenyl (PCB) were minimal in this system under all exposure scenarios.

Percutaneous absorption of topically applied permethrin and *N,N*-diethyl-*m*-toluamide (DEET), two chemical entities putatively involved in the Gulf War Syndrome, was modulated by co-exposure to one another, as well as simultaneous exposure to topical jet fuels, sulfur mustard or organophosphates (Baynes *et al.*, 2002; Riviere *et al.*, 2002, 2003). The highest flux of labeled permethrin was observed when pyridostigmine and the organophosphate nerve agent simulant DFP was infused into the *in vitro* and *ex vivo* models, an experimental manipulation which also blunted inflammatory mediator release

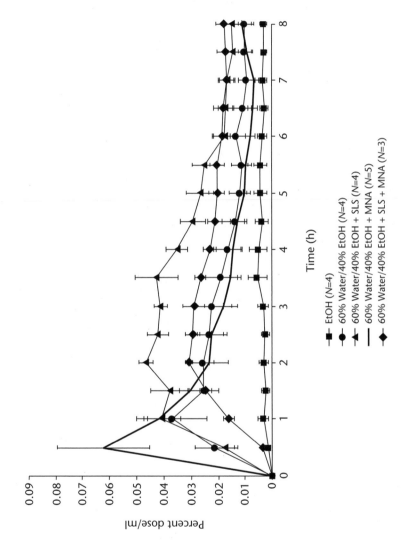

Figure 3.2: IPPSF perfusate absorption profiles of PCP (mean ± SEM).

simultaneously assessed (Monteiro-Riviere *et al.*, 2003). This later observation highlights the importance of both topical and systemic chemical exposures to modulate absorption of marker compounds.

3.4 CONCLUSIONS

This brief review clearly demonstrates that dermal absorption of a chemical administered in a complex chemical mixture of even 3–4 components, cannot be predicted from simpler exposure scenarios. However, in some cases, certain additives have consistent effects across mixtures (e.g. sodium lauryl sulfate, stannous chloride) due to a consistent mechanism of action. This approach to predict the effect of a complex mixture is to define the components based on their potential mechanism of action relative to modulating absorption. Use of multiple levels of experimental models facilitates this endeavor. Precise definition and quantitation of such interactions would allow for the development of complex interactive dermatopharmacokinetic models. (Williams *et al.*, 1996).

However, the picture is not as clear as this conclusion implies. The effect of components on marker absorption are dependent upon the chemical properties of the marker being studied, thus PCP behaved differently than PCB or TCB. Similarly, component effects on parathion and benzidine were different. It is theoretically feasible that some mixture components, such as classical enhancers like oleic acid, might induce what amounts to a phase-transition in the stratum corneum lipids which would totally change the types of interactions seen with other mixture components. This would be an example of emergent behavior, a phenomenon that would make extrapolations from experimental studies or simpler mixture exposures problematic. Evidence of this was seen in the parathion mixture experiments where certain combinations resulted in a great enhancement of treatment variance, an indicator that the system was no longer stable.

The risk assessment of topical chemical mixtures is a research and toxicological exposure paradigm which will become increasingly important as occupational and environmental problems become more common. Interactions should be defined in specific physical chemical and biological terms so that methods to integrate findings across studies can be developed. Model systems should not be over-interpreted, and caution must be exercised when extrapolating from simple *in vitro* models up the ladder of biological complexity.

REFERENCES

ABOU-HADEED, A.H., EL-TAWIL, O.S., SKOWRONSKI, G.A. and ABDEL-RAHMAN, M.S. (1998) The role of oestradiol on the dermal penetration of phenol, alone or in a mixture, in ovariectomized rats. *Toxicol In Vitro* **12**, 611–618.

ALLEN, D.G., RIVIERE, J.E. and MONTEIRO-RIVIERE, N.A. (2000) Induction of early biomarkers of inflammation produced by keratinocytes exposed to jet fuels Jet-A, JP-8, and JP-8(100). *J. Biochem. Molecular Toxicol.* **14**, 231–237.

BARRY, B.W. (2001) Novel mechanisms and devices to enable successful transdermal drug delivery. *Eur. J. Pharm. Sci.* **14**, 101–114.

BAR-YUM, Y. (1997) *Dynamic of Complex Systems*. Reading, MA: Addison-Wesley.

BAYNES, R.E., BROWNIE, C., FREEMAN, H. and RIVIERE, J.E. (1996) *In vitro* percutaneous absorption of benzidine in complex mechanistically defined chemical mixtures. *Toxicol. Appl. Pharmacol.* **141**, 497–506.

BAYNES, R.E., BROOKS, J.D., BUDSABA, K., SMITH, C.E. and RIVIERE, J.E. (2001) Mixture effects of JP-8 additives on the dermal disposition of jet fuel components. *Toxicol. Appl. Pharmacol.* **175**, 269–281.

BAYNES, R.E., MONTEIRO-RIVIERE, N.A. and RIVIERE, J.E. (2002) Pyridostigmine bromide modulates the dermal disposition of C-14 permethrin *Toxicol. Appl. Pharmacol.* **181**, 164–173.

BLISS, C.I. (1939) The toxicity of poisons applied jointly. *Ann. Appl. Biol.* **26**, 585–615.

BORGERT, C.J., PRICE, B., WELLS, C.S. and SIMON, G.S. (2001) Evaluating chemical interaction studies for mixture risk assessment. *Human Ecol. Risk Assessment* **7**, 259–306.

BRONAUGH, R.L. and STEWART, R.F. (1985) Methods for *in vitro* percutaneous absorption studies. V. Permeation through damaged skin. *J. Pharm. Sci.* **74**, 1062–1066.

BRONAUGH, R.L., STEWART, R.F. and STROM, J.E. (1989) Extent of cutaneous metabolism during percutaneous absorption of xenobiotics. *Toxicol. Appl. Pharmacol.* **99**, 534–543.

BUDSABA, K., SMITH, C.E. and RIVIERE, J.E. (2000) Compass Plots: A combination of star plot and analysis of means to visualize significant interactions in complex toxicology studies. *Toxicol. Methods* **10**, 313–332.

CHRIST, D.D. (2001) Commentary: Cassette Dosing Pharmacokinetics: Valuable Tool or Flawed Science? *Drug. Metabol. Disposit.* **29**, 935.

■ CHAPTER 3 ■

ELIAS, P.M. and FEINGOLD, K.R. (1992) Lipids and the epidermal water barrier: metabolism, regulation, and pathophysiology. *Sem. Dermatol.* **11**, 176–182.

GROTEN, J.P., FERON, V.J. and SÜHNEL, J. (2001). Toxicology of simple and complex mixtures. *TRENDS Pharmacol. Sci.* **22**, 316–322.

HADDAD, S., BÉLIVEAU, M., TARDIF, R. and KRISHNAN, K. (2001) A PBPK modeling-based approach to account for interactions in the health risk assessment of chemical mixtures. *Toxicological Sci.* **63**, 125–131.

HADDAD, S., CHAREST-TARDIF, G., TARDIF, R. and KRISHNAN, K. (2000) Validation of a physiological modeling framework for simulating the toxicokinetics of chemicals in mixtures. *Toxicol. Appl. Pharmacol.* **167**, 199–209.

IDSON, B. (1983) Vehicle effects in percutaneous absorption. *Drug Metab. Rev.* **14**, 207–222.

LUGER, T.A. and SCHWARZ, T. (1990) Evidence for an epidermal cytokine network. *J. Invest. Dermatol.* **95**, 104–110S.

MONTEIRO-RIVIERE, N.A., BAYNES, R.E. and RIVIERE, J.E. (2003) Pyridostigmine bromide modulates topical irritant-induced cytokine release from human epidermal keratinocytes and isolated perfused porcine skin. *Toxicology* **183**, 15–28.

MONTEIRO-RIVIERE, N.A., INMAN, A.O., MAK, V., WERTZ, P. and RIVIERE, J.E. (2001) Effects of selective lipid extraction from different body regions on epidermal barrier function. *Pharm. Res.* **18**, 992–998.

MORGAN, E.T. (2001) Regulation of cytochrome P450 by inflammatory mediators: Why and how? *Drug Metab. Disposit.* **29**, 207–212.

MOSER, K., KRIWET, K., KALIA, Y.N. and GUY, R.H. (2001) Enhanced skin permeation of a lipophilic drug using supersaturated formulations. *J. Contr. Release* **73**, 245–253.

MUKHTAR, H. (1992) *Pharmacology of the Skin.* Boca Raton, FL: CRC Press.

POHL, H.R., HANSEN, H. and SELENE J. and CHOU, C.H. (1997) Public health guidance values for chemical mixtures: Current practice and future directions. *Reg. Toxicol. Pharmacol.* **26**, 322–329.

QIAO, G.L., BROOKS, J.D., BAYNES, R.E., MONTEIRO-RIVIERE, N.A., WILLIAMS, P.L. and RIVIERE, J.E. (1996) The use of mechanistically defined chemical mixtures (MDCM) to assess component effects on the percutaneous absorption and cutaneous disposition of topically-exposed chemicals. I. Studies with parathion mixtures in isolated perfused porcine skin. *Toxicol. Appl. Pharmacol.* **141**, 473–486.

RASTOGI, S.K. and SINGH, J. (2001) Lipid extraction and transport of hydrophilic solutes through porcine epidermis. *Int. J. Pharm.* **225**, 75–82.

REIFENRATH, W.G., KEMPPAINEN, B.W. and PALMER, W.G. 1996. An *in vitro* pig skin model for predicting human skin penetration and irritation potential. In TUMBLESON, M.E. and SCHOOK, L.B. (Eds): *Advances in Swine in Biomedical Research, Vol. II.* New York: Plenum Press, 459–474.

RIVIERE, J.E., BAYNES, R.E., BROOKS, J.D., YEATTS, J.L. and MONTEIRO-RIVIERE, N.A. (2003) Percutaneous absorption of topical diethyl-m-toluamiode (DEET): Effects of exposure variables and coadministered toxicants. *J. Toxicol. Environ. Health. A.* **66**, 131–151.

RIVIERE, J.E., MONTEIRO-RIVIERE, N.A. and BAYNES, R.E. (2002) Gulf War Illness-related exposure factors influencing topical absorption of ^{14}C-permethrin. *Toxicol. Letters* **135**, 61–71.

RIVIERE, J.E., QIAO, G., BAYNES, R.E., BROOKS, J.D. and MUMTAZ, M. (2001) Mixture component effects on the *in vitro* dermal absorption of penta-chlorophenol. *Arch. Toxicol.* **75**, 329–334.

RIVIERE, J.E. and WILLIAMS, P.L. (1992) Pharmacokinetic implications of changing blood flow to the skin. *J. Pharm. Sci.* **81**, 601–602.

WHITE, R.E. and MANITPISITKUL, P. (2001) Pharmacokinetic theory of cassette dosing in drug discovery. *Drug. Metabol. Disposit.* **29**, 957–966.

WILHELM, K.P., SURBER, C. and MAIBACH, H.I. (1991) Effects of sodium lauryl sulfate-induced skin irritation on *in vitro* percutaneous penetration of four drugs. *J. Invest. Dermatol.* **97**, 927–932.

WILLIAMS, A.C. and BARRY, B.W. (1998) Chemical penetration enhancement: possibilities and problems. In Roberts, M.S. and Walters, K.A. (Eds.) *Dermal Absorption and Toxicity Assessment* New York: Marcel Dekker, 297–312.

WILLIAMS, P.L. and RIVIERE, J.E. (1993) Model describing transdermal ionto-phoretic delivery of lidocaine incorporating consideration of cutaneous microvascular state. *J. Pharm. Sci.* **82**, 1080–1084.

WILLIAMS, P.L., THOMPSON, D., QIAO, G.L., MONTEIRO-RIVIERE, N.A., BAYNES, R.E. and RIVIERE, J.E. (1996) The use of mechanistically defined chemical mixtures (MDCM) to assess component effects on the percutaneous absorption and cutaneous disposition of topically-exposed chemicals. II. Development of a general dermatopharmacokinetic model for use in risk assessment. *Toxicol. Appl. Pharmacol.* **141**, 487–496.

YANG, R.S.H. (1994) *Toxicology of Chemical Mixtures* San Diego: Academic Press.

■ CHAPTER 3 ■

Anatomical Factors Affecting Barrier Function

NANCY A MONTEIRO-RIVIERE

Contents

4.1 Introduction

4.2 General characteristics

4.3 Dermis

4.4 Regional and species differences

4.5 Hair follicles

4.6 Blood flow

4.7 Aging

4.8 Diseases

4.9 Conclusions

4.1 INTRODUCTION

Dermatotoxicology is the branch of science dealing with the assessment of responses of the skin to specific toxicants. It is thought that the primary function of skin is a barrier between the well-regulated "milieu interieur" and the outside environment. This may give one the impression that the structure of skin is simple and solely focused on its barrier properties. Past research in percutaneous absorption and dermatotoxicology has reinforced this view. However, more recent research in percutaneous absorption and dermal toxicology now take into consideration the possibility that additional anatomical factors may also affect the barrier function of skin, thereby altering the rate of absorption. Many earlier model systems used to evaluate percutaneous absorption were primitive and not capable of modeling all of these factors. Therefore, it is the purpose of this chapter to illustrate to scientists working in this field the complexity of the integument and how anatomical structures within the skin contribute to and influence its barrier function.

4.2 GENERAL CHARACTERISTICS

Skin is a complex, integrated, dynamic organ that has many functions (Table 4.1) that go far beyond its role as a barrier to the environment. Although metabolism and drug biotransformation are important, the reader is directed to the chapters on this subject in the present text. Skin (derived from the Latin meaning *roof)* is the largest organ of the body and is anatomically divided into the epidermis, which is the outermost layer, and the underlying dermis (Figure 4.1). The epidermis consists of a stratified squamous keratinized epithelium derived from ectoderm in which 80 percent of the cells are keratinocytes. Other cell types such as the melanocytes (pigment formation), Langerhans cells (immunological function), and Merkel cells (sensory perception) represent the nonkeratinocytes. The epidermis undergoes an orderly pattern of proliferation, differentiation, and keratinization. However, these processes are not fully understood. In addition, the epidermis can become specialized to form skin appendages such as hair, sebaceous and sweat glands, feathers, horn, digital organs (hoof, claw, nail), and specialized glandular structures.

The human epidermis consists of four to five cell layers depending on the body site. The first layer, the stratum basale is a single layer of cuboidal to columnar shaped cells that are attached laterally to adjacent cells by desmosomes and to the irregular basement membrane by hemidesmosomes. The basal

TABLE 4.1:

Functions of skin

Environmental barrier
- Diffusion barrier
- Metabolic barrier

Temperature regulation
- Regulation of blood flow
- Hair and fur
- Sweating

Immunological affector and effector axis

Mechanical support

Neurosensory reception

Endocrine

Apocrine/eccrine/sebaceous glandular secretion

Metabolism
- Keratin
- Collagen
- Melanin
- Lipid
- Carbohydrate
- Respiration
- Biotransformation
- Vitamin D

Source: Monteiro-Riviere (1991).

cell population is heterogeneous in that there are two morphologically distinct types. The first can function as stem cells and have the ability to divide and produce new cells, whereas the second serves to anchor the epidermis to the basement membrane (Lavker and Sun, 1982, 1983). The second outer layer is the stratum spinosum or "prickle cell layer," which consists of several layers of irregular polyhedral cells. These cells are connected to the stratum basale cells below and to the adjacent spinosum cells by desmosomes. The most prominent feature in this layer are the tonofilaments. Along with desmosomes, tight junctions (zona occludens) may connect cells to one another. It is in the uppermost layers of the stratum spinosum, that membrane coating or lamellar granules first appear. The third layer is the stratum granulosum that consists of several layers of flattened cells laying parallel to the epidermal-dermal junction. Irregularly shaped, nonmembrane bound electron dense keratohyalin granules are present and contain a structural protein known as profilaggrin, a precursor of filaggrin. It has been speculated that these granules are involved in keratinization and formation of the barrier function of the skin.

The lamellar or membrane coating granules (Odland bodies, lamellated bodies) containing stacks of lamellar disks are found within the stratum

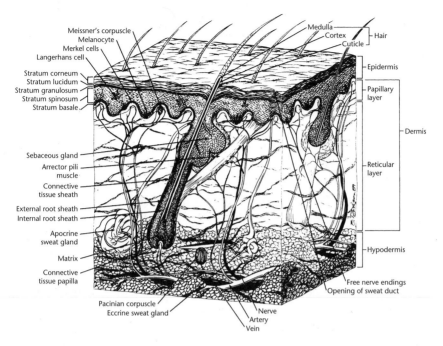

Figure 4.1: Schematic diagram illustrating the structure of mammalian skin (human and animal) from various regions of the body. (Reprinted from Monteiro-Riviere (1991)).

granulosum and increase in number and size as they approach the surface. As epidermal differentiation progresses, the lipid is synthesized and packaged into lamellar granules. These granules fuse with the cell membrane to release their lipid contents by exocytosis into the intercellular space between the stratum granulosum and stratum corneum layers (Yardley and Summerly, 1981; Matolsty, 1976). The granules then undergo a biochemical and physical change to form the lipid sheets that constitute the permeability barrier. Extraction of lipids in skin has shown that the epidermal lipid composition dramatically changes as the keratinocytes differentiate. Lipid composition of the epidermis may consist of phospholipids, glucosylceramides, ceramides, cholesterol, free fatty acids, triacylglycerols, and sphingosine (Downing, 1992; Swartzendruber *et al.*, 1989).

In exceptionally thick skin and hairless regions of the body such as the plantar and palmar surfaces, a stratum lucidum layer is present. This is a thin, translucent, homogeneous line between the stratum granulosum and stratum corneum which consists of fully keratinized, closely compacted, dense cells which lack nuclei and cytoplasmic organelles. This translucent area contains a semifluid substance known as eleiden, which is similar to keratin but has a different staining pattern as well as different protein bound phospholipids (Leeson and Leeson, 1976). The outermost and final layer is the stratum corneum, which consists of several layers of completely keratinized dead cells, devoid of nuclei and cytoplasmic organelles, that are constantly being shed. The most superficial layer of the stratum corneum is sometimes referred to as the stratum disjunctum. The thickness of the stratum corneum and/or number of cell layers varies depending on site and species (Monteiro-Riviere et al., 1990). It is this layer that provides an efficient barrier against transcutaneous water loss. Predominantly, it is the intercellular lipids, arranged into lamellar sheets, that constitute the epidermal permeability barrier. Ruthenium tetroxide post-fixation allows the visualization of these lipid lamellae at the ultrastructural layer (Swartzendruber, 1992). The number of lamellae may vary within the same tissue specimen. In some areas, it consists of a pattern of alternating electron-dense and electron-lucent bands which represent paired bilayers formed from fused lamellar granule disks as postulated by Landmann (Landmann, 1986; Swartzendruber et al., 1987, 1989; Madison et al., 1987).

It is widely acknowledged that the rate limiting barrier to the absorption of most topically applied chemicals is the stratum corneum. Anatomical factors discussed such as the number of epidermal cell layers and the thickness of the stratum corneum may be parameters that modulate absorption. However, with knowledge that the pathway through the stratum corneum is via the intercellular lipids, the real resistance to absorption should relate to the length of this pathway. This has been clearly visualized using mercuric chloride staining in passive (Bodde et al., 1991) and iontophoretic (Monteiro-Riviere et al., 1994) drug delivery. Extraction of epidermal lipids using organic solvents reduces barrier function (Monteiro-Riviere et al., 2001, Hadgraft, 2001). The length is a function of the geometry of the packing of the cells in the stratum corneum. The major route of a compound is via the intercellular bilipid channels, so the absorption of a compound should be based on its diffusion path length (300–500 µm) not the actual thickness. Previous authors have described this spatial organization of vertical columns of interdigitating stratum corneum cells as resembling a tetrakaidecahedron. This 14-sided polygonal structure provides a minimum surface-volume ratio which allows for space to be filled by packing without interstices (Menton, 1976 a,b; Mackenzie, 1975). Therefore, the length is a function of the number of cell layers, overall thickness, the cell size and the tortuosity of this pathway (Williams and Riviere, 1995).

As cells move outward from the basal layer, they undergo keratinization, which is the process by which epidermal cells differentiate. After the basal cells undergo mitosis, they migrate upward, increase in size, and produce large numbers of differentiation products (tonofilaments, keratohyalin granules, and lamellated bodies). Then the nuclei and organelles disintegrate, the filaments and keratohyalin arrange themselves into bundles, and the lamellated granules discharge their contents into the intercellular space coating the cells. The endpoint of this keratinization process is a nonviable, protein rich terminally differentiated cell with a thicker plasmalemma, containing fibrous keratin and keratohyalin, surrounded by the extracellular lipid matrix. This forms the so called "brick and mortar" arrangement which is the morphological basis for the heterogeneous, two compartment stratum corneum model (Elias, 1983).

The basement membrane is synthesized by the basal cells and separates the epithelium from the underlying connective tissue. It is a thin extracellular matrix that is complex and highly organized structure of large macromolecules. By transmission electron microscopy, the cutaneous basement membrane is composed of four major components: 1) the cell membrane of the basal epithelial cell, 2) an electron lucent area beneath the plasma membrane called the lamina lucida, 3) an electron dense area beneath the lamina lucida called the lamina densa, and 4) the sub-basal lamina containing anchoring fibrils, microfibril-like elements, and single collagen fibers (Briggaman and Wheeler, 1975). In addition to this ultrastructural characterization, new epidermal–dermal junction biochemical components are constantly being identified and characterized. Representative examples of the most common ones include type IV collagen, laminin, entactin/nidogen, bullous pemphigoid antigen, heparan sulfate proteoglycan, fibronectin, GB3 (Nicein, BM-600, epiligrin), L3d (Type VII), 19-DEJ-1 (Uncein), epidermolysis bullosa acquisita, and the list is still growing (Timpl *et al.*, 1983; Woodley *et al.*, 1984; Verrando *et al.*,1987; Fine *et al.*, 1989; Rusenko *et al.*, 1989; Briggaman, 1990). Many functions have been attributed to the basement membrane including a role in maintaining epidermal–dermal adhesion, and acting as a selective barrier between the epidermis and the dermis which restricts some molecules and permits the passage of others. In disease, they can also serve as a target for both immunologic and nonimmunologic injury.

4.3 DERMIS

The dermis lies beneath the basement membrane and consists primarily of dense irregular connective tissue within a matrix of collagen, elastic, and reticular fibers and embedded in an amorphous ground substance made up of various types of proteoglycans. The predominant cell types of the dermis are fibroblasts, mast cells, and macrophages. In addition, plasma cells, fat cells, chromatophores, and extravasated leukocytes are often found. Blood vessels, lymphatics, and nerves traverse through the dermis along with glandular structures such as sebaceous, sweat glands and hair follicles. There are two types of sweat glands in humans, eccrine and apocrine. The eccrine gland is found over the entire body, except for a few areas where the apocrine gland may dominate (e.g. axilla, areola, pubis, perianal, eyelid, and external auditory meatus). In contrast, the apocrine gland is found over the entire body surface in hairy mammals and most carnivores. The papillary layer, the most superficial layer of the dermis, conforms to the stratum basal layer and consists of loose connective tissue that blends into the deeper reticular layer which consists of dense connective tissue. The hypodermis or subcutaneous layer is beneath the dermis and anchors the dermis to the underlying muscle or bone.

4.4 REGIONAL AND SPECIES DIFFERENCES

Studies in dermatology, cutaneous pharmacology, and toxicology involve experiments in which skin from different animal species and body regions are utilized. However, differences in stratum corneum thickness or number of cell layers must not be overlooked because they may affect barrier function. Table 4.2 summarizes the thickness of the nonviable stratum corneum and viable

TABLE 4.2:
Comparative thickness of the epidermis and number of cell layers from the back of nine species.

	Epidermis (µm)	Stratum corneum (µm)	Number of cell layers (µm)
Cat	12.97±0.93	5.84±1.02	1.28±0.13
Cow	36.76±2.95	8.65±1.17	2.22±0.11
Dog	21.16±2.55	5.56±0.85	1.89±0.16
Horse	33.59±2.16	7.26±1.04	2.50±0.25
Monkey	26.87±3.14	12.05±2.30	2.67±0.24
Mouse	13.32±1.19	2.90±0.12	1.75±0.08
Pig	51.89±1.49	12.28±0.72	3.94±0.13
Rabbit	10.85±1.00	6.56±0.37	1.22±0.11
Rat	21.66±2.23	5.00±0.85	1.83±0.17

Paraffin sections stained with hematoxylin and eosin; $n=6$, mean ± S.E.
Source: Monteiro-Riviere et al. (1990).

epidermis and the number of cell layers from the back (thoracolumbar area) of nine species used in dermatology research (Monteiro-Riviere *et al.*, 1990). This finding confirms that skin thickness of the back was different across these species suggesting that body site alone is not a sufficient factor to insure successful interspecies extrapolations. For more detailed information regarding thickness of other body site measurements of these nine species see Monteiro-Riviere *et al.*, 1990. Some studies report differences in human skin but the database has only been collected at a few specific body sites (Blair, 1968). Measurements have been done on the number of cell layers at different sites and different ages in humans and showed considerable variation in different areas of the body (Southwood, 1955; Rushmer *et al.*, 1966). In general, data on the thickness of the stratum corneum is limited. Studies with human skin show the stratum corneum in a given region is variable in both thickness and number of cell layers and that the sample length of the stratum corneum measured from a region is not consistent in thickness and number of cell layers (Holbrook and Odland, 1974).

Regional variations have been shown to affect percutaneous penetration in man (Feldmann and Maibach, 1967; Maibach *et al.*, 1971; Wester *et al.*, 1980; Wester and Maibach, 1983). Studies with radiolabeled pesticides, parathion, malathion, and carbaryl were used to explore the permeability at 13 different anatomic sites in man. The palms and forearm showed a similar penetration rate but the abdomen and the dorsum of the hand had twice the penetration compared to the forearm (Maibach *et al.*, 1971). Variations in percutaneous penetration of ^{14}C hydrocortisone demonstrates the rate of absorption through back skin was more rapid than the flexor surfaces of the forearm (Feldmann and Maibach, 1967). Additional, studies using steady-state diffusion cells to investigate the absorption of phenol, methanol, octanol, caffeine and aspirin through abdominal skin have shown that permeability of human abdominal skin within and between individuals was less variable than from other anatomic sites (Southwell *et al.*, 1984). Similar studies have been conducted in other species. In the pig, absorption of topically applied parathion was greater for the back than the abdomen (Qiao *et al.*, 1994). The extent and pattern of biotransformation was also different between these two sites (Qiao and Riviere, 1995). For parathion absorption, the ventral abdomen most closely resembles the human ventral forearm. The percutaneous absorption of methyl salicylate and the nerve agent VX was significantly greater when applied to the ear versus the epigastrium of pigs (Duncan *et al.*, 2002). This finding questions the validity of using pig ears as an *in vitro* model to predict human absorption, and underscores the importance of anatomical differences in skin from different body regions on chemical absorption. Unfortunately, similar data is not available for many other compounds and species combinations.

Regional differences in total lipid content and in lipid composition may occur within the stratum corneum at different anatomical sites. Sphingolipids and cholesterol are higher in the palmar and plantar stratum corneum than in the extensor surfaces of the extremities (Lampe et al., 1983). The distribution of lipids in nonkeratinized buccal epithelium is different due to the higher water permeability than in keratinized areas. Buccal epithelium contains gluco-sylceramides, acylceramides, small amounts of ceramides, but no acylgluco-sylceramides (Squier and Hall, 1985). In keratinized and nonkeratinized porcine oral epithelia, phospholipids are present in greater amounts than in the epidermis (Wertz, 1986). Also, there are differences in lipid composition in different species. Squalene is the major component in human skin, while most animal species have substantial amounts of diester waxes (Nicolaides et al., 1968). For an excellent review on the structure and function of mammalian epidermal lipids, see Wertz and Downing, 1991.

Species differences in absorption for numerous chemicals have been well studied and adequately reviewed elsewhere (Wester and Maibach, 1975a, 1975b, 1976, 1977). In general the best animal models for human absorption are the domestic pig and the non-human primate. Evaluation of skin permeability was also performed on various animals by comparing the percutaneous penetration of nine radiolabeled compounds. Statistically significant correlations to human data were obtained for the weanling pig and human skin grafted nude mouse models. In contrast, significant correlations were not obtained in the hairless dog, pig skin grafted nude mouse, and the nude mouse (Reifenrath et al., 1984).

Differences in the permeability of nicorandil, a coronary vasodilator, was determined in six different species (hairless mouse, hairless rat, guinea pig, dog, pig, and human) with the pig and human being similar. It was suggested that the difference in permeability could be explained by the differences in species specific skin surface lipids that may also affect the partitioning of nicorandil from the vehicle to the stratum corneum (Sato et al., 1991). These findings support the use of the pig as an optimal animal model for predicting human absorption.

Lipid extraction can have a profound effect by removing the essential lipids that are necessary for barrier function (Hadgraft, 2001; Monteiro-Riviere et al., 2001). The technique of altering the lipid composition has been applied to modulate skin permeability. Removal of lipids within the stratum corneum causes an increase in transepidermal water loss (TEWL) and also allows for an increase in the penetration of compounds. This enhancement of a compound is the basis for more efficient delivery of therapeutic compounds. Extraction of lipids from pig skin in three different body regions; the abdominal, inguinal, and back using three different solvent extraction procedures or tape stripping demonstrated the mean total lipid concentration depended on the type of extraction solvents and body region. This was reproducible across sites and regions. Relative proportions individual lipids extracted were similar across the three body regions but higher concentrations of total lipids were extracted from the back (Monteiro-Riviere *et al.*, 2001).

4.5 HAIR FOLLICLES

The basic architecture of the integument is similar in all mammals. However, structural differences in the arrangement of hair follicles and hair follicle density exists between domestic and laboratory animals. The hair density in pig and human is sparse compared to that of the rodent. The skin from the back of pigs and from the abdomen of humans have 11 ± 1 hair follicles/cm^2, in comparisons to the back of the rat with 289 ± 21, the mouse with 658 ± 38 and the hairless mouse with 75 ± 6 (Bronaugh *et al.*, 1982). For a comprehensive review of hair follicle arrangement and microscopic anatomy of the integument in different domestic species see Monteiro-Riviere *et al.* (1993) and Monteiro-Riviere (1991).

Hair follicles, sebaceous and sweat glands are often envisioned as special channels through the stratum corneum that facilitate absorption of topical compounds, thus bypassing the rate limiting stratum corneum barrier. Controversy exists over the significance of these hair follicle pathways in percutaneous absorption. The comparative permeability of human and animal skin may be related to diffusion of compounds through appendages in the skin. Numerous studies have been designed to test this hypothesis. One must always remember that even when a compound traverses the skin via hair follicles, passage through the stratum corneum still occurs. It is probable that any increase in absorption attributed to the appendages probably results from the increased surface area seen in the attending invaginations of the stratum corneum, therefore areas covered with hair have a greater skin surface area available for transdermal absorption.

Hair follicle rich areas such as the scalp, angle of jaw, post-auricular area, and forehead have been shown to allow greater penetration of some pesticides (Maibach *et al.*, 1971). The importance of hair follicles in percutaneous absorption was evaluated in a model of regrown skin without hair follicles dorsally on the hairless rat. Diffusion cell studies were used to compare the absorption of tritiated hydrocortisone, niflumic acid, caffeine, and p-aminobenzoic acid in intact and appendage free skin. These studies confirmed a higher rate of diffusion in intact skin and suggested that hair follicles acted as the major absorption pathway (Illel *et al.*, 1991). Other investigators have also studied this phenomenon. Flow through organ culture studies were performed on normal haired and hairless mice with benzo[a]pyrene and testosterone. The overall permeation of testosterone was greater than that of benzo[a]pyrene, and showed no strain differences. However, benzo[a]pyrene absorption was higher in the haired mice than the hairless mice.

Additional studies of three phenotypic hair density variants, suggests that the permeability of both compounds was the highest in the haired phenotype, lowest in the hairless phenotype, and intermediate in the fuzzy-haired animal. They concluded that transappendageal penetration contributes significantly to overall skin absorption (Kao *et al.*,1988). Hence, regional distribution of skin appendages could influence absorption of some compounds. Absorption of estradiol and progesterone was studied on normal and appendage free (scar) hairless rats to determine if differences were due to lack of appendageal structures or modification of blood flow. Concentration of both steroids was significantly higher in normal than in scar tissue (Hueber *et al.*, 1994a). They also compared the absorption of estradiol, hydrocortisone, progesterone, and testosterone through scar skin (without hair follicles, sebaceous and sweat glands) from the abdomen or mammary areas of humans. Again, absorption was significantly higher in normal than in scar tissue. Based on these findings, hair follicles and sebaceous glands may constitute a route for penetration for these steroids (Hueber *et al.*, 1994b). Another study tested the appendageal density and absorption of the vasodilator methyl nicotinate, on the forehead, forearm, and palms of humans. Penetration was the greatest on the forehead, intermediate on the forearm, and least through the palms. They also concluded that there was a correlation between methyl nicotinate absorption and appendageal density (Tur *et al.*, 1991). Other investigators have found that the penetration process of a compound is dependent on the phase of the hair growth cycle and amount of sebum production (Lademann *et al.*, 2001)

However, there is another interpretation to these data. In areas with dense hair, there is little interfollicular regions of skin. Therefore, compound has to penetrate hair follicles. This factor, coupled with the increased stratum corneum surface area associated with the invaginations of follicles, may explain the enhanced penetration seen in hairy skin. In summary, hair follicle density, stratum corneum thickness, number of cell layers, and lipid composition are important structural variables to be considered when comparing absorption across different body sites or species

4.6 BLOOD FLOW

The complexity of blood vessels in the skin is limited to the dermis for the epidermis is avascular. Large arteries arise from a network in the subcutaneous layer which send some of their branches to the superficial and deep dermis. The superficial arteries traverse through the dermis and send smaller branches that supply hair follicles, sebaceous and sweat glands. A network of smaller arteries, the rete subpapillare (horizontal plexus), run between the papillary and reticular layers. Small arterioles from this plexus supply the capillary loops (subepidermal plexus) in the dermal papillary layer. Beneath the basement membrane, capillary beds are present in the matrix of hair follicles and around sebaceous and sweat glands. In specific body sites (fingertips, toes, lips, and nose), alternative channels called arteriovenous anastomoses or shunts are present which allow blood to be passed from the arteriole to the venule. When connective tissue surrounds such a vascular structure it is referred to as a glomus, which functions in regulation of body temperature and peripheral blood circulation. For a complete understanding about the cutaneous vasculature see Ryan, 1991.

Most research models in dermatology, cutaneous pharmacology, and reconstructive surgery have been on animals. It is important to be aware of the anatomic and physiologic differences in blood flow between species and sites within species before the variable of blood flow can be used to explain percutaneous absorption. In humans, laser Doppler velocimetry (LDV) is often used to assess cutaneous blood flow. LDV is an accepted non-invasive technique that assesses relative cutaneous capillary blood perfusion (Holloway and Watkins, 1977; Young *et al.*, 1985; Fischer *et al.*, 1983). It has been used to assess the vascular response in man to acute inflammation (Holloway, 1980; Ross *et al.*, 1987; Serup and Staberg, 1985), heat (Holloway, 1980), ultraviolet light (Young *et al.*,1985; Frodin *et al.*, 1988), corticosteroids (Bisgaard *et al.*, 1986), nitroglycerin (Sundberg, 1984), minoxidil (Wester *et al.*, 1984), to determine depths of superficial, deep dermal and subdermal burns (Micheels *et al.*, 1984; Alsbjorn *et al.*, 1984), as well as to evaluate donor sites in reconstructive surgery (Goldberg *et al.*, 1990).

CHAPTER 4

Skin blood flow measurements using LDV at various sites in humans showed interindividual and spatial variations (Tur *et al.*, 1983). The magnitude of cutaneous blood flow and epidermal thickness has been postulated to explain the regional differences in percutaneous absorption between body sites in humans and animals. A comprehensive study comparing the histologic thickness (Table 4.2) and laser Doppler blood flow measurements (Table 4.3) was performed at five cutaneous sites (buttocks, ear, humeroscapular joint, thoracolumbar junction, and abdomen) in nine species (cat, cow, dog, horse, monkey, mouse, pig, rabbit, rat) to determine the correlation of blood flow and thickness. These studies strongly suggested that LDV blood flow and skin thickness did not correlate across species and body sites but are independent variables that must be evaluated separately in dermatology, pharmacology and toxicology studies (Monteiro-Riviere *et al.*, 1990).

The role of the cutaneous vasculature was studied in the topical delivery of ^{3}H piroxicam, a nonsteroidal antiinflammatory drug. Dermal penetration of ^{3}H piroxicam gel was evaluated by *in vitro* diffusion cells and *in vivo* (pigs) at two different tissue beds, one that is vascularized by direct cutaneous and the other by musculocutaneous arteries. The *in vitro* fluxes were identical indicating a similar rate of stratum corneum and epidermal absorption, however more extensive and deeper tissue penetration was noted at the musculocutaneous sites. This suggests that the vascular anatomy is important in determining the extent of dermal penetration (Monteiro-Riviere *et al.*, 1993). Other studies also

TABLE 4.3:

Blood flow measurements (ml/min/100g) of comparative species at five cutaneous sites (Mean±SE).

Species	BUT	EAR	HSJ	TLJ	VAB
Cat	1.82±0.59	6.46±2.30	1.86±0.70	2.39±0.35	6.19±0.94
Cow	6.03±1.84	6.98±2.19	5.51±2.32	5.49±1.49	10.49±2.13
Dog	2.21±0.67	5.21±1.53	5.52±1.31	1.94±0.27	8.78±1.40
Horse	3.16±1.22	—	6.76±1.49	2.99±0.86	8.90±1.46
Monkey	3.12±0.58	20.93±5.37	8.49±3.28	2.40±0.82	3.58±0.41
Mouse	3.88±0.92	1.41±0.48	10.10±3.51	20.56±4.69	36.85±8.14
Pig	3.08±0.48	11.70±3.02	6.75±2.09	2.97±0.56	10.68±2.14
Rabbit	3.55±0.93	8.38±1.53	5.38±1.06	5.46±0.94	17.34±6.31
Rat	4.20±1.05	9.13±4.97	6.22±1.47	9.56±2.17	11.35±5.53

But = buttocks; Ear = pinnae; HSJ = humeroscapular joint; TLS = thoracolumbar junction; VAB = ventral abdomen.

Source: Monteiro-Riviere *et al.* (1990).

implied that topical administration in male rats resulted in a high concentration of the drug in the underlying vasculature which could not be attributed to redistribution via the systemic circulation (McNeill *et al.*, 1992). Thus, the cutaneous vasculature does not function as an infinite sink that removes all topically applied drugs to the systemic circulation (Riviere and Williams, 1992). This mechanism of drug delivery has been alluded to by other investigators (Wada *et al.*, 1982; Torrent *et al.*, 1988; Guy and Maibach, 1983). Also, we have demonstrated that local modulation of the vasculature by co-iontophoresis of vasoactive compounds could affect drug distribution to the underlying tissue (Riviere *et al.*, 1991). All of these studies suggest a major role for the cutaneous vasculature in modulating absorption and dermal penetration of some topically applied drugs.

4.7 AGING

The anatomical and physiological changes in skin associated with aging may also affect the barrier function. Some of the major problems that complicate the understanding of aged skin is the ability to differentiate actinically damaged from chronically aged or age-related changes due to environmental influences (e.g. chronic sun exposure, cold, wind, low humidity, chemical exposure, or physical trauma), maturation process (e.g. newborn to adult), diseases, or hormonal changes associated with menopause.

Aging skin is usually generalized by a wrinkled and dry appearance. However, the microscopic changes in the epidermis associated with aging include flattening of the epidermal–dermal junction, retraction of epidermal down-growths, thinness, reduction in number and output of sweat glands, and a more heterogeneous basal cell population (Rapaport, 1973; Lavker, 1979; Hull and Warfel, 1983; Gilchrest, 1984; Kligman *et al.*, 1985; Lavker *et al.*, 1986; Lavker *et al.*, 1987; Kligman and Balin, 1989). Numerous ultrastructural changes have also been documented in the dermis of aged skin. These include changes in the architecture of the elastic fiber framework (Lavker, 1979; Montagna and Carlisle, 1979), dermal shrinkage (Evans *et al.*, 1943), elastic fiber disintegration, thickening and clumping (Braverman and Fonferko,1982a), progressive rise in the modulus of elasticity (Grahame and Holt, 1969), decrease in collagen content (Branchet *et al.*, 1991), modification of collagen from fascicular to granular (Pieraggi *et al.*, 1984), and a decrease in tensile strength (Vogel, 1983). Also, thickening of the vascular wall vessels (Braverman and Fonferko, 1982b), loss of melanocytes in the hair bulb, and fewer glands were observed (Gilchrest, 1984).

CHAPTER 4

The general morphological organization and thickness of the stratum corneum in humans do not change with age (Lavker, 1979; Christophers and Kligman, 1965), but the lipid content and intercellular cohesion in the stratum corneum decreases with age (Levesque *et al.*, 1984). Thin layer chromatography and photodensitometry were used to study inter-individual differences in fatty acid composition of skin surface lipids. Both age and sex were significant factors (Nazzaro-Porro *et al.*, 1979). Stratum corneum hydration parameters remain unchanged or slightly decreased with age (Potts *et al.*, 1984) Premenopausal women tend to have smaller corneocytes than post-menopausal woman (Fluhr *et al.*, 2001). All of these alterations may alter the clearance and absorption of transdermally absorbed compounds through and from the skin. This can best be illustrated with a few examples.

A dose response study of 14 different pesticides on young and adult female rats showed significant age-dependent differences in skin penetration in 11 pesticides (Hall *et al.*, 1988). A decrease in dermal absorption of some chemicals in the aged may be due to morphological differences in blood flow (Christophers and Kligman, 1965). Studies in male rats 1 to 24 months and mice 1 to 22 months of age showed that blood flow in mice increased between at 1–2 months, remained constant to 19 months, then increased at 22 months; but the blood flow in rats was constant except at 2 months. Also, the number of viable epidermal layers in mice were constant, while in rats it decreased with age. Epidermal thickness in both mice and rats decreased from 2–3 months. Dermal thickness decreased from 3–22 months in mice, and increased in rats from 1–2 months (Monteiro-Riviere *et al.*, 1991). Other studies have shown a decrease in the dermal absorption of Evans blue dye in old rats as compared to middle-aged rats (Kohn, 1969). Cardiac output declines with age and the pattern of blood flow distribution also changes with the proportion of cardiac output received by the kidneys, skin, gastrointestinal tract and liver decreasing in older rats (Yates and Hiley, 1979). Therefore, reductions in blood flow could alter the distribution of compounds to and from these tissues. Age difference in blood flow can occur and should be considered when evaluating cutaneous toxicity studies in different aged animals.

A decrease was observed in TCDD (2,3,7,8-tetrachlorodibenzo-p-dioxin) and 4 PeCDF (2,3,4,7,8-pentachlorodibenzofuran) absorption in older rats compared to 10 week old rats (Banks *et al.*, 1990). TCDD absorption decreased from 3–5 weeks in rats (Jackson *et al.*, 1990). The decreased absorption of these compounds in older animals could be explained by decreased clearance from the application site due to reduced perfusion seen in rats older than 2 months.

Maturational changes in the dermal absorption of TCDD in rats also indicated that TCDD is absorbed to a greater degree in young animals and a significant decrease in potential for systemic exposure occurs during maturation and aging (Anderson *et al.*, 1993). Age related differences in the absorption of 14 different pesticides studied in 1 and 3-month old rats showed an increase in some compounds and a decrease in others (Shah *et al.*, 1987). Therefore, the physiological and physiochemical properties (e.g. lipophilicity, molecular size) of the compound may be as important in assessing percutaneous absorption in aged animals as anatomical or physiological differences. Other investigators studied the pharmacodynamic measurements of methyl nicotinate in aged individuals and showed no differences between young (20–34 years) and old (64–86 years) populations (Roskos *et al.*, 1990). Studies with testosterone, estradiol, hydrocortisone and benzoic acid in young controls (18–35), young old (65–75 years) and old-old (> 75 years) humans showed different patterns depending upon the compound. For estradiol, absorption in the old-old group was less than in the other two populations. For hydrocortisone and benzoic acid, absorption in the young was greater than both elderly groups. In contrast, testosterone was lowest in the young-old group (Roskos *et al.*, 1986). These studies showed a tendency for decreased absorption with most compounds with advancing age.

Another study evaluating tri-N-propyl phosphate (TNPP) in *in vitro* human skin from various anatomic sites ranging from 3 to 57 years showed a decrease in permeability with increased age (Marzulli, 1962). Studies involving the percutaneous absorption of 2-sec-butyl-4,6-dinitrophenol (dinoseb) in relation to age and dosage in *in vitro* and *in vivo* rat skin showed that dermal absorption in young rats was less than in adults at all doses studied (Hall *et al.*, 1992). These studies have many additional variables making simple extrapolations difficult. For examples, hair follicle growth cycle and body site were significant factors in hydrocortisone absorption studies in rats (Behl *et al.*, 1984). Many studies do not control for these factors. Therefore, in most studies conducted to date, age is an important multi-faceted factor involving many biological processess (e.g. altered lipid composition, blood flow) which produce compound dependent effects. These factors must be taken into account when interpreting any study.

4.8 DISEASES

Skin permeability may be increased or decreased depending on the condition of the skin. Common diseases such as psoriasis may influence absorption. Psoriasis may be defined as having an accelerated rate of epidermal cell

■ CHAPTER 4 ■

replication, a decrease in tonofilaments and keratohyalin granules, a disordered, loosely and irregularly stacked stratum corneum, and tortuous and dilated capillary loops (Braverman *et al.*, 1972). These abnormal capillaries (e.g. large lumen, fenestrations between endothelial cells, and multilayered basement membrane) may have an affect on blood flow to skin. In addition, intercellular ionic calcium distribution is different in psoriatic skin which could alter lipid permeability (Menon and Elias, 1991). For example, hydrocortisone has been shown to increase absorption in psoriatic skin (Schaefer *et al.*, 1977; Zesch *et al.*, 1975).

In addition, other skin diseases such as essential fatty acid deficiency and ichthyosis may have an effect on compound penetration. Epidermal barrrier function is altered by abnormal lipid composition in non-eczematous atopic dry skin (Fartasch *et al.*, 1992). Any disease process which altered an anatomical factor discussed above would be expected to modulate chemical percutaneous absorption. The challenge to researchers is to define the specific factor which has the greatest impact on a specific chemical's toxicology or clinical efficacy.

4.9 CONCLUSIONS

This chapter should provide the reader with a brief introduction to the effects of anatomy on percutaneous absorption which is summarized in Figure 4.2. There are numerous factors which must be taken into consideration when designing experiments or interpreting data. Many different processes such as aging, disease, or chemical damage may affect specific anatomical components of skin. Anatomy is a useful framework upon which to classify the various biological processes which may be affected. The critical anatomical variables that are important for influencing the absorption of compounds across the skin include those factors governing the length of the intercellular pathway (thickness, cell layers, cell size and tortuosity), lipid composition of this medium, potential appendageal shortcuts (hair follicle density, sebaceous and sweat glands), and the nature and density of the underlying dermal circulation. A knowledge of how a process such as aging or disease affects each structure's integrity, then gives one a perspective on how the absorption of a chemical may be modified. Changes in these factors secondary to species, body regions, age, or disease would be expected to affect overall absorption. A major complication in most cases, is that more than one component is altered and the effect observed is very dependent upon the specific chemical's physiochemistry.

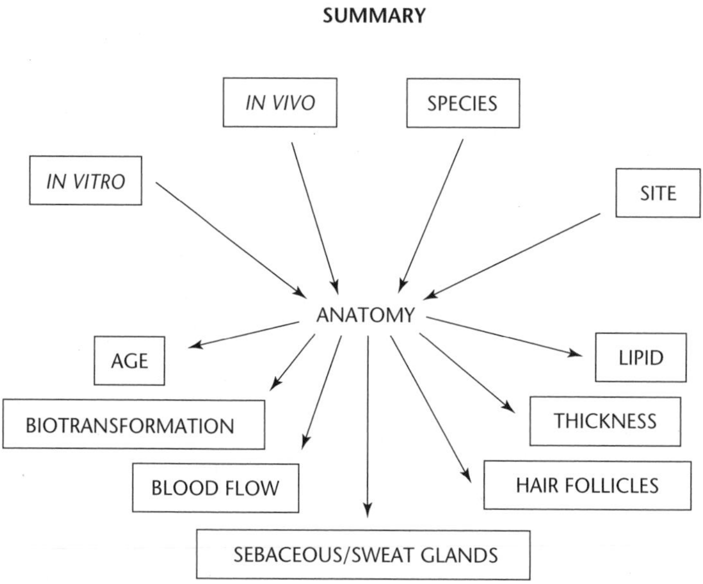

SUMMARY

Figure 4.2: Overall summary depicting the anatomical factors that can influence absorption.

REFERENCES

ALSBJORN, B, MICHEELS, J. and SORENSEN, B. (1984) Laser Doppler flowmetry measurements of superficial dermal, deep dermal and subdermal burns. *Scand. J. Reconstr. Surg.* **18**, 75–79.

ANDERSON, Y.B., JACKSON, J.A. and BIRNBAUM, L.S. (1993) Maturational changes in dermal absorption of 2, 3, 7, 8-tetrachlorodibenzo-*p*-dioxin (TCDD) in Fischer 344 rats. *Toxicol. Appl. Pharm.* **119**, 214–220.

BANKS, Y.B., BREWSTER, D.W. and BIRNBAUM, L.S. (1990) Age-related changes in dermal absorption of 2, 3, 7, 8-tetrachlorodibenzo-*p*-dioxin and 2, 3, 4, 7, 8-pentachlorodibenzofuran. *Fundam. Appl. Toxicol.* **15**, 163–173.

BEHL, C.R., FLYNN, G.L., LINN, E.E. and SMITH, W.M. (1984) Percutaneous absorption of corticosteroids: Age, site, and skin-sectioning influences on rates of permeation of hairless mouse skin by hydrocortisone. *J. Pharm. Sci.* **73**, 1287–1290.

BISGAARD, H., KRISTENSEN, J.K. and SONDERGAARD, J. (1986) A new technique for

CHAPTER 4

ranking vascular corticosteroid effects in humans using laser Doppler velocimetry. *J. Invest. Dermatol.* **86**, 275–278.

BLAIR, C. (1968) Morphology and thickness of the human stratum corneum. *Br. J. Dermatol.* **80**, 430–436.

BODDE, H.E., DE HAAN, F.H.N., KORNET, L., CRAANE-VANHINSBERG, W.H.M. and SALOMONS, M.A. (1991) Transdermal iontophoresis of mercuric chloride *in vitro:* electron microscopic visualization of pathways. *Proc. Int. Symp. Control. Rel. Bioact. Mater.* **18**, 301–302.

BRANCHET, M.C., BOISNIC, S., FRANCES, C., LESTY, C. and ROBERT, L. (1991) Morphometric analysis of dermal collagen fibers in normal human skin as a function of age. *Arch. Gerontol. Geriatr.* **13**, 1–14.

BRAVERMAN, I.M., COHEN, I. and O'KEEFE, G.O. (1972) Metabolic and ultra-structural studies in a patient with pustular psoriasis. *Arch. Dermatol.* **105**, 189–196.

BRAVERMAN, I.M. and FONFERKO, E. (1982a) Studies in cutaneous aging: I. The elastic fiber network. *J. Invest. Dermatol.* **78**, 434–443.

BRAVERMAN, I.M. and FONFERKO, E. (1982b) Studies in cutaneous aging: II. The micro-vasculature. *J. Invest. Dermatol.* **78**, 444–448.

BRIGGAMAN, R.A. (1990) Epidermal-dermal junction: Structure, composition, function and disease relationships. *Prog. Dermatol.* **24**, 1–8.

BRIGGAMAN, R. and WHEELER, C. E. (1975) The epidermal-dermal junction. *J. Invest. Dermatol.* **65**, 71–84.

BRONAUGH, R.L., STEWART, R.F. and CONGDON, E.R. (1982) Methods for *in vitro* percutaneous absorption studies. II. Animal models for human skin. *Toxicol. Appl. Pharmacol.* **62**, 481–488.

CHRISTOPHERS, E. and KLIGMAN, A.M. (1965) Percutaneous absorption in aged skin. In Montagna, W. (ed.) *Advances in Biology of Skin,* Oxford: Pergammon Press, pp. 163–175.

DOWNING, D.T. (1992) Lipid and protein structures in the permeability barrier of mammalian epidermis. *J. Lipid Res.* **33**, 301–313.

DUNCAN, E.J.S., BROWN, A., LUNDY, P., SAWYER, T.W., HAMILTON, M., HILL, I. and CONLEY, J.D. (2002) Percutaneous absorption of methyl salicylate and VX in domestic swine. *J. Appl. Toxicol.* **22**, 141–148.

ELIAS, P.M. (1983) Epidermal lipids, barrier function, and desquamation. *J. Invest. Dermatol.* **80**, 44–49.

EVANS, R., COWDRY, E.V. and NIELSON, P.E. (1943) Ageing of human skin. I. Influence of dermal shrinkage on appearance of the epidermis in young and old fixed tissues. *Anat. Rec.* **86**, 545–565.

FARTASCH, M., BASSUKAS, I.D. and DIEPGEN, T.L. (1992) Disturbed extruding mechanism of lamellar bodies in dry non-eczematous skin of atopics. *Br. J. Dermatol.* **127**, 221–227.

FELDMAN, R.J. and MAIBACH, H.I. (1967) Regional variation in percutaneous penetration of 14C cortisol in man. *J. Invest. Dermatol.* **48**, 181–183.

FINE, J.D., HORIGUCHI, Y., JESTER, J. and COUCHMAN, J.R. (1989) Detection and partial characterization of a midlamina lucida-hemidesmosome-associated antigen (19-DEJ-1) present within human skin. *J. Invest. Dermatol.* **92**, 825–830.

FISCHER, J.C., PARKER, P.M. and SHAW, W.W. (1983) Comparison of two laser Doppler flowmeters for the monitoring of dermal blood flow. *Microsurg.* **4**, 164–170.

FLUHR, J.W., PELOSI, A., LAZZERINI, S. and DIKSTOIN, S. (2001) Differences in corneocytes surface area in pre and post menopausal women. *Skin Pharmacol. Appl. Skin Physiol.* **14** (suppl 1): 10–16.

FRODIN, T., MOLIN, L. and SKOGH, M. (1988) Effects of single doses of UVA, UVB, and UVC on skin blood flow, water content, and barrier function measured by laser Doppler flowmetry, optothermal infrared spectrometry and evaporimetry. *Photodermatol.* **5**, 187–195.

GILCHREST, B. A. (1984) Age-associated changes in normal skin. In Gilchrest, B. A. (ed.) *Skin and the Aging Process*, Boca Raton: CRC Press, 17–35.

GRAHAME, R. and HOLT, P.J.L. (1969) The influence of ageing on the *in vivo* elasticity of human skin. *Gerontol.* **15**, 121–139.

GOLDBERG, J. SEPKA, R.S., PERONA, B.P., PENDERSON, W.C. and KLITZMAN, B. (1990) Laser Doppler blood flow measurements of common cutaneous donor sites for reconstructive surgery. *Plast. Reconst. Surg.* **85**, 581–586.

GUY, R.H. and MAIBACH, H.I. (1983) Drug delivery to local subcutaneous structures following topical administration. *J. Pharm. Sci.* **72**, 1375–1380.

HADGRAFT, J. (2001) Modulation of the barrier function of skin. *Skin Pharmacol Appl Skin Physiol.* **14** (suppl 1): 72–81.

HALL, L.L., FISHER, H.L., SUMLER, M.R., HUGHES, M.F. and SHAH, P.V. (1992) Age-related percutaneous penetration of 2-sec-butyl-4,6-dinitrophenol (Dinoseb) in rats. *Fundam. Appl. Toxicol.* **19**, 258–267.

CHAPTER 4

HALL, L.L., FISHER, H.L., SUMLER, M.R., MONROE, R.J., CHERNOFF, N. and SHAH, P.V. (1988) Dose response of skin absorption in young and adult rats. In MANSDORF, S. Z., SAGER, R. and NIELSEN, A. P. (eds) *Performance of Protective Clothing: Second Symposium*, Philadelphia: American Society for Testing and Materials, 177–194.

HOLBROOK, K.A. and ODLAND, G.F. (1974) Regional differences in the thickness (cell layers) of the human stratum corneum: An ultrastructural analysis. *J. Invest. Dermatol.* **62**, 415–422.

HOLLOWAY, G.A. (1980) Cutaneous blood flow responses to injection trauma measured by laser Doppler velocimetry. *J. Invest. Dermatol.* **74**, 1–4.

HOLLOWAY, G.A. and WATKINS, D.W. (1977) Laser Doppler measurement of cutaneous blood flow. *J. Invest. Dermatol.* **69**, 306–309.

HUEBER, F., BESNARD, M., SCHAEFER, H. and WEPIERRE, J. (1994a) Percutaneous absorption of estradiol and progesterone in normal and appendage-free skin of the hairless rat: Lack of importance of nutritional blood flow. *Skin Pharmacol.* **7**, 245–256.

HUEBER, F., SCHAEFER, H. and WEPIERRE, J. (1994b) Role of transepidermal and transfollicular routes in percutaneous absorption of steroids: *In vitro* studies on human skin. *Skin Pharmacol.* **7**, 237–244.

HULL, M.T. and WARFEL, K.A. (1983) Age-related changes in the cutaneous basal lamina: Scanning electron microscopic study. *J. Invest. Dermatol.* **81**, 378–380.

ILLEL, B., SCHAEFER, H., WEPIERRE, J. and DOUCET, O. (1991) Follicles play an important role in percutaneous absorption. *J. Pharm. Sci.* **80**, 424–427.

JACKSON, J.A., BANKS, Y.B. and BIRMBAUM, L.S. (1990) Maximal dermal absorption of TCDD occurs in weanling rats. *Toxicologist.* **10**, 309.

KLIGMAN, A.M. and BALIN, A.K. (1989) Aging of human skin. In BALIN, A.K. and KLIGMAN, A.M. (eds) *Aging and Skin*, New York: Raven Press, 1–42.

KLIGMAN, A.M., GROVE, G.L. and BALIN, A.K. (1985) Aging of human skin. In FINCH, C. E. and SCHNEIDER, E. L. (eds) *Handbook of the Biology of Aging*, New York: Van Nostrand Reinhold Co., 820–841.

KAO, J., HALL, J. and HELMAN, G. (1988) *In vitro* percutaneous absorption in mouse skin: Influence of skin appendages. *Toxicol. Appl. Pharmacol.* **94**, 93–103.

KOHN, R.R. (1969) Age variation in rat skin permeability. *Proc. Soc. Exp. Biol. Med.* **131**, 521–522.

LAMPE, M.A., WILLIAMS, M.L. and ELIAS, P.M. (1983) Human epidermal lipids: Characterization and modulations during differentiation. *J. Lipid Res.* **24**, 131–140.

LADEMANN, J., OTBERG, N., RICHTER, H., WEIGMANN H.J., LINDERMAN, U., SCHAEFER, H. and STERRY, W. (2001) Investigation of follicular penetration of topically applied substances. *Skin Pharmacol Appl Skin Physiol.* **14** (suppl 1): 17–22.

LANDMANN, L. (1986) Epidermal permeability barrier: Transformation of lamellar granule-disks into intercellular sheets by a membrane-fusion process, a freeze-fracture study. *J. Invest. Dermatol.* **87**, 202–209.

LAVKER, R.M. (1979) Structural alterations in exposed and unexposed aged skin. *J. Invest. Dermatol.* **73**, 59–66.

LAVKER, R.M. and SUN, T.T. (1982) Heterogeneity in epidermal basal keratinocytes: Morphological and functional correlations. *Science.* **215**, 1239–1241.

LAVKER, R.M. and SUN, T.T. (1983) Epidermal stem cells. *J. Invest. Dermatol.* **81**, 121s-127s.

LAVKER, R.M., ZHENG, P. and DONG, G. (1986) Morphology of aged skin. *Dermatol. Clin.* **4**, 379–389.

LAVKER, R.M., ZHENG, P. and DONG, G. (1987) Aged skin: A study by light, transmission electron, and scanning electron microscopy. *J. Invest. Dermatol.* **88**, 44s-51s.

LEESON, C.R. and LEESON, T.S. (1976) *Histology,* 3rd ed. Philadelphia: W.B. Saunders.

LEVEQUE, J.L., CORCUFF, P., DE RIGALE, J. and AGACHE, P. (1984) *In vivo* studies of the evolution of physical properties of the human skin with age. *Int. J. Dermatol.* **23**, 322–329.

MACKENZIE, I.C. (1975) Ordered structure of the epidermis. *J. Invest. Dermatol.* **65**, 45–51.

MADISON, K.C., SWARTZENDRUBER, D.C. and WERTZ, P.W. (1987) Presence of intact intercellular lipid lamellae in the upper layers of the stratum corneum. *J. Invest. Dermatol.* **88**, 714–718.

MAIBACH, H.I., FELDMANN, R.J., MITBY, T.H. and SERAT, W.F. (1971) Regional variation in percutaneous penetration in man: Pesticides. *Arch. Environ. Health.* **23**, 208–211.

MARZULLI, F.N. (1962) Barriers to skin penetration. *J. Invest. Dermatol.* **39**, 387–390.

CHAPTER 4

MATOLSTY, A.G. (1976) Keratinization. *J. Invest. Dermatol.* **67**, 20–25.

MCNEILL, S.C., POTTS, R.O. and FRANCOEUR, M.L. (1992) Local enhanced topical delivery of drugs: Does it truly exist? *J. Pharm Res.* **9**, 1422–1427.

MENTON, G.K. (1976a) A liquid film model of tetrakaidecahedral packing to account for the establishment of epidermal layers. *J. Invest. Dermatol.* **66**, 283–291.

MENTON, G.K. (1976b) A minimum-surface mechanism to account for the organization of cells into columns in the mammalian epidermis. *Am. J. Anat.* **145**, 1–22.

MENON, G.K. and ELIAS, P.M. (1991) Ultrastructural localization of calcium in psoriatic and normal human epidermis. *Arch. Dermatol.* **127**, 57–63.

MICHEELS, J., ALSBJORN, B. and SORENSEN, B. (1984) Clinical use of laser Doppler flowmetry in a burns unit. *Scand. J. Reconstr. Surg.* **18**, 65–73.

MONTAGNA, W. and CARLISLE, K. (1979) Structural changes in aging human skin. *J. Invest. Dermatol.* **73**, 47–53.

MONTEIRO-RIVIERE, N.A. (1991) Comparative anatomy, physiology, and biochemistry of mammalian skin. In HOBSON, D.W. (ed.) *Dermal and Ocular Toxicology: Fundamentals and Methods,* Boca Raton: CRC Press, 3–71.

MONTEIRO-RIVIERE, N.A., BANKS, Y.B. and BIRNBAUM, L.S. (1991) Laser Doppler measurements of cutaneous blood flow in ageing mice and rats. *Toxicol. Letters.* **57**, 329–338.

MONTEIRO-RIVIERE, N.A., BRISTOL, D. G., MANNING, T.O., ROGERS, R.A. and RIVIERE, J.E. (1990) Interspecies and interregional analysis of the comparative histologic thickness and laser Doppler blood flow measurements at five cutaneous sites in nine species. *J. Invest. Dermatol.* **95**, 582–586.

MONTEIRO-RIVIERE, N.A., INMAN, A.O., RIVIERE, J.E., MCNEILL, S.C. and FRANCOEUR, M.L. (1993) Topical penetration of piroxicam is dependent on the distribution of the local cutaneous vasculature. *Pharm. Res.* **10**, 1326–1331.

MONTEIRO-RIVIERE, N.A., STINSON, A.W. and CALHOUN, H.L. (1993) Integument. In DELLMAN, H. D. (ed.) *Textbook of Veterinary Histology,* 4th ed., Philadelphia: Lea and Febiger, 285–312.

MONTEIRO-RIVIERE, N.A., INMAN, A.O. and RIVIERE, J.E. (1994) Identification of the pathway of iontophoretic drug delivery: light and ultrastructural studies using mercuric chloride in pigs. *Pharm. Res.* **11**, 251–256.

MONTEIRO-RIVIERE, N.A., INMAN, A.O., MAK, V., WERTZ, P. and RIVIERE, J.E. (2001) Effect of selective lipid extraction from different body regions on epidermal barrier function. *Pharm. Res.* **18**, 992–998.

NAZZARO-PORRO, M., PASSI, S., BONIFORTI, L. and BELSITO, F. (1979) Effects of aging on fatty acids in skin surface lipids. *J. Invest. Dermatol.* **73**, 112–117.

NICOLAIDES, N., FU, H. C. and RICE, G.R. (1968) The skin surface lipids of man compared with those of eighteen species of animals. *J. Invest. Dermatol.* **51**, 83–89.

PIERAGGI, M.T., JULIAN, M. and BOUISSOU, H. (1984) Fibroblast changes in cutaneous ageing. *Virchows Arch. (Pathol. Anat.).* **402**, 275–287.

POTTS, R.O., BURAS, E.M and CHRISMAN, D.A. (1984) Changes with age in the moisture content of human skin. *J. Invest. Dermatol.* **82**, 97–100.

QIAO, G.L. and RIVIERE, J.E. (1995) Significant effects of application site and occlusion on the pharmacokinetics of cutaneous penetration and biotransformation of parathion *in vivo* in swine. *J. Pharm. Sci.* **84**, 425–432.

QIAO, G.L., WILLIAMS, P.L. and RIVIERE, J.E. (1994) Percutaneous absorption, biotransformation, and systemic disposition of parathion *in vivo* in swine. I. Comprehensive pharmacokinetic model. *Drug Metab. Dispos.* **22**, 459–471.

RAPAPORT, M. (1973) The aging skin. *J. Am. Geriatrics Soc.* **21**, 206–207.

REIFENRATH, W.G., CHELLQUIST, E.M., SHIPWASH, E.A., JEDERBERG, W.W. and KRUEGER, G.G. (1984) Percutaneous penetration in the hairless dog, weanling pig and grafted athymic nude mouse: Evaluation of models for predicting skin penetration in man. *Brit. J. Dermatol.* **111**, 123–135.

RIVIERE, J.E., MONTEIRO-RIVIERE, N.A. and INMAN, A.O. (1992) Determination of lidocaine concentrations in skin after transdermal iontophoresis: Effects of vasoactive drugs. *Pharm. Sci.* **9**, 211–214.

RIVIERE, J.E., SAGE, B.S. and WILLIAMS, P.L. (1991) The effects of vasoactive drugs on transdermal lidocaine iontophoresis. *J. Pharm. Sci.* **80**, 615–620.

RIVIERE, J.E. and WILLIAMS, P.L. (1992) Pharmacokinetic implications of changing blood flow in skin. *J. Pharm. Sci.* **81**, 601–602.

ROSKOS, K.V., BIRCHER, A.J., MAIBACH, H.I. and GUY, R.H. (1990) Pharmacodynamic measurements of methyl nicotinate percutaneous absorption: The effect of aging on microcirculation. *Br. J. Dermatol.* **122**, 165–171.

ROSKOS, K.V., GUY, R.H. and MAIBACH, H.I. (1986) Percutaneous absorption in the aged. *Dermatol. Clin.* **4**, 455–465.

■ CHAPTER 4 ■

Ross, E.V., BADAME, A.J. and DALE, S.E. (1987) Meat tenderizer in the acute treatment of imported fire ant stings. *J. Am. Acad. Dermatol.* **16**, 1189–1192.

RUSENKO, K.W., GAMMON, W.R., FINE, J.D. and BRIGGAMAN, R.A. (1989) The carboxyl-terminal domain of type VII collagen is present at the basement membrane in recessive dystrophic epidermolysis bullosa. *J. Invest. Dermatol.* **92**, 623–627.

RUSHMER, R.F., BUETTNER, K.J.K., SHORT, J.M. and ODLAND, G.F. (1966) The skin. *Science.* **154**, 343–348.

RYAN, T.J. (1991) Cutaneous circulation. In GOLDSMITH, L.A. (ed.) *Physiology, Biochemistry, and Molecular Biology of the Skin,* 2d edition, New York: Oxford University Press, 1019–1084.

SATO, K, SUGIBAYASHI, K. and MORIMOTO, Y. (1991) Species differences in percutaneous absorption of nicorandil. *J. Pharm. Sci.* **80**, 104–107.

SCHAEFER, H., ZESCH, A. and STÜTTGEN, G. (1977) Penetration, permeation and absorption of triamcinolone acetonide in normal and psoriatic skin. *Arch. Dermatol. Res.* **258**, 241–249.

SERUP, J. and STABERG, B. (1985) Qualification of weal reactions with laser Doppler flowmetry. *Allergy.* **40**, 233–237.

SHAH, P.V., FISHER, H.L., SUMLER, M.R., MONROE, R.J., CHERNOFF, N. and HALL, L. L. (1987) Comparison of the penetration of fourteen pesticides through the skin of young and adult rats. *J. Toxicol. Environ. Health.* **21**, 353–366.

SOUTHWELL, D., BARRY, B.W. and WOODFORD, R. (1984) Variations in permeability of human skin within and between specimens. *Int. J. Pharm.* **18**, 299–309.

SOUTHWOOD, W.F.W. (1955) The thickness of the skin. *Plas. Recon. Surg.* **15**, 423–429.

SQUIER, C.A. and HALL, B.K. (1985) The permeability of skin and oral mucosa to water and horseradish peroxidase as related to the thickness of the permeability barrier. *J. Invest. Dermatol.* **84**, 176–179.

SUNDBERG, S. (1984) Acute effects and long-term variations in skin blood flow measured with laser Doppler flowmetry. *Scand. J. Clin. Lab Invest.* **44**, 341–345.

SWARTZENDRUBER, D.C. (1992) Studies of epidermal lipids using electron microscopy. *Sem. Dermatol.* **11**, 157–161.

SWARTZENDRUBER, D.C., WERTZ, P.W., MADISON, K.C. and DOWNING, D.T. (1987) Evidence that the corneocyte has a chemically bound lipid envelope. *J. Invest. Dermatol.* **88**, 709–713.

SWARTZENDRUBER, D.C., WERTZ, P.W., KITKO, D.J., MADISON, K.C. and DOWNING, D.T. (1989) Molecular models of the intercellular lipid lamellae in mammalian stratum corneum. *J. Invest. Dermatol.* **92**, 251–257.

TIMPL, R., DZIADEK, M., FUJIWARA, S., NOWACK, H. and WICK, G. (1983) Nidogen: A new, self-aggregating basement membrane protein. *Eur. J. Biochem.* **137**, 455–465.

TORRENT, J., IZQUIERDO, I., BARBANOJ, M.J., MORENO, J., LAUROBA, J. and JANE, F. (1988) Anti-inflammatory activity of piroxicam after oral and topical administration on an ultraviolet-induced erythema model in man. *Curr. Ther. Res.* **44**, 340–347.

TUR, E., TUR, M., MAIBACH, H.I. and GUY, R.H. (1983) Basal perfusion of the cutaneous microcirculation: Measurements as a function of anatomic position. *J. Invest. Dermatol.* **81**, 442–446.

TUR, E., MAIBACH, H.I. and GUY, R.H. (1991) Percutaneous penetration of methyl nicotinate at three anatomic sites: Evidence for an appendageal contribution to transport? *Skin Pharmacol.* **4**, 230–234.

VERRANDO, P., HSI, B.L., YEH, C.J., PISANI, A., SERIEYS, N. and ORTONNE, J.P. (1987) Monoclonal antibody GB3, a new probe for the study of human basement membranes and hemidesmosomes. *Exp. Cell Res.* **170**, 116–128.

VOGEL, H.G. (1983) Effects of age on the biomechanical and biochemical properties of rat and human skin. *J. Soc. Cosmet. Chem.* **34**, 453–463.

WADA, Y., ETOH, Y., OHIRA, A., KIMATA, H., KOIDE, T., ISHIHAMA, H. and MIZUSHIMA, Y. (1982) Percutaneous absorption and anti-inflammatory activity of indomethacin in ointment. *J. Pharm. Pharmacol.* **34**, 467–468.

WERTZ, P.W. (1986) Lipids of keratinizing tissues. In MATOLTSY, A.G. and RICHARDS, K.S. (eds) *Biology of the Integument,* Berlin: Springer-Verlag, 815–823.

WERTZ, P.W. and DOWNING, D.T. (1991) Epidermal lipids. In Goldsmith, L. A. (ed.) *Physiology, Biochemistry, and Molecular Biology of the Skin,* 2d edition, New York: Oxford University Press, 205–236.

WESTER, R.C. and MAIBACH, H.I. (1975a) Percutaneous absorption in the rhesus monkey compared to man. *Toxicol. Appl. Pharmacol.* **32**, 394–398.

WESTER, R.C. and MAIBACH, H.I. (1975b) Rhesus monkey as a model for percutaneous absorption. In MAIBACH, H. (ed.) *Animal Models in Dermatology,* New York: Churchill-Livingstone, 133–137.

■ CHAPTER 4 ■

WESTER, R.C. and MAIBACH, H.I. (1976) Relationship of topical dose and percutaneous absorption in rhesus monkey and man. *J. Invest. Dermatol.* **67**, 518–520.

WESTER, R.C. and MAIBACH, H.I. (1977) Percutaneous absorption in man and animal: A perspective. In DRILL, V. and LAZAR, P. (eds) *Cutaneous Toxicity*, New York: Academic Press, 111–126.

WESTER, R.C., NOONAN, P.K. and MAIBACH, H.I. (1980) Variations in percutaneous absorption of testosterone in the rhesus monkey due to anatomic site of application and frequency of application. *Arch. Dermatol. Res.* **267**, 229–235.

WESTER, R.C. and MAIBACH, H.I. (1983) Cutaneous pharmacokinetics: 10 steps to percutaneous absorption. *Drug Metab. Rev.* **14**, 169–205.

WESTER, R.C., MAIBACH, H.I., GUY, R.H. and NOVAK, E. (1984) Minoxidil stimulates cutaneous blood flow in human balding scalps: Pharmaco-dynamics measured by laser Doppler velocimetry and photopulse plethys-mography. *J. Invest. Dermatol.* **82**, 515–517.

WILLIAMS, P.L., RIVIERE, J.E. (1995) A biophysically based dermatopharmaco-kinetic compartmental model for quantifying percutaneous penetration and absorption of topically applied agents. I. Theory. *J. Pharm. Sci.* **84**, 599–608.

WOODLEY, D.T., BRIGGAMAN, R.A., O'KEFFE, E.J., INMAN, A.O., QUEEN, L.L. and GAMMON, W.R. (1984) Identification of the skin basement-membrane autoantigen in epidermolysis bullosa acquisita. *N. Engl. J. Med.* **310**, 1007–1013.

YARDLEY, H.J. and SUMMERLY, R. (1981) Lipid composition and metabolism in normal and diseased epidermis. *Pharmacol. Ther.* **13**, 357–383.

YATES, M.S. and HILEY, C.R. (1979) The effect of age on cardiac output and its distribution in the rat. *Experientia.* **35**, 78–79.

YOUNG, A.R., GUY, R.H. and MAIBACH, H.I. (1985) Laser Doppler velocimetry to quantify UV-B induced increase in human skin blood flow. *Photochem. Photobiol.* **42**, 385–390.

ZESCH, A., SCHAEFER, H. and HOFFMAN, W. (1975) Penetration of radioactive hydrocortisone in human skin from various ointment bases. II. In vivo experiments. *Arch. Dermatol. Res.* **252**, 245–256.

Percutaneous Absorption: Role of Lipids

PHILIP W WERTZ

Contents

5.1 Implication of stratum corneum lipids in permeability barrier function

5.2 Alteration of lipids with differentiation

5.3 Lamellar granules

5.4 Lipid envelope

5.5 Chemical structure of the stratum corneum lipids

5.6 Ultrastructure of the intercellular spaces of the stratum corneum

5.1 IMPLICATION OF STRATUM CORNEUM LIPIDS IN PERMEABILITY BARRIER FUNCTION

Experiments performed in the early 1950s in which the effects of organic solvents on permeability of the skin were studied implicated stratum corneum lipids in the function of the permeability barrier (Berenson and Burch, 1951; Blank, 1952). However, little further progress was made until 1973, when two breakthroughs were reported. Through the use of electron dense water soluble tracers, Squier (1973) was able to demonstrate by transmission electron microscopy that the permeability barrier starts at the bottom of the stratum corneum, where the contents of the lamellar granules are extruded. These studies also indicated that all layers of stratum corneum contribute to barrier function. In this same year, Breathnach *et al.* (1973) demonstrated by freeze fracture electron microscopy that the intercellular spaces of the stratum corneum contain multiple stacked, broad lipid sheets. These findings were further elaborated by Elias and Friend (1975). In the scenario that emerged from this body of work lipids accumulate in lamellar granules, and are extruded into the intercellular spaces in the upper granular layer. After extrusion, the short stacks of lipid lamellae are transformed into multiple broad lipid sheets which fill most of the intercellular spaces throughout the stratum corneum. It is this lamellar lipid in the intercellular spaces that determines the permeability of the stratum corneum.

CHAPTER 5

5.2 ALTERATION OF LIPIDS WITH DIFFERENTIATION

Basal keratinocytes, like most mammalian cells, contain phospholipids and cholesterol as the principal lipids; however, as epidermal keratinocytes undergo differentiation there are dramatic alterations of lipid composition (Yardley and Summerly, 1981). In addition to more phospholipids, the differentiating cells synthesize a great deal of ceramides, glucosylceramides and cholesterol. In the final stages of the differentiation program the phospholipids are broken down and the glycolipids are deglycosylated, leaving ceramides, cholesterol and fatty acids as the principal lipids of the stratum corneum (Wertz and Downing, 1989a). These are the lipids that form the intercellular lamellae. It is remarkable that unlike most biological membranes, the intercellular lamellae do not contain phospholipids.

5.3   LAMELLAR GRANULES

Much of the lipid that accumulates during epidermal differentiation is packaged into lamellar granules (Landmann, 1988). This small organelle is round to ovoid in shape, approximately 0.2 μm in diameter, and consists of one or several stacks of lamellar disks surrounded by a bounding membrane. The lamellar disks are thought to be flattened lipid vesicles.

Several investigators have examined the lipid composition of isolated lamellar granules, and have found the major lipid classes to be phospholipids, cholesterol and glucosylceramides (Wertz *et al.*, 1984; Freinkel and Traczyk, 1985; Grayson *et al.*, 1985). One unusual glycolipid associated with lamellar granules consists of 30- through 34-carbon ω-hydroxyacids amide linked to sphingosine with glucose β-glycosidically attached to the primary hydroxyl group of the long-chain base and linoleic acid ester-linked to the ω-hydroxyl group (Wertz and Downing, 1983a; Abraham *et al.*, 1985). The ω-hydroxyacyl portion of this molecule is of sufficient length to span a typical lipid bilayer, and it has been proposed that the linoleate could insert into an adjacent bilayer, thus riveting the two together (Wertz and Downing, 1982). This sort of interaction could promote the flattening and stacking of lipid vesicles to produce the stacks of disks found within the lamellar granules. It has also been suggested that only about one-third of the acylglucosylceramide is associated with the internal lamellae, while the other two-thirds is in the bounding membrane (Wertz, 1992, 1996).

5.4   LIPID ENVELOPE

When the bounding membrane of the lamellar granule fuses into the cell plasma membrane, much lipid including acylglucosylceramide is introduced to the cell periphery. At about this same time, a thick band of protein is deposited on the inner aspect of the plasma membrane (Rice and Green, 1977, 1979; Mehrel *et al.*, 1990), and this protein becomes cross-linked via isopeptide (Abernathy *et al.*, 1977; Rice and Green, 1977) and disulfide linkages (Polakowska and Goldsmith, 1991). The glucose is removed from the acylglucosylceramide through the action of a glucocerebrosidase (Wertz and Downing, 1989b). The linoleate is removed and possibly recycled (Madison *et al.*, 1989), and the remaining ω-hydroxyceramide becomes attached through ester linkages to the outer surface of the cross-linked protein (Wertz and Downing, 1987). The amount of this covalently bound lipid is just sufficient to provide a mono-molecular coating over the entire surface of the cornified cell (Wertz and

Downing, 1987; Swartzendruber *et al.*, 1987). In the porcine model there is one ω-hydroxyceramide which contains sphingosine as the base (Wertz and Downing, 1987); however, in human stratum corneum, there is a second covalently bound ω-hydroxyceramide (Wertz *et al.*, 1989) that contains 6-hydroxysphingosine (Robson *et al.*, 1994). It appears that transglutaminase 1 may be responsible for attachment of the ω-hydroxyceramide molecules to involucrin in the envelope (Nemes *et al.*, 1999).

5.5 CHEMICAL STRUCTURES OF THE STRATUM CORNEUM LIPIDS

Representative structures of the major stratum corneum lipids are presented in Figure 5.1. The ceramides consist of six chromatographically distinguishable fractions and together make up 50 percent of the stratum corneum lipid mass (Wertz and Downing, 1983b and 1989a). The least polar ceramide, ceramide 1, is derived from the above mentioned acylglucosylceramide, and may serve as a molecular rivet in stabilizing the multilamellar sheets within the intercellular spaces. Ceramide 2 consists of mainly 24- through 28-carbon fatty acids amide-linked to sphingosines. Ceramide 3 contains the same range of fatty acids, but they are here amide-linked to phytosphingosines. Ceramides 4 and 5 both contain α-hydroxyacids amide-linked to sphingosines. They differ in that ceramide 4 contains 24- through 28-carbon hydroxyacids, whereas ceramide 5 contains mainly the 16-carbon α-hydroxypalmitic acid. Ceramide 6 consists of α-hydroxyacids amide-linked to phytosphingosines. Cholesterol, a ubiquitous membrane lipid, comprises 25 percent of the stratum corneum lipid mass (Yardley and Summerly, 1981; Wertz and Downing, 1989a). The free fatty acids comprise 10 percent of the stratum corneum lipid (Yardley and Summerly, 1981; Wertz and Downing, 1989a), and like those from ceramides 2 and 3, are mainly 24- through 28-carbon saturates. It is noteworthy that with the exception of the linoleate tail of ceramide 1 for which a special function has been proposed, all of the aliphatic chains in the stratum corneum lipids are straight with no methyl branches or cis double bonds, and the polar head groups are minimal. These structural features should favor formation of highly ordered, probably gel phase membrane domains, and this expectation is supported by infrared (Potts and Francoeur, 1993), X-ray and thermal studies (Bouwstra *et al.*, 1991).

The ceramide structures presented in Figure 5.1 were originally determined for porcine epidermis (Wertz and Downing, 1983b); however all of the same ceramides are present in human epidermis (Wertz *et al.*, 1985, 1987). More

CHAPTER 5

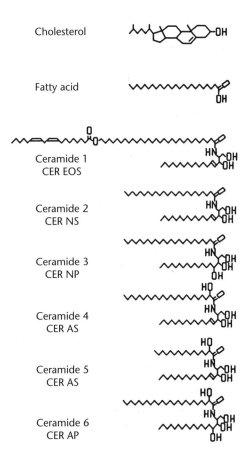

Cholesterol

Fatty acid

Ceramide 1
CER EOS

Ceramide 2
CER NS

Ceramide 3
CER NP

Ceramide 4
CER AS

Ceramide 5
CER AS

Ceramide 6
CER AP

Figure 5.1: Representative structures of the major stratum corneum lipids.

recent studies have revealed an additional series of ceramides in human stratum corneum in which the long-chain base is 6-hydroxysphingosine (Robson *et al.*, 1994; Stewart and Downing, 1999) One of these additional human ceramides contains normal fatty acids, a second consists of α-hydroxyacids, and there is a minor amount of an acylceramide analogous to ceramide 1 but containing containing 6-hydroxysphingosine. In addition, an acylceramide containin phytosphingosine as the base component has recently been identified (Ponec *et al.*, 2003).

Because of the additional ceramides in human stratum corneum and the fact that they do not all separate into discreet chromatographic fractions, the nomenclature system based on chromatographic fraction numbers is no longer adequate. A system of ceramide nomenclature proposed by Motta *et al.* (1993) is increasingly coming into use. Within this system the amide-linked fatty acid is designated by N, A or O, for normal fatty acids, α-hydroxyacids and ω-hydroxyacids, respectively. Similarly, the base component is designated as S, P or H for sphingosine, phytosphingosine and 6-hydroxysphingosine, respectively. If an ester-linked fatty acid is also present this is designated with a prefix E. Thus, ceramide 1 from Figure 5.1 would be CER EOS. Ceramide 2 would be represented as CER NS, and so on, as shown in Figure 5.1.

5.6 ULTRASTRUCTURE OF THE INTERCELLULAR SPACES OF THE STRATUM CORNEUM

Although the intercellular lamellae of the stratum corneum could be detected by the freeze fracture method (Breathnach *et al.*, 1973), this technique provides relatively little information.

Until the recent introduction of ruthenium tetroxide as a post-fixative for the preparation of samples (Madison *et al.*, 1987), the intercellular lamellae could not be visualized by transmission electron microscopy, and it was proposed that the lipids were removed during sample processing (Elias *et al.*, 1988). However, it is now known that this is not the case. The stratum corneum lipids, as appropriate for materials that interface with the external environment, are relatively chemically inert, and do not react appreciably with osmium tetroxide used for routine fixation. This difficulty was overcome by substitution of the stronger oxidizing agent, ruthenium tetroxide. With this reagent the intercellular lamellae can be routinely visualized as shown in Figure 5.2. The first lucent band adjacent to the electron dense protein band of the cornified envelope is the covalently attached lipid. The central pair of bilayers is produced by edge-to-edge fusion of flattened lipid vesicles extruded from the lamellar granules (Landmann, 1988). The narrow lucent bands intervening between the central pair of bilayers and the covalently bound lipid layers are thought to be formed by eversion of sphingosine chains from the covalently bound hydroxyceramides and fatty chains from ceramides (Swartzendruber *et al.*, 1989), including linoleate from ceramide 1 (Wertz, 1996), from the central bilayers to form an interdigitated zipper-like framework (Swartzendruber *et al.*, 1989; Wertz, 1996). Space vacated by everted chains and remaining within the framework are filled in by free lipids. Essentially the same model for the broad-narrow-broad repeat units has been arrived at independently in an attempt to explain the 13 nm repeat seen in X-ray diffraction studies (Bouwstra *et al.*, 2000, 2002).

■ CHAPTER 5 ■

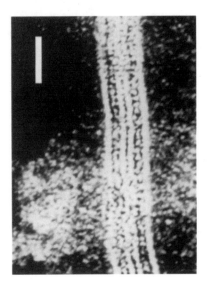

Figure 5.2: Transmission electron micrograph of stratum corneum after fixation with ruthenium tetroxide. Modified from Swartzendruber *et al.* (1989). Bar = 25 nm.

Although the three lucent banded patterns near the ends of the cells and the six lucent band patterns between the flat surfaces of adjacent corneocytes are the most frequent lamellar arrangements seen in normal epidermal stratum corneum, the number and arrangement of lamellae is highly variable, and caution should be taken in comparing intercellular material in normal verses diseased or experimentally manipulated stratum corneum.

REFERENCES

ABERNATHY. J.L., HILL, R.L. and GOLDSMITH, L.A. (1977) ε-(γ-Glutamyl) lysine cross-links in human stratum corneum. *J. Biol. Chem.* **252**, 1837–1839.

ABRAHAM, W., WERTZ, P.W. and DOWNING, D.T. (1985) Linoleate-rich acyl-glucosylceramides from pig epidermis: structure determination by proton magnetic resonance. *J. Lipid Res.* **26**, 761–766.

BERENSON, G.S. and BURCH, G.E. (1951) Studies of diffusion of water through dead human skin: The effect of different environmental states and of chemical alterations of the epidermis. *Amer. J. Trop. Med.* **31**, 842–853.

BLANK, I.H. (1952) Factors which influence the water content of the stratum corneum. *J. Invest. Dermatol.* **18**, 433–440.

BOWSTRA, J.A., GOORIS, G.S., VAN DER SPEK, J.A. and BRAS, W. (1991) Structural investigations of human stratum corneum by small-angle X-ray scattering. *J. Invest. Dermatol.* **97**, 1005–1012.

BOUWSTRA, J.A., DUBBELAAR, F.E., GOORIS, G.S., PONEC, M. (2000) The lipid organization of the skin barrier. *Acta Dermato. Venereol.* **208**, 23–30.

BOUWSTRA, J.A., GOORIS, G.S., DUBBELAAR, F.E.R., PONEC, M. (2002) Phase behavior of stratum corneum lipid mixtures based on human ceramides: The role of natural and synthetic ceramide 1. *J. Invest. Dermatol.* **118**, 606–617.

BREATHNACH, A.S., GOODMAN, T., STOLINSKI, C. and GROSS, M. (1973) Freeze fracture replication of cells of stratum corneum of human epidermis. *J. Anat.* **114**, 65–81.

ELIAS, P.M. and FRIEND, D.S. (1975) The permeability barrier in mammalian epidermis. *J. Cell Biol.* **65**, 180–191.

ELIAS, P.M., MENON, G.K., GRAYSON, S. and BROWN, B.E. (1988) Membrane structural alterations in murine stratum corneum: Relationships to the localization of polar lipids and phospholipases. *J. Invest. Dermatol.* **91**, 3–10.

FREINKEL, R.K. and TRACZYK, T.N. (1985) Lipid composition and acid hydrolase content of lamellar granules of fetal rat epidermis. *J. Invest. Dermatol.* **85**, 295–298.

GRAYSON, S., JOHNSON-WINEGAR, A.G., WINTRAUB, B.U., ISSEROFF, R.R., EPSTEIN, E.H. and ELIAS, P.M. (1985) Lamellar body-enriched fractions from neonatal mice: Preparative techniques and partial characterization. *J. Invest. Dermatol.* **85**, 289–294.

LANDMANN, L. (1988) The epidermal permeability barrier. *Anat. Embryol.* **178**, 1–13.

MADISON, K.C., SWARTZENDRUBER, D.C., WERTZ, P.W. and DOWNING, D.T. (1987) Presence of intact intercellular lamellae in the upper layers of the stratum corneum. *J. Invest. Dermatol.* **88**, 714–718.

MADISON, K.C., SWARTZENDRUBER, D.C., WERTZ, P.W. and DOWNING, D.T. (1989) Murine keratinocyte cultures grown at the air/medium interface synthesize stratum corneum lipids and "recycle" linoleate during differentiation. *J. Invest. Dermatol.* **93**, 10–17.

MEHREL, T., HOHL, D., ROTHNAGEL, J.A., LONGLEY, M.A., BUNDMAN, D., CHENG, C., LICHTI, U., BISHER, M.E., STEVEN, A.C., STEINERT, P.M., YUSPA, S.H. and ROOP, D.R. (1990) Identification of a major keratinocyte cell envelope protein, loricrin. *Cell* **61**, 1103–1112.

■ CHAPTER 5 ■

MOTTA, S.M., MONTI, M., SESANA, S., CAPUTO, R.,CARELLI, S., GHIDONI, R. (1993) Ceramide composition of the psoriatic scale. *Biochim. Biophys. Acta.* **1182**, 147–151.

NEMES, Z., MAREKOV, L.N., FESUS, L., STEINERT, P.M. (1999) A novel function for transglutaminase 1: attachment of long-chain omega-hydroxyceramides to involucrin by ester bond formation. *Proc. Nat. Acad. Sci. USA.* **96**, 8402–8407.

POLAKOWSKA, R.R. and GOLDSMITH, L.A. (1991) The cell envelope and trans-glutaminases. In GOLDSMITH, L.A. (ed.) *Physiology, Biochemistry and Molecular Biology of the Skin*, New York: Oxford University Press, 168–204.

PONEC, M., WEERHEIM, A., LANKHORST, P., WERTZ, P.W. (2003) New acylcera-mide in native and reconstructed epidermis. *J. Invest. Dermatol.* **120**, 581–588.

POTTS, R.O. and FRANCOEUR, M.L. (1993) Infrared spectroscopy of stratum corneum lipids: *in vitro* results and their relevance to permeability. In Walters, K.A. and Hadgraft, J. (eds) *Pharmaceutical Skin Penetration Enhancement*, New York: Marcel Dekker, 269–292.

RICE, R.H. and GREEN, H. (1977) The cornified envelope of terminally differen-tiated human epidermal keratinocytes consists of cross-linked protein. *Cell* **11**, 417–422.

RICE, R.H. and GREEN, H. (1979) Presence in human epidermal cells of a soluble protein precursor of the cross-linked envelope: activation of the cross-linking by calcium ions. *Cell* **18**, 681–694.

ROBSON,K.J., STEWART, M.E., MICHELSEN, S., LAZO, N.D., DOWNING, D.T. (1994) 6-Hydroxy-4-sphingenine in human epidermal ceramides. *J. Lipid Res.* **35**, 2060–2068.

SQUIER, C.A. (1973) The permeability of keratinized and nonkeratinized oral epithelium to horseradish peroxidase. *J. Ultrastruct. Res.* **43**, 160–177.

STEWART, M.E., DOWNING, D.T. (1999) A new 6-hydroxy-4-sphingenine-containing ceramide in human skin. *J. Lipid Res.* **40**, 1434–1439.

SWARTZENDRUBER, D.C., WERTZ, P.W., MADISON, K.C. and DOWNING, D.T. (1987) Evidence that the corneocyte has a chemically bound lipid envelope. *J. Invest. Dermatol.* **88**, 709–713.

SWARTZENDRUBER, D.C., WERTZ, P.W., KITKO, D.J., MADISON, K.C. and DOWNING, D.T. (1989) Molecular models of the intercellular lipid lamellae in mammalian stratum corneum. *J. Invest. Dermatol.* **92**, 251–257.

WERTZ, P.W. (1992) Epidermal lipids. *Semin. Dermatol.* **11**, 106–113.

WERTZ, P.W. (1996) Integral lipids of hair and stratum corneum. In ZAHN, H. and JOLLES, P. (eds), *Hair: Biology And Structure*, Basel: Birkhauser Verlag, 227–238.

WERTZ, P.W. and DOWNING, D.T. (1982) Glycolipids in mammalian epidermis: structure and function in the water barrier. *Science* **217**, 1261–1262.

WERTZ, P.W. and DOWNING, D.T. (1983a) Acylglucosylceramides of pig epidermis: structure determination. *J. Lipid Res.* **24**, 753–758.

WERTZ, P.W. and DOWNING, D.T. (1983b) Ceramides of pig epidermis: structure determination. *J. Lipid Res.* **24**, 759–765.

WERTZ, P.W. and DOWNING, D.T. (1987) Covalently bound ω-hydroxyacyl-sphingosine in the stratum corneum. *Biochim. Biophys. Acta* **917**, 108–111.

WERTZ, P.W. and DOWNING, D.T. (1989a) Stratum corneum: biological and biochemical considerations. In HADGRAFT, J. and GUY, R.H. (eds) *Transdermal Drug Delivery*, New York and Basel: Marcel Dekker Inc., 1–22.

WERTZ, P.W. and DOWNING, D.T. (1989b) β-Glucosidase activity in porcine epidermis. *Biochim. Biophys. Acta* **1001**, 115–119.

WERTZ, P.W., MIETHKE, M.C., LONG, S.A., STRAUSS, J.S., DOWNING, D.T. (1985) The composition of ceramides from human stratum corneum and from comedones. *J. Invest. Dermatol.* **84**, 410–412.

WERTZ, P.W., SWARTZENDRUBER, D.T., MADISON, K.C., DOWNING, D.T. (1987) Composition and morphology of epidermal cyst lipids. *J. Invest. Dermatol.* **89**, 419–425.

WERTZ, P.W., MADISON, K.C., DOWNING, D.T. (1989) Covalently bound lipids of human stratum corneum. *J. Invest. Dermatol.* **91**, 109–111.

YARDLEY, H.J. and SUMMERLY, R. (1981) Lipid composition and metabolism in normal and diseased epidermis. *Pharmacology & Therapeutics* **13**, 357–383.

■ CHAPTER 5 ■

Percutaneous Absorption

Short-Term Exposure, Lag Time, Multiple Exposures, Model Variations, and Absorption from Clothing

RONALD C WESTER AND HOWARD I MAIBACH

Contents

6.1   Introduction

6.2   Short-term exposure to hazardous chemicals

6.3   Lag time

6.4   Multiple exposure in the same day

6.5   Multiple dosing: azone self-enhanced
       percutaneous absorption

6.6   Individual variation: *in vitro* human skin

6.7   Models: *in vitro* and *in vivo*

6.8   Percutaneous absorption from chemicals in
       clothing

6.9   Human *in vivo* percutaneous absorption

6.10 Discussion

6.1 INTRODUCTION

The area of percutaneous absorption has been established as a significant part of dermatotoxicology. Human health risk assessment includes an estimate for percutaneous absorption where dermal exposure is involved. Some estimate of percent dose absorbed or steady-state absorption (flux) is included. Behind these generated numbers lies the question of validation. Human exposure is a risk endpoint, and if a model is used, that model should be validated for humans *in vivo*. Second, there is the question of relevance of the particular risk assessment situation to the provided percutaneous absorption data. For example, is an absorption estimate derived over a long period of exposure applicable to a short exposure period? (There are some examples where this is not the case.) Also, multiple exposures (daily or weekly) can exceed single exposure estimates in some situations. Third, some limitations (lag time, lipophilicity) to the *in vitro* diffusion model are shown. Finally, the data showing skin delivery and percutaneous absorption of chemicals from clothing fabric are discussed. The overall interest is relevant and validates percutaneous absorption data and proper data interpretation.

6.2 SHORT-TERM EXPOSURE TO HAZARDOUS CHEMICALS

Exposure to hazardous chemicals in water during a bath or swim is on the order of 30 min to an hour. Some tasks at work or in the home where exposure may occur can be of the same length of time. A hazardous spill is usually washed with soap and water within this time frame. The standard work day is 8 h, punctuated with breaks during this time period. Assessment of skin absorption in the laboratory is usually in the magnitude of 24 h, or some steady-state rate achieved in the course of 24+ h of exposure. Linearity in skin absorption is assumed, and the appropriate calculations to the desired time period are made.

Table 6.1 shows that the *in vivo* percutaneous absorption for a 24-h exposure is 51 percent of the dose of benzo[a]pyrene and 18.9 percent of the dose for DDT. To simulate short-term exposure, human skin was dosed and the skin surface washed with soap and water after 25 min of dosing. The receptor fluid contained, as expected, no chemical, However, the skin was assayed and benzo[a]pyrene levels were at 5.1 percent and DDT levels were at 16.7 percent (the same as for 24-h exposure). In the short 25-min exposure, sufficient chemical had partitioned from the skin surface into the interior, or was so

TABLE 6.1:

Short-term wash recovery for benzo[a]pyrene and DDT: 25-min exposure versus 24-hr exposure.

	Percent dose		
	Short exposure (25 min). *in vitro*		
Chemical	Receptor fluid	Skin	Long exposure (24 h), *in vivo*
Benzo[a]pyrene	0.00 ± 0.00	5.1 ± 2.1	51.0 ± 22.0
DDT	0.00 ± 0.00	16.7 ± 13.2	18.9 ± 9.4

Note. *In vitro* the chemical in acetone vehicle was dosed on human skin, then washed with soap and water after a 25-min period. The *in vivo* studies were 24-h exposure with acetone vehicle dosing.

bound that soap and water wash did not remove the chemical (Wester *et al.*, 1990).

In the course of studying cadmium skin absorption, short-term exposure to human skin *in vitro* was examined. This study simulated a 30-min exposure of human skin to cadmium in water (swim, bath) followed by a soap and water surface wash. Table 6.2 shows that with 30-min exposure only, receptor fluid (human plasma) contained no cadmium (0.0 percent) but that skin content was 2.3 percent of the dose. To determine if cadmium would migrate from the skin into the plasma receptor fluid (and thus be systemically absorbed chemical)

TABLE 6.2:

Exposure of cadmium in water to human skin for 30 min followed by skin surface wash with soap and water and then 48-h perfusion with human plasma

	Percentage dose	
Treatment	Skin content	Plasma receptor fluid
30-min Exposure only	2.3 ± 3.3	0.0 ± 0.0
30-min Exposure followed by 48-h perfusion	2.7 ± 2.2	0.6 ± 0.8
Statistics	$p = 0.77$	$p = 0.04^a$

Note: $n = 9$ (3 human skin sources × 3 replicates each). This study simutates a 30-min exposure of human skin to cadmium in water (swim, bath) followed by a soap-and-water surface wash. Cadmiun is able to bind to human skin in the 30-min exposure time and then be absorbed into the body during the remainder of the day.

[a]Statistically significant difference.

TABLE 6.3:

Effect of exposure time on mercury percutaneous absorption *in vitro* in human skin

Time/treatment	Percent dose	
	Receptor fluid	Skin content
30 min Only ($n = 9$)	0.01 ± 0.00^a	5.5 ± 5.2^{ab}
30 min Followed by 48-h perfusion ($n = 9$)	0.09 ± 0.05^{ab}	6.3 ± 4.9^{ab}
24-h ($n = 6$)	0.06 ± 0.03^b	35.4 ± 15.2^a

[a] Significant difference ($p < .05$ or greater).
[b] Nonsignificant difference.

some skin samples were further perfused for an additional 48 h. Some cadmium in the skin did migrate into the plasma perfusate (0.6 percent; statistically significant at $p = .04$) (Wester *et al* ., 1992b).

Table 6.3 shows the effect of exposure time on mercury ($HgCl_2$) in water as percutaneous absorption *in vitro* in human skin. With 24 h of exposure, receptor fluid accumulation was 0.06 percent: however, skin content was 35.4 percent. Human skin has great attraction for mercury in water. Similar to the study just cited, mercury was applied to human skin for 30 min and the skin was washed with soap and water. Mercury was at low levels in receptor fluid 0.01 percent) but skin content was a robust 5.5 percent. Continued perfusion increased receptor fluid content to 0.09 percent (statistically significant difference $p <$ .05). In other words, the mercury quickly partitioned into human skin, and then was slowly absorbed into the perfusate (body).

In each of the cases cited (DDT, benzo[a]pyrene, cadmium, mercury), the chemical exhibited a capacity to quickly partition into human skin with short-term exposure of 30 min.

6.3   LAG TIME

There is a calculation from *in vitro* diffusion studies also called the lag time. A line is drawn along an area of steady-state absorption to the abscissa (horizontal sequence of time) and the intercept with the abscissa is the lag time. This *in vitro* diffusion parameter should not be confused with the actual time that a chemical is needed for percutaneous absorption *in vivo*. Table 6.4 gives the flux and lag time for hydroquinone *in vitro* percutaneous absorption in human skin dosed with a 2 percent hydroquinone cream. The lag time is 8 h. The same

TABLE 6.4:

Parameters of *in vitro* hydroquinone percutaneous absorption in human skin

Treatment	Flux (μg/h cm^2)	Lag time (h)
HQ cream	2.94	7.99
HQ cream + inhibitor	2.93	8.03

Note. In vivo in human volunteers hydroquinone is readily detected in blood within 30 min following topical application. The 8-h *in vitro* diffusion lag time has no relevance to actual *in vivo* percutaneous absorption.

hydroquinone dose/vehicle was topically applied to human volunteers and hydroquinone was detected in blood within 30 min. Therefore, the 8-h *in vitro* diffusion lag time has no relevance to actual *in vivo* percutaneous absorption. The lag time is simply an artificial derivation of the *in vitro* diffusion system.

Laser Doppler velocimetry (LDV) is able to detect changes in human skin blood flow. Topical application of methyl nicotinate (a vasodilator) in human volunteers causes changes in skin blood flow within 2 min (Wester and Maibach, 1984) (Figure 6.1).

The endpoint for *in vivo* percutaneous absorption is the blood (systemic) in the microcirculation in the upper dermis at the epidermal junction. *In vitro* diffusion adds some dermis and solubility and detection sensitivity limits the process.

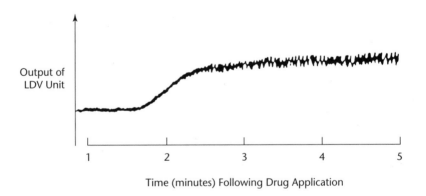

Figure 6.1: Laser Doppler velocimetry (LDV) measures human skin blood flow *in vivo*. Methyl nicotinate was able to penetrate and cause a pharmacological reaction in 2 min. This shows that *in vivo* percutaneous absorption can be rapid.

6.4 MULTIPLE EXPOSURE IN THE SAME DAY

On a historic and empiric basis, topical applications of hydrocortisone and other corticosteroids frequently use repeated, rather than single, bolus applications of drug to the skin. It is commonly assumed that multiple applications of hydrocortisone effectively increase its bioavailability and absorption. A long-term, multiple-dose rhesus monkey study by Wester *et al.* (1980) indicated that this was true. However, short-term experiments in the rhesus monkey by Wester *et al.* (1977) and long-term pharmacokinetic assays by Bucks *et al.* (1985) did not show an increase in hydrocortisone absorption following multiple dosing. An investigation was designed to determine if multiple-dose therapy (dosing the same site three times in the same day) would increase drug bioavailability in human skin. The study was done *in vivo* using male volunteers (from whom informed consent had been obtained) and *in vitro* with human skin. Hydrocortisone was in either a solvent (acetone) vehicle or in a cream base vehicle

In each *in vivo* procedure in this crossover study, the subjects were healthy male volunteers, 25–85 yr old, from whom informed consent has been obtained. The treatments were performed on two adjacent sites on each forearm. Each site received a different treatment: each was performed 2–3 wk apart, alternating forearms between the treatments to allow for systemic and dermal clearance of residual hydrocortisone and radioactivity. The dosing sequence was as follows:

Treatment	Dose per application (μg/cm^2)	Cumulative dose (μg/cm^2)	Total vehicle volume (μl) Acetone	Cream
1[a]	13.33	13.33	20	100
2[b]	40.00	40.00	20	100
3[c]	13.33	40.00	60	100

[a]Single dose of 13.33 μg/cm^2, administered in 20 μl of vehicle.
[b]Single dose of 40.0 μg/cm^2, administered in 20 μl of vehicle.
[c]Three serial 13.33 μg/cm^2 doses each administered in 20 μl of vehicle (total 60 μg).

In vitro, three separate human donor skin sources with replicates per each experiment were used. Small cells were of the flow-through design with 1 cm^2 surface area. Buffered saline at a rate of 1.25 ml/h (1 reservoir volume) served as a receptor fluid. Human cadaver skin was dermatomed to 500 μm and stored refrigerated at 4°C in Eagle's minimum essential medium. The skin was used within 5 d. This preservation/use regimen follows that used by the human skin

TABLE 6.5:

Predicted and observed hydrocortisone absorption: *in vivo*

		Hydrocortisone absorbed ($\mu g/cm^2$)	
Vehicle	Dosing sequence	Predicted	Observed
Acetone[a]	13.3 $\mu g/cm^2 \times 1$	—	0.056 ± 0.073
	40.0 $\mu g/cm^2 \times 1$	0.168[e]	0.140 ± 0.136[c]
	13.3 $\mu g/cm^2 \times 1$	0.168	0.372 ± 0.304[c]
Cream[b]	13.3 $\mu g/cm^2 \times 1$	—	0.31 ± 0.43
	40.0 $\mu g/cm^2 \times 1$	0.93[e]	0.91 ± 1.55[d]
	13.3 $\mu g/cm^2 \times 1$	0.93	1.74 ± 0.93[d]

Note: Different volunteers were used for each formulation: therefore, comparison of absolute bioavailability across vehicle is not justified.
[a]$n = 6$; Mean $\pm$ SD.
[b]$n = 5$; Mean $\pm$ SD.
[c]Statistically different ($p < .05$), paired t-test.
[d]Statistically different ($p < .006$), paired t-test.
[e]0.168 $\mu g/cm^2$ is $3 \times$ the measured value of 0.056 $\mu g/cm^2$ is $3 \times$ the measured value of 0.31 $\mu g/cm^2$.

transplant bank. Radiolabeled hydrocortisone in either acetone or cream base vehicle was applied to the skin per the study design.

Table 6.5 shows that *in vivo* the multiple dose ($\times 3$) significantly increased hydrocortisone percutaneous absorption for acetone vehicle ($p < .05$) and for the cream vehicle ($p < .006$). Statistically, *in vitro* (Table 6.6) there was no difference with multiple dose: however, the trend was the same as with *in vivo*. Figures 6.2 and 6.3 show the enhanced absorption *in vivo* from the acetone vehicle and the cream vehicle.

This study suggests that triple therapy in humans may have some advantage (Melendres *et al.*, 1992). If increased bioavailability is desired, then multiple-application therapy may be the answer, if patient convenience is not an issue. Our data suggest the possibility that increased bioavailability is related to reapplication of vehicle; hence, a case may be made for increasing hydro-cortisone bioavailability merely by applying serial doses of vehicle to a previously applied single dose of hydrocortisone at the skin surface. Such an experiment would verify if the solvent–vehicle effect was the only component by which multiple application of hydrocortisone in acetone increased its bioavailability in human skin. The cream vehicle was equal in amount for each treatment. Reapplication of cream in triple therapy may have "activated" any hydrocortisone bound up in stratum corneum reservoir.

From a toxicological viewpoint, a question remains as to whether multiple exposure during the day will differ from a single continuous exposure. Also,

TABLE 6.6:

Predicted and observed hydrocortisone absorption: *in vitro*

Vehicle	Dosing sequence	Hydrocortisone ($\mu g/cm^2$) Receptor fluid Predict	Observe	Skin Predict	Observe
Acetone[a]	$13.3\ \mu g/cm^2 \times 1$	—	0.13 ± 0.05	—	0.87 ± 0.23
	$40.0\ \mu g/cm^2 \times 1$	0.39^b	0.35 ± 0.22	2.61^b	2.21 ± 2.05
	$13.3\ \mu g/cm^2 \times 1$	0.39	0.55 ± 0.75	2.61	2.84 ± 2.05
Cream[a]	$13.3\ \mu g/cm^2 \times 1$	—	0.53 ± 0.029	—	0.30 ± 0.24
	$40.0\ \mu g/cm^2 \times 1$	0.16^b	0.23 ± 0.03	0.90^b	0.86 ± 0.53
	$13.3\ \mu g/cm^2 \times 3$	0.16	0.27 ± 0.21	0.90	1.19 ± 0.43

[a] $n = 3$; Mean ± SD
[b] $0.39\ \mu g/cm^2$ is $3 \times$ the measured value of $0.13\ \mu g/cm^2$; $0.16\ \mu g/cm^2$ is $3 \times$ the measured value of $0.053\ \mu g/cm^2$: $2.61\ \mu g/cm^2$ is $3 \times$ the measured value of 0.87 $\mu g/cm^2$: $0.91\ \mu g/cm^2$ is $3 \times$ the measured value of $0.30\ \mu g/cm^2$.

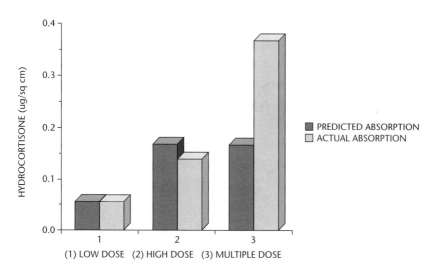

Figure 6.2: Hydrocortisone *in vivo* percutaneous absorption in human with acetone vehicle and single and multiple dosing. The multiple dosing (triple therapy) exceeded predicted absorption and was statistically ($p < .006$) greater than the single high dose.

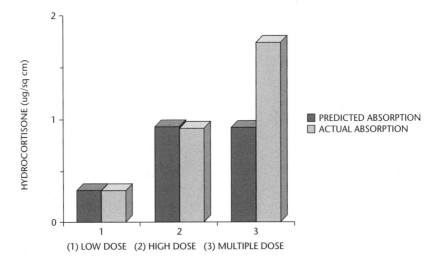

Figure 6.3: Hydrocortisone *in vivo* percutaneous absorption in human with cream vehicle and single and multiple dosing. The multiple dosing (triple therapy) exceeded predicted absorption and was statistically (*p* < .006) greater than the single high dose.

will varying conditions affect absorption (sweat or rainfall "activating" the absorption system as suggested by increased vehicle situation)?

6.5 MULTIPLE DOSING: AZONE SELF-ENHANCED PERCUTANEOUS ABSORPTION

Azone (1-dodecylazacycloheptan-2-one) is an agent that has been shown to enhance percutaneous absorption of drugs. Azone is thought to act by partitioning into skin lipid bilayers and thereby disrupting the structure. An open-label study was done with 9 volunteers (2 males, 7 females; aged 51–76 yr) in which Azone cream (1.6 percent; 100 mg) was topically dosed on a 5 × 10 cm area of the ventral forearm for 21 consecutive days. On d 1, 8, and 15, the Azone cream contained 47 µCi of [^{14}C]Azone. The skin application site was washed with soap and water after each 24-h dosing. Percutaneous absorption was determined by urinary radioactivity excretion. The [^{14}C]Azone was ring labeled [^{14}C]-2-cycloheptan. Radiochemical purity was >98.6 percent and cold Azone purity was 99 percent. Percutaneous absorption of the first dose (d 1) was 1.84 ± 1.56 percent (SD) of applied amount for 24-h skin application time. Day 8 percutaneous absorption, after repeated application, increased significantly ($p < .002$) to 2.76 ± 1.91 percent. Day 15 percutaneous absorption after continued repeated application stayed the same at 2.72 ± 1.21 percent. In humans, repeated application of Azone results in an initial self-absorption enhancement, probably due to its mechanism of action. However, steady-state percutaneous absorption of Azone is established after this initial change. Thus, Azone can enhance its own absorption as well as that of other compounds (Figure 6.4) (Wester *et al.*, 1993b).

6.6 INDIVIDUAL VARIATION: *IN VITRO* HUMAN SKIN

It is well understood that chemical trials are designed with multiple volunteers to account for individual subject variation. This extends to *in vivo* percutaneous absorption where individual subject variability has been demonstrated (Wester and Maibach, 1985). This subject variation also extends to *in vitro* human skin samples (Wester and Maibach, 1991). Table 6.7 shows the *in vitro* percutaneous absorption of vitamin E acetate through human skin *in vitro*. Percent doses

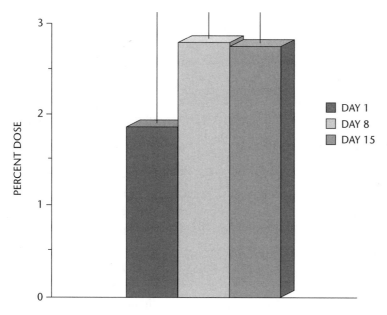

Figure 6.4: Azone *in vivo* in humans is able to enhance its own percutaneous absorption (d 1–8) until steady-state absorption is reached (d 1–15).

TABLE 6.7:

In vitro percutaneous absorption of vitamin E acetate into and through human skin

	Percent dose absorbed		
	Receptor fluid	Skin content	Surface wash
	Formula A		
Skin source			
1	0.34	0.55	74.9
2	0.39	0.66	75.6
3	0.47	4.08	89.1
4	1.30	0.96	110.0
Mean ± SD	0.63 ± 0.45[a]	1.56 ± 1.69[b]	87.4 ± 16.4
	Formula B		
Skin source			
1	0.24	0.38	—
2	0.40	0.64	107.1
3	0.41	4.80	98.1
4	2.09	1.16	106.2
Mean ± SD	0.78 ± 0.87[a]	1.74 ± 2.06[b]	103.8 ± 5.0

[a]$p = .53$ (Nonsignificant; paired *t*-test).
[b]$p = .42$ (Nonsignificant; paired *t*-test).

absorbed for two formulations, A and B, are shown for 24-h receptor fluid accumulation and for skin content (skin digested and assayed at 24-h time point). Assay of skin surface soap and water wash at the end of the 24-h period gives dose accountability.

The two formulations were the same except for slight variation in pH. Statistically ,there was no difference in absorption between the two formulations. However, a careful examination of the individual values in Table 6.7 shows consistency within individuals. Analysis of variance (ANOVA) for individual variation showed statistical significance for receptor fluid ($p = .02$) and skin content ($p = .000$) (Figure 6.5); therefore, when comparing treatments for *in vitro* percutaneous absorption, it is recommended that each treatment be a part of each skin source. Table 6.8 outlines a study based upon this.

6.7 MODELS: *IN VITRO* AND *IN VIVO*

Models are substitutes, and in the case of percutaneous absorption, the model substitutes for *in vivo* percutaneous absorption in humans. Models need to be validated, as shown for the rhesus monkey in Table 6.9. A popular substitute

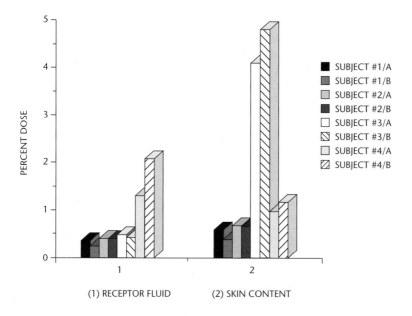

Figure 6.5: *In vitro* percutaneous absorption of vitamin E acetate in human skin. Note that individual variation is consistent between formulations A and B.

TABLE 6.8:

Study design for *in vitro* percutaneous absorption

Human skin source	Treatments					
	A	B	C	D	E	F
1	X	X	X	X	X	X
2	X	X	X	X	X	X
3	X	X	X	X	X	X
4	X	X	X	X	X	X

Note: A-F can be separate treatment, or replicates of treatments. If necessary or desired, human skin sources can be extended beyond 4.

for humans *in vivo* is the use of human skin *in vitro*. Table 6.10 gives the *in vitro* percutaneous absorption of several chemicals, expressed as percent dose accumulated in receptor fluid for 24 h, and the skin chemical content at that time frame. For DDT, benzo[a]pyrene, chlordane, pentachlorophenol, and polychlorinated biphenyls (PCBs), there is negligible receptor fluid accumulation (Wester *et al.*, 1990, 1992a, 1993b, 1993d). A basic rule on *in vitro* percutaneous absorption is that solubility of chemical in receptor fluid not be

TABLE 6.9:

In vivo percutaneous absorption in rhesus monkey and human
(% dose absorbed)

Compound	Rhesus monkey	Human
2,4-Dinitrochlorobenzene	52 ± 4	54 ± 6
Nitrobenzene	4 ± 1	2 ± 1
Cortisone	5 ± 3	3 ± 2
Testosterone	18 ± 10	13 ± 3
Hydrocortisone	3 ± 1	2 ± 2
Benzoic acid	60 ± 8	43 ± 16
Diethyl maleate	68 ± 7	54 ± 7
DDT	19 ± 9	10 ± 4
Retinoic acid	2 ± 1	1 ± 0.2
2, 4-D	9 ± 2	6 ± 2

Note: These are data collected over the years from many laboratories. The rhesus monkey is a good animal model to predict potential percutaneous absorption in humans.

TABLE 6.10:

In vitro versus *in vivo* percutaneous absorption

Contpound	Vehicle	Percent dose		*In vivo*
		In vitro		
		Skin	Receptor fluid	
DDT	Acetone	18.1 ± 13.4	0.08 ± 0.02	18.9 ± 9.4
Benzo[a]pyrene	Acetone	23.7 ± 9.7	0.09 ± 0.06	51.0 ± 22.0
Chlordane	Acetone	10.8 ± 8.2	0.07 ± 0.06	6.0 ± 2.8
Pentachlorophenol	Acetone	3.7 ± 1.7	0.6 ± 0.09	29.2 ± 5.8
PCBs (1242)	Acetone	—[a]	—[a]	21.4 ± 8.5
	TCB	—[a]	—[a]	18.0 ± 3.8
	Mineral oil	10.0 ± 16.5	0.1 ± 0.07	20.8 ± 8.5
PCBs (1254)	Acetone	—[a]	—[a]	—[a]
	TCB	—[a]	—[a]	14.6 ± 3.6
	Mineral oil	6.4 ± 6.3	0.3 ± 0.6	20.8 ± 8.3
2,4-D	Acetone	—[a]	—[a]	8.6 ± 2.1
Arsenic	Water	1.0 ± 1.0	0.9 ± 1.1	2.0 ± 1.2
Cadmium	Water	6.7 ± 4.8	0.4 ± 0.2	—[a]
Mercury	Water	28.5 ± 6.3	0.07 ± 0.01	—[a]

[a]Study was not done.

the limiting step. Table 6.11 shows that these chemicals have high log *P* values. For example, a log *P* of 6.91 (DDT) means that when DDT is introduced into an equal amount of octanol and water, 6,910,000 molecules will end up in the octanol and 1 molecule will be in the water. The stratum corneum is lipophilic,

TABLE 6.11:
Octanol/water partition coefficients of compounds

Compound	log P
DDT	6.91
Benzo[a]pyrene	5.97
Chlordane	5.58
Pentachlorophenol	5.12
2,4-D	· 2.81
PCBs mixture	4.80
Aroclor 1242	
Aroclor 1254	(high log P)

so there is a tendency for chemicals to stay in skin and not partition into water-based receptor fluid. In Table 6.10 the skin content of chemical is better than that of receptor fluid, and somewhat predictive of *in vivo* absorption, but not in all cases (pentachlorophenol, PCBs) (Wester *et al.*, 1990, 1992a, 1992b, 1993a, 1993b, 1993d).

6.8 PERCUTANEOUS ABSORPTION FROM CHEMICALS IN CLOTHING

Chemicals in cloth cause cutaneous effects. For example, Hatch and Maibach (1986) reported that chemicals added to cloth in 10 finish categories (dye, wrinkle resistance, water repellancy, soil release, and so on) caused irritant and allergic contact dermatitis, atopic dermatitis exacerbation, and urticarial and phototoxic skin responses. This is qualitative information that chemicals will transfer from cloth to skin *in vivo* in humans. Quantitative data are lacking. Snodgrass (1992) studied permethrin transfer from treated cloth to rabbit skin *in vivo*. Transfer was quantitative but less than expected. Interestingly, permethrin remained within the cloth after detergent laundering.

In other studies (Quan *et al.*, 1994), *in vitro* percutaneous absorption of glyphosate and malathion through human skin were decreased when added to cloth (the cloth then placed on the skin) and this absorption decreased as time passed over 48 h (Table 6.12). It is assumed that with time the chemical will sequester into deep empty spaces of the fabric, (or some type of bonding is established between chemical and fabric. When water was added to glyphosate/cloth and water/ethanol to malathion/cloth, the percutaneous absorption increased (malathion to levels from solution). This perhaps reflects clinical

TABLE 6.12:

In vitro percutaneous absorption of glyphosate and malathion from cloth through human skin

Chemical	Donor conditions	Treatment	Percent dose absorbed
Glyphosate	1% Solution (water)	None	1.42 ± 0.25
	1% Solution on cloth	0 h	0.74 ± 0.26
	1% Solution on cloth	24 h	0.08 ± 0.01
	1% Solution on cloth	48 h	0.08 ± 0.01
	1% Solution on cloth	Add water	0.36 ± 0.07
Malathion	1% Solution (water/ethanol)	None	8.77 ± 1.43
	1% Solution on cloth	0 h	3.92 ± 0.49
	1% Solution on cloth	24 h	0.62 ± 0.11
	1% Solution on cloth	48 h	0.60 ± 0.14
	1% Solution on cloth	Add water/ethanol	7.34 ± 0.61

Note: Both glyphosate and malathion in solution (treatment = none) are absorbed through human skin. Glyphosate and malathion on cotton cloth show some absorption into skin, depending upon time chemical was added to cloth treatment = 0 h, 24 h, 48 h). When the cloth was wetted (treatment = add water or add water/ethanol), the transfer of glyphosate and malathion from cloth to human akin was increased. This suggests that sweating, skin oil, or even rain may facilitate transfer of chemicals from cloth to skin.

situations where dermatitis occurs most frequently to human sweating areas (axilla, crotch).

6.9 HUMAN *IN VIVO* PERCUTANEOUS ABSORPTION

6.9.1 Diazinon

Diazinon is an organophosphorus insecticide that, through general use, comes into contact with human skin. To investigate its percutaneous absorption, human volunteers were exposed for 24 h to ^{14}C-labeled diazinon applied in acetone solution (2 µg/cm^2) to the forearm or abdomen, or in lanolin wool grease (1.47 µg/cm^2) to the abdomen (Table 6.13). Complete void urine samples were collected daily for 7 d. Percutaneous absorption ranged from 2.87 ± 1.16 percent (mean ± SD, $n = 6$) to 3.85 ± 2.16 percent of the applied amount, and there were no statistically significant differences with regard to site or vehicle of application. In rhesus monkeys, over the 7 d after iv dosing (2.1 µCi [^{14}C]diazinon, 31.8 µg), a total of 55.8 ± 68 percent ($n = 4$) of the dose was excreted in the urine, and 22.6 ± 5.2 percent was eliminated in the feces (78.4

TABLE 6.13:

Percutaneous absorption of diazinon in humans

Skin site	Vehicle	Percutaneous absorption (% of dose)[a]
Forearm	Acetone	3.85 ± 2.16
Abdomen	Acetone	3.24 ± 1.94
Abdomen	Lanolin	2.87 ± 1.16

[a]Mean ± SD for six volunteers per group, calculated from human urinary ^{14}C disposition corrected for incomplete/other route excretion with the monkey urinary disposition after iv dosing.

percent total accountability). In *in vitro* percutaneous absorption studies with human abdominal skin, 14.1 ± 9.2 percent of the applied dose accumulated in the receptor fluid over 24 h of exposure to 0.25 µg/cm^2 (acetone vehicle). The calculated mass absorbed was the same (0.035 µg/cm^2) for both *in vitro* and *in vivo* absorption through human skin (Wester *et al.*, 1993c).

6.9.2 Pyrethrin and Piperonyl Butoxide

In order to determine the human *in vivo* percutaneous absorption, a commercial formulation containing either [^{14}C]pyrethrin (3.8 mCi/mmol) or [^{14}C]piperonyl butoxide (3.4 mCi/mmol) was applied to the ventral forearm of six human volunteers (Table 6.14). The formulation contained 0.3 percent pyrethrin or 3.0 percent piperonyl butoxide. Spreadability studies showed that concentrations

TABLE 6.14:

Percutaneous absorption of pyrethrin and piperonyl butoxide from human forearm and calculated from human scalp

Subject	Dose absorbed (%)				
	Pyrethrin		Piperonyl butoxide	
	Forearm	Scalp[a]	Forearm	Scalp[a]
1	1.4	5.6	2.8	1.2
2	1.6	6.4	1.8	7.2
3	2.0	8.0	2.8	11.2
4	0.6	2.4	1.8	7.2
5	1.6	6.4	1.4	5.6
6	4.1	16.4	1.8	7.2
Mean ± SD	1.9 ± 1.2	7.5 ± 4.7	2.1 ± 0.6	8.3 ± 2.4

[a] Scalp is assumed to have four-fold absorption greater than forearm.

of 5.5 µg pyrethrin/cm^2 and 75.8 µg piperonyl butoxide/cm^2 (used in this study) would be consistent with levels found in actual use. The forearms were thoroughly cleansed with soap and water 30 min after application (as recommended for actual use). Percutaneous absorption was determined by urinary cumulative excretion following dose application. With a 7-d urinary accumulation, 1.9 ± 1.2 percent (SD) of the dose of pyrethrin and 2.1 ± 0.6 percent of the piperonyl butoxide applied was absorbed through the forearm skin. One hour after application, blood samples contained no detectable radioactivity. The percutaneous absorption of pyrethrin and piperonyl butoxide from the scalp was calculated to be 7.5 percent of the applied dose for pyrethrin and 8.3 percent for piperonyl butoxide. The calculated half-life of ^{14}C excretion was 50 h for pyrethrin and 32 h for piperonyl butoxide. The data should be of relevance to risk assessment where extrapolating animal data to humans (Wester *et at.*, 1994b).

6.9.3   Isofenphos

Studies were done to determine the percutaneous absorption of isofenphos in human volunteers from whom informed consent had been obtained. *In vivo* absorption in humans was 3.6 ± 3.6 percent of applied dose for 24-h exposure and 3.6 ± 0.5 percent for 72-h exposure (Table 6.15). Skin wash recovery data showed that isofenphos evaporates from *in vivo* skin during the absorption process; the surface dose is minimal (<1 percent) by 24 h. Skin stripping showed no residual isofenphos in stratum corneum. This explains the similar absorption for 24- and 72-h prewash exposures. Skin surface recovery *in vivo* with soap and water was 61.4 ± 10.4 percent for the first dosing time (15 min). Time-recovery response declined with time to 0.5 ± 0.2 percent at 24h. *In vitro* absorption

TABLE 16.15:

In vivo percutaneous absorption of isofenphos in humans

| Subject | Percentage dose absorbed[a] | |
	24-h Exposure	72-h Exposure
1	1.18	4.12
2	1.93	3.86
3	2.47	3.01
4	8.94	3.56
Mean ± SD	3.63 ± 3.58	3.64 ± 0.48

[a]Percentage dose absorbed = [(urinary ^{14}C excretion for topical/urinary ^{14}C excretion for iv)] × 100.

TABLE 6.16:

In vitro percutaneous absorption of isofenphos with human skin

Human plasma receptor fluid	Average percentage applied dose[a]		
	Skin	Surface wash	Total
2.5 ± 2.0	6.5 ± 2.4	79.7 ± 2.2	88.7 ± 4.6

[a]Means ± standard deviation for four replicates.

utilizing flow-through diffusion methodology with human cadaver skin and human plasma receptor fluid gave 2.5 ± 2.0 percent dose absorbed, an amount similar to *in vivo* studies (Table 6.16). An additional 6.5 ± 24 percent was recovered in the skin samples (total of 9 percent). Skin surface wash at 24 h recovered 79.7 ± 2.2 percent and skin content was 6.5 ± 2.4 percent (total dose accountability of 88.7 ± 4.6 percent). Thus, isofenphos was available for absorption during the whole dosing period. Neither *in vitro* absorption nor *in vitro* evaporation studies predicted the potential skin evaporation of isofenphos. Published dermal studies in the rat had predicted isofenphos absorption at 47 percent of applied dose (12-fold greater than actual in humans). Subsequent toxicokinetic modeling predicted possible concern with the use of isofenphos. This is an example where the choice of the rat produced a nonrelevant absorption prediction. *In vivo* studies in human volunteers seem more relevant for predicting percutaneous absorption in humans (Wester *et al.*, 1992c).

6.10 DISCUSSION

This chapter provides examples and discussion of information relating to relevance and validation of percutaneous absorption for risk assessment. The assessment of short-term exposure may be missed with some conventional calculations of percutaneous absorption such as conventional flux value (or modeled flux value) and lag time. *In vivo*, a chemical can rapidly partition into skin during a bath or swim (time period on the order of an hour or less). Interpretation of an artificial (due to *in vitro* diffusion system) lag time may eliminate that rapid uptake. Or a conventional flux rate, where linearity over time is scaled back to 30 min of exposure, may underestimate the actual exposure.

The other points raised in this chapter concern multiple exposures and absorption from nonformulated media (e.g., cloth/fabric). The question to be asked is, does the study design used to produce the (percutaneous absorption)

■ CHAPTER 6 ■

data reflect the problem/risk assessment that is being investigated? A firmer understanding of these specific issues is needed, as well as more substantive methods of designing and interpreting clinically relevant situtations.

6.10 REFERENCES

BUCKS, D.A.W., MAIBACH, H.I., and GUY, R.H. (1985) Percutaneous absorption of steroids: Effect of repeated applications. *J. Pharm. Sci.* **74**, 1337.

HATCH. K.L., and MAIBACH, H.I. (1986) Textile chemical finish dermatitis. *Contact Dermatitis* **14**, 1–13.

MELENDRES, J.L., BUCKS, D.A.W., CAMEL, E., WESTER, R.C., and MAIBACH, H.I., (1992) *In vivo* percutaneous absorption of hydrocortisone: Multiple-application dosing in man. *Pharm. Res.* **9**, 1164.

QUAN, D, MAIBACH, H.I., WESTER, R.C. (1994) *In vitro* percutaneous absorption of glyphosate and malathion across cotton sheets into human skin. *Toxicologist* **14**, 107.

SNODGRASS, H.L. (1992) Permethrin transfer from treated cloth to the skin surface: Potential for exposure in humans. *J. Toxicol. Environ. Health* **35**, 912–915.

WESTER, R.C., and MAIBACH, H.I. (1984) Advances in percutaneous absorption. In DRILL, V. and LAZAR, P. (eds), *Cutaneous Toxicity*, New York: Raven Press, 29–40.

WESTER, R.C., and MAIBACH, H.I. (1985) Dermatopharmacokinetics in clinical dermatology. In BRANOUGH, R. and MAIBACH, H.I. (eds), *Percutaneous Absorption*, New York: Marcel Dekker, 125–132.

WESTER, R.C., and MAIBACH, H.I. (1991) Individual and regional variation with *in vitro* percutaneous absorption. In BRONAUGH, R. and MAIBACH, H. (eds), *In Vitro Percutaneous Absorption*, Boca Raton, FL: CRC Press, 25–30.

WESTER, R.C., NOONAN, P.K., and MAIBACH, H.I. (1977) Frequency of application on percutaneous absorption of hydrocortisone. *Arch. Dermatol.* **113**, 620–622.

WESTER, R.C., NOONAN, P.K. and MAIBACH, H.I. (1980) Percutaneous absorption of hydrocortisone increases significantly with long-term administration: *In vivo* studies in Rhesus monkey. *Arch Dermatol.* **116**, 186–188.

WESTER, R.C., MAIBACH, H.I., BUCKS, D.A.W., SEDIK. L., MELENDRES, J., LIAO C., and DIZIO, S. (1990) Percutaneous absorption of [^{14}C] DDT and [^{14}C] benzo[a]pyrene from soil. *Fundam. Appl. Toxicol.* **15**, 510–516.

WESTER, R.C., MAIBACH, H.I., SEDIK, L., MELENDRES, J., LIAO, C.L., and DiZIO, S. (1992a) Percutaneous absorption of [^{14}C]chlordane from soil. *Toxicol. Environ. Health.* **35**, 269–277.

WESTER, R.C., MAIBACH. H.I., SEDIK, L., MELENDRES, J., DiZIO. S., and WADE, M. (1992b) *In Vitro* percutaneous absorption of cadmium from water and soil into human skin. *Fundam. Appl. Toxicol.* **19**, 1–5.

WESTER, R.C., MAIBACH. H.I., MELENDRES, J.L., SEDIK. L., KNAAK, J., and WANG, R. (1992c) *In vivo* and *in vitro* percutaneous absorption and skin evaporation of isofenphos in man. *Fundam. Appl. Toxicol.* **19**, 521–526.

WESTER, R.C., MAIBACH, H.I., SEDIK, L., MELENDRES, J., WADE, M., and DiZIO, S. (1993a) *In vitro* a percutaneous absorption of pentachlorophenol from soil. *Fundam. Appl. Toxicol.* **19**, 68–71.

WESTER, R.C., MAIBACH, H.I., SEDIK, L., MELENDRES, J., and Wade, M. (1993b) *In vivo* and *in vitro* percutaneous absorption and skin decontamination of arsenic from water and soil. *Fundam. Appl. Toxicol.* **20**, 336–340.

WESTER, R.C., MAIBACH, H.I., SEDIK, L., MELENDRES, J., and RUSSELL, I. (1993c) Absorption of diazinon in man. *Food Chem. Toxicol.* **31**, 569–572.

WESTER, R.C., MAIBACH, H.I., SEDIK, L., MELENDRES, J., and Wade, M. (1993d) Percutaneous absorption of PCBs from soil: *in vivo* rhesus monkey, *in vitro* human skin, and binding to powdered human stratum corneum. *J. Toxicol. Environ. Health* **39**, 375–382.

WESTER, R.C., MELENDRES, J., SEDIK, L., and MAIBACH, H.I. (1994a) Percutaneous absorption of azone following single and multiple doses to human volunteers. *J. Pharm. Sci.* **83**, 124–25.

WESTER, R.C., BUCKS, D.A.W., and MAIBACH, H.I. (1994b) Human *in vivo* percutaneous absorption of pyrethrin and piperonyl butoxide. *Food Chem. Toxicol.* **32**, 51–53.

CHAPTER 6

Chemical Partitioning into Powdered Human Stratum Corneum

A Useful *In Vitro* Model for Studying Interaction of Chemical and Human Skin

XIAOYING HUI, RONALD C WESTER, HONGBO ZHAI, AND HOWARD I MAIBACH

Contents

7.1 Introduction

7.2 PHSC and physical–chemical properties of stratum corneum

7.3 PHSC and chemical partitioning

7.4 PHSC and percutaneous absorption

7.5 PHSC and the skin barrier function

7.6 PHSC and diseased skin

7.7 PHSC and environmentally hazardous chemicals

7.8 PHSC and chemical decontamination

7.9 PHSC and enhanced topical formulation

7.10 PHSC and QSAR predictive modeling

7.11 Discussion

7.1 INTRODUCTION

Chemical delivery/absorption into and through the skin is important in both dermato-pharmacology and dermato-toxicology. The human stratum corneum is the first layer of the skin, and constitutes a rate-limiting barrier to the transport of most chemicals across the skin (Blank, 1965). Chemicals must first partition into the stratum corneum before entering the deeper layers of the skin, the epidermis and the dermis, to reach the vascular system. Chemical partitioning proceeds much faster than complete diffusion through the whole stratum corneum, and the process quickly reaches equilibrium (Scheuplein and Bronaugh, 1985). In addition to binding within the stratum corneum, a chemical can also be retained within the stratum corneum as a reservoir (Zatz, 1993). Thus, understanding the process of chemical partitioning into the stratum corneum becomes important in developing an insight into its barrier properties and transport mechanisms.

Human stratum corneum has been used for decades as an *in vitro* model to explore both percutaneous absorption and the risks associated with dermal exposure (Surber *et al.*, 1990a; Potts and Guy, 1992). The human stratum corneum includes the horny pads of palms and soles (callus), and the membranous stratum corneum covering the remainder of the body (Barry, 1983). The traditional method of preparation is via physical–chemical and enzymological processes to separate the membranous layers of the stratum corneum from whole skin (Juhlin and Shelly, 1977; Knufson *et al.*, 1985). However, it is time consuming and, in some cases, it is difficult to control the size and thickness of a sheet of stratum corneum. Moreover, it is often difficult to locate a suitable skin source.

Powdered human stratum corneum (PHSC) prepared from callus (sole) is thus substituted for the intact membranous stratum corneum. Podiatrists routinely remove and discard PHSC from the human foot, so it is easily obtained. The callus can be cut easily and quickly into smaller pieces, and ground with dry ice to form a powder. In our laboratory, PHSC particle sizes between 180 μm to 300 μm were selected with the aid of a suitable sieve. Because a corneocyte is only about 0.5 μm thick and about 30 μm to 40 μm long, the selected PHSC contains both intact corneocytes and intercellular medium structures, and thus retains its original physical-biochemical properties. More-over, the greater surface area of the PHSC enhances solute penetration. In a typical experimental procedure, a test chemical in a transport vehicle—water— is mixed with the PHSC, and the mixture is incubated. After a pre-determined

CHAPTER 7

time period, a solution is separated from the PHSC by centrifugation, and samples are measured (Hui *et al.*, 2000).

This chapter reviews powdered human stratum corneum as an *in vitro* model for studying chemical interaction with human skin, with reference to studies conducted in our laboratory over recent decades. The results demonstrate that powdered human stratum corneum (callus) offers an experimentally easy *in vitro* model for the determination of chemical partitioning into the SC and may be useful in many skin research areas.

7.2 PHSC AND PHYSICAL-CHEMICAL PROPERTIES OF STRATUM CORNEUM

The callus is derived from human stratum corneum, and thus should retain some of its physical and chemical characteristics (Wester *et al.*, 1987). Stratum corneum lipid plays an important role in the determination of skin functions. However, the average lipid content of the SC varies regionally, from 2.0, 4.3, 6.5, to 7.2 weight percent of dry stratum corneum from plantar, leg, abdomen and face, respectively (Lampe *et al.*, 1983). Table 7.1 shows that the average lipid content of the dry PHSC samples derived from various regions was 2.29 ± 0.25 weight percent after extraction. This result is consistent with that in human plantar as determined by Lampe *et al.* (1983).

TABLE 7.1:

Lipid content and water uptake of powdered human stratum corneum

Stratum corneum source	Lipid content (% w/w dry PHSC)	Water uptake (µg/mg dry PHSC)			
		Untreated PHSC	Delipidized PHSC		
			Lipid[a]	Protein[b]	Total
1	2.38	495.85	26.44	452.40	478.84
2	2.21	452.49	39.26	364.96	404.22
3	2.39	585.62	23.09	498.40	521.49
4	2.69	554.27	40.05	492.31	532.36
5	2.08	490.04	49.86	363.30	413.16
6	2.01	381.61	14.82	324.18	339.00
Mean	2.29	493.31	32.26	415.92	448.18
SD	0.25	72.66	12.97	74.50	75.47

a: Lipid part extracted from the PHSC.
b: Rest part of the PHSC after lipid extraction.

The water content of the SC is of importance in maintaining stratum corneum flexibility. Three possible mechanisms of water absorption and/or retention capacity of the SC have been suggested: (i) Imokawa *et al.* (1986) suggested that stratum corneum lipids play a critical role because their removal by the application of acetone/ether decreased absorption/retention capacity. (ii) Friberg *et al.* (1992), however, considered that protein might also play an important role in stratum corneum water retention. They found that the additional water absorbed after re-aggregation of equilibrated lipids and proteins was equally partitioned between the protein and the natural lipid fraction of the human stratum corneum. (iii) Middleton (1968) considered that water-soluble substances were responsible for water retention and for most of the extensibility of the corneum. He found that powdered stratum corneum—but not the intact corneum extracted by water—exhibited lower water retention capacity. He suggested that the powdering procedure ruptures the walls of the corneum cells and allows water to extract the water-soluble substances without a prior solvent extraction. We measured the water retention capacities of untreated PHSC, delipidized PHSC (as the protein fraction), and the lipid content, by measuring the amount of [3H]-water (μg equivalent) per mg PHSC after equilibration. As shown in Table 7.1, no statistical differences ($p > 0.05$) were observed for untreated PHSC, delipidized PHSC, and the combination of delipidized PHSC and the lipid content. The PHSC can absorb up to 49 percent by weight of dry untreated PHSC (Table 7.1), which is consistent with literature reports. Middleton (1968) found that the amount of water bound to intact, small pieces and powdered Guinea-pig footpad stratum corneum was 40 percent, 40 percent, and 43 percent of dry corneum weight. Leveque and Rasseneur (1988) demonstrated that the human stratum corneum was able to absorb water up to 50 percent of its dry weight. Our results (Table 7.1) suggest that the protein domain of the PHSC plays an important role in the absorption of water. Depletion of the PHSC lipid content did not affect water retention (Hui *et al.*, 1975, 2000).

7.3 PHSC AND CHEMICAL PARTITIONING

Table 7.2 shows the effect of varying initial chemical concentrations on the PC PHSC/w of these compounds (Hui *et al.*, 1993). Under fixed experimental conditions—2 hours' incubation time and 350°C incubation temperature—the concentration required to attain a peak value of the partition coefficient varied from chemical to chemical. After reaching the maximum, increases in the

CHAPTER 7

TABLE 7.2:

Effect of initial aqueous phase chemical concentration on powdered human callus/water partition coefficient

Chemical[b] (log $PC_{o/w}$)	Concentration (%, w/v)	Partition coefficient[a] (Mean)	(S.D.)
Dopamine	0.23	5.42	0.22
(−3.40)	0.46	6.04	0.28
	0.92	5.74	0.28
Glycine	0.05	0.36	0.01
(−3.20)	0.10	0.40	0.02
Urea	0.03	0.26	0.02
(-2.11)	0.06	0.15	0.02
	0.12	0.17	0.02
Glyphosate	0.02	0.79	0.04
(−1.70)	0.04	0.68	0.04
	0.08	0.70	0.01
Theophylline	0.18	0.37	0.02
(−0.76)	0.36	0.43	0.03
	0.54	0.42	0.02
Aminopyrine	0.07	0.44	0.09
(0.84)	0.14	0.46	0.03
Hydrocortisone	0.09	0.37	0.01
(1.61)	0.18	0.34	0.01
	0.36	0.29	0.02
Malathion	0.47	0.50	0.09
(2.36)	0.94	0.40	0.03
	1.88	0.53	0.04
Atrazine	0.09	0.53	0.06
(2.75)	0.14	0.59	0.07
	0.19	0.58	0.03
2,4-D	0.27	7.52	0.81
(2.81)	0.54	7.53	1.01
	0.82	8.39	1.67
Alachlor	0.32	1.11	0.05
(3.52)	0.64	1.08	0.04
	1.28	1.96	0.15
PCB	0.04	1237.61	145.52
(6.40)	0.08	1325.44	167.03
	0.16	1442.72	181.40

a: PC PHSC/water represent the mean of each test ($n = 5$) +/- S.D (Hui *et al.*, 1993).
b: Log PC (O/w) was cited Hansch and Leo (1979).

chemical concentration in the vehicle did not increase the PC value; rather, it slightly decreased or was maintained at approximately the same level. This is consistent with the results of Surber *et al.* (1990 a, b) on whole stratum corneum. Chemical partitioning from the vehicle into the SC involves processes in which molecular binding occurs at certain sites of the SC, as well as simple partitioning. Equilibration of partitioning is largely dependent on the saturation of the chemical binding sites of the SC (Surber *et al.*, 1990a; Rieger, 1993). The results also indicate that, under a given experimental conditions, the maximum degree of partitioning was compound specific. As the SC contains protein, lipids, and various lower molecular weight substances with widely differing properties, the many available binding sites display different selective affinities with each chemical. Thus, the degree of maximum binding or of equilibration varies naturally with molecular structure (Rieger, 1993). This result demonstrated that the solubility limit of a compound in the SC was important in determining the degree of partitioning, as suggested by Potts and Guy (1992). On the basis of the solubility limit of a chemical, the absorption process of water soluble or lipid soluble substances was controlled by the protein domain or the lipid domain, respectively or a combination of two (Raykar *et al.*, 1988). Since the lipophilicity of the lipid domain in the SC is much higher than that of water, a lipophilic compound would partition into the SC in preference to water. Thus, when water is employed as the vehicle, the PC PHSC/w increases with increasing lipophilicity of solute (Scheuplein and Bronaugh, 1983). Conversely, the protein domain of the SC is significantly more polar than octanol and governs the absorption of hydrophilic chemicals (Raykar *et al.*, 1988). For very lipophilic compounds, low solubility in water rather than increased solubility in the SC can be an important factor (Scheuplein and Bronaugh, 1983). Moreover, in addition to partitioning into these two domains, some amount of chemicals may be taken into the SC as the result of water hydration. This is the "sponge domain", named by Raykar *et al.* (1988). They assume that this water, having the properties of bulk water, carries an amount of solute into the SC equal to the amount of solute in the same volume of bathing solution. Therefore, for hydrophilic compounds and some lower lipophilic compounds, the partitioning process may include both the protein domain and sponge domain.

7.4 PHSC AND PERCUTANEOUS ABSORPTION

To evaluate sensitivity of this in the *in vitro* PHSC model, we examined chemical partitioning into the PHSC as well as that *in vitro* percutaneous absorption in

TABLE 7.3:

In vivo percutaneous absorption of *p*-nitroaniline in the rhesus monkey following 30-minute exposure to surface water: comparisons to *in vitro* binding and absorption

Phenomenon	Percent dose absorbed/bound[a]
In vivo percutaneous absorption, rhesus monkey	4.1 ± 2.3
In vitro percutaneous absorption, human skin	5.2 ± 1.6
In vitro binding, powdered human stratum corneum	2.5 ± 1.1

a: Each number represents the mean ± S.D. of four samples.

human skin, and *in vivo* percutaneous absorption in the Rhesus monkey. Table 7.3 shows that the *in vivo* percutaneous absorption of nitroaniline from surface water following 30-min exposure was 4.1 ± 2.3 percent of the applied dose. This is comparable with the 5.2 ± 1.6 percent for *in vitro* absorption with human cadaver skin and the 2.5 ± 1.1 percent bound to PHSC. Wester *et al.* (1987) suggest that this methodology—the systems tested, binding to PHSC, and *in vitro* and *in vivo* absorption—can be used to predict the burden on the human body imposed by bathing or swimming.

7.5 PHSC AND THE SKIN BARRIER FUNCTION

The barrier function of the stratum corneum is attributed to its multilayered wall-like structure, in which terminally differentiated keratin-rich epidermal cells (corneocytes) are embedded in an intercellular lipid-rich matrix. Any physical factor or chemical reagent that interacts with this two-compartment structure can affect the skin barrier function. Barry (1983) described how certain compounds and mechanical trauma can easily dissociate callus cells and readily dissolve their membranes. Thus the amount of protein (keratin) released from the stratum corneum after chemical exposure may be a measure of the solvent potential of the chemical. To evaluate this hypothesis, a test chemical in water is mixed with PHSC and incubated. After a pre-determined time period, a solution is separated from the PHSC by centrifugation. The protein (keratin) content of the solution is then measured. Table 7.4 shows the amount of protein released from the PHSC after incubation with glycolic acid, sodium hydroxide, or water alone, at different time points. Sodium hydroxide has a pronounced ability to release protein from PHSC. This ability increases with increasing

TABLE 7.4:

Protein releasing from PHSC following chemical/water exposure

Test chemicals	Protein content (mg/4 ml)[a]		
	10 min	40 min	24 hr
Glycolic acid	0.093	0.175	0.173
	(0.026)	(0.029)	(0.041)
Sodium hydroxide	0.419	0.739	5.148
	(0.054)	(0.301)	(1.692)
Water	0.002	0.135	0.077
	(0.014)	(0.043)	(0.021)

a: Each number represents the mean (S.D.) of six samples.

incubation time. The results suggest that the PHSC model constitutes a vehicle to probe the barrier nature of the stratum corneum and the chemical interactions with the PHSC.

7.6 PHSC AND DISEASED SKIN

PHSC has potential application in medical treatment. For instance, a set of vehicles can be screened to determine which vehicle most readily releases a given drug into the stratum corneum. This information would assist in the determination of the most effective approaches to drug delivery via the skin. Furthermore, diseases involving the stratum corneum can be studied using PHSC. An example is Table 7.5, the partitioning of hydrocortisone from normal and psoriatic PHSC. In this case, we have shown that there is no difference in partitioning between normal and psoriatic PHSC. It should be noted that there is no difference between *in vivo* percutaneous absorption of hydrocortisone in normal volunteers and that in psoriatic patients (Wester *et al.*, 1983).

7.7 PHSC AND ENVIRONMENTALLY HAZARDOUS CHEMICALS

The leaching of environmentally hazardous chemicals from soil and their absorption by the skin of a human body is a major concern. Knowledge of the extent and degree of such absorption will aid in determining the potential health hazards of polluted soil. Our laboratory's interest is in the potential percutaneous absorption of contaminants from soil. Soil can be readily mixed

TABLE 7.5:

Aqueous partition coefficient of hydrocortisone with normal and psoriatic stratum corneum

Stratum corneum type	Partition coefficient[a]	
	Mean	S.E.
Normal sheet (abdominal)	1.04	0.88
Normal powdered (plantar)	1.70	0.47
Psoriatic	1.94	0.42

a: No statistical significant ($P > 0.05$).

with PHSC, but centrifugation does not separate the two. However, centrifugation readily separates PHSC from any liquid, to varying degrees. Thus, the partition coefficients of various liquids may be determined relative to a common third liquid. These relative partitions can then be compared to those of other compounds and to skin absorption values (Wester *et al.*, 1992, 1993a, b) to evaluate the degree of hazard. We have determined such coefficients for several environmentally hazardous chemicals partitioning from soil into PHSC (Table 7.6).

7.8 PHSC AND CHEMICAL DECONTAMINATION

Our laboratory uses the PHSC model to determine which chemicals might be able to remove (decontaminate) hazardous chemicals from human skin. A contaminant chemical is mixed with PHSC, and the decontaminant effects of a series of possible decontaminants measured. The liquid decontaminant is mixed with contaminated PHSC and, after a pre-determined time period, a solution is separated from the PHSC by centrifugation. The content of the

TABLE 7.6:

Partition coefficients of four environmental hazardous chemicals in PHSC/water and soil/water

Test chemicals	Partition coefficient	
	PHSC	Soil
Arsenic	1.1×10^4	2.4×10^4
Cadmium chloride	3.6×10^1	1.0×10^5
Arodor 1242	2.6	1.7
Arodor 1254	2.9	2.0

TABLE 7.7:

Decontaminants selection to remove environmental hazardous chemical (alachlor) from human skin[a]

	[14C]-Alachlor (% dose)
PHSC	90.3 ± 1.2
Alachlor in Lasso supernatant	5.1 ± 1.2
Water only wash of PHSC	4.6 ± 1.3
10% Soap and water wash	77.2 ± 5.7
50% Soap and water wash	90.0 ± 0.5

a: [14C]-Alachlor in Lasso EC formulation (1:20 dilution) mixed with powdered human stratum corneum, let set for 30 min, then centrifuged. Stratum corneum wash with (1) water only, (2) 10% soap water, and (3) 50% soap and water.

solution is a measure of decontaminant's potential. This is shown in Table 7.7, which demonstrates that alachlor readily contaminates PHSC. Water alone removes only a small portion of the alachlor. However, a 10 percent soap solution removes a larger portion of the alachlor, and 50 percent soap solution removes most of it. Perhaps this is an elegant way to show that soapy water is effective in washing one's hands. However, it does illustrate the use of PHSC to determine the effectiveness of skin decontamination (Scheuplein and Blank. 1973).

7.9 PHSC AND ENHANCED TOPICAL FORMULATION

Macromolecules have attracted interest as potential drug entities, and as modulators to percutaneous delivery systems. Two macromolecular polymers (MW 2081 and 2565) were developed to hold cosmetics and drugs to the skin surface by altering the initial chemical and skin partitioning. The effect of these polymers on the partition coefficient of estradiol with PHSC and water was determined in our laboratory. As shown in Table 7.8, the polymer L had no effect on the estradiol PC between PHSC and water. The polymer H, however, showed a significant increase ($P < 0.01$) in log PC for estradiol concentrations of 2.8 mg/ml and 0.25 mg/ml. This increase was dependent upon the polymer concentration (Wester *et al.*, 2002). The results suggest that the PHSC model can help in the development and selection of enhanced transdermal delivery systems.

TABLE 7.8:

Effect of two polymers (L and H) on the estradiol PC between PHSC and water

Test formulation and Polymer concentration	Log PC PHSC/water (Mean ± SD, $n=5$) Estradiol concentration (µg/ml)		
	2.8	0.028	0.028
Polymer H (Hydrophilic polymer)			
10%	2.31 ± 0.22^a	2.36 ± 0.14^a	2.13 ± 0.07^a
5%	1.93 ± 0.10^b	2.06 ± 0.21^b	1.94 ± 0.06^b
1%	1.71 ± 0.10	1.61 ± 0.19	1.59 ± 0.26
Polymer L (Lipophilic polymer)			
10%	1.74 ± 0.10	1.65 ± 0.07	1.61 ± 0.14
5%	1.70 ± 0.20	1.62 ± 0.17	1.65 ± 0.09
1%	1.59 ± 0.19	1.57 ± 0.15	1.71 ± 0.07
Control (no polymer)	1.62 ± 0.14	1.68 ± 0.11	1.71 ± 0.13

a: Statistically significantly different from control ($P < 0.01$).
b: Statistically significantly different from control ($P < 0.05$).

7.10 PHSC AND QSAR PREDICTIVE MODELING

Many experiments have been conducted to predict chemical partitioning into the stratum corneum *in vitro*. However, most were based on quantitative structure–activity relationships (QSARs) or related chemicals to determine the partitioning process, and few studies focus on structurally unrelated chemicals (13). Since the range of molecular structure and physicochemical properties is very broad, any predictive model must address a broad scope of partitioning behavior.

This study assesses the relationship of a number of chemicals with a broad scope of physicochemical properties in the partitioning mechanism between PHSC and water. Uniqueness and experimental accuracy are added by using PHSC. The experimental approach is designed to determine how the PC PHSC/w is affected by (1) chemical concentration, (2) incubation time, and (3) chemical lipophilicity (or hydrophilicity), and other factors. These parameters are used to develop an *in vitro* model that will aid in the prediction of chemical dermal exposure to hazardous chemicals.

Figure 7.1 describes a smooth, partially curvilinear relationship between the log PC PHSC/w and the log PC o/w of a number of chemicals. The lipophilicities

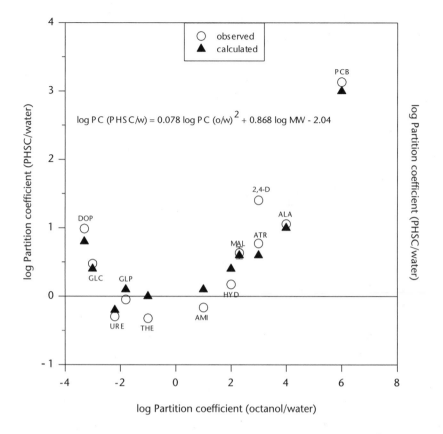

Figure 7.1: Correlation of the logarithm of stratum corneum/water partition coefficients (log PC sc/w) and logarithm of octanol/water partition coefficients of the 12 test chemicals.

Open symbols expressed as observed values and each represented the mean of a test chemical +/- S.D. (*n*=5).

Close symbols expressed as calculated values by Eq. (3). DOP = dopamin; GLC = glycine; URE = urea; GLP = glyphosate; THE = theophylline; AMI = aminopyrine; HYD = hydrocortisone; MAL = malathion; ATR = atrazine; 2,4-D = 2,4-dichlorophenoxyacetic acid; ALA = alachlor; PCB = polychlorinated biphenyls.

and hydrophilicities of compounds were defined as log PC o/w larger or smaller than 0, respectively. For lipophilic chemicals, such as aminopyrine, hydrocortisone, malathion, atrazine, 2,4-D, alachlor, and PCB, the logarithms of PHSC/water partition coefficients are proportional to the logarithms of the octanol/water partition coefficients.

■ CHAPTER 7 ■

■ 117

$$\log PC\ PHSC/w = 0.59 \log PC\ o/w - 0.72 \tag{1}$$

Student T values: 9.93

$n = 7$ $r^2 = 0.95$ $s = 0.26$ $F = 98.61$

For hydrophilic chemicals, such as theophylline, glyphosate, urea, glycine, and dopamine, the log PC PHSC/w values are approximately and inversely proportional to log PC o/w.

$$\log PC\ PHSC/w = -0.60 \log PC\ o/w - 0.27 \tag{2}$$

Student T value: −4.86

$n = 5$ $r^2 = 0.88$ $s = 0.26$ $F = 23.61$

However, the overall relationship of the PC PHSC/w of these chemicals and their PC o/w is non-linear. This non-linear relationship is adequately described by the follow equation:

$$\log PC\ PHSC/w = 0.078 \log PC\ o/w^2 + 0.868 \log MW - 2.04 \tag{3}$$

Student T values: 8.29   2.04

$n = 12$ $r^2 = 0.90$ $s = 0.33$ $F = 42.59$

The logarithm of molecular weight (MW) gave a stronger correlation in this regression than MW ($T = 1.55$) itself. In Figure 7.1, the calculated log PC PHSC/w (Y estimate) values are compared to the corresponding observed values for these chemicals. As shown, the calculated values are acceptably close to the observed values. The correspondence with minimal scatter suggests that this equation would be useful in predicting *in vitro* partitioning in the PHSC for important environmental chemicals (Hui *et al.*, 1993).

7.11   DISCUSSION

A new *in vitro* model employing powdered human stratum corneum (callus) to investigate the interaction between chemicals and human skin has been developed in our laboratory. The powdered human stratum corneum (callus) offers an experimentally easy *in vitro* model for the determination of chemical partitioning from water into the SC. Due to the heterogeneous nature of the SC, the number and affinity of the SC binding sites may vary from chemical to chemical, depending upon molecular structure. For most lipophilic compounds, the PC PHSC/w were governed by the lipid domain, whereas PCs of the more hydrophilic compounds are determined by the protein domain and possibly, by the sponge domain (Raykar *et al.*, 1988). These relationships can be expressed by the log PC PHSC/w of these chemicals as a function of the corresponding square of log PC o/w and log MW (Eq. (3)), which is useful in predicting various chemical partitionings into the SC *in vitro*. However, a disadvantage in using the human callus is that it may display some differences in water and chemical permeation when compared with membranous stratum corneum (Barry, 1983).

This chapter has summarized a variety of potential applications for PHSC, ranging from basic science to applications in medicine and environmental impact studies. PHSC, imagination, and a balanced study design can add to scientific knowledge.

REFERENCES

BARRY, B.W. (1983) Structure, function, diseases, and topical treatment of human skin. In BARRY, B. W. (ed.) *Dermatological Formulations: Percutaneous Absorption*, New York: Marcel Dekker, Inc., 1–48.

BLANK, I.H. (1965) Cutaneous barriers. *J. Invest. Dermatol.* **45**, 249–256.

FRIBERG, S.E., KAYALI, I., SUHERY, T., RHEIN, L.D. and SIMION, F.A. (1992) Water uptake into stratum corneum: partition between lipids and proteins. *J. Dispersion Science and Technology* **13**(3), 337–347.

HANSCH, C. and LEO, A. (eds) (1979) *Substituent Constants for Correlation Analysis in Chemistry and Biology*, New York: John Wiley.

HUI, X., WESTER, R.C., MAIBACH, H.I. and MAGEE, P.S. (1995) Partitioning of chemicals from water into powdered human stratum corneum (cells): a model study. *In Vitro Toxicology* **8**(2), 159–167.

HUI, X., WESTER, R.C., MAIBACH, H.I. and MAGEE, P.S. (2000) Chemical partitioning into powdered human stratum corneum (callus). In MAIBACH, H.I. (ed.) *Toxicology of Skin*. Philadelphia, PA: Taylor & Francis, 159–178.

IMOKAWA, G., AKASAKI, S., HATTORI, M. and YOSHIZUKA, N. (1986) Selective recovery of deranged water-holding properties by stratum corneum lipids. *J. Investigative Dermatology*. **87**(6), 758–761.

JUHLIN, L. and SHELLY, W.B. (1977) New staining techniques for the Langerhans cell. *Acta Dermatol. (Stockholm)* **57**, 289–296.

■ CHAPTER 7 ■

KNUTSON, K., POTTS, R.O., GUZEK, D.B., GOLDEN, G.M., MCKIE, J.E., HIGUCHI, W.J. and HIGUCHI, W.I. (1985) Macro and molecular physical chemical considerations in understanding drug transport in the stratum corneum. *J. Contr. Rel.* **2**, 67–68.

LAMPE, M.A., BURLINGAME, A.L., WHITNEY, J., WILLIAMS, M.L., BROWN, B.E., ROITMEN, E. and ELIAS, P.M. (1983) Human stratum corneum lipids: characterization and regional variations. *J. Lipid Res.* **24**,120–130.

LEVEQUE, J.L. and RASSENEUR, L. (1988) Mechanical properties of stratum corneum: influence of water and lipids. In MARKS, R.M., BARTON, S.P. and EDWARDS, C. (eds) *The Physical Nature of the Skin*. Norwell, MA, USA: Norwell. Chapter 17.

MIDDLETON, J.D. (1968) The mechanism of water binding in stratum corneum. *Brit J. Derm.* **80**, 437–450.

POTTS, R.O. and GUY, R.H. (1992) Predicting skin permeability. *Pharmaceut Res.* **9**(5), 663–669.

RAYKAR, P.V., FUNG, M.C. and ANDERSON, B.D. (1988) The role of protein and lipid domains in the uptake of solutes of human stratum corneum. *Pharmaceutical Res.* **5**(3), 140–150.

RIEGER, M. (1993) Factors affecting sorption of topically applied substances. In: ZATZ, J.L. (ed.) *Skin Permeation Fundamentals and Application*. Wheaten: Allured Publishing Co., 33–72.

SCHEUPLEIN R.J. and BLANK, I.H. (1973) Mechanisms of percutaneous absorption, IV. Penetration of nonelectrolytes (alcohols) from aqueous solutions and from pure liquids. *J. Invest. Dermatol.* **60**, 286.

SCHEUPLEIN, R.J. and BRONAUGH, R.L. (1983) Percutaneous absorption. In: GOLDSMITH L.A. (ed.) *Biochemistry and Physiology of the Skin*. vol. 1, Oxford: Oxford University Press, 1255–1294.

SURBER, C., WILHELM, K.P., HORI, M., MAIBACH, H.I., HALL L. and GUY, R.H. (1990a) Optimization of topical therapy: partitioning of drugs into stratum corneum. *Pharmceut Res.* **7**(12), 1320–1324.

SURBER, C., WILHELM, K.P., MAIBACH, H.I., HALL L. and GUY, R.H. (1990b) Partitioning of chemicals into human stratum corneum: implications for risk assessment following dermal exposure. *Fundamental and Applied Toxicology* **15**, 99–107.

WESTER, R.C. and MAIBACH, H.I. (1983) Dermatopharmacokinetics in clinical dermatology. *Seminars in Dermatology* **2**(2), 81–84.

WESTER, R.C., MOBAYEN, M. and MAIBACH, H.I. (1987) *In vivo* and *in vitro* absorption and binding to powdered stratum corneum as methods to evaluate skin absorption of environmental chemical contaminants from ground and surface water. *J. Toxicol. and Environ. Health* **21**, 367–374.

WESTER, R.C., MAIBACH, H.I., SEDIK, L., MELENDRES, J., DI ZIO, S. and WADE, M. (1992) *In vitro* percutaneous absorption of cadmium from water and soil into human skin, *Fundam. Appl. Toxicol.* **19**, 1–5.

WESTER, R.C., MAIBACH, H.I., SEDIK, L., MELENDRES, J. and WADE, M. (1993a) *In vitro* percutaneous absorption and skin decontamination of arsenic from water and soil, *Fundam. Appl. Toxicol.* **20**, 336.

WESTER, R.C., MAIBACH, H.I., SEDIK, L. and MELENDRES, J. (1993b) Percutaneous absorption of PCBs from soil: *in vivo* rhesus monkey, *in vitro* human skin, and binding to powdered human stratum. *J. Toxicol. and Environ. Health* **39**, 375–382.

WESTER, R.C., HUI, X., HEWITT, P.G., HOSTYNET, J., KRAUSER, S., CHAN, T. and MAIBACH, H.I. (2002) Polymers effect on estradiol coefficient between powdered human stratum corneum and water. *J. Pharmaceutical Sciences* **91**, 2642–2645.

ZATZ, J.L. (1993) Scratching the surface: rationale approaches to skin permeation. In: Zatz, J.L. (ed.) *Skin Permeation Fundamentals and Application.* Wheaten: Allured Publishing Co., 11–32.

■ CHAPTER 7 ■

Sensitive Skin

HARALD LÖFFLER, JÚN ARAMAKI, ISAAK EFFENDY
AND HOWARD I MAIBACH

Contents

8.1   Introduction

8.2   Findings in individuals with self-reported
sensitive skin

8.3   Findings in populations with a different
"sensitive skin"

8.4   Definition of terms concerning skin
susceptibility

8.1 INTRODUCTION

Today, hardly any cosmetic preparation without the label "for sensitive skin" can be found. Indeed, what is "sensitive skin"?

For many patients, "sensitive skin" stands in general for allergic reactions to common contact allergens, e.g., nickel (de Lacharriere *et al.*, 2001; Francomano *et al.*, 2000). Their main problems are eczematous skin reactions due to contact (e.g., in costume jewelry), or by ingestion of food, followed by hematogenic eczema (Hindsen *et al.*, 2001). Other patients which are particularly affected by the problem of "sensitive skin" are atopic individuals (Amin and Maibach, 1996; Basketter *et al.*, 1996; Löffler and Effendy, 1999; Mills and Berger, 1991; Tupker *et al.*, 1995a). These individuals develop atopic dermatitis caused by numerous triggers. Exogenous triggers (e.g., chemical or mechanical irritation, allergens, climatic conditions, wrong skin care, nutrition) are for these patients as relevant as endogenous ones (e.g., psychological stress, endogenous eruption, predisposition to dry, xerotic skin) (Diepgen *et al.*, 1989; Tupker *et al.*, 1995a; Tupker *et al.*, 1995b). The atopic individual describes his skin in the symptom free intervals as a "sensitive skin" which can be transformed by a combination of the mentioned triggers to a clinically visible atopic eczema. Indeed, many patients with acute eczematous problems complain about "sensitive skin." This is so far understandable, since all kinds of eczema are frequently accompanied by a skin barrier disruption leading to the so-called "sensitive skin," since due to this barrier disruption or even slight irritations (hand washing) may lead to a clinically visible skin reaction (e.g., worsening of the underlying dermatitis) (Effendy *et al.*, 1996). Such a skin reaction may concern individuals with rosacea, irritant dermatitis, nummular eczema and exsiccation eczema as well (Meding *et al.*, 2001).

Another group complaining about "sensitive skin" are subjects with non-visible skin changes, or with a normal unimpaired skin. But, these individuals claim of skin symptoms after otherwise harmless affections of the skin, like the use of cosmetics, sun, wind, clothes, etc. However, some claim "sensitive skin" even without any known exogenous influences (Table 8.1).

Hence, a closer definition of the term "sensitive skin" is needed to avoid the mix-up of different entities of skin diseases and skin non-diseases (Maibach *et al.*, 1989). The first group with "sensitive skin" showing indeed clinical signs which can be detected by visual evaluation or by measurement of skin physiological parameters. The complaints concern all manifestations (clinical signs) of dermatitis (Table 8.1) and can be accompanied by any of the symptoms

TABLE 8.1:

Signs and symptoms of "sensitive skin"

Signs of "sensitive skin"	Symptoms of "sensitive skin"
erosion	burning
erythema	itching
excoriations	pain
hyperkeratosis	tickling
infiltration	tightening
lichenifications	smarting
oozing	
papules	
rhagaden	
vesicules	
xerosis	

(second row of Table 8.1). On the other hand, there is also a group complaining about "sensitive skin" without any clinical detectable skin changes (only the second row of Table 8.1).

8.2 FINDINGS IN INDIVIDUALS WITH A SELF REPORTED SENSITIVE SKIN

The explanation for the visible symptoms in the group claiming about "sensitive skin" is founded in their skin precondition (e.g., dermatitis) and may be manifested in any degree of skin irritation. Whilst non-visible symptoms are hard to explain, even though they are important for their epidemiology: The number of individuals stating their skin as "sensitive" is high and is estimated at 50 percent with a clear dominance of women (Willis *et al.*, 2001). A common statement of these individuals is that they have discomfort when using some cosmetic products (Willis *et al.*, 2001). It is difficult to verify such complains using objective reproducible methods. Recently, we investigated whether "sensitive skin" is a result of different anatomic or biophysical skin conditions (which can be evaluated by bioengineering methods) or, perhaps, the consequence of a different perception of skin sensations (Löffler *et al.*, 2001).

A questionnaire was completed by 420 volunteers, recruited in a mobile center for skin problems throughout Germany. This questionnaire dealt with various influencing factors concerning skin susceptibility and "skin sensitivity" (Table 8.2). Atopy scores according to Diepgen *et al.* (1989) and skin type according to Fitzpatrick (1988) were evaluated. In addition, patch testing with

TABLE 8.2:

Questionnaire for estimation of "sensitive skin", see (Löffler *et al.*, 2001)

Question	Possible answers
General skin susceptibility	1–4 Scale:
Skin susceptibility in summer	1: no
Skin susceptibility in winter	2: moderate
Skin sensitivity to sun rays	3: strong
Skin susceptibility to sheep wool	4: severe
Skin susceptibility to cosmetics, soaps, deodorants or perfume	
Skin dryness	
Signs of skin susceptibility	Itching, burning, reddening, tension, development of eczema, other
Localization	Hands, face, other
Flexural eczema	yes or no
Eczema of hands or face	
Itching during sweating	
Itching during contact to sheep wool	
Allergy against nickel	

an anionic detergent (0.5 percent sodium lauryl sulfate, SLS) for 24 h (Effendy and Löffler, 1996) was conducted on the forearm of 152 volunteers. Evaluation was performed by measurement of transepidermal water loss (TEWL) with TEWAMETER TM 210, cutaneous blood flow with Laser Doppler (LD) PF 5010 using an integrating probe (probe 413) and skin hydration with Corneometer CM 820.

Willis (Willis *et al.*, 2001) found that almost 50 percent of volunteers estimated their skin sensitivity as strong or severe. However, the reason for their "sensitive skin" is difficult to define. One reason may be an atopic constitution. Indeed, we found a significant correlation between "sensitive skin" and atopy score. Hence, the subgroup of atopic patients are mostly included in the group of volunteers with "sensitive skin." The majority of the volunteers with a "sensitive skin" had, however, no atopic constitution. But they chose nearly every possible trigger for worsening of their "sensitive skin" like sheep wool, cosmetics, soaps, deodorants, perfume or sun rays. Interestingly, the skin suscep-tibility has been related to sun ray exposure, but there was no correlation to the Fitzpatrick skin type. It appears that without any differentiation every proposed influence was chosen by people with a "sensitive skin," however, objectivability is missing.

Mostly, non-objectivable terms were used to describe the problem with "sensitive skin," e.g. feelings of tension, burning or reddening, but exactly defined and objectivable skin problems, like eczema, were not associated with the degree of "sensitive skin." This underlines again the diversity between the subjects with visible symptoms, like eczema, and patients with subjective non-visible skin problems. This is supported by other investigators (Berg and Axelson, 1990) who also found a minimal correlation between objective skin findings and subjective complaints about skin symptoms.

In accordance with these findings, no changes in biophysical functions have been found in the group with the "sensitive skin," neither basal nor after SLS testing. In general, there was no correlation between the degree of self-estimated skin sensitivity and every single measured parameter. It therefore seems that the "sensitive skin" is a non-objectivable estimation, probably influenced by the individual education and possibly by the mass media. Furthermore, it seems indeed to be fashionable to have a "sensitive skin," particularly for women and men of "modern society." Although previously changes in biophysical skin functions in the elderly has been found (Cua et al., 1990), there was no correlation between complaints about "sensitive skin" and age of the subjects. This indicates, that the estimation of a "sensitive skin" is a complaint independent of age.

However, there are arguments that a "sensitive skin" does exist. One is the finding that individuals with a "sensitive skin" might be detectable by a stinging-test and rather not by a skin irritation-test. On the other hand, there are individuals who state their skin as sensitive but react normally in the stinging-test and in the SLS patch test (Basketter and Griffiths, 1993; Lammintausta et al., 1988; Seidenari et al., 1998).

Aramaki et al. (2002) investigated a population known to have a very "sensitive skin", namely Japanese individuals. The rate of reported skin problems with cosmetics for Caucasians is estimated with 12 percent (Willis et al., 2001). Rapaport measured the skin irritation caused by cosmetical products in Caucasian versus Japanese subjects (Rapaport, 1984). He reported a generally greater cumulative response of Japanese subjects. Moreover, Japanese had a far higher incidence of adverse skin effects (and resulting in drop outs) in clinical trials (Tadaki et al., 1993). Most of these adverse skin effects are just subjective sensations as described in Table 8.1 row 2. Whether the difference in skin susceptibility between Caucasian and Japanese are only a subjective or objective nature was the aim of one of our studies where besides of a standard SLS patch test, a stinging-test was performed (Aramaki et al., 2002).

8.3 FINDINGS IN POPULATIONS WITH A DIFFERENT "SENSITIVE SKIN"

In this experimental prospective study, we investigated the skin susceptibility of 22 Japanese and 22 German women, all living in Germany (Aramaki *et al.*, 2002). A 24 h patch test with 0.25 percent and 0.5 percent SLS was performed on the forearm. Skin reactions were evaluated by measurement of TEWL and cutaneous blood flow with a Laser Doppler (LD) Flowmeter by use of an integrating probe. Stratum corneum hydration was measured with a corneometer, sebum levels determined using Sebumeter, the content of melanin and hemoglobin (erythema) in the skin were detected employing a Mexameter. In a second part of the study, 18 of the Japanese and 20 of the German women were tested with lactic acid (stinging test). Ten percent lactic acid was applied to one cheek and pure water was applied as a control to the other. The subjects cleaned up the facial area below the eyes with soap and water at least 3 hours earlier. The subjects evaluated their sensations for tightness, burning, itching and stinging. Subjective sensations were described every 2, 4 and 5 min by using a 4-point scale (0–3) (Christensen and Kligman, 1996) and a visual analog scale (Scott and Huskisson, 1976). Before and after application, the skin color reaction was measured with a Minolta Chromameter CR-300.

After SLS 0.5 percent and 0.25 percent we found significantly higher values in Corneometrie-measurement only in Japanese women. This might be due to the habit of applying ointment on the body which is far more common in Japanese women than in German women (and which might influence the measurement even when 24 h before evaluation no application of cosmetics was allowed). All other measured parameters showed no difference between the two tested population indicating that the objective skin irritability to detergents is similar in Japanese and German women. This is supported by investigations which has shown that the corneocyte size and spontaneous desquamation of Asians, Afro-Americans and Caucasians are similar (Robinson, 2000) and that the neuroanatomy of the skin, certainly relevant to the issue of neurosensory irritation, indicates no racial differences in epidermal innervation between Caucasians, Chinese, and Japanese (Reilly *et al.*, 1997). Reported differences between ceramides in the epidermis are, obviously, not relevant for the skin barrier function and therefore for the skin irritability.

When the objective skin irritability of Japanese and German women is the same, the higher incidence of adverse skin effects against cosmetics are probably founded in a different perception of the skin. If it is true, then we probably can

CHAPTER 8

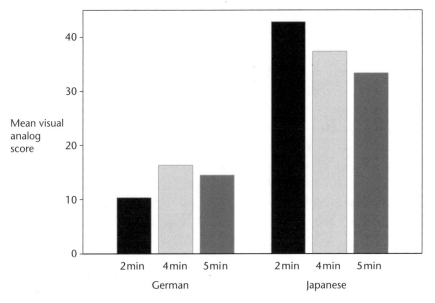

Figure 8.1: Mean value of difference between stinging-sensations after lactid acid and after water, evaluation after 2, 4 and 5 minutes (according to (Aramaki, *et al.*, 2002).

find an increased reactivity of Japanese to the stinging-test. Indeed, we found that the self reported sensitivity rate of Japanese was higher than that of German women (Figure 8.1) (Aramaki *et al.*, 2002).

Moreover, Japanese felt stinging immediately, whereas German women felt stinging somewhat later. This may be due to the assumption that (Kompaore *et al.*, 1993) Asian skin is more permeable to water than Caucasian skin and that several chemicals, like benzoic acid, caffeine and acetylsalicylic acid showed an increase percutaneous absorption in Asians relative to Caucasians (Lotte *et al.*, 1993). These findings suggest that objective findings in skin permeability may be the reason for the "sensitive skin" of Japanese women. However, there is a certain difference in the culture and education between Japan and Germany. In Japan femininity is more desirable for women than in western countries, leading to a desirable "vulnerable" and "female" behavior. In this female role expectation a dainty woman is expected to have a "sensitive skin" and problems with many cosmetics. However, it is hard to say whether the "sensitive skin" of Japanese women is caused by different cultural assessment of discomfort or by differences in penetration speed.

Even in these considerations about "sensitive skin" in Japanese and German women, the mix-up between different meanings of "sensitive skin" has become obvious. Is "sensitive skin" objective or subjective, which parameters will define it? Hence, a better definition of all kinds of skin susceptibility is needed.

8.4 DEFINITION OF TERMS CONCERNING SKIN SUSCEPTIBILITY

As the term "sensitive skin" is extensively used by the cosmetic industry (and subsequently by many consumers) it should be used with caution in medical literature. We propose the following classification of skin irritancy (Table 8.3).

People with "sensitive skin" are only individuals who stated their skin as sensitive. There is no possibility to prove the statement with objective methods, because the skin may have normal biophysiological skin parameters and may react to stinging tests.

If such individuals react repeatedly to a skin test with sensation induced by chemical irritants (like lactic acid), they are identified as a "stinger." It can be assumed that these individuals have indeed an increase in unpleasant skin sensations after use of otherwise well tolerated skin products.

If, however, individuals do have an increased skin susceptibility to irritation caused by chemical irritants (like detergents), which can objectively be measured using bioengineering methods, they are identified as individuals with an "irritable skin."

This classification might be of relevance in discriminating individuals with a higher risk of developing skin irritation, particularly on the hands (Effendy et al., 1995; Lee and Maibach, 1995; Löffler et al., 1996; 1999).

■ CHAPTER 8 ■

TABLE 8.3:

Definition of terms concerning skin susceptibility

Term	Definition	Objective findings
Sensitive skin	Individuals, who stated their skin as more sensitive than average	None
Irritable skin	Individuals, who objectively develop a stronger skin reaction to an irritant than average	Enhanced values of bio-engineering evaluation methods
Stinger	Individuals, who react reproducible positive in a test with a sensation inducing chemical	Reproducible positive skin stinging-test

With this classification it can be stated that there is neither any significant correlation nor any significant coincidence between individuals with a "sensitive skin" and individuals with an "irritable skin." Only a minority of individuals with a "sensitive skin" or an "irritable skin" can be identified as "stingers" (Basketter and Griffiths, 1993; Coverly *et al.*, 1998; Löffler *et al.*, 2001; Simion *et al.*, 1995). Hence, if the patient states "I have a very sensitive skin," he does not give you any important information, but is telling you that he cares about his skin.

REFERENCES

AMIN, S. and MAIBACH, H.I. (1996) Cosmetic intolerance syndrome: pathophysiology and management. *Cosmet. Dermatol.* **9**, 34–42.

ARAMAKI, J., KAWANA, S., EFFENDY, I., HAPPLE, R. and LÖFFLER, H. (2002) Differences of skin irritation between Japanese and European women. *Br. J. Dermatol.* **146**, 1052–1056.

BASKETTER, D., BLAIKIE, L. and REYNOLDS, F. (1996) The impact of atopic status on a predictive human test of skin irritation potential. *Contact Dermatitis* **35**, 33–39.

BASKETTER, D.A. and GRIFFITHS, H.A. (1993) A study of the relationship between susceptibility to skin stinging and skin irritation. *Contact Dermatitis* **29**, 185–188.

BERG, M. and AXELSON, O. (1990) Evaluation of a questionnaire for facial skin complaints related to work at visual display units. *Contact Dermatitis* **22**, 71–77.

CHRISTENSEN, M. and KLIGMAN, A.M. (1996) An improved procedure for conducting lactic acid stinging tests on facial skin. *J. Soc Chem* **47**, 1–11.

COVERLY, J., PETERS, L., WHITTLE, E. and BASKETTER, D.A. (1998) Susceptibility to skin stinging, non-immunologic contact urticaria and acute skin irritation; is there a relationship? *Contact Dermatitis* **38**, 90–95.

CUA, A.B., WILHELM, K.P. and MAIBACH, H.I. (1990) Cutaneous sodium lauryl sulfate irritation potential: Age and regional variability. *Br. J. Dermatol.* **123**, 607–613.

DE LACHARRIERE, O., JOURDAIN, R., BASTIEN, P. and GARRIGUE, J.L. (2001) Sensitive skin is not a subclinical expression of contact allergy. *Contact Dermatitis* **44**, 131–132.

DIEPGEN, T.L., FARTASCH, M. and HORNSTEIN, O.P. (1989) Evaluation and relevance of atopic basic and minor features in patients with atopic dermatitis and in the general population. *Acta Derm. Venereol.* Suppl. **144**, 50–54.

EFFENDY, I. and LÖFFLER, H. (1996) Experiences with patch testing with sodium lauryl sulfate as a tool predicting human skin susceptibility. *Skin Research and Technology* **2**, 252.

EFFENDY, I., LÖFFLER, H. and MAIBACH, H.I. (1995) Baseline transepidermal water loss in patients with acute and healed irritant contact dermatitis. *Contact Dermatitis* **33**, 371–374.

EFFENDY, I., WELTFRIEND, S., PATIL, S. and MAIBACH, H.I. (1996) Differential irritant skin responses to topical retinoic acid and sodium lauryl sulfate: alone and in crossover design. *Br. J. Dermatol.* **134**, 424–430.

FITZPATRICK, T.B. 1988. The validity and practicality of sun-reactive skin types I through VI. *Arch Dermatol* 124, 869–871.

FRANCOMANO, M., BERTONI, L. and SEIDENARI, S. (2000) Sensitive skin as subclinical expression of contact allergy to nickel sulfate. *Contact Dermatitis* **42**, 169–170.

HINDSEN, M., BRUZE, M. and CHRISTENSEN, O.B. (2001) Flare-up reactions after oral challenge with nickel in relation to challenge dose and intensity and time of previous patch test reactions. *J. Am. Acad. Dermatol.* **44**, 616–623.

KOMPAORE, F., MARTY, J.P. and DUPONT, C. (1993) *In vivo* evaluation of the stratum corneum barrier function in blacks, Caucasians and Asians with two noninvasive methods. *Skin Pharmacol* **6**, 200–207.

LAMMINTAUSTA, K., MAIBACH, H.I. and WILSON, D. (1988) Mechanisms of subjective (sensory) irritation. Propensity to non-immunologic contact urticaria and objective irritation in stingers. *Derm. Beruf. Umwelt.* **36**, 45–49.

LEE, C.H. and MAIBACH, H.I. (1995) The sodium lauryl sulfate model: An overview. *Contact Dermatitis* **33**, 1–7.

LÖFFLER, H., DICKEL, H., KUSS, O., DIEPGEN, T.L. and EFFENDY, I. (2001) Characteristics of self-estimated enhanced skin susceptibility. *Acta Derm. Venereol.* **81**, 343–346.

LÖFFLER, H. and EFFENDY, I. (1999) Skin susceptibility of atopic individuals. *Contact Dermatitis* **40**, 239–242.

LÖFFLER, H., EFFENDY, I. and HAPPLE, R. (1996) The sodium lauryl sulfate test. A noninvasive functional evaluation of skin hypersensitivity. *Hautarzt* **47**, 832–838.

CHAPTER 8

LÖFFLER, H., EFFENDY, I. and HAPPLE, R. (1999) Patch testing with sodium lauryl sulfate: benefits and drawbacks in research and practice. *Hautarzt* **50**, 769–778.

LOTTE, C., WESTER, R.C., ROUGIER, A. and MAIBACH, H.I. (1993) Racial differences in the *in vivo* percutaneous absorption of some organic compounds: a comparison between black, Caucasian and Asian subjects. *Arch. Dermatol. Res.* **284**, 456–459.

MAIBACH, H.I., LAMMINTAUSTA, K., BERARDESCA, E. and FREEMAN, S. (1989) Tendency to irritation: sensitive skin. *J. Am. Acad. Dermatol.* **21**, 833–835.

MEDING, B., LIDEN, C. and BERGLIND, N. (2001) Self-diagnosed dermatitis in adults. Results from a population survey in Stockholm. *Contact Dermatitis* **45**, 341–345.

MILLS, O.H., JR. and BERGER, R.S. (1991) Defining the susceptibility of acne-prone and sensitive skin populations to extrinsic factors. *Dermatol. Clin.* **9**, 93–98.

RAPAPORT, M.J. (1984) Patch testing in Japanese subjects. *Contact Dermatitis* **11**, 93–97.

REILLY, D.M., FERDINANDO, D., JOHNSTON, C., SHAW, C., BUCHANAN, K.D. and GREEN, M.R. (1997) The epidermal nerve fibre network: characterization of nerve fibres in human skin by confocal microscopy and assessment of racial variations. *Br. J. Dermatol.* **137**, 163–170.

ROBINSON, M. K. (2000) Racial differences in acute and cumulative skin irritation responses between Caucasian and Asian populations. *Contact Dermatitis* **42**, 134–143.

SCOTT, J. and HUSKISSON, E.C. (1976) Graphic representation of pain. *Pain* **2**, 175–184.

SEIDENARI, S., FRANCOMANO, M. and MANTOVANI, L. (1998) Baseline biophysical parameters in subjects with sensitive skin. *Contact Dermatitis* **38**, 311–315.

SIMION, F.A., RHEIN, L.D., MORRISON, B.M., JR., SCALA, D.D., SALKO, D.M., KLIGMAN, A.M. and GROVE, G.L. (1995) Self-perceived sensory responses to soap and synthetic detergent bars correlate with clinical signs of irritation. *J. Am. Acad. Dermatol.* **32**, 205–211.

TADAKI, T., WATANABE, M., KUMASAKA, K., TANITA, Y., KATO, T., TAGAMI, H., HORII, I., YOKOI, T., NAKAYAMA, Y. and KLIGMAN, A.M. (1993) The effect of topical tretinoin on the photodamaged skin of the Japanese. *Tohoku J. Exp. Med.* **169**, 131–139.

TUPKER, R.A., COENRAADS, P.J., FIDLER, V., DE JONG, M.C., VAN DER MEER, J.B. and DE MONCHY, J.G. (1995a) Irritant susceptibility and weal and flare reactions to bioactive agents in atopic dermatitis: I. Influence of disease severity. *Br. J. Dermatol.* **133**, 358–364.

TUPKER, R.A., COENRAADS, P.J., FIDLER, V., DE JONG, M.C., VAN DER MEER, J.B. and DE MONCHY, J.G. (1995b) Irritant susceptibility and weal and flare reactions to bioactive agents in atopic dermatitis: II. Influence of season. *Br. J. Dermatol.* **133**, 365–370.

WILLIS, C.M., SHAW, S., DE LACHARRIERE, O., BAVEREL, M., REICHE, L., JOURDAIN, R., BASTIEN, P. and WILKINSON, J.D. (2001) Sensitive skin: an epidemiological study. *Br. J. Dermatol.* **145**, 258–263.

CHAPTER 8

Transdermal Drug Delivery System — An Overview

CHERYL LEVIN AND HOWARD I MAIBACH

Contents

9.1   Introduction

9.2   Percutaneous Drug Absorption

9.3   Transdermal drug delivery devices

9.4   Advantages of transdermal drug delivery

9.5   Disadvantages of transdermal drug delivery

9.6   Adverse reactions to transdermal systems—
       general

9.7   Local effects

9.8   Systemic/immunologic

9.9   Prophylactic measures to decrease ACD
       incidence

9.10   Future

9.1 INTRODUCTION

The skin is a seemingly impermeable barrier with its primary function to protect against entry of foreign agents into the body. However, recent research has demonstrated that intact skin may be used as a route of administration for systemic delivery of simple potent drug molecules through a transdermal patch. The first US-approved transdermal patch was introduced in 1981 for scopolamine. In the past two decades, another seven drugs have been introduced to the US market, namely nitroglycerin, clonidine, estradiol, nicotine, fentanyl, testosterone and most recently a combination estrogen/progesterone system (Hogan and Cottam, 1991). Many more transdermal drug delivery systems (TDDS) are currently under investigation, including timolol, propranolol, insulin and prostaglandin patches.

9.2 PERCUTANEOUS DRUG ABSORPTION

The skin's uppermost layer of epithelium, the stratum corneum (SC), is the rate-limiting barrier to percutaneous drug transport. In fact, it is significantly more impermeable than the gastrointestinal, vaginal, nasal, buccal or rectal epithelial barriers. The SC, which is comprised of approximately 40 percent lipids, 40 percent protein, and only 20 percent water, is generally only permeable to small, lipophilic molecules (Elias and Feingold, 1988). This is because lipophilic drugs may dissolute into intercellular lipids around the cells of the SC and thus easily pass through the SC barrier. Hydrophilic molecules, on the other hand, must route through openings within hair follicles and sebaceous glands. These pores comprise only about 1 percent of the total skin surface, severely limiting the amount of hydrophilic drug absorption (Kitson and Thewalt, 2000).

Once a drug is able to cross the SC, it is relatively easy to permeate the deeper epithelial and dermal layers and become systemically absorbed. The challenge in transdermal drug delivery is systemic absorption in a safe, controllable and therapeutic fashion without permanently reducing the efficacy of the skin barrier (Berti and Lipsky, 1995). Rate and extent of drug absorption must be tightly controlled in order to successfully achieve these goals. Factors, such as the thickness of the SC in a body region (Ya-Xian *et al.*, 1999) (SC is thicker on the palmar and plantar regions and thinner on the postauricular, axillary and scalp) and formulation of vehicle are instrumental in designing the appropriate patch. In general, drugs that have been successfully designed for a transdermal system are small, of low molecular weight, high potency, and moderate

CHAPTER 9

lipophilicity (because they must get through the hydrophilic epithelial and dermal layers) (Ogiso and Tanino, 2000; Kalia and Guy, 2001).

9.3 TRANSDERMAL DRUG DELIVERY DEVICES

There are currently two types of transdermal drug delivery devices—matrix-controlled and membrane (reservoir)-controlled (Figures 9.1 and 9.2) (Ranade, 1991). The matrix-controlled device incorporates a drug-in-polymer matrix layer between frontal and backing layers, where the matrix binds to the drug and controls its rate of release from the skin. In the reservoir system, there is a rate-controlling membrane present between the drug matrix and the adhesive layer, which controls the rate of drug release. In both systems, the rate of drug permeation is greater than the permeation rate across the skin. This provides drug uptake at a predetermined rate that is independent of patient skin variability (Ansel and Allen, 1999).

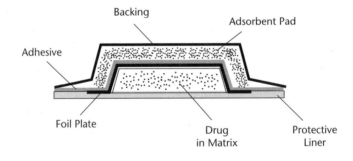

Figure 9.1: Matrix-controlled Device

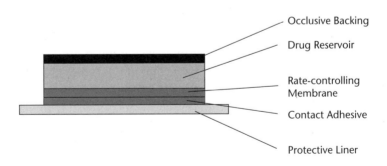

Figure 9.2: Membrane-controlled Device

TABLE 9.1:

Typical formulations in transdermal delivery
(Physicians Desk Reference 2000)

Drug	Typical Formulation
Scopolamine	Scopolamine 1.5 mg base
Clonidine	Clonidine 0.1 mg, 0.2 mg, or 0.3 mg tablets
Nitroglycerin	Nitroglycerin 0.1 mg, 0.2 mg, 0.3 mg, 0.4 mg, 0.6 mg, or 0.8 mg per hour
Nicotine	Nicotine—three steps of 21 mg, 14 mg, and 7 mg per hour Or Nicotine 15 mg in 16 hours
Estradiol	Estradiol 0.025 mg, 0.05 mg, 0.075 mg, or 0.1 mg per day
Estradiol/Progestin	Estradiol/Progestin 0.05/0.14 mg per day Or Estradiol/Progestin 0.05/0.25 mg per day
Testosterone	Testosterone 2.5 mg, 4 mg, 5 mg or 6 mg per day
Fentanyl	Fentanyl 2.5 mg, 5 mg, 7.5 mg, or 10 mg per hour

The advantage of the membrane-controlled system is that it provides a true constant (zero-order) release of drug from the system irrespective of the amount of drug remaining in the patch. In the matrix system, the rate of release is dependent upon the matrix bound to the drug. As drug is depleted from the system, there is a slight decline in the release rate when using the matrix system. This is because drug in the surface layers has already permeated and the remaining drug must diffuse a longer distance through the matrix in order to penetrate the skin. With well-designed matrix systems this rate is insignificant. A disadvantage of the reservoir system is that drug molecules may saturate the rate-controlling membrane and thereby cause a "burst effect" whereby the patch initially releases too much drug into the system and potentially causes toxicity. Of course, the burst effect may be advantageous for drugs that normally exhibit a long lag time between patch application and therapeutic effect (Ranade and Hollinger, 1996; Kydonieus, 1992).

9.4 ADVANTAGES OF TRANSDERMAL DRUG DELIVERY

Transdermal drug delivery avoids the gastrointestinal and hepatic first-pass metabolism and thereby increases drug bioavailability in comparison to oral formulations. Another important advantage of the transdermal drug delivery system is the elimination of the generally observed "peaks" and "valleys" in

CHAPTER 9

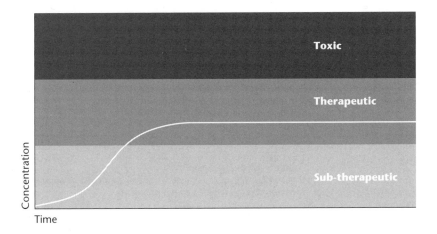

Figure 9.3: Concentration profiles

the plasma drug concentration profile observed in patients receiving oral drug delivery formulations (Kydonieus, 1992). With the appropriate TD-DDS the drug input rate into the blood-stream can be controlled to stay in the therapeutic region, potentially avoiding toxic or sub-therapeutic drug plasma levels. In addition, transdermal systems also reduce the frequency of drug administration and some allow for multiday continuous drug delivery. These factors may improve patient compliance (Bronaugh and Maibach, 1999).

9.5   DISADVANTAGES OF TRANSDERMAL DRUG DELIVERY

The main disadvantage to the use of transdermal drug delivery is in its limitations. The stratum corneum is an excellent barrier and therefore only small, highly potent molecules with moderate lipophilicity will be candidates for transdermal delivery (Bronaugh and Maibach, 1999). In addition, there is the potential for a long lag time between patch application and effect of drug, which is a disadvantage when immediate drug action is needed. Depending upon the circumstance, it may be necessary to supplement with oral medication during the initial patch application. Other disadvantages include variable intra and interindividual percutaneous absorption efficiency, variable adhesion to different skin types and a limited time that the patch can be affixed. Finally, transdermal drug delivery systems are currently only developed when conventional administration has serious limitations. This is because transdermal systems are costly and involve complex technology to develop the system.

9.6 ADVERSE REACTIONS TO TRANSDERMAL SYSTEMS—GENERAL

The adverse reactions due to transdermal systems may be classified into two broad categories; local irritation due to the patch itself or a systemic, immunologic reaction to the components of the patch (Maibach, 1992).

9.7 LOCAL EFFECTS

9.7.1 Occlusion

Transdermal drug delivery systems are occlusively applied to the skin for 1–7 days (Brown and Langer, 1988). Occlusion enhances skin hydration by allowing eccrine sweat glands and water vapor to accumulate on the skin's surface (Hurkmans *et al.*, 1985). Hydration enhances skin absorption of compound but may also lead to adverse effects, such as miliaria rubra, caused by sweat duct occlusion. In miliaria rubra, sweat infiltrates below the epidermis and results in pruritic erythematous papulovesicles (Hurkmans *et al.*, 1985). Generally, the miliaria rubra is limited to the application site and resolves within one day. Treatments for miliaria rubra include topical steroids to reduce the associated itching, and increased fluid intake to maintain homeostasis in the body. In order to prevent miliaria from occurring, transdermal patches are not reapplied to the same site following a 1–7 day course. Transdermals should not be given for more than 7 days at a time.

9.7.2 Erythema

Transient mild to moderate erythema occurs in most patients. Removal of the pressure-sensitive adhesive is responsible for the erythematous skin response (Fisher, 1984).

9.7.3 Irritant Contact Dermatitis

There is an increased risk of developing irritant contact dermatitis (ICD) proportional to the increased occlusive period of the patch. Additionally, irritant

CHAPTER 9

dermatitis may occur if the transdermal system is repeatedly applied to the same skin site.

9.7.4 Miscellaneous

Scopolamine patches have been implicated in causing anisocoria in several patients when they are inadvertently transferred to another site (Carlston, 1982; McCrary and Webb, 1982). A nitroglycerin disk was implicated in causing a second-degree burn on a patient's chest, in one case report (Murray, 1984). Person-to-person transfer of transdermal therapeutic systems may cause toxicity in the recipient (Wick *et al.*, 1989). This is most likely to occur when the TTD has been applied for a long time to one site. The longer the application period of the transdermal drug delivery system, the lower the skin adhesion and the more likely the system will become dislocated inadvertently.

9.8 SYSTEMIC/IMMUNOLOGIC

The most common type of hypersensitivity reaction to the transdermal drug delivery system is an allergic contact dermatitis. Generally, the reaction is in response to a component of the drug or the adhesive background in the transdermal system (Nieboer *et al.*, 1987); the reaction is prevalent during any stage of drug use. Lanolin, a vehicular ingredient in many of the transdermal ointments, is one of the primary accountable agents. Patches applied to thin skinned areas, such as the postauricular region (scopolamine) or the scrotal area (testosterone) are more likely to cause ACD. Sensitization is also promoted in response to local irritation (resulting from prolonged occlusion) as well as oily, inflamed, broken, calloused or occluded (Dwyer and Forsyth, 1994) (Nieboer *et al.*, 1987) skin. Lack of patient compliance with regard to applying the patch to the designated site, applying the patch for a designated period of time, or rotating patch application sites may also lead to skin sensitization. The skin hypersensitivity reaction is generally manifest as a rash accompanied by redness, burning, itching, heat and swelling. If the reaction persists, the therapeutic system should be discontinued.

9.9 PROPHYLACTIC MEASURES TO DECREASE ACD INCIDENCE

Allergic contact dermatitis from transdermal drug delivery systems is one of the limiting factors in patient compliance. Some prophylactic measures that should/ are being taken to decrease the incidence of ACD include limiting patch application time and rotating the patch site.

Improved predictive tests of sensitization should be developed for each of the therapeutic systems. In the development of clonidine, standard predictive tests indicated that it was not an allergen; however, when marketed, many users developed allergic contact dermatitis. Currently, mouse strains are being developed as an alternative to the standard guinea pig model (Kalish *et al.* 1996). Robinson and Cruze used guinea pig models and a local lymph node assay (LLNA) in mouse models to aid in the detection of weak allergens (Robinson and Sozeri, 1990). Through Vitamin A supplementation and the introduction of chronic conditions, they were able to detect contact sensitization of clonidine in both mice and guinea pigs. Other predictive models have analyzed the electrophiles within various haptens, such as scopolamine and clonidine and their relationship with nucleophilic groups of skin protein to form antigens (Benezra, 1991).

Contact sensitization from transdermal d-chlorpheniramine and benzoyl peroxide were reduced when hydrocortisone was coadministered (Amkraut *et al.*, 1996). Additionally, when applied prior to the transdermal patch, ion channel modulators, such as ethacrynic acid, have been found to prevent sensitization in mice (Kalish *et al.*, 1997; Wille *et al.*, 1999). The potential role of corticosteroids and ion channel modulators in the prevention of contact sensitization from TTS should be further investigated and better defined.

Additionally, minimizing reapplication to the same application site (Hogan and Cottam, 1991) and maintaining caution when performing oral provocation tests (Vermeer, 1991) would help to reduce the induction of allergic contact dermatitis among TTS users.

9.10 FUTURE

The advantages associated with TTS, including avoidance of the first-pass metabolism, elimination of "peaks and valleys" and improved patient compliance, have led to continual interest in the development of new transdermal systems. Some transdermal systems that may be available in the US in the

■ CHAPTER 9 ■

near future include insulin (Sen *et al.*, 2002) and asthma (Kato *et al.*, 2002) medication.

The current transdermal delivery systems are useful for delivering small, lipophilic molecules through the skin. However, there are many compounds that do not meet these requirements. New techniques are being developed to allow the transfer of hydrophilic, charged drugs through the skin. "Active" transdermal drug delivery involves utilizing external driving forces on the stratum corneum in order to allow penetration of the molecule of interest (Barry, 2001).

Electrically-assisted methods include iontophoresis, phonophoresis, electroporation, magnetophoresis and photochemical waves. Iontophoresis passes an electric current through the skin and thereby provides the driving force to enable penetration of ions into the skin (Singh *et al.*, 1995). The development of transdermal insulin may require the use of iontophoresis (Rastogi and Singh, 2002). Phonophoresis utilizes ultrasound energy to enhance drug penetration. Higher frequency energy enables greater penetration but also is associated with greater adverse events. Electroporation uses strong, brief pulses of electric current to punch holes in the stratum corneum. These holes close 1 to 30 minutes following the electrical stimulus (Banga and Prausntiz, 1998). Electroporation coupled with iontophoresis may be helpful in the delivery of some drugs (Badkar *et al.*, 1999). The application of high gradient magnetic fields and vibrational forces to biological systems is termed magnetophoresis. Magnetophoresis may be effective in the delivery of terbutaline sulfate (TS), a drug widely used for the treatment of acute and chronic bronchitis patients (Narasimha and Shobha Rani, 1999). Laser-induced stress waves, known as photochemical waves, may also be of benefit in drug delivery.

Hydrating agents and chemical enhancers (Smith and Maibach, 1995) also increase pore size to enhance drug delivery. Moisturizers are the primary hydrating agents. There are numerous chemical enhancers, including benzalkonium chloride, oleyl alcohol and alphaterpineol (Monti *et al.*, 2001; Sinha and Kaur, 2000). Transdermal delivery may be most improved utilizing a combination of chemical enhancers and electically-assisted devices (Terahara *et al.*, 2002).

The stratum corneum may also be removed or bypassed utilizing ablation, microneedles or follicular delivery. Pulsed CO_2 lasers are used in tissue ablation to damage the skin. Microneedle enhanced transdermal drug delivery also damages the skin by creating channels for drug diffusion across the stratum corneum. The existing needles are 150 microns long and leave holes about one micron in diameter when removed from the skin. Originally developed for the microelectronics industry, the tiny needles can avoid causing pain because they penetrate only the outermost layer of skin that contains no nerve endings (Henry *et al.*, 1998). Follicular media include liposomes, ethosomes, transfersomes and niosomes. While passive transdermal systems have been on the market for more than twenty years, active transdermal systems are still not available for clinical use. Further clinical trials are needed to evaluate the safety and efficacy of the active transdermal products.

REFERENCES

AMKRAUT, A., JORDAN, W.P., *et al.* (1996) Effect of coadministration of corticosteroids on the development of contact sensitization. *J. Am. Acad. Dermatol.* **35**, 27–31.

ANSEL, H. and ALLEN, L.J. (1999) *Pharmaceutical Dosage Forms and Drug Delivery Systems*, 7th edn. New York, Williams and Wilkins.

BADKAR, A., BETAGERI, G., HOFFMAN, G.A. and BANGA, A.K. (1999) Enhancement of transdermal iontophoretic delivery of a liposomal formulation of colchicine by electroporation. *Drug Delivery*, **6**, 111–115.

BANGA, A. and PRAUSNTIZ, M. (1998) Assessing the potential of skin electroporation for the delivery of protein- and gene-based drugs, *Trends Biotechnol.* **16**, 408–412.

BARRY, B. (2001) Novel mechanisms and devices to enable successful transdermal drug delivery. *Eur. J. Pharm. Sci.* **14**(2), 101–114.

BENEZRA, C. (1991) Structure-activity relationships of skin haptens with a closer look at compounds used in transdermal devices. *J. Controlled Release.* **15**, 267–270.

BERTI, J. and LIPSKY, J. (1995) Transcutaneous drug delivery: a practical review. *Mayo Clin. Proc.* **70**(6), 581–586.

BRONAUGH, R. and MAIBACH, H. (1999) *Percutaneous Absorption: Drugs Cosmetics Mechanisms Methodology*, New York: Marcel Dekker.

BROWN, L. and LANGER, R. (1988) Transdermal delivery of drugs. *Annu. Rev. Med.* **39**, 221–229.

CARLSTON, J. (1982) Unilateral dilated pupil from scopolamine disk. *J. Am. Med. Assoc.* **248**, 31.

CHAPTER 9

DWYER, C. and FORSYTH, A. (1994) Allergic contact dermatitis from methacrylates in a nicotine transdermal patch. *Contact Derm.* **30**, 309–310.

ELIAS, P. and FEINGOLD, K. (1988) Lipid-related barriers and gradients in the epidermis. *Ann. NY Acad. Sci.* **548**, 4–13.

FISHER, A. (1984) Dermatitis due to therapeutic systems. *Cutis.* **34**, 526–531.

HENRY, S., MCALLISTER, D., ALLEN, M.G. and PRAUSNITZ, M.R. (1998) Microfabricated microneedles: a novel approach to transdermal drug delivery. *J. Pharm. Sci.* **87**(8), 922–925.

HOGAN, D. and COTTAM, J. (1991) Dermatological aspects of transdermal drug delivery systems. In *Dermatotoxicology.* Marzulli, F. and Maibach, H. (eds) Washington DC: Taylor & Francis.

HURKMANS, M., BODDE, H., VAN DRIEL, L.M.J., VAN DOORNE, H. and JUNGINGER, H.E. (1985) Skin irritation caused by transdermal drug delivery systems during long-term (5 day) application. *Br. J. Dermatol.* **112**, 461–476.

KALIA, Y. and GUY, R. (2001) Modeling transdermal drug release. *Adv. Drug Deliv. Rev.* **48**(2–3), 159–172.

KALISH, R., WOOD, J., KYDONIEUS, A. and WILLE, J.J (1997) Prevention of contact hypersensitivity to topically applied drugs by ethacrynic acid: Potential application to transdermal drug delivery. *J. Controlled Release.* **48**, 79–87.

KALISH, R., WOOD, J.A., WILLE, J.J., KYDONIEUS, A. (1996) Sensitization of mice to topically applied drugs: albuterol, chlorpheniramine, clonidine and nadolol. *Contact Derm.* **35**(2), 76–82.

KATO, H., NAGATA, O., *et al.* (2002) [Development of transdermal formulation of tulobuterol for the treatment of bronchial asthma] (in Japanese). *Yakugaku Zasshi.* **122**(1), 57–69.

KITSON, N. and THEWALT, J. (2000) Hypothesis: the epidermal permeability barrier is a porous medium. *Acta Derm. Venereol. Suppl. (Stockh.).* **208**, 12–15.

KYDONIEUS, A. (1992) *Treatise on Controlled Drug Delivery: Fundamentals, Optimization and Applications*, New York, NY: Marcel Dekker.

MAIBACH, H. (1992) Cutaneous adverse reactions to transdermal delivery systems—mechanisms and prevention. *Acta Pharm. Nord.* **4**(2), 125.

MCCRARY, J. and WEBB, N. (1982) Anisocoria from scopolamine patches. *JAMA*, **243**, 353–354.

MONTI, D., GIANNELLI, R., et al. (2001) Comparison of the effect of ultrasound and of chemical enhancers on transdermal permeation of caffeine and morphine through hairless mouse skin in vitro. Int. J. Pharm. 229(1–2), 131–137.

MURRAY, K. (1984) Hazards of microwave ovens to transdermal delivery systems. N. Engl. J. Med. 310, 721.

NARASIMHA, M.S. and SHOBHA RANI, R. (1999) Effect of magnetic field on the permeation of salbutamol sulfate and terbutaline sulfate. Indian Drugs. 36, 663–664.

NIEBOER, C., BRUYNZEEL, D., et al. (1987) The effect of occlusion of the skin with transdermal therapeutic system on Langerhans cells and the induction of skin irritation. Arch. Dermatol. 123, 1499–1502.

OGISO, T. and TANINO, T. (2000) [Transdermal delivery of drugs and enhancement of percutaneous absorption] (in Japanese). Yakugaku Zasshi. 120(4), 328–338.

RANADE, V. (1991) Drug delivery systems. 6. Transdermal drug delivery. J. Clin. Pharmacol. 31(5), 401–418.

RANADE, V. and HOLLINGER, M. (1996) Drug Delivery Systems. Boca Raton: CRC Press.

RASTOGI, S. and SINGH, J. (2002) Transepidermal transport enhancement of insulin by lipid extraction and iontophoresis. Pharm Res. 19(4), 427–433.

ROBINSON, M. and SOZERI, T. (1990) Immunosuppressive effects of clonidine on the induction of contact sensitization in the balb/c mouse. J. Invest. Dermatol. 95(5), 587–591.

SEN, A., DALY, M., et al. (2002) Transdermal insulin delivery using lipid enhanced electroporation. Biochim. Biophys. Acta. 1564(1), 5–8.

SINGH, P., ANLIKER, M., et al. (1995) Facilitated drug delivery during transdermal iontophoresis. Curr. Prob. Dermatol. 22, 184–188.

SINHA, V. and KAUR, M. (2000) Permeation enhancers for transdermal drug delivery. Drug Dev. Ind. Pharm. 26(11), 1131–1140.

SMITH, E. W. and MAIBACH, H. (1995) Percutaneous Penetration Enhancers, Boca Raton: CRC Press.

TERAHARA, T., MITRAGOTRI, S., and LANGER, R. (2002) Porous resins as a cavitation enhancer for low-frequency sonophoresis. J. Pharm. Sci. Technol. 91(3), 753–759.

CHAPTER 9

VERMEER, B. (1991) Skin irritation and sensitization. *J. Controlled Release*, **15**, 261–266.

WICK, K., WICK, S., *et al.* (1989) Adhesion-to-skin performance of a new transdermal nitroglycerin adhesive patch. *Clin. Ther.* **11**, 417–424.

WILLE, J., KYDONIEUS, A., and KALISH, R.S. (1999) Several different ion channel modulators abrogate contact hypersensitivity in mice. *Skin Pharmacol. Appl. Skin Physiol.* **12**, 12–17.

YA-XIAN, Z., SUETAKE, T. and TAGAMI, H. (1999) Number of cell layers of the stratum corneum in normal skin—relationship to the anatomical location on the body, age, sex and physical parameters, *Arch. Dermatol. Res.* **291**(10), 555–559.

Iontophoresis

ANGELA N ANIGBOGU
AND HOWARD I MAIBACH

Contents

10.1 Introduction and historical perspectives

10.2 Theory

10.3 Iontophoresis devices and experiment parameters

10.4 Pathways of ion transport

10.5 Factors affecting iontophoretic drug delivery

10.6 *In vitro-in vivo* correlation

10.7 Advantages of iontophoresis

10.8 Problems associated with iontophoresis

10.9 Applications of iontophoresis in dermatology

10.10 Conclusion

10.1   INTRODUCTION AND HISTORICAL PERSPECTIVES

The skin has long been used as a site for drug administration of therapeutic agents for localized pharmacological actions (Kastrip and Boyd, 1983). Drug delivery through the skin for systemic effects, though limited, is a well-established branch of pharmaceutics. The stratum corneum, the outermost layer of the skin offers excellent barrier properties to applied substances thus limiting the number of drug candidates for passive transdermal delivery to usually small, potent and lipophilic compounds. Physical and chemical techniques have been used to improve the permeability of the skin to applied substances. Dermal iontophoresis is one of such physical techniques.

A Greek physician, Aetius, first prescribed shock from electric fish for the treatment of gout more than 1000 years ago and since then the use of electric current to introduce drugs into the body has intrigued scientists. Iontophoresis was first introduced by Pivati to treat arthritis in the 1740s (Licht, 1983) and Palaprat claimed in 1833 to have been able to deliver iodine directly to tissues by means of electric current (Jones, 1907).

Iontophoresis may be defined as the facilitated transport of ions of soluble salts across membranes under the influence of an applied electric field. The technique temporarily lost its importance partly because it was not well understood and partly due to safety considerations. Munch earlier demonstrated the systemic application of this technique in 1879, when strychnine delivered under the positive electrode in rabbit killed the animal within 15 minutes of current passage. Leduc (1900) described some of the earliest systematic experiments outlining the usefulness of iontophoresis in systemic drug delivery. He placed a solution of strychnine sulfate (positively charged strychnine ion) in the positive electrode (anode) of an iontophoresis set up on one rabbit with the negative electrode filled with water and a solution of potassium cyanide (negatively charged cyanide ion) in the negative electrode (cathode) of a set up on another rabbit with the positive electrode filled with water. The animals were connected and when a constant current of 40–50 mA was applied, both animals died due to strychnine and cyanide poisoning respectively. In a subsequent experiment reversing the polarity of the delivery electrodes (i.e. strychnine in the cathode and cyanide in the anode), neither animal died demonstrating that in the first case, the electric current delivered the lethal ions.

Since the early years, there has been a resurgence of interest in iontophoresis. Gibson and Cooke (1959) used iontophoretic delivery of pilocarpine to induce sweating and the procedure is now used for the diagnosis of cystic fibrosis. Iontophoresis has been used for the treatment of palmoplantar hyperhydrosis. In addition to this and other local applications of the technique, the present focus of research and development efforts on iontophoresis is for systemic drug delivery. With interest in controlled drug delivery surfacing in the last two decades, and the inability to deliver a great number of drugs especially proteins and peptides passively, iontophoresis appears to be particularly attractive and holds great commercial promise for non-invasive rate-controlled transdermal drug delivery of a wide array of drugs including hydrophilic, charged and high molecular weight compounds all of which would not permeate the skin by passive diffusion.

10.2 THEORY

Biological tissues including skin consist of membrane barriers made up of lipids and proteins. Transport through these membranes is better suited to un-ionized than ionized compounds. Many potential drug candidates are ionized at skin pH (4–5) and cannot therefore be transported across membranes passively. As stated previously, the stratum corneum provides an excellent barrier to transport across the skin. In addition, passive diffusion depends on a concentration gradient across the membrane. Membrane transport of drugs can be facilitated by the application of an external energy source (active transport).

Iontophoresis by utilizing electric current provides an excellent source of this external energy. It operates on the general principles of electricity, i.e. opposite charges attract and like charges repel. Thus if the drug of interest is cationic, for delivery across the skin, it is placed in the anode reservoir. When a voltage is applied, the positively charged drug is repelled from the anode through the skin and into the systemic circulation. Conversely, an anionic drug is placed in the cathode reservoir. The transport of neutral and uncharged molecules can also be facilitated by iontophoresis by the process of electroosmosis (Gangarosa et al., 1980). Figure 10.1 is an illustration of an iontophoretic set-up.

In this section, the underlying principles of iontophoretic transport will be described briefly. The Nernst-Planck flux equation as applied in iontophoresis provides that the flux of an ion across a membrane under the influence of an applied charge is due to a combination of iontophoretic (electrical potential difference), diffusive (increased skin permeability induced by the applied field) and electroosmotic (current-induced water transport) components (Schultz, 1980).

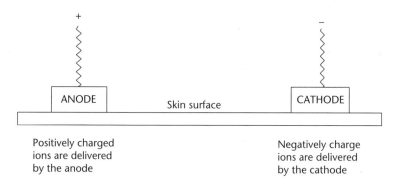

Figure 10.1: A schematic illustration of transdermal iontophoresis.

$$J_{ion} = J_e + J_p + J_c \tag{1}$$

where J_e is the flux due to electrical potential difference and is given by:

$$J_e = \frac{Z_i D_i F}{RT} C_i \frac{\partial E}{\partial x} \tag{2}$$

and J_p is the flux due to passive delivery and is given by:

$$J_p = K_s D_s \frac{\partial C}{\partial x} \tag{3}$$

and J_c is the flux due to electroosmosis or convective transport and is given by:

$$J_c = kC_s I \tag{4}$$

where Z_i is the valence of the ionic species, D_i is the diffusivity of the ionic species, i in the skin, F is the Faraday constant, T is the absolute temperature, and R is the gas constant, ∂E, ∂x is the electrical potential gradient across the skin, C_i is the donor concentration of the ionic species, K_s is the partition coefficient between donor solution and stratum corneum, D_s is the diffusivity across the skin, ∂C, ∂x is the concentration gradient across the skin, C_s is the concentration in the skin, I is the current density, k is the proportionality constant (Chien *et al.*, 1990).

In iontophoretic drug delivery, the major contribution to the overall flux of a compound would be that due to electrical potential gradient (electro-migration). The contribution to the flux due to electroosmosis is likely to be

■ CHAPTER 10 ■

small (Srinivasan *et al.*, 1989) and Roberts *et al.* (1990) have suggested that only about 5 percent of the overall flux is due to convective solvent flow. In the anodal iontophoresis of lidocaine hydrochloride, electromigration was shown to contribute approximately 90 percent of the total flux (Marro *et al.*, 2001a). Electroosmosis is always in the direction as the flow of the counterions. Human skin is negatively charged at pH above 4 and the counterions are positive ions and therefore, electroosmotic flow would occur from anode to cathode.

The Goldman constant field approximation is used to facilitate the integration of Eq. (1) to give an enhancement factor E (relative to passive flux) and which is given by Srinivasan *et al.* (1989):

$$E = (Flux_{ionto} / Flux_{pass}) = \frac{-K}{1 - \exp(K)} \tag{5}$$

where

$$K = \frac{Z_i F \Delta E}{RT} \tag{6}$$

At high voltages, deviations from the predictions based on Eq. (5) have been known to occur (Srinivasan *et al.*, 1989; Kasting and Keister, 1989).

Whereas the Nernst-Planck equation when applied to iontophoresis describes the flux of a drug through a membrane under the influence of applied potential, Faraday's law describes flux in terms of electric current flowing in the circuit. Applying Faraday's law therefore, the mass of substance transported in an aqueous solution is proportional to the charge applied (this is the product of current and time). The flux of a compound transported across the skin (J_{trans}) is thus given by:

$$J_{trans} = \frac{t}{zF} I \tag{7}$$

where t is transport number of the compound, z is charge on the drug, F is Faraday's constant and is equal to 96,500 C mole^{-1} and I is the current density (A/cm^2). In iontophoresis, all ions in a formulation as well as ions in the skin carry a fraction of the applied electric current. The most important ions for consideration, are however, those of the drug of interest with transport number t, which is defined as the fraction of the total current carried by the drug and is given by:

$$t = \frac{z^2 mc}{\sum_i z_i^2 m_i c_i}$$ (8)

where z is the charge of the drug, m is the ionic mobility, c is concentration of the ion and i is all the ions in the system. In theory therefore, if the mobility of a drug in the skin is known, the iontophoretic flux can be predicted. In practice, however, it is not easy to estimate the skin mobility of a drug and free solution mobility is thus usually used as an approximation (Singh *et al.*, 1997).

10.3 IONTOPHORESIS DEVICES AND EXPERIMENT PARAMETERS

10.3.1 *In vitro*

As the technique is still in development, there are relatively few descriptions in the literature of different apparatuses used in *in vitro* iontophoresis experiments. Examples include (Molitor, 1943; Burnette and Marrero, 1986; Bellantone *et al.*, 1986; Masada *et al.*, 1989; Green *et al.*, 1991; Thysman *et al.*, 1991; Chang and Banga, 1998). Usually these involve modifications of the two-compartment *in vitro* passive diffusion set-up. Two electrodes connected to a power supply are used, and in some instances, one is inserted in each compartment separated by the mounted skin and voltage or current measurements are made between the electrodes. In other instances using vertical flow through diffusion cells, a horizontally mounted piece of skin separates the positive and negative electrode chambers with the epidermal side of the skin from the receptor phase bathing the dermal side.

A four-electrode potentiostat system designed to maintain a constant voltage drop across a membrane in a two-chamber diffusion cell has been described by Masada *et al.* (1989). As with passive diffusion studies, the whole assembly is kept at 37°C with the aid of a constant-temperature water bath in order to maintain the skin surface temperature at 32°C.

In all constructs, the receiver compartment medium is usually stirred with the aid of magnetic bar stirrers. The electrodes usually consist of platinum wires or silver/silver chloride. Cationic drugs are placed under the anode electrode in the donor compartment with the cathode in the receiver compartment and the opposite is true of anionic drugs. Pulsed or constant current may be applied.

Regardless of the type of electrodes and cells used, the same principles and transport mechanisms apply. Bellatone *et al.* (1986) demonstrated that diffusion

■ CHAPTER 10 ■

cell type had little impact on the diffusion of benzoate ions across hairless mouse skin. Similarly, Kumar *et al.* (1992) have shown that cell design was not a factor in the delivery of an analogue of growth hormone releasing factor *in vitro* across hairless guinea pig skin by iontophoresis.

10.3.2 *In vivo*

Devices used in iontophoresis are designed for rate-controlled delivery of therapeutic agents. The devices used *in vivo* vary in complexity from those that use household current to battery-and-rheostat type to modern electronic circuit devices (Singh and Maibach, 1993). Essentially, they consist of a power source to provide current, anode and cathode reservoirs. The reservoir electrodes usually consist of a small metal plate over which a moist material preferably a pad or gauze is overlaid and this portion comes in direct contact with the skin. During use, an indifferent electrode (without drug) is placed some distance from the active electrode. Regardless of design, the most important considerations in choosing an iontophoretic device include safety and comfort of patients, cost, ease of operation, reliability, size and therefore portability.

Generally, they are operated at a constant voltage allowing the current to be varied for patient comfort and compliance over a given period. As with *in vitro* apparatuses, various devices have been described for use in iontophoresis *in vivo* (Molitor and Fernandez, 1939; Barner, 1961; Rapperport *et al.*, 1965). Rattenbury and Worthy, 1996 described systems used in the UK. Hidrex (Gessellschaft für Medizin and Technik, Wuppertal, Germany) has been described by Hölzle and Alberti, (1987). Phipps *et al.*, (1989) described a custom-made battery operated device with two hydrogel electrodes for *in vivo* delivery of pyridostigmine. These devices deliver direct steady current, which have been postulated to be responsible for skin irritation arising from iontophoresis due to continuous electric polarization. To minimize this, others advocate devices delivering pulsed current such as has been used to administer catecholamines to dogs (Sanderson *et al.*, 1987). In furtherance of this argument, two delivery systems using pulsed direct current have been described, one being the Advance Depolarizing Pulse Iontophoretic System (ADIS-4030) designed to continuously deliver drugs under constant pulsed current Application (Okabe *et al.*, 1986). The other, the Transdermal Periodic Iontophoretic System (TPIS) delivers pulsed direct current with combinations of frequency, waveform, on/off ratio and current density for a programmed treatment duration (Chien *et al.*, 1990).

Available in the US is a portable battery operated power supply unit called a

Phoresor® (Dermion Drug Delivery Research, Salt Lake City, Utah, USA) and is suitable for home use.

The US Food and Drug Administration has categorized iontophoretic devices into those for specialized uses (Class II) and others (Class III) (Tyle, 1986). These include Drionic® (General Medical Company, Los Angeles, CA, USA), Macroduct (Wescor Inc., Logan, UT, USA), Iontophor-PM (Life-Tech Inc., Houston, TX, USA), Model IPS-25 (Farrall Instruments Inc., Grand Island, NE, USA), Electro-Medicator (Medtherm Corporation, Huntrille, AL, USA), Dagan® (Dagan Corporation, MN, USA), Desensitron II® (Parkell, Farmingdale, NY, USA).

10.3.1 Choice of Electrode Materials in Iontophoresis

Platinum electrodes or patches consisting of zinc/zinc chloride or silver/silver chloride electrodes are used. The choice of electrode material depends on several factors including good conductivity, malleability and the ability to maintain a stable pH. In addition, the electrodes should not produce gaseous by-products and must be safe to be used on the skin. Silver/silver chloride electrodes also referred to as reversible electrodes are made from a metal in contact with solution of its own ions (Boucsein, 1992) and are the most commonly used as they satisfy these requirements. At the anode, silver under the influence of an applied electric field is oxidized and reacts with chloride to form silver chloride. At the cathode, silver chloride is reduced to silver with the liberation of chloride ions. These electrodes are thus stable. They should however be thoroughly cleaned after use and rinsed with distilled water. When not in use for prolonged periods, it is advisable to store the electrodes dry.

Platinum electrodes though used are less desirable in some situations than silver/silver chloride electrodes because with prolonged use of platinum electrodes, there is oxidation of water to oxygen gas and hydronium ions. This was demonstrated by Phipps et al. (1989) in anodal delivery of lithium across hydrogel membranes. The efficiency of delivery achieved using platinum electrodes was 20 percent compared to 37 percent when silver anode was used instead.

Careful selection of the electrode used to deliver a particular drug is also important. For instance, dexamethasone sodium phosphate can be delivered under the anode electrode by electro-osmosis. However considering that electro-osmosis contributes a small fraction to the overall iontophoretic transport of any given drug, cathodal iontophoresis should therefore be considered. It is in fact known that the delivery efficiency of dexamethasone sodium phosphate

CHAPTER 10

by iontophoresis from the cathode is far greater than from the anode. It has been suggested that for monovalent ions with Stoke's radii larger than 1 nm, electroosmotic flow may be the dominant transport mechanism. In addition, for large anions or negatively charged protein, electroosmotic flow from the anode may be more efficient than cathodal electromigration (Pikal, 2001).

10.3.2 Animal Models

The ultimate goal of any research done in the field of iontophoresis is the application in humans for drug delivery. For obvious reasons, animals and not human subjects are the first choice for experimental purposes. There is no consensus as to which of the animal models used in passive uptake studies is suitable for iontophoresis. Hairless mouse has been the most commonly used model e.g. (Bellantone *et al.*, 1986). Other models which have been investigated include hairless guinea pig (Walberg, 1970), dog (McEvan-Jenkinson *et al.*, 1974), furry rat (Siddiqui *et al.*, 1987), pig (Monteiro-Riviere, 1991), hairless rat (Thysman and Preat, 1993), Rabbit (Lau *et al.*, 1994; Anigbogu *et al.*, 2000). Phipps *et al.*, (1989) found no differences in the fluxes of lithium and pyridostigmine through human, pig and rabbit skin *in vitro*. There is therefore the need to establish which model closely resembles human skin for both penetration and toxicological studies. Recently, Marro *et al.*, 2001 evaluated the suitability of porcine skin as a model for human skin in iontophoretic studies by comparing the anode-to-cathode and cathode-to-anode delivery of mannitol through both skin types at different pH. They concluded that the isoelectric points, 4.4 for pig skin and 4.8 for human skin were close enough and that pig skin showed the same pH-dependent perselectivity for mannitol as did human skin and would therefore be an appropriate model for human skin.

10.4 PATHWAYS OF ION TRANSPORT

The predominant pathway for ion transport through the skin remains controversial. Appendages: sweat ducts and hair follicles are thought to be the major pathway for iontophoretic transport through the skin (Grimnes, 1984; Burnette, 1989). This is obviously so in the use of pilocarpine for the diagnosis of cystic fibrosis. Abramson and Gorin (1940) showed that charged dyes delivered iontophoretically produced a dotlike pattern on human skin and the dots were identified as sweat glands. Papa and Kligman (1966) observed a direct link between methylene blue staining of the skin and the location of sweat ducts.

Monteiro-Riviere (1991) demonstrated the appendageal pathway for the iontophoretic delivery of mercuric chloride. Cullander and Guy (1991) using a vibrating probe electrode identified the largest currents to be in the area of residual hairs. Laser scanning confocal microscopy has been used to elucidate the pathway for the iontophoretic transport of Fe^{2+} and Fe^{3+} ions (Cullander, 1992) as being the sweat glands, hair follicles and sebaceous glands. Based on these and other studies, the sweat ducts and glands, however, appear to be more important than hair follicles in the transport of ions through the shunts. A schematic of the routes of ion transport across the skin is shown in Figure 10.2.

It is however not correct to assume that all charged transport takes place through the appendages. Walberg (1968) demonstrated that Na^+ and Hg^{2+} could penetrate through guinea pig skin in areas devoid of sweat glands and hair follicles. Millard and Barry (1988) compared the iontophoretic delivery of water and glutamic acid through full thickness human skin and shed snakeskin, which is largely devoid of sweat glands and hair follicles. Iontophoresis was shown to

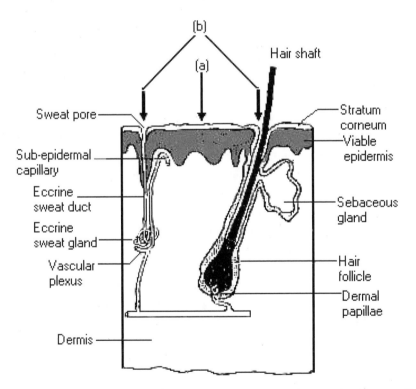

Figure 10.2: A schematic representation of human skin showing the (a) intercellular and (b) appendageal pathways for ion transport during iontophoresis.

CHAPTER 10

increase the delivery of both materials through snakeskin. Sharata and Burnette, (1989) showed that mercuric and nickel ions can diffuse passively between the keratinocytes. Jadoul *et al.* (1996) concluded from results of Fourier transform Infrared spectroscopy (FTIR) and small angle x-ray scattering (SAXS) studies on isolated rat and human cadaver skin following prolonged *in vitro* iontophoresis that iontophoresis transport is related to lipid bilayer stacking disorganization.

10.5 FACTORS AFFECTING IONTOPHORETIC DRUG ADMINISTRATION

Several factors come into play when considering iontophoresis for drug delivery. These include the physicochemical properties of the drug in question: the charge, molecular size and concentration; formulation parameters: choice of vehicle, pH range in which drug is ionic, presence of competing or parasitic ions, viscosity or mobility; Others include physiologic considerations such as appropriate skin site for application; instrumentation, e.g. type of current source, pulsed or constant, current density. This list is by no means exhaustive but includes some of the more critical factors, which will be considered briefly in this section.

10.5.1 pH

Transdermal iontophoresis achieves the transport of drug molecules into and through the skin under the influence of an applied electric field. This means that the drug candidate should be charged to allow for delivery in therapeutically relevant levels through the skin. The optimum pH for delivery of a drug by iontophoresis is that at which it exists predominantly in the ionic form. This has been demonstrated by Siddiqui *et al.* (1985, 1989). The pH of peptides, proteins and other amphoteric substances characterized by their isoelectric point is of particular significance, i.e. a pH above which the molecule is anionic and below which it is cationic. For instance, the skin permeability of insulin has been shown to be greater at a pH below its isoelectric point (Siddiqui *et al.*, 1987). Furthermore, the pH gradient encountered in the skin is an important factor in iontophoretic transport. The pH of the skin ranges from 4–6 on the outside to about 7.3 in the viable tissues. If at any time the drug encounters an environment in which it becomes uncharged, its transport becomes impeded. Thus for a molecule to be delivered efficiently by iontophoresis, it must remain charged during its transport into and through the skin. For proteins and peptides, iontophoretic transport may be limited to those with isoelectric points below 4 or above 7.3.

10.5.2 Molecular size

The molecular size of the compound of interest is crucial in predicting the efficiency of its iontophoretic delivery (Srinivasan *et al.*, 1989, 1990; Yoshida and Roberts, 1993). Generally, monovalent positively charged drugs are delivered with greater efficiency by iontophoresis than monovalent negatively charged anions. This has been ascribed to the net negative charge on the skin. The greater the molecular size, the lower the permeability coefficient. Nevertheless, high molecular weight proteins and peptide drugs with molecular weight 3000–5000 daltons have been delivered effectively by iontophoresis.

10.5.3 Concentration

The concentration of the drug in the formulation also affects the flux achieved by iontophoresis. There abound in the literature insurmountable evidence that increasing the concentration of drug in the donor compartment increases proportionately, the flux of the compound e.g. Arginine-Vasopressin (Lelawongs *et al.*, 1989), butyrate (DelTerzo *et al.*, 1989) and diclofenac (Koizumi *et al.*, 1990). A linear relationship between concentration of drug in the donor solution and flux has been established for gonadotropin releasing hormone (GnRH) and sodium benzoate with flux increasing linearly with increasing concentration (Bellantone *et al.*, 1986). With some drugs, however, increasing the concentration in the donor solution beyond a certain point appears not to further increase the flux. This was demonstrated for methylphenidate the steady-state flux of which was found to increase with concentration up to 0.1M (Singh *et al.*, 1997). It was shown recently that increasing the concentration of methotrexate in hydrogels did not further improve the effectiveness of delivery by iontophoresis (Alvarez-Figueroa and Blanco-Méndez, 2001).

10.5.4 Competing ions

The fraction of current carried by each type of ion in solution is called the transference or transport number. When a migrating ion carries 100 percent of the current through the membrane, its rate of transport is maximal and its transport number is unity. In order to control the pH of the donor solution, buffers are often employed. The buffers, however, introduce extraneous ions, which may be of a different type but are of the same charge as the drug ion. These are called co-ions and are usually more mobile than the drug ion. The co-ions reduce the fraction of current carried by the drug ion thus resulting in a diminished transdermal flux of the drug. Some workers also employ antioxidants and antimicrobials which themselves contain co-ions. In addition to these, co-ions can also be introduced from reactions occurring at the electrodes if for example platinum is the conducting material. Hydrolysis of water occurs resulting in the generation of hydronium ion at the anode and hydroxyl ion at the cathode. Reducing the amount of competing ions in the drug donor solution will increase the transport efficiency of the drug ions but as there are also endogenous ions in the skin, e.g. sodium, potassium, chloride, bicarbonate, lactate, etc. which carry an appreciable fraction of the ionic current (Phipps and Gyory, 1992), the transport number of any drug will always be less than unity. Marro *et al.* (2001b) concluded that the mole fraction of drug relative to competing ions of similar polarity was the determinant of the extent to which it can carry charge across the skin during iontophoresis.

10.5.5 Current

A linear relationship has been established between the iontophoretic fluxes of a number of compounds and the current applied. Examples include lithium (Phipps *et al.*, 1989), thyrotropin releasing hormone (Burnette and Marrero, 1986), mannitol (Burnette and Ongpipattanakul, 1987), gonadotropin releasing hormone (Miller *et al.*, 1990), verapamil (Wearley and Chien, 1989). Tissue distribution of phosphorus following iontophoretic delivery was shown to be proportional to current density (O'Malley and Oester, 1955). This relationship between skin flux and applied current is closely related to fall in skin resistance. As shown in Figure 10.3, the greater the applied current, the lower the steady state skin resistance achieved (Anigbogu *et al.*, 2000). This relationship is however seen not to be linear at current densities above 2 mA/cm^2. The rate of transfer of ketoprofen from skin to cutaneous blood in rats has been found to be proportional to applied electric current with the enhancement ratios compared to passive delivery being 17 and 73 respectively for 0.14 and 0.70 A/cm^2 (Tashiro *et al.*, 2000). Plasma and tissue levels of diclofenac sodium in rabbit were found to be proportional to applied current density (Hui *et al.*, 2001) and at up to 0.5 mA/cm^2 of current for 6 hours in the presence of drug, rabbit skin showed no significant irritation. The limiting factor especially in

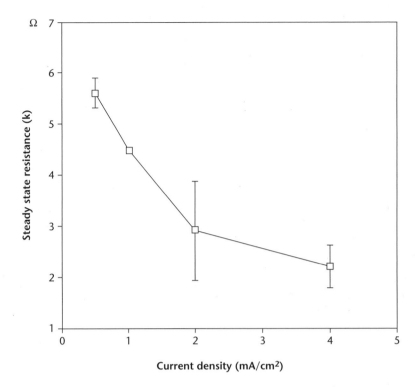

Figure 10.3: Apparent steady-state skin resistance as a function of current density. Area of Application = 1 cm², Duration = 1 h, Electrolyte in patch = 0.15 M NaCl, pH = 7.

humans, however, is safety, comfort and acceptability. The upper limit of current tolerable to humans is thought to be 0.5 mA/cm² (Abramson and Gorin, 1941; Ledger, 1992). Increasing the surface area of the electrodes allows for increasing current and therefore improving the delivery of some drugs. This is, however, not a linear relationship and may not apply to all drugs (Phipps *et al.*, 1989). In terms of skin barrier properties, it has recently been suggested that the fall in skin impedance following iontophoresis does not necessarily represent damage to the barrier but rather is a response to the relevant electrical potential and ion concentration gradients involved in iontophoresis (Curdy *et al.*, 2002).

10.5.6   Species, sex and site

Iontophoretic deliveries of lithium and pyridostigmine have been found to be comparable in pig, rabbit and human skin (Phipps *et al.*, 1989). Burnette and Ongpipattanakul, (1987) found the iontophoretic fluxes of sodium chloride and mannitol through thigh skin from male and female cadavers to be comparable. Successive iontophoretic delivery of iodine through the same knee in a human volunteer resulted in a constant uptake (Puttemans *et al.*, 1982). Iontophoresis therefore decreases the intra- and intersubject variability as well as influence of site usually observed with passive diffusion. Further studies need to be done, however, to establish the degree to which factors such as race, age, skin thickness, hydration and status of the skin (healthy or diseased) affect iontophoretic drug delivery. Skin tolerability of electric current appears to be species dependent. Rabbit, which is normally reactive to applied chemicals and is used commonly in Draize skin irritation test tolerated 1 mA/cm^2 current for up to 1 h without irritation as opposed to human skin for which the upper limit is 0.5 mA/cm^2 (Anigbogu *et al.*, 2000). However, the same study found skin irritation in rabbit to be tied to applied current density or treatment duration with currents greater than 1 mA/cm^2 applied for periods of 30 minutes or greater or 1 mA/cm^2 for application times greater than 1 h producing irritation.

10.5.7   Continuous versus Pulsed Current

Whether pulsed or continuous direct current should be used, is one of the controversies that exist in the field of iontophoresis. Continuous direct current causes skin polarization with time and this reduces the efficiency of delivery. This can be avoided by using pulsed direct current i.e. direct current delivered periodically. During the "off-period," the skin becomes depolarized returning to near its original state. Chien and co-workers (1989) applying the same current density (0.22 mA/cm^2) over the same 40 minute period, were able to deliver a two-fold level of vasopressin *in vivo* in rabbits using pulsed current from the Transdermal periodic Iontophoretic System (TIPS) described earlier compared to the Phoresor® system which delivers constant direct current. They also showed a peak plasma insulin level in 30 minutes in diabetic rabbits using TIPS (1 mA, 40 min) compared to 1–2 h for the Phoresor® system (4 mA, 80 min). Ion transport using pulsed current may, however, be affected by the frequency. If the frequency is high, the efficiency of pulsed delivery is reduced (Bagniefski and Burnette, 1990). While Lui *et al.* (1988) observed a greater blood glucose reduction in diabetic rats using 2 kHz compared to 1 kHz, Haga *et al.* (1997) found no significant difference in the decrease in blood glucose levels when frequency was changed from 1 to 2 kHz, in the same species. More studies need to be done to explain these discrepancies in results from different studies.

10.6 *IN VITRO-IN VIVO* CORRELATION

We recently compared the pharmacokinetic and local tissue disposition of diclofenac sodium delivered iontophoresis and i.v. infusion (Hui *et al.*, 2001) (as shown in Figure 10.4). Within 30 minutes of turning on the current, same plasma concentration was achieved by 0.2 mA/cm² current as the i.v. infusion which at later time points produced plasma concentrations surpassing iontophoresis under this conditions at all other time points up to 6 hours. On the other hand, iontophoresis of diclofenac sodium at 0.5 mA/cm² achieved superior plasma concentration than i.v. infusion from the time the current was initiated till the end of the treatment period. The peak plasma concentration

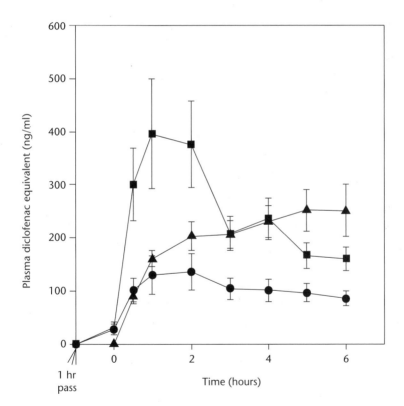

Figure 10.4: Plasma Diclofenac sodium concentrations (mean ± SEM, *n* = 4) over time in rabbit following iv infusion (Dose = 1.25 mg at 0.2 mg/h) and transdermal iontophoresis (Donor concentration = 7 mg/ml; pH = 7.4. Key: ▲ iv infusion, ● 0.2 mA/cm², ■ 0.5 mA/cm².

■ CHAPTER 10 ■

observed between 1–2h during 6 hours of iontophoresis was 132 and 371 µg/L with current densities of 0.2 and 0.5 mA/cm² respectively. The iontophoretic delivery rates calculated using the C_{max} values from the iontophoresis results and clearance values from the i.v. infusion data were 0.027 and 0.074 mg/(cm²h⁻¹) for 0.2 and 0.5 mA/cm² respectively. The *in vivo* delivery efficiency for diclofenac sodium in rabbit was 0.15 mg/mA.h, a value double that of unpublished data obtained *in vitro* with hairless mouse skin. Bearing in mind differences in experimental conditions and species differences the *in vitro* and *in vivo* data appear realistic. More studies need to be done in this area.

10.7 ADVANTAGES OF IONTOPHORESIS

Considering the complexity of iontophoresis compared to traditional dosage forms such as tablets, liquids, injections, ointments and even passive transdermal patches, it must have advantages to enjoy a resurgence of interest.

Transdermal iontophoresis shares many of the advantages of passive transdermal drug delivery including the bypass of hepatic first-pass metabolism, avoidance of gut irritation, controlled drug delivery, and ease of termination of drug-input when necessary. An important consideration is patient compliance. The dosage regimens of many pharmacologic agents available for delivery through other routes pose a challenge to patients. An example is the need to take with or without food, dosing frequency (e.g. to be taken every 4–6 hours), etc. In addition, the injectable route is particularly uncomfortable to many patients. Many drugs which are available for systemic therapy cannot be delivered through many of the existing traditional dosage forms as they are subject to extensive hepatic first pass metabolism and variable gut absorption. Many drugs including new biotech drugs (proteins, peptides, oligonucleosides, etc.) (Meyer, 1988; Merino *et al.*, 1997) and local anesthetics such as lidocaine (Gangarosa, 1981) which would have to be injected to derive maximum benefit have been delivered efficiently using iontophoresis.

Since the rate of drug delivery is generally proportional to the applied current, the rate of input can therefore be preprogrammed on an individual basis (Banga and Chien, 1988). The controllability of the device would eliminate the peaks and troughs in blood levels seen with oral dosing and injections. Patients can titrate their intake of drugs as required.

10.8 PROBLEMS ASSOCIATED WITH IONTOPHORESIS

Only a fraction of the charge introduced in iontophoresis is delivered suggesting that iontophoresis is not necessarily as efficient as theoretically proposed (Sage and Riviere, 1992).

Of more serious consideration, however, are the unwanted skin effects of iontophoresis arising from the system itself and/or drug formulation. Typically, side effects of iontophoresis with low voltage electrodes, properly used are minimal but, nevertheless, must be considered. These include itching, erythema, edema, small punctate lesions and sometimes burns. A slight feeling of warmth and tingling is generally associated with iontophoresis (Kellog *et al.*, 1989; Zeltzer *et al.*, 1991; Ledger, 1992; Maloney *et al.*, 1992). Erythema is also commonly reported and is thought to arise from skin polarization associated with continuous direct current. To minimize this, pulsed direct current has been advocated. Electric shock can occur when high current density is directed at the skin. To minimize this, the current should be increased slowly from zero to the maximum desired current level acceptable to the patient. Similarly, at the end of the procedure, current should be returned from the maximum to zero in a stepwise manner. The effect of current on nerve fibers is thought to be responsible for the itching, tingling and erythema.

The histological and functional changes that occur in animal skin following iontophoresis have been studied. Under similar delivery conditions (i.e. drug concentration, current density and duration) as are used in humans, Moteiro-Riviere, (1990) studied structural changes in porcine skin following iontophoresis of lidocaine. Light microscopy revealed epidermal changes. He, however, noted that similar changes were not observed following iontophoresis of other compounds suggesting the effects were largely due to the lidocaine rather than the electric current. Cho and Kitamura (1988) iontophoresing lidocaine through the tympanic membrane of the guinea pig, observed a loss of adhesion of the epidermis to underlying connective tissue and retraction of non-cornified epidermal cells. Jadoul *et al.* (1996) used Fourier transform infrared spectroscopy (FTIR) and small angle x-ray scattering (SAXS) to study isolated rat skin and human skin from cadaver following prolonged iontophoresis. While FTIR revealed transient increases in the hydration of the outer layers of the stratum corneum but no increase in lipid fluidity, SAXS showed that iontophoresis induced a disorganization of the lipid layers. This was also reversible within days of the procedure. Using wide-angle x-ray scattering (WAXS), the authors did not find evidence of modification of the intralamellar crystalline packing of lipids nor of keratin.

The answer to what should be the upper limit of current tolerable to humans is not very straightforward, as what may be just discernible to one patient may be uncomfortable to another. Generally, however, 0.5 mA/cm^2 is cited (e.g. Abramson and Gorin, 1941; Banga and Chien, 1988; Ledger, 1992). Molitor and Fernandez (1939) found that the greater the surface area of the electrode, the larger the tolerable current but the relationship is curvilinear. Small punctate lesions are associated with electric current traveling through a path of least resistance in the skin. Common sense thus dictates that iontophoresis not be used on skin showing signs of damage. Pain and burns arising from iontophoresis are linked to electrochemical reactions which occur at the electrodes and involve the electrolysis of water to generate hydronium and hydroxyl ions resulting in pH changes (Sanderson et al., 1989). Much earlier, however, Molitor and Fernandez (1939) using continuous flow electrodes which did not generate hydroxyl and hydronium ions and therefore did not produce any pH changes, showed that burns could not solely be related to pH changes.

Erythema is the most common side effect associated with iontophoresis and could be due to non-specific skin irritation such as that which occur with the delivery of an irritant drug. Erythema may be due to a direct effect of electric current on blood vessels and/or current induced release of histamine, prostaglandins or other neurotransmitters leading to local vasodilatation of the affected area. It has also been suggested that electric current can stimulate specific classes of noiceptors, the C-fibers causing them to release the potent vasodilators, substance P and calcitonin gene-related peptide (CGRP) (Brain and Edwardson, 1989; Dalsgaard et al., 1989). Whatever the cause of the erythema, it is usually transient and not associated with any permanent changes in the skin.

Delayed-type contact sensitivity to components of the iontophoresis system, electrodes, electrode gels, etc. (Fisher, 1978; Zugerman, 1982; Schwartz and Clendenning, 1988) or to the drug being delivered (Teyssandier et al., 1977; Holdiness, 1989) have been reported.

Another consideration in choosing iontophoresis for drug delivery is cost. Iontophoresis requires a power source to supply electrical energy. Even though the power requirement for a unit delivery may be small, repeated applications would require a considerable investment in battery supply. Better batteries than those currently used need to be developed.

An important consideration in the use of iontophoresis for drug delivery especially for unstable compounds is whether they are delivered intact or degraded. This has recently been addressed by Brand *et al.* (2001) who delivered antisense, phosphorothioate oligonucleotides into rats by iontophoresis. They were able to measure the decline in CYP3A2 levels suggesting that the antisense agent was successfully delivered in sufficient therapeutic amounts and intact.

Iontophoresis is contraindicated in patients with high susceptibility to applied currents and in patients with known hypersensisitivity to the drug in question. Iontophoresis should be avoided in patients with electrically sensitive implants such as pacemakers. To improve acceptability by both prescribers and patients, more studies need to be done in the field of iontophoresis to minimize unwanted side effects and improve safety.

10.9 APPLICATIONS OF IONTOPHORESIS IN DERMATOLOGY

In the past, iontophoresis was found useful in local delivery of pharmacologic agents. Iontophoresis has been used for the treatment of various dermatologic conditions including lupus vulgaris using zinc. Before the advent of antibiotics, infections were treated by the iontophoresis of metals, e.g. the treatment of streptococcal infections with copper sulfate. Other conditions that have benefited from the use of iontophoresis include lichen planus, scleroderma, plantar warts, hyperhydrosis, infected burn wounds, achieving local anesthesia. Bursitis and other musculoskeletal conditions have been treated with iontophoresed corticoids (Harris, 1982). Summaries of dermatologic applications of iontophoresis have been made by Sloan and Soltani (1986) and Singh and Maibach (1994). Of greater interest in this era is the use of iontophoresis for controlled systemic drug delivery and for targeting deep tissue penetration. Recently, "reverse iontophoresis" involving the extraction of material from the body for the purposes of clinical chemistry has been described (Guy, 1995; Guy *et al.*, 1996). Although glucose is not charged, iontophoresis can markedly increase its passage across the skin by electroosmosis (Merino *et al.*, 1997; Tierney *et al.*, 2000) and this has been applied for the non-invasive monitoring of diabetics' blood sugar levels (Tamada *et al.*, 1995; Svedman and Svedman, 1997; Tierney *et al.*, 2001a, b; Potts *et al.*, 2002). In addition to drug delivery, with the availability of sensitive assay methods, iontophoresis is thus being touted as a diagnostic tool. The "Glucowatch® Biographer" was in fact approved by the Food and Drug Administration in 2001 and launched in the US in April 2002.

CHAPTER 10

10.10 CONCLUSIONS

A large number of drugs generated by the biotech industry today consist of proteins, peptides and oligonucleotides, which at present can only be delivered by the injection route. In addition, many of the old drugs already in use have the same dosage form requirements with its associated problems. Iontophoresis provides an attractive alternative to the existing dosage forms in delivering these drugs both for local as well as systemic indications. The fact that it could allow for a programmable rate-controlled delivery of drugs is particularly relevant. With the approval of the Glucowatch® Biographer, it is more likely in the future that iontophoresis will be used as a diagnostic tool for other disease conditions. Like any new technology, more work is needed to clearly define the parameters that would maximize the safety, acceptability and efficiency of iontophoresis as a dosage form.

REFERENCES

ABRAMSON, H.A. and GORIN, M.H. (1940) Skin reactions. IX. The electrophoretic demonstration of the patent pores of the living human skin; its relation to the charge of the skin. *J. Phys. Chem.*, **44**, 1094–102.

ABRAMSON, H.A. and GORIN, M.H. (1941) Skin reactions: X. Preseasonal treatment of hay fever by electrophoresis of ragweed pollen extracts into the skin: Preliminary report. *J. Allergy.*, **12**, 169–75.

ALVAREZ-FIGUEROA, M.J. and BLANCO-MENDÉZ, J. (2001) Transdermal delivery of methotrexate: iontophoretic delivery from hydrogels and passive delivery from microemulsions. *Int. J. Pharm.*, **215**, 57–65.

ANIGBOGU, A., PATIL, S., SINGH, P., LIU, P., DIHN, S. and MAIBACH, H. (2000) An *in vivo* investigation of the rabbit skin responses to transdermal iontophoresis. *Int. J. Pharm.*, **200**, 195–206.

BAGNIEFSKI, T. and BURNETTE, R.R. (1990) A comparison of pulsed and continuous current iontophoresis. *J. Control. Rel.*, **11**, 113–122.

BANGA, A. and CHIEN, Y.W. (1988) Iontophoretic delivery of drugs: Fundamentals, developments and biomedical applications. *J. Control. Rel.*, **7**, 1–24.

BARNER, H.B. (1961) Cataphoresis in demabrasion tatooing. *Plast. Reconstr. Surg.* **27**, 613–617.

BELLANTONE, N.H., RIM, S., FRANCOUER, M.L. and RASADI, B. (1986) Enhanced percutaneous absorption via iontophoresis I; Evaluation of an *in vitro* system and transport of model compounds. *Int. J. Pharm.*, **30**, 63–72.

BOUCSEIN, W. (1992) *Electrochemical Activity.* New York: Plenum Press.

BRAND, R.M., HANNAH, T.L., NORRIS, J. and IVERSEN, P.L. (2001) Transdermal delivery of antisense oligonucleotides can induce changes in gene expression *in vivo. Antisense and Nucleic Acid Drug Dev.*, **11**, 1–6.

BRAIN, S.D. and EDWARDSON, J.A. (1989) Neuropeptides and the skin. In GREAVES, M.W. and SHUSTER, S. (eds) *Pharmacology of the Skin I.* Berlin: Springer Verlag, 409–422.

BURNETTE, R.R. (1989) Iontophoresis. In HADGRAFT, J. and GUY, R.H. (eds) *Transdermal Drug Delivery.* New York: Marcel Dekker, 247–291.

BURNETTE, R. and MARRERO, D. (1986) Comparison between the iontophoretic and passive transport of thyrotropin releasing hormone across excised nude mouse skin. *J. Pharm. Sci.*, **75**, 738–743.

BURNETTE, R.R. and ONGPIPATTANAKUL, B. (1987) Characterization of the perselective properties of excised human skin during iontophoresis. *J. Pharm. Sci.*, **77**, 132–137.

CHANG, S. and BANGA, A.K. (1998) Transdermal iontophoretic delivery of hydrocortisone from cyclodextrin solutions. *J. Pharm. Pharmacol.*, **50**, 635–640.

CHIEN, Y.W., LELAWONGS, P., SIDDIQUI, O., SUN, Y. and SHI, W.M. (1990) Facilitated transdermal delivery of therapeutic peptides and proteins by iontophoretic delivery of devices. *J. Control. Rel.*, **13**, 263–278.

CHO, Y.B. and KITAMURA, K. (1988) Short-term effects of iontophoresis on the structure of the guinea pig tympanic membrane. *Acta Otolaryngol. (Stockh.)*, **106**, 161–170.

CURDY, C., KALIA, Y.N. and GUY, R.H. (2002) Post-iontophoresis recovery of human skin impedance *in vivo. Eur. J. Pharm. Biopharm.*, **53**, 15–21.

CULLANDER, C. (1992) What are the pathways of iontophoretic current flow through mammalian skin? *Adv. Drug Del. Rev.*, **9**, 119–135.

CULLANDER, C. and GUY, R.H. (1991) Sites of iontophoretic current flow into the skin: identification and characterization with the vibrating probe electrode. *J. Invest. Dermatol.*, **97**, 55–64.

DALSGAARD, C.J., JERNBECK, J., STAINS, W., KJARTANSSON, J., HAEGERSTRAND, A., HÖKFELT, T., BRODIN, E., CUELLO, A.C. and BROWN, J.C. (1989) Calcitonin gene-related peptide-like immunoreactivity in nerve fibers in human skin. *Histochemistry*, **91**, 35–38.

DELTERZO, S., BEHL, C.R. and NASH, R.A. (1989) Iontophoretic transport of a homologous series of ionized and non-ionized model compounds: Influence of hydrophobicity and mechanistic interpretation. *Pharm. Res.*, 6, 89–90.

FISHER, A.A. (1978) Dermatitis associated with transcutaneous electrical nerve stimualtion. *Cutis.*, 21, 24–47.

GANGAROSA, L.P. (1981) Defining a practical solution for iontophoretic local anesthesia of skin. *Methods Fund. Exp. Clin. Pharmacol.*, 3, 83–94.

GANGAROSA, L.P., PARK, N.H., WIGGINS, C.A. and HILL, J.M. (1980) Increased penetration of nonelectrolytes into hairless mouse skin during iontophoretic water transport (iontohydrokinesis). *J. Pharmacol. Exp. Ther.*, 212, 377–381.

GIBSON, L.E. and COOKE, R.E. (1959) A test for the concentration of electrolytes in sweat in cystic fibrosis of the pancreas utilizing pilocarpine by iontophoresis. *Pediatrics*, 23, 545–549.

GREEN, P.G., HINZ, R.S., CULLANDER, C., YAMANE, G and GUY, R.H. (1991) Iontophoretic delivery of amino acids and amino acid derivatives across the skin *in vitro*. *Pharm. Res.*, 8, 1113–1120.

GRIMNES, S. (1984) Pathways of ionic flow through the human skin *in vivo*. *Acta Derm. Venereol. (Stockh.)*, 64, 93–98.

GUY, R.H. (1995) A sweeter life for diabetics? *Nature Med.*, 1, 1132–1133.

GUY, R.H., POTS, R.O. and TAMADA, J.A. (1996) Non-invasive techniques for *in vivo* glucose sensing. *Diabetes, Nutrition and Metabolism*, 9, 42–46.

HAGA, M., AKATAMI, M., KIKUCHI, J., UENO, Y. and HAYASHI, M. (1997) Transdermal iontophoretic delivery of insulin using a photoetched micro-device. *J. Control. Rel.*, 43, 139–149.

HARRIS, P.R. (1982) Iontophoresis: Clinical research in musculoskeletal inflammatory conditions. *J. Orth. Sport Phy. Ther.*, 4, 109–112.

HOLDINESS, M.R. (1989) A review of contact dermatitis associated with transdermal therapeutic systems. *Contact Dermatitis.*, 20, 3–9.

HÖLZLE, E. and ALBERTI, N. (1987) Long-term efficacy and side effects of tap water iontophoresis of palmoplantar hyperhydrosis-the usefulness of home therapy. *Dermatologica.*, 175, 126–135.

HUI, X., ANIGBOGU, A., SINGH, P., XIONG, G., POBLETE, N., LUI, P. and MAIBACH, H.I. (2001) Pharmacokinetic and local tissue disposition of [^{14}C]-Sodium diclofenac following iontophoresis and systemic administration in rabbits. *J. Pharm. Sci.*, 90, 1269–1276.

JADOUL, A., DOUCET, J., DURAND, D. and PREAT, V. (1996) Modifications induced on stratum corneum structure after *in vitro* iontophoresis: ATR-FTIR and X-ray scattering studies. *J. Control. Rel.*, **42**, 165–173.

JONES, H.L. (1907) The principles of ionic medication. *Proc. Royal Soc. Med.*, **1**, 65–82.

KASTING, G.B. and KEISTER, J.C. (1989) Application of electrodiffusion theory for a homogeneous membrane to iontophoretic transport through skin. *J. Control. Rel.*, **8**, 195–210.

KASTRIP, E.K. and BOYD, J.R. (1983) *Drug: Facts and Comparisons*. St. Louis: Lippincott.

KELLOG, D.L., JOHNSON, J.M. and KOSIBA, W.A. (1989) Selective abolition of adrenergic vasoconstrictor responses in skin by local iontophoresis by bretylium. *Am. J. Physiol.*, **257**, H1599–H1606.

KOIZUMI, T., KAKEMI, M., KATAYAMA, K., INADA, H., SUDEJI, K. and KAWASAKI, M. (1990) Transfer of diclofenac sodium across excised guinea pig skin on high-frequency pulse iontophoresis II. Factors affecting steady-state transport rate. *Chem. Pharm. Bull.*, **38**, 1022–1023.

KUMAR, S., CHAR, H., PATEL, S., PIEMONTESES, D., IQBAL, K., MALICK, A.W., NEUGROSCHEL, E. and BEHL, C.R. (1992) Effect of iontophoresis on *in vitro* skin permeation of an analogue of growth hormone releasing factor in the hairless guinea pig model. *J. Pharm. Sci.*, **8**, 635–639.

LAU, D.T., SHARKEY, J.W., PETRYK, L., MANCUSO, F.A., YU, Z. and TSE, F.L.S. (1994) Effect of current magnetude and drug concentration on iontophoretic delivery of octreotide acetate (sandostatin) in the rabbit. *Pharm. Res.*, **11**, 1742–1746.

LEDGER, P.W. (1992) Skin biological issues in electrically enhanced transdermal delivery. *Adv. Drug Del. Rev.*, **9**, 289–307.

LEDUC, S. (1900) Introduction of medicinal substances into the depth of tissues by electric current. *Ann D'electrobiol.*, **3**, 545–560.

LELAWONGS, P., LIU, J.C., SIDDIQUI, O. and CHIEN, Y.W. (1989) Transdermal iontophoretic delivery of arginine-vasopressin (I): Physicochemical considerations. *Int. J. Pharm.*, **56**, 13–22.

LICHT, S. (1983) History of electrotherapy. In STILLWELL, G.K. (ed.) *Therapeutic Electricity and Ultraviolet Radiation*, Baltimore: Williams and Wilkins, 1–64.

LIU, J.C., SUN, O., SIDDIQUI, O., CHIEN, Y.W., SHI, W.M. and LI, J. (1988) Blood glucose control in diabetic rats by transdermal iontophoretic delivery of insulin. *Int. J. Pharm.*, **44**, 197–204.

CHAPTER 10

MALONEY, J.M., BEZZANT, J.L., STEPHEN, R.L. and PETELENTZ, T.J. (1992) Ionto-phoretic administration of lidocaine anesthesia in office practice: An appraisal. *J. Dermatol. Surg. Oncol.*, **18**, 937–940.

MARRO, D., GUY, R.H. and DELGADO-CHARRO, M. (2001) Characterization of the iontophoretic permselectivity properties of human and pig skin. *J. Control. Rel.*, **70**, 213–217.

MARRO, D., DELGADO-CHARRO, M. and GUY, R.H. (2001a) Contributions of electromigration and electroosmosis to iontophoretic drug delivery. *Pharm. Res.*, **18**, 1701–1708.

MARRO, D., DELGADO-CHARRO, M. and GUY, R.H. (2001b) Optimizing ionto-phoretic delivery: Identification and distribution of the charge-carrying species. *Pharm. Res.*, **18**, 1709–1713.

MASADA, T., HIGUCHI, W.I., SRINIVASAN, V., ROHR, U., FOX, J., BEHL, C.R. and PONS, S. (1989) Examination of iontophoretic transport of drugs across skin: Baseline studies with the four electrode system. *Int. J. Pharm.*, **49**, 57–62.

MCEVAN-JENKINSON, D., MCLEON, J.A. and WALTON, G.S. (1974) The potential use of iontophoresis in the treatment of skin disorders. *Vet. Rec.*, **94**, 8–11.

MERINO, V., KALIA, Y.N. and GUY, R.H. (1997) Transdermal therapy and diagnosis by iontophoresis. *Trends Biotechnol.*, **15**, 288–290.

MEYER, R.B. (1988) Successful transdermal administration of therapeutic doses of a polypeptide to normal human volunteers. *Clin. Pharmacol. Ther.*, **44**, 607–612.

MILLARD, J. and BARRY, B.W. (1988) The iontophoresis of water and glutamic acid across full thickness human skin and shed snake skin. *J. Pharm. Pharmacol.*, **40**(suppl.), 41.

MILLER, L.L., KOLASKIE, C.J., SMITH, G.A. and RIVIERE, J. (1990) Transdermal iontophoresis of gonadotropin releasing hormone (LHRH) and two analogues. *J. Pharm. Sci.*, **79**, 490–493.

MOLITOR, H. (1943) Pharmacologic aspects of drug administration by ion-transfer. *The Merck Report.*, January, 22–29.

MOLITOR, H. and FERNANDEZ, L. (1939) Studies on iontophoresis. I. Experimental studies on the causes and prevention of burns. *Am. J. Med. Sci.*, **198**, 778–785.

MONTEIRO-RIVIERE, N.A. (1990) Altered epidermal morphology secondary to lidocaine iontophoresis: *in vivo* and *in vitro* studies in porcine skin. *Fundam. Appl. Toxicol.*,**15**, 174–175.

MONTEIRO-RIVIERE, N.A. (1991) Identification of the pathway of transdermal iontophoretic drug delivery: ultrastructural studies using mercuric chloride *in vivo* in pigs. *Pharm. Res.*, **8**, S41.

OKABE, K., YAMAGUCHI, H. and KAWAI, Y. (1986) New iontophoretic transdermal administration of the betablocker metoprolol. *J. Control. Rel.*, **4**, 79–85.

O'MALLEY, E.P. and OESTER, Y.T. (1955) Influence of some physical chemical factors on iontophoresis using radio isotopes. *Arch. Phys. Med. Rehabil.*, **36**, 310–316.

PAPA, C.M. and KLIGMAN, A.M. (1966) Mechanism of eccrine anhydrosis. *J. Invest. Dermatol.*, **47**, 1–9.

PHIPPS, J.B. and GYORY, J.R. (1992) Transdermal ion migration. *Adv. Drug Del. Rev.*, **9**, 137–176.

PHIPPS, J.B., PADMANABHAN, R.V. and LATTIN, G.A. (1989) Iontophoretic delivery of model inorganic and drug ions. *J. Pharm. Sci.*, **78**, 365–369.

PIKAL, M.J. (2001) The role of electroosmotic flow in transdermal iontophoresis. *Adv. Drug Del. Rev.*, **46**, 281–305.

POTTS, R.O., TIERNEY, M.J. and TAMADA, J.A. (2002) Glucose monitoring by reverse iontophoresis. *Diab. Met. Res. and Rev.*, **18**(Suppl. 1), 49–53.

PUTTEMANS, F.J.M., MASSART, D.L., GILLES, F., LIEVENS, P.C. and JONCKEER, M.H. (1982) Iontophoresis: Mechanism of action studied by potentiometry and x-ray fluorescence. *Arch. Phys. Med. Med. Rehabil.*, **63**, 176–180.

RAPPERPORT, A.S., LARSON, D.L., HENGES, D.F., LYNCH, J.B., BLOCKER, T.G. JR. and LEWIS, R.S. (1965) Iontophoresis. A method of antibiotic administration in the burn patient. *Plast. Reconstr. Surg.* **36**, 547–552.

RATTENBURY, J.M. and WORTHY, E. (1996) Is the sweat test safe? Some instances of burns received during pilocarpine iontophoresis. *Ann. Clin. Biochem.*, **33**, 456–458.

ROBERTS, M.S., SINGH, J., YOSHIDA, N.H. and CURRIES, K.I. (1990) Iontophoretic transport of selected solutes through human epidermis. In SCOTT, R.C., GUY, R.H. and HADGRAFT, J. (eds) *Prediction of Percutaneous Absorption*. London: IBC Technical Services, 230–241.

SAGE, B.H. and RIVIERE, J.E. (1992) Model systems in iontophoresis-transport efficacy. *Adv. Drug. Del. Rev.*, **9**, 265–287.

SANDERSON, J.E., CALDWELL, R.W., HSIAO, J. DISON, R. and TUTTLE, R.R. (1987) Noninvasive delivery of a novel ionotropic catecholamine: Iontophoretic versus intravenous infusion in dogs. *J. Pharm. Sci.*, **76**, 215–218.

SANDERSON, J.E., DE RIEL, S. and DIXON, R. (1989) Iontophoretic delivery of nonpeptide drugs: formulation optimization for maximum skin permeability. *J. Pharm. Sci.*, **78**, 361–364.

SCHULTZ, S.G. (1980) Basic Principles of Membrane Transport. New York: Cambridge University Press, pp. 21–30.

SCHWARTZ, B.K. and CLENDENNING, W.E. (1988) Allergic contact dermatitis from hydroxypropyl cellulose in a transdermal estradiol patch. *Contact Dermatitis*, **18**, 106–107.

SHARATA, H. and BURNETTE, R.R. (1989) Percutaneous absorption of electron-dense ions across normal and chemically perturbed skin. *J. Pharm. Sci.*, **77**, 27–32.

SIDDIQUI, O., ROBERTS, M.S. and POLACK, A.E. (1985) The effect of iontophoresis and vehicle pH on the *in vitro* permeation of lignocaine through human stratum corneum. *J. Pharm. Pharmacol.*, **37**, 732–735.

SIDDIQUI, O. ROBERTS, M.S. and POLACK, A.E. (1989) Iontophoretic transport of weak electrolytes through excised human stratum corneum. *J. Pharm. Pharmacol.*, **41**, 430–432.

SIDDIQUI, O., SUN, Y., LIU, J.C. and CHIEN, Y.W. (1987) Facilitated transdermal transport of insulin. *J. Pharm. Sci.*, **76**, 341–345.

SINGH, J. and MAIBACH, H.I. (1993) Topical iontophoretic drug delivery *in vivo*: Historical development, devices and future perspectives. *Dermatol.*, **187**, 235–238.

SINGH, P. and MAIBACH, H.I. (1994) Iontophoresis in drug delivery: Basic principles and applications. *Crit. Rev. Ther. Drug Carr. Sys.*, **11**, 161–213.

SINGH, P., BONIELLO, S., LIU, P. and DIHN, S. (1997) Iontophoretic transdermal delivery of methylphenidate hydrochloride. *Pharm. Res.*, **14**(suppl), 309–310.

SLOAN, J.B. and SOLTANI, K. (1986) Iontophoresis in dermatology. *J. Am. Acad. Dermatol.*, **15**, 671–684.

SRINIVASAN, V., HIGUCHI, W.I., SIMS, S.M.,GHANEM, A.H., BEHL, C.R. and PONS, S. (1989) Transdermal iontophoretic drug delivery: Mechanistic analysis and application to polypeptide delivery. *J. Pharm. Sci.*, **78**, 370–375.

SRINIVASAN, V., SU, M-H., HIGUCHI, W.I., SIMS, S.M.,GHANEM, A.H. and BEHL, C.R. (1990) Iontophoresis of polypeptides: effects of ethanol pretreatment of human skin. *Int. J. Pharm.*, **79**, 588–591.

SVEDMAN, P. and SVEDMAN, C. (1997) Skin mini-erosion sampling technique: feasibility study with regard to serial glucose measurement. *Pharm. Res.*, **15**, 883–888.

TAMADA, J., BOHANNON, N.J.V. and POTTS, R.O. (1995) Measurement of glucose in diabetic subjects using noninvasive transdermal extraction. *Nature Med.*, **1**, 1198–1201.

TASHIRO, Y., KATO, Y, HAYAKAWA, E. and ITO, K. (2000) Iontophoretic transdermal delivery of ketoprofen: effect of iontophoresis on drug transfer from skin to cutaneous blood. *Biol. Pharm. Bull.*, **23**, 1486–1490.

TEYSSANDIER, M.J., BRIFFOD, P. and ZIEGLER, G. (1977) Interêt de la dielectolyse de ketoprofene en heumalogie et en petite traumalogie. *Sci. Med.*, **8**, 157–162.

THYSMAN, S. and PREAT, V. (1993) *In vivo* iontophoresis of fentanyl and sufentanyl in rats: Pharmacokinetics and Acute Antinoiceptive effects. *Anesth Analg.*, **77**, 61–66.

THYSMAN, S., PREAT, V. and ROLAND, M. (1991) Factors affecting iontophoretic mobility of metoprolol. *J. Pharm. Sci.*, **81**, 670–675.

TIERNEY, M.J., KIM, H.L., BURNS, M.D., TAMADA, J.A. and POTTS, R.O. (2000) Electroanalysis of glucose in transcutaneously extracted samples. *Electroanalysis*, **12**, 666–671.

TIERNEY, M.J., TAMADA, J.A., POTTS, R.O., JOVANOVIC, L., GARG, S. and THE CYGNUS RESEARCH TEAM (2001a) Evaluation of Glucowatch Biographer: A continual, non-invasive, Glucose Monitor for patients with diabetes. *Biosensors and Bioelectronics*, **16**, 621–629.

TIERNEY, M.J., TAMADA, J.A. and POTTS, R.O. (2001b) A non-invasive glucose monitor: The Glucowatch® Biographer. *The Biochemist*, **23**, 17–19.

TYLE, P. (1986) Iontophoretic devices for drug delivery. *Pharm. Res.*, **3**, 318–326.

WALBERG, J.E. (1968) Transepidermal or transfollicular absorption. *Acta Derm. Venereol. (Stockh.)*, **48**, 336–344.

WALBERG, J.E. (1970) Skin clearance of iontophoretically administered chromium (51Cr) and sodium (22Na) ions in the guinea pig. *Acta Derm. Venereol. (Stockh.)*, **50**, 255–262.

WEARLEY, L.L. and CHIEN, Y.W. (1989) Iontophoretic transdermal permeation of verapamil II: Factors affecting the reversibility of skin permeability. *J.Control. Rel.*, **9**, 231–281.

CHAPTER 10

YOSHIDA, N.H. and ROBERTS, M.S. (1993) Solute molecular size and transdermal iontophoresis across excised human skin. *J. Control. Rel.*, **25**, 177–195.

ZELTZER, L., REGALADO, M., NITCHTER, L.S., BARTON, D., JENNINGS, S. and PITT, L. (1991) Iontophoresis versus subcutaneous injection: A comparison of the two methods of local anesthesia in children. *Pain*, **44**, 73–84.

ZUGERMAN, C. (1982) Dermatitis from transcutaneous electrical nerve stimulation. *J. Am. Acad. Dermatol.*, **6**, 936–939.

Irritant Dermatitis (Irritation)

SARA WELTFRIEND, MICHAL RAMON AND
HOWARD I MAIBACH

Contents

11.1 Clinical aspects

11.2 Localization of irritant contact dermatitis

11.3 External factors

11.4 Predisposing factors

11.5 Predictive irritancy testing

11.6 Histology, histopathology, and pathology

11.7 Mechanism of irritant dermatitis

11.8 Treatment

11.1 CLINICAL ASPECTS

Irritation, or irritant dermatitis, previously considered a monomorphous process, is now understood to be a complex biologic syndrome, with a diverse pathophysiology, natural history, and clinical appearance. Thus, the clinical appearance of irritant contact dermatitis varies depending on multiple external and internal factors. The exact mechanisms of irritant action are incompletely understood, but it seems likely that there is an immunologic-like component to the irritant response. The actual types, with reference to major characteristics in the clinical appearance, are listed in Table 11.1.

11.1.1 Acute irritant dermatitis (primary irritation)

When exposure is sufficient and the offending agent is potent, such as acids or alkaline solutions, classic symptoms of acute skin irritation are seen. Contact with a strong primary irritant is often accidental, and an acute irritant dermatitis is elicited in almost anyone independent of constitutional susceptibility. This classic, acutely developing dermatitis usually heals soon after exposure. The healing of acute irritant dermatitis is described as a *decrescendo phenomenon*,

TABLE 11.1:

Clinical classification of irritation

Irritation	Onset	Prognosis
1. Acute (primary) irritant dermatitis	acute, often single exposure	good
2. Irritant reaction	acute, often multiple exposures	good
3. Delayed acute irritant dermatitis	delayed, 12–24 h or longer	good
4. Subjective irritation	acute	excellent
5. Suberythematous (suberythematous) irritation	slowly developing	variable
6. Cumulative irritant contact dermatitis	slowly developing (weeks to months)	variable
7. Traumiterative dermatitis	slowly developing (weeks to months)	variable
8. Traumatic irritant dermatitis	slowly developing following trauma	variable
9. Pustular and acneiform dermatitis	moderate-slow developing (weeks to months)	variable
10. Exsiccation eczematoid	moderate-slow developing (weeks to months)	variable
11. Friction dermatitis	moderate-slow developing (weeks to months)	variable

where the irritant reaction quickly peaks and then immediately begins to heal upon removal of irritant. In unusual cases the dermatitis may persist for months after exposure, followed by complete resolution. The availability of the material Safety Data Sheet and data from the single-application Draize rabbit test combined with activities of industrial hygienists and other informed personnel greatly decreased the frequency of such dermatitis in industry. Further educational efforts and appropriate industrial engineering should make this form of irritation a rarity.

11.1.2 Delayed, acute irritant contact dermatitis

Some chemicals like anthralin (dithranol), benzalkonium chloride and hydrofluoric acid are chemicals which may elicit a retarded inflammatory response, so that inflammation is not seen until 8–24 h or more after exposure (Malten *et al.*, 1979; Lovell *et al.*, 1985) (Table 11.2). Except for the delayed onset, the clinical appearance and course resemble those of acute irritant contact dermatitis. The delayed acute irritant dermatitis, because of its delayed onset, is often confused with allergic contact dermatitis; appropriately performed diagnostic patch tests easily separate the two.

11.1.3 Irritant reaction

Individuals extensively exposed to irritants, in the first months of exposure, often develop erythematous, chapped skin on the dorsum of the hands and fingers. This irritant reaction (Fregert, 1981; Griffiths and Wilkinson, 1985; Hjorth and Avnstorp, 1986) may be considered a pre-eczematous expression

TABLE 11.2:
Chemicals inducing delayed acute irritation

Anthralin
Bis(2-chloroethyl)sulfide
Butanedioldiacrylate
Dichloro(2-chlorovinyl)arsine
Epichlorhydrin
Ethylene oxide
Hydrofluoric acid
Hexanedioldiacrylate
Hydroxypropylacrylate
Podophyllin
Propane sulfone

of acute skin irritation. It is frequently seen in hairdressers and variable wet work-performing employees repeatedly exposed. Repeated irritant reactions sometimes lead to contact dermatitis, with good prognosis, although chronic contact dermatitis may also develop.

11.1.4 Subjective/sensory irritation

Subjective irritation is experienced by some individuals ("stingers") in contact with certain chemicals (Frosch and Kligman, 1982; Lammintausta *et al.*, 1988b). Itching, stinging, or tingling is experienced, for example, from skin contact with lactic acid, which is a model for nonvisible cutaneous irritation. The threshold for this reaction varies between subjects, independent of susceptibility to other irritation types. The quality as well as the concentration of the exposing agent is also important, and neural pathways may be contributory, but the pathomechanism is unknown. Some sensory irritation may be subclinical contact urticaria. Screening raw ingredients and final formulations in the guinea pig ear swelling test (Lahti and Maibach, 1985) or the human forehead assay allows us to minimize the amount of subclinical contact urticaria. Although subjective irritation may have a neural component, some studies suggest that the blood vessel may be more responsive in "stingers" than nonstingers (Lammintausta *et al.*, 1988b; Berardesca *et al.*, 1991). At least 10 percent of women complain of stinging with certain facial products; thus, further work is needed to develop a strategy to overcome this type of discomfort.

11.1.5 Suberythematous irritation

In the early stages of skin irritation, subtle skin damage may occur without visible inflammation. As a correlate of nonvisible irritation, objectively registered alterations in the damaged epidermis have been reported (Berardesca and Maibach, 1988a, b; van der Valk *et al.*, 1985; Lammintausta *et al.*, 1988b; Charbonnier *et al.*, 2001). Common symptoms of suberythematous irritation include burning, itching or stinging. Consumer dissatisfaction with many chemicals may result from exposure to this low-grade irritation; thus the patient feels more than the physician observes. It is customary in Japan to screen new chemicals, cosmetics, and textiles for subtle signs of stratum corneum damage, employing replicas of stratum corneum (the Kawai method) (Kawai, 1971).

11.1.6   Cumulative irritant dermatitis

Multiple subthreshhold skin insults induced by repeated applications of weak irritants may lead to cumulative cutaneous irritation. In cumulative cutaneous irritation, the frequency of exposure is too high in relation to the skin recovery time. Acute irritant skin reaction is not seen in the majority of patients, but mild or moderate invisible skin changes. Repeated skin exposures and minor reactions lead to a manifest dermatitis when the irritant load exceeds the threshold for visible effects. The development of a cumulative irritant dermatitis was carefully documented by Malten and den Arend (1978) and Malten *et al.* (1979). Classic signs are erythema and increasing dryness, followed by hyperkeratosis with frequent cracking and occasional erythema.Cumulative irritant dermatitis is the most common type of irritant contact dermatitis. This syndrome may develop after days, weeks, or years of subtle exposure to chemical substances. Variation in individual susceptibility increases the multiplicity of clinical findings. Delayed onset and variable attack lead to confusion with allergic contact dermatitis. To rule out allergic etiology, appropriate diagnostic patch testing is indicated. Models of cumulative irritant dermatitis have been developed (Freeman and Maibach, 1988; Widmer *et al.*, 1994) (Figure 11.1).

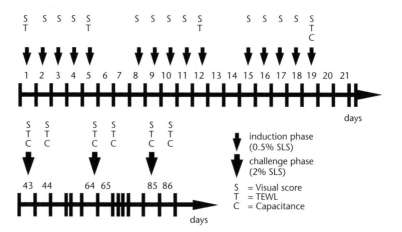

Figure 11.1: Schematic display of the experimental protocol. The arrows refer to time of dosing.
Adapted from Widmer *et al.* (1994).

11.1.7 Traumiterative irritant dermatitis

Traumiterative irritant dermatitis in the older German literature ("traumiterative" = traumas repeating) (von Hagerman, 1957; Agrup, 1969), is a consequence of too frequent repetition of one impairing factor. This syndrome and cumulative irritant dermatitis are very similar clinically.

11.1.8 Traumatic irritant dermatitis

Traumatic irritant dermatitis develops after acute skin trauma. The skin does not completely heal, but erythema, vesicles and/or vesicopapules, and scaling appear. The clinical course later resembles nummular (coin-shaped) dermatitis. This may occur after burns or lacerations and after acute irritant dermatitis: It may be compounded by a concurrent allergen exposure. The healing period is generally prolonged. Often these patients are considered to have a factitial dermatitis because of a healing phase followed by exacerbation. Although factitial (unnatural) aspects may occur in some patients, this peculiar form of irritation appears to be a disease *sui generis*. Its chronicity and recalcitrance to therapy provides a challenge to both patient and physician. We have no information explaining why the occasional patient develops this phenomenon, and how this patient differs from the general population. Many such patients are considered factitial in origin if the dermatologist is unaware of the syndrome.

11.1.9 Pustular and acneiform irritant dermatitis

Pustular and acneiform irritant dermatitis may develop from exposure to metals, oils and greases, tar, asphalt, chlorinated naphthalenes, and polyhalogenated naphthalenes (Wahlberg and Maibach, 1981, 1982, Fischer and Rystedt, 1985, Dooms-Goossens *et al.*, 1986). In occupational exposure, only a minority of subjects develop pustular or acneiform dermatitis. Thus, the development of this type of irritant contact dermatitis appears to be dependent on both constitutional and chemical factors. Cosmetic dermatitis commonly assumes this morphology.

11.1.10 Exsiccation eczematoid

Exsiccation eczematoid is seen mainly in elderly individuals during the winter months, when humidity is low. Patients suffer from intensive itching, and their

■ CHAPTER 11 ■

skin appears dry with ichthyosiform scaling. The condition is thought to be due to a decrease in skin surface lipid and persistence of both peripheral and non-peripheral corneodesmosomes in the upper stratum corneum (Simon *et al.*, 2001). In severe cases a reduction of skin content of amino-acid due to low profilaggrin biosynthesis was found (Horii *et al.*, 1989).

11.1.11   Friction dermatitis

This is sometimes seen on the hands and knees in the workplace, and results from frictional trauma. The syndrome has been characterized by Susten (1985).

In addition to the usual clinical features of dermatitis, the clinical presentations vary according to the irritant in question (Table 11.3). Ulcerative lesions can

TABLE 11.3:
Clinical features that may suggest the etiology of irritant contact dermatitis

Ulcerations:
> Strong acids, especially chromic, hydrofluoric, nitric, hydrochloric, sulphuric. Strong alkalis, especially calcium oxide, sodium hydroxide, potassium hydroxide, ammonium hydroxide, calcium hydroxide, sodium metasilicate, sodium silicate, potassium cyanide, trisodium phosphate. Salts, especially arsenic trioxide, dichromates. Solvents, especially acrylonitrile, carbon bisulfide. Gases, especially ethylene oxide, acrylonitrile.

Folliculitis and acneiform:
> Arsenic trioxide, glass fibers, oils and greases, tar, asphalt. Chlorinated naphthalenes, polyhalogenated biphenyls and others.

Miliaria:
> Occlusive clothing and dressing, adhesive tape, ultraviolet, infrared, aluminum chloride.

Pigmentary alterations:
> Hyperpigmentation, any irritant or allergen, especially phototoxic agents such as psoralens, tar, asphalt, phototoxic plants, others. Metals, such as inorganic arsenic (systemically), silver, gold, bismuth, mercury. Radiation, ultraviolet, infrared, microwave, ionizing. Hypopigmentation, p-tert-amylphenol, p-tert-butylphenol, hydroquinone, monobenzyl ethyl hydroquinone, monomethyl hydroquinone ether, p-tert-catechol, p-cresol, 3-hydroxyanisole, butylated hydroxyanisole, 1-tert-butyl-3 ,4-catechol, 1-isopropyl-3, 4-catechol, 4-hydroxypropriophenone.

Alopecia:
> Borax, chloroprene dimmers.

Urticaria:
> Numerous chemicals, cosmetics, animal products, foods, plants, textile, woods.

Granulomas:
> Keratin, silica, beryllium, talc, cotton fibers, bacteria, fungi, parasites, and parasite parts.

develop from skin contact with strong acids or strong alkalis. Calcium oxide and calcium hydroxide, sodium hydroxide, sodium metasilicate and sodium silicate, potassium cyanide, and trisodium phosphate may induce strong cutaneous irritation with ulcerations. Chrome ulcers are the most common type of cutaneous ulcers induced by irritation of dichromates. Compounds of beryllium, arsenic, or cadmium are also capable of inducing strong irritation and ulcers. Solvents such as acrylonitrile and carbon bisulfide as well as gaseous ethylene oxide are examples of contactants that may induce ulceration in certain occupations. Cutaneous ulcerations develop from the direct corrosive and necrotizing effect of the chemical on the living tissue. Exposed areas, where both friction and chemical irritation are associated, are most susceptible for ulcers; minor preceding trauma in the exposed skin increases the risk. The ulcerations tend to be deeper, with an undermined thickened border, and the exudate under the covering crusts predisposes to infection. Cutaneous granulomas are considered a variant of irritant contact dermatitis when caused by a biologically inactive substance inoculated into the skin. A granuloma appears as a focal, tumid lesion persisting chronically in its primary site. It is subjectively symptomless. Macrophages respond with phagocytosis to the foreign body inoculation, and even giant cells may be seen (Epstein, 1983). Powders, lead, and metals such as metallic mercury, beryllium, and silica are examples of substances that elicit toxic skin granulomas (Kresbach *et al.*, 1971). Miliaria is induced by aluminum chloride, hyperpigmentation by heavy metals and hypopigmentation by chemicals such as p-tert-butylphenol (O'Malley *et al.*, 1988).

11.2 LOCALIZATION OF IRRITANT CONTACT DERMATITIS

In irritant contact dermatitis the exposed sites are first affected. The dorsal and lateral aspects of the hands and fingers have the greatest contact with chemical irritants. Thick stratum corneum provides better protection for palms in most occupations. Other unidentified factors may also protect the palms and soles. The degree of protection may be greater than what might be expected from decreases in skin penetration. Some compounds are almost as permeable through the palm as the forearm (Feldmann and Maibach, 1967a, b). Dermatitis on the anterior thighs, upper back, axillary areas, and feet may be due to an irritant in clothing. When dermatitis is observed on the face, under the collar or belt, or in the flexures, airborne irritants (e.g., dust) may be involved.

11.3 EXTERNAL FACTORS

The onset and development of irritant contact dermatitis depend on external factors, such as characteristics of the molecule, exposure time, cumulative effect with other irritants, and environmental conditions.

11.3.1 Irritants

Many chemicals qualify as irritant when the exposing dose is high (Kligman and Wooding, 1967) (Figure 11.2). Molecular size, ionization, polarization, fat solubility, and other factors that are important in skin penetration are also important in cutaneous irritation. The threshold of strength and quality of irritation depends on the physicochemical properties of the substance.

11.3.2 Exposure

The absorbed dose may vary when the substance is suspended in different vehicles (Cooper, 1985; Gummer, 1985). The solubility of the irritant in the vehicle and the inherent irritancy of the vehicle have an impact on each reaction (Flannigan and Tucker, 1985). The effective tissue dose depends on concentration, volume, application time, and duration on and in the skin. Long exposure time and large volume increase penetration, thus, greater response may be expected (Aramaki *et al.*, 2001). If exposure is repeated, the recovery from previous exposure(s) affects the subsequent response. Sometimes a shorter, repeated exposure leads to a lengthened recovery period (Malten and den Arend, 1978). This was demonstrated in experimental studies with dimethyl sulfoxide (DMSO). Intermittent application leads to a different response as compared with one lengthened application (Lammintausta *et al.*, 1988a). These experimental observations are consistent with the multiple clinical appearances of cumulative irritant dermatitis.

11.3.3 Multiple simultaneous exposures

Simultaneous or subsequent exposure may lead to an additive effect and increased reaction, although each chemical alone would elicit only a minor reaction, or none. On the other hand, subsequent exposure may lead to a decreased response. For instance, exposure to a detergent and then to a soap led to a response less than exposure to a detergent alone. The detergent was washed

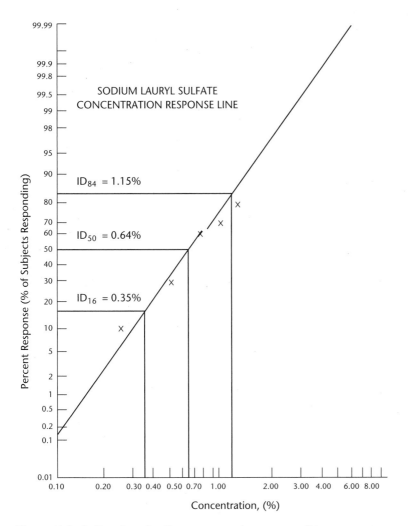

Figure 11.2: Sodium lauryl sulfate concentration response line. Adapted from Kligman and Wooding (1967).

away by the subsequent soap exposure (Malten, 1981). Furthermore, when benzalkonium chloride, a cationic surfactant was applied to skin exposed to sodium dodecyl sulfate, an anionic surfactant, the resulting irritant reaction was attenuated (McFadden *et al.*, 2000). The outcome of multiple, subsequent, or simultaneous exposures is some-times unexpected (Lammintausta *et al.*, 1987a) and rules must be sought (Pittz *et al.*, 1985).

A "crossover" phenomenon between two distinct irritants has been also suggested. In this study human volunteers were irritated first with retinoic acid

(RA), then with sodium lauryl sulfate (SLS). Alternatively, SLS was applied the first day and RA the following day. The serial application of SLS/RA caused considerably more erythema, more scaling, higher transepidermal water loss (TEWL) values and decreased stratum corneum hydration than the serial application of RA/SLS or the effect of the individual components alone (Effendy et al., 1996). A pharmacological synergism or antagonism between the compounds may explain this phenomenon. Alternatively, the effects of one agent may result in a change in the percutaneous penetration kinetics of the other. Subsequently, when SLS and toluene were concurrently applied, significantly stronger effects were noted than twice daily application of SLS or toluene alone (Wigger-Alberti et al., 2000).

11.3.4 Environmental factors

Low environmental humidity enhances irritability: skin tests with irritants produce more and stronger reactions in winter when the weather is cool, windy, and dry (Hannuksela et al., 1975). It also produces variable irritation symptoms: itching and erythema associated with whealing or erythema and scaling (Rycroft, 1981). Stronger reactions to SLS were found during the winter than the summer as indicated by visual scorring and by measurements of TEWL (Agner and Serup, 1989). Temperature may be important, with warm temperatures generally more damaging than cool (Rothenborg et al., 1977). Warm citral perfume produced more irritation than citral at lower temperature, and warm temperature increased also skin irritation induced by surfactant (Berardesca, 1995). Furthermore, in vitro penetration of SLS increased with increasing temperature (Emilson et al., 1993). It is well known that water temperature influences the irritant capacity of a detergent. Higher ionic content and higher temperature were found to be determinative for the irritant potential (Clarys et al., 1997). Changes in temperature may be an important means for prevention of irritant contact dermatitis (Ohlenschlaeger, 1996). UVB diminished immediate reactions induced by phenol and DMSO and delayed reactions from SLS and DMSO (Larmi et al., 1989). Occlusion enhances stratum corneum hydration and often increases percutaneous absorption and acute irritation (Table 11.4). On the other hand, it compromises skin barrier function by impairing passive transepidermal water loss (TEWL) at the application site. Thus, skin reactions frequently become stronger when the chemical is applied under occlusion (van der Valk et al., 1989a), providing a humid environment that minimizes evaporation and makes the stratum corneum more permeable.

TABLE 11.4:

Effect of duration of occlusion on percutaneous absorption of malathion in humans

Duration (h)	Absorption (%)
0[a]	9.6
0.5	7.3
1	12.7
2	16.6
4	24.2
8	38.8
24	62.8

[a] Immediate wash with soap and water. From Feldmann and Maibach (1974).

Gloves and clothing increase the susceptibility for irritant dermatitis. Frequent changes of these articles is important, to minimize the humid and occlusive environment. Occlusion alone may produce cytological damage to the skin that had been termed hydration dermatitis by Kligman. Stratum corneum lipids are implicated as an important determinant in water-retaining properties and the barier function. A seasonal comparison of the total lipid amounts extracted from the stripped stratum corneum revealed an increased level in summer, while ceramides were slightly increased in winter compared with summer (Yoshikawa et al., 1994).

11.3.5 Airborne irritation

Airborne irritation dermatitis is located most commonly in exposed skin areas, such as the face, hands, and arms (Lachapelle, 1986). Volatile chemicals and dusts are common sources of exposure, but even sharp particles in dust may induce lesions (Table 11.5). Airborne irritation is a type of exposure in which physical sources of irritation frequently exacerbate the response with an additive influence. For instance, sunlight, wind, and cold air are additive to chemical exposure. Depending on the occupational situation, multiple environmental and occupational irritants may induce airborne irritation (Dooms-Goossens et al., 1986).

CHAPTER 11

TABLE 11.5:
Common airborne irritants

Volatile substances
 Acids and alkalis, ammonia
 Cleaning products
 Formaldehyde
 Industrial solvents
 Noncarbon required (NCR) paper
 Epoxy resins
Foams (e.g., insulation foams in urea-formaldehyde process)
Powders
 Aluminum
 Anhydrous calcium silicate
 Cement
 Cleaning products
 Metallic oxides
Particles
 Tree-sawing particles
 Wool
 Plastics, dry
 Particles from plants
 Stone particles in mining

11.4 PREDISPOSING FACTORS

11.4.1 Methodological aspects

Although irritant contact dermatitis accounts for most occupational skin diseases and many non-occupational eczemas are exclusively or partially induced by irritation, in-depth investigation of irritant contact dermatitis is rare. Individual susceptibility to chemicals has been studied by documenting skin reactivity to model irritants. The intensity of the wheal created by DMSO, the time required to raise a blister (MBT) after cutaneous application of aluminum hydroxide solution and reactivity to SLS are examples of objective methods that have been used (Frosch, 1985). Stinging occurs with certain test substances (e.g., lactic acid), and clinical experiments provide some information about individual susceptibility (Frosch and Kligman, 1982). A method for quantifying interindividual differences in stratum corneum barrier function was described (Wilhelm *et al.*, 1990). This assay showed a high correlation between subjects developing increased water loss after application of sodium hydroxide and propensity for SLS damage (Figure 11.3). An increased baseline TEWL in patients with acute and healed irritant contact dermatitis was also

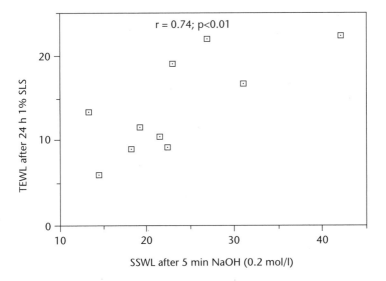

Figure 11.3: Relationship between skin surface water loss (SSWL), 5 min after a
5-min NaOH (0.2 mol/L)
Application, and transepidermal water loss (TEWL) after a 24h SLS patch test.
A significant linear correlation was observed between the two exposures
(*n* = 10 volunteers).
Adapted from Wilhelm *et al.* (1990).

noted (Effendy *et al.*, 1995). Later on, an association between reactivity to an
irritant and the likelihood of positive elicitation reactions to lower hapten
concentrations was noted (Smith *et al.*, 2002). These simple approaches
provided a first step toward a preemployment test for irritant dermatitis
potential. Recently, a nonatopic genetic marker for irritant susceptibility in
normal individuals was described. In this study, an association of TNF α gene
polymorphism at position –308 with susceptibility to irritant dermatitis was
noted (Allen *et al.*, 2000). However, despite important steps taken in the
investigation of the pathogenesis of irritant contact dermatitis, no experimental
design has proved entirely successful for the clinical evaluation of individual
susceptibility.

The main factors that influence individual proclivity are age, race, sex, site
and history of dermatitis.

11.4.2 Regional anatomic differences

Skin permeability is variable in different skin sites, being generally greatest in
thin skin areas (Cronin and Stoughton, 1962; Feldmann and Maibach, 1967a,b;

Tur *et al.*, 1985; Wester and Maibach, 1985, 1989), corresponding association between permeability, skin thickness, and skin irritation is expected, but direct correlation is lacking (Figure 11.4). Regional variation has been studied comparing the whealing response a variation of immediate irritation to DMSO and measuring differences in minimal blistering time (MBT) after topical ammonium hydroxide application in different skin sites (Frosch and Kligman, 1982). Both tests showed the mandibular area to be most reactive, followed by the upper back, forearm, lower leg, and palm. With DMSO whealing, the forehead was more sensitive than the back, the antecubital area reaction preceded that of the rest of the upper extremity, and the wrist was more sensitive than the leg. In patch testing, the irritant benzalkonium chloride and several allergens produced maximal reactivity in the upper back (Magnusson and Hersle, 1965), particularly the middle scapula (Flannigan *et al.*, 1984). The greater reactivity may be related to pressure in this area when sleeping (von Hornstein and Kienlein-Kletschka, 1982; Gollhausen and Kligman, 1985). TEWL measurements after exposure to SLS revealed the thigh as the most vulnerable site followed by the upper arm, abdomen, upper back, dorsal and volar forearm, postauricular and ankle, with the palm as the least vulnerable location (Cua *et al.*, 1990). In a similar study of the volar surface of the forearm the potential

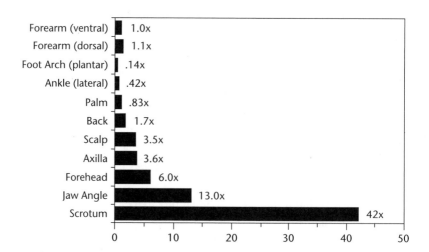

Figure 11.4: Anatomic regional variation of percutaneous absorption. This is the relative amount of hydrocortisone absorption from different sites. Skin thickness differences alone do not explain marked differences in flux.
Adapted from Feldmann and Maibach (1967b).

for irritation increased from the wrist to the cubital fossa (van der Valk, 1989b). Vulvar skin was significantly more reactive than the forearm to benzalkonium chloride (17 percent) and maleic acid (20 percent) (Britz and Maibach, 1979; Oriba *et al.*, 1989) (Figure 11.5). However, no differences were found between vulvar and forearm skin when sodium lauryl sulfate was applied at various concentrations (Elsner *et al.*, 1990). On the other hand, it is often noted in clinical occupational dermatology that male genitalia are affected in occupational irritant dermatitis. Since cutaneous irritant responses to various irritants might be mediated by distinctly different pathophysiological pathways regional susceptibility to diverse irritants vary accordingly (Patrick *et al.*, 1985). Additionally, stratum corneum barrier properties have been associated with stratum corneum lipid composition, regions with higher neutral lipids and lower sphingolipids are generally associated with superior barrier properties (Lampe *et al.*, 1983). Certain "inherent" differences between different skin sites in irritation reactivity may also exist.

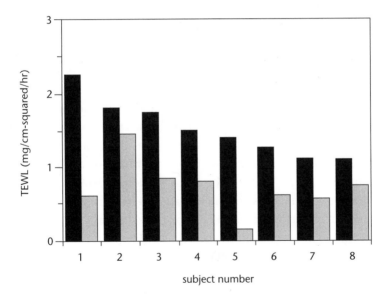

Figure 11.5: Transepidermal water loss from vulva and forearm. The black column is the vulva and the shaded column is the forearm. Note that the vulva is more permeable to water loss than the forearm: however, the ratio of the two is highly variable.
Adapted from Oriba *et al.* (1989).

■ CHAPTER 11 ■

11.4.3 Age

The threshold for skin irritation is decreased in babies, who develop dermatitis from irritation that does not occur in adult skin (Jordan and Blaney, 1982). Except for structural and functional immaturity of infant's skin, other factors (intestinal *Candida albicans*, low frequency of diaper changes) are contributory (Seymour *et al.*, 1987). Children below the age of 8 years are generally considered more susceptible to skin irritation (Mobly and Mansman, 1974; Epstein, 1971; Fisher, 1975), irritation susceptibility gradually decreases after this age. Maibach and Boisits (1982) define this data base; unfortunately, despite extensive chemical exposure of infants and children, our experimental evidence is lacking because of methodologic problems and limited data. Studies in newborn infants showed high and variable TEWL in the first 4 hours after birth settling to a constant level thereafter (Rutter, 1978), and newborn term infants have less TEWL than adults (Cunico *et al.*, 1977). No differences in baseline TEWL were demonstrable between young and old individuals (Thune *et al.*, 1988; Roskos, 1989; Wilhelm and Maibach, 1989). However, elderly subjects reacted to skin irritants less sharply and more slowly than younger individuals (Grove *et al.*, 1981; Lejman *et al.*, 1984; Schwindt *et al.*, 1998; Robinson, 2002), the difference was particularly significant in sites characterized by low TEWL under basal conditions (Cua *et al.*, 1990) (Table 11.6).When premenopausal and postmenopausal women were compared, age related differences were apparent in the forearm skin, but not the vulva (Elsner *et al.*, 1990). A corresponding alteration occurred with regard to cutaneous reactivity to allergens. With ammonium hydroxide skin tests, older subjects had a shorter reaction time (MBT, minimal blistering time), whereas the time needed to develop a tense blister was longer (Frosch and Kligman, 1977a), and a longer time was also needed for the resorption of a wheal elicited by saline injection (Kligman, 1976). Age-associated alterations in skin reactivity may be related to altered cutaneous penetration, although contradictory results have been reported (Christophers and Kligman, 1965; Tagami, 1971; DeSalva and Thompson, 1965; Guy *et al.*, 1985, Roskos *et al.*, 1990). Alterations in structural lipids (Elias, 1981), in cell composition (Gilchrest *et al.*, 1982) and renewal (Baker and Blair, 1968; Roberts and Marks, 1980) are reported in association with structural alteration (Montaga and Carlisle, 1979; Holzle *et al.*, 1986). Finally, the effects of stratum corneum hydration on irritancy potential is probably non-contributory, baseline capacitance did not differ between age groups on most regions (Cua *et al.*, 1990). Thus, age-associated alterations in cutaneous reactivity are expected; however, the subject requires more investigation.

TABLE 11.6:

SLS-irritant patch test reactions: Transepidermal water loss measurements (TEWL, $g/m^2/h$)

Region	Young	Old	Significance
Forehead			
Control	7.1±1.1	4.8±1.7	NS
SLS	15.8±2.1	14.1±5.0[a]	NS
Upper arm			
Control	3.8±0.7	1.8±0.6	$p < .05$
SLS	17.0±5.2[a]	4.6±1.6[a]	$p < .05$
Volar forearm			
Control	5.0±1.4	2.3±0.8	NS
SLS	13.3±4.5	5.3±1.9[a]	NS
Dorsal forearm			
Control	3.8±0.7	2.1±0.8	NS
SLS	11.6±2.8[a]	4.2±1.5[a]	$p < .05$
Postauricular			
Control	6.1±0.8	6.6±2.3	NS
SLS	11.4±2.3[a]	11.6±4.1[a]	NS
Palm			
Control	31.0±7.7	26.2±9.3	NS
SLS	26.9±4.0	22.5±8.0	NS
Abdomen			
Control	5.4±0.9	1.9±0.7	$p < .01$
SLS	20.0±4.7[a]	5.1±1.8[a]	$p < .01$
Upper back			
Control	5.6±1.2	3.3±1.2	NS
SLS	18.2±3.5[a]	6.6±2.3[a]	$p < .02$
Thigh			
Control	5.1±1.6	2.2±0.8	NS
SLS	24.6±7.6[a]	7.1±2.5[a]	$p < .05$
Ankle			
Control	6.2±1.7	2.5±0.9	NS
SLS	6.5±1.8	3.7±1.3	NS

Note. SLS, sodium lauryl sulfate. From Cua *et al.* (1990).
[a] Differences were compared between control and SLS-treated sites.
NS, not significant ($p < .05$).

11.4.4 Race

It is difficult to compare irritant reactions in white and black skin. Results based on traditional visual grading suggest an equal or lesser susceptibility of black skin to develop irritation from chemicals (Weigand and Gaylor, 1974; Anderson and Maibach, 1979). Use of alternative evaluative techniques, including laser Doppler flowmetry (LDF), and transepidermal water loss (TEWL) tend to support this conclusion. However, a few studies have shown slight but significant increases in methyl-nicotinate-induced blood flow in Caucasians versus blacks (Guy *et al.*, 1985) or non-significant differences in SLS induced blood flow in blacks versus Caucasians (Berardesca *et al.*, 1988a). Baseline TEWL measurements were significantly higher in Asian subjects and black subjects compared with white subjects. No baseline differences were seen between black and Asian subjects (Kompaore *et al.*, 1993). On the other hand, no difference was found in this parameter when African black subjects were compared with white European subjects or among other racial groups studied (DeLuca *et al.*, 1983; Pinnagoda *et al.*, 1990). Blacks and Hispanics showed higher TEWL responses after SLS (Berardesca *et al.*, 1988a,b) and *in vitro* TEWL differences between blacks and whites have also been reported (Wilson *et al.*, 1988). In a similar study, Chinese have been found to be more sensitive than Malays but no significant differences were found between Chinese and Indians or between Malays and Indians (Goh and Chia, 1988). Differences in vasodilatation induced by methyl nicotinate were also noted (Guy *et al.*, 1985; Gean *et al.*, 1984). Rapaport using a 21-day cumulative irritation test protocol found a generally greater cumulative response to SLS and several consumer product formulations among the Japanese subjects (Rapaport,1984). Similar notifications appeared in the Japanese literature, Ishihara reported a greater patch test reactivity to cosmetic products among female Japanese (Ishihara *et al.*, 1986) and a higher level of intolerance among Japanese subjects to topical tretinoin cream was also noted (Tadaki *et al.*, 1993). Recently, an international dose-response study with the anionic surfactant SLS at different concentrations was conducted under Unilever's direction. In this study the German population tended to be the most responsive and the Asian population was no more reactive than the Caucasians (Basketter *et al.*, 1996a). However, studying populations in different geographic locations and at different times of the year creates difficulties in the interpretation of the data. Robinson analysing skin reactivity between human subpopulations compiled results from nine acute irritation patch test studies, conducted at three test facilities over a 5-year period. For three irritant test chemicals, 20 percent sodium dodecyl sulfate, 100 percent decanol and 10 percent acetic acid an increased reactivity for Asian versus Caucasian subjects was noted (Robinson, 2002). Cutaneous erythema induced by methacholine injections was compared in Warain Indians, Tibetans, and Caucasians. Caucasians reacted to the greatest degree (Buckley *et al.*, 1985), and associations between skin irritation and cholinergic reactivity may exist (Berardesca and Maibach, 1988).

11.4.5 Gender

There is a common perception that women are more prone to skin irritation than men (Agrup, 1969; Lantinga *et al.*, 1984; Rystedt, 1985). However, in a recent study male subjects were found to be directionally or significantly more reactive than females, to each of the four irritants tested (Robinson, 2002). Female skin seems to elicit more tape irritation (Wagner and Porschel, 1962; Magnusson and Hillgren, 1962). Whereas, skin tests with surfactants, have not experimentally documented a difference in most studies (Bjornberg, 1975; Lammintausta *et al.*, 1987b; Goh and Chia, 1988, Meding, 2000). The increased occurrence of irritant contact dermatitis in females may be related to the more extensive exposure to irritants and wet work. A minimal relationship between gender and constitutional skin irritability is supported by the fact that the female preponderance in the irritant contact dermatitis populations does not hold true for all geographic areas (Olumide, 1987).

11.4.6 Previous and preexisting skin diseases

Patients with atopic dermatitis are alleged to have defective skin barrier function, both in irritated and normal looking skin. Itchy and dry atopic skin has been connected with an increased risk for developing hand dermatitis (Lammintausta and Kalimo, 1981; Rystedt, 1985). Reduced capacity to bind water has been related to atopic skin (Werner *et al.*, 1982), which in noneczematous sites demonstrates greater TEWL than does nonatopic skin, and stratum corneum water content may even be increased (Finlay *et al.*, 1980; Al Jaber and Marks, 1984; Gloor *et al.*, 1981). The response to SLS was statistically significantly increased in atopics compared to controls, when evaluated by visual scoring and skin thickness (Agner, 1991), and increased water loss with detergent patch tests were also reported (van der Valk *et al.*, 1985, Goh, 1997). When different concentrations of SLS were tested, a higher percentage of positive results and a significantly greater intensity of response to SLS were noted in the atopic dermatitis group than in controls; the same result was demonstrated in atopic allergic rhinitis patients without dermatitis (Nassif *et al.*, 1994). Whereas, in patients with past history of atopic dermatitis the responsiveness to SLS was not increased (Agner, 1991). Basketter noted a statistically higher reaction of atopic skin only to 20 percent sodium dodecyl sulfate, however, 35 percent cocotrimethyl ammonium chloride and 10 percent hydrochloric acid failed to provoke significantly different irritation in atopics compared to

CHAPTER 11

controls (Basketter *et al.*, 1996b). Later on, the relative reactivity of an apparently normal skin in atopic and non-atopic groups was studied. SLS was applied at a range of concentrations and exposure times. At various time points, the irritation response was measured by visual assessment, chromametry, laser Doppler flowmetry and TEWL. Using all of the methods of assessment, the reactions in atopics were similar to or a little less than those seen in non-atopics (Basketter *et al.*, 1998). However, when different irritants were used, higher levels of TEWL in apparently normal skin of atopic patients were found (Tupker *et al.*, 1990). Hannuksela and Hannuksela data suggested that different methods of application, like open application and plastic chamber, may produce dichoto-mous results (Hannuksela and Hannuksela, 1995). Tanaka evaluating the recovery of barrier function of stratum corneum after its tap stripping, found no differences in the response to mechanical irritation on atopic skin compared to controls (Tanaka *et al.*, 1997). Ichthyosis vulgaris is sometimes seen in association with atopic dermatitis; in ichthyosis vulgaris, patients' irritant reactivity has been shown to be increased to alkali irritants (Ziierz *et al.*, 1960). Seborrheic skin has not been shown to possess increased susceptibility to skin irritants; reports and interpretations are contradictory (Holland, 1958; Vickers, 1962; von Hornstein *et al.*, 1986), whereas after exposure to SLS the blood flux was significantly greater in patients with seborrheic dermatitis (Cowley and Farr, 1992). Clinical experience suggests that some increased irritability is associated with a seborrheic constitution in certain subjects. This may be true in certain geographic areas, where environmental humidity is low in the winter in relation to the cold temperatures.

Different methods have been used in studies on skin irritability in psoriatic individuals. Those studies revealed decreased and increased irritant reactivity (Kingston and Marks, 1983; Maurice and Greaves, 1983; Lawrence *et al.*, 1984; MacDonalds and Marks, 1986) when anthralin (dithranol) irritancy was the main interest. Psoriatic skin is particularly irritable in certain individuals (Epstein and Maibach, 1985), and the development of psoriatic lesions in irritation sites (Koebner phenomenon) is often seen.

In the presence of eczema, the threshold for skin irritation is decreased (Mitchell, 1981; Bruynzeel *et al.*, 1983; Bruynzeel and Maibach, 1986; Agner, 1991). A whole-body examination of employees sometimes reveals nummular lesions or other constitutional eczema symptoms. Such a clinical finding may suggest increased skin irritability in different locations. Pompholyx (dyshidrosis) type dermatitis is harmful. As a constitutional eczema, it probably increases skin irritability in general. These patients often have difficulty wearing gloves, since phompholyx is made worse by occlusion. A history of contact dermatitis may be important when susceptibility to irritant contact dermatitis is evaluated (Nilsson *et al.*, 1985; Lammintausta *et al.*, 1988a). Although increased irritability has been hard to demonstrate (Lammintausta *et al.*, 1988a) further improvement of methodological equipment in the bioengineering industry should make this possible.

11.5 PREDICTIVE IRRITANCY TESTING

Predictive irritancy testing involves specific tests for the irritant potential of individual chemicals as well as tests for individual susceptibility to irritation.

11.5.1 Predictive testing for chemical irritant potential

Predictive testing is widely performed to determine the irritant potential of various chemicals. The most popular methods are bioassays with human or animal subjects. Most procedures employ a single application of a test substance, with evaluation of the response in 24–48 h. The oldest of these assays is the Draize rabbit test, in which test substances are applied for 24 h under occlusion to abraded and nonabraded skin. While this procedure detects severe irritants for human skin, it is unsatisfactory for mild to moderate irritants (Phillips *et al.*, 1972). Numerous modifications adaptable to special situations have been developed. The reader is referred to the National Research Council (1977) special publication that discusses the principles and practices involved. Because of species variability, correlation of irritancy studies of animal skin with human skin has not been entirely satisfactory. A rabbit cumulative irritancy test has been described that compares favorably with a cumulative human irritancy assay (Marzulli and Maibach, 1975; Steinberg *et al.*, 1975). Bioassays involving human subjects are patterned after those involving animal models. Frosch and Kligman (1977b) introduced a chamber scarification test, which enhances the capacity to detect mild irritants. The forearm is scarified in a crisscross pattern; the suspected irritant is applied to this area in a large aluminum chamber once daily for 3 days. To date, bioassays have utilized visible degrees of erythema and edema as indices of irritancy; this method is simple and convenient. The development of physical techniques for measuring subtle degrees of noninflammatory skin damage has improved our understanding of this area. Skin permeability to water vapor (transepidermal water loss) was the first physical measurement to be used for this purpose. Early investigations clearly established that chemicals that provoked inflammation increased transepidermal water loss (Spruit, 1970, 1971; Rollins, 1978). Malten and Thiele (1973) subsequently showed that increases in transepidermal water loss occurred *before* visible inflammation when ionic, polar, water-soluble substances (e.g., sodium hydroxide, soaps, detergents) were used as irritants. Malten and den Arend (1978) showed that an un-ionized, polar irritant (dimethyl sulfoxide) did not provoke increased water vapor loss until visible inflammation had already occurred. Similarly, two un-ionized nonpolar (water-insoluble) irritants, hexanediol diacrylate and butanediol diacrylate, did not provoke increased skin water vapor loss until visible inflammation occurred (Malten *et al.*, 1979). Thus, transepidermal water loss measurements may detect the irritant capacity of certain chemicals in the absence of visible inflammation, but possibly only for ionizable, polar, watersoluble substances.

Measurements of the electrical impedance (resistance) of human skin also detect subtle degrees of skin damage before skin inflammation occurs (Thiele and Malten, 1973). This method has the advantage over water loss measurements that it is capable of detecting subtle changes produced by un-ionizable or nonpolar substances as well as ionizable, polar ones (Malten *et al.*, 1979).

Measurements of carbon dioxide emission from human skin have been developed (Malten and Thiele, 1973). Rates of carbon dioxide emission from irritated skin increase roughly in proportion to the degree of irritation (Thiele, 1974).

Electrolyte flux through the skin barrier may be measured with the aid of ion-specific skin electrodes (Grice *et al.*, 1975; Anjo *et al.*, 1978). Measurements of chloride ion flux through psoriatic or eczematous skin indicate that, despite the dramatic increases in permeability to water vapor, the electrolyte barrier remains relatively intact (Grice *et al.*, 1975). Chloride ion flux may provide another noninflammatory index of cutaneous irritation. A potassium ion electron has been of value in quantifying potassium flux postdamage (Lo *et al.*, 1990).

In vitro skin irritation tests are being developed in the hope that the methods of analysis can be more predictive of actual human response and will provide an objective quantifiable means of determining the irritancy potential of a substance. In addition *in vitro* testing could be designed to provide insight into the specific action of a toxicant on the epidermis and the actual mechanism of damage. Proposed *in vitro* tests for irritation are based on cell cytotoxicity, inflammatory or immune system response, alterations of cellular or tissue physiology, cell morphology, biochemical end points and structure activity analysis. The published methods examine toxic effects on keratinocyte and other cell cultures, multilayered "skin equivalents" the chorioallantoic membrane of fertilized eggs, irritant-sensitive microorganisms and a keratin/collagen-reagent system membrane that mimics skin response to irritants (Table 11.7) (Bulich, 1981; Silverman, 1983; Borenfreund, 1984; Luepke, 1986; Enslein *et al.*, 1987; Gordon, 1989; Parce, 1989; Stephens, 1990; Benassi *et al.*, 1999; Wilhelm *et al.*, 2001). Rougier *et al.* details this rapidly enlarging field (Rougier *et al.*, 1994).

11.5.2 Predictive testing for susceptibility to irritation

The ability to predict which individuals are more prone to irritant skin reactions has practical significance as a preemployment screening test. The ability of

TABLE 11.7:

In vitro irritation systems

Method	System	Principle	Toxicity assessment
"Testskin"	Synthetic human epithelium to skin	Histologically, physiologically similar mediators	Morphologic changes inflammatory
Microphysiometer	Cell culture	pH monitored as an indicator of metabolism	Decreased metabolism
Neutral red dye assay	Cell culture	Dye uptake by viable cells measured spectrophotometrically	Cell death
"Microtox"	Luminiscent bacteria	Only viable bacteria luminesce	Organism death
Tetrahymena thermophilia	Protozoa	Motility	Decreased motility
Chorioallantoic membrane	Fertilized egg membrane vasculature	Vasculature changes	Damage to vasculature
"Skintex" (MB/PM) System	Keratine/collagen matrix linked to dye	Dye released and turbidity are measured spectrophotometrically	Increased dye turbidity reflects membrane disruption
Computer-based structure-activity relationships (SAR)	Computer analysis	Computer modeling of similar compounds with a given irritation potential	Irritation prediction based on structural analysis

Note. From Bason and Maibach (1992).

the skin to neutralize solutions of sodium hydroxide was first proposed as a screening test for susceptibility to irritation by Gross *et al.* (1954). Bjornberg (1974) reviewed previous attempts to predict general susceptibility by determining irritant responses to selected irritants. He was unable to corroborate early claims that inability to neutralize alkaline solutions, decreased resistance to alkaline irritation, or that increased susceptibility to common experimental irritants could be used to predict susceptibility to irritations in a preemployment setting. Frosch and Kligman (1977a) used the length of time to slight blister formation after experimental exposure to ammonium hydroxide as a predictive index. They found that short times were highly correlated with the intensity of inflammation produced by irritating concentrations of SLS. They also found that patients with atopic dermatitis (who were presumably more susceptible to irritation) had shorter times to blister formation than controls (Frosch, 1978). Wilhelm utilized sodium hydroxide to produce TEWL as a measure of skin damage. This assay shows a high correlation between subjects developing increased water loss after application of sodium hydroxide and a propensity for SLS damage (Wilhelm *et al.*, 1990). Effendy showed increased baseline TEWL in patients with acute and healed irritant contact dermatitis (Effendy *et al.*, 1995). Later on, an association between reactivity to an irritant and the likelihood of positive elicitation reactions to lower hapten concentrations was noted (Smith *et al.*, 2002). These simple approaches provided a first step toward a preemployment test for irritant dermatitis potential. Recently, a nonatopic genetic marker for irritant susceptibility in normal individuals was described by Allen *et al.* In this work an association of TNF α gene polymorphism at position −308 with susceptibility to irritant contact dermatitis was found (Allen *et al.*, 2000). As functional polymorphisms in cytokine genes may affect responses to irritants, future studies may contribute to identifying individuals at risk of developing irritant contact dermatitis.

11.6 HISTOLOGY, HISTOPATHOLOGY, AND PATHOLOGY

Irritant contact dermatitis, being a heterogenous disease caused by different compounds cannot be characterized on the basis of histologic findings. The histology is different in acute and chronic contact dermatitis. The degree and severity of the dermatitis and the interval between the onset and the actual time of biopsy influence the histological findings. If the acute irritant or toxic skin reaction is strong, vesicles may be seen. In the vesicle, a mixture of neutrophils and lymphocytes is seen. In initial acute irritant contact dermatitis, dermal changes may be absent or minimal. Dermal infiltrates appear and increase during the first day of the developing dermatitis. The cell infiltrates in irritant and allergic contact dermatitis are not significantly or diagnostically different. In chronic irritant contact dermatitis, scaling, hyperkeratosis, and lichenification are apparent in older skin lesions, often resembling neuro-dermatitis. In addition the effects of irritants on epidermal structures are influenced by the different chemical properties of molecules. Irritants, such as surfactants, removed skin lipids and keratins (Berardesca *et al.*, 1993), organic solvents damage cell membranes, and other compounds, such as anthralin, induce direct cytotoxic damage of keratinocytes (Willis *et al.*, 1989; Landman *et al.*, 1990). The inflammatory cell response has been characterized in guinea pigs treated with toxic croton oil or repeated sodium lauryl sulfate (SLS) applications. In both reactions monocyte counts were increased, even as compared with an allergic reaction. The heterogeneous monocyte group, however, consisted of lymphocytes, fibroblasts, and monocytes. Only a minority of basophils was seen, less than in allergic contact reactions. Mast cells were also slightly increased, suggesting some association between nonimmunologic contact urticaria and an acute irritant contact reaction (Anderson *et al.*, 1988). SLS and alkyl dimethyl benzammonium chloride (ADBC) were shown to enhance the migration of polymorphonuclear leukocytes. SLS and ADBC also induced the secretion of preformed mediators, such as histamine and lysozymal enzyme beta-G from the cells (Frosch and Czarnetzki, 1987). Wide variation in the inhibitory response was documented for cutaneous inflammation elicited by different irritants, whether induction was by histamine antagonists, prosta-glandin and kinin synthesis inhibitors, or neutropenia-inducing agents (Patrick *et al.*, 1987). Exposure to DMSO or SLS induced a small increase in lymph node cell proliferation compared with aqueous solution alone, examined in the murine local lymph node assay (LLNA). Exposure to SLS in DMSO or metal salts in DMSO or SLS caused a significant increase in LNC proliferation (Ikarashi *et al.*, 1993). Langerhans cells, are actively involved, both in allergic and irritant reactions. Application of irritants to human skin *in vivo* resulted in a progressive depletion in the number and function of antigen-presenting cells (Lisby *et al.*, 1989; Mikulowska *et al.*, 1996; Forsey *et al.*, 1998). Identical composition of peripheral T lymphocytes, associated with peripheral HLA-DR (histocompati-bility locus A) positive macrophages and Langerhans cells, was seen in irritant and allergic contact dermatitis (Scheynius *et al.*, 1984; Ferguson *et al.*, 1985). In the lymphocyte population, helper/inducer lymphocytes exceed the number of

CHAPTER 11

T-suppression/ cytotoxic cells (Scheynius *et al.*, 1984; Avnstorp *et al.*, 1987). In irritant contact dermatitis, keratinocytes have been demonstrated to express major histocompatibility complex (MHC) class II antigens concerned with the antigen presentation and the elicitation of the T-lymphocyte-dependent immune response (Gawkrodger *et al.*, 1987). These antigens were expressed by the keratinocytes in both allergic and irritant contact dermatitis.

Recent interest has concentrated on cytokines. Cytokines are a heterogeneous group of peptides, released from a variety of cells in the skin, that play a pivotal role in immune and inflammatory reactions. Studies of irritant reactions have noted that almost all of the cytokines previously linked to allergic reactions are found in irritant reactions. The role of cytokines in irritant reactions is discussed extensively by Effendy and Maibach in Chapter 20.

11.7 MECHANISM OF IRRITANT DERMATITIS

Irritant dermatitis is a multifaceted disease previously thought as non-immunologic inflammatory reaction. However, a growing body of evidence suggests that immunologic mechanisms may also in part underlie the pathogenesis of irritant contact dermatitis. Irritants, such as surfactants, remove skin lipids and keratins (Berardesca *et al.*, 1993), organic solvents damage cell membranes, and other compounds, such as anthralin, induce direct cytotoxic damage of keratinocytes (Willis *et al.*, 1989; Landman *et al.*, 1990). As different irritants with different chemical properties of molecules, produce different effects on epidermal structures, it seems likely that there are many routes by which irritant dermatitis may be arrived at. However, all irritants bear in common the same pathophysiological changes including: skin barrier disruption by chemical stimuli or mechanical trauma, cellular epidermal damage and release of proinflammatory mediators particularly cytokines, all of which are interlinked. Disruption of the barrier leads to perturbation or disruption of the lipid bilayers of the epidermis associated with loss of cohesion of corneocytes and desquamation with increased TEWL. Exposure to the irritant SLS alters the synthesis of new lipids, which in turn leads to disturbance of lamellar body lipid extrusion (Fartasch *et al.*, 1998). Acetone or tape stripping causes increased keratinocyte proliferation in the basal cell layer (Grubauer *et al.*, 1989). Disruption of the barrier leads also to release of cytokines such as interleukin (IL)-1 α, IL-1 β and tumor necrosis factor (TNF) α. Furthermore, when the barrier is disrupted, the entry of chemicals into the epidermis is facilitated, leading to structural changes in keratinocytes and further cytokine release. Among the pro-inflammatory cytokines which have been found to be released are interleukin (IL)-1 α, tumor necrosis factor (TNF) α, IL-6, IL-8, granulocyte-macrophage colony-stimulating factor (GM-CSF) and T-cell-derived cytokines, including IL-2 and interferon-γ (Wood *et al.*, 1992; Ulfgren *et al.*, 2000). CD 36 expression is ALSO increased by certain irritants (SLS and propylene glycol) that induce hyperproliferative effect (Willis *et al.*, 1991). Keratinocyte involvement is not confined to the production and release of cytokines but extends to the up-regulation and expression of immune-associated adhesion molecules. These molecules include intercellular adhesion molecule –1 (ICAM-1) that bind to lymphocyte function associated antigen-1 (LFA –1) positive leukocytes (Willis *et al.*, 1991). Finally, class II major histocompatibility complex (MHC) molecule HLA-DR expression by keratinocytes in some irritant reactions has been also described (Brasch *et al.*, 1992).

Recently, there is increasing evidence that oxidative stress plays a role in the pathogenesis of acute irritant contact dermatitis. The effect of irritant chemicals on the anti-oxidant enzyme systems in the skin has been examined using quantitative immunocytochemistry. Following topical application of dithranol and SLS, reduced levels of Cu, Zn-superoxide dismutase enzyme (Willis *et al.*, 1998), and changing levels of two classes of glutathione S-transferase (Willis *et al.*, 2001) were noted.

It has been well documented that irritants increase epidermal turnover (Fisher and Maibach, 1975). Damage to the barrier, with removal of intercellular lipids, increases TEWL, which stimulates lipid synthesis and promotes barrier restoration. Acetone or tape stripping causes increased keratinocyte proliferation in the basal cell layer (Grubauer *et al.*, 1989). The possible mechanisms include production of cytokines: IL –1α, IL-1β, TNF-α, IL-6, IL-8 and 12-HETE, which have been shown to induce epidermal hyperplasia; disruption of cell membrane structure with damage to keratinocytes may cause reduction in availability of adenyl cyclase, leading to reduction in cAMP and increased cell division; involvement of ornithine decarboxylase (ODC), an intracellular enzyme, believed to influence the kinetics of proliferation (Marks *et al.*, 1979; Berardesca, 1994).

11.8 TREATMENT

Avoiding the irritants and individual skin protection remains the basis of treating irritant contact dermatitis. Distilled water and physiologic saline compresses enhanced resolution of experimentally-induced irritant contact dermatitis. While the exact mechanism is unknown, the compresses may

CHAPTER 11

provide a moist environment for the healing of irritation (Levin *et al.*, 2001). Additionally, the hygroscopic effect of water may increase the capacity for intracellular moisture retention. Sea water or its components significantly inhibited the increase of TEWL and the decrease of capacitance, after open application of 2 percent SLS for 10 min (Yoshizawa *et al.*, 2001). Cool compresses of either Burrow's solution, saline, silver nitrate or water may reduce the inflammation and skin surface temperature associated with the irritant reaction (Levin *et al.*, 2001). Recently, the anti-irritative effect of 0.5 percent methyl-rosaniline chloride (Gentian violet) was also noted (Gloor and Wolnicki, 2001).

To maintain normal hydration of the stratum corneum moisturizers are frequently used. Moisturizers may contain humectants of low molecular weight and lipids. Humectants, such as lactic acid, urea, glycerin, pyrrolidone carboxylic acid (PCA) and salts, probably exert their effect by attracting water, and thereby increasing hydration (Zhai *et al.*, 1998). The lipids contained within the moisturizer, such as petrolatum, beeswax, lanolin and various oils, may act as emulsifiers, improving the skin barrier in irritated skin, possibly by influencing the structure of the epidermal membrane lipids (Loden, 1997). Moisturizers may prevent absorption of exogenous substances and accelerate barrier recovery by diffusing into the delipidized stratum corneum (Ghadially *et al.*, 1992). In normal skin, only repeated application of a moisturizer produced a significant increase in conductance for at least 1 week post-treatment (Serup *et al.*, 1989). Unfortunately, specific moisturizers may make the skin more susceptibile to irritation (Held and Agner, 2001).

Topical corticoids are widely utilized to treat irritant contact dermatitis, its use is still controversial. In theory, the anti-inflammatory properties of corticoids could improve the dermatitis, however their anti-proliferative effects might slow recovery of the skin barrier and allow further penetration of irritants. Corticoids were associated with no or possibly a negative effect in treating cumulative irritant contact dermatitis (van der Valk *et al.*, 1989c; Le *et al.*, 1997), and recently, corticosteroids of low- and medium-potency were also found ineffective in treating surfactant-induced acute irritant dermatitis (Levin *et al.*, 2001).

Macrolide antibiotics may improve dermatitis by suppressing the immune response. Tacrolimus (FK506) was first isolated from the soil microorganism Streptomyces tsukubaensis.This drug was also shown to inhibit calcium-dependent events mediated by calcineurin, such as IL-2 gene transcription, nitric oxidase synthase activation, cell degranulation, and apoptosis (Thomson *et al.*, 1995). However, when the anti-inflammatory activity of FK 506 was evaluated in a human skin inflammation model, FK 506 was shown to enhance experimentally induced irritant contact dermatitis and not to accelerate healing of irritant contact dermatitis (Fuchs *et al.*, 2002).

Autooxidative tissue damage may occur in the case of irritant contact dermatitis. The flavonoids have been considered to possess antioxidant and anti-inflammatory activities. However, when quercetin, a bioflavonoid was applied topically the recovery of barrier function and erythema caused by SLS was not increased (Katsarou *et al.*, 2000).

Ultraviolet (UV) exposure increase the capacity to resist irritation in the skin. This effect appears to be nonspecific (Thorvaldsen and Volden, 1980). When the acute phase of an irritant contact dermatitis is over and relapses are expected, repeated UV exposures may elicit nonspecific "desensitization" in the skin, increasing the capacity to avoid relapses. Alterations at the cellular level, in cell surface proteins, and in the release of inflammatory mediators probably contribute to the therapeutic benefit achieved by UV therapies (Denig *et al.*, 1998). Both UVB and PUVA may alter the immune system by decreasing the density of HLA-DR-positive epidermal Langerhans cells (Rosen *et al.*, 1989). Furthermore, PUVA may induce DNA/RNA damage in cells and thereby lead to a transient suppression of cellular proliferation Jampel *et al.*, 1991). Finally, UVB-initiated dimmers may also lead to an observed immune suppression (Vink *et al.*, 1997).

REFERENCES

AGNER, T. and SERUP, Z. (1989) Seasonal variation of skin resistance to irritants. *Br. J. Dermatol.*, **121**, 323–328.

AGNER, T. (1991) Skin susceptibility in uninvolved skin of hand eczema patients and healthy controls. *Br J. Dermatol*, **125**, 140–146.

AGRUP, G. (1969) Hand eczema and other dermatoses in South Sweden (Thesis). *Acta Dermatol. Venereol. [Suppl.] (Stockh.)*, **49**, 61.

AL JABER, H. and MARKS, R. (1984) Studies of the clinically uninvolved skin in patients with dermatitis. *Br. J. Dermatol.*, **111**, 437–443.

ALLEN, M.H., WAKELIN, S.H., HOLLOWAY, D., LISBY, S., BAADSGAARD, O., BARKER, J.N. and McFADDEN, J.P. (2000) Association of TNF alpha gene polymorphism at position –308 with susceptibility to irritant contact dermatitis. *Immunogenetics*, **51**(3), 201–205.

ANDERSEN, K.E. and MAIBACH, H.I. (1979) Black and white human skin differences. *J. Am. Acad. Dermatol.*, **1**, 276–228.

CHAPTER 11

ANDERSEN, K.E., SJOLIN, K.E. and SOELGAARD, P. (1988) Acute irritant contact folliculitis in a galvanize, European Symposium on Contact Dermatitis, Heidelberg, May 27–29, p. 62.

ANJO, D.M., CUNICO, R.L. and MAIBACH, H.I. (1978) Transepidermal chloride diffusion in man. *Clin. Res.*, **26**, 208A.

ARAMAKI, J., LOFFLER, C., KAWANA, S., EFFENDY, I., HAPPLE, R. and LOFFLER, H. (2001) Irritant patch test with SLS: interrelation between concentration and exposure time. *British J. Dermatol.*, **145**(5), 704–708.

AVNSTORP, C., RALFKIAER, E., JORGENSEN, J. and WANTZIN, G.L. (1987) Sequential immunophenotypic study of lymphoid infiltrate in allergic and irritant reactions. *Contact Dermatitis*, **16**, 239–245.

BAKER, H. and BLAIR, C.P. (1968) Cell replacement in the human stratum corneum in old age. *Br. J. of Dermatol.*, **80**, 367–372.

BASKETTER, D.A., GRIFFITHS, H.A., WANG, X.M., WILHELM, K.P and McFADDEN, J. (1996a) Individual, ethnic and seasonal variability in irritant susceptibility of skin: The implications for a predictive human patch test. *Contact Dermatitis*, **35**, 208–213.

BASKETTER, D.A., BLAIKIE, L. and REYNOLDS, F. (1996b) The impact of atopic status on a predictive human test of skin irritation potential. *Contact Dermatitis*, **35**, 33–39.

BASKETTER, D.A., MIETTINEN, J. and LAHTI, A. (1998) Acute irritant reactivity to sodium lauryl sulfate in atopics and non-atopics. *Contact Dermatitis*, **38**(5), 253–257.

BENASSI, L., BERTAZZONI, G., SEIDENARI, S. (1999) *In vitro* testing of tensides employing monolayer cultures: a comparison with results of patch tests on human volunteers. *Contact Dermatitis*, **40**, 38–44.

BERARDESCA, E. and MAIBACH, H.I. (1988a) Racial differences in sodium lauryl sulfate induced cutaneous irritation: Black and white. *Contact Dermatitis*, **18**, 65–70.

BERARDESCA, E. and MAIBACH, H.I. (1988b) Sodium-lauryl-sulfate-induced cutaneous irritation. Comparison of white and hispanic subjects. *Contact Dermatitis*, **19**, 136–140.

BERARDESCA, E., CESPA, M., FARINELLI, N., RABBIOSI, G. and MAIBACH, H.I. (1991) *In vivo* transcutaneous penetration of nicotinates and sensitive skin. *Contact Dermatitis*, **25**, 35-38.

BERARDESCA, E. and ELSNER, P. and DISTANTE, F. (1994) The modulation of skin irritation. *Contact Dermatitis*, **31**, 281–287.

BERARDESCA, E., VIGNOLI,G.P., DISTANTE, F., BRIZZI, P. and RABBIOSI, G. (1995) Effect of water temperature on surfactant induced skin irritation. *Contact Dermatitis*, **32**(2), 83–87.

BJORNBERG, A. (1974) Skin reactions to primary irritations and predisposition to eczema. *Br. J. Dermatol.*, **91**(4), 425.

BJORNBERG, A. (1975) Skin reactions to primary irritants in men and women. *Acta Derm. Venereol. (Stockh.)*, **55**, 191–194.

BORENFREUND, E. and PUERNER, J.A. (1984) A simple quantitative procedure using monolayer cultures for cytotoxicity assays. *J. of Tissue Culture Methods*, **9**, 7–9.

BRASCH, J., BUGARD, J. and STERRY, W. (1992) Common pathogenetic pathways in Allergic and Irritant Contact Dermatitis. *J. Inves. Dermatol.*, **98**, 166–170.

BRITZ, M.B. and MAIBACH, H.I. (1979) Human cutaneous vulvar reactivity to irritants. *Contact Dermatitis*, **5**, 375–377.

BRUYNZEEL, D.P., VAN KETEL, W.G. and SCHEPER, R.J. (1983) Angry back of the excited skin syndrome: A prospective study. *J. Am. Acad. Dermatol.*, **8**, 392–397.

BRUYNZEEL, D.P. and MAIBACH, H.I. (1986) Excited skin syndrome (angry back). *Arch. Dermatol.*, **12**, 323–328.

BUCKLEY, C.E.III, LARRICK, J.W. and KAPLAN, J.E. (1985) Population differences in cutaneous metacholine reactivity and circulating IgE concentrations. *J. Allergy Clin. Immunol.*, **76**, 847–854.

BULICH, A.A., GREENE, M.W. and ISENBERG, D.L. (1981) Reliability of bacterial luminescence assay for determination of the toxicity of pure compounds and complex effluents Aquatic Toxicology and Hazard Assessment, 4th Conference, BRAMSON, D.R. and DICKSON, K.L. (eds), Philadelphia: American Society for Testing and Materials (ASTM737) pp. 338–347.

CHARBONNIER, JR V., MORRISON, B.M., PAYE, M. and MAIBACH, H.I. (2001) Subclinical, non-erythematous irritation with an open assay model (washing): sodium lauryl sulfate (SLS) versus sodium laureth sulfate (SLES). *Food Chem. Toxicol.*, **39**, 279–286.

CHRISTOPHERS, E. and KLIGMAN, A.M. (1965) Percutaneous absorption in aged skin. In MONTAGNA, E. (ed.) *Advances in the Biology of the Skin*, Oxford: Pergamon Press, 160–179.

CHAPTER 11

CLARYS, P., MANOU, I. and BAREL, A.O. (1997) Influence of temperature on irritation in the hand/forearm immersion test. *Contact Dermatitis*, **36**(5), 240–243.

COOPER, E.R. (1985) Vehicle effects on skin penetration. In MAIBACH, H.I. and BRONAUGH, R.L. (eds) *Percutaneous Absorption*, New York: Marcel Dekker, 525–530.

COWLEY, N.C. and FARR, P.M. (1992) A dose-response study of irritant reactions to sodium lauryl sulfate in patients with seborrheic dermatitis and atopic eczema. *Acta Derm. Venereol. (Stockh.)*, **72**, 432–435.

CRONIN, E. and STOUGHTON, R.B.L. (1962) Percutaneous absorption: regional variations and the effect of hydration and epidermal stripping. *Br. J. Dermatol.*, **74**, 7265–7272.

CUA, A.B., WILHELM, K.P. and MAIBACH, H.I. (1990) Cutaneous sodium lauryl sulfate irritation potential: age and regional variability. *Br. J. Dermatol.*, **123**, 607–613.

CUNICO, R.L., MAIBACH, H.I. and BLOOM, E. (1977) Skin barrier properties in the newborn. Transepidermal water loss and carbon dioxide emission rates. *Biol. Neonate*, **32**, 177–182.

DELUCA, R., BALESTRIER, A. and DINLE, Y. (1983) Measurements of cutaneous evaporation. 6. Cutaneous water loss in the people of Somalia. *Boll. Soc. Ital. Biol. Sper.*, **59**, 1499–1501.

DENIG, N., HOKE, A.W. and MAIBACH, H.I. (1998) Irritant contact dermatitis. *Postgrad. Med.*, **103**, 199–213.

DESALVA, S.J. and THOMPSON, G. (1965) Na22CI skin clearance in humans and its relation to skin age. *J. Invest. Dermatol.*, **45**, 315–318.

DOOMS-GOOSSENS, E., DELUSSCHENE, K.M., GEVERS, D.M., DUPREE, K.M., DEGREEF, H.J. LONCKE, J.P. and SNAUWAERT, J.E. (1986) Contact dermatitis caused by airborne irritant. *J. Am. Acad. Dermatol.*, **15**, 1–10.

EFFENDY, I., LOEFFLER, H., MAIBACH, H.I. (1995) Baseline transepidermal water loss in patients with acute and healed irritant contact dermatitis. *Contact Dermatitis*, **33**(6), 371–374.

EFFENDY, I., WELTFRIEND, S., PATIL, S. and MAIBACH, H.I. (1996) Differential irritant skin responses to topical retinoic acid and sodium lauryl sulfate: alone and in crossover design. *Br. J. Dermatol.*, **134**, 424–430.

ELIAS, P.M. (1981) Lipids and the epidermal permeability barrier. *Arch. Dermatol. Res.*, **270**, 95–117.

ELSNER, P., WILHELM, D. and MAIBACH, H.I. (1990) Sodium lauryl sulfate-induced irritant contact dermatitis in vulvar and forearm skin of premenopausal and postmenopausal women. *J. Am. Acad. Dermatol.*, **23**, 648–652.

EMILSON, A., LINDBERG, M. and FORSLIND, B. (1993) The importance effect on *in vitro* penetration of sodium lauryl sulfate and nickel chloride through human skin. *Acta Derm Venereol (Stockh.)*, **73**, 203-207.

ENSLEIN, K., BORGSTEDT, H.H., BLAKE, B.W. and HART, J.B. (1987) Prediction of rabbit skin irritation severity by structure-activity relationships. *In Vitro Toxicol.*, **1**, 129–147.

EPSTEIN, E. (1971) Contact dermatitis in children. *Pediatr. Clin. North. Am.*, **18**, 839–852.

EPSTEIN, W.L. (1983) Cutaneous granulomas as a toxicologic problem. In MARZULLI, F.M. and MAIBACH, H.I. (eds) *Dermatotoxicology*, 2nd ed., New York: Hemisphere, 533–545.

EPSTEIN, E. and MAIBACH, H.I. (1985) Eczematous psoriasis: what is it? In ROENIGK, H.H. JR. and MAIBACH, H.I. (eds) *Psoriasis*, New York: Marcel Dekker, 9–14.

FARTASCH, M., SCHRETZ, E. and DIEPGEN, T. (1998) Characterisation of detergent-induced barrier alteration. *J. Invest. Dermatol.*, 3(suppl.), 121–127.

FELDMANN, R. and MAIBACH, H.I. (1967a) Regional variation in percutaneous penetration. *Int. J. Dermatol.*, **48**, 1813–1819.

FELDMANN, R.J. and MAIBACH, H.I. (1967b) Regional variations in percutaneous absorption of C-cortisol in man. *J. Invest Dermatol.*, **48**, 181–183.

FELDMANN, R.J. and MAIBACH, H.I. (1974) Systemic absorption of pesticides through the skin of man. Occupational Exposure to Pesticides: Report to the Federal Working Group on Pest Management from the Task Group on Occupational Exposure to Pesticides, Appendix B, pp. 120–127.

FERGUSON, J., GIBBS, J.H. and SWANSON BECK, J. (1985) Lymphocyte subsets and Langerhans cells in allergic and irritant patch test reactions: Histometric studies. *Contact Dermatitis*, **13**, 166–174.

FINLAY, A.Y., NOCHOLLS, S., KING, C.S. and MARKS, R. (1980) The "dry" non-eczematous skin associated with atopic eczema. *Br. J. Dermatol.*, **102**, 249–256.

FISHER, A.A. (1975) Childhood allergic contact dermatitis. *Cutis*, **15**, 635–645.

FISHER, L.B. and MAIBACH, H.I. (1975) Effect of some irritants on human epidermal mitosis. *Contact Dermatitis*, **1**, 273–276.

FISCHER, T. and RYSTEDT, I. (1985) False positive, follicular and irritants patch test reactions to metal salts. *Contact Dermatitis,* 12, 93–98.

FLANNIGAN, S.A., SMITH, R.E. and MCGOVERN, J.P. (1984) Intraregional variation between contact irritant patch test sites. *Contact Dermatitis,* 10, 123–124.

FLANNIGAN, S.A. and TUCKER, S.B. (1985) Influence of the vehicle on irritant contact dermatitis. *Contact Dermatitis,* 12, 177–178.

FORSEY, R.J., SHAHIDULLAH, H., SANDS, C., MCVITTIE, E., ALDRIDGE, R.D., HUNTER, J.A. and HOWIE, S.E. (1998) Epidermal Langerhans cell apoptosis is induced *in vivo* by nonanoic acid but not by sodium lauryl sulfate. *Br. J. Dermatol.,* 139(3), 453–461.

FREEMAN, S. and MAIBACH, H.I. (1988) Study of irritant contact dermatitis produced by repeat patch test with sodium lauryl sulfate and assessed by visual methods, transepidermal water loss, and laser Doppler velocimetry. *J. Am. Acad. Dermatol.,* 19, 496–502.

FREGERT, S.F. (1981) Irritant contact dermatitis. In Fregert, S.F. (ed.) *Manual of Contact Dermatitis,* 2nd ed., Copenhagen: Munksgaard, 55–62.

FROSCH, P.J. and KLIGMAN, A.M. (1977) Rapid blister formation in human skin with ammonium hydroxide. *Br. J. Dermatol.,* 96, 461–473.

FROSCH, P.J. and KLIGMAN, A.M. (1978) An improved procedure for assaying irritants. The scarification test. *Curr. Probl. Dermatol.* 7, 69–79.

FROSCH, P.J. and KLIGMAN, A.M. (1982) Recognition of chemically vulnerable and delicate skin. In *Principles of Cosmetics for Dermatologists,* St. Louis: C.V. Mosby, 287–296.

FROSCH, P.J. (1985), Hautirritation und empfindliche Haut (Thesis), pp. 1–118. Grosse Scripta 7, Berlin: Grosse Verlag.

FROSCH, P.J. and CZARNETZKI, B.M. (1987) Surfactants cause *in vitro* chemotaxis and chemokinesis of human neutrophils. *J. Invest. Dermatol.,* 88, 525–555. Presented before the Society of Investigative Dermatology, San Francisco.

FUCHS, M., SCHLIEMANN-WILLERS, S., HEINEMANN, C., ELSNER, P. (2002) Tacrolimus enhances irritation in a 5-day human irritancy *in vivo* model. *Contact Dermatitis,* 46, 290–294.

GAWKRODGER, D.J., CARR, M.M., MCVITTIE, E., GUY, K. and HUNTER, J.A. (1987) Keratinocyte expression MCH class III antigens in allergic sensitization and challenge reactions and in irritant contact dermatitis. *J. Invest. Dermatol.,* 88, 11–20.

GILCHREST, B.A., MURPHY, G.F. and SOTTER, N.A. (1982) Effects of chronologic aging and ultraviolet irradiation on Langerhans cells in human skin. *J. Invest. Dermatol.*, **79**, 85–88.

GEAN, C.J., TUR, E., MAIBACH, H.I. and GUY, R.H. (1984) Cutaneous responses to topical methyl nicotinate in black, oriental, and caucasian subjects. *Arch. Dermatol. Res.*, **281**, 95–98.

GHADIALLY, R., HALKIER-SORENSEN, L. and ELIAS, P. (1992) Effects of petrolatum on stratum corneum structure and function *J. Am. Acad. Dermatol.*, **26**, 387–96.

GLOOR, M. and HEYMAN, B. and STUHLERT, T. (1981) Infrared spectrocopic determination of water content of the horny layer in healthy subjects and in patients suffering from atopic dermatitis *Arch. Dermatol. Res.*, **271**, 429–458.

GLOOR, M., WOLNICKI, D. (2001) Anti-irritative effect of methylrosaniline chloride (Gentian violet) *Dermatology*, **203**(4), 325–328.

GOH, C.L. and CHIA, S.E. (1988) Skin irritability to sodium lauryl sulfate—as measured by skin water vapour loss—by sex and race *Clin. Exp. Dermatol.*, **13**, 16–19.

GOH, C.L. (1997) Comparing skin irritancy in atopics and non atopics to sodium lauryl sulfate and benzalkonium chloride by using TEWL measurements. *Environ. Dermatol.*, **4**, 30–32.

GOLLHAUSEN, R. and KLIGMAN, A.M. (1985) Effects of pressure on contact dermatitis. *Am. J. Ind. Med.*, **8**, 323–328.

GORDON, V.C., KELLY, C.P. and BERGMAN, H.C. (1989) Skintex: An *in vitro* method for determining dermal irritation, Abstr 5th Int. Congress Toxicol. p. 123.

GRICE, K., SATTAR, H. and BAKER, H. (1973) The cutaneous barrier to salts and water in psoriasis and in normal skin. *Br. J. Dermatol.*, **88**, 459–463.

GRICE, K., SATTAR, H., CASEY, T. and BAKER, H. (1975) An evaluation of Na+, Cl-, and pH ion-specific electrodes in the study of the electrolyte contents of epidermal transudate and sweat. *Br. J. Dermatol.*, **92**, 511–518.

GRIFFITHS, W.A.D. and WILKINSON, D.S. (1985) Primary irritants and solvents. In GRIFFITHS, W.D. and WILKINSON, D.S. (eds) *Essentials of Industrial Dermatology*, Oxford: Blackwell Scientific, 58–72.

GROSS, P., BLADE, M.O., CHESTER, J. and SLOANE, M.B. (1954) Dermatitis of housewives as a variation of nummular eczema. A study of pH of the skin and alkali neutralization by the Burckhart technique. Further advances in therapy and prophylaxis. *Arch. Dermatol.*, **70**, 94.

GROVE, G. L., LAVKER, R.M., HOELZLE, E., and KLIGMAN, A.M. (1981) Use of nonintrusive tests to monitor age-associated changes in human skin. *J. Soc. Cosmet. Chem.,* **32,** 15–26.

GRUBAUER, G., ELIAS, P.M. and FEINGOLD, K.R. (1989) Transepidermal water loss: the signal for recovery of barrier structure and function. *J. Lipid Res.,* **30,** 323–333.

GUMMER, C.L. (1985) Vehicles as penetration enhancers. In MAIBACH, H.I. and BRONAUGH, R.L. (eds) *Percutaneous Absorption,* New York: Marcel Dekker, 561–570.

GUY, R.H., TUR, E., BJERKE, S., MAIBACH, H.I. (1985) Are there age and racial differences in methyl-nicotinate-induced vasodilatation in human skin? *J. Am. Acad. Dermatol.,* **12,** 1001–1006.

HANNUKSELA, M., PIRILA, V. and SALO, O.P. (1975) Skin reactions to propylene glycol. *Contact Dermatitis,* **1,** 112–116.

HANNUKSELA, A. and HANNUKSELA, M. (1995) Irritant effects of a detergent in wash and chamber tests. *Contact Dermatitis,* **32,** 163–166.

HELD, E. and AGNER, T. (2001) Effect of moisturizers on skin susceptibility to irritants. *Acta Derm. Venereol.,* **81,** 104–107.

HJORTH, N. and AVNSTORP, C. (1986) Rehabilitation in hand eczema. *Derm Beruf Umwelt,* **34,** 74–76.

HOLLAND, B.D. (1958) Occupational dermatoses—Predisposing and direct causes *JAMA,* **167,** 2203–2205.

HOLZLE, E., PLEWIG, G. and LEDOLTER, A. (1986) Corneocyte exfoliative cytology: A model to study normal and diseased stratum corneum. In MARKS, R. and PLEWIG, G. (eds) *Skin Models,* New York: Springer Verlag, 183–193.

HORII, I., NAKAYAMA, Y., OBATA, M. and TAGAMI, H. (1989) (Stratum corneum hydration and amino acid content in xerotic skin *Br. J. Dermatol.,* **121**(5), 587–592.

IKARASHI, Y., TSUKAMOTO, Y., TSUCHIYA, T. and NAKAMURA, A. (1993) Influence of irritants on lymph node cell proliferation and the detection of contact sensitivity to metal salts in the murine local lymph node assay. *Contact Dermatitis,* **29,** 128–132.

ISHIHARA, M., TAKASE, Y., HAYAKAWA, R., NISHIKAWA, T., NIIMURA, M. and TOKUDA, Y. (1986) Skin problems caused by cosmetics and quasidrugs: Report by six university hospitals to Ministry of Health and Welfare. *Skin Research (Hifu),* **28,** 80–85.

JAMPEL, R.M., FARMER, E.R., VOGELSANG, G.B., WINGARD, J., SANTOS, G.W. and MORISON, W.L. (1991) Puva therapy for chronic cutaneous graft-vs-host disease. *Arch. Dermatol.*, **127**, 1673–1678.

JORDAN, W.E. and BLANEY, T.L. (1982) Factors influencing infant diaper dermatitis. In MAIBACH, H.I. and BOISITS, E.K. (eds) *Neonatal Skin*, New York: Marcel Dekker, 205–221.

KATSAROU, A., DAVOY, E., XENOS, K., ARMENAKA, M. and THEOHARIDES, T.C. (2000) Effect of an antioxidant (quercetin) on sodium-lauryl-sulfate-induced skin irritation. *Contact Dermatitis*, **42**, 85–89.

KAWAI, K. (1971) Study of determination method of patch test based on microscopical observation. *Acta Derm (Kyoto)*, **66**, 161–182.

KINGSTON, T. and MARKS, R. (1983) Irritant reactions to dithranol in normal subjects and in psoriatic patients. *Br. J. Dermatol.*, **108**, 307–313.

KLIGMAN, A.M. and WOODING, W.A. (1967) A method for the measurement and evaluation of irritants on human skin. *J. Invest. Dermatol.*, **49**, 78–94.

KLIGMAN, A.M. (1976) Perspectives and problems in cutaneous gerontology. *J. Invest. Dermatol.*, **73**, 39–46.

KOMPAORE, F., MARTY, J.P. and DUPONT C. (1993) *In vivo* evaluation of the stratum corneum barrier function in blacks, Caucasians and Asians with two non-invasive methods. *Skin Pharmacol.*, **6**, 200–7.

KRESBACH, H., KARL, H. and WAWSCHINK, O. (1971) Cutaneous mercury granuloma. *Berufsdermatoisen*, **18**, 173–186.

LACHAPELLE, J.M. (1986) Industrial airborne irritant or allergic contact dermatitis. *Contact Dermatitis*, **14**, 137–145.

LAHTI, A. and MAIBACH, H.I. (1985) Guinea pig ear swelling test as an animal model for nonimmunologic contact urticaria. In MAIBACH, H.I. and LOWE, N.I. (eds) *Models in Dermatology*, vol. II, New York: Karger, 356–359.

LAMMINTAUSTA, K. and KALIMO, K. (1981) Atopy and hand dermatitis in hospital wet work. *Contact Dermatitis*, **7**, 301–308.

LAMMINTAUSTA, K., MAIBACH, H.I. and WILSON, D. (1987a) Human cutaneous irritation: induced hyperreactivity. *Contact Dermatitis*, **17**, 193–198.

LAMMINTAUSTA, K., MAIBACH, H.I. and WILSON, D. (1987b) Irritant reactivity in males and females. *Contact Dermatitis*, **17**, 276–280.

LAMMINTAUSTA, K., MAIBACH, H.I. and WILSON, D. (1988a) Susceptibility to cumulative and acute irritant dermatitis. An experimental approach in human volunteers. *Contact Dermatitis*, **19**, 84–90.

CHAPTER 11

LAMMINTAUSTA, K., MAIBACH, H.I. and WILSON, D. (1988b) Mechanisms of subjective (sensory) irritation propensity to nonimmunologic contact urticaria and objective irritation in stingers. *Derm. Beruf Umwelt,* 36, 45–49.

LAMPE, M.A., BURLINGAME, A.L. and WHITNEY, J., WILLIAMS, M.L., BROWN, B.E., ROITMAN, E. and ELIAS, P.M. (1983) Human stratum corneum lipids: characterization and regional variation. *J. Lipid Res.,* 24, 120–130.

LANDMAN, G., FARMER, E.R. and HOOD, A.F. (1990) The pathophysiology of irritant contact dermatitis. In JACKSON E.M., GOLDNER R. (eds) *Irritant Contact Dermatitis.* New York: Marcel Dekker, 67–77.

LANTINGA, H., NATER, J.P. and COENRAADS, P.J. (1984) Prevalence, incidence and course of eczema on the hand and forearm in a sample of the general population. *Contact Dermatitis,* 10, 135–139.

LARMI, E., LAHTI, A. and HANNUKSELA, M. (1989) Effect of ultraviolet B on nonimmunologic contact reactions induced by dimethyl sulphoxide, phenol and sodium lauryl sulfate. *Photodermatology,* 6, 258–262.

LAWRENCE, C.M., HOWEL, C. and SCHESTER, S. (1984) The inflammatory response to anthralin. *Clin. Exp. Dermatol.,* 9(4), 336.

LE, T.K.M., DEMON, P. SCHALKWIJK, J. and VAN DER VALK, P.G. (1997) Effect of a topical corticosteroid, a retinoid and a vitamin D3 derivative on sodium dodecyl sulfate induced skin irritation. *Contact Dermatitis,* 37, 19–26.

LEJMAN, E., STOUDEMAYER, T., GROVE, G. and KLIGMAN, A.M. (1984) Age differences in poison ivy dermatitis. *Contact Dermatitis,* 11, 163–167.

LEVIN, C.Y. and MAIBACH, H.I. (2001) Do cool water or physiologic saline compresses enhance resolution of experimentally-induced irritant contact dermatitis? *Contact Dermatitis,* 45(3), 146–150.

LEVIN, C., ZHAI, H., BASHIR, S., CHEW, A.L., ANIGBOGA, A., STERN, R. and MAIBACH, H.I. (2001) Efficacy of corticosteroids in acute experimental irritant contact dermatitis? *Skin Res. Technol,* 7(4), 214–218.

LISBY, S., BAADSGAARD, O., COOPER, K.D. and VEJLSGAARD, G.L. (1989) Decreased number and function of antigen-presenting cells in the skin following application of irritant agents: relevance for skin cancer? *J. Invest. Dermatol.,* 92(6), 842–847.

LO, J.S., ORIBA, H.A., MAIBACH, H.I. and BAILIN, P.L. (1990) Transepidermal potassium ion, chloride ion, and water flux across delipidized and cellophane tapestripped skin. *Dermatologica,* 180, 66–68.

LODEN, M. (1997) Barrier recovery and influence of irritant stimuli in skin treated with a moisturizing cream. *Contact Dermatitis,* **36,** 256–260.

LOVELL, C.R., RYCROFT, R.C.G., WILLIAMS, D.M.J. and HAMLIN, J.W. (1985) Contact dermatitis from the irritancy (immediate and delayed) and allergenicity of hydroxy acrylate. *Contact Dermatitis,* **12,** 117–118.

MACDONALDS, K.J.S. and MARKS, J. (1986) Short contact anthralin in the treatment of psoriasis: A study of different contact times. *Br. J. Dermatol.,* **114,** 235–239.

MCFADDEN, J.P., HOLLOWAY D.B., WHITTLE E.G., BASKETTER D.A. (2000) Benzalkonium chloride neutralizes the irritant effect of sodium dodecyl sulfate. *Contact Dermatitis,* **43**(5), 264–266.

MAGNUSSON, B. and HERSLE, K. (1965) Patch test methods: Regional variation of patch test responses. *Acta Derm. Venereol. (Stockh.),* **45,** 22–25.

MAGNUSSON, B. and HILLGREN, L. (1962) Skin irritating and adhesive characteristics of some different adhesive tapes. *Acta Derm. Venereol. (Stockh.),* **42,** 463–472.

MAIBACH, H.I. and BOISITS, E.K. (eds) (1982) *Neonatal Skin: Structure and Function,* New York: Marcell Dekker.

MALTEN, K.E. and THIELE, F.A.J. (1973) Evaluation of skin damage. II. Water loss and carbon dioxide release measurements related to skin resistance measurements. *Br. J. Dermatol.,* **89**(6), 565–569.

MALTEN, K.E. and DEN AREND, J. (1978) Topical toxicity of various concentrations of DMSO recorded with impedance measurements and water vapour loss measurements. *Contact Dermatitis,* **4,** 80–92.

MALTEN, K.E., DEN AREND, J. and WIGGERS, R.E. (1979) Delayed irritation: hexanediol diacrylate and butanediol diacrylate. *Contact Dermatitis,* **5,** 178–184.

MALTEN, K.E. (1981) Thoughts on irritant contact dermatitis. *Contact Dermatitis,* **7,** 238–247.

MARKS, F., BERTSCH, S. and FURSTENBURGER, G. (1979) Ornithin decarboxylase activity, cell proliferation,and tumor promotion in mouse epidermis *in vivo. Cancer Res,* **39,** 4183–4188.

MARZULLI, F.N. and MAIBACH, H.I. (1975) The rabbit as a model for evaluating skin irritants: A comparison of results in animals and man using repeated skin exposures. *Food Cosmet. Toxicol.,* **13**(5), 533–540.

■ CHAPTER 11 ■

MAURICE, P.D.L. and GREAVES, M.W. (1983) Relationship between skin type and erythema response to anthralin. *Br. J. Dermatol.,* **109**, 337–341.

MEDING, B. (2000) Differences between the sexes with regard to work-related skin disease. *Contact Dermatitis,* **43**, 65–71.

MIKULOWSKA, A. and ANDERSSON, A. (1996) Sodium lauryl sulfate effect on the density of epidermal Langerhans cells. Evaluation of different test models. *Contact Dermatitis,* **34**(6), 397–401.

MITCHELL, J.C. (1981) Angry back syndrome. *Contact Dermatitis,* **7**, 359–360.

MOBLY, S.L. and MANSMANN, H.C. (1974) Current status of skin testing in children with contact dermatitis. *Cutis,* **13**, 995–1000.

MONTAGA, W. and CARLISLE, K. (1979) Structural changes in aging human skin. *J. Invest. Dermatol.,* **73**, 47–53.

NASSIF, A., CHAN, S., STORRS, F. and HANIFIN, J.M. (1994) Abnormal skin irritancy in atopic dermatitis and in atopy without dermatitis. *Arch. Dermatol.,* **130**(11), 533–540.

National Research Council (1977) *Principles and Procedures for Evaluating the Toxicity of Household Substances,* Washington, DC: National Academy of Sciences.

NILSSON, E., MIKAELSSON, B. and ANDERSSON, S. (1985) Atopy, occupation and domestic work as risk factors for hand eczema in hospital workers. *Contact Dermatitis,* **13**, 216–223.

OHLENSCHLAEGER, J., FRIDBERG, J., RAMSING, D. and AGNER, T. (1996) Temperature dependency of skin susceptibility to water and detergents. *Acta Dermatol. Venerol.,* **76**(4), 274–276.

OLUMIDE, G. (1987) Contact dermatitis in Nigeria. II. Hand dermatitis in men. *Contact Dermatitis,* **17**, 136–138.

O'MALLEY, M.A., MATHIAS, C.G., PRIDDY, M., MOLINA, D., GROTE, A.A. and HALPERIN, W.E. (1988) Occupational vitiligo due to unsuspected presence of phenolic antioxidant byproducts in commercial bulk rubber. *J. Occup. Med.* **30**(6), 512–516.

ORIBA, H.A., ELSNER, P. and MAIBACH, H.I. (1989) Vulvar physiology. *Semin. Dermatol.,* **8**, 2–6.

OSBORNE, R. and PERKINS, M.A. (1994) An approach for development of alternative test methods based on mechanisms of skin irritation. *Food Chem. Toxicol.,* **32**(2), 133–142.

PARCE, J.W., OWICKI, J.C., KEROSO, K.M. SIGAL, G.B., WADA, H.G., MUIR, V.C., BOUSSE, L.J., ROSS, K.L., SIKIC, B.I. and MCCONNELL, H.M. (1989) Detection of cell-affecting agents with silicon biosensor. *Science*, **246**, 243–247.

PATRICK, E., BURKHALTER, A. and MAIBACH, H.I. (1985) Recent investigations of mechanisms of chemically induced skin irritation in laboratory mice. *J. Invest. Dermatol.*, **88**, 245–315.

PHILLIPS, L., STEINBERG, M., MAIBACH, H.I. and AKERS, W.A. (1972) A comparison of rabbit and human skin responses to certain irritants. *Toxicol. Appl. Pharmacol.*, **21**(37), 369–382.

PINNAGODA, J., TUPKER, R.A., AGNER, T., SERUP, J. (1990) Guidelines for transepidermal water loss (TEWL) measurement. *Contact Dermatitis*, **22**, 164–178.

PITTZ, E.P., SMORBECK, R.V. and RIEGER, M.M. (1985) An animal test procedure for the simultaneous assessment of irritancy and efficacy of skin care products. In MAIBACH, H.I. and LOWE, N.J. (eds) *Models in Dermatology*, vol. II, New York: S. Karger, 209–224.

RAPAPORT, M.J. (1984) Patch testing in Japanese subjects. *Contact Dermatitis*, **11**, 93–97.

ROBERTS, D. and MARKS, R. (1980) The determination of regional and age variations in the rate of desquamation: A comparison of four techniques. *J. Invest. Dermatol.*, **74**, 13–16.

ROBINSON, M.K. (2002) Population differences in acute skin irritation responses. Race, sex, age, sensitive skin and repeat subject comparisons. *Contact Dermatitis*, **46**(2), 86–93.

ROLLINS, T.G. (1978) From xerosis to nummular dermatitis: The dehydration dermatosis. *J. Am. Med Assoc.*, **206**, 637.

ROSEN, K., JONTELL, M., MOBACKEN, H. and ROSDAHL, I. (1989) Epidermal Langerhans cells in chronic eczematous dermatitis of the palms treated with PUVA and UVB *Acta Derm. Venereol.*, **69**, 200–205.

ROSKOS, K.V. (1989) The effect of skin aging on the penetration of chemicals through human skin (dissertation). San Francisco, University of California San Francisco.

ROSKOS, K.V., BIRCHER, A.J., MAIBACH, H.I. and GUY, R.H. (1990) Pharmacodynamic measurements of methyl nicotinate percutaneous absorption: the effect of aging on microcirculation. *Br. J. Dermatol.*, **122**, 165–171.

ROTHENBORG, H. W., MENNE, T. and SJOLIN, K. E. (1977) Temperature dependent primary irritant dermatitis from lemon perfume. *Contact Dermatitis*, **1**, 37–48.

ROUGIER, A., GOLDBERG, G. and MAIBACH, H.I. (1994) *In Vitro Irritation.* New York: M. Liebert.

RUTTER, N. (1978) Evaporative water loss from the skin of newborn infants. *J. Physiol. (Lond.),* **276**, 51.

RYCROFT, R.J.G. (1981) Occupational dermatoses from warm dry air. *Br. J. Dermatol.,* **105**(Suppl.) (21), 29–34.

RYSTEDT, I. (1985) Factors influencing the occurrence of hand eczema in adults with a history of atopic dermatitis in childhood. *Contact Dermatitis,* **12**, 247–254.

SCHEYNIUS, A., FISCHER, T., FORSUM, U. KLARESKOG, L. (1984) Phenotypic characterization in situ of inflammatory cells in allergic and irritant contact dermatitis in man *Clin. Exp. Immunol.,* **55**, 81–90.

SCHWINDT, D.A., WILHELM, K.P., MILLER, D.L. and MAIBACH, H.I. (1998) Cumulative irritation in older and younger skin: a comparison. *Acta Derm. Venereol.,* **78**(4), 279–283.

SERUP, J., WINTHER, A. and BLICHMANN, C.W. (1989) Effects of repeated application of a moisturizer. *Acta Derm. Venereol.,* **69**, 457–459.

SEYMOUR, J.L., KESWICH, B.H., HANIFIN, J.M., JORDAN, W.P. and MILLIGAN, M.C. (1987) Clinical effects of diaper types on the skin of normal infants and infants with atopic dermatitis. *J. Am. Acad. Dermatol.,* **17**, 988–997.

SILVERMAN, J. (1983) Preliminary findings on the use of Protozoa (Tetrahymena thermophila) as models for ocular irritation testing in rabbits. *Lab. Anim. Sci.,* **33**, 56–58.

SIMON, M., BERNARD, D., MINODO, A.M. (2001) Persistence of both peripheral and non-peripheral corneodesmosomes in the upper stratum corneum of winter xerosis skin versus only peripheral in normal skin. *J. Invest. Dermatol.,* **116**(1), 23–30).

SMITH, H.R., KELLY, D.A., YOUNG, A.R., BASKETTER, D.B. and McFADDEN, J.P. (2002) Relationship between 2,4-dinitrochlorobenzene elicitation responses and individual irritant threshold. *Contact Dermatitis,* **46**(2), 97–100.

SPRUIT, D. (1970) Evaluation of skin function by the alkali application technique. *Curr. Probl. Dermatol.,* **3**, 148.

STEINBERG, M., AKERS, W.A., WEEKS, M., McCREESH, A.H. and MAIBACH, H.I. (1975) A comparison of test techniques based on rabbit and human skin responses to irritants with recommendations regarding the evaluation of mildly or moderately irritating compounds. In MAIBACH, H.I. (ed.) *Animal Models in Dermatology,* New York: Churchill Livingstone, 1–11.

SUSTEN, A.S. (1985) The chronic effects of mechanical trauma to the skin: A review of the literature. *Am. J. of Indust Med,* **8**, 281–288.

TADAKI ,T., WATANABE, M., KUMASAKA, K., TANITA, Y., KATO, T., TAGAMI, H., HORII, I., YOKOI, T., NAKAYAMA, Y. and KLIGMAN, A.M. (1993) The effect of topical tretinoin on the photodamaged skin of the Japanese. *Tohoku J. Exp. Med.,* **169**, 131–139.

TAGAMI, H. (1971) Functional characteristics of aged skin. *Acta Derm. Venereol. (Stockh.),* **66**, 19–21.

TANAKA, M., ZHEN, Y.X. and TAGAMI, H. (1997) Normal recovery of the stratum corneum barrier function following damage induced by Tape stripping in patients with atopic dermatitis. *Br. J. of Dermatol.,* **136**, 966–967.

THIELE, F.A.J. and MALTEN, K.E. (1973) Evaluation of skin damage I. Skin resistance measurements with alternative current impedance measurements. *Br. J. Dermatol.,* **89**, 373–382.

THIELE, F.A.J. (1974) *Measurements on the Surface of the Skin,* Nijmegen, Netherlands: Drukkeij van Mammeren BV, 81.

THOMSON, A.W., BONHAM, C.A. and ZEEVI, A. (1995) Mode of action of tacrolimus (FK506): Molecular and cellular mechanism. *Ther. Drug Monit.,* **17**, 584–591.

THORVALDSEN, J. and VOLDEN, G. (1980) PUVA-induced diminution of contact allergic and irritant skin reactions. *Clin. Exp. Dermatol.,* **5**, 43–46.

THUNE, P., NILSEN, T., HANSTAD, I.K., GUSTAVSEN, T. and LOVIG DAHL, H. (1988) The water barrier function of the skin in relation to the water content of stratum corneum, PH and skin lipids: The effect of alkaline soap and syndet on dry skin in elderly, non-atopic patients. *Acta Derm. Venereol. (Stockh.),* **66**, 277–283.

TUPKER, R.A., PINNAGODA, J., COENRAADS, P.G. and NATER, J.P. (1990) Suscepti-bility to irritants: role of barrier function, skin dryness and history of atopic dermatitis. *Br. J. of Dermatol.,* **123**, 199–205.

TUR, E., MAIBACH, H.I. and GUY, R.H. (1985) Spatial variability of vasodilatation in human forearm skin. *Br. J. Dermatol.,* **113**, 197–303.

ULFGREN, A.K., KLARESKOG, L. and LINDBERG, M. (2000) An immunohisto-chemical analysis of cytokine expression in allergic and irritant contact dermatitis. *Acta Derm. Venereol.,* **80**(3), 167–170.

VAN DER VALK, P.G.M., NATER, J.P.K. and BLEUMINK, E. (1985) Vulnerability of the skin to surfactants in different groups of eczema patients and controls as measured by water vapour loss. *Clin. Exp. Dermatol.,* **10**(2), 98–103.

CHAPTER 11

VAN DER VALK, P.G.M. and MAIBACH, H.I. (1989a) Post application occlusion substantially increases the response of the skin to repeated short term SLS exposure. *Contact Dermatitis,* **21**, 335–338.

VAN DER VALK, P.G.M. and MAIBACH, H.I. (1989b) Potential for irritation increases from the wrist to the cubital fossa. *Br. J. Dermatol.,* **121**, 709–712.

VAN DER VALK, P.G.M. and MAIBACH, H.I. (1989c) Do topical corticosteroids modulate skin irritation in human beings? Assessment by transepidermal water loss and visual scoring. *J. Am. Acad. Dermatol.,* **21**, 519–522.

VICKERS, H. R. (1962) The influence of age on the onset of dermatitis in industry. Prague, Symposium Dermatologorum de Morbis Cutaneis, pp. 145–148.

VINK, A.A., MOODYCLIFFE, A.M., SHREEDHAR, V., ULLRICH, S.E., ROZA, L., YAROSH, D.B. and KRIPKE, M.L. (1997) The inhibition of antigen-presenting activity of dendritic cells resulting from UV irradiation of murine skin is restore by *in vitro* photorepair of cyclobutane pyrimidine dimmers. *Proc. Natl. Acad. Sci.,* **94**, 5255–5260.

VON HAGERMAN, G. (1957) Uber das "traumiterative" (toxische) Ekzem *Dermatologica,* **115**, 525–529.

VON HORNSTEIN, O.P., BAURLE, G. and KIENLEIN-KLETSCHKA, B.M. (1986) Prospktiv-Studie zur bedeutung konstitutioneller Parameter fur die Ekzemgenese im Friseur und Baugewerbe. *Derm. Beruf Umwell,* **33**(2), 43–498.

VON HORNSTEIN, O.P. and KIENLEIN-KLETSCHKA, B.M. (1982) Improvement of patch test allergen exposure by short-term local pressure. *Dermatologica,* **165**, 607–611.

WAGNER, G. and PORSCHEL, W. (1962) Klinisch-analytische studie zum neuro-dermatitisproblem. *Dermatologica,* **125**, 1–32.

WAHLBERG, J.E. and MAIBACH, H.I. (1981) Sterile-cutaneous pustules: A manifestation of contact pustulogens. *J. Invest Dermatol.,* **76**, 381–383.

WAHLBERG, J.E. and MAIBACH, H.I. (1982) Identification of contact pustulogens. In MARZULLI, F.N. and MAIBACH, H.I. (eds) *Dermatotoxicology,* 2nd ed., New York: Hemisphere, 627–635.

WEIGAND, D.A. and GAYLOR, J.R. (1974) Irritant reaction in Negro and Caucasian skin. *South Med. J.,* **67**, 548–551.

WERNER, Y., LINDBERG, M. and FORSLIND, B. (1982) The water binding capacity of stratum corneum in dry non-eczematous skin of atopic eczema. *Acta Derm. Venereol. (Stockh.),* **62**, 334–336.

WESTER, R.C. and MAIBACH, H.I. (1985) Dermatopharmocokinetics. In MAIBACH, H.I. and BRONAUGH, R.L. (eds) *Clinical Dermatology in Percutaneous Absorption*, New York: Marcel Dekker, 525–530.

WESTER, R.C. and MAIBACH, H.I. (1989) Regional variation in percutaneous absorption. In Bronaugh, R.L. and Maibach, H.I. (eds) *Percutaneous Absorption*, New York: Marcel Dekker.

WIDMER, J., ELSNER, P. and BURG, G. (1994) Skin irritant reactivity following experimental cumulative irritant contact dermatitis. *Contact Dermatitis*, **30**, 35–39.

WIGGER-ALBERTI, W., KREBS, A., ELSNER, P. (2000) Experimental irritant contact dermatitis due to cumulative epicutaneous exposure to sodium lauryl sulfate and toluene: single and concurrent application. *Br. J. Dermatol.*, **143**, 551–556.

WILHELM, K.P., SURBER, C. and MAIBACH, H.I. (1989) Quantification of sodium lauryl sulfate irritant dermatitis in man: comparison of four techniques: skin color reflectance, transepidermal water loss, laser Doppler flow measurement and visual scores. *Arch. Dermatol. Res.* **281**(4), 293–295.

WILHELM, K.P., PASCHE, F. and SURBER, C. (1990) Sodium hydroxide-induced subclinical irritation. *Acta Derm. Venereol. (Stockh.)*, **70**, 463–467.

WILHELM, K.P., BOTTJER, B., SIEGERS, C.P. (2001) Quantitative assessment of primary skin irritants *in vitro* in a cytotoxicity model: comparison with *in vivo* human irritation test. *Br. J. of Dermatol.*, **145**, 709–715.

WILLIS, C.M., STEPHENS, C.J.M. and WILKINSON, J.D. (1989) Epidermal damage induced by irritants in man: a light and electron microscopic study *J. Invest. Dermatol.*, **92**, 695–699.

WILLIS, C.M., STEPHENS, C.J.M.and WILKINSON, J.D. (1991) Selective expression of immune associated surface antigens by keratinocytes in irritant contact dermatitis. *J. Invest. Dermatol.*, **96**, 505–511.

WILLIS, C.M., BRITTON, L.E., REICHE, L. and WILKINSON, J.D. (2001) Reduced levels of glutathione S-transferases in patch test reactions to dithranol and sodium lauryl sulfate as demonstrated by quantitative immunocyto-chemistry: evidence for oxidative stress in acute irritant contact dermatitis. *Eur J. Dermatol.*, 11(2), 99–104.

WILSON, D., BERARDESCA, E. and MAIBACH, H.I. (1988) *In vitro* transepidermal water loss: differences between black and white human skin. *Br. J. Dermatol.*, **119**, 647–652.

CHAPTER 11

WOOD, L.C., JACKSON, S.M., ELIAS, P.M., GRUNFELD, C. and FEINGOLD, K.R. (1992) Cutaneous barrier pertubation stimulates cytokine production in the epidermis of mice. *J. Clin. Invest.,* **90**, 482–487.

WORTH, A.P. and CRONIN, M.T. (2001) Prediction models for eye irritation potential based on end points of the HETCAM and neutral uptake test. *In Vitr. Mol. Toxicol.* **14**(3), 143–156.

YOSHIKAWA, N., IMOKAWA, G., AKIMOTO, K. JIN, K., HIGAKI, Y. and KAWASHIMA, M. (1994) Regional analysis of ceramides within the stratum corneum in relation to seasonal changes. *Dermatology,* **188**, 207–214.

YOSHIZAWA, Y., TANOJO, H., KIM, S.J., MAIBACH, H.I. (2001) Sea water or its components alter experimental irritant dermatitis in man. *Skin Res. Technol.,* **7**(1), 36–39.

ZHAI, H. and MAIBACH, H.I. (1998) Moisturizers in preventing irritant contact dermatitis: an overview. *Contact Dermatitis,* **38**, 241–244.

ZIIERZ, P., KIESSLING, W. and BERG, A. (1960) Experimentelle Prufung der Hautfunktion bei Ichthyosis Vulgaris. *Arch. Klin. Exp. Dermatol.,* **209**, 592.

12

Allergic Contact Dermatitis

FRANCIS N MARZULLI AND HOWARD I MAIBACH

Contact dermatitis, an inflammatory skin disease characterized by itching, redness, and skin lesions, is caused by skin contact with either an irritant or an allergenic chemical. Acute irritant contact dermatitis arises on first contact with an adequate concentration of a direct-acting cytotoxic chemical. On the other hand, allergic contact dermatitis (ACD) usually arises following more than one skin contact (induction and elicitation) with an allergenic chemical. The skin response of ACD is delayed, immunologically mediated, and consists of varying degrees of erythema, edema, and vesiculation. In the Gell and Coombs system (1968) it is classified as a cell-mediated, tuberculin-like, Type IV allergy.

The best known example of ACD is the linear vesicular skin response that is often seen hours after contact with poison ivy, at which time itching is a prominent symptomatic feature.

Allergenic chemicals penetrate the skin as small molecules (usually <400 MW), and they are incompletely allergenic (haptens) until they bind to protein and form a complete allergen.

In ACD, the first significant exposure to a haptenic chemical activates the immune system (induction) and sensitizes the skin. After sensitization (which takes a few days to a few weeks), subsequent antigenic exposures result in the evocation of an altered ("allergic") skin response (elicitation), that is, one that is more pronounced than the original response. In order for sensitization to take place, the allergenic chemical must first penetrate the skin, so that it can reach and interact with key elements of the underlying immune system. A certain level of allergen entry must be achieved that represents a threshold for triggering the immune system. The threshold can be reached following a single skin exposure to a sufficiently high amount or concentration of allergenic chemical, or after contact with a large area of skin, or as a consequence of repeated skin applications.

Once the allergenic chemical has abrogated the horny barrier layer of skin and entered the viable layer of the epidermis, it makes contact and binds with Langerhans cells. These are dendritic cells that direct the allergen to a regional lymph node where interaction with T lymphocytes is followed by replication of sensitized T lymphocytes and expansion of the sensitized T-lymphocyte population, completing the induction phase of the sensitization process.

In the sensitized individual, the next contact with the allergenic chemical results in the elicitation of a hypersensitive skin response that is due to a reaction between circulating sensitized lymphocytes and allergen at the skin site where allergen has entered the living epidermis.

The term allergy was coined by von Pirquet in 1910; however, our present understanding of events of the sensitization process probably began to unfold after the patch test was developed by Jadassohn (1895). This test was intended to clinically duplicate contact allergy on a small scale by applying a suspect chemical to the skin of a sensitized patient (under occlusion) to confirm its allergenic potential.

The next important episode involved the passive transfer of immediate-type allergy by the Prausnitz-Kustner reaction (1921). This consisted of injecting blood serum from an allergic person into the skin of a normal person, making the injected site reactive to the injected allergen.

Landsteiner and Jacobs (1936) demonstrated that delayed-type reactions could be induced by intradermal injection of certain allergens.

Another important finding was that of Landsteiner and Chase (1942) that lymphocytes become sensitized during the development of ACD.

Other early historical events were reviewed in the 50th anniversary issue of the *Journal of Allergy and Clinical Immunology* (Allergy, 1979).

The development of predictive and diagnostic human and guinea pig tests for skin sensitization focused further attention on ACD (Schwartz, 1941), as did regulatory and legal requirements for evaluating drug and cosmetic safety (Draize, 1959).

Early in the study of ACD, humans were the primary investigative test species. Later, guinea pigs were added as the animal model of choice. More recently the mouse has been used extensively.

Concordance of developments in genetics and molecular biology, based on mouse studies, with the entry of the mouse as a test species for ACD potential led ultimately to the finding that cytokines play a role in both irritant dermatitis and ACD. A detailed interpretation of cellular and molecular events of ACD is given in Sauder and Pastore (1993).

Entrance of an irritant or allergenic chemical into the epidermis signals the release of a cascade of cytokines from affected keratinocytes, suggesting a key role for keratinocytes in these inflammatory processes. It is not yet clear how cytokines differ qualitatively and quantitatively during ACD and irritant reactions, but this is likely to be an important area of future research.

While foundations for the overall picture of events of ACD appear secure, the future may unhinge some present interpretations of the details.

Keratinocytes comprise the main cellular composition of the human epidermis. They are involved in synthesis of various cytokines during both normal and abnormal cell functions. Cytokines are regulatory proteins that mediate cell communication, and include interleukins, growth factors, colony-stimulating factors, and interferons. When keratinocytes are damaged during contact with irritant or allergenic compounds, various inflammatory elements, including cytokines, adhesion molecules, and chemotactic factors, are released (Barker *et al.*, 1991; Kupper, 1989). Current research interest in this area has sparked a continuously expanding literature.

A number of studies have been conducted to investigate the activation sequence following keratinocyte damage. In one such study (Willis *et al.*, 1989), 10 healthy human volunteers were patch tested with 6 structurally unrelated irritants, and their skins were biopsied 48 h later and examined by light and electron microscopy. Keratinocytes were damaged in distinctly different patterns, and mononuclear cells were the predominant infiltration response.

It is virtually impossible to distinguish irritant dermatitis from ACD with precision, on gross and even microscopic inspection. Recently, Brasch *et al.* (1992) reported an attempt to find a distinction between the two dermatides. Topically applied sodium lauryl sulfate (SLS), an irritant chemical, was administered to seven sensitized subjects along with the allergenic chemical, on two separate test skin sites, in order to produce experimental irritant and allergic contact dermatitis on a small scale. Both skin sites responded similarly in clinical appearance, histology, and immunohistology. A large battery of monoclonal antibodies directed against numerous surface, intracellular, and nuclear antigens failed to uncover a difference between the irritant and the allergic sites by these immunostaining techniques.

The finding that cytokines are released during the ACD process opens the way to the ultimate development of a specific test to differentiate ACD from irritant dermatitis (Enk and Katz, 1992; Paludan and Thestrup-Pederson, 1992).

Some commonly encountered allergens that have been reported by members of the North American Contact Dermatitis Research Group during diagnostic studies of clinical patients include (Storrs *et al.*, 1989) balsam of Peru, benzocaine, benzoyl peroxide, black rubber paraphenylenediamine mix, caine mix minus benzocaine, carba mix, cinnamic alcohol, cinnamic aldehyde, dibucaine, cyclomethycaine sulfate, epoxy resin, ethylenediamine dihydro-chloride, eugenol, formaldehyde, hydroxycitronellal, imidazolidinyl urea, isoeugenol, lanolin alcohol, mercapto rubber mix, mercaptobenzothiazole, neomycin sulfate, nickel sulfate, oak moss, *p*-tertiary butylphenol formaldehyde resin, potassium dichromate, *p*-phenylene diamine, quaternium-15, rosin (colophony), tetracaine, thimerosol, and thiuram rubber mix.

■ CHAPTER 12 ■

Vehicle and preservative allergens include ammoniated mercury, benzo-phenone, 2-bromo-2-nitropropane 1, 3-diol (bronopol), captan, chloroaceta-mide, *p*-chloro-*m*-cresol, chloroxylenol, diazolidinyl urea, dichlorophene, DMDM hydantoin, Kathon CG, paraben mix, polythylene glycol, *o*-phenylphenol, propylene glycol, sorbic acid, and Tween 85.

Cosmetic injury reports to the Office of Cosmetics and Colors, FDA (1988–1993), are similar to preceding years when fragrances and preservatives were established as the most common sensitizers in cosmetics.

Among the newer preservative chemicals that may sensitize are methyldibro-moglutaronitrile and phenoxyethanol (Euxyl K 400). Dibenzoyl methanes in addition to PABA (*para*-aminoben-zoic acid) are among the newer sunscreens that are potential allergens (Brancaccio, 1992). Furthermore, glyceryl mono-thioglycolate is a sensitizer in hair products; nicotine is in transdermal therapeutic systems; and corticosteroids such as hydrocortisone are of increasing concern as sensitizers (Brancaccio, 1992).

Natural rubber latex, now widely used in surgical gloves and in condoms, is producing allergic reactions in epidemic proportions.

Additional useful information relating to the allergenic potential of specific chemicals is published in other scientific journals.

The Cosmetic Ingredient Review Committee of the Cosmetic, Toiletry and Fragrance Association has published 22 special issues of the *Journal of the American College of Toxicology* that contain information on skin sensitization and other safety data on cosmetic ingredients beginning in 1982.

The Research Institute for Fragrance Material has published sensitization data on chemicals that have been proposed for use as fragrance ingredients and are in *Food and Chemical Toxicology.*

REFERENCES

ALLERGY, a historical review. (1979) *J. Allergy Clin. Immunol.* (50th Anniversary Issue, 1929–1979) **64**(5).

BARKER, J.N.W.N., MITRA, R.S., GRIFFITHS, C.E.M., DIXIT, V. M., and NICKOLOFF, B.J. (1991) Keratinocytes as initiators of inflammation. *The Lancet* **337**, 221–215.

BRANCACCIO, R.R. (1992) Three cosmetic preservatives. *Am. J. Contact Dermatis.* **4**, 55–57.

BRASCH, J., BURGARD, J., and STERRY, W. (1992) Common pathogenetic pathways in allergic and irritant contact dermatitis. *J. Invest. Dermatol.* **98**, 166–170.

DRAIZE, J. (1959) Dermal toxicity. In *Appraisal of the Safety of Chemicals in Foods, Drugs, and Cosmetics*, Austin, TX: Association of Food and Drug Officials of the United States, Texas State Department of Health, 46–49.

ENK, A.H., and Katz, S.(1992) Early events in the induction phase of contact sensitivity. *Soc. Invest. Dermatol.* **99**, 39S–41S.

GELL, P.G.H., and Coombs, R.R.A. (1968) *Clinical Aspects of Immunology*, 2nd ed., Oxford: Blackwell.

JADASSOHN, J. 1895. Zur Kenntnis der medikamentosen dermatosen. In JARISCH, A. and NEISSER, A. (eds) *Verh. Dtsch. Derm Gesellschaft. V. Kongress*, 103–129.

KUPPER, T.S. (1989) Mechanisms of cutaneous inflammation. *Arch. Dermatol.* **125**, 1406–1412.

LANDSTEINER, K., and CHASE, M.W. (1941) Studies on the sensitization of animals with simple chemical compounds. *J. Exp. Biol. Med.* **73**, 431.

LANDSTEINER, K., and CHASE, M.W. (1942) Experiments on transfer of cutaneous sensitivity to simple compounds. *Proc. Soc. Exp. Biol. Med.* **49**, 688.

LANDSTEINER, K., and JACOBS, J.L. (1936) Studies on the sensitization of animals with simple chemical compounds. *J. Exp. Biol. Med.* **64**, 625–639.

OFFICE of COSMETICS and COLORS, FDA. (1988–1993) Cosmetic Injury Reports from consumers, as reported to the Office of Cosmetics and Colors, FDA.

PALUDAN, K., and THESTRUP-PEDERSEN, (1992) Use of the polymerase chain reaction in quantification of interleukin 8 mRNA in minute epidermal samples. *Soc. Invest. Dermatol.* **99**, 830–835.

PRAUSNITZ, C., and KUSTNER, H. (1921/1968). Studies on supersensitivity, transl. from the German original article by C. Prausnitz. In GELL, P.G.H. and COOMBS, R.R.A., (eds) *Clinical Aspects of Immunology*, Oxford: Blackwell.

SAUDER, D., and PASTORE, S. (1993). Cytokines in contact dermatitis. *Am. J. Contact Derm.* **4**, 215–224.

SCHWARTZ, L. (1941) Dermatitis from new synthetic resin fabric finishes. *J. Invest. Dermatol.* **4**, 459–470.

STORRS, F.J., ROSENTHAL, L.E., ADAMS, R.M., CLENDENNING, W., EMMETT, E.A., FISHER, A.A., LARSEN, W.G., MAIBACH, H.I., RIETSCHEL, R.L., SCHORR, W.F. *et. al.* (1989) Prevalence and relevance of allergic reactions in patients patch-tested in North America—1984 to 1985. *J. Am. Acad. Dermatol.* **20**, 1038–1045.

VON PIRQUET, C. (1910) *Allergie*. Berlin: Julius Springer.

WILLIS, C. M., STEPHENS, J. M., and WILKINSON, J. (1989) Epidermal damage induced by irritants in man: Light and electron microscopic study. *J. Invest. Dermatol.* **93**, 695–700.

■ CHAPTER 12 ■

Irritant Contact Dermatitis versus Allergic Contact Dermatitis

IRIS S ALE AND HOWARD I MAIBACH

Contents

13.1 Introduction

13.2 Clinical diagnosis

13.3 Histological and immunohistochemical studies

13.4 Cytokines

13.5 Allergens and irritants in immunotoxicology testing

13.6 Conclusions

13.1 INTRODUCTION

Topical exposure to a variety of xenobiotics may result in irritant contact dermatitis (ICD) as well as allergic contact dermatitis (ACD), both in animals and humans. ICD and ACD may have clinical, histological and immuno-histochemical similarities (Lammintausta and Maibach, 1990; Patil and Maibach, 1994; Brasch et al., 1992; Scheynius et al., 1984), but the immuno-logical mechanisms that underlie both types of response are thought to be essentially different. Allergic contact hypersensitivity has been considered a prototype of cutaneous delayed-type hypersensitivity reaction, requiring the activation and clonal expansion of allergen-responsive T-lymphocytes. The cutaneous inflammatory response is thus orchestrated by primed memory T-cells. In contrast, ICD has been defined as local inflammatory reaction following a single or repeated exposure to an irritant, which is an agent producing direct toxic insult to the cutaneous cells (Mathias and Maibach, 1978). Irritants are believed to initiate the immune cascade independently of the antigen presentation pathway, by inducing proinflammatory mediators that directly recruit and activate T-lymphocytes. Irritant reactions do not result in the induction of antigen-specific memory T-cells, and are considered as the result of a primarily nonimmunological damage to the skin. However, as new information becomes available, the distinction between immunological and nonimmunological events becomes progressively blurred, and it is now apparent that allergic and irritant contact reactions have at least partially overlapping pathophysiology and share common effector pathways (Brand et al., 1996; Effendy et al., 2000; Mohamadzadeh et al., 1994). Moreover, many chemicals that are capable of behaving as contact allergens have also irritant properties, frequently disregarded because their allergenic potential dominates their toxicity profile. Indeed, it is believed that irritancy promotes allergic sensitization to some degree, even if the mechanisms underlying this interaction are only partially known. The "danger signal" hypothesis (Matzinger, 1998) suggests that the immune responses can be induced by danger signals released by tissues undergoing stress, damage or abnormal death. In this context, an antigenic signal will produce sensitization only in the presence of a danger signal; in its absence tolerance will occur. Irritancy may represent a "danger signal" for the immune system as direct toxic damage of dendritic cells (DC) or other cells (principally keratinocytes) and cytokine release may activate the DC and therefore, predispose to allergic sensitization (Gallucci and Matzinger, 2001; McFadden and Basketter, 2000). In fact, as most allergens have irritant

■ CHAPTER 13 ■

properties, both the antigenic and "danger" signals arise from the hapten (Smith *et al.*, 2002).

The basis for a diagnosis of either irritant contact dermatitis (ICD) or allergic contact dermatitis (ACD) is mainly established by considering the morphology of the clinical lesions, assessing the relationship between the putative exposure and the time course of the dermatitis, as well as performing appropriate diagnostic testing. Differentiation between ICD and ACD is frequently difficult in the clinical setting. This represents a considerable predicament, in view of the high frequency of these entities and their impact in the patients' quality of life. Discriminating between allergens and irritants is also crucial in toxicological research. Major efforts have been made to identify histological, immunohisto-chemical and immunological changes allowing for a clear-cut distinction between allergen and irritant treatments. Such information will enhance our understanding of the molecular processes involved in ICD and ACD and may provide a mechanistic basis for designed refined *in vivo* and *in vitro* models to be applied in toxicological testing.

13.2 CLINICAL DIAGNOSIS

Irritant dermatitis is not a single clinical entity but rather a heterogeneous spectrum of disorders (Table 13.1) with diverse pathophysiology and a broad range of clinical and histological features (Berardesca, 1997). The diagnosis of acute ICD to strong skin irritant agents is usually straightforward, because the rapid onset of skin lesions after exposure points to the causative agent. On the other hand, subacute or chronic contact dermatitis, frequently appears as an eczematous condition without a readily apparent cause. In these circumstances the clinician must go through a decision process to discriminate between ICD, ACD or other eczematous conditions. Differentiation between chronic ICD and ACD is frequently impossible on the basis of macroscopic or microscopic morphology (Table 13.2). The clinical picture in both conditions may include erythema, lichenification, excoriations, scaling and hyperkeratosis. ICD lesions are usually sharply demarcated and confined to the contact area whilst in ACD, lesions are poorly circumscribed and frequently disseminated. However, ICD lesions may disseminate depending on the characteristics of the exposure. Irritant reactions were believed to be unspecific and reproducible in all exposed subjects in contradistinction with the uniqueness and specificity of allergic reactions. Yet, different irritants produce inflammation by different mechanisms and through different mediators. The effects of irritants on cutaneous targets

TABLE 13.1:

Clinical spectrum of irritant contact dermatitis

Type of irritation	Onset and Type of Exposure	Clinical Characteristics
Acute ICD	Acute. Often single exposure to a strong irritant	Erythema, edema, weeping, vesicles, bullae, necrosis
Irritant reaction-ICD	Develops in weeks to months. Often multiple exposure	Erythema, papules, dryness, scaling
Acute Delayed ICD	Delayed onset of clinical lesions: 8–24 h or more	Erythema, papules, vesicles, bullae
Cumulative ICD	Develops slowly: months to years—Multiple exposure to a variety of agents	Erythema, papules, dryness, scaling, fissuring, lichenification
Traumiterative ICD	Develops slowly: months to years—Multiple exposure to a single agent	Erythema, papules, dryness, scaling, fissuring, lichenification
Traumatic Irritant Dermatitis	Develops in weeks after skin trauma	Erythema, papules, bullae, dryness, scaling, fissuring, lichenification, callus
Pustular and Acneiform Dermatitis	Develops in weeks to months—Exposure to special agents	Papules, pustules, comedones
Exsiccation Eczematide	Develops in weeks—Multiple exposure	Dryness, scaling, fissuring
Nonerythematous Irritation	Variable onset	Dryness, scaling
Subjective	Variable onset—Exposure to special agents	Non-visible changes

■
CHAPTER 13
■

depend on several factors, such as the type of chemical, concentration, mode of exposure, concomitant environmental factors, and individual susceptibility (Lammintausta *et al.*, 1987; Berardesca and Maibach, 1988; Lammintausta and Maibach, 1988; Wilhelm and Maibach, 1990; Patil and Maibach, 1994; Judge *et al.*, 1996; Rietschel, 1997). Irritant thresholds and dose responses vary considerably among individuals when tested with a low concentrated or mild irritant and also in the same individual over time (Judge *et al.*, 1996).

Concerning the timing of the dermatitis, features claimed helpful in distinguishing irritant dermatitis include: cutaneous reaction upon first exposure— at least with potent irritants—and rapid onset of dermatitis after exposure. In ACD two phases are required: an induction phase, during which sensitization is acquired, followed by elicitation of a cutaneous inflammatory reaction in subsequent exposures. Usually, the induction phase does not result in clinical

TABLE 13.2:
Clinical and histological differences between ICD and ACD

	ICD	ACD
Clinical characteristics	Acute lesions: Erythema, oedema, oozing sometimes vesicles and bullae. Ulceration, necrosis and pustules may be seen Chronic lesions: May be indistinguishable of ACD, including hyperkeratosis, fissuring, redness, chapping, glazed or scalded appearance of the skin.	Acute lesions: Erythema, edema, vesicles, oozing Intense vesiculation increases the suspicion of ACD Pustules, necrosis or ulceration are rarely seen Chronic lesions: May be indistinguishable of ACD. Vesiculation may not be present
	Lesions are characteristically circumscribed to the contact area. Usually there is absence of distant lesions, but sometimes dermatitis may be generalized depending on the nature of the exposure.	Clinical lesions are stronger in the contact area but their limits are usually ill defined. Dissemination of the dermatitis with distant lesions may occur.
	Lesions may appear after first exposure (at least with strong irritants)	A phase of induction (sensitization) without clinical signs is required. Clinical lesions appear after subsequent challenges. However, exposure to a strong allergen may serve as both induction and elicitation of contact sensitivity
	In acute ICD lesions usually appear rapidly, in minutes to few hours after exposure, and are characterized by the "decrescendo phenomenon," the reaction reaches its peak quickly, and then heals However delayed-onset reactions can be seen (12 to 24 h or more after exposure)	Lesions usually appear 24–72 hours after the last exposure to the causative agent, but they may develop as early as five hours or as late as 7 days after exposure Allergic reactions are characterized by the "crescendo phenomenon."
	Symptoms of acute ICD are burning, stinging, pain and soreness of the skin (pruritus may be present).	Pruritus is the main symptom of ACD.
Histological characteristics	Greater pleomorphism than ACD Moderate spongiosis, intracellular edema (ballooning), exocytosis Diffuse distribution of the inflammatory infiltrate in epidermis. Occasionally, neutrophil-rich infiltrates Pustulation and necrosis may develop.	Less pleomorphism than ICD Spongiosis with microvesicles predominate Focal distribution of the inflammatory infiltrate in epidermis Pustulation and necrosis are rare

skin lesions, probably due to the low numbers of responder T-lymhocytes present. Subsequent challenges, resulting in clonal T-cell expansion and representation of the antigen to already primed (memory) T-cells may induce an enhanced inflammatory response eliciting the clinical dermatitis. However, a potent allergen may induce both sensitization and elicitation phases through a single exposure. Acute ICD develops rapidly after exposure, whilst ACD lesions usually appear 24 to 96 hours after the last exposure to the causative agent, depending on the characteristics of the sensitizer, the conditions of exposure and the individual susceptibility.

Patch testing is applied to make the distinction between ACD and ICD in clinical settings. The morphology and kinetics of the response is important when assessing patch test reactions. The irritant reaction usually reaches its peak quickly after exposure, and then starts to heal; this is called the *decrescendo* phenomenon. Allergic reactions are characteristically delayed, reaching their maximum at approximately 72 to 96 hours (*crescendo* phenomenon). However, some irritants may elicit a delayed inflammatory response, and visible inflammation is not seen until 24 hours or even more after exposure (Malten *et al.*, 1979; Bruynzeel *et al.*, 1982; Lammintausta and Maibach, 1990; Reiche *et al.*, 1998).

13.3 HISTOLOGICAL AND IMMUNOHISTOCHEMICAL STUDIES

Cellular changes that take place during the development of ACD and ICD, including modifications in the morphological appearance, proliferative state and cell kinetics have been evaluated in an attempt to discriminate between both disorders.

ICD shows much greater histological pleomorphism than ACD (Table 13.2). Irritants produce a wide range of histopathological changes as a consequence of their different mechanism of action and chemical interaction with the skin components. Lesions will also vary according to concentration of the irritant, type and duration of the exposure, and individual reactivity of the skin (Patrick *et al.*, 1985; Willis *et al.*, 1988, 1992; Lachapelle 1995). ACD is a spongiotic dermatitide and the histology varies depending on the evolutive stage. Early allergic reactions are characterized by dermal inflammatory infiltrates around the dilated venules of the superficial plexus, edema and spongiosis. The inflammatory infiltrate in the epidermis characteristically adopt a focal distribution (Avnstorp *et al.*, 1987). Fully developed spongiosis becomes organized in

CHAPTER 13

focal microvesicles. If the process evolves more slowly, the spongiosis propels the epidermis to become hyperplastic. Rubbing and scratching will cause lichenification with acanthosis and hyperkeratosis. In time, slowly evolving lesions of ACD become less spongiotic and more psoriasiform. In late lesions of ACD there is almost no spongiosis. ICD also shows a perivascular inflammatory infiltrate in the dermis. In epidermis, the inflammatory infiltrate characteristically adopts a more widespread, diffuse distribution. There may be some spongiosis, but it is habitually associated with ballooning of epidermal cells (intracellular edema), a phenomenon characterized by abundant, pale-staining cytoplasm of keratinocytes. In addition, the intraepidermal vesicles often develop into vesiculo-pustules and there is dermal and epidermal infiltration of neutrophilic granulocytes (Avnstorp, 1988). Strong irritants may induce necrosis of keratinocytes. Chronic ICD is usually indistinguishable of chronic ACD, showing thickening of the epidermis and hyperkeratosis.

It has been suggested that spongiosis may be specific of allergic reactions. In a comparative light microscopic study, early allergic patch test responses (6 to 8 h after challenge) were characterized by follicular spongiosis, while clinically equipotent irritant reactions induced by sodium lauryl sulfate (SLS) showed no significant changes (Vestergaard *et al.*, 1999). However, spongiosis has been observed after challenge with other irritants, such as benzalkonium chloride, croton oil and dithranol (Willis *et al.*, 1989).

Avnstorp *et al.* (1988) selected 17 histological variables for establishing the differential diagnosis between irritant and allergic reactions. In ACD reactions, the focal disposition of the inflammatory infiltrate in epidermis was found to be significantly different from disperse distribution in ICD reactions. Necrosis was a significant feature in the diagnosis of irritant reactions, as it was the finding of neutrophilic granulocytes infiltrating the dermal stroma. Statistical analysis by correlation of the selected variables gave a diagnostic specificity of 87 percent and a sensitivity of 81 percent for allergic reactions. In irritant reactions the specificity was 100 percent but the sensitivity was only 46 percent. By multiple regression analysis, an index could be calculated: 4 × necrosis − 3 × edema −2. Subzero values denoted irritancy, whilst values above zero indicated allergy.

Both allergic and irritant challenges induce epidermal proliferation, however the dynamics are different. Irritant reactions to SLS induced a statistically significant increase in epidermal volume at 24 and 72 hours after challenge, compared to 0 and 6 hours ($p < 0.003$ and $p < 0.001$ respectively), whereas the increase in the epidermal volume in allergic reactions to nickel sulfate was not noted until 72 hours after challenge, compared with 0, 6 hours ($p < 0.001$) and 24 hours ($p < 0.004$) (Emilson *et al.*, 1998). Le *et al.* (1995) observed that challenge with the irritant SLS induced a higher and earlier increase in the number of cycling epidermal cells, and the maximum proliferation was reached four days after challenge. In comparison, allergic reactions showed a gradual increase in proliferating cells until a peak was attained on day five. Similarly, the expression of keratin 16 (K16), a molecule that is present in the suprabasal epidermis under hyperproliferative conditions, and involucrin, a marker of terminal differentiation, increased rapidly following challenge with SLS, reaching a peak after three days and fading thereafter, whilst allergic reactions exhibited a more delayed response reaching a maximum after four days. A positive CD36 (OKM5) expression was found both in irritant and allergic patch tests (Vestergaard *et al.*, 1995). It has been postulated that there may possibly be a connection between OKM5 expression in the stratum granulosum and the proliferative state of the epidermis (Willis *et al.*, 1991).

Concerning the cells of the inflammatory infiltrate, identical composition of peripheral T-lymphocytes, associated with peripheral HLA-DR positive macrophages and Langerhans cells is observed in irritant and allergic contact dermatitis (Scheynius *et al.*, 1984; Ferguson *et al.*, 1984; Brasch *et al.*, 1992; Ranki *et al.*, 1983). In the lymphocyte population, helper/induced T-lymphocytes exceed the number of suppressor/cytotoxic cells in both types of reaction. (Scheynius *et al.* 1984; Avnstorp *et al.*, 1987). The number of infiltrating cells was larger in biopsies from allergic reactions induced by nickel sulfate than in irritant reactions induced by SLS. However, the kinetics of the cell responses, the phenotypes of the inflammatory cells, their allocation and spatial relationship was comparable (Scheynius, 1984). Similar findings were reported by Gawkrodger *et al.* (1986) although slight differences in the spatial distribution between both types of reactions were observed. Dermal infiltrates were larger in the allergic reactions, but epidermal invasiveness was greater in the irritant reactions. At the single-cell level, the expression of very late activation antigen (VLA) molecules, lymphocyte function associated molecule-1 (LFA-1), CD44 and intercellular adhesion molecule-1 (ICAM-1) was similar in both groups. The endothelial cells in allergic reactions showed a stronger expression of vascular cell adhesion molecule-1 (VCAM-1), endothelial leucocyte adhesion molecule-1 (ELAM-1) and ICAM-1 compared to irritant reactions (Wahbi *et al.*, 1996).

Using laser scanning microscopy and indirect immunofluorescence (Emilson *et al.*, 1998) evaluated the epidermal expression of human leucocyte antigen (HLA)-DR and the invariant chain reactivity associated with antigen processing

CHAPTER 13

and presentation in allergic and irritant reactions. No significant change in the epidermal volume of HLA-DR reactivity was found in both types of reactions, nor was any significant change in the epidermal volume of invariant change reactivity in the allergic reactions. In the irritant reactions, however, there was a significant decrease in the epidermal volume of invariant chain reactivity from 24 to 72 h. Also, 72 h irritant reactions had a significantly lower epidermal volume of invariant chain reactivity compared with allergic reactions. This decline might reflect an epitope-induced alteration by irritants or a down-regulated biosynthesis of the invariant chain due to variance in local cytokine production between both types of inflammatory reactions.

Using confocal and electron microscopy (Rizova *et al.*, 1999) showed that freshly-isolated human Langerhans cells (LCs) pre-incubated with contact sensitizers internalized the HLA-DR molecules preferentially in lysosomes situated near the nucleus, whereas the irritant-treated or not treated LCs internalized these molecules in small prelysosomes located near the cell membrane.

13.4 CYTOKINES

Cytokines comprise an intriguing group of primarily locally active peptide regulatory factors (PRF) whose biological significance is beginning to be recognized. Cytokines qualified as possible candidate molecules involved in directing and modulating primary immune responses in the skin, regulating the activation, proliferation and differentiation on several target cells. Numerous studies have investigated whether there were differences in the cytokine expression between allergic and irritant reactions, which might in turn reflect different pathogenic mechanisms acting in both types of inflammatory responses. Until now, the results have been conflictive and did not provide clear-cut differences (Tables 13.3 and 13.4).

Cytokines and epidermal LC play a critical role in the initiation phase of contact sensitivity reactions in the skin. LC are antigen-presenting cells required for development of primary and secondary immune responses in skin. Following exposure to contact allergens, a substantial diminution in LCs' number in the skin and accumulation in the draining lymph nodes as dendritic cells (DC) is perceived. The immunostimulatory capacity of antigen-presenting cells in ACD is acquired as they migrate from the skin and accumulate in the skin lymph nodes. Functional maturation of LC is associated with phenotypic changes in surface determinants including increased expression of the MHC class II (Ia) antigen and co-stimulatory molecules, which will in turn enhance its capacity

TABLE 13.3:
Cytokines, chemokines and growth factors profiles in ICD and ACD (human studies)

Expression	ICD	ACD	Reference
IL-1α	Upregulated	Upregulated	Hoefakker *et al.* (1995); Ulfgren *et al.* (2000); Enk *et al.* (1993a); Hunziker *et al.* (1992)
IL-1β	Upregulated (or not altered)	Upregulated	Rambukkana *et al.* (1996); Brand *et al.* (1996)
IL-2	Upregulated (or not altered)	Upregulated	Hoefakker *et al.* (1995); Ulfgren *et al.* (2000); Ryan and Gerberick (1999); Hunziker *et al.* (1992)
IL-4	Not altered (or upregulated)	Upregulated at 24 h	Ryan and Gerberick (1999)
IL-6	Upregulated	Upregulated	Ulfgren *et al.* (2000); Hunziker *et al.* (1992); Hoefakker *et al.* (1995)
IL-8	Upregulated	Upregulated	Wilmer *et al.* (1994); Mohamadzadeh *et al.* (1994)
IL-10	Not altered (or upregulated)		Ulfgren *et al.* (2000); Brand *et al.* (1997); Ryan and Gerberick (1999)
TNF-α	Upregulated (or not altered)	Upregulated	Hoefakker *et al.* (1995); Hunziker *et al.* (1992)
IFN-γ	Upregulated	Upregulated	Pichowski *et al.* (2000); Hoefakker *et al.* (1995)
IP-10, IP-9	Not altered	Upregulated	Flier *et al.* (1999)
MIF	Not altered	Upregulated	Flier *et al.* (1999)
GM-CSF	Upregulated	Upregulated	Hunziker *et al.* (1992)

CHAPTER 13

to form stable clusters with lymphocytes. It is believed that such changes are induced by IL-1, GM-CSF and other cytokines, after a signal for migration is provided by TNF-α (Kimber and Cumberbatch, 1992; Kimber *et al.*, 1995). Some studies (Gawkrodger *et al.*, 1986; Willis *et al.*, 1986; Marks *et al.*, 1987) have showed that LC migrate from the epidermis in the irritant reactions. The absolute and relative number of LC has been demonstrated to dramatically increase in the late phase of the SLS-induced irritant reactions in human skin lymph. Even after topical treatment with clobetasol propionate and when the clinical signs of ICD had disappeared, the LC output still markedly exceeded the basal values (Brand *et al.*, 1992, 1993, 1995a). It has been postulated that SLS may directly activate the production of cytokines such as tumor necrosis factor (TNF)-α by keratinocytes, which in turn will facilitate the effect of

TABLE 13.4:

Cytokines, chemokines and growth factors profiles in ICD and ACD (murine studies)

Expression	ICD	ACD	Reference
IL-1α	Upregulated	Upregulated	Cumberbatch *et al.* (2000); Enk and Katz (1995); Kermani, Flint and Hotchkiss (2000); Kondo *et al.* (1994); Haas *et al.* (1992)
IL-1β	Upregulated (or not altered)	Upregulated	Cumberbatch *et al.* (2002); Enk and Katz (1995); Kondo *et al.* (1994)
IL-2	Upregulated (or not altered)	Upregulated	Enk and Katz (1993)
IL-6	Upregulated		Kondo et al. (1994)
IL-10	Upregulated	Upregulated	Enk and Katz (1993); Kondo *et al.* (1994)
TNF-α	Upregulated	Upregulated	Enk and Katz (1992); Enk and Katz (1995); Kondo *et al.* (1994); Haas *et al.* (1992)
IFN-γ	Upregulated	Upregulated	Enk and Katz (1992)
IP-10, IP-9	Not altered	Upregulated	Enk and Katz (1992)
MIP 2	Upregulated (or not altered)	Upregulated	Enk and Katz (1992); Enk and Katz (1993)
GM-CSF	Upregulated (or not altered)	Upregulated	Enk and Katz (1992); Kondo *et al.* (1994)

interleukin (IL)-1α increasing the migration of epidermal LC toward the skin lymph (Kimber and Cumberbatch, 1992; Cumberbatch *et al.*, 2002). The phenotypic characteristics of DC collected in draining lymph nodes in response to oxazolone and SLS were similar with respect to the membrane determinants major histocompatibility complex (MHC) class II, B7–1, B7–2, and ICAM-1 (Cumberbatch *et al.*, 2002). In addition (Brand *et al.*, 1995a, b) observed cell rosettes in the lymph draining the skin in the late phase of a SLS-induced irritant reactions in human volunteers, that showed a central LC with three to five peripherals, in part activated, T-cells, as well as gap junction-like structures between both cell types.

It was postulated that the induction of LC migration in response to contact allergens required two different signals: one provided by TNF-α, an inducible product of epidermal keratinocytes, and the other by IL-1β produced by LC. Both cytokines induced LC activation, characterized by the acquisition of a more dendritic morphology and the increased expression of Ia molecules, as well as migration of LC from the epidermis and accumulation in the skin draining lymph nodes as DC (Cumberbatch *et al.*, 1997a). Changes in both parameters were induced more rapidly following intradermal administration of TNF-α, yet, the reduction in the number of LC in the epidermis was more persistent after treatment with IL-1β. Using neutralizing anti-TNF-α and anti-IL-1β antibodies, administered by intraperitoneal injection prior to skin sensitization with oxazolone in mice, (Cumberbatch *et al.*, 1997b) observed a marked decrease in the number of DC in the draining lymph nodes. It was demonstrated also that anti-IL-1β inhibited TNF-α induced LC migration and DC accumulation. Likewise, the stimulation of LC migration produced by IL-1β was inhibited by previous treatment with anti-TNF-α. In short-term human skin organ cultures (Rambukkana *et al.*, 1996) demonstrated expression of IL-1β protein in LC after treatment with allergens, but not with irritants. In skin explants incubated with human recombinant (hr) cytokines, hrIL-1β, but not other hr cytokines, such as IL-1α, TNF-α, granulocyte-macrophage colony-stimulating factor (GM-CSF) or IL-6, induced the LC migration within and out from the epidermis. Pre-incubation of skin explants with neutralizing IL-1β antibodies, but not antibodies to IL-1α, TNF-α, or GM-CSF, significantly prevented the allergen-induced migration of LC. Similarly, (Cumberbatch *et al.*, 2002) showed that LC migration following skin sensitization with oxazolone in mice required IL-1β, but was independent of a requirement for IL-1α. In contrast, LC migration from the epidermis and accumulation as DC in the draining skin lymph nodes following treatment with SLS required IL-1α and not IL-1β. These data suggest that contact sensitization and skin irritation make use of subtly different cytokine networks in the regulation of LC migration, both involving TNF-α but requiring different IL-1 isoforms (Cumberbatch *et al.*, 2002). Enk and Katz (1992) demonstrated that the increase in the levels of IL-1β mRNA was one of the earliest manifestations of LC activation, occurring within 15 min after exposure to contact allergens. When intradermally injected into the ears of BALB/c mice, IL-1 beta mimicked the changes produced by topically applied allergen (3 percent trinitrochlorobenzene-TNCB) on the morphologic, phenotypic, and functional levels. IL-1β (but not IL-1 α or TNF-α) produced a 5- to 100- fold increase in the mRNA signals for IL-1 α, IL-1β, macrophage inflammatory protein (MIP)-2, IL-10, TNF-α, and major histocompatibility complex (MHC) class II (I-A α), and enhanced the expression of LC MHC class II. In addition, when a monoclonal antibody anti-mIL-1 β was injected into the skin prior to TNCB treatment, sensitization to this allergen was prevented, whilst the injection of anti-mIL-1α mAb was without effect (Enk *et al.*, 1993a). These authors observed

■ CHAPTER 13 ■

that TNF-α, interferon (IFN)-γ and GM-CSF mRNAs were upregulated after the application of SLS, tolerogens, and the allergens TNCB, dinitrofluorobenzene (DNFB) and dinitrochlorobenzene (DNCB) in BALB/c mice. However, MHC class II (I-Aα), IL-1α, IL-1β, IFN-induced protein (IP)-10, and macrophage inflammatory protein (MIP)-2 mRNAs were upregulated only after allergen treatment. Depletion of specific cell populations demonstrated that LC were the primary source of the IL-1β and the MHC class II (I-Aα) mRNAs, keratinocytes were the primary source of TNF-α, IL-1-α, IP-10, and MIP-2, and T-lymphocytes were the source of IFN-γ (Enk and Katz, 1992). Analysis of murine skin homogenates after treatment with oxazolone demonstrated an increase in IL-1β expression 30 minutes after treatment with oxazolone followed by a decrease below the detection limit at 2 hours. IL-1β expression returns to the constitutive low levels at 4 and 24 hours (Kermani *et al.*, 2000). Pichowski *et al.* (2000) studied the mRNA expression for IL-1β in blood-derived dendritic cells, cultured in the presence of DNFB, SLS or vehicle. A two- to threefold increase in IL-1β mRNA was observed in cells derived from three of eight DNFB-treated donors, whereas SLS treatment did not induce IL-1β mRNA expression in the cells of any of the donors investigated. According with these results, dendritic cell-derived IL-1β was deemed to be a key cytokine with a critical role in the initiation of contact allergic reactions in skin (Enk and Katz, 1992; Enk *et al.*, 1993a; Knop and Enk, 1995; Rambukkana *et al.*, 1996; Cumberbatch *et al.*, 2002).

In contrast with these observations, Brand *et al.* (1996) observed that the protein levels of IL-1β in human skin lymph increased in the course of both, irritant and allergic contact dermatitis and therefore did not allow discriminating between them. In a similar study, Hunziker *et al.* (1992) observed an 8–10-fold increase of TNF-α and IL-6 and a delayed 2–3-fold increase of IL-1β, IL-2, IL-2 receptors and GM-CSF in the lymph draining an ICD site. Kondo *et al.* (1994) observed that treatment with SLS in BALB/c mice upregulated not only the expression of TNF-α and GM-CSF, as reported by Enk and Katz (1992), but also IL-1β, IL-6 and IL-10 mRNA at 24 hours after treatment. Also, IL-1α was elevated during the first 3 hours after SLS treatment followed by suppression thereafter. IL-1α was produced in a dose-dependent manner by SLS on HaCaT monolayers (Whittle *et al.*, 1995). The production of IL-1α, TNF-α, IL-2 and IFN-γ was equally upregulated during both, allergic reactions to epoxy resin 1 percent and formaldehyde 1 percent, and irritant reactions to SLS 10 percent and formaldehyde 8 percent after 48 hours application in healthy volunteers, making impossible to discriminate between both types of reaction (Hoefakker *et al.*, 1995). Similarly, Ulfgren *et al.* (2000) observed that the cytokine profile in contact allergic skin reactions to nickel and irritant reactions to SLS 6 hours after challenge was similar. At 72 hours, the dermal cells expressed Il-1α, IL-1β, IL-2, IL-4, IL-6 and IL-10 in both types of inflammatory reactions. However, staining for the IL-1 receptor antagonist was more prominent in the dermis at the late stages of the allergic reaction and the inflammatory mononuclear infiltrate showed a more prominent interferon (IFN)-γ staining in the irritant reactions.

In cultured human keratinocytes, different irritants, i.e. SLS, phenol and croton oil, as well as the allergen dinitrofluorobenzene (DNFB) induced the production and intracellular accumulation of IL-1α and IL-8 (Wilmer *et al.*, 1994). Similarly, the expression of IL-8 gene by human keratinocytes was significantly increased by SLS and the allergens 2,4 DNFB and 3-n-pentadecylcatechol (Mohamadzadeh *et al.*, 1994).

Interleukin-10 has been considered a down regulatory molecule in contact hypersensitivity, as it prevented the expression of co-stimulatory molecules in the surface of LC, thus inhibiting LC accessory cell function (Enk *et al.*, 1993b; Knop and Enk, 1995; Enk and Katz, 1995, Ferguson *et al.* 1994). Intradermal injection of IL-10 before application of the allergen induces allergen-specific tolerance *in vivo*. Brand *et al.* (1997) observed that the IL-10 levels in lymph derived from irritant reactions and primary sensitization of allergic contact dermatitis were similar to those obtained from normal skin, remaining below 4.4 pg/ml. In contrast, the IL-10 levels increased manifold, both in the primary allergic reaction (928.5 pg/ml) and the elicitation of allergic contact dermatitis (124 pg/ml). In addition, the IL-10 mRNA signal, was markedly stronger in lymph and epidermal blister cells from the elicitation reactions as compared to the signal in lymph cells derived from normal skin and from the primary sensitization of allergic reactions. Similarly, Ryan and Gerberick (1999) observed stronger mRNA expression of IL-10, IL-4 and IL-2 in allergic patch test reactions (rhus) compared to the minimal expression observed in irritant reactions induced by SLS and vehicle.

Using an in situ hybridization technique, Flier *et al.* (1999) detected a time-dependent increase of mRNA expression for the chemokine IP-10 as well as the related CXCR3 activating chemokines, Mif and IP-9 in seven of nine contact allergic reactions, but not in SLS-induced irritant reactions, at least in the first 72 hours. Expression of chemokine mRNA was more apparent at 48–72 hours after challenge and roughly correlated with the clinical reaction and the density of the infiltrates. Additionally, up to 50 percent of the infiltrating cells in allergic contact dermatitis expressed CXCR3, the receptor for IP-10, Mif, and IP-9, which is nearly exclusively expressed on activated T-cells. In contrast

■ CHAPTER 13 ■

CXCR3 expression was found in only 20 percent of irritant reactions. The differential expression of IP-10 in human irritant and allergic contact dermatitis is consistent with the results of previous studies in mice (Enk and Katz, 1992) and suggests that this chemokine intervenes in the generation of the inflammatory infiltrate in allergic contact dermatitis (ACD), but not in SLS-induced irritant reactions. Hence, expression of these chemokines may represent an important feature for differentiation between allergic and irritant reactions. In addition, ICAM-1 expression by keratinocytes was only found in allergic reactions correlating with chemokine expression (Flier *et al.* 1999). Since the expression of CXC chemokines, ICAM-1 and HLA-DR is induced by IFN-γ, the authors assumed that their observations could be explained by the local presence of IFN-γ in ACD reactions. Expression of ICAM-1 in keratinocytes was found in 55 percent of allergic patch tests and in only 10 percent of irritant patch tests to SLS by Verheyen *et al.* (1995). Likewise, Vejlsgaard *et al.* (1989) reported that ICAM-1 expression can be found in allergic reactions but it did not occur in irritant reactions induced by SLS or croton oil. These results agree with the concept that ICAM-1 plays a role in the specific immune response by facilitating the antigen presentation and/or lymphocytic infiltration. However, Willis *et al.* (1991) showed an upregulation of ICAM-1 expression by keratinocytes, in correlation with expression of LFA-1 positive leukocytes after application of irritants such as SLS and croton oil, indicating that ICAM-1 induction may not be restricted to diseases characterized by antigen presentation. Ballmer-Weber *et al.* (1997) measured the concentration of the following soluble adhesion molecules (sAM): sICAM-1, soluble vascular cell adhesion molecule-1 (sVCAM-1) and E-selectin (sE-selectin) in human skin lymph derived from normal untreated skin, ICD and the induction and elicitation phases of ACD. A marked increase in the sAM levels to about three times the baseline values was seen in lymph draining the skin in the elicitation phase of ACD. A slight increase was seen after day 9 in the induction phase and no changes were observed in the irritant reactions.

In summary, even if cytokines play a major role in the pathogenic mechanisms of inflammatory skin diseases, present knowledge of the complex interactions of cytokines and cellular targets does not allow for identification of a specific "fingerprint" pattern of cytokine production that clearly distinguish allergic from irritant reactions.

13.5 ALLERGENS AND IRRITANTS IN IMMUNOTOXICOLOGY TESTING

During the past two decades growing interest arose in developing improved toxicological methods for differentially diagnosing contact allergic reactions from contact irritant reactions in humans. The majority of tests for predicting allergenicity of chemicals use guinea pigs or mice with biphasic protocols, comprising a sensitization phase (induction) and an elicitation phase (challenge) (Buehler, 1965; Magnusson and Kligman, 1969; Maurer et al., 1980). In guinea pig models, such as the guinea pig maximization test, Buehler's occluded patch test, or the optimization test, contact reactivity is assessed mainly by a subjective local erythema score and determined by the frequency of animals exhibiting a positive response. In the challenge-induced mouse ear swelling test (MEST), induration is the predominant feature of the positive allergic reaction. To avoid false-positive results, challenge must be performed with a concentration of the test material that is unable to provoke skin irritation in nonsensitized controls. It is possible, therefore, with highly irritant materials that the concentrations selected for challenge are below those necessary to elicit a contact hypersensitivity reaction. More recently, the murine local lymph node assay (LLNA), was described as an alternative method for the detection of moderate or strong contact sensitizers. In contrast to guinea pig models and the MEST, the LLNA is based upon the detection of a primary immune response as a function of the cell proliferation in the draining lymph nodes after epicutaneous exposure to materials (Kimber et al., 1986; Kimber and Weisenberger, 1989; Basketter et al., 1991, 1994). Although the LLNA was first described to selectively detect allergic skin immune responses, recent studies showed that many irritant compounds like sodium dodecyl sulfate (SDS), chloroform/methanol, triton X-100, croton oil, benzalkonium chloride, salicylic acid, dimethyl sulfoxide, among others, also induce node cell proliferation not distinguishable from the results with low-grade or moderate irritants (Montelius et al., 1994; Ikarashi et al., 1993; Homey et al., 1998). Therefore, irritant substances could be wrongly classified as allergens, or the allergenicity of substances with both allergenic and irritant properties could be overestimated.

To differentiate the cellular and molecular events elicited by allergens and irritants, (Sikorski et al., 1996) performed a phenotypic analysis of lymphocyte subsets in the draining lymph nodes after topical treatment. The expression of CD3, CD4, CD8, and B220 was evaluated by flow cytometry. The allergens oxazolone and TNCB and the irritant benzalkonium chloride, increased the

CHAPTER 13

total number of T- and B-lymphocytes in comparison with vehicle. In allergen treated mice, a preferential increase in B-lymphocytes, as seen by an increase in B220+ cells, was apparent in comparison with those treated with irritant and vehicle. This increase was consistently more prominent when stronger sensitizers and/or higher concentrations were used. Specific markers of antigen-induced T-cell activation were also examined (Gerberick *et al.*, 1997). CD62L (L-selectin) and CD44 (H-CAM) expression was selectively modulated after treatment with the contact allergen TNCB when compared with the irritant benzalkonium chloride or the vehicle control. Mice treated with dinitro-chlorobenzene (DNCB) also had an increase in the percentage of CD4+ cells expressing CD62L^{lo}CD44^{hi} that were dose dependent and peaked at 72 hours after the final allergen treatment. In addition, increases in the percentage of CD8+ cells expressing CD62L^{lo}CD44^{hi} were observed with allergens, including DNCB, oxazolone and hexylcinnamic aldehyde, but not with irritants (Gerberick *et al.* 1997). Homey *et al.* (1998) observed that topical treatment with allergens (1 percent oxazolone) strongly induced the activation markers CD25 and CD69 on CD4+ and CD8+ lymph node cells, whereas irritants (croton oil) induced only marginal upregulation. Furthermore, treatment with oxazolone resulted in an expansion of I-A+/B220+ and a significant upregulation of CD69 on I-A+ lymph node cells. In contrast, croton oil treatment resulted in only a minor increase of both I-A+/B220+ and CD69/I-A+ lymph node cell subpopulations. Differences were considered to be qualitative rather than quantitative, since the analyses were performed with oxazolone and croton oil concentrations that induced comparable lymph node cells count indices. The upregulation of CD69 on I-A+ lymph node cells, confirming antigen-specific sensitization, was the most prominent marker for differentiation between the reaction patterns of oxazolone and croton oil. Phenotypic analyses of the CD69/I-A+ lymph node cells revealed them to be predominantly B220+ cells. Thus, examination of cellular phenotypic changes by flow cytometry demonstrates to be valuable in differentiating between allergic and irritant responses in the draining lymph nodes of mice.

Further criteria for the differentiation between allergens and irritants using a modified LLNA were proposed by Homey *et al.* (1998). They postulated that contact allergens induce activation and proliferation of skin-draining lymph node cells with only marginal skin inflammation, whereas irritants predominantly induce skin inflammation and, as a result, generate lymph node cell proliferation. Therefore, a differentiation index (DI) was developed considering the relationship between local draining lymph node activation (calculated as a percentage of the maximal increase in lymph node cell count index) and skin inflammation (calculated as a percentage of maximal ear swelling). DI values > 1 indicated an allergic reaction pattern, whereas DI values < 1 denoted an irritant response. The sensitizing potential of oxazolone was clearly confirmed eliciting a DI ranging from 2.5 to 16.6 in three different experiments. In contrast, the irritant croton oil produced a DI varying from 0.7 to 0.8 (Homey *et al.*, 1988).

An increased understanding of the immunologic events that mediate and regulate allergic and irritant skin responses may provide a mechanistic basis for development of more objective and accurate *in vivo* and *in vitro* models of immunotoxicology testing.

13.6 CONCLUSIONS

The current understanding of mechanisms of both irritant and allergic dermatitis does not allow for establishing pertinent and practical criteria for a clear-cut differentiation between them. Although the pathways for ICD and ACD are distinctly defined, there seems to exist an overlapping and inter-connected cellular and molecular network between both types of contact dermatitis. Therefore, differences between irritants and allergens are more conceptual than verifiable.

Further understanding of the molecular pathways in contact dermatitis would be significant in dermatological practice, as well as in clinical and toxicological research.

REFERENCES

Avnstorp, C., Balslev, E. and Thomsen, H.K. (1988) The occurrence of different morphological parameters in allergic and irritant patch tests reactions. In Frosch, P.J., Dooms-Goosens, A., Lachapelle, J.M., Rycroft, R.J.G. and Scheper, R.J. (eds) *Current Topics in Contact Dermatitis*. Berlin-Heidelberg-New York-London: Springer-Verlag, 38–41.

Avnstorp, C., Ralflkiaer, E., Jorgensen, J. and Wantzin, G.L. (1987) Sequential immunophenotypic study of lymphoid infiltrate in allergic and irritant reactions. *Contact Dermatitis* 16(5), 239–245.

Ballmer-Weber, B.K., Braathen, L.R. and Brand, C.U. (1997). SICAM-1, sE-selectin and sVCAM-1 are constitutively present in human skin lymph and increased in allergic contact dermatitis. *Arch. Dermatol. Res.* 289(5), 251–255

CHAPTER 13

BARKER, J.N.W.N., MITRA, R.S., GRIFFITHS, C.E., DIXIT, V.M., NICKOLOFF, B.J. (1991) Keratinocytes as initiators of inflammation. *Lancet* **337**(8735), 211–214.

BASKETTER, D.A., SCHOLES, E.W., KIMBER, I., BOTHAM, P.A., HILTON, J., MILLER, K., ROBBINS, M.C., HARRISON, P.T.C. and WAITE, S.J. (1991). Interlaboratory evaluation of the local lymph node assay with 25 chemicals and comparison with guinea pig test data. *Toxicology Methods* **1**, 30–43.

BASKETTER, D.A., SCHOLES, E.W. and KIMBER, I. (1994). The performance of the local lymph node assay with chemicals identified as contact allergens in the human maximization test. *Food Chem. Toxicol.* **32**, 543–547.

BERARDESCA, E. (1997). What's new in irritant dermatitis. *Clin. Dermatol.* **15**(4), 561–563.

BERARDESCA, E. and MAIBACH, H.I. (1988) Racial differences in sodium lauryl sulfate induced cutaneous irritation: black and white. *Contact Dermatitis* **18**, 65–70.

BRAND, C.U., HUNZIKER, T. and BRAATHEN, L.R. (1992). Studies on human skin lymph containing Langerhans cells from sodium lauryl sulfate contact dermatitis. *J. Invest. Dermatol.* **99**(5), 109S–110S.

BRAND, C.U., HUNZIKER, T., LIMAT, A. and BRAATHEN, L.R. (1993). Large increase of Langerhans cells in human skin lymph derived from irritant contact dermatitis. *Br. J. Dermatol.* **128**(2), 184–188.

BRAND, C.U., HUNZIKER, T., SCHAFFNER, T., LIMAT, A., GERBER, H.A. and BRAATHEN, L.R. (1995a) Activated immunocompetent cells in human skin lymph derived from irritant contact dermatitis: an immunomorphological study. *Br. J. Dermatol.* **132**(1), 39–45.

BRAND, C.U., HUNZIKER, T., GERBER, H.A., SCHAFFNER, T., LIMAT, A. and BRAATHEN, L.R. (1995b) Rosettes of Langerhans cells and activated T-cells in human skin lymph derived from irritant dermatitis. *Adv. Exp. Med. Biol.* **378**, 527–529.

BRAND, C.U., HUNZIKER, T., YAWALKAR, N. and BRAATHEN, L.R. (1996) IL-1 beta protein in human skin lymph does not discriminate allergic from irritant contact dermatitis. *Contact Dermatitis* **35**(3), 152–156.

BRAND, C.U., YAWALKAR, N., HUNZIKER, T. and BRAATHEN, L.R. (1997) Human skin lymph derived from irritant and allergic contact dermatitis: interleukin 10 is increased selectively in elicitation reactions. *Dermatology* **194**(3), 221–228.

BRASCH, J., BUGARD, J. and STERRY, W. (1992) Common pathogenetic pathways in allergic and irritant contact dermatitis. *J. Invest. Dermatol.* **98**(2), 166–170.

BRUYNZEEL, D.P., VAN KETEL, W.G., SCHEPER, R.J. and VON BLOMBERG-VAN DER FLIER, B.M. (1982) Delayed time course of irritation by sodium lauryl sulfate: observations on threshold reactions. *Contact Dermatitis* **8**(4), 236–239.

BUEHLER, E.V. (1965) Delayed contact sensitivity in the guinea pig. *Arch. Dermatol.* **91**, 171–177.

CUMBERBATCH, M., DEARMAN, R.J., GROVES, R.W., ANTONOPOULOS, C. and KIMBER, I. (2002). Differential regulation of epidermal Langerhans cell migration by interleukins (IL)-1 alpha and IL-1 beta during irritant- and allergen-induced cutaneous immune responses. *Toxicol. Appl. Pharmacol.* **182**(2), 126–135.

CUMBERBATCH, M., DEARMAN, R.J. and KIMBER, I. (1997a). Interleukin 1 beta and the stimulation of Langerhans cell migration: comparisons with tumor necrosis factor alpha. *Arch. Dermatol. Res.* **289**(5), 277–284.

CUMBERBATCH, M., DEARMAN, R.J. and KIMBER, I. (1997b). Langerhans cells require signals from both tumor necrosis factor-alpha and interleukin-1 beta for migration. *Immunology* **92**(3), 388–395.

EFFENDY, I. and MAIBACH, H.I. (2001). Cytokines and Irritant Dermatitis Syndrome. In MAIBACH, H.I. (ed.) *Toxicology of Skin*, Philadelphia; Hove, Sussex: Taylor & Francis, 85–104.

EFFENDY, I., LOFFLER, H. and MAIBACH, H.I. (2000) Epidermal cytokines in murine cutaneous irritant responses. *J. Appl. Toxicol.* **20**(4), 335–341.

EMILSON, A., LINDBERG, M. and SCHEYNIUS, A. (1998) Differential epidermal expression of the invariant chain in allergic and irritant contact dermatitis. *Acta Derm. Venereol.* **78**(6), 402–407.

ENK, A.H. and KATZ, S.I. (1992) Early molecular events in the induction phase of contact sensitivity. *Proc. Natl. Acad. Sci. USA* **89**(4), 1398–1402.

ENK, A.H. and KATZ, S.I. (1995) Contact sensitivity as a model for T-cell activation in skin. *J. Invest. Dermatol.* **105**(1 Suppl), 80S–83S.

ENK, A.H., ANGELONI, V.L., UDEY, M.C. and KATZ, S.I. (1993a) Inhibition of Langerhans cells antigen-presenting function by IL-10. A role for IL-10 in induction of tolerance. *J. Immunol.* **151**(5), 2390–2398.

ENK, A.H., ANGELONI, V.L., UDEY, M.C. and KATZ, S.I. (1993b) An essential role for Langerhans cell-derived IL-beta in the initiation of primary immune responses in skin. *J. Immunol.* **150**(9), 3698–3704.

■ CHAPTER 13 ■

FERGUSON, T.A., DUBE, P. and GRIFFITH, T.S. (1994). Regulation of contact hypersensitivity by interleukin 10. *J. Exp. Med.* **179**(5), 1597–1604.

FLIER, J., BOORSMA, D.M., BRUYNZEEL, D.P., VAN BEEK, P.J., STOOF, T.J. SCHEPER, R.J., WILLEMZE, R. and TENSEN, C.P. (1999) The CXCR3 activating chemokines IP-10, Mig, and IP-9 are expressed in allergic but not in irritant patch test reactions. *J. Invest. Dermatol.* **113**(4), 574–578.

GALLUCCI, S. and MATZINGER, P. (2001). Danger signals: SOS to the immune system. *Curr. Opin. Immunol.* **13**(1), 114–119.

GAWKRODGER, D.J., MCVITTIE, E., CARR, M.M., ROSS, J.A. and HUNTER, J.A. (1986) Phenotypic characterization of the early cellular responses in allergic and irritant contact dermatitis. *Clin. Exp. Immunol.* **66**(3), 590–598.

GERBERICK, G.F., CRUSE, L.W., MILLER, C.M., SIKORSKI, E.E. and RIDDER, G.M. (1997). Selective modulation of T-cell memory markers CD62L and CD44 on murine draining lymph node cells following allergen and irritant treatment. *Toxicol. Appl. Pharmacol.* **146**, 1–10.

HAAS, J., LIPKOW, T., MOHAMADZADEH, M., KOLDE, G. and KNOP, J. (1992). Induction of inflammatory cytokines in murine keratinocytes upon *in vivo* stimulation with contact sensitizers and tolerizing analogues. *Exp. Dermatol.* **1**, 76–83.

HOEFAKKER, S., CAUBO, M., VAN'T ERVE, E.H., ROGGEVEEN, M.J., BOERSMA, W.J., VAN JOOST, T., NOTTEN, W.R. and CLAASSEN, E. (1995) *In vivo* cytokine profiles in allergic and irritant contact dermatitis. *Contact Dermatitis* **33**(4), 258–266.

HOMEY, B., VON SCHILLING, C., BLÜMEL, J., SCHUPPE, H-C., RUZICKA, T., AHR, H.J., LEHMANN, P. and VOHR, H-W. (1998) An integrated model for the differentiation of chemical-induced allergic and irritant skin reactions. *Toxicol. Appl. Pharmacol.* **153**, 83–94.

HUNZIKER, T., BRAND, C.U., KAPP, A., WAELTI, E.R. and BRAATHEN, L.R. (1992) Increased levels of inflammatory cytokines in human skin lymph derived from sodium lauryl sulfate-induced contact dermatitis. *Br. J. Dermatol.* **127**(3), 254–257.

IKARASHI, Y., TSUKAMOTO, Y., TSUCHIYA, T. and NAKAMURA, A. (1993). Influence of irritants on lymph node cell proliferation and the detection of contact sensitivity to metal salts in the murine local lymph node assay. *Contact Dermatitis* **29**, 128–132.

JUDGE, M.R., GRIFFITHS, H.A. and BASKETTER, D.A. (1996) Variation in response of human skin to irritant challenge. *Contact Dermatitis* **34**, 115–117.

KERMANI, F., FLINT, M.S. and HOTCHKISS, S.A. (2000) Induction and localization of cutaneous interleukin-1 beta mRNA during contact sensitization. *Toxicol. Appl. Pharmacol.* **169**(3), 231–237.

KIMBER, I. and CUMBERBATCH, M. (1992). Stimulation of Langerhans cell migration by tumor necrosis factor alpha (TNF-alpha). *J. Invest. Dermatol.* **99**, 498–503.

KIMBER, I. and WEISENBERGER, C. (1989). A murine local lymph node assay for the identification of contact allergens. *Arch. Toxicol.* **63**, 274–282.

KIMBER, I., MITCHELL, J.A. and GRIFFIN, A.C. (1986). Development of a murine local lymph node assay for the determination of sensitizing potential. *Food. Chem. Toxicol.* **24**, 585–586.

KIMBER, I., HOLLIDAY, M.R. and DEARMAN, R.J. (1995). Cytokine regulation of chemical sensitization. *Toxicol. Lett.* **82–83**, 491–496.

KNOP, J. and ENK, A.H. (1995). Cellular and molecular mechanisms in the induction phase of contact sensitivity. *Int. Arch. Allergy Immunol.* **107**(1–3), 231–232.

KONDO, S., PASTORE, S., SHIVJI, G.M., McKENZIE, R.C. and SAUDER, D.N. (1994). Characterization of epidermal cytokine profiles in sensitization and elicitation phases of allergic contact dermatitis as well as irritant contact dermatitis in mouse skin. *Lymphokine, Cytokine Res.* **13**(6), 367–375.

LACHAPELLE, J.M. (1995) Histopathological and immunohistopathological features of irritant and allergic contact dermatitis. In: RYCROFT, R.J.G., MENNÉ, T. and FROSCH, P.J. (eds). *Textbook of Contact Dermatitis*. Berlin-Heidelberg-New York: Springer, 91–101.

LAMMINTAUSTA, K. and MAIBACH, H.I. (1990) Contact dermatitis due to irritation: general principles, etiology and histology. In: Adams, R.M. (ed.) *Occupational Skin Disease*, Philadelphia: Saunders; 1–15.

LAMMINTAUSTA, K. and MAIBACH, H.I. (1988) Exogenous and endogenous factors in skin irritation. *Int. J. Dermatol.* **27**, 213–222.

LAMMINTAUSTA, K., MAIBACH, H.I. and WILSON, D. (1987) Irritant reactivity in males and females. *Contact Dermatitis* **17**, 276–280.

LE, T.K., VAN DER VALK, P.G., SCHALKWIJK, J. and VAN DER KERKHOF, P.C. (1995) Changes in epidermal proliferation and differentiation in allergic and irritant contact dermatitis reactions. *Br. J. Dermatol.* **133**(2), 236–240.

MAGNUSSON, B. and KLIGMAN, A.M. (1969) The identification of contact allergens by the animal assay, guinea pig maximization test method. *J. Invest. Dermatol.* **52**, 268–276.

CHAPTER 13

MALTEN, K.E., DEN AREND, J.A. and WIGGERS, R.E. (1979) Delayed irritation: hexanediol diacrylate and butanediol diacrylate. *Contact Dermatitis* **3**, 178–184.

MARKS, J.G., JR., ZAINO, R.J., BRESSLER, M.F. and WILLIAMS, J.V. (1987). Changes in lymphocyte and Langerhans cell populations in allergic and irritant contact dermatitis. *Int. J. Dermatol.* **26**(6), 354–357.

MATHIAS, C.G. and MAIBACH, H.I. (1978) Dermatotoxicology Monographs I. Cutaneous irritation: Factors influencing the response to irritants. *Clin. Toxicol.* **13**, 399–415.

MATZINGER, P. (1998) An innate sense of danger. *Semin. Immunol.* 10, 399–415.

MAURER, T., WEIRICH, E.G. and HESS, R. (1980) The optimization test in guinea pig in relation with other predictive sensitization methods. *Toxicology* **15**, 163–171.

MCFADDEN, J.P. and BASKETTER, D.A. (2000). Contact allergy, irritancy and "danger." *Contact Dermatitis* **42**(3), 123–127.

MCKENZIE, R.C. and SAUDER, D.N. (1990) The role of keratinocyte cytokines in inflammation and immunity. *J. Invest. Dermatol.* **95**, 105S-107S.

MOHAMADZADEH, M., MÜLLER, M., HULTSCH, T., ENK, A., SALOGA, J. and KNOP, J. (1994) Enhanced expression of IL-8 in normal human keratinocytes and human keratinocyte cell line HaCaT *in vitro* after stimulation with contact sensitizers, tolerogens and irritants. *Exp. Dermatol.* **3**, 298–303.

MONTELIUS, J., WAHLKVIST, H., BOMAN, A., FERNSTROM, P., GRABERGS, L. and WAHLBERG, J.E. (1994). Experience with the murine local lymph node assay: Inability to discriminate between allergens and irritants. *Acta Derm. Venereol.* **74**(1), 22–27.

NICKOLOFF, B.J. and NAIDU, Y. (1994) Perturbation of epidermal barrier function correlates with initiation of cytokine cascade in human skin. *J. Am. Acad. Dermatol.* **30**, 535–546.

PASTORE, S., SHIVJI, G.M., KONDO, S., KONO, T., MCKENZIE, R.C., SEGAL, L., SOMERS, D. and SAUNDER, D.N. (1995) Effects of contact sensitizers neomycin sulfate, benzocaine and 2–4 dinitrobenzene l-sulfonate, sodium salt on viability, membrane integrity and IL-1 alpha mRNA expression of cultured normal human keratinocytes. *Food Chem. Toxicol.* **33**, 57–68.

PATIL, S. and MAIBACH, H.I. (1994) Effect of age and sex on the elicitation of irritant contact dermatitis. *Contact Dermatitis* **30**, 257–264.

PATRICK, E., MAIBACH, H.I. and BURKHALTER, A.(1985) Mechanisms of chemically induced skin irritation: I. Studies of time course, dose response, and components of inflammation in the laboratory mouse. *Toxicol. Appl. Pharmacol.* **81**, 476–490.

PICHOWSKI, J.S., CUMBERBATCH, M., BASKETTER, D.A. and KIMBER, I. (2000) Investigation of induced changes in interleukin 1beta mRNA expression by cultured human dendritic cells as *in vitro* approach to skin sensitization testing. *Toxicol. In Vitro* **14**(4), 351–360.

RAMBUKKANA, A., PISTOOR, F.H., BOS, J.D., KAPSENBERG, M.L. and DAS, P.K. (1996) Effect of contact allergens on human Langerhans cells in skin organ culture: migration, modulation of cell surface molecules, and early expression of interleukin-1 beta protein. *Lab. Invest.* **74**(2), 422–436.

RANKI, A., KANERVA, L., FORSTROM, L., KONTTINEN, Y. and MUSTAKALLIO, K.K. (1983) T and B lymphocytes, macrophages and Langerhans cells during the contact allergic and irritant skin reactions in man. *Acta Derm. Venereol.* **63**(5), 376–383.

REICHE, L., WILLIS, C., WILKINSON, J., SHAW, S. and DE LACHARRIERE, O. (1998) Clinical morphology of sodium lauryl sulfate (SLS) and nonanoic acid (NAA) irritant patch test reactions at 48 h and 96 h in 152 subjects. *Contact Dermatitis* **39**(5), 240–243.

RIETSCHEL, R.L. (1997). Mechanism in irritant contact dermatitis. *Clin. Dermatol.* **15**(4), 557–559.

RIZOVA, H., CARAYON, P., BARBIER, A., LACHERETZ, F., DUBERTRET, L. and MICHEL, L. (1999) Contact allergens, but not irritants, alter receptor-mediated endocytosis by human epidermal Langerhans cells. *Br. J. Dermatol.* **140**(2), 200–209.

RYAN, C.A. and GERBERICK, G.F. (1999) Cytokine mRNA expression in human epidermis after patch test treatment with rhus and sodium lauryl sulfate. *Am. J. Contact Dermat.* **10**(3), 127–135.

SCHEYNIUS, A. and FISHER, T. (1986). Phenotypic difference between allergic and irritant patch test reactions in man. *Contact Dermatitis* **14**, 297–302.

SCHEYNIUS, A., FISCHER, T. and FORSUM, U. (1984) Phenotypic characterization of in situ inflammatory cells in allergic and irritant dermatitis in man. *Clin. Exp. Immunol.* **55**(1), 81–90.

SIKORSKI, E.E., GERBERICK, G.F., RYAN, C.A., MILLER, C.M. and RIDDER, G.M. (1996). Phenotypic analysis of lymphocyte subpopulations in lymph nodes draining the ear following exposure to contact allergens and irritants. *Fundam. Appl. Toxicol.* **34**, 25–35.

SMITH, H.R., BASKETTER, D.A. and MCFADDEN, J.P. (2002). Irritant dermatitis, irritancy and its role in allergic contact dermatitis. *Clin. Exp. Dermatol.* **27**(2), 138–146.

ULFGREN, A.K., KLARESKOG, L. and LINDBERG, M. (2000) An immunohisto-chemical analysis of cytokine expression in allergic and irritant contact dermatitis. *Acta Derm. Venereol.* **80**(3), 167–170.

VEJLSGAARD, G.L., RALFKIAER, E., AVNSTORP, C., CZAJKWOSKI, M., MARLIN, S. and ROTHLEIN, R. (1989) Kinetics characterization of intercellular adhesion molecule-1 (ICAM-1) expression on keratinocytes in various inflammatory skin lesions and malignant cutaneous lymphomas. *J. Am. Acad. Dermatol.* **20**, 782–790.

VERHEYEN, A., MATTHIEU, L., LAMBERT, J., VAN MARCK, E. and DOCKX, P. (1995) An immunohistochemical study of contact irritant and contact allergic patch tests. In ELSNER, P. and MAIBACH, H.I. (eds) *Irritant Dermatitis. New Clinical and Experimental Aspects: Current Problems in Dermatology*, Vol. 23. Basel-Paris-London-New York: Karger, 108–113.

VESTERGAARD, L., CLEMMENSEN, O.J., SORENSEN, F.B. and ANDERSEN, K.E. (1999) Histological distinction between early allergic and irritant patch test reactions: follicular spongiosis may be characteristic of early contact dermatitis. *Contact Dermatitis* **41**(4), 207–210.

WAHBI, A., MARCUSSON, J.A. and SUNDQVIST, K.G. (1996) Expression of adhesion molecules and their ligands in contact allergy. *Exp. Dermatol.* **5**(1), 12–19.

WHITTLE, E., CARTER, J., WOLFREYS, A., *et al.* (1995). HaCaT-derived cytokine response to noxious agents (abstract). *J. Invest. Dermatol.* **104**, 562 (abstract).

WILHELM, K.P. and MAIBACH, H.I. (1990) Susceptibility to irritant dermatitis induced by sodium lauryl sulfate. *J. Am. Acad. Dermatol.* **23**(1), 122–124.

WILLIS, C.M., STEPHENS, C.J. and WILKINSON, J.D. (1992) Differential effects of structurally unrelated chemical irritants on the density of proliferating keratinocytes in 48 h patch test reactions. *J. Invest. Dermatol.* **99**(4), 449–453.

WILLIS, C., STEPHENS, C.J.M. and WILKINSON, D. (1991) Selective expression of immune-associated surface antigens by keratinocytes in irritant dermatitis. *J. Invest. Dermatol.* **96**(4), 505–511.

WILLIS, C., STEPHENS, C.J.M. and WILKINSON, D. (1989) Epidermal damage induced by irritants in man: A light and electron microscopic study. *J. Invest. Dermatol.* **93**, 695–699.

WILLIS, C., STEPHENS, C.J.M. and WILKINSON, D. (1988) Preliminary findings on the patterns of epidermal damage induced by irritants in man. In FROSCH, P.J., DOOMS-GOOSENS, A., LACHAPELLE, J.M., RYCROFT, R.J.G. and SCHEPER, R.J. (eds) *Current Topics in Contact Dermatitis*. Berlin-Heidelberg-New York-London: Springer-Verlag, 42–45.

WILLIS, C.M., YOUNG, E., BRANDON, D.R. and WILKINSON, J.D. (1986). Immuno-pathological and ultraestructural findings in human allergic and irritant contact dermatitis. *Br. J. Dermatol.* **115**, 305–316.

WILMER, J.L., BURLESON, F.G., KAYAMA, F., KANNO, J. and LUSTER, M.I. (1994) Cytokine induction in human epidermal keratinocytes exposed to contact irritants and its relation to chemical-induced inflammation in mouse skin. *J. Invest. Dermatol.* **102**, 915–922.

■ CHAPTER 13 ■

Molecular Basis of Allergic Contact Dermatitis

JEAN-PIERRE LEPOITTEVIN AND VALÉRIE BERL

Contents

14.1 Introduction

14.2 Some chemical reminders

14.3 Principal electrophilic chemical groups present in contact allergens

14.4 Back to contact allergy

14.5 The hapten–protein bond: covalent or noncovalent?

14.6 Metabolism and prohaptens

14.7 Haptens and cross-allergy

14.8 Conclusion

14.1 INTRODUCTION

Among the pathological conditions in which chemistry plays an especially important role is contact allergy (Lepoittevin *et al.*, 1998) and chemical reactions/interactions are involved throughout the biological process that will result in the patient developing delayed hypersensitivity. Thus, the crossing of the cutaneous barrier is mainly controlled by the physicochemical properties of the allergen (molecular volume and lipophilicity). The formation of the hapten–protein complex, which involves the formation of new chemical bonds, is driven by molecular orbital properties. Finally, the recognition between the antigen and the receptors on T-lymphocytes can be explained by a discipline undergoing rapid development, that of supramolecular chemistry.

Recently, there has been a major step forward in our understanding of the molecular basis of hapten recognition by T-cells. Nevertheless, this does not eliminate the need to understand the characteristics of the preceding processes, as it is true that the properties of a chemical are implicit in its molecular structure.

To cause sensitization, a compound has to penetrate the skin (Roberts and Walters, 1998), where it may be metabolized (Hotchkiss, 1998), and react with Langerhans cell surface proteins to form new chemical structures that are recognized as foreign. We discuss in this chapter the way low-molecular-weight chemicals can react with skin proteins to form complete antigens and how these structures could be recognized by T-cell receptors.

■ CHAPTER 14 ■

14.2 SOME CHEMICAL REMINDERS

Haptens (small molecules with a molecular weight less than 1000 Da) can interact with biological macromolecules by mechanisms leading to the formation of bonds of various strengths. These bonds, known as chemical bonds, are the result of electronic interactions between atoms and are characterized by the energy involved. This reflects the bond stability as this amount of energy must be provided to break the link between the two atoms. In general, a distinction is made between so-called weak interactions, involving energy levels from a few calories to around 12 kcal/mol, and strong interactions, covalent or coordinate bonds, with energies ranging from 50 to 100 kcal/mol.

14.2.1 Weak interactions

Weak interactions are normally grouped into three main categories: hydrophobic bonds, dipolar bonds, and certain ionic bonds. Although these weak interactions involve modest energy levels and produce structures of low stability, they are nonetheless of great biological importance, as they control virtually all the phenomena of interaction between receptors and substrates.

Hydrophobic bonds represent the ability of organic molecules to organize themselves in water so as to minimize the contact area that they expose to the aqueous solvent. It is, for exemple, by such means that hydrophobic molecules insert themselves into the phospholipid bilayers of cell membranes and into the hydrophobic regions of proteins or membrane receptors. These hydrophobic bonds, which involve energies of the order of 10–20 cal/Å^2/mol, seem, nevertheless, to play an important role in allergies to very lipophilic products (Darley *et al.*, 1977), such as the allergens from poison ivy (*Rhus radicans* L.) or poison oak (*Rhus diversiloba* T.). This could also be of importance for the interactions of haptens with the lipophilic domains of antigen-presenting cells.

Dipolar bonds are electrostatic interactions between permanent or induced dipoles. The electron clouds do not always have a uniform charge density (these variations result from the structure of the molecule), and the zones of high electron density can interact electrostatically with zones of low electron density (permanent dipoles). Electron clouds can also be deformed and polarized as they approach one another, thus creating induced dipoles. These interactions between dipoles, also known as van der Waals bonding, involve energies of the order of 50–500 cal/mol. Hydrogen bond is a special case of dipolar interaction and they occur between a hydrogen atom, bound to an electron-withdrawing atom, and an electron-rich atom. The energy of such bonds can be as high as 5 kcal/mol.

Ionic bonds are based on electrostatic interactions between preexisting and generally localized charges on organic molecules or minerals. Such interactions occur, for example, between the charged amino acids in proteins and are therefore important in recognition phenomena.

14.2.2 Strong interactions

Covalent bonds, result when two atoms share a pair of electrons, and are classically represented in chemical formulas by dashes. They involve energies of the order of 50–100 kcal/mol and are therefore very stable compared with the weak interactions. The two electrons required for bond formation can be contributed by both partners, which is called a radical reaction, or can be provided by one of the atoms, which is especially electron rich, and shared with an electron-poor atom; this case is referred to as a reaction between a *nucleophile* (electron rich) and an *electrophile* (electron poor) center. These two terms, nucleophile and electrophile, represent the capacity of a molecule, or rather an atom of this molecule, to donate or accept electrons to form a covalent bonding. Nucleophilic centers are rich in electrons and therefore partially negatively charged, while electrophilic centers, deficient in electrons, are partially positively charged.

Coordinate bonds are another type of relatively strong bond, comparable to covalent bonds; this occurs between metals or metal salts and electron-rich atoms (mainly heteroatoms, such as nitrogen or oxygen). These interactions permit these electron-rich groups or ligands to transfer part of their electron density to the metal and increase its stability. Coordinate bonds are characterized by the number of ligands and by a geometry characteristic both of the metal and of its oxidation degree (Figure 14.1). For example, cobalt(II) (Co^{2+}) is characterized by a tetrahedral arrangement, nickel (II) (Ni^{2+}) by a square planar tetra coordinated arrangement, and chromium(III) (Cr^{3+}) by a six-ligand octahedral arrangement. The number of ligands and the geometry of these coordination complexes determine whether the metals are allergenic and control cross-reactions.

CHAPTER 14

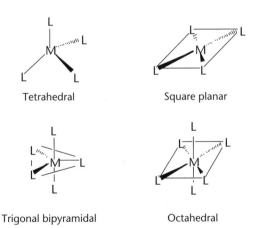

| Tetrahedral | Square planar |

| Trigonal bipyramidal | Octahedral |

Figure 14.1: Examples of geometry for coordinate bonds.

14.2.3   Mechanisms of bond formation

The main mechanisms for the formation of covalent bonds involved in contact allergy can be grouped into three main categories: nucleophilic substitutions, on either a saturated or unsaturated center, and nucleophilic additions.

Nucleophilic substitution on a saturated center (Figure 14.2) involves the attack by an electron rich nucleophile on an electron-poor electrophilic center. As the electrophilic carbon already has four single bonds, a new bond can only be formed if one of the existing bonds is broken. The overall effect will therefore be a substitution of one of the groups (the leaving group) by the nucleophile.

A *nucleophilic substitution* reaction can also take place at an *unsaturated center* (a carbon with one or more multiple bonds). In this case, although the overall result is again a substitution, the mechanism is slightly different. The presence

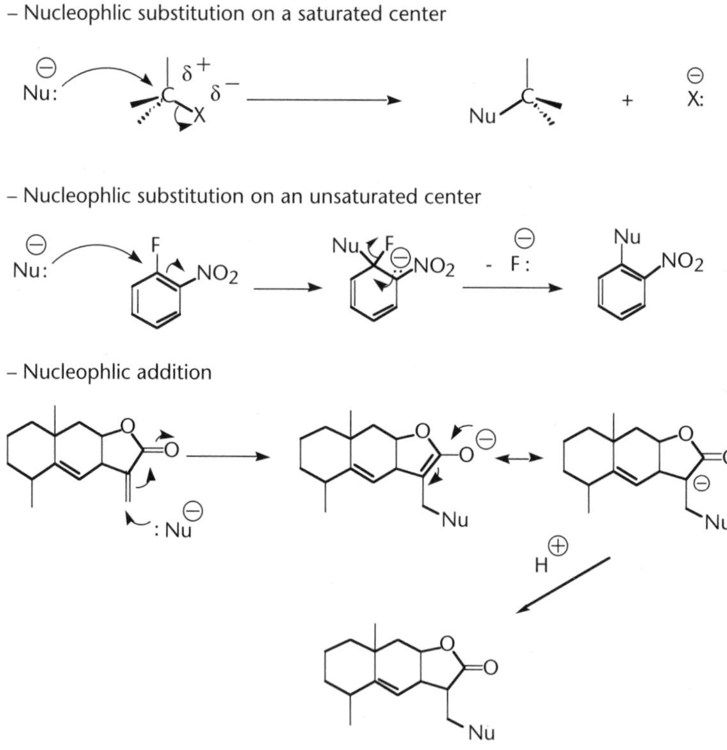

Figure 14.2: Principal mechanisms of covalent bond formation in contact allergy.

of a multiple bond allows the formation of a saturated intermediate and the subsequent reformation of the multiple bond, permitted by the departure of a leaving group, resulting in the substitution product. This mechanism is illustrated in the aromatic series in which it is all the more favored by attracting groups (e.g. nitro), which stabilize the intermediate.

Nucleophilic addition is simply the addition (with no leaving group) of a nucleophilic atom to an unsaturated electrophilic center (containing one or more multiple bonds). This mechanism is very similar to the first stage of nucleophilic substitution on an unsaturated center, but the absence of a leaving group rules out the reformation of the multiple bond. A saturated compound is thus produced.

14.3 PRINCIPAL ELECTROPHILIC CHEMICAL GROUPS PRESENT IN CONTACT ALLERGENS

Many chemical groups have electrophilic properties and are thus able to react with various nucleophiles to form covalent bonds. Table 14.1 shows those chemical groups most frequently found in contact allergens and the mechanism by which they react with nucleophilic groups. The previously defined three main types of mechanism, nucleophilic substitution on a saturated center (e.g., alkyl halides and epoxides), nucleophilic substitution on an unsaturated center (aromatic halides or esters), and nucleophilic addition (carbonyl derivatives and α,β-unsaturated systems), can be seen.

14.4 BACK TO CONTACT ALLERGY

If we consider biological systems from a chemical viewpoint, it becomes apparent that a very large proportion of structures, especially nucleic acids and proteins, contain many electron-rich groups (those containing nitrogen, phosphorus, oxygen, or sulfur). We can thus consider biological systems as being overall nucleophilic. It is therefore not surprising that many biological mechanisms are disturbed on contact with electrophilic chemical substances. Depending on the site of action of these electrophilic molecules, the effect can be mutagenic (Frierson *et al.*, 1986), toxic (Guengerich and Liebler, 1985), or allergenic if the target is the epidermis. In proteins, the side chains of many amino acids contain electron-rich groups capable of reacting with allergens (Figure 14.3). Lysine and cysteine are those most often cited, but other amino acids containing nucleophilic heteroatoms, such as histidine, methionine, and

TABLE 14.1:

Principal electrophilic groups seen in contact allergy, with mechanisms of reaction and the products.

Group	Name	Reaction mechanism	Product
R-CH$_2$-X X = Cl, Br, I	Alkyl halide	Nucleophilic substitution on a saturated center	Nu-CH$_2$-R
 X = F, Cl, Br, I	Aryl halide	Nucleophilic substitution on an unsaturated center	
	Aldehyde; R' = H Ketone, R' = alkyl ou aryl	Nucleophilic addition	
	Ester; R' = OR Amide; R' = NHR	Nucleophilic substitution on an unsaturated center	
	Epoxide	Nucleophilic substitution on a saturated center	
	Lactone; X = O Lactame; X = NH	Nucleophilic substitution on an unsaturated center	
 R = H, R, OR	Aldehyde or ketone α,β-unsaturated	Nucleophilic addition	
	p-quinone	Nucleophilic addition	
	o-quinone	Nucleophilic addition	
Ni^{++}, Co^{++}, Cr^{IV}	Metal salts	Coordinate bonds	

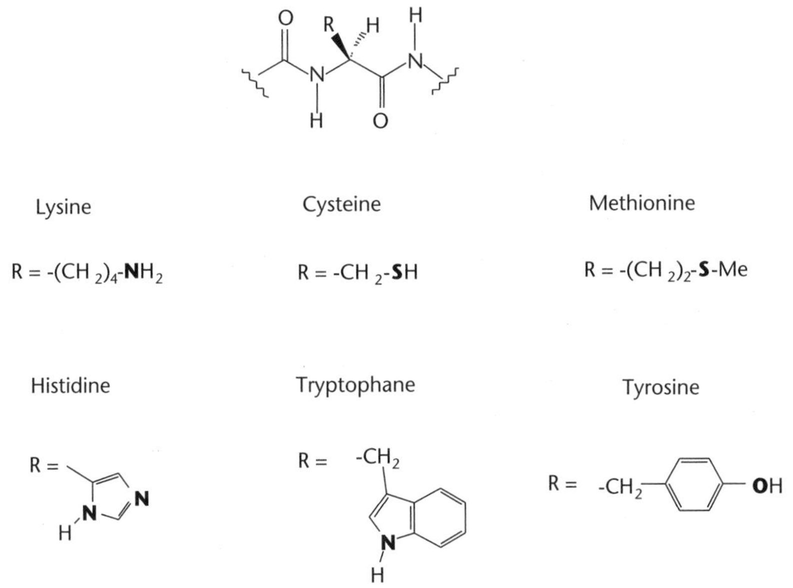

Lysine

Cysteine

Methionine

R = -(CH$_2$)$_4$-**NH**$_2$

R = -CH$_2$-**SH**

R = -(CH$_2$)$_2$-**S**-Me

Histidine

Tryptophane

Tyrosine

R =

R = -CH$_2$

R = -CH$_2$—⟨ ⟩—**OH**

Figure 14.3: Principal nucleophilic residues in proteins.

tyrosine, can react with electrophiles (Means and Feeney, 1971). Thus, it has been shown by nuclear magnetic resonance (NMR) studies that nickel sulfate, for example, was interacting with histidine residues of peptides (Romagnoli *et al.*, 1991) and that methyl alkanesulfonates, allergenic methylating agents, were mainly reacting with histidine and to a less extent with lysine, methionine, cysteine, and tyrosine (Lepoittevin and Benezra, 1992). If we consider the chemical structure of some allergens (Figure 14.4) in the light of the chemical principles already outlined, it is easy to understand that all of these molecules will be able to react with biological nucleophiles. The so formed extremely stable covalent bonds could then lead to the triggering of delayed hypersensitivity. Again, the previously described three main types of mechanism for the formation of covalent bonds are seen; the arrows indicate the reactive center of each molecule.

14.4.1 Chemical selectivity of haptens for amino acids

A direct consequence of the diversity of hapten-protein interactions is the existence of selectivity for amino acid modifications. For example, we have shown that the α-methylene-γ-butyrolactones, the major allergens of plants of

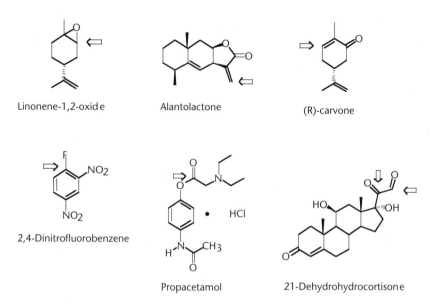

Linonene-1,2-oxide   Alantolactone   (R)-carvone

2,4-Dinitrofluorobenzene

Propacetamol   21-Dehydrohydrocortisone

Figure 14.4: Examples of sensitizing molecules. The electrophilic center is indicated by an arrow.

the Asteraceae family, principally modify lysine residues (Franot *et al.*, 1993). It has also been shown that not all modifications were antigenic and that the sensitization potential of a molecule is probably more related to its ability to modify some specific residues rather than to modify a large number of amino acids. Thus, the difference in sensitizing potential of two sultone derivatives, an alkenylsultone (a strong sensitizer) and an alkylsultone (a weak sensitizer), which differ only by the presence of a double bond, could be rather explained by the selective modification of lysine residues by the strong sensitizer than by the many tyrosine residues modified by both derivatives (Meschkat, 2001a, b).

A direct consequence of hapten selectivity for amino acids is the existence of differences in the modification sites of proteins and in the density of these modifications. These differences, initially purely chemical, seem increasingly to have a major impact on the response of the immune system. The selectivity of the sites of haptenization is directly involved in the selection of the peptide fragments that are presented by the APC to the T-cells and thus in the selection of T-cell receptors. This selectivity also indirectly controls the level of haptenization of the protein, or proteins. It appears that the epitope density on the surface of the APC directly or indirectly directs the immune response toward Th1 or Th2, high epitope densities directing the response toward Th1 and low densities toward Th2 (Hosken *et al.*, 1995). It is reasonable to ask if this selection of response profile, related to epitope density and thus to hapten reactivity, might not explain, for example, the observed differences between respiratory and skin allergens.

In recent years, the radical mechanism has gained increased interest in the discussion of the mechanism of hapten-protein binding. This mechanism, which has never been firmly established, has been postulated to explain, for example, the allergenic potential of eugenol versus iso-eugenol (Barratt, 1992). More recently, studies indicating that radical reactions were important for haptens containing allylic hydroperoxide groups have been published (Lepoittevin and Karlberg, 1994; Giménez-Arnau *et al.*, 2002).

14.5 THE HAPTEN–PROTEIN BOND: COVALENT OR NONCOVALENT?

In biology, few phenomena are irreversible, with the majority being controlled by equilibria. It is easy to understand that the more stable the hapten–protein complex, the greater is the possibility of the immune system being able to process the immunological information, resulting in allergy. Given this, we can understand why the very strong and difficult-to-reverse covalent bond produces a maximal biological efficacy. It is therefore natural that it is this type of bond that is found in the majority of cases of allergy. However, it would be incorrect to think that only covalent bonds result in allergy. In the case of metal salts, the formation of a covalent bond is impossible, and it is clear that a sufficiently stable coordination complex must be formed between the metal salt and the electron-rich residues of proteins (Polak and Frey, 1973; Hutchinson *et al.*, 1975). These coordinate complexes are therefore sufficiently stable, and the protein modification sufficiently important, to lead to allergy (Sinigaglia, 1994).

14.6 METABOLISM AND PROHAPTENS

Far from being an inert tissue, the skin is the site of many metabolic processes, which can result in structural modification of xenobiotics that penetrate into it. These metabolic processes, primarily intended for the elimination of foreign molecules during detoxification, can, in certain cases, convert harmless molecules into derivatives with electrophilic, and therefore allergenic, properties. The metabolic processes are mainly based on oxidation reactions via extremely powerful enzymatic hydroxylation systems, such as the cytochrome P-450 enzymes (Mansuy, 1985), but monoamine oxidases, which convert amines to aldehydes, and peroxidases seem to play an important role in the metabolism of haptens. When activated by the production of hydrogen peroxide during the oxidative stress following the introduction of a xenobiotic into the skin, peroxidases convert the electron-rich aromatic derivatives (aminated or hydroxylated) into quinones, which are powerful electrophiles. In this way, it has been proposed that the long-chain catechols, responsible for the severe allergies to poison ivy (*Rhus radicans* L.) and poison oak (*Rhus diversiloba* T.), could be oxidized *in vivo* to the highly reactive orthoquinones (Dupuis, 1979) (Figure 14.5). The same applies to paraphenylenediamine or hydroquinone derivatives, such as the allergens from *Phacelia crenulata* Torr. (Reynolds and Rodriguez, 1981), which are converted into electrophilic paraquinones. Metabolic reactions involving enzymatic hydrolyses can also occur in the skin. It is thus that the tuliposides A and B, found in the bulb of the tulip (*Tulipa gesneriana* L.), are hydrolyzed, releasing the actual allergens, tulipalines A and B (Bergmann *et al.*, 1967).

All these molecules, which have themselves no electrophilic properties and cannot therefore be haptens but which can be metabolized to haptens, are

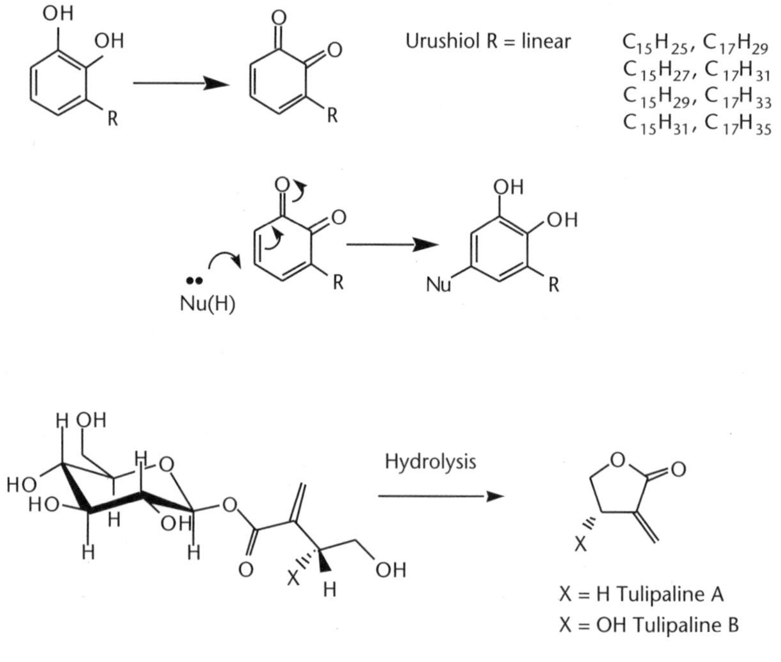

Figure 14.5: Examples of prohapten metabolism.

referred to as prohaptens (Landsteiner and Jacobs, 1936; Dupuis and Benezra, 1982) and play an important role in contact allergy because of their number and their highly reactive nature. The fact that the structure of the metabolized molecule can be far removed from the structure of the initial molecule can make allergologic investigations even more difficult.

Nonenzymatic processes, such as reaction with atmospheric oxygen or ultraviolet irradiation, can also induce changes in the chemical structure of molecules. Many terpenes spontaneously auto-oxidize in air, producing allergizing derivatives. In the 1950s it was found that allergenic activity of turpentine was mainly due to hydroperoxides of one of the monoterpene Δ^3-carene (Hellerstrom *et al.*, 1955). This is also the case for abietic acid, the main constituent of colophony, which is converted into the highly reactive substance hydroperoxide (Karlberg, 1988) by contact with air (Figure 14.6). Such an auto-oxidation mechanism has also been demonstrated for another monoterpene, *d*-limonene, found in citrus fruits. *d*-Limonene itself is not allergenic, but at air exposure hydroperoxides, epoxides, and ketones are formed that are strong allergens (Karlberg *et al.*, 1994).

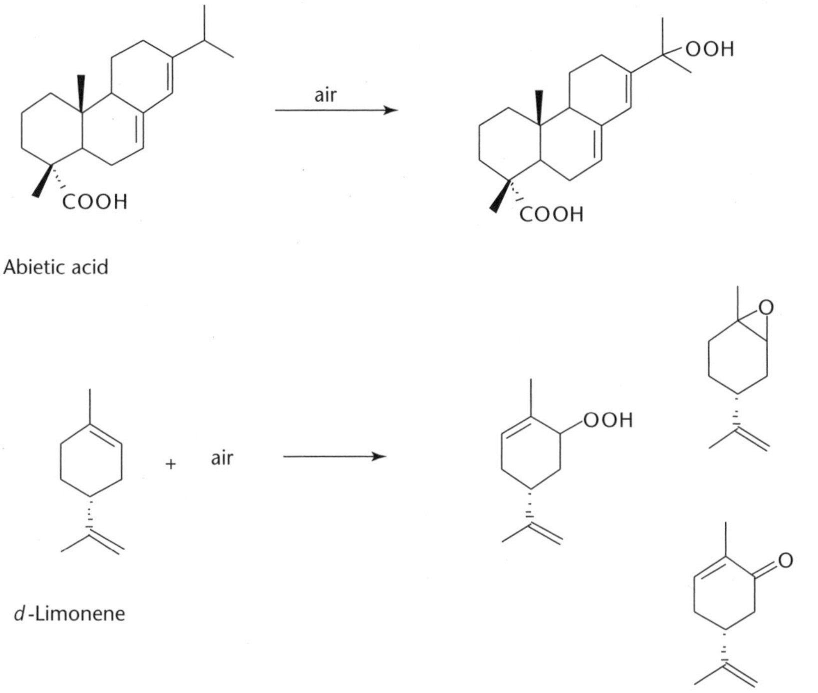

Figure 14.6: Examples of chemical modification by reaction with air.

14.7 HAPTENS AND CROSS-ALLERGY

The factors that control molecular recognition during the elicitation stage are primarily the nature of the chemical group and the compatibility of the spatial geometry. Although the first factor (the identity of the chemical group) is very important and serves to define what are commonly called the group allergies, it cannot account for all structure-activity relationships. Receptor molecules are highly sensitive to volume and shape, and molecules must have a similar size and spatial geometry to be recognized by the same receptor. Thus, even though the molecules tulipaline A or B and alantolactone (the allergen of *Inula helenium* L.) bear the same chemical group, α-methylene-β-butyrolactone, they cannot give rise to cross-allergenic reactions, as their spatial volumes are too different. In contrast, isoalantolactone and alantolactone produce a cross-allergic reaction (Stampf *et al.* 1982), since they share a homologous chemical group and spatial volume. The term cross-allergy is often misused and should be restricted to the well-defined cases that can be called the true cross-allergies (Baer, 1954; Benezra and Maibach, 1984).

True cross-allergy between a sensitizer A and a triggering agent B can be interpreted in various ways:

- A and B are chemically and structurally similar.
- A is metabolized to a compound that is similar to B.
- B is metabolized to a compound that is similar to A.
- A and B are metabolized to similar compounds.

The identification of cross-allergenic responses can be especially difficult, particularly in humans, in whom the possibility of co- or polysensitization should never be ruled out. In addition, the metabolism of molecules can be very complex, and two molecules with a priori little in common can be converted to derivatives that have a similar structure. Thus, derivatives of hydroquinones and *p*-phenylenediamines can be converted into benzoquinone derivatives. It is therefore dangerous to draw conclusions from tests without knowing how the substances used are liable to be metabolized. Many reactions described as demonstrating cross-allergy are, without doubt, due to co-sensitization (Benezra and Maibach, 1984). Experimental studies in animals are often the only means of being really certain of what happens during recognition. The concept of the prohapten is very important in the interpretation of results in allergy. As the structure of the metabolized molecule can sometimes be very different from that of the initial molecule, it can be difficult to establish similarities of chemical groups and structure.

14.7.1 Molecular modeling as a tool for cross-reactivity analysis

In the last few years, molecular modeling has been shown to be a powerful tool in studies of conformation-dependent drug-receptor interactions and structure-activity relationship analysis (Cohen *et al.*, 1990). Despite the great potential of this technique, few attempts to analyze cross-reaction patterns in the field of allergic contact dermatitis have yet been reported. One reason may be the heterogeneous population of patients with heterogeneous clinical histories, in which it is somewhat difficult to distinguish between actual cross-reaction and concomitant sensitization. A second reason is that, to be effective, structure-activity relationship studies need data for a wide range of molecules. The clinical investigation of contact dermatitis to corticosteroids, in which a large number of related substances are tested on a large number of patients, represents a good opportunity to carry out such a structure-activity study. From the statistical analysis of the clinical data, it is now possible to advance an experimentally supported hypothesis for cross-reaction patterns. Coopman *et al.* (1989) hypothesized that cross-reactions occur primarily within certain groups of corticosteroids. They distinguished four groups, group A consisting of hydrocortisone, tixocortol pivalate, and related compounds, group B consisting of triamcinolone acetonide, amcinonide, and related compounds, group C consisting of betamethasone, dexamethasone, and related compounds, and group D consisting of esters such as hydrocortisone-17-butyrate and clobetasone-17-butyrate (Figure 14.7). It is now possible to correlate this with conformational characteristics and to establish a molecular basis for cross-reaction patterns in patient sensitized to corticosteroids. This could be invaluable in the prediction of potential cross-reactions to new molecules.

14.7.2 Example of conformational analysis. Cross-reaction to corticosteroids

The conformation of corticosteroids from groups A, B, C, and D was analyzed (Lepoittevin *et al.*, 1995). This study was based on two hypotheses. The first was that all corticosteroids should interact with proteins in a very similar way. All corticosteroid molecules were designed to interact with the same type of

■ CHAPTER 14 ■

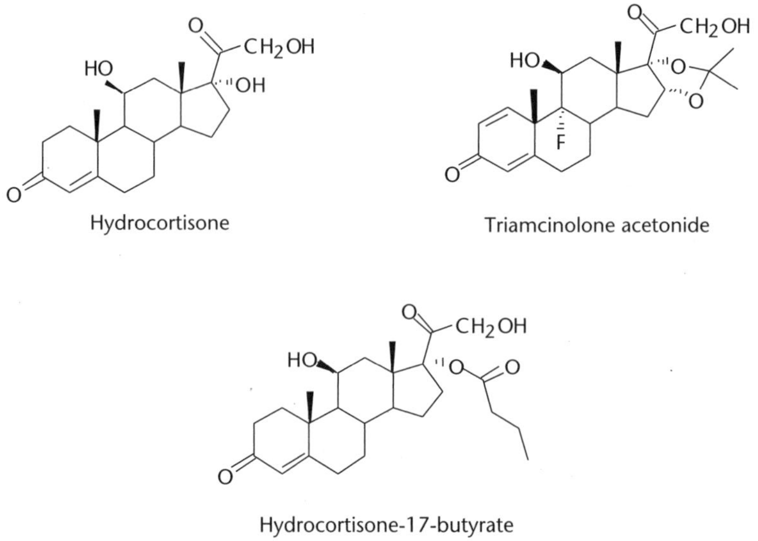

Hydrocortisone

Triamcinolone acetonide

Hydrocortisone-17-butyrate

Figure 14.7: Chemical structure of hydrocortisone (group A), triamcinolone acetonide (group B), and hydrocortisone 17-butyrate (group D).

receptors, and thus should be more or less metabolized in similar ways. The second hypothesis, based on chemical observations, was that esters at position 21 are readily hydrolyzed to give the free alcohol while esters at position 17 are more resistant to hydrolysis, due to a strong steric hindrance. Thus, for example, tixocortol pivalate was considered as tixocortol with a free thiol group at position 21, and alclometasone 17,21-dipropionate was considered as alclometasone 17-propionate.

All molecules were drawn from energy-minimized building blocks and were then submitted to a multiconformational analysis in order to achieve the most energetically stable conformation. These conformations were then compared for analogies or differences in the van der Waals volumes that define the electronic shape of the molecule. As expected from the hypothesis, significant group-specific characteristics of volume and shape were found for molecules of group A, B, and D but not for molecules of group C (Figure 14.8).

In terms of molecular characteristics, the existence of groups A, B, and D, as defined by the analysis of cross-reaction patterns in patients sensitized to corticosteroids, is fully supported by the conformational analysis of these molecules. Molecules of the same group have very similar spatial structures, explaining the cross-reactions observed. In addition, molecules from one group

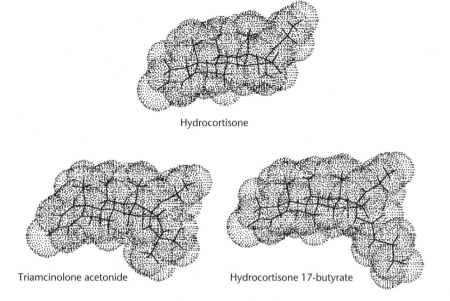

Hydrocortisone

Triamcinolone acetonide   Hydrocortisone 17-butyrate

Figure 14.8: Electronic shape of corticosteroids of group A, B and D.

are sufficiently different from molecules of another group to explain the lack of cross-reactions observed between groups A, B, and D.

The volume occupied by specific groups on the α face of ring D seems to be critical for the molecular recognition of corticosteroids by receptors of immunocompetent cells, while modifications of other parts of the molecule seem to have little effects on the recognition patterns. As shown in Figure 14.8, each group represents a well-defined, characteristic shape that can be very useful for the prediction of potential cross-reactions of new corticosteroid molecules.

14.8 CONCLUSION

The principles that we have just discussed permit a rational approach to the phenomena of contact allergy, but, in actual fact, we often have available only indirect evidence suggestive of one mechanism or another. Although the chemical bases for hapten–protein interactions can be checked in the laboratory by the use of nucleophilic amino acids, small peptides, and model proteins, and although a certain number of steps can be checked, at the present time, no method is available to follow a hapten step by step during the entire immunological process leading to contact allergy. Many points await investigation, but in many cases a "chemical" analysis of the problem does allow us to understand and to foresee cross-allergies and thus to warn the patient about structurally related products.

REFERENCES

BAER, R.L. (1954) Cross-sensitization phenomena, in MACKENNA, R.M.B. (ed.) *Modern Trends in Dermatology*, London: Butterworth.

BARRATT, M.D. and BASKETTER, D.A. (1992) Possible origin of the skin senstization potential of eugenol and related compounds, *Contact Dermatitis* **27**, 98–104.

BENEZRA, C. and MAIBACH, H. (1984) True cross-sensitization, false cross-sensitization and otherwise, *Contact Dermatitis* **11**, 65–69.

BERGMANN, H.H., BEIJERSBERGEN, J.C.H., OVEREEM, J.C. and SIJPESTEIJN, A.K. (1967) Isolation and identification of α-methylene-β-butyrolactone: A fungitoxic substance from tulips, *Rec. Trav. Chim. Pays-Bas* **86**, 709–713.

COHEN, N.C., BLANEY, J.M., HUMBLET, C., GUND, P. and BARRY, D.C. (1990) Molecular modeling software and methods for medicinal chemistry, *J. Med. Chem.* **33**, 883–984.

COOPMAN, S., DEGREEF, H. and DOOMS-GOOSSENS. A. (1989) Identification of cross-reaction patterns in allergic contact dermatitis from topical corticosteroids, *Br. J. Dermatol.* **121**, 27–34.

DARLEY, M.O., POST, W. and MUNTER, R.L. (1977) Induction of cell-mediated immunity to chemically modified antigens in guinea pigs, *J. Immunol.* **118**, 963–970.

DUPUIS, G. (1979) Studies of poison ivy. *In vitro* lymphocytes transformation by urushiol protein conjugates, *Br. J. Dermatol.* **101**, 617–624.

DUPUIS, G. and BENEZRA, C. (eds) (1982) *Allergic Contact Dermatitis to Simple Chemicals*, New York: Marcel Dekker.

FRANOT, C., BENEZRA, C. and LEPOITTEVIN, J.-P. (1993) Synthesis and interaction studies of 13C labeled lactone derivatives with a model protein using ^{13}C NMR, *Biorg Med Chem* **1**, 389–397.

FRIERSON, M.R., KLOPMAN, G. and ROSENKRANZ, H.S. (1986) Structure activity relationship among mutagens and carcinogens: A review, *Environ. Mutagen.* **8**, 283–327.

GIMÉNEZ ARNAU, E., HABERKORN, L., GROSSI, L. and LEPOITTEVIN, J.-P. (2002) Identification of alkyl radicals derived from an allergenic cyclic tertiary allylic hydroperoxide by combined use of radical trapping and ESR studies *Tetrahedron* **58**, 5535–5545.

GUENGERICH, F.P. and LIEBLER, D.C. (1985) Enzymatic activation of chemicals, *CRC Crit. Rev. Toxicol.* **14**, 259–307.

HELLERSTROM, S., THYRESSON, N., BLOHM, S.-G. and WIDMARK, G. (1955) On the nature of eczematogenic component of oxidized Δ^3-carene *J. Invest. Dermatol.* **24**, 217–224.

HOSKEN, N.A., SHIBUYA, K., HEATH, A.W., MURPHY, K.M., O'GARRA, A. (1995) The effect of antigen dose on CD4+ T helper cell phenotype development in a T cell receptor-alpha beta-transgenic model, *J. Exp Med* **182**, 1579–1584.

HOTCHKISS, S.A.M. (1998) Dermal metabolism in Roberts, M.S. and Walters, K.A. (eds) *Dermal absorption and toxicity assessment; Drugs and pharmaceutical sciences, Vol. 91*, New York: Marcel Dekker.

HUTCHINSON, F., MCLEOD, T.M. and RAFFLE, E.J. (1975) Nickel hypersensitivity. Nickel binding to aminoacids and lymphocytes *Br. J. Dermatol.* **93**, 557–561.

KARLBERG, A.-T. (1988) Contact allergy to colophony. Chemical identification of allergens. Sensitization experiments and clinical experiments *Acta Dermato-Venereol.* **68**(Suppl. 139), 1–43.

KARLBERG, A.-T., SHAO, L. P., NILSSON, U., GÄFVERT, E. and NILSSON, J.L.G. (1994) Hydroperoxides in oxidized d-limonene identified as potent contact allergens, *Arch. Dermatol. Res.* **286**, 97–103.

LANDSTEINER, K. and JACOBS, J.L. (1936) Studies on the sensitization of animals with simple chemicals, *J. Exp. Med.* **64**, 625–639.

LEPOITTEVIN, J.-P., BASKETTER, D.A., GOOSSENS, A. and KARLBERG A.-T. (eds) (1998) *Allergic Contact Dermatitis: The Molecular Basis*, Berlin, Heidelberg, New York: Springer.

LEPOITTEVIN, J.-P. and BENEZRA, C. (1992) ^{13}C enriched methyl alkanesulfonates: New lipophilic methylating agents for the identification of nucleophilic amino acids of proteins by NMR, *Tetrahedron Lett.* **33**, 3875–3878.

LEPOITTEVIN, J.-P. and KARLBERG, A.-T. (1994) Interaction of allergenic hydroperoxides with proteins: A radical mechanism? *Chem. Res. Toxicol.* **7**, 130-133.

LEPOITTEVIN, J.-P., DRIEGHE, J. and DOOMS-GOOSSENS, A. (1995) Studies in patients with corticosteroid contact allergy: Understanding cross-reactivity among different steroids *Arch. Dermatol.* **131**, 31–37.

■ CHAPTER 14 ■

MANSUY, D. (1985) Particular ability of cytochrome P450 to form reactive intermediates and metabolites, in Siest, G. (ed.) *Drug Metabolism: Molecular Approaches and Pharmacological Implications*, New York: Pergamon.

MEANS, G.E. and FEENEY, R.E. (1971) *Chemical Modification of Proteins*, San Francisco: Holden Day.

MESCHKAT, E., BARRATT, M.D. and LEPOITTEVIN, J.-P. (2001a) Studies of the chemical selectivity of hapten, reactivity, and skin sensitization potency. 1. Synthesis and studies on the reactivity toward model nucleophiles of the 13C-labeled skin sensitizers hex-1-ene- and hexane-1,3-sultones, *Chem. Res. Toxicol.* **14**, 110–117.

MESCHKAT, E., BARRATT, M.D. and LEPOITTEVIN, J.-P. (2001b) Studies of the chemical selectivity of hapten, reactivity, and skin sensitization potency. 2. NMR studies of the covalent binding of the 13C-labeled skin sensitizers 2-[13C]- and 3-[13C]hex-1-ene- and 3-[13C]hexane-1,3-sultones to human serum albumin, *Chem. Res. Toxicol.* **14**, 118–126.

POLAK, L. and FREY, J.R. (1973) Studies on contact hypersensitivity to chromium in the guinea pig *Int. Arch. Allergy Appl. Immunol.* **44**, 51–61.

REYNOLDS, G. and RODRIGUEZ, E. (1981) Prenylated hydroquinones: Contact allergens from trichomes of Phacelia minor and P. parryi, *Phytochemistry* **20**, 1365–1366.

ROBERTS, M.S. and WALTERS, K.A. (eds) (1998) *Dermal Absorption and Toxicity Assessment*, New York: Marcel Dekker.

ROMAGNOLI, P., LABAHRDT, A. M. and SINIGAGLIA, F. (1991) Selective interaction of nickel with an MHC bound peptide, *EMBO J.* **10**, 1303–1306.

SINIGAGLIA, F. (1994) The molecular basis of metal recognition by T cells, *J. Invest. Dermatol.* **102**, 398–401.

STAMPF, J.-L., BENEZRA, C., KLECAK, G., GELEICK, H., SCHULZ, K. H. and HAUSEN, B. (1982) The sensitization capacity of helenin and two of its main constituents, the sesquiterpene lactones, alantolactones and isoalantolactone, *Contact Dermatitis* **8**, 16–24.

Systemic Contact Dermatitis

**NIELS K VEIEN, TORKIL MENNÉ,
AND HOWARD I MAIBACH**

Contents

15.1 Introduction

15.2 Immunology/mechanism

15.3 Clinical features

15.4 Medicaments

15.5 Nickel

15.6 Chromium, cobalt and other metals

15.7 Other contact allergens

15.8 Risk assessment-oriented studies

15.9 Diagnosis

15.1 INTRODUCTION

Systemic contact dermatitis is an inflammatory skin disease that may occur in contact-sensitized individuals when these persons are exposed to the hapten orally, transcutaneously, intravenously or by inhalation. The entity can present with clinically characteristic features or be clinically indistinguishable from other types of contact dermatitis. Contact sensitization to ubiquitous haptens is common. In a recent Danish population-based study 15.2 percent reacted to one or more of the haptens in the Standard patch test series (Nielsen *et al.*, 2001). The total number of individuals at risk of developing a systemic contact dermatitis reaction is therefore large. Systemic contact dermatitis from medicaments is a well-established entity. There is increasing evidence for similar reactions from plant derivatives and metals such as nickel (Hindsén, 2001).

The first description of systemic contact dermatitis can probably be ascribed to the pioneering British dermatologist Thomas Bateman (Shelley and Crissey, 1970). His description of the mercury eczema called eczema rubrum is similar to what we today describe as the baboon syndrome:

> Eczema rubrum is preceded by a sense of stiffness, burning, heat and itching in the part where it commences, most frequently the upper and inner surface of the thighs and about the scrotum in men, but sometimes it appears first in the groins, axillae or in the bends of the arms, on the wrists and hands or on the neck.

In the twentieth century the systemic spread of nickel dermatitis was described by Schittenhelm and Stockinger in Kiel in 1925. By patch testing nickel-sensitive workers with nickel sulfate, they observed the spread of dermatitis and flares in the original areas of contact dermatitis. Similar clinical features have been seen in large groups of carefully evaluated nickel-sensitive patients (Calnan, 1956; Marcussen, 1957). The literature on systemic contact dermatitis is now comprehensive. Reviews include Veien *et al.* (1990) and Menné *et al.* (1994).

15.2 IMMUNOLOGY/MECHANISM

Systemic contact dermatitis may start a few hours or 1 to 2 days after experimental provocation, suggesting that more than one type of immunological reaction is involved. The local flare-up reaction has been studied experimentally in both humans and in animals. Christensen *et al.* (1981) studied flare-up reactions in 4- to 7-week-old positive nickel patch tests in five nickel sensitive

■ CHAPTER 15 ■

patients after oral provocation with 5.6 mg nickel. The histology was that of acute dermatitis. Direct immunofluorescence examination for deposits of IgG, IgA, IgM, complement 3, and fibrinogen was negative. A few sensitized T-cells can remain in the skin for months (Scheper *et al.*, 1983; Yamashita *et al.*, 1989). Systemic exposure to haptens can activate sensitized T-cells in sites of previous contact dermatitis and initiate the inflammatory response.

The investigation of lymphocyte subsets in the gastrointestinal mucosa and in blood before and after oral challenge with nickel in nickel-sensitized women showed a reduction of CD4+ cells, CD4+CD45Ro+ cells and CD8+ cells in the peripheral blood of women with evidence of systemic contact dermatitis. Oral challenge with nickel induced maturation of naive T cells into memory cells that tended to accumulate in the intestinal mucosa (di Gioacchino, 2000).

Möller *et al.*, 1998 challenged 10 gold allergic patients with an intramuscular dose of gold and saw a flare-up of 1-week-old gold patch test reactions in all of them. Five also experienced a maculo-papular rash, and four had transient fever. Plasma levels of TNF-α, IL-1ra and sTNF-R1 and C-reactive protein were increased, particularly in those with fever.

In a later study of 20 gold and 28 nickel-allergic patients challenged orally with nickel and gold in a double-blind, double-dummy fashion, 3 of 9 nickel-sensitive patients reacted to 2.5 mg nickel, while none reacted to gold. Six of 10 gold-allergic patients reacted to 10 mg gold sodium thiomalate, none of them reacted to nickel. TNF-R1 was increased in the plasma of nickel-sensitive patients challenged with nickel, while TNF-R1, TNF-α and IL-1 were increased in gold-sensitive patients challenged with gold (Möller, 1999a).

The mechanism behind skin symptoms unrelated to previous contact dermatitis sites has been minimally evaluated. Veien *et al.* (1979) investigated 14 patients with positive nickel patch tests and severe dermatitis. All were challenged orally with 2.5 mg nickel. After 6–12 h, five developed widespread erythema. No clinical dermatitis developed in the erythematous areas. In a passive immunodiffusion assay three of the five demonstrated precipitating antibodies in their sera against a nickel-albumin complex. The same phenomenon was observed by Polak and Turk (1968a, b) in chromium-sensitized guinea pigs. As in humans, the response started 6–8 h after a chromate injection. Histopathology 24 h after the challenge showed a marked dilatation of the capillaries in the upper dermis. The authors suggested that circulating immune complexes were the triggering mechanism.

Van Hoogstraten *et al.* (1992) demonstrated antigen specific tolerance to nickel and chromate in guinea pigs. Administration of the allergens to the oral mucosa proved the most effective means of inducing tolerance. Prior to this study the same author conducted a retrospective clinical study of the risk of nickel sensitization from pierced ears in patients who did or did not wear dental braces. It was shown that fewer cases of nickel sensitization were seen when dental braces were fitted before ear piercing, than when the braces were fitted after ear piercing (Van Hoogstraten et al., 1991). These findings have been confirmed by Mørtz in a study of 13–15 year-old girls (Mørtz, 1999).

It has also been shown that giving repeated oral doses of nickel to nickel-sensitive patients gradually reduces the severity of flares of dermatitis seen after oral challenge with nickel (Sjövall et al., 1987). It is possible that the repeated doses of nickel decrease the intestinal absorption of the metal (Santucci et al., 1994).

Hyposensitization to poison ivy was observed in 9 of 13 poison-ivy-sensitive workers who were exposed to dust from cashew nut shells. The route of hyposensitization was thought to be gastrointestinal from swallowed dust (Reginella et al., 1989).

A patient was successfully hyposensitized to *Parthenium hysterophorus* by the oral route of exposure (Srinivas et al., 1988).

Twenty parthenium-sensitive patients were hyposensitized orally for 12 weeks with ether extracts of parthenium. Fourteen completed the procedure and improved. Six stopped due to aggravation of their dermatitis. Seven of the 14 were followed for a year. Four of them had recurrences within 2 months (Handa et al., 2001).

Two patients with chrysanthemum dermatitis were successfully hyposensitized using chrysanthemum juice for 21 days. Aggravation of the dermatitis was seen initially in both patients. The patients remained clear of dermatitis for more than 2 years (Mori et al., 2000).

15.3 CLINICAL FEATURES

The clinical symptoms related to systemic contact dermatitis are summarized in Table 15.1. The symptoms usually appear exclusively on the skin but general symptoms are occasionally seen. Knowledge of the clinical symptoms stems from clinical observations and experimental oral challenge studies.

Flare-up reactions in the primary site of dermatitis or previously positive patch-test sites raise the suspicion of systemic contact dermatitis (Ekelund and Möller, 1969; Christensen and Möller, 1975; Menné and Weismann, 1984; Hindsén, 2001). Flare-up of previously positive patch-test sites following

■ CHAPTER 15 ■

TABLE 15.1:

Clinical aspects of systemic contact dermatitis reactions

Dermatitis in areas of previous exposure
Flare-up of previous dermatitis
Flare-up of previously positive patch test sites
Skin symptoms in previously unaffected skin
Vesicular hand eczema
Flexural dermatitis
The baboon syndrome
Maculo-papular rash
Vasculitis-like lesions
General symptoms
Headache
Malaise
Arthralgia
Diarrhea and vomiting

ingestion of the hapten is a fascinating and specific sign of systemic contact dermatitis. It is seen in relation to systemic contact dermatitis from medicaments and in experimental oral provocation studies. Such flares of patch test sites have not been a feature of the clinical spectrum of systemic contact dermatitis. This symptom is hapten specific and can be seen years after the original patch testing. Christensen *et al.* (1981) and later Hindsén *et al.* (2001) examined the specificity of this symptom in nickel-sensitive individuals. Positive patch tests to nickel and to the primary irritant sodium lauryl sulfate were made on previously unaffected skin areas. After several weeks the individuals were given an oral nickel dose. A flare of dermatitis was seen at the nickel patch-test site, but not at the site of irritant dermatitis.

Vesicular hand eczema (pompholyx or dyshidrotic eczema) (Veien and Menné, 1993), a pruritic eruption on the palms, volar aspects and sides of the fingers and occasionally the plantar aspects of the feet, presents with deep-seated vesicles and sparse or no erythema. If the distal dorsal aspects of the fingers are involved, transversal ridging of the fingernails can be a consequence. Recurrent, vesicular hand eczema is a common clinical manifestation of hand eczema and can have many different causes. It is a frequent symptom seen in systemic contact dermatitis.

Erythema or a flare of dermatitis in the elbow and/or the knee flexures is a common symptom of systemic contact dermatitis. It is difficult to distinguish from the early lesions of atopic dermatitis. Flexual psoriasis can be a Köbner phenomenon associated with systemic contact dermatitis.

The baboon syndrome (Andersen *et al.*, 1984) is a well-demarcated eruption on the buttocks, in the genital area and in a V-shape on the inner thighs with a color ranging from dark violet to pink. It may occupy the whole area or only part of it. Nakayama *et al.* (1983) described the same syndrome as mercury exanthema, and Shelley and Shelley (1987) described it as a nonpigmented fixed drug eruption with a distinctive pattern. In the latter publication, no mention is made of patch test results. Based on case stories, the patients may have had systemic contact dermatitis. Even extensive patch testing fails to confirm the diagnosis of systemic contact dermatitis in some patients who present with features of the baboon syndrome.

A non-specific maculo-papular rash is often part of a systemic contact dermatitis reaction. Even cases of vasculitis presenting as palpable purpura have been seen (Veien and Krogdahl, 1989).

In relation to oral provocation with nickel or medicaments, general symptoms such as headache and malaise have occasionaly been seen in sensitized individuals. In neomycin- (Ekelund and Möller, 1969) and chromate-sensitive patients (Kaaber and Veien, 1977), oral provocation with the hapten has caused nausea, vomiting, and diarrhea. A few patients have complained of arthralgia. The available information on the general symptoms observed in relation to the systemic contact dermatitis reaction is anecdotal and deserves systematic documentation.

15.4 MEDICAMENTS

15.4.1 Antibiotics

Neomycin and bacitracin are widely used topical antibiotics. Contact allergy to these compounds is particularly frequent (4 percent to 8 percent) in patients with leg ulcers. Ekelund and Möller (1969) challenged 12 leg-ulcer patients sensitive to neomycin with an oral dose of the hapten. Ten of the 12 had a reaction. Five had flares of their original dermatitis; six had flares at the sites of previously positive patch tests. Three developed vesicular hand eczema for the first time. Four experienced various gastrointestinal symptoms. Some surgeons use oral neomycin prior to colon surgery. Even if neomycin is poorly absorbed from the gastrointestinal tract, severe systemic contact dermatitis might occur in neomycin-sensitive individuals (Menné and Weismann, 1984).

Contact sensitivity to penicillin was previously common, and flares of dermatitis have been seen in sensitized persons following exposure to traces of

■ CHAPTER 15 ■

penicillin in milk (Vickers *et al.*, 1958). Contact sensitivity and systemic contact dermatitis caused by penicillin can still occur after the topical use of the drug in the middle ear, in the peritoneum during abdominal surgery (Andersen *et al.*, 1984), or after occupational exposure. Tagami *et al.* described a patient with toxic epidermal necrolysis after the systemic administration of ampicillin and reviewed 10 other patch-test proven cases of dermatitis of similar morphology caused by various medications (Tagami *et al.*, 1983).

Penicillin, ampillin/amoxicillin and erythromycin have been described as causes of systemic contact dermatitis with baboon-like clinical features (Llamazares, 2000; Goossens *et al.*, 1997).

Systemic contact dermatitis was seen in nurses occupationally sensitized to streptomycin (Wilson, 1958) when attempts were made to induce tolerance by subsequent systemic exposure to the drug.

During World War II, sulfonamides were used extensively for the treatment of wounds. Later systemic use of sulfonamides in sensitized individuals caused dose-dependent flares of dermatitis. The persons who had the most pronounced reactions were those most sensitive to sulfonamides (Park, 1943).

Systemic contact dermatitis caused by pristinamycine and gentamicin has also been described (Bernard *et al.*, 1988; Ghadially and Ramsay, 1988).

15.4.2 Antihistamines

The pharmacological effectiveness of topically applied antihistamines is questionable. Antihistamines derived from ethanolamine and ethylenediamine are the most common contact-sensitizing antihistamines in the United States (Fisher, 1976). Ethylenediamine-based antihistamines may elicit systemic contact dermatitis in patients sensitized to ethylenediamine. Aminophylline, which contains theophylline and ethylenediamine, may elicit reactions in ethylenediamine-sensitized patients (Provost and Jilson, 1967; Guin *et al.*, 1999).

Much of the knowledge in this field is based on anecdotal therapeutic accidents. In view of the large number of persons who are contact-sensitized to ethylenediamine, incidents of systemic contact dermatitis to ethylenediamine derivatives must be considered rare.

15.4.3 *Para*-amino compounds

Sidi and Dobkevitch-Morrill (1951) studied cross reactions between *para*-amino compounds. Systemic reactions were seen after oral challenge with procaine in

TABLE 15.2:
Oral challenge with sulfonyl urea hypoglycemic drugs in sulfanilamide-sensitive patients

Substance	Allergen dose	Duration of treatment	Response
Carbutamide	500 mg	Single exposure	7/25
Tolbutamide	500 mg	Single exposure	3/11
Chlorpropamide	500 mg	Single exposure	1(1?)/20

sulfonamide-sensitive patients, after challenge with *p*-aminophenylsulfamide in procaine-sensitive patients, and after challenge with *p*-aminophenylsulfamide and procaine in *p*-phenylenediamine-sensitive patients.

Oral challenge with the sulfonyl urea hypoglycemic drugs in patients sensitized to *para*-amino compounds (sulfanilamide, paraphenylenediamine, and benzocaine) resulted in flare-up reactions in sulfanilamide-sensitive patients, but not in *para*-phenylenediamine and benzocaine-sensitive patients (Table 15.2). Oral challenge with tartrazine (20 mg) and saccarine (150 mg) in patients sensitized to *para*-amino compounds and sulfonamide did not produce any flare-up reactions (Angelini and Meneghini, 1981; Angelini *et al.*, 1982).

15.4.4 Corticosteroids

Contact allergy to glucocorticoids is not uncommon in patients with eczematous skin diseases (Lauerma, 1992). The frequency seems to vary from center to center depending on local prescribing habits, degree of patient selections, and the diagnostic method used.

Patch testing with topical corticosteroids has not yet been standardized with regard to patch test concentrations and vehicles. Intradermal testing may offer additional diagnostic possibilities.

Patients sensitized to hydrocortisone may react with systemic contact dermatitis when provoked orally with 100–200 mg hydrocortisone (Lauerma *et al.*, 1991; Torres *et al.*, 1993). These authors also investigated whether cortisol produced in the adrenals (i.e., hydrocortisone) could provoke systemic contact dermatitis. In a placebo-controlled study, a patient was challenged with an adrenocorticotropic hormone (ACTH) stimulation test. A skin rash similar to that seen after oral hydrocortisone developed after 8 h.

Räsänen and Hasan (1993) studied five patients who developed rashes when treated with systemic or intralesional hydrocortisone. They recommend patch testing and intradermal testing to make the diagnosis of systemic hydrocortisone sensitivity and, if these tests fail, an oral challenge.

Whitmore (1995) reviewed 16 studies with a total of 24 patients who had systemic contact dermatitis from corticosteroids. Typical clinical features were exanthema, localized dermatitis, generalized dermatitis and purpura. Onset was often hours to days following ingestion of the corticosteroids.

As a part of her thesis on corticosteroid allergy, Isaksson (2000) challenged 15 budesonide-sensitive patients with 100 and 800 μg budesonide or placebo by inhalation. Four of seven challenged with budesonide had reactivation of previously positive patch test sites as well as papular exanthema and/or a flare-up of previous dermatitis.

15.4.5 Miscellaneous medications

Antabuse (tetraethylthiuram disulfide) is of particular interest, since it can cause systemic contact dermatitis in three ways. Antabuse is used in the manufacture of rubber as a fungicide and in the treatment of chronic alcoholism. In patients sensitized to thiurams from the use of rubber gloves, systemic exposure to Antabuse can give rise to systemic contact dermatitis (Pirilä, 1957). Subcutaneous implantation of Antabuse led to contact sensitization in two patients. Subsequent oral challenge with the hapten produced a flare-up reaction in one of the two patients (Lachapelle, 1975). A similar patient was described by Kiec-Swierczynska et al. (2000). Severe recall dermatitis of the penis was seen in a thiuram-sensitive patient after Antabuse treatment. He had been sensitized by the use of a rubber condom (Fisher, 1989). Antabuse also induces a systemic contact reaction by an entirely different mechanism. As Antabuse and its metabolites are strong metal-chelating substances, they can cause systemic contact reactions in nickel and cobalt-sensitive patients via a pharmacological interaction in a dose-dependent manner (Kaaber et al., 1979; Kaaber et al., 1983; Veien, 1987; Klein and Fowler, 1992).

Experimental oral challenge with 1 mg nickel before and during disulfiram treatment of a nickel-allergic patient showed greatly increased urinary nickel excretion during disulfiram treatment. A corresponding flare-up of dermatitis was seen (Hindsén et al., 1995).

The antitumor antibiotic mitomycin C is used for the treatment of superficial bladder cancer. Colver et al. (1990) demonstrated delayed-type hypersensitivity in 13 of 26 patients who had received mitomycin installations by applying the allergen as a patch test (Colver et al., 1990). De Groot and Conemans (1991) reported six cases where intravesical administration of the drug resulted in a systemic contact dermatitis reaction including vesicular eczema of the hands and feet and/or dermatitis of the buttocks and genital area. A more widespread rash was eventually seen.

Calkin and Maibach (1993) reviewed delayed hypersensitivity to drugs and mentioned several patients who had positive patch tests to drugs and reactions to oral challenge with the same substances.

Other medications associated with systemic contact dermatitis are listed in Table 15.3.

15.5 NICKEL

Contact sensitivity to nickel is common, particularly among young females (Nielsen and Menné, 1992). Nickel-sensitive individuals seem to run an increased risk of developing hand eczema, particularly of the vesicular type (Wilkinson and Wilkinson, 1989). Christensen and Möller (1975) showed that oral intake of nickel induces a systemic contact dermatitis reaction in nickel sensitive individuals. This observation led to intense research in the area of nickel dermatitis and systemic contact dermatitis (Menné and Maibach, 1991; Fowler, 1990).

Daily nickel intake varies from 100 to 800 μg (Biego et al., 1998). The highest nickel content is found in vegetables, nuts, whole wheat or rye bread, shellfish, and cocoa. Nickel exposure from drinking water, air pollution and cigarettes is usually negligible, although exceptions occur (Grandjean et al., 1989).

Certain makes of electric kettles and coffee machines and some glazed tea mugs may release significant amounts of nickel (Berg et al., 2000; Ajmal et al., 1997). Stainless steel cooking utensils contribute little to total nickel intake (Flint, 1995). Intravenous fluids may be contaminated with 100–200 μg nickel per liter (Sunderman, 1983).

Only 1–10 percent of ingested nickel is absorbed. Nickel absorption varies greatly. Ingestion of 12 μg Ni/kg 1 h prior to eating a 1400 kJ portion of scrambled eggs gave a 13-fold higher serum concentration of nickel compared with the simultaneous ingestion of nickel and scrambled eggs (Nielsen et al., 1999). Both fecal nickel excretion and urinary nickel excretion can be used as parameters of systemic nickel exposure. The nickel concentration in sweat is high, ranging from seven to 270 μg nickel per liter (Grandjean et al., 1989; Hohnadel et al., 1973; Christensen et al., 1979).

Christensen and Möller (1975) challenged 12 nickel-sensitive female patients with an oral dose of 5.6 mg nickel given as nickel sulfate. Nine of the patients

TABLE 15.3:

Medicaments that have caused systemic contact dermatitis *

Acetylsalicylic acid (Hindson, 1977)
Aminophylline
5-aminosalicylic acid (Gallo and Parodi, 2002)
Amlexanox (Hayakawa, et al., 1992)
Ampicillin
Antihistamines
Butylated hydroxy anisole (BHA), butylated hydroxy toluene (BHT)
Cinchocaine (Erdmann et al., 2001)
Clobazam (Machet, et al., 1992)
Codeine (De Groot and Conemans, 1986)
Corticosteroids
Diclofenac (Alonso et al., 2000)
Dimethyl sulfoxide (Nishimura et al., 1988)
Ephedrine (Audicana et al., 1991)
Epsilon-aminocaproic acid (Villarreal, 1999)
Erythromycin (Redondo, 1994)
Estradiol (Gonçalo, et al., 1999)
Gentamycin
Hydromorphone (de Cuyper and Goeteyn, 1992)
Hydroxyquinoline (Ekelund and Möller, 1969)
Immunoglobulins (Barbaud et al., 1999)
8-methoxypsoralen (Ravenscroft, et al., 2001)
Mitomycin C
Neomycin (Menné and Weismann, 1984)
Norfloxacin (Silvestre et al., 1998)
Nystatin (Lechner et al., 1987; Copper et al., 1999)
Panthothenic acid (Hemmer et al., 1997)
Parabens (Kleinhans and Knoth, 1979)
Penicillin
Phenobarbitol (Pigatto et al., 1987)
Pristinamycine
Pseudoephedrine (Tomb et al., 1991; Sánchez et al., 2000)
Pyrazinobutanzone (Bris et al., 1992)
Resorcinol (Barbaud et al., 2001)
Streptomycin
Sulfonamides
Tetraaethylthiuram disulfide (Antabuse®)
Vitamin B_1 (Hjorth, 1958)
Vitamin C (Metz et al., 1980)

* Only references not mentioned in the text are given in the table.

developed flares of the dermatitis with crops of vesicles on the hands. The reaction appeared within 2–16 h after ingestion. This observation has been confirmed (Table 15.4), and there is a marked dose-response relationship. Only a few nickel-sensitive patients react to oral doses of less than 1.25 mg of nickel, while most react to doses of 5.6 mg. A positive challenge test includes one or more of the previously described symptoms.

TABLE 15.4:

Challenge studies in nickel-sensitive patients with an oral dose of nickel given as the sulfate

Author	Type of study	Allergen dose (elementary nickel)	Duration of dosing	Response frequency
Christensen and Möller (1975)	Double blind	5.6 mg	Single exposure	9/12
Kaaber et al. (1978)	Double blind	2.5 mg	Single exposure	17/28
Kaaber et al. (1979)	Double blind	0.6 mg	Single exposure	1/11
		1.2 mg	Single exposure	1/11
		2.5 mg	Single exposure	9/11
Veien et al. (1979)	Open	4.0 mg	Single exposure	4/7
Jordan and King (1979)	Double blind	0.5 mg	Two repeated days	1/10
Cronin et al. (1980)	Open	0.6 mg	Single exposure	1/5
		1.25 mg	Single exposure	4/5
		2.50 mg	Single exposure	5/5
Burrows et al. (1981)	Double blind	2.0 mg	Two repeated days	9/22
		4.0 mg	Two repeated days	8/22
Goitre et al. (1981)	Open	4.4 mg	Single exposure	2/2
Percegueiro and Brandao (1982)	Single blind	2.8 mg 5.6 mg	Repeated dose	34/43
Sertoli et al. (1985)	Open	2.2 mg	Single exposure	13/20
Gawkrodger et al. (1986)	Double blind	0.4 mg	Two repeated days	5/10
		2.5 mg	Two repeated days	5/10
		5.6 mg	Single dose	6/6
Veien et al. (1987)	Double blind	2.5 mg	Single exposure	55/131
Santucci et al. (1988)	Open	2.2 mg	Single exposure	18/25
Hindsén (2001)	Double blind	1.0 mg		2/10
		3.0 mg		9/9

The flares seen at former nickel patch-test sites are also dose-dependent and are correlated to the intensity of the previous patch test reaction and to the length of time since patch testing (Hindsén et al., 2001).

Hindsén et al. (1994) suggested that atopics absorb nickel more readily than non-atopics and that systemic nickel dermatitis should be looked for in atopics with nickel allergy.

There was rapid elimination of nickel in the urine after i.m. injection of nickel in hamsters, while elimination after cutaneous application of nickel was slow. Keratinocytes retained nickel much longer than did fibroblasts (Lacy et al., 1996).

The clinical implication of these findings is uncertain (Burrows, 1992; Möller, 1993). The nickel doses used in the challenge studies often exceed the amount

CHAPTER 15

of nickel in a normal daily diet. In experimental studies, we have often observed flare-up reactions at sites of previously positive nickel patch tests. This phenomenon has not been observed in clinical practice. After oral challenge with 0.6–5.6 mg nickel typically given as nickel sulfate, a non-physiologically high concentration of urinary nickel was observed on the days following the challenge (20–200 µg nickel/L). In two studies (Menné and Thorboe, 1976; De Yongh *et al.*, 1978) involving a small number of patients, higher nickel excretion in the urine tended to be related to active hand dermatitis, but the urinary nickel levels were much lower than the concentrations measured on the days following oral nickel challenge.

These observations do not exclude the possibility that systemic exposure to nickel is important for the chronicity of hand eczema related to nickel sensitivity. Undoubtedly, the daily nickel intake will sometimes exceed 0.6 mg, and two of five patients reacted to this dose in a study carried out by Cronin *et al.* (1980). A rather unpleasant diet with a high nickel content has been shown to increase the activity of chronic nickel dermatitis (Nielsen *et al.*, 1990). A diet with low nickel content may diminish the activity of hand eczema in some nickel-sensitive patients (Veien *et al.*, 1993b), and a flare of hand eczema has been seen in patients who abandoned such a diet (Veien *et al.*, 1985a).

Dietary intervention controlled the dermatitis of 44 of 112 nickel-sensitive patients and all except one patient who responded to the diet reacted to a placebo-controlled oral challenge with 2.23–4.47 mg nickel. The clinical manifestations were pruritic dermatoses, atopic dermatitis and urticaria (Antico and Soana, 1999).

The inhalation of nickel while working in an electroplating plant caused a nickel-sensitive man to develop a widespread rash that cleared after disulfiram treatment and a low-nickel diet (Candura *et al.*, 2001).

A nickel-sensitive woman who took two ampoules of Oligosol® per day or the equivalent of a daily intake of 145.2 µg nickel per day had generalized dermatitis that cleared when Oligosol® was discontinued (el Sayed *et al.*, 1996). A study by Christensen *et al.* (1999) showed that Danish nickel-sensitive patients had lower serum nickel than controls. This appeared to be because the diet of the former had a lower nickel content.

If nickel is given intravenously to nickel-sensitive patients, 1–3 µg can elicit a severe systemic contact dermatitis reaction. This has been observed in patients treated with intravenous infusions through cannulas that released traces of nickel and in patients treated with hemodialysis (Stoddard, 1960; Smeenk and Teunissen, 1977; Olerud *et al.*, 1984). This difference between oral and intravenous challenge doses indicates that very small variations in the amount of nickel in the skin may cause flares of dermatitis.

Nickel binds to a variety of naturally occurring proteins and amino acids (Nieboer *et al.*, 1984). Thus, flares of dermatitis in nickel-sensitive patients may not always be caused by increased oral exposure to nickel but could be elicited by metabolic and pharmacological reactions. Interaction between nickel and zinc formed the basis for an open treatment trial in which 15 nickel-sensitive patients participated. The dermatitis of most of the patients for whom this assay was carried out improved or cleared, and their urinary nickel excretion was reduced (Santucci *et al.*, 1999).

15.6 CHROMIUM, COBALT AND OTHER METALS

Sidi and Melki (1954) suggested that oral dichromate ingestion in chromate-sensitive patients might be of importance for the chronicity of their dermatitis. This hypothesis has been tested in the studies listed in Table 15.5. Fregert (1965) challenged five chromate-sensitive patients with 0.05 mg chromium given as potassium dichromate. Within 2 h they developed severe vesiculation of the palms. One of the patients experienced acute exacerbation of generalized dermatitis. Schleiff (1968) observed flares of chromate dermatitis in 20 patients challenged with 1–10 mg potassium dichromate contained in a homeopathic drug. Some of the patients also experienced flares in previously positive dichromate patch test sites.

Kaaber and Veien (1977) studied the significance of the oral intake of dichromate by chromate-sensitive patients in a double-blind study. Thirty-one

TABLE 15.5:
Challenge studies in chromate-sensitive patients with an oral dose of chromium given as potassium dichromate

Author	Type of study	Allergen dose (given as the metal chromium)	Duration of dosing	Response frequency
Fregert (1965)	Open	0.05 mg	Single exposure	5/5
Scheiff (1968)	Open	1–10 mg	Single exposure	20/20
Kaaber and Veien (1977)	Double blind	2.5 mg	Single exposure	11/31
Goitre *et al.* (1982)	Open	7.1–14.2 mg	Repeated exposure	1/1
Veien *et al.* (1994)	Double blind	2.5 mg	Single exposure	17/30

* 11 patients with pompholyx.

patients were challenged orally with 2.5 mg chromium given as potassium dichromate and a placebo tablet. Nine of the 11 patients with vesicular hand eczema reacted with a flare of dermatitis within one or two days but did not react to the placebo. Three patients experienced vomiting, abdominal pain, and/or transient diarrhea after the chromate challenge, but not after challenge with the placebo.

A systemic contact dermatitis reaction to chromium has been seen after inhalation of welding fumes containing chromium (Shelley, 1964), after the ingestion of a homeopathic drug (van Ulsen *et al.*, 1988) and after a nutritional supplement with chromium picolate (Fowler, 2000).

Compared to chromium and nickel, cobalt is well absorbed from the gastrointestinal tract. This makes cobalt-sensitive individuals candidates for further study of the possible existence of systemic contact dermatitis caused by this metal (Veien *et al.*, 1987a). In a double-blind study, 6 of 9 patients with positive patch tests to cobalt reacted to oral challenge with 1 mg cobalt given as 4.75 mg cobalt chloride (Veien *et al.*, 1995). Most of the patients had recurrent vesicular hand dermatitis. Glendenning (1971) observed a 49-year-old housewife with persistent eczema of the palms and isolated cobalt allergy. After the removal of metal dentures made of a cobalt-chromium alloy (Vitallium), the dermatitis cleared. The patient had not had symptoms of stomatitis. After removal of the prosthesis, she noticed a return of her appetite, the loss of which had been a definite symptom during the entire disease period.

Flare of cobalt dermatitis has been seen as a recall phenomenon in chronic alcoholics treated with tetraethylthiuram disulfide (Menné, 1985).

Systemically aggravated contact dermatitis has been caused by aluminum in toothpaste in children who have been sensitized to aluminium in vaccines (Veien *et al.*, 1993a).

There have been several reports of widespread exanthema or multiforme-like erythema in patients with positive patch tests to mercury compounds (Nakayama *et al.*, 1984). Vena *et al.* (1994) described nine such patients, seven of whom also had systemic symptoms such as malaise, pyrexia and leukocytosis. The sensitization was induced by an antiparasitic powder that was thought to cause systemic contact dermatitis after inhalation. Mercury in homeopathic medicine caused baboon syndrome in a 5-year-old girl (Audicana *et al.*, 2001). Another route of systemic exposure is via dental treatment following the drilling of amalgam fillings. Following such treatment, a widespread maculopapular rash was seen in one mercury-sensitive patient (Aberer, 1993), two patients developed nummular dermatitis (Adachi *et al.*, 2000), while another had flexural dermatitis (White and Smith, 1984) and one also had a flare of dermatitis at the site of a 4-week-old patch test to mercury (Veien, 1990). Flexural dermatitis is another manifestation of systemic dermatitis in mercury-sensitive patients. A baboon-like syndrome has also been seen (Pambor and Timmel, 1989; Faria and de Freitas, 1992; Zimmer *et al.*, 1997).

A careful study of the concentration of mercury in saliva, feces, blood, plasma and urine showed increased levels of mercury in saliva, blood and feces during the first week after the removal of amalgam fillings. After removal of all the amalgam fillings, plasma Hg concentrations fell to 40 percent of the pre-treatment level (Ekstrand *et al.*, 1998).

Systemic contact dermatitis from implanted metals are rare with the currently employed technology within orthopedic surgery.

Case reports indicate that systemic contact dermatitis may still occur in a sensitized patient after the insertion of a metal prosthesis. Giménez-Arnau *et al.* (2000) reported widespread dermatitis in a nickel- and cobalt-sensitive woman whose aortic aneurism was repaired with a stent containing nickel and titanium.

A nickel-sensitive man developed vesicular hand dermatitis after his ankle fracture was repaired with plates containing 14 percent nickel. The dermatitis improved after the plate was removed (Kanerva and Förström, 2001).

Orthodontic appliances have been seen to cause urticaria and dermatitis in nickel-sensitive persons (de Silva and Doherty, 2000; Kerosuo and Kanerva, 1997; Fernández-Redondo *et al.*, 1998). In some nickel-sensitive patients the diagnosis has required oral challenge with the metals nickel, cobalt and chromium (Veien *et al.*, 1994).

Gold has become a common contact allergen in several centers. Möller *et al.* (1996) challenged 20 gold-sensitive patients with sodium thiomalate or placebo. One of 10 who received the active compound experienced flare-up of a previous contact dermatitis site. All 10 patients experienced a flare-up of their previous gold patch test sites, and several patients had toxicoderma-like symptoms. In a later study, Möller *et al.* (1999b) saw a flare-up of previously positive gold patch test sites and transient fever in five of five gold-sensitive patients. Russell *et al.* (1997) reported three patients who developed lichenoid dermatitis after drinking liquor containing gold.

15.7 OTHER CONTACT ALLERGENS

Kligman (1958a) attempted to hyposensitize persons with *Rhus* dermatitis by giving increasing amounts of the allergen in oral doses. Half of the moderately

CHAPTER 15

to severely sensitive patients experienced either pruritus or a rash; 10 percent of the patients experienced flares of their dermatitis at sites of previously healed contact dermatitis. Flares of vesicular hand eczema and erythema multiforme were rare. Pruritus ani occurred in 10 percent of the highly sensitive individuals. Severe systemic contact dermatitis was described in *Rhus*-sensitive patients who had eaten cashew nuts (Ratner *et al.*, 1974). The allergen in cashew nut shells cross-reacts with the poison ivy allergen, which explains the reactions (Kligman, 1958b).

Sporadic cases of cashew nut dermatitis caused by the presence of shell fragments among edible nuts have been described. A case of perianal dermatitis occurred after the ingestion of cashew nut butter (Rosen and Fordice, 1994). A baboon-like eruption occurred 36 h after the ingestion of a pesto sauce containing cashew nuts (Hamilton and Zug, 1998).

The lacquer tree contains antigens related to those found in poison ivy and cashew nuts. Thirty-one patients with systemic contact dermatitis were seen following the ingestion of lacquer. A widespread erythematous, maculopapular eruption was the most common clinical symptom. Some patients experienced abdominal pain, nausea, vomiting and chills (Park *et al.*, 2000).

Systemic contact dermatitis has been seen in patients sensitive to balsam of Peru which contains naturally occurring flavors. The perfume mixture may be a better indicator of sensitivity to spices than balsam of Peru (van der Akker *et al.*, 1990). Hjorth (1965) observed systemic contact dermatitis in balsam of Peru-sensitive patients who had eaten flavored icecream and orange marmalade. Veien *et al.* (1985b) challenged 17 patients sensitive to balsam of Peru with an oral dose of 1 g of balsam of Peru. Ten patients reacted to balsam of Peru and one to a placebo.

Hausen (2001a) reviewed 102 patients sensitive to balsam of Peru. Ninety-three reacted to one or more of 19 constituents. Eight who had reactions to coniferyl benzoate and benzyl alchohol had systemic contact dermatitis. Three of these patients had hand eczema and three had widespread dermatitis.

Based on questionnaires mailed to the patients 1–2 years after the initiation of diet treatment Veien *et al.* (1996a) reviewed 46 balsam-sensitive patients who had been asked to reduce their dietary intake of balsams. Sixteen of 22 (73 percent) who had reacted to 1 g balsam of Peru in a placebo-controlled oral challenge had benefit from a low-balsam diet compared to 3 of 10 (30 percent) who had shown no reaction to the oral challenge. Nine of 14 (64 percent) who were placed on a low-balsam diet, but who were not challenged orally, benefited from a low-balsam diet.

Salam and Fowler (2001) studied 71 perfume and/or balsam-sensitive patients retrospectively. The dermatitis of 21 of 45 patients who followed a low-balsam diet improved or cleared. The most common sites of dermatitis were the hands, face and anogenital region. The most commonly implicated foods were tomato, citrus and spices.

Niinimäki (1995) challenged 22 patients orally with balsam of Peru in a placebo-controlled study. Eight patients reacted to balsam of Peru but not to the placebo, while four reacted to both balsam of Peru and the placebo or only to the placebo. Aggravation of vesicular hand eczema was the most common clinical response. Similarly, Niinimäki (1984) challenged 71 patients sensitive to balsam of Peru with spices. Seven had positive reactions to the challenge. Most had vesicular hand eczema.

A 56-year-old woman had dermatitis on the fingers of both hands, and patch testing showed a + reaction to balsam of Peru and a +++ reaction to coniferyl benzoate. Her hand eczema cleared after she stopped smoking and drinking 3 L of Coca-Cola® per day (Hausen, 2001b).

The dermatitis of two balsam of Peru-patients cleared after a reduction in the intake of plant extracts (le Sellin, 1998).

A patient sensitive to balsam of Peru and to rosin experienced a flare of hand eczema and widespread dermatitis after dental work involving the filling of a root canal with rosin (Bruze, 1994).

Dooms-Goossens *et al.* (1990) described systemic contact dermatitis caused by the ingestion of spices in a patient with a positive patch test to nutmeg and in two patients sensitive to plants of the composita family after the ingestion of laurel. Sesquiterpene lactones found in compositae caused systemic contact dermatitis in a patient following the ingestion of lettuce (Oliwiecki *et al.*, 1991).

Goldenrod in an oral medication (Urodyn®) caused systemic contact dermatitis in a 52-year-old man (Schätzle *et al.*, 1998).

German chamomile tea caused a widespread eruption and anal pruritus in a 26-year-old woman who was sensitive to sesquiterpene lactone (Rodríguez-Serna *et al.*, 1998).

Inhalation of the allergen costus resinoid caused a baboon-like eruption in a sesquiterpene lactone-sensitive woman (le Coz and Lepoittevin, 2001).

A 45-year-old man developed widespread dermatitis after the ingestion of tea tree oil to which he had previously had a positive patch test (De Groot and Weyland, 1992).

Kava extract caused systemic contact dermatitis in one patient (Suus and Lehmann, 1996).

Garlic has been shown to cause systemic contact dermatitis with vesicular hand eczema as the clinical manifestation. The dermatitis could be reproduced by placebo-controlled oral challenge (Burden *et al.*, 1994). Ingestion of garlic has also caused systemic contact dermatitis in the elbow flexures and periorbitally (Pereira *et al.*, 2002).

Cutaneous reactions following the ingestion of alcoholic beverages were reviewed by Ophaswongse and Maibach (1994). Both immediate-type and delayed-type hypersensitivity reactions causing systemic contact dermatitis were described. One patient became sensitized to ethanol in an estrogen transcutaneous delivery system. She developed widespread exanthema after the ingestion of alcoholic beverages (Grebe *et al.*, 1993).

The antioxidant butylated hydroxyanisole, which is used both in cosmetics and in foods, can cause systemic contact dermatitis (Roed-Petersen and Hjorth, 1976), as can substances as diverse as formaldehyde (Bahmer and Koch, 1994) and ethyl ethoxymethylene cyanoacetate (Hsu *et al.*, 1992).

Preservatives such as sorbic acid have caused systemic contact dermatitis presenting clinically as hand eczema (Raison-Peyron *et al.*, 2000; Dejobert *et al.*, 2001).

Parabens have been suspected as the cause of systemic contact dermatitis. However, only two of 14 paraben-sensitive patients experienced flares of their dermatitis after placebo-controlled oral challenge with 200 mg methyl and propyl parahydroxybenzoate. Both patients who reacted to the challenge had vesicular hand eczema (Veien *et al.* 1996b).

15.8 RISK ASSESSMENT-ORIENTED STUDIES

While the risk of systemic contact dermatitis from drugs can be assessed, it is more difficult to carry out similar studies on ubiquitous contact allergens such as metals and naturally occurring flavors. In spite of intensive research on the significance of orally ingested nickel in nickel-sensitive individuals, we are unable to give firm advice concerning the oral dose that would represent a hazard for the wide range of nickel-sensitive individuals. Many variables, such as the route of administration, bioavailability, individual sensitivity to nickel, interaction with naturally occurring amino acids and interaction with drugs must be considered. A number of as yet unknown factors could influence nickel metabolism. Furthermore, immunological reactivity to nickel can change with time and can be influenced by sex hormones and the development of tolerance.

It is important to recognize that this area of research is extremely complex and that much well-controlled research is still needed.

With regard to medicaments, it is possible to perform well-controlled oral challenge studies in sensitized individuals. The beta-adrenergic blocking agent alprenolol is a potent contact sensitizer. Ekenvall and Forsbeck (1978) identified 14 workers employed in the pharmaceutical industry who were contact-sensitized to this compound. Oral challenge with a therapeutic dose (100 mg) led to a flare in one worker, who experienced pruritus and widespread dermatitis.

Merthiolate is a preservative widely used in sera and vaccines. Förström *et al.* (1980) investigated 45 merthiolate contact-sensitive persons to evaluate the risk of a single therapeutic dose of 0.5 ml of a 0.01 percent merthiolate solution given subcutaneously. Only one of the 45 patients developed a systemic contact dermatitis reaction. Aberer (1991) did not observe any reactions in a similar study involving 12 patients.

Maibach (1987) studied a group of patients who had discontinued the use of transdermal clonidine because of dermatitis. Of 52 patients with positive patch tests to clonidine, 29 were challenged orally with a therapeutic dose of the substance. Only one patient reacted with a flare-up at the site of the original dermatitis.

Propylene glycol is used as a vehicle in topical medications and cosmetics and as a food additive. Propylene glycol is both a sensitizer and a primary irritant. Hannuksela and Förström (1978) challenged 10 contact-sensitized individuals with two to 15 ml propylene glycol. Eight reacted with exanthema 3–16 h after the ingestion.

15.9 DIAGNOSIS

Systemic contact dermatitis can occur in patients who are contact sensitized to haptens if these patients are then exposed systemically to the same hapten. The number of persons who will actually react to a systemic exposure depends on the dose administered and for nickel to the strength of the patch test reaction and the time elapsed since patch testing (Hindsén, 2001). According to the available literature, particularly from experimental nickel challenge studies and challenge studies with medicaments, the dose needed to produce such systemic contact dermatitis reactions is relatively large. The number of patients with systemic contact dermatitis seen in clinical practice is low compared to the number of patients with allergic and irritant contact dermatitis (Veien *et al.*, 1987b). In spite of the fact that systemic contact dermatitis is relatively rare, it

■ CHAPTER 15 ■

is important to identify this type of reaction to provide optimal management of the individual patient. The diagnosis rests upon patch testing and oral challenge studies. Severe reactions are exceptional. To our knowledge severe or lethal anaphylactic reactions have not occurred after accidental or experimental oral challenge of patients with allergic contact dermatitis.

REFERENCES

ABERER, W. (1991) Vaccinations despite thiomersal sensitivity. *Contact Dermatitis* **24**, 6–10.

ABERER, W. (1993) Amalgam-Füllungen bei Amalgam-Allergie. *Dermatosen* **41**, 188–190.

ADACHI, A., HORIKAWA, T., TAKASHIMA, T., et al. (2000) Mercury-induced nummular dermatitis. *J. Am. Acad. Dermatol.* **43**, 383–385.

AJMAL, M., KHAN, A., NOMANI, A.A., et al. (1997) Heavy metals: leaching from glazed surfaces of tea mugs. *Sci. Total Environ.* **207**, 49–54.

ALONSO, R., ENRIQUE, E. and CISTERÓ, A. (2000) Positive patch test to diclofenac in Stevens-Johnson syndrome. *Contact Dermatitis* **42**, 367.

ANDERSEN, K.E., HJORTH, N. and MENNÉ, T. (1984) The baboon syndrome: Systemically induced allergic contact dermatitis. *Contact Dermatitis* **10**, 97–101.

ANGELINI, G. and MENEGHINI, C.L. (1981) Oral tests in contact allergy to para-amino compounds. *Contact Dermatitis* **7**, 311–314.

ANGELINI, G., VENA, G.A., AND MENEGHINI, C.L. (1982) Allergia da contatto e reazioni secondrie ad additivi alimentari. *G. It. Derm. Venereol.* **117**, 195–198.

ANTICO, A. and SOANA, R. (1999) Chronic allergic-like dermatopathies in nickel-sensitive patients. Results of dietary restrictions and challenge with nickel salts. *Allergy and Asthma Proc.* **20**, 235–242.

AUDICANA, M., URRUTIA, I., ECHECHIPIA, S., MUNOZ, D. and FERNANDEZ DE CORRES, L. (1991) Sensitization to ephedrine in oral anticatarrhal drugs. *Contact Dermatitis* **24**, 223–239.

AUDICANA M., BERNEDO, N., GONZALEZ, I., MUNOZ, D., FERNANDEZ, E. and GASTAMINZA, G. (2001) An unusual case of baboon syndrome due to mercury present in a homeopathic medicine. *Contact Dermatitis* **45**, 185.

BAGOT, M., TERKI, N. and BACHA, S. (1999) Désensibilisation *per os* dans l'eczéma de contact au nickel: étude clinico-biologique en double insu contre placebo. *Ann. Dermatol. Venereol.* **26**, 502–504.

BAHMER, F.A. and KOCH, P. (1994) Formaldehyd-induzierte Erythema multiforme-artige Reaktion bei einen Sektionsgehilfen. *Dermatosen* **42**, 71–73.

BARBAUD, A., TRECHOT, P., GRANEL, F., *et al.* (1999) A baboon syndrome induced by intravenous human immunoglobulin. A report of a case and immunological analysis. *Dermatology* **199**, 258–260.

BARBAUD, A., REICHERT-PENETRAT, S., TRECHOT, P., *et al.* (2001) Sensitization to resorcinol in a prescription verrucide preparation. . . . unusual systemic clinical features and prevalence. *Ann. Dermatol. Venereol.* **128**, 615–618.

BERG, T., PETERSEN, A., ALSIN, G., *et al.* (2000) The release of nickel and other trace elements from electric kettles and coffee machines. *Food Additives and Contaminants* **17**, 189–196.

BERNARD, P., FAYOL, J. and BONNAFOUX, A. (1988) Toxidermies apres prise orale de pristinamycine. *Ann. Dermatol. Venereol.* 115, 63–66.

BIEGO, G.H., JOYEUX, M., HARTEMANN, P., *et al.* (1998) Daily intake of essential minerals and metallic micropollutants from foods in France. *Sci. Total Environ.* **217**, 27–36.

BRIS, J.M.D., MONTANES, M.A., CANDELA and M.S., DIEZ, A.G. (1992) Contact sensitivity to pyrazinobutazone (Carudol^R) with positive oral provocation test. *Contact Dermatitis* **26**, 355–356.

BRUZE, M. (1994) Systemically induced contact dermatitis from dental rosin. *Scand. J. Dent. Res.* **102**, 376–378.

BURDEN, A.D., WILKINSON, S.M., BECK, M.H., and CHALMERS, R.J.G. (1994) Garlic-induced systemic contact dermatitis. *Contact Dermatitis* 30, 299–325.

BURROWS, D., CRESWELL, S. and MERRET, J.D. (1981) Nickel, hands and hip prostheses. *Br. J. Dermatol.* **105**, 437–444.

BURROWS, D. (1992) Is systemic nickel important? *J. Am. Acad. Dermatol.* **26**, 632–635.

CALKIN, J.M. and MAIBACH, H.I. (1993) Delayed hypersensitivity drug reactions diagnosed by patch testing. *Contact Dermatitis* **29**, 223–233.

CALNAN, C.D. (1956) Nickel dermatitis. *Br. J. Derm.* **68**, 229–236.

CANDURA, S.M., LOCATELLI, C., BUTERA, R., MANZO, L., GATTI, A. and FASOLA, D. (2001) Widespread nickel dermatitis from inhalation. *Contact Dermatitis* **45**, 174–175.

CHRISTENSEN, J.M., KRISTIANSEN, J., NIELSEN, N.H., *et al.* (1999) Nickel concentrations in serum and urine of patients with nickel eczema. *Toxicology Letters* **108**, 185–189.

■ CHAPTER 15 ■

CHRISTENSEN, O.B. and MÖLLER, H. (1975) External and internal exposure to the antigen in the hand eczema of nickel allergy. *Contact Dermatitis* 1, 136–141.

CHRISTENSEN, O.B., MÖLLER, H., ANDRATHO, L., and LAGESSON, V. (1979) Nickel concentration of blood, urine and sweat after oral administration. *Contact Dermatitis* 5, 312–316.

CHRISTENSEN, O.B., LINDSTRÖM, G.C., LÖFBERG, H., and MÖLLER, H. (1981) Micromorphology and specificity of orally induced flare-up reactions in nickel-sensitive patients. *Acta Dermato-Venereol. (Stockh.)* 61, 505–510.

COLVER, G.B., INGLIS, J.A., McVITTIE, E. *et al.* (1990) Dermatitis due to intra-vesical mitomycin C: A delayed-type hypersensitivity reaction? *Br. J. Dermatol.* 122, 217–224.

COOPER, S.M., REED, J. and SHAW, S. (1999) Systemic reaction to nystatin. *Contact Dermatitis* 41, 345–346.

CRONIN, E. (1980) Reactions to the systemic absorption of contact allergens. In CRONIN, E. (ed.) *Contact Dermatitis*, London: Churchill Livingstone, 26–29.

CRONIN, E., DI MICHIEL, A.D. and BROWN, S.S. (1980) Oral challenge in nickel-sensitive women with hand eczema. In BROWN, S. and SUNDERMAN, F.W. JR. (eds) *Nickel Toxicology*, New York: Academic Press, 149–155.

DE CUYPER, C. and GOETEYN, M. (1992) Systemic contact dermatitis from subcutaneous hydromorphone. *Contact Dermatitis* 27, 220–223.

DE GROOT, A.C. and CONEMANS, J. (1986) Allergic urticarial rash from oral codeine. *Contact Dermatitis* 14, 209–214.

DE GROOT, A.C. and CONEMANS, J.M.H. (1991) Systemic allergic contact dermatitis from intravesical installation of the antitumor antibiotic mitomycin C. *Contact Dermatitis* 24, 201–209.

DE GROOT, A.C. and WEYLAND, J.W. (1992) Systemic contact dermatitis from tea tree oil. *Contact Dermatitis* 27, 279–280.

DE SILVA B.D. and DOHERTY, V.R. (2000) Nickel allergy from orthodontic appliances. *Contact Dermatitis* 42, 102–103.

DE YONGH, G.F., SPRUIT, D., BONGAARDS, P.J.M. *et al.* (1978) Factors influencing nickel dermatitis I. *Contact Dermatitis* 4, 142–148.

DEJOBERT Y., DELAPORTE, E., PIETTE, F. and THOMAS, P. (2001) Vesicular eczema and systemic contact dermatitis from sorbic acid. *Contact Dermatitis* 45, 291.

DI GIOACCHINO, M., BOSCOLO, P., CAVALLUCCI, E., *et al.* (2000) Lymphocyte subset changes in blood and gastrointestinal mucosa after oral nickel challenge in nickel-sensitized women. *Contact Dermatitis* 43, 206–211.

DOOMS-GOOSSENS, A., DUBELLOY, R. and DEGREEF, H. (1990) Contact and systemic contact-type dermatitis to spices. *Dermatologic Clinics* **8**, 89–93.

EKELUND, A-G. and MÖLLER, H. (1969) Oral provocation in eczematous contact allergy to neomycin and hydroxyquinolines. *Acta Dermato-Venereol. (Stockh.)* **49**, 422–426.

EKENVALL, L., FORSBECK, M. (1978) Contact eczema produced by a beta-adrenergic blocking agent (alprenolol). *Contact Dermatitis* **4**, 190–194.

EKSTRAND, J., BJÖRKMAN, L, EDLUND, C., and SANDBORG-ENGLUND, G. (1998) Toxicological aspects on the release and systemic uptake of mercury from dental amalgam. *Eur. J. Oral Sci.* **106**, 678–686.

EL SAYED, R., GARIGUE, J., SANS, B., *et al.* (1996) Generalized eczema elicited by trace elements in a nickel-sensitized patient. *Contact Dermatitis* **35**, 123–124.

ERDMANN, S.M., SACHS, B. and MERK, H.F. (2001) Systemic contact dermatitis from cinchocaine. *Contact Dermatitis* **44**, 260–261.

FARIA, A. and DE FREITAS, C. (1992) Systemic contact dermatitis due to mercury. *Contact Dermatitis* **27**, 110–132.

FERNÁNDEZ-REDONDO, V., GOMEZ-CENTENO, P. and TORIBIO, J. (1998) Chronic urticaria from a dental bridge. *Contact Dermatitis* **38**, 178–179.

FISHER, A.A. (1976) Antihistamine dermatitis. *Cutis* **18**, 329–336.

FISHER, A.A. (1986) Systemic contact-type dermatitis. In FISHER, A.A. (ed.) *Contact Dermatitis*, Philadelphia: Lea and Febiger, 119–131.

FISHER, A.A. (1989) Unusual condom dermatitis. *Cutis* **44**, 365–366.

FOWLER, J.F. (1990) Allergic contact dermatitis to metals. *Am. J. Contact Dermatitis* **1**, 212–223.

FOWLER, J.F., Jr. (2000) Systemic contact dermatitis caused by oral chromium picolinate. *Cutis* **65**, 116.

FLINT, G.N. and PACKIRISAMY, S. (1995) Systemic nickel: the contribution made by stainless-steel cooking utensils. *Contact Dermatitis* **32**, 218–224.

FREGERT, S. (1965) Sensitization to hexa- and trivalent chromium. In *Phemphigus. Occupational dermatosis due to chemical sensitization*, pp. 50–55. Budapest: Hungarian Dermatological Society.

FÖRSTRÖM, L., HANNUKSELA, M., KOUSA, M. and LEHMUSKALLIO, E. (1980) Merthiolate hypersensitivity and vaccines. *Contact Dermatitis* **6**, 241–245.

GALLO, R. and PARODI, A. (2002) Baboon syndrome from 5-aminosalicylic acid. *Contact Dermatitis* **46**, 110.

CHAPTER 15

GAWKRODGER, D.J., COOK, S.W., FELL, G.S., *et al.* (1986) Nickel dermatitis: the reaction to oral nickel challenge. *Br. J. Dermatol.* **115**, 33–38.

GHADIALLY, R. and RAMSAY, C.A. (1988) Gentamicin: Systemic exposure to a contact allergen. *J. Am. Acad. Dermatol.* **19**, 428–430.

GIMÉNEZ-ARNAU, A., RIAMBAU, V., SERRA-BALDRICH, E. and CAMARASA, J.G. (2000) Metal-induced generalized pruriginous dermatitis and endovascular surgery. *Contact Dermatitis* **43**, 35–40.

GLENDENNING, E.W. (1971) Allergy to cobalt in metal dentures as cause of hand dermatitis. *Contact Dermatitis Newsletter* **10**, 225–226.

GOITRE, M., BEDELLO, P.O. and CANE, D. (1981) Su due casi di dermatite da nickel. *G. It. Dermatol. Venereol.* **116**, 43–45.

GOITRE, M., BEDELLO, P.G. and CANE, D. (1982) Chromium dermatitis and oral administration of the metal. *Contact Dermatitis* **8**, 208–209.

GONÇALO, M., OLIVEIRA, H.S., MONTEIRO, C., *et al.* (1999) Allergic and systemic contact dermatitis from estradiol. *Contact Dermatitis* **40**, 58–59.

GOOSSENS, C., SASS, U. and SONG, M. (1997) Baboon syndrome. *Dermatology* **194**, 421–422.

GRANDJEAN, P., NIELSEN, G.D. and ANDERSEN, O. (1989) Human nickel exposure and chemobiokinetics. In MAIBACH, H.I. and MENNÉ, T. (eds) *Nickel and the skin: Immunology and toxicology,* Boca Raton, FL: CRC Press, 9–34.

GREBE, S.K.G., ADAMS, J.D. and FEEK, C.M. (1993) Systemic sensitization to ethanol by transdermal estrogen patches. *Arch. Dermatol.* **129**, 379–380.

GUIN, J.D., FIELDS, P. and THOMAS, K.L. (1999) Baboon syndrome from i.v. aminophylline in a patient allergic to ethylenediamine. *Contact Dermatitis* **40**, 170–171.

HAMILTON, T.K. and ZUG, K.A. (1998) Systemic contact dermatitis to raw cashew nuts in a pesto sauce. *Am. J. Contact Dermatitis* **9**, 51–54.

HANDA, S., SAHOO, B. and SHARMA V.K. (2001) Oral hyposensitization in patients with contact dermatitis from *Parthenium hysterophorus. Contact Dermatitis* **44**, 279–282.

HANNUKSELA, M. and FÖRSTRÖM, L. (1978) Reactions to peroral propylene glycol. *Contact Dermatitis* **4**, 41–45.

HAUSEN, B.M. (2001a) Contact allergy to balsam of Peru. II. Patch test results in 102 patients with selected balsam of Peru constituents. *Am. J. Contact Dermatitis* **12**, 93–102.

HAUSEN, B.M. (2001b) Rauchen, Süssigkeiten, Perubalsam—ein Circulus vitiosus? *Akt. Dermatol.* **27**, 136–143.

HAYAKAWA, R., OGINO, Y., ARIS, K. and MATSUNAGA, K. (1992) Systemic contact dermatitis due to amlexanox. *Contact Dermatitis* **27**, 122–123.

HEMMER, W., BRACUN, R., WOLF-ABDOLVAHAB, S., *et al.* (1997) Maintenance of hand eczema by oral pantothenic acid in a patient sensitized to dexpanthenol. *Contact Dermatitis* **37**, 51.

HINDSÉN, M., CHRISTENSEN, O.B. and MÖLLER, H. (1994) Nickel levels in serum and urine in five different groups of eczema patients following oral ingestion of nickel. *Acta Dermato-Venereol. (Stockh.)* **74**, 176–178.

HINDSÉN, M., MÖLLER, H. and BERGLUND, M. (1995) Orally provoked urinary nickel excretion during disulfiram treatment. *Am. J. Contact Dermatitis* **6**, 225–227.

HINDSÉN, M., BRUZE, M. and CHRISTENSEN, O.B. (2001) Flare-up reactions after oral challenge with nickel in relation to challenge dose and intensity and time of previous patch test reactions. *J. Am. Acad. Dermatol.* **44**, 616–623.

HINDSON, C. (1977) Contact eczema from methyl salicylate reproduced by oral aspirin/acetylsalicylic acid. *Contact Dermatitis* **3**, 348–349.

HJORTH, N. (1958) Contact dermatitis from vitamin B (thiamine). *J. Invest. Dermatol.* **30**, 261–264.

HJORTH, N. (1965) Allergy to balsams. *Spectrum Int.* **7**, 97–101.

HOHNADEL, D.C., SUNDERMAN, F.W., JR., NECKAY, M.W. and MCNEELY, M.D. (1973) Atomic absorption spectrometry of nickel, copper, zinc, and lead in sweat collected from healthy subjects during sauna bathing. *Clin. Chem.* **19**, 1288–1292.

HSU, C.-K., SUN, C.-C., SU, M-S., KUO, E.-F. and WU, Y.-C. (1992) Systemic contact allergy from occupational contact with ethyl ethoxymethylene cyanoacetate. *Contact Dermatitis* **27**, 58–59.

ISAKSSON, M. (2000) Clincial and experimental studies in corticosteroid contact allergy. (Thesis). Malmö, Sweden: Dept. of Dermatology, University Hospital.

JORDAN, W.P. and KING, S.E. (1979) Nickel feeding in nickel-sensitive patients with hand eczema. *J. Am. Acad. Dermatol.* **1**, 506–508.

KAABER, K. and VEIEN, N.K. (1977) The significance of chromate ingestion in patients allergic to chromate. *Acta Dermato-Venereol.* **57**, 321–323.

KAABER, K., VEIEN, N.K. and TJELL, J.C. (1978) Low nickel diet in the treatment of patients with chronic nickel dermatitis. *Br. J. Dermatol.* **98**, 197–201.

KAABER, K., MENNÉ, T., TJELL, J.C. and VEIENE, N. (1979) Antabuse treatment of nickel dermatitis. Chelation—a new principle in the treatment of nickel dermatitis. *Contact Dermatitis* **5**, 221–228.

KAABER, K., MENNÉ, T., VEIEN, N.K. *et al.* (1983) Treatment of nickel dermatitis with Antabuse®, a double blind study. *Contact Dermatitis* **9**, 297–299.

KANERVA, L. and FÖRSTRÖM, L. (2001) Allergic nickel and chromate hand dermatitis induced by orthopaedic metal implant. *Contact Dermatitis* **44**, 103–104.

KEROSUO, H. and KANERVA, L. (1997) Systemic contact dermatitis caused by nickel in a stainless steel orthodontic appliance. *Contact Dermatitis* **36**, 112–113.

KIEC-SWIERCZYNSKA, M., KRECISZ, B. and FABICKA, B. (2000) Systemic contact dermatitis from implanted disulfiram. *Contact Dermatitis* **43**, 246–247.

KLEIN, L.R. and FOWLER, J.F. (1992) Nickel dermatitis recall during therapy for alcohol abuse. *J. Am. Acad. Dermatol.* **26**, 645–646.

KLEINHANS, D. and KNOTH, W. (1979) Paraben Kontakt Allergie mit enteraler Provokation. *Z. Haut* **48**, 699–701.

KLIGMAN, A.M. (1958a) Hyposensitization against *Rhus* dermatitis. *Arch. Dermatol.* **78**, 47–72.

KLIGMAN, A.M. (1958b) Cashew nut shell oil for hyposensitization against *Rhus* dermatitis. *Arch. Dermatol.* **78**, 359–363.

LACHAPELLE, J.M. (1975) Allergic "contact" dermatitis from disulfiram implants. *Contact Dermatitis* **1**, 218–220.

LACY, S.A., MERRITT, K., BROWN, S.A. and PURYEAR, A. (1996) Distribution of nickel and cobalt following dermal and systemic administration with *in vitro* and *in vivo* studies. *J. Biomed. Mater. Res.* **32**, 279–283.

LAUERMA, A.I., REITAMO, S. and MAIBACH, H.I. (1991) Systemic hydrocortizone/cortisol induces allergic skin reactions in presensitized subjects. *J. Am. Acad. Dermatol.* **24**, 182–185.

LAUERMA, A.I. (1992) Contact hypersensitivity to glucocortico steroids. *Am. J. Contact Dermatol.* **3**, 112–132.

LE COZ, C.-J. and LEPOITTEVIN, J.-P. (2001) Occupational erythema-multiforme-like dermatitis from sensitization to costus resinoid, followed by flare-up and systemic contact dermatitis from β-cyclocostunolide in a chemistry student. *Contact Dermatitis* **44**, 310–311.

LE SELLIN, J. (1998) Dermatoses de contact systémiques. *Allergie et Immunologie* 30, 157–158.

LECHNER, T., GRYNTZMAN, B. and BÄURLE, G. (1987) Hämatogenes allergische Kontaktekszem nach oraler Gabe von Nystatin. *Mycosen* 30, 143–146.

LLAMAZARES, A. A. (2000) Flare-up of skin tests to amoxycillin and ampicillin. *Contact Dermatitis* 42, 166.

MACHET, L., VAILLANT, L., DARDAINE, V. and LORETTE, G. (1992) Patch testing with clobazom: Relapse of generalized drug eruption. *Contact Dermatitis* 26, 347–348.

MAIBACH, H.I. (1987) Oral substitution in patients sensitized by transdermal clonidine treatment. *Contact Dermatitis* 16, 1–9.

MARCUSSEN, P.V. (1957) Spread of nickel dermatitis. *Dermatologica*, 115, 596–607.

MENNÉ, T. and THORBOE, A. (1976) Nickel dermatitis—nickel excretion. *Contact Dermatitis* 2, 353–354.

MENNÉ, T. and WEISMANN, K. (1984) Hämatogenes Kontakteksem nach oraler Gabe von Neomycin. *Der Hautarzt* 35, 319–320.

MENNÉ, T. (1985) Flare-up of cobalt dermatitis from Antabuse® treatment. *Contact Dermatitis* 12, 53.

MENNÉ, T. and MAIBACH, H.I. (1991) Systemic contact-type dermatitis. In Marzulli, F.N. and Maibach, H.I. (eds) *Dermatotoxicology*, New York: Hemisphere, 453–472.

MENNÉ, T., VEIEN, N., SJØLIN, K.-N. *et al.* (1994) Systemic contact dermatitis. *Am. J. Contact Dermatitis* 5, 1–12.

METZ, J., HUNDERTMARK, U. and PEVNY, I. (1980) Vitamin C allergy of the delayed type. *Contact Dermatitis* 6, 172–174.

MÖLLER, H. (1993) Yes, systemic nickel is probably important! *J. Am. Acad. Dermatol.* 28, 511–512.

MÖLLER, H., BJORKNER, B. and BRUZE, M. (1996) Clinical reactions to systemic provocation with gold sodium thiomalate in patients with contact allergy to gold. *Br. J. Dermatol.* 135, 423–427.

MÖLLER, H., OHLSSON, K., LINDER, C., BJORKNER, V. and BRUZE, M. (1998) Cytokines and acute phase reactants during flare-up of contact allergy to gold. *Am. J. Contact Dermatitis* 9, 15–22.

MÖLLER, H., OHLSSON, K., LINDER, C., *et al.* (1999a) The flare-up reactions after systemic provocation in contact allergy to nickel and gold. *Contact Dermatitis* 40, 200–204.

■ CHAPTER 15 ■

MÖLLER, H., BJÖRKNER, B., BRUZE, M. *et al.*, (1999b) Laser Doppler perfusion imaging for the documentation of flare-up in contact allergy to gold. *Contact Dermatitis* **41**, 131–13.

MORI Y., SON, S., MURAKAMI, K., *et al.* (2000) Two cases of chrysanthemum dermatitis—successful oral tolerance induction using chrysanthemum juice. *Environ. Dermatol.* **7**, 223–229.

MORRIS, D.L. (1998) Intradermal testing and sublingual desensitization for nickel. *Cutis* **61**, 129–132.

MØRTZ, C.G. (1999) The prevalence of atopic dermatitis, hand eczema, allergic contact dermatitis, type IV and type I sensitisation in 8th grade school children in Odense. (Thesis). Odense, Denmark: University of Southern Denmark.

NAKAYAMA, H., NIKI, F., SHONO, M. and HADA, S. (1983) Mercury Exanthem. *Contact Dermatitis* **9**, 411–417.

NAKAYAMA, H., SHONO, M. and HADA, S. (1984) Mercury exanthem. *J. Am. Acad. Dermatol.* **11**, 137–139.

NIEBOER, E., STAFFORD, A.R., EVANS, S.L., *et al.* (1984) Cellular binding and/or uptake of nickel (II) ions. In SUNDERMAN, J.R. (ed.) *Nickel in the human environment*, Lyon: IARC Scientific Publication **53**, 321–333.

NIELSEN, G.D., JEPSEN, L.V., JØRGENSEN, P.J., GRANDJEAN, P. and BRANDRUP, F. (1990) Nickel-sensitive patients with vesicular hand eczema: oral challenge with a diet naturally high in nickel. *Br. J. Dermatol.* **122**, 299–308.

NIELSEN, G.D., SØDERBERG, U., JØRGENSEN, P.J., *et al.* (1999) Absorption and retention of nickel from drinking water in relation to food intake and nickel sensitivity. *Toxicol. Appl. Pharmacol.* **154**, 67–54.

NIELSEN, N.H. and MENNÉ, T. (1992) Allergic contact senstization in an unselected Danish population. *Acta Dermato-Venereol. (Stockh.)* **72**, 456–460.

NIELSEN, N.H., LINNEBERG, A., MENNÉ, T., MADSEN, F., FRØLUND, L., DIRKSEN, A. and JØRGENSEN, T. (2001) Allergic contact sensitization in an adult Danish population: Two cross-sectional surveys eight years apart. *Acta Dermato-Venereol. (Stockh.)* **81**, 31–34.

NIINIMÄKI, A. (1984) Delayed-type allergy to spices. *Contact Dermatitis* **11**, 34–40.

NIINIMÄKI, A. (1995) Double-blind placebo-controlled peroral challenges in patients with delayed-type allergy to balsam of Peru. *Contact Dermatitis* **33**, 78–83.

NISHIMURA, M., TAKANO, Y. and YOSHITANI, S. (1988) Systemic contact dermatitis medicamentosa occurring after intravesical dimethyl sulfoxide treatment for interstitial cystitis. *Arch. Dermatol.* **124**, 182–183.

OLERUD, J.E., LEE, M.Y., ULVELLI, D.A. *et al.* (1984) Presumptive nickel dermatitis from hemodialysis. *Arch. Dermatol.* **120**, 1066–1068.

OLIWIECKI, S., BECK, M.H. and HAUSEN, B.M. (1991) Composite dermatitis aggravated by eating lettuce. *Contact Dermatitis* **24**, 318–319.

OPHASWONGSE, S. and MAIBACH, H.I. (1994) Alcohol dermatitis: Allergic contact dermatitis and contact urticaria syndrome. A review. *Contact Dermatitis* **30**, 1–6.

PAMBOR, M. and TIMMEL, A. (1989) Mercury dermatitis. *Contact Dermatitis* **20**, 157.

PANHANS-GROSS, A., GALL, H.I. and PETER R.-U. (1999) Baboon syndrome after oral penicillin. *Contact Dermatitis* **41**, 352–353.

PANZANI, R.C., SCHIAVINO, D., NUCERA, E., PELLEGRINO, S., FAIS, G., SCHINCO, G. and PATRIARCA, G. (1995) Oral hyposensitization to nickel allergy: Preliminary clinical results. *Int. Arch. Allergy Immunol.* **107**, 251–254.

PARK, R.G. (1943) Cutaneous hypersensitivity to sulphonamides. *Br. Med. J.* **2**, 69–72.

PARK, S.D., LEE, S.-W., CHUN, J.-H. *et al.* (2000) Clinical features of 31 patients with systemic contact dermatitis due to the ingestion of *Rhus* (lacquer). *Br. J. Dermatol.* **142**, 937–942.

PERCEGUEIRO, M. and BRANDAO, M. (1982) Administracao oral de niquel en individuos sensibilizados. *Med. Cut. I.L.A.* **10**, 295–298.

PEREIRA, F., HATIA, M. and CARDOSO, J. (2002) Systemic contact dermatitis from diallyl disulfide. *Contact Dermatitis* **46**, 124.

PIGATTO, P.D., MORELLI, M., POTENGHI, M.M., MOZZANICA, N. and ALTOMARE, G.F. (1987) Phenobarbital-induced allergic dermatitis. *Contact Dermatitis* **16**, 279.

PIRILÄ, V. (1957) Dermatitis due to rubber. *Acta Dermato-Venereol. (Stockh.)* **11**, 252–255.

POLAK, L. and TURK, J.L. (1968a) Studies on the effect of systemic administration of sensitizers in guinea-pigs with contact sensitivity to inorganic metal compounds. *Clin. Exp. Immunol.* **3**, 245–251.

■ CHAPTER 15 ■

POLAK, L. and TURK, J.L. (1968b) Studies on the effects of systemic administration of sensitizers in guinea-pigs with contact sensitivity to inorganic metal compounds. *Clin. Exp. Immunol.* **3**, 253–262.

PROVOST, T.T. and JILSON, O.F. (1967) Ethylenediamine contact dermatitis. *Arch. Dermatol.* **96**, 231–234.

PRYSTOVSKY, S.D., ALLEN, A.M., SMITH, R.W., NONOMURA, J.H., ODOM, R.B. and AKERS, W.A. (1979) Allergic contact hypersensitivity to nickel, neomycin, ethylenediamine and benzocaine. *Arch. Dermatol.* **115**, 959–962.

RAISON-PEYRON, N., MEYNADIER, J.M. and MEYNADIER, J. (2000) Sorbic acid: an unusual cause of systemic contact dermatitis in an infant. *Contact Dermatitis* **43**, 247–248.

RÄSÄNEN, L. and HASAN, T. (1993) Allergy to systemic and intralesional corticosteroids. *Br. J. Dermatol.* **128**, 407–411.

RATNER, J.H., SPENCER, S.K. and GRAINGE, J.M. (1974) Cashew nut dermatitis. *Arch. Dermatol.* **110**, 921–923.

RAVENSCROFT, J., GOULDEN, V. and WILKINSON, M. (2001) Systemic allergic contact dermatitis to 8-methoxypsoralen (8-MOP). *J. Am. Acad. Dermatol.* **45**, S218–S219.

REDONDO, V.F., CASAS, L., TABOADA, M. and TORIBIO, J. (1994) Systemic contact dermatitis from erythromycin. *Contact Dermatitis* **30**, 311.

REGINELLA, R.F., FAIRFIELD, J.C. and MARKS, J.G., JR. (1989) Hyposensitization to poison ivy after working in a cashew nut shell oil processing factory. *Contact Dermatitis* **20**, 274–279.

RODRÍGUEZ-SERNA, M., SÁNCHEZ-MOTILLA, M.M., RAMÓN, R. and ALIAGA, A. (1998) Allergic and systemic contact dermatitis from *Matricaria chamomilla* tea. *Contact Dermatitis* **39**, 192–209.

ROED-PETERSEN, J. and HJORTH, N. (1976) Contact dermatitis from antioxidants. *Br. J. Dermatol.* **94**, 233–241.

ROSEN, T. and FORDICE, D.B. (1994) Cashew nut dermatitis. *South. Med. J.* **87**, 543–546.

RUSSELL, M.A., LANGLEY, M., TRUETT, A.P. *et al.* (1997) Lichenoid dermatitis after consumption of gold-containing liquor. *J. Am. Acad. Dermatol.* **36**, 841–844.

SALAM, T.N. and FOWLER, J.F. JR. (2001) Balsam-related systemic contact dermatitis. *J. Am. Acad. Dermatol.* **45**, 377–381.

SÁNCHEZ, T.S., SÁNCHEZ-PÉREZ, J., ARAGÜÉS, M. *et al.* (2000) Flare-up reaction of pseudoephedrine baboon syndrome after positive patch test. *Contact Dermatitis* 42, 312–313.

SANTUCCI, B., CRISTAUDO, A., CANNISTRACI, C. *et al.* (1988) Nickel sensitivity— Effects of prolonged oral intake of the element. *Contact Dermatitis* 19, 202–205.

SANTUCCI, B., MANNA, F., CANNISTRACI, C., CRISTAUDO, A., CAPPARELLA, R., BOLASCO and A., PICARDO, M. (1994) Serum and urine concentrations in nickel-sensitive patients after prolonged oral administration. *Contact Dermatitis* 30, 97–101.

SANTUCCI, B., CRISTAUDO, A., MEHRABAN, M., VALENZANO, C., CAMERA, E. and PICARDO, M. (1999) $ZnSO_4$ treatment of $NiSO_4$-positive patients. *Contact Dermatitis* 40, 281–281.

SCHÄTZLE, M., AGATHOS, M. and BREIT, R. (1998) Allergic contact dermatitis from goldenrod (*Herba solidaginis*) after systemic administration. *Contact Dermatitis* 39, 271–272.

SCHEPER, R.J., VON BLOMBERG, B.E.N., BOERRIGTER, *et al.* (1983) Induction of local memory in the skin. Role of local T cell retention. *Clin. Exp. Immunol.* 51, 141–151.

SCHITTENHELM, A. and STOCKINGER, W. (1925) Über die Idiosynkrasie gegen Nickel (Nickel-krätze) und ihre Beziehung zur Anaphylaxie. *Z. Gesamte Exp. Med.* 45, 58–74.

SCHLEIFF, P. (1968) Provocation des Chromatekzems zu Testswechen durch interne Chromzufur. *Hautarzt* 19, 209–210.

SERTOLI, A., LOMBARDI, P., FRANCALANCI, S., *et al.* (1985) Effetto della somministrazione orale de apteni in soggetti sensibilizzati affetti da eczema allergizo da contatto. *G. It. Dermatol. Venereol.* 120, 207–218.

SHELLEY, W. B. (1964) Chromium in welding fumes as a cause of eczematous hand eruption. *J. Am. Med. Assoc.* 189, 772–773.

SHELLEY, W.B. and CRISSEY, J.T. (1970) Thomas Bateman. In SHELLEY, W.B. and CRISSEY, J.T. (eds) *Classics in Clinical Dermatology*, Springfield IL: Charles C. Thomas, 22.

SHELLEY, W.B. and SHELLEY, E.D. (1987) Nonpigmented fixed drug eruption as a distrinctive reaction pattern: Examples caused by sensitivity to pseudoephedrine hydrochloride and tetrahydrozoline. *J. Am. Acad. Dermatol.* 17, 403–407.

SIDI, E. and DOBKEVITCH-MORRILL, S. (1951) The injection and ingestion test in cross-sensitization to the para group. *J. Invest. Dermatol.* 16, 299–310.

■ CHAPTER 15 ■

SIDI, E. and MELKI, G.R. (1954) Rapport entre dermatitis de cause externe et sensibilisation par voi interne. *Sem. Hop. Paris* **30**, 1560–1565.

SILVESTRE, J.F., ALFONSO, R., MORAGON, M., RAMON, R. and BOTELLA, R. (1998) Systemic contact dermatitis due to norfloxacin with a positive patch test to quinoline mix. *Contact Dermatitis* **39**, 83.

SJÖVALL, P., CHRISTENSEN, O.B. and MÖLLER, H. (1987) Oral hyposensitization in nickel allergy. *J. Am. Acad. Dermatol.* **17**, 774–778.

SMEENK, G. and TEUNISSEN, P.C. (1977) Allergische reacties op nikkel uit infusietoedieningssystemen. *Ned. Tijdschr. Geneeskd.* **121**, 4–9.

SRINIVAS, C.R., KRUPASHANKAR, D.S., SINGH, K.K., BALACHANDRAN, C. and SHENOI, S.D. (1988) Oral hyposensitization in *Parthenium* dermatitis. *Contact Dermatitis* **18**, 242–243.

STODDARD, J.C. (1960) Nickel sensitivity as a cause of infusious reaction. *Lancet* **ii**, 741–742.

SUNDERMAN, F.W. Jr. (1983) Potential toxicity from nickel contamination of intravenous fluids. *Ann. Clin. Lab. Sci.* **13**, 1–4.

SUSS, R. and LEHMANN, P. (1996) Hamatogenes Kontaktekzem durch pflanzliche Medikamente am Beispiel des Kavawurzel-extraktes. *Hautarzt.* **47**, 459–461.

TAGAMI, H., TETANTA, K. and IWATAKI, K. (1983) Delayed hypersensitivity in ampicillin-induced toxic epidermal necrolysis. *Arch. Dermatol.* **119**, 910–913.

TOMB, R., LEPOITTEVIN, J.P., ESPINASSONZE, F., HEID, E. and FOUSSEREAU, J. (1991) Systemic contact dermatitis from psoeudoephedrine. *Contact Dermatitis* **24**, 86–88.

TORRES, V., TAVARES-BELLO, R., MELO, H. and SOARES, A.P. (1993) Systemic contact dermatitis from hydrocortisone. *Contact Dermatitis* **29**, 106.

VAN DER AKKER, TH.W., ROESYANTO-MAHADI, I.D., VAN TOORENENBERGEN, A.W. and VAN JOOST, TH. (1990) Contact allergy to spices. *Contact Dermatitis* **22**, 267–272.

VAN ULSEN, J., STOLZ, E. and VAN JOOST, TH. (1988) Chromate dermatitis from a homeopathic drug. *Contact Dermatitis* **18**, 56–57.

VAN HOOGSTRATEN, I.M.W., ANDERSEN, K.E., VON BLOMBERG, B.M.E., BODEN, D., BRUYNZEEL, D.P., BURROWS, D., CAMARASA, J.G., DOOMS-GOOSSENS, A., KRALL, G., LAHTI, A., MENNÉ, T., RYCROFT, R.J.G., SHAW, S., TODD, D., VREEBURG, K.J.J., WILKINSON, J.D. and SCHEPER, R.J. (1991) Reduced frequency of nickel allergy upon oral nickel contact at an early age. *Clin. Exp. Immunol.* **85**, 441–445.

VAN HOOGSTRATEN, I.M.W., BODEN, D., VON BLOMBERG, M.E., KRAAL, G. and SCHEPER, R.J. (1992) Persistent immune tolerance to nickel and chromium by oral administration prior to cutaneous sensitization. *J. Invest. Dermatol.* **99**, 607–616.

VEIEN, N.K. (1987) Cutaneous side effects of Antabuse® in nickel allergic patients treated for alcoholism. *Boll. Dermato. Allergol. Prof.* **2**, 139–144.

VEIEN, N.K. (1990) Stomatitis and systemic dermatitis from mercury in amalgam dental restorations. *Dermatologic Clinics* **8**, 157–160.

VEIEN, N.K., KAABER, K. (1979) Nickel, cobalt and chromium sensitivity in patients with pompholyx (dyshidrotic eczema). *Contact Dermatitis* **5**, 371–374.

VEIEN, N.K. and MENNÉ, T. (1993) Acute and recurrent vesicular hand dermatitis (pompholyx), In MENNÉ, T. and MAIBACH, H.I. (eds) *Hand eczema*, Boca Raton, FL: CRC Press, 57–73.

VEIEN, N.K., CHRISTIANSEN, A.H., SVEJGAARD, E. and KAABER, K. (1979) Antibodies against nickel albumin in rabbits and man. *Contact Dermatitis* **5**, 378–382.

VEIEN, N.K., HATTEL, T. and JUSTESEN, O. and NØRHOLM, A. (1985a) Dietary treatment of nickel dermatitis. *Acta Dermato-Venereol.* **65**, 138–142.

VEIEN, N.K., HATTEL, T., JUSTESEN, O. and NØRHOLM, A. (1985b) Oral challenge with balsam of Peru. *Contact Dermatitis* **12**, 104–107.

VEIEN, N. K., HATTEL, T., JUSTESEN, O. and NØRHOLM, A. (1987a) Oral challenge with nickel and cobalt in patients with positive patch tests to nickel and/or cobalt. *Acta Dermato-Venereol.* **67**, 321–325.

VEIEN, N.K., HATTEL, T., JUSTENSEN, O. and NØRHOLM, A. (1987b) Diagnostic procedures for eczema patients. *Contact Dermatitis* **17**, 35–40.

VEIEN, N.K. and KROGDAHL, A. (1989) Is nickel vasculitis a clinical entity? In FROSCH, P., DOOMS-GOOSSENS, A., LACHAPELLE, J.M., RYCROFT, R.J.G. and SCHEPER, R.J. (eds) *Current Topics in Contact Dermatitis*, Heidelberg: Springer-Verlag, 172–177.

VEIEN, N.K., MENNÉ, T. and MAIBACH, H.I. (1990) Systemically induced allergic contact dermatitis. In MENNÉ, T. and MAIBACH, H.I. (eds) *Exogenous dermatosis: Environmental dermatitis*, Boca Raton, FL: CRC-Press, 267–283.

VEIEN, N.K., HATTEL, T., LAURBERG, G. (1993a) Systemically aggravated contact dermatitis caused by aluminium in tooth paste. *Contact Dermatitis* **28**, 199–200.

VEIEN, N.K., HATTEL, T., LAURBERG, G. (1993b) Low nickel diet: An open, prospective trial. *J. Am. Acad. Dermatol.* **29**, 1002–1007.

VEIEN, N.K., BORCHORST, E., HATTEL, T., LAURBERG, G. (1994) Stomatitis or systemically-induced contact dermatitis from metal wire in orthodontic materials. *Contact Dermatitis* **30**, 210–211.

■ CHAPTER 15 ■

VEIEN, N.K., HATTEL, T., LAURBERG, G. (1994) Chromate-allergic patients challenged orally with potassium dichromate. *Contact Dermatitis* **31**, 137–139.

VEIEN, N.K., HATTEL, T., LAURBERG, G. (1995) Placebo-controlled oral challenge with cobalt in patients with positive patch tests to cobalt. *Contact Dermatitis.* **33**, 54–55.

VEIEN, N.K., HATTEL, T. and LAURBERG, G. (1996a) Can oral challenge with balsam of Peru Predict possible benefit from a low-balsam diet? *Am. J. Contact Dermatitis* **7**, 84–87.

VEIEN, N.K., HATTEL, T. and LAURBERG, G. (1996b) Oral challenge with parabens in paraben-sensitive patients. *Contact Dermatitis* **34**, 433.

VENA, G. A., FOTI, C., GRANDOLFO, M. and ANGELINI, G. (1994) Mercury exanthem. *Contact Dermatitis* **31**, 214–216.

VICKERS, H.R., BAGRATUNI, L. and ALEXANDER, S. (1958) Dermatitis caused by penicillin in milk. *Lancet* **i**, 351–352.

VILLARREAL, O. (1999) Systemic dermatitis with eosinophilia due to epsilon-aminocaproic acid. *Contact Dermatitis* **40**, 114.

WHITE, I.R. and SMITH, B.G.N. (1984) Dental amalgam dermatitis. *Br. Dent. J.* **156**, 258–259.

WHITMORE, S.E. (1995) Delayed systemic allergic reactions to corticosteroids. *Contact Dermatitis* **32**, 193–198.

WILKINSON, D.S. and WILKINSON, J.D. (1989) Nickel allergy and hand eczema. In MENNÉ, T. and MAIBACH, H.I. (eds) *Nickel and the Skin: Immunology and Toxicology*, Boca Raton, FL: CRC Press, 133–165.

WILSON, H.T.H. (1958) Streptomycin dermatitis in nurses. *Br. Med. J.* **1**, 1378–1382.

YAMASHITA, N., NATSUAKI, M. and SAGAMIS, S. (1989) Flare-up reactions on murine contact hypersensitivity. I. Description of an experimental model: Rechallenge system. *Immunology* **67**, 365–369.

YSART, G., MILLER, P., CROASDALE, M. *et al.* (2000) 1997 UK total diet study—dietary exposures to aluminium, arsenic, cadmium, chromium, copper, lead, mercury, nickel, selenium, tin and zinc. *Food Additives and Contaminants* **17**, 775–786.

ZIMMER, J., GRANGE, F., STRAUB, P. *et al.* (1997) Erytheme mercuriel apres exposition accidentelle a des vapeurs de mercure. *Ann. Med. Interne Paris* **148**, 317–320.

Permeability of Human Skin to Metals and Paths for Their Diffusion

16

JURIJ J. HOSTÝNEK

Contents

16.1 Introduction

16.2 Factors affecting dermal absorption of metals

16.3 Routes for skin absorption of metals

16.4 Descriptors of skin permeability

16.5 Absorption determined through stratum corneum analysis

16.6 Summary

16.1   INTRODUCTION

Metals and their compounds are ubiquitous in the environment, on the earth's surface and underground. Those which are water soluble are constantly dissolved by atmospheric factors (precipitation, run-off) and by hydrothermal, subterranean currents; they are ultimately transported into the vast bodies of water of the seas and lakes and thus removed from significant human contact. Those which remain in the lithosphere are relatively harmless due to their low solubility and thus bioavailability. In contrast it is the anthropogenic forms of many metals which pose an increasing threat to living organisms. Generated by large-scale industrial activities, they are not only dispersed throughout the environment, but also accumulated in concentrated form in waste sites representing hazardous foci.

Exposure in industrial processing as well as emissions and waste sites thus constitute a human health risk, both in an occupational setting and in normal everyday activities among the general population. According to EPA's Toxic Release Inventory for the year 2000, metal mining accounted for 47 percent of releases to air, water and land (7.10 billion lb), and of the bioaccumulative releases, mercury and mercury compounds accounted for 36 percent of the total 12.1 million lb. Besides respiratory and gastrointestinal exposure, traditionally a prime concern in toxicology, also skin contact more recently has gained recognition as an important port of entry for xenobiotics into the living organism. Cases of morbidity and mortality due to exposure of the skin to toxic agents has contributed to such a shift in attention. Absorption of the neurotoxic cleansing agent hexachlorophene through the skin of neonates and babies in France resulted in the death due to cerebral edema of some 40 children after mothers applied an antibacterial-containing talcum on their skin, besides further dozens of hospitalized cases (Plueckhahn *et al.*, 1978); dimethylmercury, an organomercury compound with unknown skin absorption data was apparently absorbed transdermally after gloved-skin contact with milliliter amounts of the substance, resulting in the fatality of a university scientist (Smith, 1997; Toribara *et al.*, 1997).

The skin is permeable to a wide range of chemicals; it can function as a potential reservoir for their accumulation, as well as for their slow release. Over recent years skin diffusivity of organic chemical structures has proven amenable to mathematical modeling, and their bioavailability has become predictable with increasing accuracy using mathematical models to describe quantitative structure-permeability relationships (Flynn, 1990; Potts and Guy, 1992, 1995). Metal compounds, however, defy such modeling and predictability; this is especially true for strongly electropositive metals as they avidly react with electronegative constituents they encounter along the path of diffusion through the skin. A number of confounding factors come into play expressing their idiosyncrasy, which impact both rate and route of skin penetration the importance of which is not estimable with our present knowledge. What complicates the picture further is the interdependence between these multiple factors. Those which have an obvious bearing on the process of metal diffusion are listed in Table 16.1 to illustrate the variables which have to be taken into account if one were to formulate an algorithm predictive of their penetration through biological membranes for purposes of dermal exposure assessment (Table 16.1). The factors perceived as critical for skin diffusion have been divided into two groups: those proper to the metals themselves, the exogenous factors, and those inherent in the barrier tissue as part of the target organism itself, the endogenous factors. These factors are briefly presented below, illustrated with typical case observations.

16.2 FACTORS AFFECTING DERMAL ABSORPTION OF METALS

16.2.1 Exogenous factors

Dose

Review of data assembled on diffusivity of metals so far, and particularly of the transition metals, shows that their diffusion is not necessarily dose-related; this

TABLE 16.1:

Factors in metal absorption

Exogenous factors	Endogenous factors
Dose	Age of skin—*in vivo* or *in vitro*
Vehicle	Anatomical site
Counter ion and molecular volume	Homeostatic controls
Nature of chemical bond	Skin tissue section
Valence	Red / Ox metabolism
Protein reactivity	
Depot formation	
Solubility	
pH dependence	
Time of diffusion	

appears to be one of several effects attributable to the electron-seeking or electrophilic properties which causes them to form stable bonds with proteins of the skin. In some cases, absorption at first increases with increasing dose, then reaches a plateau value and decreases again with a further increase in concentration, as was recorded for sodium chromate with guinea pig skin *in vivo* (Wahlberg and Skog, 1963). For others, such as potassium chromate on human epidermis *in vitro*, absorption steadily decreased with increasing dose (Fitzgerald and Brooks, 1979).

Vehicle

A factor for consideration when choosing a vehicle for percutaneous penetration studies is the effect the solvent will have on the skin membrane and thus its barrier properties, as well on the solubility of the permeant.

Petrolatum for instance is a poor solvent for metal salts, where the permeant remains suspended as fine particles affording less than ideal uniformity in skin contact, but on the other hand has an occlusive effect which would increase skin hydration and thus promote diffusion of a hydrophilic compound. Another solvent which enhances penetration is dimethylsulfoxide (DMSO). It appears to modify intercellular solute diffusion to include the transcellular path (Sharata and Burnette, 1988).

Counter ion and molecular volume

Intuitively, size of permeant is critical for its rate of diffusion through biological membranes, aside from other factors which may play a part in the process. A measure of the effect of the counter ion is the degree of irritancy (and thereby diffusivity) certain metals salts have on contact with the skin, investigated with nickel and chromium with the purpose of optimizing skin patch test materials for immunological diagnostic testing (Shabalina and Spiridonova, 1988; Wahlberg, 1990, 1996; Lansdown, 1991).

Nature of chemical bond and polarity

To the degree to which metals form compounds ranging from inorganic (ionic) to organic ligands, bonds increasingly assume covalent character and their penetration characteristics become similar to those of common organic non-electrolytes. The lipophilic category, mainly alkyl and aryl derivatives of the

■ CHAPTER 16 ■

more toxic metals thus represent a major risk in chemicals manufacture due to their ease of skin penetration. Extreme examples of skin diffusivity on either end of the scale are the hair darkening agent, lead acetate, and the lubricant lead naphthenate, both listed in Tables 16.2 and 16.3. In the latter, the covalent bond between the metal and the organic moiety determines the ease of penetration, a risk particularly in the industry where such lubricants are manufactured.

Valence

The outer electron shell of elements expresses their valence, determines their size and electropositivity. As a consequence these two associated factors effectively determine diffusivity: degree of steric hindrance retarding penetration, and bond formation with electronegative molecular functions in proteins which result in deposits.

A twenty-fold increase in the concentration of chromic sulfate {Cr(III)} containing the bulky sulfate ligand was required to achieve the same degree of

TABLE 16.2:

Experimentally measured non-electrolyte Kps in human skin

Non-electrolyte	$10^4 \times Kp$ (cm/h)	Reference
Toluene	1,000	Dutkiewitz and Tyras (1968)
Styrene	700	Dutkiewitz and Tyras (1968)
Benzene	100	Blank and McAuliffe (1985)
Methanol	20	Southwell et al. (1984)
Water	10	Bronaugh et al. (1986)
Ethanol	8	Scheuplein and Blank (1973)

TABLE 16.3:

Experimentally measured electrolyte Kps in human skin

Electrolyte	$10^4 \times Kp$ (cm/h)	Reference
Lead naphthenate	23	Rasetti et al. (1961)
Potassium dichromate	0.1	Gammelgaard et al. (1992)
Chromic nitrate	0.013	Gammelgaard et al. (1992)
1% Nickel chloride	0.007	Tanojo et al. (2001)
Lead acetate	0.005	Moore et al. (1980)
Mercuric acetate	0.001	Marzulli and Brown (1972)

cutaneous contact sensitization as with potassium chromate {Cr(VI)} (van Neer, 1965). On the other hand, the same degree of contact sensitivity resulted from the intradermal application of either potassium dichromate or chromic sulfate at equivalent concentrations, evidence that the SC barrier was the limiting factor for the diffusion either of the chromium compounds and their reaching the immunocompetent cells in the epidermis (van Neer, 1963).

Protein reactivity and depot formation

Metal-protein bonds are typically formed with aluminum, silver, mercury, chromium, arsenic, and nickel, and also with proteins designed to selectively retain specific metals: metallothioneins binding to copper, zinc, cadmium or iron. Deposits are seen to form in all strata of the skin and they can be reversible or irreversible in nature. Examples of the first kind are essential elements subject to homeostatic control, e.g., zinc retained by metallothionein, released upon physiological demand (Burch *et al.*, 1975). Aluminum, chromium, and mercury are metals belonging to the second group, where non-specific binding causes protein denaturation forming permanent depots in the epidermis; these appear to be mainly subject to the counter-current effect of continuous sloughing of the outer layers, which over time release significant amounts of the metals absorbed. This was convincingly demonstrated for mercury absorbed in the skin (Hursh *et al.*, 1989).

CHAPTER 16

Solubility and pH dependence

Changes in pH can affect the penetration of certain electrolytes, due to changes in their solubility or complex formation. Diffusivity of chromium (VI)-oxo complexes can vary widely and ranges over more than an order of magnitude as, dependent upon pH, Cr(VI) exists in either the chromate CrO_4 (pH >6) or the bulkier dichromate Cr_2O_4 form (pH = 2–6).

pH dependence of zinc oxide absorption was demonstrated by Ågren; at a pH of 5.4 *in vitro*, uptake of the compound through human skin was 21 times greater than at pH 7.4 (Ågren, 1990).

Time interval

Permeation constants can depend on the time span examined in diffusion experiments. Measured *in vitro*, after initial dosing they change due to the gradual build-up of the secondary barrier over time; the Kp gets smaller the longer the diffusion experiment continues.

With mercuric chloride *in vitro* on whole-thickness human skin, the effect of time post-application was the most influential variable for absorption rate, with the greatest Kp in the first measurement period (0–5 hours), decreasing in each successive period. In a similar experiment also cobalt chloride showed highest permeation values in the first 5 h of exposure (Wahlberg, 1965).

16.2.2 Endogenous factors

Age of skin

The permeability of the skin for xenobiotics appears to change with advancing age, according to most observations in a decreasing mode. This is attributed to a diminishing blood supply and also to decreasing lipid content of aging skin (Roskos *et al.*, 1989). Own investigation of skin permeability to a nickel salt and a nickel soap using dermatomed skin under identical experimental conditions confirmed the decreasing trend in skin diffusivity with age, specifically between skin from a young (age 14) versus an older source (age 67). While the ratios of diffusivity values for salt and soap remained the same, the rate of nickel diffusion was over two orders of magnitude slower in the older skin (unpublished data).

Anatomical site

Anatomical differences in accumulation and penetration of xenobiotics in the skin, for metals in particular, have been noted repeatedly, with the decreasing rank order of permeability described as: scrotum–forehead–postauricular–abdomen–forearm–leg–back (Rougier *et al.*, 1986; Wester and Maibach, 1980; Wahlberg, 1996). This appears due in part to regional SC thickness and shunt density, but mainly to intercellular lipid composition which plays a pivotal role in diffusion (Loth *et al.*, 2000). Since penetration of electrolytes appears to occur mainly through the skin's appendages, diffusion in hairy areas may be at an advantage, although absorption was also observed through the palm of the hands devoid of hair follicles; route of diffusion there were probably the sweat ducts (Feldmann and Maibach, 1967). Practical importance of such site differences becomes obvious in patch testing for diagnosis of allergic sensitization. False-negative reactions may result when hypersensitive subjects are patch tested on the less penetrable skin on the back rather than on the antecubital fossa on the arm (Basketter and Allenby, 1990; Seidenari *et al.*, 1996a, b; Simonetti *et al.*, 1998).

Homeostatic controls

Essential elements such as sodium, calcium, zinc, or copper are subject to homeostatic control which regulate body burdens, and also appear to maintain natural balances of such elements in the skin. Such controls also prevent undue losses of essential elements due to perspiration or natural exfoliation by recirculating them in the superficial strata of the skin (Cage and Dobson, 1965; Warner *et al.*, 1988). They can also act as surveillance sequestering toxic levels of certain metals, e.g., cadmium or copper, complexing them with metal-binding proteins such as metallothioneins and coeruloplasmin. Particularly *in vivo* dermal absorption experiments thus should consider such natural processes which may antagonize passive diffusion leading to erroneous conclusions, or the uncertainties observed for cutaneous penetration as in the case of zinc.

Skin layers

The different strata of the skin: stratum corneum, epidermis, full thickness skin or dermatomed skin—used for *in vitro* diffusion experiments adds to the variables which often makes data generated by different research groups irreconcilable. Thus, *in vitro* measurement of nickel chloride diffusion ranged from a minimum Kp of 6.8×10^{-7} cm/h in the SC (Tanojo *et al.*, 2001) to a maximum seen in dermatomed skin with the Kp of 9.8×10^{-3}, a rate which is three orders of magnitude higher (Hostýnek and Reifenrath, 2002).

Oxidation and reduction of xenobiotics in the skin

There is evidence that points to a change of metal valence in situ in the process of diffusion. Oxidation of some metals was observed to lead to enhanced immunogenicity, reduction to a discoloration of the skin due to accumulation of the element in the metallic state.

Chromium applied on the skin as chromate or dichromate {Cr(VI)} is reduced to chromic ion {Cr(III)} by tissue proteins containing sulfhydryl groups (Little *et al.*, 1996).

■ CHAPTER 16 ■

The observation was made in humans that nickel allergic hypersensitivity develops more readily on exposure of irritated skin than from application on intact, normal skin. Experiments conducted in animals by Artik *et al.* to test the hypothesis that the immunogenic activity of nickel is enhanced when Ni(II) is oxidized in transit through the skin to the more reactive Ni(III) or Ni(IV) species. Such bio-oxidation was assumed to occur through endogenous reactive oxygen in the form of hydrogen peroxide or hypochlorite present in inflamed skin (Artik *et al.*, 1999).

Reduction of metals in the skin or also of those occurring throughout the organism becomes evident as they accumulate in the superficial strata of the skin, resulting in discoloration characteristic for metals like arsenic, silver, or mercury.

16.3 ROUTES FOR SKIN ABSORPTION OF METALS

Metals and other solid, particulate matter are not expected to penetrate the intact stratum corneum barrier, the first line of the human defense against xenobiotics. For diffusion to occur, such materials must either come in contact with the skin as pre-formed solutions, or become soluble by action of chemical agents present on the skin surface. Besides water, sweat components are mainly chloride ion, butyric, pyruvic and lactic acid, urocanic and pyrrolidone carboxylic acid and, most importantly for metal dissolution, free fatty acids (Elias, 1983; Lampe *et al.*, 1983; Schurer and Elias, 1991). With evidence so far gathered on the process of xenobiotic diffusion into and through the skin, three different penetration pathways appear available, applicable also to metal derivatives: the intercellular, the transcellular and the appendageal penetration routes.

Base metals in particular, applied as pre-formed ions or oxidized by surface exudates on the skin (Hostýnek and Reifenrath, 2002) can readily form ionized water soluble salts as chlorides, as well as lipophilic compounds (soaps), e.g., with fatty acids present on the skin, and use any or all of the three avenues.

a) Depending on the polarity of the ion pair formed, shunts consisting of the hair follicles and sweat ducts which transverse all the layers of the epidermis and reach into the dermis serve for relatively rapid passage of hydrophilic (ionized) salts as an early stage event. They constitute relatively large openings through which diffusion can occur if two principal conditions are met: sweat is present to serve as an aqueous diffusion medium, and the outflow of sweat is significant. Poral diffusion of ions was demonstrated using high current flow in ionto-phoresis (Scheuplein and Blank, 1971; Guy and Maibach, 1984; Burnette and Ongpipattanakul, 1988; Hadgraft, 1989; Cullander, 1991, 1992; Potts and Guy, 1992) and observations made using autoradiography or micro-PIXE analysis (Odintsova, 1975; Lloyd, 1980; Bos *et al.*, 1985). Ductal penetration of the skin was also investigated histologically for certain metals, particularly for aluminum and zirconium, with the intent of demonstrating their relative antiperspirant effectiveness through emphraxis or ductal closure (Reller and Luedders, 1983). Sweat duct plugs isolated from aluminum chlorohydrate (ACH)-inhibited sweat glands of human forearm skin have been analyzed using Fourier transform infrared spectroscopy. Thereby it was established that epidermal cells in the sweat duct migrate toward the ductal lumen, keratinize and desquamate into the lumen, binding irreversibly to aluminum chloro-hydrate (ACH). Metal hydroxide masses have been observed as far down as the secretory coil. Histological examination by transmission electron microscopy and fluorescence microscopy of skin treated with ACH revealed an obstructive, aluminum-rich, electron-dense mass within the sweat gland duct, typically at the level of the stratum granulosum, and occasionally as deep as the upper layers of the viable epidermis and the Malpighian layer (Quatrale *et al.*, 1981). Considerable experimental data indicated that the depth of sweat duct pene-tration is significantly dependent upon ionic mobility (i.e., size) and electronic charge of the metal. In this context, salts of Zn, Cr, Fe, Ti, In, Ga, Sn, Mg, Cu, Be, and Sc were also found to diffuse through shunts (Lyon and Klotz, 1958; Fiedler, 1968).

That penetration of electrolytes through sweat ducts can occur within 1–5 minutes following exposure, with no comparable transport via the transcellular path observable in that time span, was noted by several investigators (Abramson and Gorin, 1940; MacKee *et al.*, 1945; Shelley and Melton, 1949). Selective poral transit by nickel also became manifest clinically, observed as follicular inflammation or punctate erythema in consequence of patch testing with the metal's salts (Fischer and Rystedt, 1985; Menné and Calvin, 1993; Kanerva and Estlander, 1995).

b) Such initial, rapid diffusion is followed by the slower, potentially more important intercellular diffusion along the all-enveloping, continuous lipid bilayer. For any appreciable penetration to occur, charged, electrophilic and thus protein-bound molecules such as zinc are likely to follow that intercellular

CHAPTER 16

path. The lipid pathway for nickel salt diffusion was demonstrated by evaluating skin susceptibility to challenge with nickel chloride in allergic subjects. Pre-treatment of the skin with a lipid-rich moisturizer increased reactions to exposure as compared with non-treated skin. Such reduction in threshold values for elicitation of allergic reactions following supply of lipids is an indication of the route chosen by the immunogenic hapten (Zachariae *et al.*, 2002). There is evidence for the formation of fatty acid soaps by metals in contact with the skin (Hostýnek *et al.*, 2001b). and it appears reasonable to postulate that metal ion pairs with a predominantly covalent bond which they form with fatty acids will preferably partition into the intercellular, lipophilic environment of the stratum corneum.

c) The third route, transcellular (stratum corneum) diffusion, would appear to have marginal toxicological importance; particularly absorption of electro-positive metals is limited to the outermost layers of the SC which consists of hydrophilic and lipophilic domains, and possibly in the epithelium of appendages, where they form deposits with protein and can act as a dynamic reservoir. Such depot formation can become visible with some metals, and often is described in the literature, e.g., as calcinosis cutis (calcium), chrysiasis (gold), argyria (silver), haemochromatosis (iron), saturnism (lead), hydrargyrosis cutis (mercury), or as an icteroid discoloration (selenium).

16.4 DESCRIPTORS OF SKIN PERMEABILITY

16.4.1 The permeation coefficient Kp and Fick's first law of membrane diffusion

The most commonly used quantitative *in vitro* technique for determining the percutaneous absorption, describing it as the Permeation Coefficient Kp involves placing a piece of excised skin in a two-chamber diffusion cell. The solute passes from the fixed higher concentration medium in the donor chamber by passive diffusion into the less concentrated solution in the receptor chamber. The advantage of such diffusion experiments lies in the standardized expression of quantitative results when Fick's first law of diffusion is applicable (Fick, 1855). Formulated to characterize passive diffusion of compounds across membranes in general, Fick's law has been shown to also apply to passive diffusion of xenobiotics through the SC of the skin, and with certain restrictions also applicable to the skin's permeability for metal compounds. That law states that, if the permeation process from an "infinite" reservoir reaches the point of steady state equilibrium, i.e., the concentrations in the donor and receptor phases remain constant over time, the measured steady-state flux Jss describes the amount of permeant per unit time and area, usually expressed as mg/h/cm^2. The permeability coefficient or permeation constant Kp, typically in cm/h, is then calculated from the Jss value divided by ΔC, the concentration gradient between donor and acceptor phase. In a diffusion experiment conducted under dynamic conditions, i.e., where the permeant reaching the receptor fluid is constantly removed, C in the receptor compartment is zero, and the resulting calculation then becomes

Kp = Jss / C.

The technique is easily standardized and allows the determination of Kp through skin or other membranes as long as the barrier properties are not affected by either permeant or carrier solvent. That implies that the permeant, in this case the metallic ion, may not react with barrier material thereby changing barrier permeability. Since heavy metals are electrophilic and avidly bind to electron-rich moieties present in epidermal tissue, such as oxygen, nitrogen or sulfur, this prejudices the general validity of Kp values (see below). Nevertheless, flux values for metal compounds *in vitro*, if obtained under conditions of steady state from an "infinite" reservoir and normalized for concentration, are so far the most frequently measured and best descriptor available for the skin penetration of such metals also, and the calculated Kp serves as a convenient parameter for putting their diffusion in context with that of other, more conforming permeants. Such a scale of diffusion constants is presented in Tables 16.2 and 16.3, expressing depth of permeation per unit of time (here in cm/h).

Using *in vitro* experimentation with electropositive metals it may not be possible to attain steady state diffusion in the conventional sense due to long-time retention of the permeant in the barrier material (induction period); the Kp is then arrived at from permeant identified quantitatively in the barrier strata (epidermis or dermis).

Typically, diffusivity of ionized metal salts is several orders of magnitude lower than that measured for organic compounds of intermediate polarity and molecular weight. The permeability coefficients (Kp) for a number of organic compounds and metal salts are listed in Tables 16.2 and 16.3 for comparison.

■ CHAPTER 16 ■

16.4.2   Percent of dose absorbed

The optimal *in vivo* method for the determination of skin absorption is the one developed by Feldmann and Maibach (1969). It yields large part of the data so far available on skin penetration by drugs and pesticides, using human volunteers or monkeys,

In human studies, following topical application of the permeant the plasma levels of test compounds are low and the use of radiolabelled compounds becomes necessary. The compound labeled with carbon-14 or tritium, or a metal isotope, is applied to the skin in a minimal volume of a volatile solvent that is left to evaporate, and the total amount of radioactivity excreted is then determined. The amount retained in the body is corrected for by determining the amount of radioactivity excreted following parenteral administration of the compound. The resulting radioactivity value is then expressed as the percent of the applied dose absorbed. Fick's postulates for membrane diffusion are not met there. A concentration of the permeant cannot be defined and neither is a steady state equilibrium observable with this method; the permeability coefficient thus cannot be calculated. Nevertheless, for purposes of risk assessment the indication of potential (whole-body) absorption is an important factor as it gives a measure for human (worst case) exposure.

16.5   ABSORPTION DETERMINED THROUGH STRATUM CORNEUM ANALYSIS

Rougier developed a predictive method by which the systemic uptake of permeant can be derived from the amount which diffuses into the stratum corneum after a limited time of exposure *in vivo* (Rougier and Lotte 1993). By that method, the chemical is dosed on the skin of animals or human volunteers, after 30 minute-contact the surface of the SC wiped clean of residual compound, and the SC removed by successive application of adhesive tape and stripping. The strippings are analyzed for chemical and from that value then the amount may be estimated which eventually will be systemically absorbed over a longer period of time. The method is only applicable to compounds of Fickian behaviour, but not for electrophilic metals which react with barrier tissue rendering in-depth diffusion unpredictable. In addition, certain metals such as copper, zinc or chromium are essential nutrients subject to homeostatic controls, which appear to determine deposition or mobilization in function of fluctuating body burdens.

In our lab SC stripping was used for other purposes, however, and applied to investigate mode of metal diffusion into the SC itself (Hostýnek *et al.*, 2001a, b). Tracing the concentration profiles of permeants in SC has been rendered facile by using that non-invasive method and by state-of-the-art analysis with inductively coupled plasma atomic emission spectroscopy (ICP AES) and inductively coupled plasma mass spectroscopy (ICP-MS). With this non-invasive method it is now possible to analyze for the presence of elements in trace amounts in skin tissues and other biological materials to a level of 0.5 ppb (0.5 µg/kg), making the use of radioisotopes unnecessary. The method makes it possible to estimate actual metal concentration profiles to the level of living epidermal tissue.

16.6 SUMMARY

Present understanding of skin penetration by metals is limited. As becomes evident from a review of the literature on skin diffusivity of metals, research so far has been scarce and has proceeded on a priority basis, investigating essential micronutrients as well as hazardous metals in the environment and industry which pose a threat to human health in general and the immune system in particular. Skin exposure to xenobiotics can result from the air, from contact with contaminated surfaces or immersion into contaminated liquids, and there still prevails a disconnect between contamination of the skin and systemic uptake of metals. Efforts toward a better understanding of the permeability of the skin to metals continue, with the objective of arriving at a robust assessment of risks to humans associated with such exposures. This review points to the complexity of the interrelations which exist between exogenous and endogenous factors; consider as an instance the many factors known to act in concert which determine skin diffusion of chromium compounds: valence, size, electropositivity, concentration, pH and polarity. Only investigation of metals and also of their compounds individually provides the basis necessary for solid risk assessment. Continued advances in this area will lead to better preventive and therapeutic measures for both workers and the general public.

REFERENCES

ABRAMSON, H.A. and GORIN, M.H. (1940) The electrophoretic demonstration of the patent pores of the living human skin in relation to the charge of the skin. *J. Phys. Chem.* **44**, 1094–1102.

ÅGREN, M.S. (1990) Percutaneous absorption of zinc from zinc oxide applied topically to intact skin in man. *Dermatologica* **180**, 36–39.

ARTIK, S., VON VULTÉE, C., GLEICHMANN, E., SCHWARZ, T. and GRIEM, P. (1999) Nickel allergy in mice: enhanced sensitization capacity of nickel at higher oxidation states. *J. Immunol.* **163**, 1143–1152.

BASKETTER, D. and ALLENBY, F. (1990) A model to simulate the effect of detergent on skin and evaluate any resulting effect on contact allergic reactions. *Contact Dermatitis* **23**, 291.

BOS, A. J., VAN DER STAP, C.C., VALKOVIC, V., VIS, R.D. and VERHEUL, H. (1985) Incorporation routes of elements into human hair; implications for hair analysis used for monitoring. *Sci. Total Environ.* **42**, 157–169.

BURCH, R.E., HAHN, H.K.J. and SULLIVAN, J.F. (1975) Newer aspects of the roles of zinc, manganese and copper in human nutrition. *Clin. Chem.* **21**, 501–520.

BURNETTE, R.R. and ONGPIPATTANAKUL, B. (1988) Location of sites of increased transport during iontophoresis. *J. Pharm. Sci.* **77**, 132–137.

CAGE, G.W. and DOBSON, R.L. (1965) Sodium secretion and reabsorption in the human eccrine sweat gland. *J. Clin. Invest.* **44**, 1270–1276.

CULLANDER, C. and GUY, R.H. (1991) Sites of iontophoretic current flow into the skin: identification and characterization with the vibrating probe electrode. *Journal of Investigative Dermatology* **97**, 55–64.

CULLANDER, C. and GUY, R.H. (1992) Visualization of iontophoretic pathways with confocal microscopy and the vibrating probe electrode. *Solid State Ionics* **53**, 197–206.

ELIAS, P. (1983) Epidermal lipids, barrier function, and desquamation. *J. Invest. Dermatol.* **80**, 44s-49s.

FELDMANN, R.J. and MAIBACH, H.I. (1967) Regional variation in percutaneous penetration of C-14 cortisol in man. *J. Invest. Dermatol.* **48**, 181–183.

FIEDLER, H.P. (1968) *Der Schweiss* (2nd edn.) Cantor (Aulendorf), 303–377.

FICK, A.E. (1855) On liquid diffusion. *Philosophical Magazine* **10**, 30–39.

FISCHER, T. and RYSTEDT, I. (1985) False-positive, follicular and irritant patch test reactions to metal salts. *Contact Dermatitis* **12**(2), 93–98.

FITZGERALD, J.J. and BROOKS, T. (1979) A new cell for *in vitro* skin permeability studies—chromium (III)/(VI) human epidermis investigations. *J. Invest. Dermatol.* **72**, 198.

FLYNN, G.L (1990) Physicochemical determinants of skin absorption. In GERRITY, T.R. and HENRY, C.J. (eds) *Principles of Route-to-Route Extrapolation for Risk Assessment.* New York: Elsevier Science Publishing Co, 93–127.

GUY, R.H. and MAIBACH, H.I. (1984) Correction factors for determining body exposure from forearm percutaneous absorption data. *J. Appl. Toxicol.* **4**, 26–28.

HADGRAFT, J., GREEN, P.G. and WOTTON, P.K. (1989) Facilitated percutaneous absorption of charged drugs. In BRONAUGH, R. and MAIBACH, H.I. *Percutaneous Absorption.* New York: Marcel Dekker, 55–64.

HOSTÝNEK, J.J., DREHER, F., PELOSI, A., ANIGBOGU, A. and MAIBACH, H.I. (2001a) Human stratum corneum adsorption of nickel salts: investigation of depth profiles by tape stripping *in vivo. Acta Derm.-Venereol. (Suppl.)* **212**, 11–18.

HOSTÝNEK, J.J., DREHER, F., PELOSI, A., ANIGBOGU, A. and MAIBACH, H.I. (2001b) Human stratum corneum penetration by nickel: *in vivo* study of depth distribution after occlusive application of the metal as powder. *Acta Derm.-Venereol. (Suppl.)* **212**, 5–10.

HOSTÝNEK, J.J. and REIFENRATH, W. (2002) Flux of nickel salts versus a nickel soap across human skin. *Perspectives in Percutaneous Penetration* **8a**, 99

HURSH, J.B., CLARKSON, T.W., MILES, E.F. and GOLDSMITH, L.A. (1989) Percutaneous absorption of mercury vapor by man. *Arch. Environ. Health* **44**, 120–127.

KANERVA, L. and ESTLANDER, T. (1995) Occupational allergic contact dermatitis asociated with curious pubic nickel dermatitis from minimal exposure. *Contact Dermatitis* **32**, 309–310.

LAMPE, M.A., BURLINGAME, A.L., WHITNEY, J., WILLIAMS, M.L., BROWN, B.E., ROITMAN, E. and ELIAS, P.M. (1983) Human stratum corneum lipids: characterization and regional variations. *J. Lipid Res.* **24**, 120–130.

LANSDOWN, A.B. (1991) Interspecies variations in reponse to topical application of selected zinc compounds. *Food. Chem. Toxicol.* **29**, 57–64.

LITTLE, M.C., GAWKRODGER, D.J. and MACNEIL, S. (1996) Chromium- and nickel-induced cytotoxicity in normal and transformed human keratinocytes: an investigation of pharmacological approaches to the prevention of Cr(VI)-induced cytotoxicity. *Br. J. Dermatol.* **134**, 199–207.

LLOYD, G.K. (1980) Dermal absorption and conjugation of nickel in relation to the induction of allergic contact dermatitis—preliminary results. In Brown, S.S. and Sunderman, F.W. (eds) *International Conference on Nickel Toxicology (2nd: 1980: Swansea, Wales),* London: Academic Press, 145–148.

LOTH, H., HAUCK, G., BORCHERT, D. and THEOBALD, F. (2000) Statistical testing of drug accumulation in skin tissues by linear regression versus contants of stratum corneum lipids. *Int. J. Pharm.* **209**, 95–108.

LYON, I. and KLOTZ, I.M. (1958) The interaction of epidermal protein with aluminum salts. *J. Am. Pharm. Assoc. Scientific Edition* **47**, 509–512.

MACKEE, G.M., SULZBERGER, M.B., HERRMANN, F. and BAER, R.L. (1945) Histologic studies on percutaneous penetration with special reference to the effect of vehicles. *J. Invest Dermatol.* **6**, 43–61.

MENNÉ, T. and CALVIN, G. (1993) Concentration threshold of non-occluded nickel exposure in nickel-sensitive individuals and controls with and without surfactant. *Contact Dermatitis* **29**, 180–184.

ODINTSOVA, N.A. (1976) Permeability of the epidermis for lead acetate according to fluorescence and electron-microscopic studies. *Vestn. Dermatol. Venerol.* **9**, 19–24.

PLUECKHAHN, V.D., BALLARD, B., BANKS, J.M., COLLINS, R.B. and FLETT, P.T. (1978) Hexachlorophene preparations in infant antiseptic skin care: benefits, risks, and the future. *Med. J. Aust.* **2**, 555–560.

POTTS, R.O. and GUY, R.H. (1992a) Predicting skin permeability. *Pharmaceutical Research* **9**, 663–669.

POTTS, R.O. and GUY, R.H. (1992b) Routes of ionic permeability through mammalian skin. *Solid State Ionics* **53**, 165–169; 663–669.

POTTS, R.O. and GUY, R.H. (1995) A predictive algorithm for skin permeability: The effects of molecular size and hydrogen bond activity. *Pharmaceutical Research* **12**(11), 1628–1633

QUATRALE, R.P., WALDMAN, A.H., ROGERS, J.G. and FELGER, C.B. (1981) The mechanism of antiperspirant action by aluminum salts. *J. Soc. Cosmet. Chem.* **32**, 67–73.

RELLER, H.H. and LUEDDERS, W.L. (1983) Mechanism of action of metal salt antiperspirants. Part 2. In MARZULLI, F.N. and MAIBACH, H.I. (eds) *Dermatotoxicology*, volume 4, Washington: Hemisphere Publishing Corporation, 18–54.

ROSKOS, K.V., MAIBACH, H.I. and GUY, R.H. (1989) The effect of aging on percutaneous absorption in man. *J. Dermatol.* **16**, 475–479.

ROUGIER, A., DUPUIS, D., LOTTE, C., ROGUET, R., WESTER, R.C. and MAIBACH, H.I. (1986) Regional variation in percutaneous absorption in man: Measurement by the stripping method. *Arch. Dermatol. Res.* **278**, 465–469.

SCHEUPLEIN, R.J. and BLANK, I.H. (1971) Permeability of the skin. *Physiol. Rev.* **51**, 707–747.

SCHURER, N.Y. and ELIAS, P.M. (1991) The biochemistry and function of stratum corneum lipids. *Adv. Lipid Res.* **24**, 27–56.

SEIDENARI, S., BELLETTI, B., MANTOVANI, L., PELLACANI, G. and PIGNATTI, M. (1996a) Comparison of 2 different methods for enhancing the reaction to nickel sulfate patch tests in negative reactors. *Contact Dermatitis* **35**, 308.

SEIDENARI, S., MOTOLESE, A. and BELLETTI, B. (1996b) Pretreatment of nickel test areas with sodium lauryl sulfate detects nickel sensitivity in subjects reacting negatively to routinely performed patch tests. *Contact Dermatitis* **34**, 88–92.

SHABALINA, L.P. and SPIRIDONOVA, V.S. (1988) Toxicity and character of the effect of some zinc compounds. *J. Hyg. Epidemiol. Microbiol. Immunol.* **32**, 397–405.

SHARATA, H.H. and BURNETTE, R.R. (1988) Effect of dipolar aprotic permeability enhancers on the basal stratum corneum. *J. Pharm. Sci.* **77**, 27–32.

SHELLEY, W.B. and MELTON, F.M. (1949) Factors accelerating the penetration of histamine through normal intact skin. *J. Invest. Dermatol.* **13**, 61–71.

SIMONETTI, V., MANZINI, B.M. and SEIDENARI, S. (1998) Patch testing with nickel sulfate: comparison between 2 nickel sulfate preparations and 2 different test sites on the back. *Contact Dermatitis* **39**, 187–191.

SMITH, S.L. (1997) An avoidable tragedy. *Occupational Hazards* **59**, 32.

TANOJO, H., HOSTÝNEK, J.J., MOUNTFORD, H.S. and MAIBACH, H.I. (2001) *In vitro* permeation of nickel salts through human stratum corneum. *Acta Derm.-Venereol. (Suppl.)* **212**, 19–23.

TORIBARA, T.Y., CLARKSON, T.W. and NIERENBERG, D.W. (1997) Chemical safety: More on working with dimethylmercury. *C. and E. News* **75**, 6.

VAN NEER, F.C.J. (1963) Sensitization of guinea pigs to chromium compounds. *Nature (Lond)* **198**, 1013.

VAN NEER, F.C.J. (1965) Reacties op intracutane injecties van drie en zeswaardige chroomverbindgen bij gesen-sibiliseerde mensen, vackens en caviae. *Ned Tijdschr Geneeskd* **109**, 1684.

WAHLBERG, J.E. (1965) Percutaneous absorption of sodium chromate (51Cr), cobaltous (58Co), and mercuric (203Hg) chlorides through excised human and guinea pig skin. *Acta Derm. Venereol. (Stockh.)* **45**, 415–426.

WAHLBERG, J.E. (1990) Nickel chloride or nickel sulfate? Irritation from patch-test preparations as assessed by laser doppler flowmetry. *Dermatol. Clin.* **8**, 41–44.

CHAPTER 16

WAHLBERG, J.E. (1996) Nickel: the search for alternative, optimal and non-irritant patch test preparations. Assessment based on laser Doppler flowmetry. *Skin Res. Technol.* **2**, 136–141.

WAHLBERG, J.E. and SKOG, E. (1963) The percutaneous absorption of sodium chromate (^{51}Cr) in the guinea pig. *Acta Derm. Venereol. (Stockh.)* **43**, 102–108.

WARNER, R.R., MYERS, M.C. and TAYLOR, D.A. (1988) Electron probe analysis of human skin: element concentration profiles. *J. Invest. Dermatol.* **90**, 78–85.

WESTER, R.C. and MAIBACH, H.I. (1980) Regional variation in percutaneous absorption. In BRONAUGH, R.L. and MAIBACH, H.I. (eds) *Percutaneous Absorption: Mechanisms-Methodology-Drug Delivery*, New York: Marcel Dekker, Inc., 111–120.

ZACHARIAE, C., HELD, E., JOHANSEN, J.D., MENNE, T. and AGNER, T. (2002) Skin susceptibility to NiCl2 after moisturizer application. *Am. J. Contact Dermat.* **13**, 97.

Photoirritation (Phototoxicity, Phototoxic Dermatitis)

FRANCIS N MARZULLI AND HOWARD I MAIBACH

Contents

17.1   Introduction

17.2   Phototoxic agents

17.3   Nonsteroidal anti-inflammatory drugs

17.4   Elements of the test for phototoxicity

17.5   Mechanisms of phototoxicity

17.6   Highlights

17.7   Conclusions

17.1 INTRODUCTION

Phototoxicity is a chemically induced nonimmunologic skin irritation requiring light (photoirritation). The skin response resembles an exaggerated sunburn. The involved chemical is photoactive, and it may enter into the skin by topical administration or it may reach the skin by the circulatory system following ingestion or parenteral administration. Some systemically administered and possibly topical chemicals may require metabolic conversion to become photoactive.

Erythema, edema, vesiculation, hyperpigmentation, and desquamation are typical phototoxic skin effects. Histamine, kinins, and arachidonic acid derivatives such as prostaglandins are products that are often released during the inflammatory processes.

Phototoxicity is mainly produced by chemicals that are activated by the ultraviolet (UV) area of the electromagnetic spectrum, which is subdivided arbitrarily into UVA (from 320 to 420 nm), UVB (from 280 to 320 nm), and UVC (below 280 nm). Thus UVA represents the less energetic portion of the UV spectrum and UVC the more energetic (cytotoxic) area. UVA in the range 320–340 nm (UVA2) is more energetic and more skin-damaging than UVA in the range 340–400 nm (UVA 1).

Tests for phototoxic potential of topically applied chemicals are usually conducted with radiation within the UVA range. Some phototoxic chemicals are activated by wavelengths in the visible spectrum (bikini dermatitis) (Hjorth and Moller, 1976), some by UVB (Jeanmougin et al., 1983), and some (doxycycline) are augmented by UVB (Bjellerup, 1986).

Accurate measurements of radiation intensity and frequency are important prerequisites for work, in phototoxicity.

Among animal models that have proven useful in predicting human phototoxicity are the mouse, rabbit, swine, guinea pig, squirrel monkey, and hamster, in that approximate order of effectiveness (Marzulli and Mailbach, 1970).

Phototoxic events are initiated when a photoactive chemical (a chemical capable of absorbing UV radiation) enters the viable elements of skin (via skin penetration or blood circulation) and becomes excited by appropriate UV radiation that penetrates skin. In some cases the photoexcited drug transfers its energy to oxygen, exciting it to the singlet oxygen state, which is cytotoxic. In other cases, oxygen may not be involved. Chlorpromazine is thought to be activated by a photodynamic process involving molecular oxygen, whereas psoralens do not require molecular oxygen to produce phototoxic effects.

Clinical identification of phototoxicity requires knowledge about skin effects of phototoxic chemicals, and clinical insight gained from practical experience. Phototoxic skin effects are characterized by erythema, vesiculation or bullae, increased skin temperature, and pruritis. This is followed later by long-lasting hyperpigmentation.

That the morphologic aspects of phototoxic skin eruptions are not always apparent was demonstrated by the frequent lack of identification in many of the earlier cases of dimethyl-*p*-aminobenzoic acid (sunscreen) dermatitis (Emmett *et al.*, 1977). However, the greatest challenge to the clinician comes from phototoxic and photoallergic dermatoses induced by oral agents.

17.2 PHOTOTOXIC AGENTS

Naturally occurring plant-derived furocoumarins, including psoralen, 5-methoxypsoralen (bergapten), 8-methoxypsoralen (xanthotoxin), angelicin, and others, constitute the most important class of phototoxic chemicals. Psoralens occur in a wide variety of plants, such as parsley, celery, and citrus fruits (Pathak, 1974; Juntilla, 1976).

The Rutaceae (common rue, gas plant, Persian limes, bergamot) and Umbelliferae (fennel, dill, wild carrot, cow parsnip) are prominent among plant families responsible for phytophotodermatitis (Juntilla, 1976). Bergapten, psoralen, and xanthotoxin are among the more commonly encountered phototoxic agents. Bergapten is the active component of bergamot oil, and is a well-known perfume ingredient whose toxic skin effects have been accorded the name berlock dermatitis. Based on results of their studies of perfume phototoxicity, Marzulli and Maibach (1970) suggested that perfume should contain no more than 0.3 percent bergamot, which is equivalent to about 0.001 percent bergapten, to avoid phototoxicity. Their work also established that bergapten was the only one of five components isolated from oil of bergamot that was responsible for phototoxic effects of the parent material. Limettin (5,7-dimethoxycoumarin), although more intensely fluorescent than bergapten, did not prove phototoxic to human skin. Bergapten phototoxicity continues to occur in some countries where bergapten-free bergamot is not used (Zaynoun *et al.*, 1981), in Norway, from contact with *Heracleum lacinatum* (Kavli *et al.*, 1983), and in Denmark from skin contact with *Heracleum mantegazzianum*, the giant hogweed (Knudsen, 1983).

Xanthotoxin (8-MOP) is effective in treating vitiligo and psoriasis by oral administration or topical application followed by exposure to UVA (PUVA phototherapy). The *Ammi majus* plant, containing xanthotoxin (8-MOP) in crude form, has been used therapeutically in Egypt since ancient times (El Mofty, 1948). However, at present, PUVA therapy is considered to have carcinogenic potential and warrants caution. Chronic use of this therapeutic regimen enhances prospects of inducing squamous-cell skin cancer, especially in young patients and in those who are genetically predisposed (Stem et al., 1979). This potential has resulted in a reduced use of PUVA phototherapy in the United States (Parrish *et al.*, 1974).

Phototoxicity reactions have been reported to psoralen-containing sweet oranges (Volden *et al.*, 1983) and to common rue (*Ruta graviolens*) (Heskel *et al.*, 1983).

Coal-tar derivatives, another important group of phototoxic agents, produce occupational contact photodermatitis in industrial workers and in road workers. Anthraquinone-based disperse blue 35 dye caused such effects in dye process workers. Radiation in the visible spectrum activates the dye (Gardiner *et al.*, 1974). Pyrene, anthracene, and fluoranthrene are strongly phototoxic to guinea pigs (Kochevar *et al.*, 1982).

Oral therapeutic use of amiodarone, a cardiac antiarrhythmic drug, has produced phototoxic effects (Chalmers *et al.*, 1982). Incidence, time course, and recovery from phototoxic effects of amiodarone in humans were studied by Rappersberger *et al.* (1989).

Quinoline antimalarials appear to be phototoxic, and some of these have been studied *in vitro* and *in vivo* (Moore and Himmens, 1982; Epling and Sibley, 1987; Ljunggren and Wirestrand, 1988).

Tetracyclines, particularly demethylchlortetracycline, but also doxycycline, chlortetracycline, and tetracycline, are phototoxic when orally ingested (Verbov, 1973; Frost *et al.*, 1972; Maibach *et al.*, 1967). Doxycycline was reported more potent than demethylchlortetractracycline or limecycline in one human study (Bjellerup and Ljunggren, 1985).

Cadmium sulfide, used in tattoos for its yellow color, may be phototoxic (Bjornberg, 1963). Thiazide diuretics were shown to have a phototoxic potential in one study (Diffey and Langtry, 1989), but thiazide-induced phototoxicity is actually rare in clinical practise.

17.3 NONSTEROIDAL ANTI-INFLAMMATORY DRUGS

Nonsteroidal anti-inflammatory drugs (NSAID) were the subject of extensive investigations for phototoxic potential following reports that benoxaprofen, a suspended British antirheumatic NSAID, has this capacity (Webster *et al.*, 1983; Allen, 1983; Stern, 1983; Anderson *et al.*, 1987). *In vitro* studies with sheep erythrocytes or human leukocytes suggested a phototoxic potential (Anderson *et al.*, 1987; Pryzbilla *et al.*, 1987).

NSAID that are structurally related to propionic acid have been shown to possess phototoxic potential, whereas certain other types of NSAID such as tenoxicam and piroxicam were not experimentally phototoxic by *in vivo* or *in vitro* test methods (Anderson *et al.*, 1987; Kaidbey and Mitchell, 1989; Western *et al.*, 1987). The propionic acid-derived NSAID produce unique immediate wheal and flare, in contrast with a much delayed exaggerated sunburn response that typifies psoralen phototoxicity.

Although piroxicam is not phototoxic under experimental conditions involving human test conditions (Kaidbey and Mitchell, 1989), it has been implicated as a possible clinical photoallergic or phototoxic photosensitizer. One explanation for the unexpected photoactivity of piroxicam in skin is that a metabolite of piroxicam is indeed phototoxic when isolated and tested on human mononuclear cells *in vitro* (Western *et al.*, 1987). These positive findings and likely explanation are related to the production of singlet oxygen, as indicated by emission at 1270 nm when the suspect metabolite was irradiated with UV *in vitro* (Western *et al.*, 1987; Kochevar, 1989).

Other propionic acid-derived NSAID associated with an immediate phototoxic response are nabumetone, naproxen, and tiaprofenic acid (Kaidbey and Mitchell, 1989; Diffey *et al.*, 1983). Carprofen (Merot *et al.*, 1983) and ketoprofen (Alomar, 1985) appear to be photoallergenic. However, further work may be needed to separate, clarify, and identify three possible outcomes—allergy, photoallergy, and phototoxicity—in studies involving NSAID.

The general area of cutaneous reactions to NSAID has been extensively reviewed by Ophaswongse and Maibach (1993).

17.4 ELEMENTS OF THE TEST FOR PHOTOTOXICITY

The test material is applied to skin of a human subject or an animal model (clipped skin of mouse, guinea pig, rabbit, or swine). After a suitable waiting period for skin absorption to take place (several minutes, depending on the rate of skin penetration), the chemical test site is irradiated with UV of appropriate wavelengths. The test site is then examined at 1, 24, 48, and 72 h for evidence of phototoxicity, such as erythema, vesiculation, bullae, and finally hyperpigmentation. A comparison is made between the skin of the test site and control sites (one without chemical and one without light).

Results are modified by factors that affect skin penetration, such as test concentration and vehicle, as well as by duration of exposure and by distance from the irradiation source to the test area.

Some photoirritants (e.g., bergapten) produce clinical phototoxicity when the photoirritant site is irradiated within minutes to 1 h after skin application; with others, irradiation is effective when administered at 24 h.

Phototoxic effects are expected when UV is directed at and absorbed by a phototoxic chemical residing in the skin. This results in a skin reaction with cellular components, such as DNA.

One of the earliest indicators of phototoxic potential was based on a paralyzing effect on the cilia of *Paramecium* from acridine plus light, reported by Oscar Raab at the close of the 19th century. This test method was later followed by a simpler test involving a lytic effect on red blood cells, as an endpoint for phototoxicity.

The subject of *in vitro* assay for phototoxic effects has recently been reviewed (Rougier *et al.*, 1994).

17.5 MECHANISMS OF PHOTOTOXICITY

The questions of site and mechanism of action of phototoxic chemicals and the importance of oxygen have been much studied. Some photoactive chemicals require oxygen to exert their phototoxic effects whereas others do not. Some photoactive chemicals act on cellular DNA, whereas others act on cellular membranes. Recent studies by Gendimenico and Kochevar (1990) have shown that acridine requires oxygen to produce a lethal (phototoxic) effect on mast cells. (Dermal mast cells are known to participate in cutaneous phototoxic responses initiated by UV and visible radiation). Many years ago, Mathews (1963) showed that toluidine blue requires oxygen to produce its lethal (phototoxic) effect on *Sarcina lutea*, however, oxygen is not needed for the phototoxic effect of 8-MOP on *S. lutea*. In addition, it was found that 8-MOP phototoxicity results in damage to cellular DNA, whereas toluidine kills by action on the cell membrane.

A more complete discussion of mechanisms of photosensitized reactions is given in Spikes (1983).

17.6 HIGHLIGHTS

Investigative studies in phototoxicity require a rudimentary understanding of what constitutes appropriate radiation sources for experimental work, as a first step. Knowledge about safety in the use of radiation equipment is equally important.

Well-calibrated equipment for measuring radiation is another prerequisite, including a recognition that with time and use, equipment changes and requires proper upkeep to ensure its quality in performance.

Filters are sometimes needed to provide an appropriate cutoff of unwanted radiation. Window glass is useful in eliminating wavelengths below 320 nm.

Natural sunlight is filtered by atmospheric oxygen, ozone, clouds, particulates, and other environmental factors including altitude, so that wavelengths below 290 nm are effectively shielded from reaching the earth's surface. Consequently, radiation sources that deliver highly energetic shorter wavelengths in the UVC range are unlikely to be useful in experimental phototoxic studies involving humans.

The radiation ranges that are of greatest biologic focus in phototoxicity studies are UVA (320–400 nm), UVB (280–320 nm), and UVC (<280 nm). As the Commision de l'Eclairage recommends 315 nm as the cutoff for UVB rather than 320 nm, it is important that the investigative photobiologist identify the system of use. However, a rationale for using 320 nm rather than 315 nm as the cutoff for UVA is given in Peak and van der Leun (1992).

The first rule of photochemistry is that cells are injured or killed when photons of radiant energy are absorbed and energy is transferred to target molecules (Spikes, 1983). Phototoxic effects are therefore produced when absorption wavelengths of the sensitizer are the same as those of the radiant energy source (Grotthus–Draper law).

DNA, RNA, deoxy—or ribodeoxynucleotides, enzymes containing such cofactors, and aromatic and cysteine residues of proteins are typical targets of UV phototoxic damage.

Oxygen may or may not participate in the production of a phototoxic event; however, when oxygen is indeed involved, it is often referred to as a photo-dynamic action.

Psoralens are among the most frequently encountered phototoxic chemicals, as they are present in many plants. Petroleum products, coal tar, cadmium sulfide, acridines, porphyrins, and other chemicals may also be implicated as causative agents for phototoxic effects. Table 17.1 provides a list of phototoxic chemicals.

TABLE 17.1:

Clemicals, plants, and drugs with phototoxic potential

Topical
    Dyes—anthraquinone, disperse blue 35, cosin, nethylene blue, rose bengal.
    toluidine blue. camiuni sulfidc in tattoos
    Fragrances—oil of bergamot
    Furocoumarins—angelicin, bergapten, psoralen, 8-methoxypsoralen. 4,5′,
    8-trimethylpsoralen
    Plant products—celery, figs, limes, hogweed, parsnips, fennel, dill
    Coal tar components—acridine, anthracene, benzopyrene, creosote,
    phenanthrene, pitch, pyridine

Systemic
    Antibiotics—griseofulvin, nalidixic acid, sulfanilamide, tetracyclines
    Chemotherapeutics—dacarbazine, 5-fluorouracil, vinblastine
    Drugs—amiodarone, chlorpromazine, chloroquin, tolbutamide
    Diuretics—hydrochlorothizide, furosemide
    Nonsteroidal antiinflammatories—benoxaprofen, naproxen, piroxicam
    Porphyrins—hematoporphyrin
    Psoralens—8-methoxypsoralen, 5-methoxypsoralen

Finally, it is suggested that investigators be complete in identifying equipment and methodology that they employ, in order to reduce some of the confusion that may enter and has already entered the literature on this subject.

17.7 CONCLUSIONS

Years of investigative efforts, along with improved methods of measuring and administering radiation, have brought considerable progress in our understanding of various aspects of phototoxic events. We appear to have identified the major chemical structures that are currently involved in producing phototoxic effects in humans. We also have gained some insight into some of the mechanisms that are involved. Nevertheless, it is always important to be flexible and aware that time may change some of our present apparently well-conceived perceptions, as it often does.

REFERENCES

ALLEN, B. (1983) Benoxaprofen and the skin. *Br. J. Dermatol.* **109**, 361–364.

ALOMAR, A. (1985) Ketoprofen photodermatitis. *Contact Dermatitis.* **12**, 112–113.

CHAPTER 17

ANDERSON, R., EFTYCHIS, H., WEINER, A., and FINDLAY, G. (1987) An in vivo and in vitro investigation of the phototoxic potential of tenoxicam, a new non-steroidal anti-intiammatory agent. *Dermatologica* **175**, 229–234.

BJELLERUP, M. (1986) Medium-wave ultraviolet radiation (UVB) is important in doxycycline photoxicity. *Acta Dermato-Venerol.* **66**, 510–5l4.

BJELLEJUP, M., and LJUNGGREN, B. (1985) Photohemolytic potency of tetracyclines. *J. Invest. Dermatol.* **83**, 179–183.

BJORNBERG, A. (1964) Reactions to light in yellow tattoos from cadmium sulfide. *Arch. Dermatol.* **88**, 267.

CHALMERS, R.J.G., MUSTON, H.L., SRINIVAS, V., and BENNETT, D.H. (1982) High incidence of amiodarone-induced photosensitivity in Northwest England. *Br. Med. J.* **31**, 285–341.

DIFFEY, B.L., and LANGTRY, J. (1989) Phototoxic potential of thiazide diuretics in normal subjects. *Arch. Dermatol.* **125**, 1355–1358.

DIFFEY, B.L., DAYMOND, T.J., and FAIRGREAVES, H. (1983) Phototoxic reactions to piroxicam, naproxen, and tiaprofenic acid. *Br. J. Rheumatol.* **22**: 239–242.

EL MOFTY, A.M. (1948) A preliminary clinical report on the treatment of leukoderma with *Ammi majus*, Linn. *J. R. Egypt Med. Assoc* **31**, 651.

EMMETT, E.A., TAPHORN, B.R., and KOMINSKY, J.R. (1977) Phototoxicity occurring during the manufacture of ultraviolet-cured ink. *Arch. Dermatol.* **113**, 770–775.

EPLING, G., and SIBLEY, M. (1987) Photosensitized lysis of red blood cells by phototoxic antimalarial compounds. *Photochem. Photobiol.* **46**, 39–43.

FROST, P., WEINSTEIN, C.D., and GOMEX, E.C. (l972) Phototoxic potential of minacycline and doxycycline. *Arch. Dermatol.* **105**, 681.

GARDINER, J.S., DICKSON, A., MACLEOD, T.M., and FRAIN-BELL, W. (1974) The investigation of photocontact dermatitis in a dye manufacturing process. *Br. J. Dermatol.* **86**, 264–271.

GENDIMENICO, G.J., and KOCHEVAR, I.E. (l990) A further characterization of acridine-photosensitized inhibition of mast cell degranulation. *Photoderm. Photoimmunol. Photomed.* **7**, 51–55.

HESKEL, N.S., AMON, R.B., STORRS, F., and WHITE, C.R. (1983) Phytophoto-dermatitis due to Ruta graviolens. *Contact Dermatitis* **9**, 278–280.

HJORTH, N., and MOLLER, H. (1976) Phototoxic textile dermatitis (bikini dermatitis). *Arch. Dermatol.* **112**, 1445–1447.

JEANMOUGIN, M., PEDREIO, J., BOUCHET, J., and CIVETTE, J. (1983) Phototoxicity of 5% benzoyl peroxide in man. Evaluation of a new methodology. *Fra-Dermatologica* **167**, 19–23.

JUNTILLA, O. (1976) Allelopathic inhibitors in seeds of *Heracleum laciniatum*. *Physiol. Plant.* **36**, 374–378.

KAIDBEY, K., and MITCHELL, F. (1989) Photosensitizing potential of certain non-steroidal anti-inflammatory agents. *Arch. Dermatol.* **125**, 783–786.

KAVLI, G., MIDELFART, G.V.K., HAUGSBO, S., and PRYTZ, J.O. (1983) Phototoxicity of *Heracleum lacinatum*. *Contact Dermatitis* **9**, 27–32.

KNUDSEN, E.A. (1983) Seasonal variations in the content of phototoxic compounds in the giant hogweed. *Contact Dermatitis* **9**, 281–284.

KOCHEVAR, I. (1989) Photoxicity of non-steroidal and anti-inflammatory drugs. *Arch. Dermatol.* **125**, 824–826.

KOCHEVAR, I., ARMSTRONG, R.B., EINBINDER, J., WALTHER, R.R., and HARBER, L. (1982) Coal tar phototoxicity: Active compounds and action spectra. *Photochem. Photobiol.* **36**, 65–69.

LJUNGGREN, B., and WIRESTRAND, L. (1988) Phototoxic properties of quinine and quinidine: Two quinoline methanol isomers. *Photodermatology* **5**, 133–138.

MAIBACH, H., SAMS, W., and EPSTEIN. J. (1967) Screening for drug toxicity by wavelengths greater than 3100 A. *Arch. Dermatol.* **95**, 12–15.

MARZULLI, F., and MAIBACH, H. (1970) Perfume phototoxicity. *J. Soc. Cosmet. Chem.* **21**, 686–715.

MATHEWS, M.M. (1963) Comparative study of lethal photosensitization of *Sarcina lutea* by 8-methoxypsoralen and by toluidine blue. *J. Bacteriol.* **85**, 322–328.

MEROT, Y., HARMS, M., and SAUVAT, J.H. (1983) Photosensibilization au carpro-fene (Imadyl): Un novel anti-inflammatoire non-steroidien. *Dermatologica* **166**, 301–307.

MOORE D.E., and HEMMENS, V.J. (1982) Photosensitization by antimalarial drugs. *Photochem. Photobiol.* **36**, 71–77.

OPHASWONGSE, S., and MAIBACH, H. (1993) Topical nonsteroidal antiin-flammatory drugs: Allergic and photoallergic contact dermatitis and phototoxicity. *Contact Dermatitis* **29**, 57–64

CHAPTER 17

PARRISH, J.A., FITZPATRICK, T.B., TANNENBAUM, L., and PATHAK, M.A. (1974) Photochemotherapy of psoriasis with oral methoxsalen and longwave ultraviolet light. *N. Engl. J. Med.* **291**, 1207–1211.

PATHAK, M. A. 1974. Phytophotodermatitis. In PATHAK, M.A., HARBER, L., SEIJI, M. and KUKITA, A. (eds) *Sunlight and Man: Normal and abnormal photobiological responses*, Tokyo: University of Tokyo Press.

PEAK, M.J., and VAN DER LEUN, J.C. (1992) Boundary between UVA and UVB. In SHIMA, A., ICHAHASHI, M., FUJIWARA, Y. and TAKEBE, H (eds) *Frontiers of Photobiology*, Int. Congress Series Amsterdam: Elsevier, 425.

PRYZBILLA, B., SCHWAB-PRYZBILLA, V., RUZICKA, T., and RING, J. (1987) Phototoxicity of non-steroidal antiinflammatory drugs demonstrated in vitro by a basophil-histamine-release test. *Photodermatology* **4**, 73–78.

RAPPERSBERGER, K., HONIGSMANN, H., ORTEL, B., TANEW, A., KONRAD, K., and WOLFF, K. (1989) Photosensitivity and hyperpigmentation in Amiodarone-treated patients: Incidence, time-course and recovery. *J. Invest. Dermatol.* **93**, 201–209.

ROUGIER, A., GOLDBERG, A., and MAIBACH, H., (eds) (1994) *In vitro skin toxicology.* New York: M. Liebert.

SPIKES J.D. (1983) Comments on light, light sources and light measurements. In DAYNES, R.A. and SPIKES, J.O. (eds) In *Experimental and clinical photoimmunology*, Vol. 1, Boca Raton, FL. CRC Press, 70–71.

STERN, R.S. (1983) Phototoxic reactions to piroxican and other nonsteroidal antiinflammatory agents. *N. Engl. J. Med.* **309**, 186–187.

STERN, R.S., THIBODEAU L.A., KLINERMAN, R.A., PARRISH, I.A., and FITZPATRICK, T.B. (1979) Risk of cutaneous carcinoma in patients treated with oral methoxsalen photochemotherapy for psoriasis. *N. Engl. J. Med.* **300**, 809–813.

VERBOV, J. (1973) Iatrogenic skin disease. *Br. J. Clin Pract.* **27**, 310–314.

VOLDEN, G., KROKAN, H., KAVLI, G., and MIDELFART, K. (1983) Phototoxic and contact toxic reactions of the exocarp of sweet oranges: A common cause of cheilitis? *Contact Dermatitis* **9**, 201–204.

WEBSTER, G., KAIDBEY, K., and KLIGNIAN, A.M. (1983) Phototoxicity from benoxaprofen: In vivo and in vitro studies. *Plotochem. Photobiol.* **36**, 59–64.

WESTERN, A., VAN CAMP, J., BENSASSON, R., LAND, E., and KOCHEVAR, I. (1987) Involvement of singlet oxygen in the phototoxicity mechanism for a metabolite of piroxicam. *Photochem. Photobiol.* **46**, 469–475.

ZAYNOUN, S., AFTIMOS, B., TENEKJIAN, K., and KURBAN, A. (1981) Berloque dermatitis—A continuing cosmetic problem. *Contact Dermatitis* **7**, 111–116.

Chemically Induced Scleroderma

GLENN G RUSSO

Contents

18.1 Introduction

18.2 Environmental agents

18.3 Occupational agents

18.4 Iatrogenic agents

18.5 Nonprescription drugs

18.1   INTRODUCTION

Exposure to environmental, occupational, and iatrogenic chemicals may sometimes be followed by scleroderma-like clinical findings whose cause and effect relationship is not easily established. This chapter reviews some chemicals that appear to suggest an association between chemical exposure and subsequent symptomatology suggestive of scleroderma.

18.2   ENVIRONMENTAL AGENTS

18.2.1   Toxic oil syndrome

In 1981, an epidermal multisystem disorder with chronic scleroderma-like cutaneous changes was linked with the ingestion of rapeseed oil that was sold as olive oil in Spain. Called the toxic oil syndrome, more than 300 deaths resulted (Phelps and Fleishmajer, 1988). The patients first presented with an acute phase of fever, pneumonitis, adenopathy, nausea, arthralgias, and pruritic exanthems (Martinez-Tello *et al.*, 1982). Eosinophilia was always present. The initial symptoms soon resolved, and an intermediate phase of intense myalgias, edema, and paresthesias of the extremities occurred. Months later, many patients, especially women, had progressive neuromuscular atrophy and paralysis, pulmonary hypertension, sicca syndrome, Raynaud's phenomenon, and alopecia. The pruritic exanthems became sclerotic, leading to a diffuse scleroderma-like picture (Martinez-Tello *et al.*, 1982). The pruritic exanthem resembles those caused by viruses and involved the abdomen, trunk, and limbs, Sometimes there was also an associated erythema multiforme or palpable purpura, Another skin eruption occurred in 10 percent of patients that consisted of yellowish or brownish papules which spared the palms and soles (Iglesias and De Morgas, 1983).

The histopathologic features have been well characterized and are caused by a multiorgan systemic vasculopathy. The chronic dermal lesions showed thickening of the collagen bundles, hyalinization, perivascular inflammation, endothelial swelling, and slight luminal obliteration (Martinez-Tello *et al.*, 1982; Fonsecaea and Soils, 1985). Toxic substances in the oil (e.g., anilides) may stimulate the proliferation of mast cells that thereby interact with fibroblasts and mediate sclerosis (Prestana and Munoz, 1982).

Others have suggested that the progressive vasculopathy primarily stimulates fibrosis, including the sclerotic changes observed clinically (Martinez-Tello *et al.*,

1982). Soon after the initial cases of toxic oil syndrome were reported, more than 3 million liters of oil were seized; however, the causative agent may be persistent in stored oils because it appears to be stable (Phelps and Fleishmajer, 1988). The contaminant found in the toxic oil has been identified as 3-phenylamino-1, 2 propanediol (D'Cruz, 2000).

18.2.2 Hexachlorobenzene

During the outbreaks of porphyria turcica due to accidentally ingested hexachlorobenzene-treated seed grain, patients were also noted to have sclerodermoid changes (Peters *et al.*, 1982: Schmid, 1960: Cripps *et al.*, 1980). It is believed that these sclerodermoid changes may have been due to the production of hyalin stimulated by the deposition of porphyrins in the skin (Cripps *et al.* 1980). The pathogenesis of the sclerodermoid changes in porphyria turcica may be related to the dermal perivascular hyalinization as a residual alteration of the abnormal accumulation of porphyrins (Torinuki *et al.*, 1989). Hexachlorobenzene is no longer produced for use as a fungicide. It is now present only as an unwelcome by-product in the manufacturing of pesticides and hydrocarbons (Burns *et al.*, 1974; Peters *et al.*, 1982). Hexachlorobenzene has a strong tendency to persist in soil and to accumulate in aquatic environments (Isensee *et al.*, 1976).

18.2.3 Urea formaldehyde foam insulation

Urea formaldehyde foam insulation may lead to a scleroderma-like syndrome that has been reported in one case. The patient, shortly after cleaning out the ceiling of his garage, developed Raynaud's phenomenon, arthritis, pulmonary fibrosis, and sclerodermatous skin changes. Dermal fibrosis was noted histologically. It is thought that urea formaldehyde foam insulation may elicit an immunologic response, which, in conjunction with genetic susceptibility, may lead to this syndrome (Rush and Chaiton, 1986). However, as only one case has been reported chance association remains a very likely explanation for its appearance.

18.3   OCCUPATIONAL AGENTS

18.3.1   Vinyl chloride disease

Some workers in the plastics industry, especially those exposed for long periods to the unreacted vinyl chloride monomer while cleaning polymerization reactors, have had a scleroderma-like illness (Meyerson and Meier, 1972). This is characterized by fatigue, Raynaud's phenomenon, shortened fingers with sclerodactyly, distinctive distal phalangeal bone resorption sparing the tufts (acro-osteolysis), facial telangiectasias, and pulmonary and hepatic fibrosis. Angiosarcoma can develop in areas of severe hepatic involvement with the added association of ethanol ingestion. The findings in the skin include plaque-like fibrotic lesions that show thickened dermal collagen histologically with perivascular lymphocytic infiltrates. Endothelial cell swelling has also been seen in the microvasculature (Meyerson and Meier, 1972; Maricq *et al.*, 1976).

Because less than 10 percent of those exposed are susceptible, immuno-genetic factors appear to be additionally important in providing for the capillary pathologic condition that may mediate vinyl chloride disease (Ward *et al.*, 1976). Cellular immune reactivity was decreased, while circulating immune complexes and human leukocyte antigen (HLA) B8 and DR3 frequency were increased in workers who experienced vinyl chloride disease (Meyerson and Meier, 1972; Veltman, 1980; Black *et al.*, 1983).

A genetic susceptibility to developing scleroderma when exposed to vinyl chloride may be a possible reason for the great difference in the reported incidences of the disease in vinyl chloride workers from various countries. For example Czirjak has pointed out that British vinyl chloride workers have a much higher frequency of developing scleroderma compared to Hungarian workers (Czirjak *et al.*, 1995).

The vascular occlusion, in particular, may stimulate new collagen synthesis through ischemia, thus producing fibrosis (Black *et al.*, 1983). However, if the level of exposure to vinyl chloride monomer is reduced in the work place, additional cases of vinyl chloride disease are less likely to occur (Maricq *et al.*, 1976).

18.3.2   Trichloroethylene and perchloroethylene

Chemically similar to vinyl chloride, trichloroethylene and perchloroethylene exposure may also lead to scleroderma-like conditions. Trichloroethylene is used as a degreasing agent which is used in clothes dry-cleaning. Upon exposure to trichloroethylene, a severe irritant contact dermatitis may occur. Characteristic features of the scleroderma like condition produced by trichloroethylene include myalgia, weakness, hepatitis, Raynaud's phenomenon, and sclero-dermoid skin tightening (Sparrow, 1977). Other symptoms which have been reported associated with prolonged trichloroethylene exposure include malabsorption syndrome, pigmentation, gynecomastia, impotency, lymph-adenopathy, peripheral neuropathy and sleepiness (Saihan et al., 1978).

Although one series of workers who developed scleroderma usually involved prolonged exposure to trichloroethylene in the range of 2 to 14 years, one woman reportedly developed acute swelling of her hands and scleroderma after only 2.5 hours of intense exposure to the chemical (Bottomlay et al., 1993). A study by Nietert and associates demonstrated a statistically significant association between organic solvents including trichloroethylene with men who had scleroderma and positivity for antitopoisomerase antibody. This association may have implications concerning the pathogenesis of scleroderma in some patients (Nitert et al., 1993). Trichloroethylene has also been implicated as a cause of localized morphea of the forearm and ankles in a female worker who was exposed to it by inhalation (Czirják et al., 1994).

Skin biopsy in trichloroethylene exposure reveals extensive dermal fibrosis extending into subcutaneous tissue consistent with scleroderma. Although sclerodermoid changes are not pathologically demonstrated in perchloro-ethylene exposure, endothelial swelling and a perivascular infiltrate have been noted (Sparrow, 1977).

The pathogenesis of trichloroethylene and perchloroethylene disease may involve the altering of proteins by these chemicals, providing for an immune response to be manifested in genetically susceptible individuals (Sparrow, 1977; Lockey et al., 1987).

18.3.3   Aromatic hydrocarbon solvents

Aromatic hydrocarbon solvents such as benzene and toluene, which are used for cleaning clothes, painting, and removing oil and grease in industry, have been associated with scleroderma-like features (Walder, 1983). These chemicals predominantly enter the body through vapor inhalation and later produce systemic manifestations. Scleroderma skin changes are limited only to areas of direct contact (Haustein and Ziegler, 1982). Aliphatic hydrocarbons may also produce scleroderma changes through either vapor exposure or direct contact (Yamakage and Ishikawa, 1982). Histologic features are consistent with scleroderma.

18.3.4 Organic solvents

A study of 21 women with systemic scleroderma revealed that eight of them were exposed to organic solvents on an occupational level (Czirják *et al.*, 1987). Other abnormalities reported in these eight patients included: hypofunction of the thyroid gland, delayed-type hypersensitivity to D-penicillamine, antimicro-tubullis antibody, and lupus anticoagulant. This study also reported that there was a slight decrease in OKT4 positive cells in the peripheral blood of the eight affected patients.

A case referent study of 21 cases of scleroderma in the province of Trento, Italy concluded that there was a statistically significant association between organic solvent exposure and the development of scleroderma. The range of exposure time to the solvents was 9 to 38 years (Bovenzi *et al.*, 1995).

The toxicity of aliphatic hydrocarbons was further demonstrated by the induction of skin changes through intraperitoneal injection in mice (Haustein and Ziegler, 1982). Solvents are constituents of paints, varnishes, lacquers, polishes, inks, adhesives, pharmaceutical products, and preservatives. If protective clothing is worn and ventilation is improved, thereby decreasing contact, disease production should be limited (Haustein and Ziegler, 1982).

Another report suggests that prolonged exposure to toluenes, toluidines, xylenes, xylidines, aniline compounds, and ethanolamine and its derivatives produced a syndrome of cold receptivity, restrictive lung defect, peripheral neuropathy, esophageal dysfunction, hypertension, monoclonal paraprotein-emia, and diffuse thickening of the skin and subcutaneous tissue, which spared the hands and feet (Bottomlay *et al.*, 1993).

18.3.5 Epoxy resins

In the early 1980s, six of 233 Japanese workers exposed to the vapor of epoxy resins used in television set transformer production were reported to have experienced fatigue, myalgia, arthralgia, erythema, and skin sclerosis (Yamakage *et al.*, 1980). The cause was ascertained to be the amine known as bis(4-amino-3-methyl-cyclohexyl)methane. Histologically, dense collagen bundles were noted in the lower dermis with superimposed glycosaminoglycan deposits and a perivascular lymphocytic infiltrate. Investigators found the full histologic picture to be more consistent with that of generalized morphea than systemic scleroderma (Yamakage *et al.*, 1980).

Heparan sulfate extracted from the glucosaminoglycans in the skin of these patients induced sclerotic changes in mice, indicating that, perhaps through faulty metabolism, the biogenic amine in eposy resins indirectly elicits the clinical syndrome observed (Ishikawa *et al.*, 1980). Further outbreaks of epoxy resin induced scleroderma have not been reported, indicating that the toxic exposure to this amine may be an incidental finding (Yamakage *et al.*, 1980).

18.3.6 meta-Phenylenediamine

Workers exposed to meta-Phenylenediamine have been reported to develop a systemic sclerosis-like disorder. These workers developed Raynaud's phenomenon, hyperpigmentation, pulmonary fibrosis, and sclerodermatous skin changes (Owens and Medsger, 1988). meta-Phenylenediamine, as a biogenic amine, most likely induces sclerodermatous changes similarly to the epoxy resins. Chemical workers exposed to large quantities appear to be at most risk.

18.3.7 Detergents

One report from Japan suggests that a patient exposed to a commercial detergent containing polyoxyethylene alkyl ether and fatty acid alkanol amide developed Raynaud's phenomenon, joint pain, and decreased ability to close his hands within 3 months after exposure (Tanaka *et al.*, 1993). By 13 months after exposure he had hardening of the skin of his trunk as well. A skin biopsy done 10 months after exposure was consistent with scleroderma.

18.3.8 Silica

Exposure to silica dust, primarily in mining in South Africa, Pennsylvania and Germany, has not been linked with pseudoscleroderma, but with true progressive systemic sclerosis (Rodnan *et al.*, 1967; Reiser and Last, 1979). Symptoms include Raynaud's phenomenon, arthritis, sclerodactyly, and other classic features of scleroderma. Silicotic lung changes frequently precede the scleroderma in those patients who are affected (Rodnan *et al.*, 1967 and Reiser Last, 1979). The pulmonary pathologic condition is consistent with progressive systemic sclerosis showing diffuse alveolar, interstitial, perivascular, and vascular fibrosis (Reiser and Last, 1979).

The role of silica in the pathogenesis of scleroderma is thought to involve the enhancement of fibroblast collagenosis, perhaps by immune adjuvantcy (Rodnan *et al.*, 1967; Reiser and Last, 1979). Whether this stems from macrophage-fibroblast interaction remains debatable.

It has been proposed that the mechanism of action of silica exposure producing progressive systemic sclerosis involves the macrophages engulfing the silica then as the macrophages die the silica is released again. IL-1 is then released which stimulates fibroblasts to increase their production of collagen. This increased collagen production leads to skin sclerosis, vascular occlusion, and fibrosis of the lungs (Yañez *et al.*, 1992). On a basic research level, Haustein and Anderegy have been able to demonstrate that silica when injected into mice can produce changes in fibroblasts and mononuclear cells which are similar to changes seen in the cells in patients with idiopathic scleroderma (Haustein and Anderegy, 1998). Studies have shown that exposure to silica can lead to the production of antinuclear antibodies, immune complexes, and damage to endothelial cells (Rustin *et al.*, 1990). The pathogenicity of silica *in vitro* and *in vivo* is related to its structure, particle size, and concentration, and its association with scleroderma is less well established than its relationship with lung disease (Rodnan *et al.*, 1967; Reiser and Last, 1979). According to investigators, the incidence of progressive systemic sclerosis in Germany is 25 times higher in workplaces where there is exposure to silica and 110 times higher for those patients with silicosis. This indicates that some immunomodulating mechanism may be operating in an adjuvant manner (Rodnan *et al.*, 1967; Reiser and Last, 1979).

A study by McHugh *et al.* demonstrated increased frequency of anti-topoisomerase antibody levels in patients with scleroderma who were exposed to silica (McHugh *et al.*, 1994). Similarly another study (Conrad *et al.*, 1995) showed an increased frequency of positive anticentromere antibody levels in men who developed scleroderma who were exposed to silica. This study also surprisingly demonstrated that there were increased anticentromere antibodies even in men who were exposed to silica at high levels while working in uranium mines and did not develop scleroderma (Conrad *et al.*, 1995).

18.3.9   Pesticides

Sclerodermatous changes have occurred in workers handling pesticides such as chlordane, heptachlor, malathion, parathion DDT, sodium dinitro-*ortho*-cresolate, and 7-chlorocylohexane. Reported patients developed Raynaud's phenomenon and sclerodermatous skin changes, but no internal involvement. Histological features are compatible with scleroderma (Jablonska, 1975).

There is a report of a 58 year old West Indian man who had a 3 month intense exposure to a herbicide which contained bromacil, diuron, and aminotriazole and then developed generalized sclerosis of his skin along with sclerodermatous symptoms of his esophagus and muscles (Dunnill and Black, 1994). The patient suffered particularly from prominent acrosclerosis of his hands which extended up his forearms. It should be noted that aminotriazole has also been reported to produce an allergic contact dermatitis in workers exposed to it (English *et al.*, 1986).

18.4 IATROGENIC AGENTS

There have been several reports of scleroderma developing between 2 and 21 years after silicone breast implantation (Sahn *et al.* 1990). Silicone fluids in breast implants are chemically known as dimethylpolysiloxane. These substances can "bleed" through the silicone envelope into surrounding tissue.

Clinical symptoms include Raynaud's phenomenon, sicca syndrome, pulmonary and gastrointestinal abnormalities, and diffuse skin sclerosis that usually begins in the upper extremities (Lilla and Vistner, 1976; Kumagai *et al.*, 1984; McCoy *et al.*, 1984; Brozenza *et al.*, 1988; Silverstein *et al.*, 1988; Spiera, 1988; McCoy *et al.*, 1989). With injection, breast masses, local erythema, and adenopathy may develop locally (McCoy *et al.*, 1984). Histopathologic examination shows thickening of collagen bundles through the dermis, sclerosis of subcutaneous fat, blood vessel dilatation, and a perivascular lymphocytic infiltrate (Lilla and Vistner, 1976; Kumagai *et al.*, 1984; McCoy *et al.*, 1984; Brozenza *et al.*, 1988; Silverstein *et al.*, 1988; Spiera, 1988; Varga *et al.*, 1989).

It has been proposed that macrophages ingest the silicone and produce silica. The presence of silica would then stimulate a more intense immunologic reaction. This would further stimulate macrophages to release transforming growth factor $-\beta$ and platelet-derived growth factor, which would then stimulate fibroblasts to produce collagen (Sahn *et al.*, 1990). Upon removal of the breast implants, some, but not all, patients show gradual improvement in the edema and firmness of their skin.

18.4.1 Bleomycin and cisplatin

Scleroderma-like changes have been reported in patients with cancers of primary gonadal origin after treatment with bleomycin and cisplatin (Nixon *et al.*, 1981; Finch *et al.*, 1980). Histopathologically, in bleomycin-induced scleroderma, the dermis shows dense collagen with areas of homogenization, particularly associated with endothelial thickening (Cohen *et al.*, 1973).

Many factors may contribute in the development of this iatrogenic syndrome. Bleomycin produces endothelial cell injury by peroxidation of the plasma membrane, which may then initiate fibrosis (Adamson and Bowden, 1974; Burkhardt and Holtje, 1976; Tom and Montgomery, 1980; Mountz *et al.*, 1983). Bleomycin has stimulated collagen synthesis by cultured normal skin fibroblasts, and may induce a lymphoproliferative response *in vitro* (Mountz *et al.*, 1983).

There is a case report describing three patients having been exposed to less than a total of 100 U total of bleomycin, developing Raynaud's phenomenon along with thickening of fingers, periungual erythema, and sclerodactyly all within six months of exposure, some as early as three months after exposure (Kerr and Spiera, 1992).

18.4.2 Pentazocine

Pentazocine, when used as an analgesic, has been linked to the development of diffuse pigmentation changes and sclerotic fibrosis around injection sites, with the formation of large, irregular ulcers (Parks *et al.*, 1971; Swanson *et al.*, 1973; Palestine *et al.*, 1980). On examination of a skin biopsy specimen, there is dermal thickening and fibrosis with an inflammatory cell infiltrate that is granulomatous in areas. Histologic examination also shows both venous and arterial small vessel thrombosis, endarteritis with endothelial hyperplasia, and lymphohistiocytic perivascular inflammation.

Pentazocine-induced fibrosis has been related to vascular ischemia, and the resultant tissue changes to pentazocine-induced vasoconstriction. Because their vasculature is already compromised, patients with diabetes may be more prone to developing these skin changes with the additive effect of pentazocine-induced vasoconstriction (Parks *et al.*, 1971; Swanson *et al.*, 1973; Palestine *et al.*, 1980).

18.4.3 Ethosuximide

Ethosuximide, an anticonvulsant, has been associated with a lupus-scleroderma syndrome in one patient (Teoh and Chan, 1975). Clinical features included fevers, arthritis, malar flush, maculopapular eruption, and widespread skin sclerosis. Histological examination revealed dermal collagen bundles to be homogeneous and hyalinized with a perivascular lymphocytic infiltrate (Teoh and Chan, 1975).

An immunopathogenetic mechanism appears evident in ethosuximide-induced scleroderma with the coincident development of lupus. Connective tissue changes may also be considered when evaluating epileptic patients with rheumatological symptoms, as well as primary connective tissue diseases (Alarcon-Segovia 1969; Teoh and Chan, 1975).

18.4.4 Penicillamine

A teenager with Wilson's disease who was treated with penicillamine developed systemic sclerosis-like lesions. Hyperpigmentation, pulmonary restriction, and proximal scleroderma were also evident (Miyagawa *et al.*, 1987).

Penicillamine has been noted to have connective tissue and autoimmune effects that may involve its relation to the development of a scleroderma like-picture (Fulghum and Katz, 1968; Hasimoto *et al.*, 1981; Walsh, 1981). As penicillamine is utilized as a treatment for progressive systemic sclerosis, its "sclerodermatous" effect is questionable in consideration of this one case.

There has also been a case of morphea-like plaques developing in a patient with rheumatoid type arthritis who had been treated with D-penicillamine at 250 mg/d for 1 year (Bernstein *et al.*, 1981).

18.4.5 Ergot methysergide

Patients with migraine headaches treated with ergot and methysergide have been linked with the development of scleroderma. Clinical manifestations noted included Raynaud's phenomenon, as well as additional features associated with progressive systemic sclerosis. Histological features were also consistent with scleroderma (Robb, 1975).

As similar vasoactive phases are involved in the pathogenesis of migraines and Raynaud's phenomenon, it would seem as though they could be linked. Perhaps ergot and methysergide perpetuate this linkage by mediating vascular hyperreactivity leading to a scleroderma-like condition (Barret and McSharry, 1975; Robb, 1975). Ergot in particular, has been shown to exacerbate Raynaud's phenomenon, and caution may be needed in treating patients with migraine headaches with these medications (Barret and McSharry, 1975; Robb, 1975; Goldberg *et al.*, 1978).

18.5 NONPRESCRIPTION DRUGS

18.5.1 Eosinophilia-myalgia syndrome

First reported in October 1989 by the Centers for Disease Control and now including more than 1500 cases, an association has been made between the ingestion of L-tryptophan and the occurrence of the eosinophilia-myalgia syndrome, which often involves sclerodermoid features (Hertzman *et al.*, 1990: Silver *et al.*, 1990). L-tryptophan is an essential amino acid that is available in dietary supplement form. It is used to treat insomnia, depression, tinnitus, and premenstrual-related symptoms. The eosinophilia-myalgia syndrome is primarily defined by severe, incapacitating myalgias and peripheral eosinophilia (Sternberg *et al.*, 1980; Centers for Disease Control, 1990a, b; Hertzman *et al.*, 1990; Silver *et al.*, 1990; Stutsker *et al.*, 1990; Varga *et al.*, 1990).

Characteristic clinical features also include arthralgias, fevers, dyspnea, edema, and macular exanthems, followed by acrally sparing sclerodermatous induration with a puckered or a peau d'orange appearance (Fishman and Russo, 1991). Eosinophilic fasciitis and papular mucinosis may also be observed (Lin *et al.*, 1992). Raynaud's phenomenon, however, is absent in this condition (Sternberg *et al.*, 1980; Centers for Disease Control, 1990a, b; Hertzman *et al.*, 1990; Silver *et al.*, 1990; Stutsker *et al.*, 1990; Varga *et al.*, 1990). On deep incisional biopsy, dermal thickening and homogenization of collagen bundles with mucin accumulation are seen replacing fat and adnexa. Blood vessel walls show thickening and endothelial swelling, and mast cells and plasma cells may be seen perivascularly and in the dermal infiltrate (Lin *et al.*, 1992). Two additional observations are minimal tissue eosinophilia, despite the extent of peripheral eosinophilia, and minimal myofiber atrophy, regeneration, or necrosis, despite the clinically significant myalgias (Kaufman *et al.*, 1990; Silver *et al.*, 1990; Lin *et al.*, 1992).

The fibrotic effects of L-tryptophan have most often been associated with its role as a precursor in two metabolic pathways: One involves the production of serotonin and the other involves the production of nicotinic acid (Hertzman *et al.*, 1990; Silver *et al.*, 1990). This is supported by the development of cutaneous

■ CHAPTER 18 ■

sclerosis in the carcinoid syndrome in which serotonin is produced in excess (Zarafonetis *et al.*, 1959). The kynurenine pathway leads to the production of nicotinic acid. A patient with progressive systemic sclerosis has been described who had an elevated urinary kynurenine level along with a partial deficiency of kynurenine hydroxylase (Zarafonetis *et al.*, 1959; Conolly *et al.*, 1990). Additionally, in a patient who received L-5-hydroxytryptophan and carbidopa both pathways may have been involved in the production of scleroderma because carbidopa can bind pyridoxal phosphate, which is a necessary co-factor in each pathway (Zarafonetis *et al.*, 1959; Conolly *et al.*, 1990). Isoniazid has been reported to have produced an apparent pyridoxal phosphate deficiency with elevated levels of urinary kynurenine and pellagra, as well as subsequent sclerodermatous changes (McConell and Cheltham, 1952). Some investigators report a possible genetic mechanism for L-tryptophan-induced fibrosis. In situ hybridizations have shown L-tryptophan to enhance expression of the collagen gene resulting in dermal and fascial fibrosis (Price *et al.*, 1967). Mast cells may mediate this interaction (Lin *et al.*, 1992; Conolly *et al.*, 1990). Finally, endothelial changes with associated vascular alterations as observed histologically may induce sclerosis (Lin *et al.*, 1992). Tryptophan is no longer widely available because it was taken off the market in November 1989 by the Food and Drug Administration. Factors such as individual susceptibility and particular preparation contaminants may explain the relatively low incidence of eosinophilia-myalgia syndrome (Centers for Disease Control, 1989). However, recent data appear to implicate a Japanese company that also produces the presumed toxin di-L-tryptophan as the source of the L-tryptophan-producing eosinophilia-myalgia syndrome (Stutsker *et al.*, 1990).

The contaminant responsible for eosinophilia-myalgia syndrome appears to have been 3-(phenylamino) alanine (D'Cruz, 2000). Philen and Hill have pointed out that the contaminants in toxic oil syndrome and eosinophilia-myalgia syndrome are chemically similar and this may explain why the two syndromes produce similar clinical features (Philen and Hill, 1993).

18.5.2 Appetite suppressants

A report out of England has proposed that the appetite suppressants diethylpropion and mazindol may induce sclerosis. Patients had taken appetite suppressants, and subsequently developed Raynaud's phenomenon, arthritis, pulmonary and gastrointestinal symptoms, and sclerodermatous skin changes (Tomlinson and Jayson, 1984). Histological examination was not performed.

The sympathomimetic properties of diethylpropion may lead to vasomotor stress, which leads to Raynaud's phenomenon and other features of skin ischemia. Diethylpropion and mazindol also have serotonergic properties that may play a role in the kynurenine and serotonin metabolism reported in other scleroderma-like conditions (Bourgeois and Aerchliman, 1991).

18.5.3 Cocaine

The association between cocaine abuse and scleroderma was suggested in two male patients (Trozak and Gould, 1984; Kerr, 1989). Common features included Raynaud's phenomenon, acral scarring, and diffuse sclerosis (Trozak and Gould, 1984). A skin biopsy specimen of one of the patients showed dermal thickening and collagen sclerosis.

An association between cocaine use and sclerodermatous changes has also been reported in four other young males (Kilaru and Kim Sequeira, 1991). All cases showed Raynaud's phenomena, sclerodactyly, skin thickening proximal to metacarpal phalangeal joints, and digital scars. It was hypothesized that the vasoconstrictive properties of cocaine may either promote or unmask an underlying propensity for scleroderma. Skin biopsy of one of the four patients demonstrated dermal thickening and collagen sclerosis (Kilaru and Kim Sequeira, 1991).

CHAPTER 18

REFERENCES

ADAMSON, I.Y. and BOWDEN D.H. (1974) The pathogenesis of bleomycin induced pulmonary fibrosis in mice. *Am. J. Pathol.* **77**, 185–198.

ALARCON-SEGOVIA, D. (1969) Drug-induced lupus syndromes. *Mayo Clin. Proc.* **44**, 664–681.

BARRET, A.M. and MCSHARRY, L. (1975) Inhibition of drug-induced anorexia in rats by methysergide. *J. Pharm. Pharmacol.* **27**, 889–895.

BERNSTEIN, R.M., ANN HALL, M. and GOSTELIEU, B.E. (1981) Morphea-like reaction to D-penicillamine therapy. *Ann. Rheum. Dis.* **40**, 42–44.

BLACK, C.M., WALKER, A.E., CATTOGGIOL, J., *et al.* (1983) Genetic susceptibility to scleroderma-like syndrome induced by vinyl chloride. *Lancet* **8**, 53–55.

BOTTOMLAY, W.W., SHEEHAN-DARE, R.A., HUGHES, P. *et al.* (1993) A sclerodermatous syndrome with unusual features following prolonged occupational exposure to organic solvents. *Br. J. Dermatol.* **128**, 203–206.

BOURGEOIS, P. and AERCHLIMANA, A. (1991) Drug-induced scleroderma. *Balliere's Clin. Rheumatol.* **5**, 13–20.

BOVENZI, M., BARBONE F., BETTA, A. *et al.* (1995) Scleroderma and occupational exposure. *Scand. J. Work Environ. Health* **21**, 289–292.

BROZENZA, S.J., FENSKE, N.A., CRUSE, W. *et al.* (1988) Human adjuvant disease following augmentation mammoplasty. *Arch Dermatol.* **124**, 1383–1386.

BURKHARDT, A. and HOLTJE, W.J. (1976) Vascular lesions following perfusion with bleomycin: Electronmicroscopic observations. *Virchows Arch. Dermatol.* **372**, 227–236.

BURNS, J.E., MILLER, F.M., GOMES, E.D. *et al.* (1974) Hexachlorobenzene exposure from contaminated DCPA in vegetable spraymen. *Arch. Environ. Health* **29**, 192–194.

CENTERS FOR DISEASE CONTROL (1989) Eosinophilia-myalgia syndrome and L-tryptophan-containing products—New Mexico, Minnesota, Oregon and New York. *Morbid. Mortal. Weekly Rep.* **38**, 785–788.

CENTERS FOR DISEASE CONTROL (1990a) Eosinophilia-myalgia syndrome—Canada. *Morbid. Mortal. Weekly Rep.* **39**, 327–337.

CENTERS FOR DISEASE CONTROL (1990b) Analysis of L-tryptophan for the etiology of eosinophilia-myalgia syndrome. *Morbid. Mortal. Weekly Rep.* **39**, 589–591.

COHEN, I.S., MOSHER, M.B., O'KEEFE, E.J. *et al.* (1973) Cutaneous toxicity of bleomycin therapy. *Arch. Dermatol.* **107**, 553–555.

CONOLLY, S.M., QUIMBY, S.R. and GRIFFING, W.L. (1990) Scleroderma and L-tryptophan: A possible explanation of the eosinophilia-myalgia syndrome. *J. Am. Acad. Dermatol.* **23**, 451–457.

CONRAD K., STAHNKE, G., LIEDVOGAL B. *et al.* (1995) Anti-CENP-B response in sera of uranium miners exposes to quartz dust and patients with possible development of systemic sclerosis. *J. Rheum.* **22**, 1286–94.

CRIPPS, D.J., GOCMAN, A. and PETERS, H.A. (1980) Porphyria turcica. *Arch. Dermatol.* **116**, 46–50.

CZIRJAK, L., CSIKI, Z., NAGG, Z. *et al.* (1995) Exposure to chemicals and systemic sclerosis (letter). *Ann. Rheum. Dis.* **54**(6), 529.

CZIRJÁK, L., DANKÓ, K., SCHLAMMADINGER, J. *et al.* (1987) Progressive Systemic Sclerosis Occurring in Patients Exposed to Chemicals. *Int. J. Dermatol.* **26**(6), 374–378.

CZIRJÁK, L., PÓCS, E., SZEGEDI, G. (1994) Localized scleroderma after exposure to organic solvents. *Dermatology* **189**, 399–401.

D'CRUZ, D. (2000) Autoimmune diseases associated with drugs, chemicals and environmental factors. *Toxicol. letters* **112–113**, 421–432.

DUNNILL, M.G.S. and BLACK, M. (1994) Sclerodermatous syndrome after occupational exposure to herbicides—response to systemic steroids. *Clin. and Exper. Dermatol.* **19**, 518–520.

ENGLISH, J.S.C., RYCROFT, R.J.G., CALNAN, C.D. (1986) Allergic contact dermatitis from aminotriazole. *Contact Derm.* **14**, 255–256.

FINCH, W.R., RODNAN, G.P., BUCKINGHAM, R.B., *et al.* (1980) Bleomycin induced scleroderma. *J. Rheumatol.* **7**, 651–659.

FISHMAN, S.J. and RUSSO, G. (1991) The toxic pseudosclerodermas. *Int. J. Dermatol.* **30**, 837–842.

FONSECA, E. and SOILS, J. (1985) Mast cells in the skin: Progressive systemic sclerosis and the toxic oil syndrome. *Ann. Intern. Med.* 102, 864–865.

FULGHUM, D.D. and KATZ, R. (1968) Penicillamine for scleroderma. *Arch. Dermatol.* **98**, 51–52.

GOLDBERG, N.C., DUNCAN, S.C. and WINKELMAN, R.K. (1978) Migraine and systemic scleroderma. *Arch. Dermatol.* **114**, 550–551.

HASIMOTO, K., MCEVOY, B. and BELCHER, R. (1981) Ultrastructure of penicillamine induced skin lesions. *J. Am. Acad. Dermatol.* **4**, 300–315.

HAUSTEIN, U.F., ANDEREGY, U. (1998) Silica-induces scleroderma: clinical and experimental aspects. *J. Rheumatol.* **25**, 1917–1926.8.

HAUSTEIN, U.F. and ZIEGLER, V. (1982) Environmentally induced systemic sclerosis-like disorders. *Int. J. Dermatol.* **24**, 147–151.

HERTZMAN, P.A., BLEVINS, W.L. and MAYER, J. (1990) Association of the eosinophilia-myalgia syndrome with the ingestion of tryptophan. *N. Engl. J. Med.* **322**, 869–873.

IGLESIAS, J.L. and DE MORGAS, J.M. (1983) The cutaneous lesions of the Spanish toxic oil syndromes. *J. Am. Acad. Dermatol.* **9**, 159–160.

ISENSEE, A.Z., HOLDEN, E.R., WOOLSEN, E.A. *et al.* (1976) Soil persistence and aquatic bioaccumulation potential of hexachlorobenzene (HCB). *J. Agric. Food Chem.* **24**, 1210–1214.

ISHIKAWA, H., YAMAKAGE, A., KITIBATAKE, M. *et al.* (1980) Detection of sclerosis-inducing glycosaminoglycan in the skin of an amine induced experimental skin sclerosis. *Dermatologica* **161**, 145–157.

CHAPTER 18

JABLONSKA, S., ed. (1975) *Scleroderma and Pseudoscleroderma*. Warsaw: Polish Medical Publishers.

KAUFMAN, L.D., SEIDMAN, R.J., PHILLIPS, M.E. *et al*. (1990) Cutaneous manifestations of the L-tryptophan associated eosinophilia-myalgia syndrome: A spectrum of sclerodermatous skin disease. *J. Am. Acad. Dermatol.* **23**, 1063–1069.

KERR, H.D. (1989) Cocaine and scleroderma. *South. Med. J.* **82**, 1275–1276.

KERR, L.D. and SPIERA, H. (1992) Scleroderma in association with the use of bleomycin: A report of 3 cases. *J. Rheumatol.* **19**, 294–296.

KHAN, M., KAPHALIA, B., PRABHAKAR, B. *et al*. (1995) Trichloroethylene-induced autoimmune response in female MRL+/+mice *Toxicol. Appl. Pharmacol.* **134**, 155–160.

KILARU, P. and KIM SEQUEIRA, W. (1991) Cocaine and scleroderma: Is there an association? *J. Rheumatol.* **18**, 1753–1755.

KUMAGAI, Y., SHIOKAWA, Y., MEDSGER, T.A., Jr. *et al*. (1984) Clinical spectrum of connective tissue disease after cosmetic surgery: Observations on 18 patients and a review of the Japanese literature. *Arthritis Rheum.* **27**, 1–12.

LILLA, J.A. and VISTNER, L.M. (1976) Long-term study of reactions to various silicone breast implants in rabbits. *Plast. Reconstr. Surg.* **57**, 637–640.

LIN, J.D., PHELPS, R.G., GORDON, M.L. *et al*. (1992) Pathological manifestations of the eosinophilia myalgia syndrome: analysis of eleven cases. *Hum. Patrhol.* **23**(4), 429–437.

LOCKEY, J.E., KELLY, C.R. and CANNON, G.W. (1987) Progressive systemic sclerosis associated with exposure to trichlorethylene. *J. Occup. Med.* **29**, 493–496.

MARICQ, H.R., JOHNSON, M.N., WHETSTONE, C.L. *et al*. (1976) Capillary abnormalities in polyvinyl chloride production workers. *J. Am. Med. Assoc.* **236**, 1368–1371.

MARTINEZ-TELLO, F.V., NAVAS-PALACIOS, T.J., RICORY, J.R. *et al*. (1982) Pathology of a new toxic syndrome caused by ingestion of adulterated oil in Spain. *Virchows Arch. Dermatol.* **397**, 261–285.

McHUGH, N.J., WHYTE, J., HARVEY, G. *et al*. (1994) Anti-topoisomerase antibodies in silica associated SSc, a model for immunity *Arthritis Rheum.* **37**, 1198–1205.

McCONELL, R.B. and CHELTHAM, H.D. (1952) Acute pellagra during isoniazid therapy. *Lancet* **2**, 959–960.

McCoy, B.J., Person, P. and Cohen, I.K. (1984) Collagen production and types in fibrous capsules around breast implants. *Plast. Reconstr. Surg.* **73**, 924–927.

Meyerson, L.B. and Meier, G.C. (1972) Cutaneous lesions in acro-osteolysis. *Arch. Dermatol.* **106**, 224–227.

Miyagawa, S., Yoshioka, A., Hatoko, M. *et al.* (1987) Systemic sclerosis-like lesions during long-term penicillamine therapy for Wilson's disease. *Br. J. Dermatol.* **116**, 95–100.

Mountz, J.D., Downs Minor, M.B., Turner, R. *et al.* (1983) Bleomycin induced cutaneous toxicity in the rat: Analysis of histopathology and ultrastructure compared with progressive systemic sclerosis. *Br. J. Dermatol.* **108**, 679–686.

Nietert P.J., Sutherland S.E., Silver R.M. *et al.* (1998) Is Occupational Organic Solvent Exposure a Risk Factor for Scleroderma. *Arthritis Rheum.* **41**, 1111–1118.

Nixon, D.W., Pirozzi, D. and York, R.M. (1981) Dermatologic changes after systemic cancer therapy. *Cutis* **27**, 181–194.

Owens, G.R. and Medsger, T.A., Jr. (1988) Systemic sclerosis secondary to occupational exposure. *Am. J. Med.* **85**, 114–116.

Palestine, R.F., Millns, J.L., Speigel, G.T. *et al.* (1980) Skin manifestations of pentazocine abuse. *J. Am. Acad. Dermatol.* **2**, 47–55.

Parks, D.L., Perry, H.O. and Muller, S.A. (1971) Cutaneous complications of pentazocine injections. *Arch. Dermatol.* **104**, 231–235.

Peters, H.A., Gocmen, A., Crippd, D.J. *et al.* (1982) Epidemiology of hexachloro-benzene-induced porphyria in Turkey. *Arch. Neurol.* **39**, 744–749.

Phelps, R.G. and Fleishmajer, R. (1988) Clinical, pathologic, and immuno-pathologic manifestations of the toxic oil syndrome. *J. Am. Acad. Dermatol.* **18**, 313–324.

Philen, R.M., Hill, R.H., Jr. (1993) 3-(phenylamine) alanine—A link between eosinophilia-myalgia syndrome and toxic oil syndrome? *Mayo Clin. Proc.* **68**, 197–200.

Prestana, A. and Munoz, E. (1982) Anilides and the Spanish toxic oil syndrome. *Nature* **298**, 608.

Price, J.M., Yero, N., Brown, R.R. *et al.* (1967) Tryptophan metabolism a hither-to unreported abnormality occurring in a family. *Arch Dermatol.* **95**, 462–472.

Reiser, K.M. and Last, J.A. (1979) Silicosis and fibrogenesis: Fact and artifact. *Toxicology* **13**, 51–72.

CHAPTER 18

ROBB, L.G. (1975) Severe vasospasm following ergot administration. *West. J. Med.* **123**, 231–235.

RODNAN, G.P., BENEDEK, T.G., MEDSGER, T.A. *et al.* (1967) The association of progressive systemic sclerosis (scleroderma) with coal miner's pneumoconiosis and other forms of silicosis. *Ann. Intern. Med.* **66**, 323–334.

RUSH, P.J. and CHAITON, A. (1986) Scleroderma, renal failure and death associated with exposure to urea formaldehyde foam insulation. *J. Rheumatol.* **13**, 475–476.

RUSTIN, M.H.A., BULL, H.A., ZIEGLER, V. *et al.* (1990) Silica-associated systemic sclerosis is clinically, serologically, and immunologically indistinguishable from idiopathic systemic sclerosis *Br. J. Dermatol.* **123**, 725–734.

SAHN, E.E., GAREN, P.D., SILVER, R.M. *et al.* (1990) Scleroderma following augmentation mammoplasty. *Arch. Dermatol.* **126**(9), 1198–1202.

SAIHAN, E.M., BURTON, J.L., HEATON, K.W. (1978) A new syndrome with pigmentation, scleroderma, gynecomastia, Raynaud's phenomenon and peripheral neuropathy *Br. J. Dermatol.* **99**, 437–440.

SCHMID, R. (1960) Cutaneous porphyrias in Turkey. *N. Engl. J. Med.* **263**, 397–398.

SILVER, R.M., HEYES, M.P. and MAIZE, J.C. (1990) Scleroderma, fascitis, and eosinophilia associated with the ingestion of tryptophan. *N. Engl. J. Med.* **32**, 874–881.

SILVERSTEIN, M.J., HANDEL, N., GAMAGAMI, P. *et al.* (1988) Breast cancer in women after augmentation mammoplasty. *Arch. Surg.* **123**, 681–685.

SPARROW, G.P. (1977) A connective tissue disorder similar to vinyl chloride disease in a patient exposed to perchloroethylene. *Clin. Exp. Dermatol.* **2**, 17–22.

SPIERA, H. (1988) Scleroderma after silicone augmentation mammoplasty. *J. Am. Med. Associ.* **260**, 236–238.

STEEN, V.D. (1999) Occupational Scleroderma. *Curr. Opin. in Rheumatol.* **11**, 490–494.

STERNBERG, E.M., VANWOERT, M.H., YOUNG, S.N. *et al.* (1980) Development of a scleroderma-like illness during therapy with L-5-hydroxytryptophan and carbidopa. *N. Engl. J. Med.* **303**, 782–787.

STUTSKER, L., HOESLY, F.C. and MILLER, L. (1990) Eosinophilia-myalgia syndrome associated with exposure to tryptophan from a single manufacturer. *J. Am. Med. Assoc.* **264**, 213–217.

SWANSON, D.W., WEDDIGE, R.L. and MORSE, R.M. (1973) Hospitalized pentazocine abusers. *Mayo Clin. Proc.* **48**, 85–93.

TANAKA, M., NIIZEKI, H., SHIMIZU, S. *et al.* (1993) Scleroderma after exposure to
domestic detergent LOC^R. *J. Rheumatol.* **20**, 1993–1994.

TEOH, P.C. and CHAN, H.L. (1975) Lupus-scleroderma syndrome induced by
ethosuximide. *Arch. Dis. Child.* **50**, 658–661.

TOM, W.M. and MONTGOMERY, M.R. (1980) Bleomycin toxicity: Alternations in
oxidative metabolism in lung and liver microsomal fractions. *Biochem.
Pharmacol.* **29**, 3239–3244.

TOMLINSON, W. and JAYSON, M.I.V. (1984) Systemic sclerosis after therapy with
appetite suppressants. *J. Rheumatol.* **11**, 254.

TORINUKI, W., KUDOH, K. and TAGAMI, H. (1989) Increased mast cell numbers
in sclerotic skin of porphyria cutanea tarda. *Dermatologica* **178**, 75–78.

TROZAK, D.J. and GOULD, W.M. (1984) Cocaine abuse and connective tissue
disease. *J. Am. Acad. Dermatol.* **10**, 525.

VARGA J., PELTONEN, J., UITTO, J. *et al.* (1990) Development of diffuse fasciitis
with eosinophilia during L-tryptophan treatment: demonstration of elevated
Type I collagen expression in affected tissues. *Ann. Intern. Med.* **112**, 344–351.

VARGA, J., SCHUMACHER, H.R. and JIMENEZ, S.A. (1989) Systemic sclerosis after
augmentation ©mammoplasty with silicone implants. *Ann. Intern. Med.* **111**,
377–383.

VELTMAN, G. (1980) Klinishe befunde und arbeitsmedizinische Aspetkete der
Vinylchlorid-Krankheit. *Dermatol. Monastschr.* **166**, 70–212.

WALDER, B.K. (1983) Do solvents cause scleroderma? *Int. J. Dermatol.* **22**, 157–158.

WALSH, J.M. (1981) Penicillamine and the SLE syndrome. *J. Rheumatol.* **8**, 155.

WARD, A.M., UDNOON, S., WATKINS, J. *et al.* (1976) Immunological mechanisms
in the pathogenesis of vinyl chloride disease. *Br. Med. J.* **1**, 936–938.

YAMAKAGE, A. and ISHIKAWA, H. (1982) Generalized morphea-like scleroderma
occurring in people exposed to organic solvents. *Dermatologica* **165**, 186–193.

YAMAKAGE, A., ISHIKAWA, H., SAITO, Y. *et al.* (1980) Occupational scleroderma-
like disorder occurring in men engaged in the polymerization of epoxy resins.
Dermatologica **161**, 33–44.

YAÑEZ DIAZ, S., MORÁN, M., UNAMUNO, P. *et al.* (1992 Silica and Trichloroethylene—Induced Progressive Systemic Sclerosis. *Dermatology* **184**, 98–102.

ZARAFONETIS, C.J.D., LORBER, S.H. and HANSON, S.M. (1959) Association of
functioning carcinoid syndrome and scleroderma. *Am. J. Med. Sci.* **236**, 1–14.

CHAPTER 18

Chemical Agents that Cause Depigmentation

LESLIE P MCCARTY[†] AND HOWARD I MAIBACH

Contents

19.1   Introduction

19.2   History

19.3   Chemical structures causing depigmentation

19.4   Repigmentation

19.5   Mechanism of action

19.6   Conclusions

[†] With acknowledgments to the late Leslie McCarty.

19.1 INTRODUCTION

Many disorders result in disturbances of pigment formation by the melanocytes (Mosher *et al.*, 1987). Hypomelanosis or a decrease in the formation of the pigment melanin may be caused by many disorders. Leukoderma, derived from the Greek terms, λευκο white + δερμα skin, due to chemical exposure has been associated with several different classes of compounds; most being phenols or thiols. These chemicals are useful as antioxidants and find utility in rubbers and plastics, in foods, and as polymerization inhibitors in monomers. Because of the widespread use of these chemicals, it is important to examine the effects of exposure and the mechanism of depigmentation.

19.2 HISTORY

Occupational leukoderma due to exposure to chemicals was first reported more than 55 years ago (Oliver *et al.*, 1939). The depigmentation, which may resemble vitiligo, was produced by the monobenzyl ether of hydroquinone (MBEH), which translocated from rubber gloves worn by workers. Once it was documented that chemical agents could depigment the skin, it became important to test them for this property, and several laboratory procedures have been developed for this purpose. The methods used for testing depigmenting chemicals have been reviewed previously (Gellin and Maibach, 1987).

19.3 CHEMICAL STRUCTURES CAUSING DEPIGMENTATION

Chemical depigmentation has been associated with a variety of compounds. Most of these materials are phenols or sulthydryl compounds, but divalent metals that bind to melanin have also been implicated. These materials are useful as antioxidants and inhibitors of polymerization. Because of these properties, they are employed in a wide variety of products and can potentially contact many people during manufacture and use. In addition, some of these agents have been applied intentionally for the purpose of lightening hyper-pigmented skin. The structures and acronyms of these materials are shown in Figure 19.1, but catechol (CAT) and phenol have not been included. MBEH has been used to intentionally depigment hyperpigmented skin in humans (Lerner and Fitzpatrick, 1953; Becker and Spencer, 1962). The results were not very satisfactory because the response had wide individual variation. Furthermore,

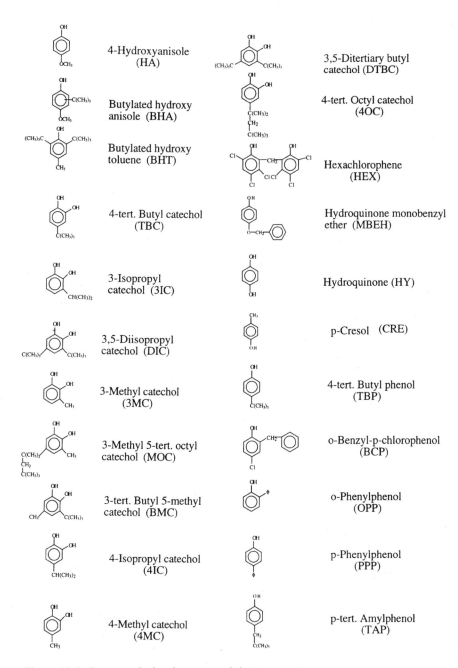

Figure 19.1: Compounds that have caused depigmentation

depigmentation occurred at sites remote from the site of application. There was no depigmentation without some evidence of inflammation. In another study, MBEH was used at 10–33 percent concentration in lotions and ointments, and was deemed to give satisfactory results when used to treat hyperpigmentation in patients (Denton *et al.*, 1952). Bleaching creams containing hydroquinone (HY) have also been reported to cause leukoderma (Fisher. 1982).

Some clinical data have been gathered from exposures to products containing depigmenting chemicals. Some ceramic lacquers contain phenolic compounds (exact structure unidentified), and one case of leukoderma has been reported from exposure to these materials (Tosti *et al.*, 1991). One case of leukoderma from contact with neoprene swim goggles has been reported (Goette, 1984), but the agent responsible was not identified. A case of hypopigmentation due to contact with phototypesetting paper containing *tert*-butyl catechol (TBC) has been described (Fardal and Gurphey, 1983). TBC is also used as an anti-oxidant in industrial lubricants, and workers who come in contact with these experience depigmentation (Gellin *et al.*, 1970). Antioxidants are added to polyethylene film, and these materials can translocate if the film is in contact with skin. Polyethylene film, used as an occlusive dressing during steroid treatment, produced two cases of leukoderma (Vollum, 1971). A case of depigmentation due to adhesive tape was described (Frenk and Kocsis, 1974), but the component in the tape was not identified because the subject refused to be tested with the individual components.

Phenols are a common ingredient in germicidal disinfectants. A study describing five cases of depigmentation in one hospital and seven in another was reported (Kahn, 1970). The antiseptic used for cleaning surfaces in the hospital contained 4.1 percent of *o*-benzyl-*p*-chlorophenol (BCP) and 3 percent 4-*tert*-butylphenol (TBP). In addition, experimental studies were carried out on five volunteers who were tested with 6 percent TBP in 70 percent ethyl alcohol applied to the upper arm under occlusion. Maximal pigment loss occurred at approximately 1 mo, and pigment returned in all subjects about 1 mo later. Another group of subjects was tested with 6 percent hexachlorophene (HEX), *o*-phenyl phenol (OPP), BCP and MBEH, and 1 per cent solitions of *tert*-amyl phenol (TAP) and BCP. Depigmentation was produced in some of the subjects by all materials with the exception of MBEH. MBEH is capable of producing depigmentation as shown by other studies where a 20 percent solution was used (Lemer and Fitzpatrick, 1953; Becker and Spencer, 1962).

Exposure to depigmenting agents can and does occur if proper handling procedures are not practiced during the manufacture. Thirteen cases of

CHAPTER 19

leukoderma have been described in workers in a plant producing OPP and
p-phenyl phenol (PPP) (Ito et al., 1968). Two cases of leukoderma in a plant
producing the monomethyl ether of hydroquinone or 4-hydroxyanisole (HA)
were described, although 169 other men in the same plant were examined and
showed no sign of depigmentation (O'Sullivan and Stevenson, 1981). HA is
used as a stabilizer of vinylidene chloride, and two cases of leukoderma have
been described in a plant where the material was being made (Chivers, 1972).
A plant making TBP had 54 of 198 men with leukoderma; the intensity of the
disorder was related to the degree of exposure (James et al., 1977). A total of nine
cases of leukoderma was seen in two plants engaged in the production of TBP,
butylated hydroxytolutene (BHT), and TBG (Romaguera and Grimalt, 1981).

In addition to the clinical observations, experimental studies have identified
many compounds that cause hypomelanosis. Laundry ink containing p-cresol
(CRE) produced depigmentation in CBA/J mice (Shelly, 1974). Thirty-three
compounds were tested in black guinea pigs (Bleehen et al., 1968). Of these, 12
compounds produced depigmentation to some degree. Those that were very
strong depigmenters were TBC, 4-isopropyl catechol (4IC), 4-methyl catechol
(4MC), and catechol itself (CAT). Some produced definite but moderate
hypopigmentation, among them, 3-isopropyl catechol (3IC), 3,5,-diisopropyl
catechol (DIC), HY, 3-methyl catechol (3MC), and 3-methyl-5-tert-octyl catechol
(MOC). Others produced definite but weak depigmentation: 3-tert-butyl 5-
methyl catechol (BMC), 3,5-ditertiary butyl catechol (DTBC), and 4-tert-octyl
catechol (4OC). Twenty-two additional compounds are listed in Table 19.1;
some produced depigmentation and others did not. It is stated that substitution
in the 4 position confers greater activity than the same substituent in the 3
position; for example, 4-methyl catechol is more potent than 3-methyl catechol.
Some, but not all, compounds containing a sulfhydryl group are capable of
producing depigmentation. β-Mercaptoethylamine hydrochloride (MEA) and
N-(2-mercaptoethyl)-dimethylamine hydrochloride (MEDA) were strong
depigmenting agents. 3-Mercaptopropyl amine hydrochloride and cystamine
hydrochloride are weak to moderate depigmenters. Sulfanilic acid, cystamine,
bis(2-amino-1-propyl)disulfide, 2-(N,N-dimethylamine)ethanethiol S-acetate,
2-mercaptopropylamine hydrochloride, and α-mercaptoacetamide were weak
depigmenters. Another study compared HQ, MEA and MEDA in black guinea
pigs (Pathak et al., 1966). There is not as clear a pattern of structure–activity
relationship among the thiols as there is with the phenols.

Another study on 23 different compounds was carried out in black guinea
pigs and black mice (Gellin et al., 1979). Strong depigmentation was found with

TABLE 19.1:

Compounds tested in black guinea pigs

Compound	Depig-menting potency	Compound	Depig-menting potency
1,2,4-Trihydroxybenzene	0 to ±	2,3,5,6-Tetrahydroxyquinone	0
2-Hydroxy- 1,4-napthoquinone	0	3,4-Dihydroxyphenylacetic acid	0
2,3-Dihydroxybenzoic acid	0	Sulfanilic acid, pH 7	0
Sulfanilic acid, pH 3.9	0	Bis(2-aminoethyl) disulfide or cystamine	0 to ±
Bis(2-amino-1-propyl) disulfide	±	2-Hydroxypyridine	0
β-Mercaptoethylamine hydrochloride (MEA)	± to + +	N-(2-Mercaptoethyl) dimethylamine hydrochloride (MEDA)	± to + +
2-Aminoethanethiol S-acetate	0	2-(N,N-Dimethylamine) ethanethio-S-acetate	±
2-Mercaptoisopropyl amine hydrochloride	0 to ±	Cystamine hydrochloride	± to +
x-Mercaptoacetic acid	0	α-Mercaptoacetamide	0 to ±
2-Ethyl-n-hexyl-diphenylmethylene cyanoacetate	0	1,3-Propane sultone	0
2,3,5,6-Tetrahydroxyquinone	0	3-Hydroxypropane sodium sulfonate	0

Note: From Bleehen *et al.* (1968). Criteria for assessing activity are as follows:
1. No visible depigmentation; skin color similar   0
2. Small spots or speckles of depigmentation   ±
3. Uniform hypopigmentation   +
4. Complete depigmentation   + +

HA, TBG, TAP, and MEBH. Moderate depigmentation was noted with HQ, TBP, phenol, and catechol. They failed to find depigmenting properties when testing butylated hydroxyanisole (BHA), BHT, octyl and propyl gallate, ethoxyquin gum guaiac, diethyl amine, hydrochloride, dilauryl thiodiproprionate, nonyl phenol, *o*-phenyl phenol, *p*-phenyl phenol, octyl phenol, nordihydroguaiarctic acid, and tocopherol. All the last mentioned compounds are used in a wide variety of products with which a large population comes in contact.

19.4   REPIGMENTATION

Repigmentation after exposure to depigmenting agents is highly variable. Aside from individual variation, it is related to the degree and length of exposure to the agent. After application of MBEH for 30 d, repigmentation occurred 1 mo after cessation of application (Denton *et al.*, 1952). After workers ceased wearing rubber gloves containing MBEH, repigmentation commenced but the degree of repigmentation is not stated (Oliver *et al.*, 1939). Black subjects tested with 20 percent or 5 percent MBEH (Lerner and Fitzpatrick, 1953) had one subject who depigmented in 1 mo and repigmentation was complete 2 mo later. A case of depigmentation resulting from rubber swim goggles containing a depigmenting agent gradually repigmented over an 8-wk period after use of the goggles was discontinued (Goette, 1984). MBEH was used to depigment black subjects, and in some, white patches remained after 2 yr and the investigators speculated it might be permanent (Becker and Spencer, 1962). Some subjects tested with TBP repigmented within 6 mo but others remained depigmented after 1 yr (Kahn, 1970). Those areas that depigmented least, repigmented first.

19.5 MECHANISM OF ACTION

The biosynthesis of melanin is a complex process that involves several steps, several of which are still not known. For example, several different protein structures can condense with indole quinone or 5-*S*-cysteinyldopa to give different colored pigments. Some of this is under genetic control and thus is different in individuals as well as species. Some of this process is shown in Figure 19.2. Pigment formation can be disrupted by interference at any of these steps.

Seven mechanisms have been suggested by which the chemical agents could be producing depigmentation (Bleehen *et al.*, 1968):

1   The agent may act selectively on a specific cell. The phenols do structurally resemble some of the intermediates involved in the synthesis of melanin, such as tyrosine or DOPA. Menter (1988) tested eight compounds as substrates for tyrosinase and found all of them to be suitable. Among them were the depigmenting agents TBC, 4MC, HA, and (BHT). The presence of DOPA-melanin enhances the action of tyrosinase on these substrates. It has been suggested that some of these products may act as antimetabolites and lead to degeneration or death of the cell (Lemer, 1971).

2   Chemical agents such as 4IC may react and tie up the active sites of tyrosinase. The molecule does not have the necessary side chain for conversion to the indole quinone and the reaction may bog down at step III in Figure 19.2.

3   The agent can inhibit the melanin formation by blocking the enzymatic oxidation of tyrosine to dopa and the subsequent conversion to melanin.

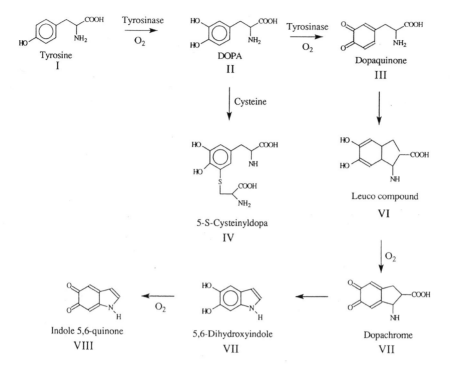

Figure 19.2: Steps in the synthesis of melanin (Lerner and Case, 1959). Indole 5,6-quinone undergoes condensation with proteins to form eumelanins, which are black or brown. The cysteine conjugate, 5-S-cysteinyldopa is further oxidized to a quinoid structure and then is conjugated with proteins to form pheomelanins, which are red or yellow in color.

Tyrosinase activity can be diminished by substrate inhibition and, since several depigmenting agents with a phenolic structure can act as substrates, this may be one mechanism (Menter, 1988; McGuire and Hendee, 1971).

4   The agent can interfere with the biosynthesis of the organelles—premelanosomes and melanosomes. Melanin is a free radical and produces a signal when analyzed by electron spin resonance. The addition of HA to the system changes and increases the signal (Riley, 1970). Free radicals are capable of generating peroxides and disrupting cell and organelle membranes by lipid peroxidation. Investigations by electron microscopy have shown disruption of melanosomes and destruction of membranous organelles in melanocytes (Jimbow *et al.*, 1974).

5   The agent can interfere with the biosynthesis of the protein (e.g., by combining with the melanocytic ribosomes, which appear to be the sites

for tyrosinase synthesis) (Jimbow et al., 1974). This may be another facet of lipid peroxidation.

6   The agent can interfere with the transfer of melanosomes to keratinocytes, either by inhibiting the arborization of melanocytic dendrites or by causing intercellular edema. Irritation plays a role in pigment loss (Gellin et al., 1979; Becker and Spencer, 1962). Irritation is accompanied by edema, so this may be a factor in depigmentation.

7   The agent can chemically alter the melanin present in the melanosomes. Because of the reducing action of some of the thiols, it appears that the dark-colored, oxidized form of melanin could be altered to the lighter-colored, reduced form. Since cysteine can condense with dopa to yield pheomelanins, it may be possible for other thiols to be involved in a similar reaction.

It has also been suggested that depigmenting agents may act as an antigen after increased cellular permeability due to inflammation. An antibody is formed and this stops the formation of melanin granules. If antigen is produced in sufficient quantities, the reticuloendothelial system could respond (Becker and Spencer, 1962). This hypothesis has not been tested but it may explain depigmentation at remote sites (Gellin et al., 1970).

Another mechanism that alters the level of glutathione reductase, which in turn affects the level of the reduced form of glutathione, may involve a change in the type of pigment produced (Yonemoto et al., 1983). Hairless mice treated with TBC showed an increase of the enzyme glutathione reductase. It was suggested that this change increases the level of reduced glutathione and in turn increases the number of pheomelanins, which are lighter in color than eumelanins.

Some important findings have been made using cultures of human melanoma cells (del Marmol et al., 1993). In this study, intracellular glutathione was depleted by treating the cells with buthionine-S-sulfoximine (BSO). Tyrosine hydroxylase activity increased in parallel with glutathione depletion. The effect of thiols on melanogenesis can occur by at least two different mechanisms. First, low-molecular-weight thiol compounds can inhibit melano-genesis by direct interaction of the thiol groups with the tyrosinase active site, thus inhibiting tyrosine hydroxylation. Second, thiol groups are able to react with L-dopaquinone to form dopa-thiol conjugates that are pheomelanogenic precursors.

19.6 CONCLUSIONS

Many chemicals have been identified as depigmenting agents from clinical observations and experimental studies. These agents fall into primarily two categories: phenols and thiols. The most potent phenols are those containing an alkyl substitution in the 4 position. Those that are most irritating to the skin have the greatest potential for depigmentation. The mechanism by which depigmentation occurs is probably related to interference with one or more of the many steps of melanin biosynthesis. It is accompanied by destruction of melanocytes and their organelles. The structure—activity relationship of the thiols is much less defined. The mechanism of action of the thiols may be related to the depletion of glutathione and/or the involvement of the thiol in the place of glutathione in the formation of melanin. Fortunately, experimental methods have been developed to test compounds for depigmenting properties. Once the potential is recognized, proper protective measures can usually be instituted to minimize human exposure. The human is more sensitive than other species, and there is a large variation in sensitivity among individuals.

REFERENCES

BECKER, S.W., and SPENCER, M.C. (1962) Evaluation of monobenzone. *J. Am. Med. Assoc.* **180**, 279–284.

BLEEHEN, S.S., PATHAK, M.A., HORI, Y., and FITZPATRICK, T.B. (1968) Depigmentation of skin with 4-isopropylcatechol, mercaptoamines, and other compounds. *J. Invest. Dermatol.* **50**, 103–117.

CHIVERS, C.P. (1972) Two cases of occupational leucoderma following contact with hydroquinone monomethyl ether. *Br. J. Ind. Med.* **29**, 105–107.

DEL MARMOL, V., SOLANO, F., SELS, A., HUEZ, G., LIBERT, A., LEJEUNE, F., and GHANEM, G. (1993) Glutathione depletion increases tyrosinase activity in human melanoma cells. *J. Invest. Dermatol.* **101**, 871–874.

DENTON, C.R., LERNER, A.B., and FITZPATRICK, T.B. (1952) Inhibition of melanin formation by chemical agents. *J. Invest. Dermatol.* **18**, 119–135.

FARDAL, R.W., and GURPHEY, E.R. (1983) Phototypesetting paper as a cause of allergic contact dermatitis in newspaper production workers. *Cutis* **31**, 509–517.

FISHER, A.A. (1982) Leukoderma from bleaching creams containing 2% hydroquinone. *Contact Dermatitis* **8**, 272–273.

FRENK, E., and KOCSIS, M. (1974) Dépigmentation due à un sparadrap. *Dermatologica* **148**, 276–284.

GELLIN, G.A., and MAIBACH, H.I. (1987) Detection of environmental depigmenting chemicals. In MARZULLI, F.N. AND MAIBACH, H.I. (eds) *Dermatotoxicology.* 3rd ed., Washington, DG: Hemisphere, 497–513.

GELLIN, G., POSSICK, P.A., and DAVIS, I.H. (1970) Occupational depigmentation due to 4-tertiarybuityl catechol (TBC). *J. Occup. Med.* **12**, 386–389.

GELLIN, G.A., MAIBACH, H.I., MISIASZEK, M.H., and RING, M. (1979) Detection of environmental depigmenting substances. *Contact Dermatitis* **5**, 201–213.

GOETTE, D.K. (1984) Raccoon-like periorbital leukoderma from contact with swim goggles. *Contact Dermatitis* **10**, 129–131.

Ito, K., NISHITANI, K., and HARA, I. (1968) A study of cases of leucomelanodermatosis due to phenyl phenol compounds. *Bull. Pharm. Res. Inst.* **76**, 5–13.

JAMES, O., MAYES, R.W., and STEVENSON, C.J. (1977) Occupational vitiligo induced by *p-tert*-butylphenol, a systemic disease? *Lancet* **II**, 1217–1219.

JIMBOW, K., OBATA, H., PATHAK, M.A., and Fitzpatrick, T.B. (1974) Mechanism of depigmentation by hydroquinone. *J. Invest. Dermatol.* **62**, 436–449.

KAHN, G. (1970) Depigmentation caused by phenolic detergent germicides. *Arch. Dermatol.* **102**, 177–187.

LERNER, A.B. (1971) On the etiology of vitiligo and gray hair. *Am. J. Med.* **51**, 141–147.

LERNER, A.B., and CASE, J.D. (1959) Pigment cell regulatory factors. *J. Invest. Dermatol.* **32**, 211–221.

LERNER, A.B., and FITZPATRICK, T.B. (1953) Treatment of melanin hyperpigmentation. *J. Am. Med. Assoc.* **152**, 577–582.

MCGUIRE, J., and HENDEE, .J. (1971) Biochemical basis for depigmentation of skin by phenolic germicides. *J. Invest. Dermatol.* **57**, 256–261.

MENTER, J.M. (1988) Mechanism of occupational leukoderma. NTIS report PB88–247986 11P. Springfield, VA.

MOSHER, D.B., FITZPATRICK, T.B., ORTONNE, J., and HORI, Y. (1987) Disorders of pigmentation. In FITZPATRICK, T., EISEN, A.Z., WOLFF, K., FREEDBERG, I.M. and AUSTEN, K.F. (eds) *Dermatology in General Medicine,* New York: McGraw-Hill, 794–876.

OLIVER, E.A., SCHWARTZ, L., and WARREN, L.H. (1939) Occupational leukoderma *J. Am. Med. Assoc.* **113**, 927–928.

O'SULLIVAN, J.J., and STEVENESON, C.J. (1981) Screening for occupational vitiligo in workers exposed to hydroquinone monomethyl ether and to paratertiary-amyl-phenol. *Br. J. Ind. Med.* **38**, 381–383.

PATHAK, M.A., FRENK, E., Szabó, G., and Fitzpatrick, T.B. (1966) Cutaneous depigmentation. *Clin. Res.* **14**, 272.

RILEY, P.A. (1970) Mechanism of pigment-cell toxicity produced by hydroxy-anisole. *J. Pathol.* **101**, 163–169.

ROMAGUERA, C., and GRIMALT, F. (1981) Occupational leukoderma and contact dermatitis from paratertiarybutylphenol. *Contact Dermatitis* **7**, 159–160.

SHELLY, W.B. (1974) *p*-Cresol: Cause of ink induced hair depigmentation in mice. *Br. J. Dermatol.* **90**, 169–174.

TOSTI, A., GADDONI, G., PIRACCINI, B.M., and DE MARIA, P. (1991) Occupational leukoderma due to phenolic compounds in the ceramics industry? *Contact Dermatitis* **25**, 67–68.

VOLLUM, D.I. (1971) Hypomelanosis from an antioxidant in polyethylene film. *Arch. Dermatol.* **104**, 70–72.

YONEMOTO, K., GELLIN, G.A., EPSTEIN, W.L., and FUKUYAMA, K. (1981) Glutathione reductase activity in skin exposed to 4-tertiary butyl catechol. *Int. Arch. Occup. Environ. Health* **51**, 341–345.

■ CHAPTER 19 ■

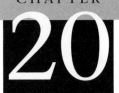

Sulfur Mustard: A Chemical Vesicant Model

FREDERICK R SIDELL, WILLIAM J SMITH,
JOHN P PETRALI, AND CHARLES G HURST

Contents

20.1 Background and military use

20.2 Toxicity

20.3 Biochemical mechanism of sulfur mustard
toxicity

20.4 Histopathology, models, and ultrastructure

20.5 Immunohistochemistry of the mustard skin
lesion

20.6 The mustard gas skin lesion and apoptosis

20.7 Clinical manifestations

20.8 Diagnosis

20.9 Management of skin lesions

20.10 Long-term effects

20.1 BACKGROUND AND MILITARY USE

On July 12, 1917, Allied troops on a battlefield near Ypres, Belgium, began noticing redness on their skin and some redness in and irritation of their eyes. At first they thought they had contacted a disease, but when the skin erythema began turning to blisters they realized that the Germans had used a new chemical agent. Because of its odor, this agent was called "mustard" by the Allies, a name that is still used 85 years later.

Mustard, actually sulfur mustard ((bis (2-chloroethyl)sulfide; 2,2'-dichloro-ethyl sulfide), became the major chemical agent of World War I and despite its late introduction into that conflict caused 75 percent of the US and 80 percent of the British chemical casualties. However, it was not usually lethal as fewer than 3 percent of these casualties died.

Mustard is a vesicant, a substance that produces blisters. Many things around us are vesicants, including energy (sunlight), plants (poison ivy), animals (some sea creatures), and chemicals.

Several decades after WWI other "mustards" were synthesized by replacing the carbon with nitrogen. These were the nitrogen mustards: (HN_1, 2,2"-dichlorotriethylamine; HN_2, bis [2-chloroethyl)] methylamine); and HN_3 (2,2"2"-trichlorotriethylamine). These were found not to be useful for the battlefield, but HN_2 known as Mustargen (Merck and Co. Inc.), became the first cancer chemotherapeutic agent.

Mustard was first synthesized in the early 1800s and was "rediscovered" several times in that century. In the early 1900s Germany recognized its potential as a battlefield agent and used it quite successfully during WWI. The Allies soon followed and by the end of the War both sides had sustained large numbers of casualties from this agent (Medema, 1986)

Since then other countries have used it, most notably by Iraq (versus Iran) and also by Japan (versus China), and by Italy (versus Ethiopia). The US has a large military stockpile of this agent as do other countries. Most casualties from mustard today are among fishermen who accidentally dredge up, mixed with their catch, shells that were dumped in the sea to destroy them (Jorgensen *et al.*, 1985) or occasionally among souvenir hunters on the battlefields of Europe (Ruhl *et al.*, 1994).

The military designation for sulfur mustard is HD or H. HD is the pure or distilled material, and H contains about 20 percent impurities. It has also been called Lost or S-Lost (for Lommell and Steinkopf, two chemists who suggested its use), "yellow cross" (for the German shell markings), and Yperite (from the site of its first) use. Mustard is an oily liquid, not a gas, and has a low volatility. Its molecular weight is 159.08, and it has a specific gravity of 1.27. A vapor density of 5.4 causes it to stay close to the ground. It freezes/melts at 57°F making it unsuitable for cold weather use. It is sometimes mixed with another agent to lower this.

20.2 TOXICITY

A 10 mcg droplet of mustard on the skin will produce a blister. This penetrates the skin quite rapidly and once in the skin it cannot be removed. The amount not absorbed will evaporate within minutes. An amount of 100 mg/kg on the skin is estimated to be lethal. Mustard is absorbed into the skin within minutes, but the clinical manifestations from this do not occur until hours later.

When discussing the vapor or gaseous form of a chemical, the term usually used is a form of the expression Ct, where C is the concentration of the material and t is a time period. In expressing concentration limits in industrial medicine, these terms are usually expressed as parts per million or billion (ppm; ppb) and time as hours. When discussing chemical warfare agents the units are almost always mcg/meter^3 and minutes.

The most sensitive part of the body to most chemical agents is the eye. A Ct of 12–70 has been estimated to be enough to damage the eye (for comparison, a Ct of "tear gas" of 5–10 will cause severe burning in the eyes). The amount of mustard vapor to cause skin redness and blistering varies greatly from one part of the body to another, with moist, warm areas being the most sensitive. The average Ct is about 200. If mustard is inhaled, a Ct of about 1500 will produce death (this is also about the lethal Ct for hydrogen cyanide).

Skin sensitivity varies from one person to another. In a group of people with similar skin pigmentation some were many-fold times more sensitive than others, and people with heavily pigmented skin were less sensitive than lighter skinned people. There is variation between non-human primates. Horses' skin is most sensitive, the skin of the guinea pig and the monkey were least sensitive, and the dog most closely demonstrated the sensitivity of humans (Marshall *et al.*, 1919).

Although it is called a "blister agent," referring to its skin damage, mustard causes severe effects in other organs. As vapor, it damages the eyes of unprotected people, causing mild to severe conjunctivitis, edema of the lids, and severe corneal damage. These effects, like all clinical effects from mustard, become apparent 2 to 24 hours after contact.

When inhaled, mustard damages the mucosa lining the respiratory tract from the nose to the most distal bronchiole, depending on the Ct inhaled. If the amount is small there may be only redness and irritation of the nose, the sinuses, and the pharynx. Larger amounts will cause, progressively, edema and irritation of the larynx, damage to the mucosa of the bronchi, and finally of the smaller airways. This mucosal inflammation may lead to pseudomembrane formation, and these tend to block airways. Again, the initial effects begin after a several hour latent period.

Mustard is most toxic to young cells, and after systemic absorption of mustard through either the lungs or the skin, the mucosa of the gastrointestinal tract and the young cells of the bone marrow are damaged. The former causes fluid loss, which may be massive. The latter stops production of the blood cells, first the white cells then the platelets and red cells. This may lead to a severe pancytopenia and death from sepsis if infection is superimposed. If death occurs, it usually takes place 5 days or more after contact with the agent.

20.3 BIOCHEMICAL MECHANISM OF SULFUR MUSTARD TOXICITY

Sulfur mustard is an alkylating agent with cytotoxic, mutagenic and vesicating potential. Its chemical reactivity is based the ability to undergo internal cyclization of an ethylene group to form a highly reactive episulfonium ion. This reactive electrophile is capable of combining with any of the numerous nucleophilic sites present in macromolecules of cells. The products of these reactions are stable adducts which can modify the normal function of the target macromolecule. Since nucleophilic sites exist in peptides, proteins, RNA, DNA, and membrane components, extensive efforts have been underway to identify the most critical biomolecular reactions leading to mustard injury.

While the chemistry of mustard interactions with cellular components is well defined, the correlation of these interactions with injury has not been made. Over the past few decades, scientists have made major advances in understanding the cellular and biochemical consequences of exposure to mustard and several hypotheses have been put forth to account for the mustard injury.

Three hypotheses, in particular, have been studied for many years and have been extensively reviewed by Papirmeister *et al.* Briefly, these are:

1 The poly(ADP-ribose) polymerase (PARP) hypothesis in which DNA strand breaks, induced by mustard, activate the nuclear enzyme PARP culminating

in metabolic disruption and protease activation in the region of the basal epidermal cells (Papirmeister *et al.*, 1985),

2   The thiol depletion hypothesis presented by Orrenius *et al.* (1987) established that menadione-induced depletion of GSH resulted in loss of protein thiols and inactivation of sulfhydryl-containing enzymes. Included in this class of proteins are the Ca^{++}/Mg^{++}-ATPases which regulate calcium homeostasis. Intracellular Ca^{++} levels would then increase resulting in activation of proteases, phospholipases, and endonucleases which could give rise to the breakdown of membranes, cytoskeleton, and DNA, resulting in cell death. Whitfield (1987) suggested that this mechanism could be activated by mustards and might be the mechanism of mustard injury. Ray *et al.* (1997) extended Whitfield's suggestion by demonstrating, in mustard exposed cells, that Ca^{2+}-activated phospholipase causes arachidonic acid release and membrane fluidity decreases.

3   In the lipid peroxidation hypothesis, (Miccadei *et al.*, 1988; Paulet, 1952) depletion of GSH allows for the formation of toxic oxidants through H_2O_2 dependent mechanisms. The oxiding species thus formed will react with membrane phospholipids to form lipid peroxides, which could in turn lead to membrane alterations and eventual breakdown of cellular membranes.

While data have been obtained for discrete elements of each of these hypotheses, a fully descriptive mechanism of mustard-induced injury has yet to be developed.

Due to the highly reactive nature of mustard, it is conceivable that the injury following tissue exposure to mustards might result from a combination of effects described in the three hypotheses above or from additional changes not yet described. The pathogenic processes seen in skin, lung, or eye may have common biochemical initiating events, but their distinct pathologies suggest that tissue specific effects may dominate once the biochemical insults develop. While much effort is being expended in developing therapeutic interventions that will limit the extent of tissue pathology, the best immediate approaches involve prevention of contact between mustard and tissues and medical procedures that ease patient trauma and discomfort.

While there is great complexity in the cellular and tissue mechanism of toxicity following exposure to mustard, significant strides have been made over the past ten years toward the development of medical countermeasures against the vesicating action of mustard. Today we know a great deal about the changes brought on by mustard and can extend the PARP hypothesis originally

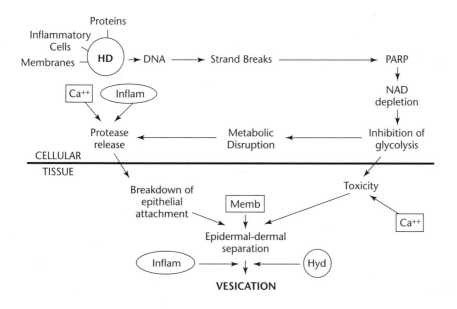

Figure 20.1: Proposed mechanism of HD action.

generated by Papirmeister (1985) to account for cellular and tissue damage to include manifestations of histopathology, as will be described in a later section. The schema shown in Figure 20.1 has been presented in several forums and has been instrumental in identifying several pharmacological approaches to the mustard injury (Table 20.1).

Over the past few years, studies have added to our understanding of the role of inflammation in the presentation of the mustard lesion (Cowan and Broomfield, 1993) the contribution of apoptotic activities to the death process following mustard exposure, (Rosenthal *et al.*, 1998) and novel approaches to

TABLE 20.1:

Strategies for pharmacologic intervention of the HD lesion

Biochemical observation	Pharmacologic strategy	Example
DNA alkylation	Intracellular scavengers	N-acetyl cysteine
DNA strand breaks	Cell cycle inhibitors	Mimosine
PARP activation	PARP inhibitors	Niacinamide
Disruption of calcium	Calcium modulators	Ca^{2+} chelators
Proteolytic activation	Protease inhibitors	Sulfonyl fluorides
Inflammation	Anti-inflammatories	Indomethacin
		Olvanil

therapy for mustard victims. (Wormser *et al.*, 2000). With the world-wide interest in the threat presented by mustard, research will solve the complex secrets of this debilitating agent, and therapies will be developed from that research.

20.4 HISTOPATHOLOGY, MODELS, AND ULTRASTRUCTURE

Human dermal exposure to the chemical warfare agent sulfar mustard results in the delayed formation of fluid-filled bullae, which are incapacitating, persistent and slow to heal. Although the exact pathogenesis of mustard skin toxicity remains investigatively elusive, morphopathological data gathered in controlled animal investigations are providing important clues as to approximate mechanisms. Typically, animal mustard skin histopathology is presented as that occurring during a prevesication period and that of a vesication period. During the first 24 h the pathology involves the latent-lethal targeting of epidermal basal cells, a disabling of hemidesmosomes, and recruitment of inflammatory cells within the dermal vasculature, all beginning 4–6 h post-exposure (prevesication), and at later time periods a progressive inflammatory edema of the lamina lucida contributing to the formation of characteristic lucidolytic microvesicles persisting at the dermal epidermal junction (vesication) (Papirmeister *et al.*, 1984, 1991). Leading contributions to this morphopathological data base have been made through the use of *in vivo* models such as human skin-grafted athymic nude mice, hairless guinea pigs, and *in vitro* systems such as cultured monotypic human cells, organotypic human epidermal models, and isolated perfused porcine skin flaps (Mershon *et al.*, 1990; Petrali *et al.*, 1991; Tyson and Frazier, 1993; Petrali and Oglesby-Megee, 1997) Additional models presently being utilized for mustard study are the domestic weanling pig and the mouse ear.

Recent *in vivo* ultrastructural studies have expanded mustard histopathological investigations to elaborate effects on subcellular entities of the basal cell and basement membrane microenvironment (Moore *et al.*, 1986; Petrali *et al.*, 1991). During prevesication, *in vivo* models persistently present subcellular injury to basal cells to the exclusion of cells of other epidermal strata. These injuries typically presenting at 6 h postexposure include condensation and margination of nuclear chromatin, dilatations of the nuclear envelope, mitochondrial swelling, disabling of desmosomes and hemidesmosomes, tonofilament condensations, widening of intercellular spaces, and plasmalemmal effects. At vesication, the cytopathology progresses to extensive paranuclear and cytoplasmic vacuolations, swollen endoplasmic reticulum, mitochondrial densities, nuclear pyknosis, cellular fragmentation, and necrosis that now involve suprabasal cells and cells of the stratum spinosum. At the dermal–epidermal junction, *in vivo* models generate characteristic microvesicles within the lamina lucida of the basement membrane, beginning at 9–12 h post-exposure. The cavities of microvesicles, formed as a consequence of basal cell pathology and disabling of anchoring filaments of hemidosmosomes, are bound by degenerating basal and epidermal cells at the roof and by the basal lamina of the basement membrane at the floor. Microvesicles rapidly become infiltrated with inflammatory cells, phagocytic cells, degenerating cells, cellular debris, and tissue fluid, all exacerbating the lesion to form pervasive lucidolytic microblisters, which cleave the epidermis from the dermis at later time periods (Figure 20.2). *In vitro* mustard studies utilizing organotypic human epidermal models and isolated perfused porcine skin flaps demonstrate similar basal-cell–epidermal cytopathology and microvesication (Petrali *et al.*, 1993; King and Monteiro-Riviere, 1990).

Ultrastructural studies of monotypic human cells in culture, such as isolated keratinocytes and lymphocytes, have added important subcellular information of mustard temporal effects on nuclei and cytoplasmic organelles, reflecting predicted and expected cellular biochemical lesions associated with mustard toxicity. A suggested and much studied mustard–biochemical lesion cascade involves activation of poly(ADP-ribose) polymerase, reduction of cellular NAD, inhibition of glycolysis, and activation of the hexose monophosphate shunt, which may stimulate release of cellular protease leading to the observed cytopathology (Papirmeister *et al.*, 1985).

20.5 IMMUNOHISTOCHEMISTRY OF THE MUSTARD SKIN LESION

Primary and/or secondary effects of mustard toxicity on specific extracellular components of the epidermal basement membrane microenvironment are being elucidated. Among these extracellular domains are structural adherent proteins known to be antigenically altered or lost to specific antisera in some clinical bullous diseases (Fine, 1987: Mutasin *et al.*, 1989; Heagerty *et al.*, 1986). Taking leads from clinical reports, our laboratory is investigating possible mustard effects on a family of epidermal adherent proteins that, if altered, may contribute to vesication or influence the repair process. Proteins selected for immunohistochemical study were laminin, type IV collagen, bullous

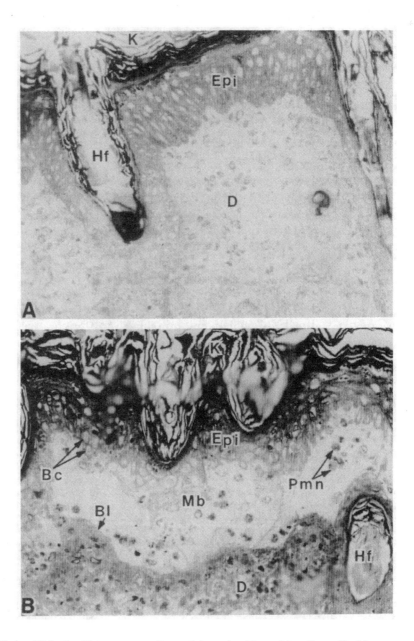

Figure 20.2: Semithin epoxy sections of dermal-epidermal junction of hairless guinea pig skin. (**A**) Nonblistered skin: epidermis (Epi), dermis (D), keratin (K), hair follicle (Hf). (**B**) Microblister cavity (Mb) infiltrated with polymorphonuclear leukocytes (Pmn) and cellular debris. The basel lamina (Bl) forms the floor of the cavity with the roof formed by degenerating basal cells (Bc) of the epidermis. Magnification 330×. From Petrali *et al.* (1990b). Reprinted with permission.

pemphigoid antigen (BPA), anchoring filament protein (GB-3, laminin-5), fibronectin, and desmosomal protein.

Of immediate interest were laminin, type IV collagen, and BPA. Laminin is a major glycoprotein of the lamina lucida and has been used immunohistochemically to anatomically describe and define boundaries of bullous lesions. Type IV collagen is a ubiquitous collagenous protein assigned to the lamina densa of basement membranes. Its immunoreactivity is used to ascertain boundaries and extent of dermal penetration of bullous lesions. BPA and its epitopes (230 kD, 180 kD) have been localized to hemidesmosomes and subadjacent regions of the lamina lucida and, diagnostically, may be absent or faintly localized in bullous diseases. Its role as an autoimmune antigen in the etiology of bullous diseases, especially bullous pemphigoid, is well documented.

To demonstrate mustard effects on basement membrane zone protein antigenicity, hairless guinea pig skin sites, exposed to 10 µl mustard vapor for 8 min, were harvested at selected postexposure times and plunged frozen unfixed into liquid freon. Cryosections were reacted with polyclonal immunoperoxidase antibody sequences appropriate for light and electron microscopic analysis (Petrali *et al.*, 1994). Results demonstrated that, compared to control levels, laminin reactivity was unchanged early during the prevesication phase but became increasingly scanty and lost during vesication. BPA immunoreactivity was suppressed during the first hours of prevesication and remained unreactive to specific antisera through vesication (Figure 20.3). Type IV collagen appeared unaltered to specific antisera throughout the toxicity. The loss of BPA immunoreactivity early during the prevesication period suggests that this protein may be conformationally changed directly by the alkylating effects of mustard. Since the association between altered BPA and bullous pemphigoid lesion is known, it may be predicted that an induced change in antigenicity may subsequently affect its adherent properties as well as promote its candidacy as an autoimmune antigen. Laminin, altered to recognition primarily during the vesication phase, may be responding secondarily to released proteases from toxic basal cells or to cellular chemical mediators of the accompanying inflammatory response, or both. Type IV collagen, remaining immunospecifically intact throughout the time course of the toxicity, correlates with the apparently maintained structural integrity of the lamina densa during the development of mustard vesication, as demonstrated by histopathological and ultrastructural study.

Although these immunohistochemical findings are qualitative and may be peculiar to the hairless guinea pig, results suggest that proteins of the basement

■ CHAPTER 20 ■

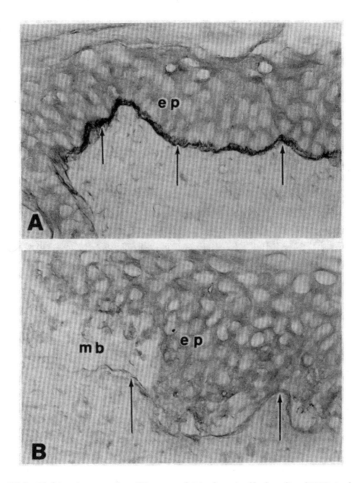

Figure 20.3: Light micrographs of immunohistochemically localized BPA in hairless guinea pig skin. (**A**) Nonexposed control skin with BPA (arrows) localized to the lamina lucida of the basement membrane; epidermis (ep). (**B**) HD-exposed skin with microblister formation (mb) and absence of BPA immunoreactivity (arrows). Magnification 330×. From Petrali *et al.* (1994) Reprinted with permission.

membrane microenvironment are affected during the development of mustard-induced skin pathology. Still to be investigated is the role of this alteration in the pathogenesis of microvesication, its influence on repair mechanisms, and its possible use in diagnostic strategies of mustard toxicity.

20.6   THE MUSTARD GAS SKIN LESION AND APOPTOSIS

Latent-lethal targeting of basal cells is an inevitable consequence of sulfur mustard skin toxicity. Although investigative studies have suggested that basal cell death is associated with cellular biochemical consequences of DNA alkylations, the totality of the cytopathogenesis of toxicity remains elusive especially when addressing mechanisms of selected epidermal basal cell death. Recent ultrastructural and immunohistochemical evidence suggests that induced apoptosis may be a factor. In a time-course study of HD exposure, hairless guinea pig [Crl: IAF(HA)-hrBr] skin sites reacted for *in situ* apoptosis using terminal deoxyribonucleotidyl transferase nick end labeling (TUNEL) immunoassay methods revealed that 18 percent and 59 percent of basal cells were involved in apoptotic pathways at 6 and 12 h postexposure respectively (Kan *et al.*, 2001). In a companion study of HD-induced apoptosis as revealed by an immunoperoxidase in situ oligo ligation procedure considered more distinquishing for cellular apoptosis versus cellular necrosis (ISOL, Intergen Co., Purchase, NY), apoptotic markers were positive in basal cells beginning at 6 h postexposure and remained distinctive up to 12 h postexposure (Petrali *et al.*, 2002; Kan *et al.*, 2003) (Figure 20.4(a) and (b)). In both studies, apoptosis was confirmed by transmission electron microscopy. These studies show that apoptosis is a factor in HD-induced skin cytopathology, with apoptosis occurring early in the toxicity and progressing to necrosis along an apoptotic-necrotic continuum.

20.7   CLINICAL MANIFESTATIONS

The biochemical effects of sulfur mustard begin very soon, seconds to a few minutes, after exposure. Clinical effects, however, are delayed or latent, one of the several characteristics that make it a dangerous warfare agent. After exposure either to vapor or liquid, there is no pain or itching, skin discoloration, or eye irritation, and the exposed person is not warned to take steps for removal. Over the following hours, the burning, itching, and erythema (redness) begin.

Erythema appears in 2–48 hours after exposure of skin to mustard. The onset is shorter and has greater severity with a larger exposure. Effects from liquid exposure appear more rapidly. And, in general, liquid burns are more severe than vapor, but everything depends on time and concentration of exposure, severity. The average time of onset is between 4 and 8 hours. Vesication

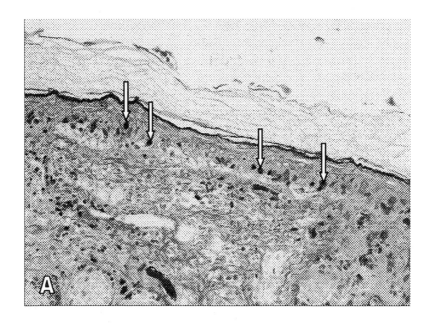

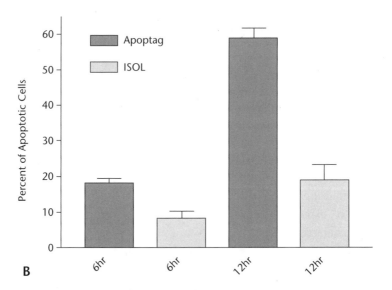

Figure 20.4: (A) HD-exposed hairless guinea pig skin with epidermal basal cells specific for apoptotic markers (arrows). (B) Incidence (percentage) of apoptotic basal cells at selected HD postexposure times.

(blistering) begins several hours after erythema develops, and blistering may not be maximal for several days. A total body skin exposure to mustard vapor may range from that of severe sunburn to life threatening, while a total body liquid skin exposure is certainly life threatening. It all depends on the total dose.

The mildest and earliest form of visible skin injury is erythema, again resembling sunburn, which is usually accompanied by pruritic (itching), burning, or stinging pain. After a small exposure, there may be no further injury. More commonly, small vesicles (blisters) will develop within or on the periphery of the erythematous areas ("string-of-pearls"), and these small vesicles will later coalesce to form central large bullae (blisters).

The typical bulla (blister) is dome-shaped, thin-walled, superficial, translucent, yellowish, and surrounded by erythema. Generally, the bulla is 0.5–5.0 cm in diameter, although it may be larger. The blister fluid is initially thin and clear or slightly straw-colored, and later is yellowish and tends to coagulate (Willems, 1989; Renshaw, 1946; Warthin, 1926). The blister fluid does not contain mustard, is not a vesicant, and presents zero hazards to others (Buscher, 1944; Vedder, 1925, J.R. Keeler, personal communication, 1990). Vapor injury, in general, equates to a first- or second-degree burn, while liquid may produce deeper damage, comparable to a third-degree burn.

After exposure to extremely high doses, such as from liquid, lesions may be characterized by a central zone of coagulation necrosis with blister formation at the periphery. These lesions are of greater severity, take longer to heal, and are more prone to secondary infection than those caused by smaller amounts of mustard (Papirmeister *et al.*, 1991).

The healing time for mustard skin lesions depends on the severity of the lesion. Erythema may heal within several days, whereas severe lesions may require several weeks to several months, depending on the anatomical site, the area of skin surface affected, the depth of the lesion, and whether the lesion was infected (Willems, 1989).

Healing of mustard skin lesions is accompanied by postinflammatory hyperpigmentation, a brownish discoloration. However, at the site of actual vesication, there may be temporary or permanent hypopigmentation from exfoliation of the pigmented layers and destruction of melanocytes (Willems, 1989; Balali-Mood and Navaeian, 1986).

CHAPTER 20

20.8 DIAGNOSIS

The skin lesions of mustard resemble those of another vesicating agent, Lewisite. Also, they may look like those of contact dermatitis from certain plants and animals, other chemicals, and clinical diseases. A history of possible exposure is very important.

The only specific laboratory tests for mustard exposure are experimental. However, studies now standardized by the military have demonstrated the presence of significant amounts of thiodiglycol, a major metabolite of mustard, in the urine of mustard casualties. This was noted in Iranian casualties (Willems *et al.*, 1985, 1988) and in a laboratory worker (Jakubowski *et al.*, 1996).

20.9 MANAGEMENT OF SKIN LESIONS

Since mustard binds so rapidly to tissue components, immediate removal of the agent and deactivation are the only effective means of preventing or decreasing tissue damage. Once the lesion develops, the goals of therapy are to keep the patient comfortable, to keep the lesion clean, and to prevent infection. The pain and itching of erythema might be relieved with a soothing calamine lotion or steroid cream (along with vigilance for secondary infection). Small blisters should be left intact, but larger ones should be unroofed (alternate therapy, sterile needle drainage leaving the blister roof intact). In either case, reddened and denuded areas should be irrigated several times daily, and a topical antibiotic cream or ointment applied liberally. Adequate amounts of systemic analgesics should be given to patients with large burned areas. Significant fluid and electrolyte therapy are required, but systemic fluid replacement is not of the magnitude seen with thermal burns (probably because mustard burns are generally more superficial). Care should be used in fluid administration, for over-hydration has resulted in pulmonary edema (Willems, 1989). Healing is prolonged compared to comparable injuries, and may be followed by pigment changes and scarring proportional to the burn depth. Skin grafting is rarely needed, but was successful in one person with a deep burn (Ruhl *et al.*, 1994).

Recent experimental studies with laser debridement of deep mustard skin wounds followed by skin grafting in weanling pigs (Graham *et al.*, 2002) have shown a significant reduction in healing time (>50 percent), with barrier function, skin color and mechanical properties returning to near-normal levels within 15 days of treatment, along with a return to normal skin architecture (mustard skin burns without debridement do not heal with normal architecture), and very little contraction of the healing area. Partial-thickness laser debridement of these deep wounds without grafting did not produce results as good as those attained through the use of grafts, but was better than no surgical treatment of the wounds.

20.10   LONG-TERM EFFECTS

Skin exposure to mustard may result in areas of hypo- or hyperpigmentation. Scarring may occur, particularly if the wound is deep. Skin cancer may develop in scarred areas (Novick *et al.*, 1977; Treves and Pack, 1930), but there seems to be little evidence that skin cancer follows a single mustard exposure.

A published study from the Institute of Medicine discusses long-term effects in skin and in other organs (Pechura and Rall, 1993).

REFERENCES

BALALI-MOOD, M. and NAVAEIAN, A. (1986) Clinical and paraclinical findings in 233 patients with sulfur mustard poisoning. *Proc. Second World Congress on New Compounds in Biological and Chemical Warfare,* pp. 464–473, Ghent, Belgium.

BUSCHER, H. (1944) *Green and Yellow Cross*. Trans. N. Conway, Cincinnati, OH; Kettering Laboratory of Applied Physiology.

COWAN, F.M. and BROOMFIELD, C.A. (1993) Putative roles of inflammation in the dermatopathology of sulfur mustard. *Cell Biol. and Toxicol.* 9, 201–213.

FINE, J. (1987) Altered skin basement membrane antigenicity in epidermolysis bulosa. *Current Prob. Dermatol.* 17, 111–126.

GRAHAM J.S., SCHOMACKER K.T., GLATTER R.D., BRISCOE C.M., BRAUE E.H. and SQUIBB K.S. (2002) Bioengineering methods employed in the study of wound healing of sulfur mustard burns. *Skin Res. Technol.* 8(1), 57–69.

HEAGERTY, A., KENNEDY, A., GUNNER, D. and EADY, R. (1986) Rapid prenatal diagnosis and exclusion of epidermolysis bullosa using novel antibody probes. *J. Invest. Dermatol.* 86, 603–607

JAKUBOWSKI, E.M., SIDELL, F.R., EVANS, R.A., CARTER, M.A., KEELER, J.R., MCMONAGLE, J.D., SWIFT, A. and DOLZINRE, T.W. (1996) Accidental human sulfur mustard exposure: Verification and uantification by monitoring thiodiglycol levels. *J. Nal. Toxicol.* (in press).

JORGENSEN, B.S., OLESEN, B. and BERNTSEN, O. (1985) Mustard gas accidents on Bornholm. *Ugreskr. Laeg.* **147**, 2251–2254.

KAN, R.K., PLEVA, C.M., HAMILTON, T.A., ANDERSON, D.R. and PETRALI, J.P. (2001) Sulfur mustard induced apoptosis in hairless guinea pig skin. *Proc. Microsc. Microanal.*, **7**(2), 654–655.

KAN, R.K., PLEVA, C.M., HAMILTON, T.A., ANDERSON, D.R. and PETRALI, J.P. (2003) Sulfur mustard-induced apoptosis in hairless guinea pig skin. *Toxicol. Pathol.*, **31**(2), 185–190.

KING, J.R. and MONTEIRO-RIVIERE, N.A. (1990) Cutaneous toxicity of 2-chloro methyl sulfidein isolater perfused porcine skin. *Toxicol. App. Pharmacol.* **104**, 167–179.

MARSHALL, E.K., JR., LYNCH, V. and SMITH, H.W. (1919) On dichlorethylsulphide (mustard gas)II. Variations in susceptibility of the skin to dichlorethylsulphide. *J. Pharmacol. Exp. Ther.* **12**, 91–301.

MEDEMA, J. (1986) Mustard gas. The science of H. *NBC Defense Technol. Int.* **1**(4), 66–71.

MERSHON, M.M., MITCHELTREE, L.W., PETRALI, J.P., BRAUE, E.H. and WADE, J.V. (1990) Hairless guinea pig bioassay models for vesicant skin exposure. *Pharm. Appl. Toxicol.* **15**, 622–630.

MICCADEI, S., KYLE, M.E., GILFOR, D. and FARBER, J.L. (1988) Toxic consequences of the abrupt depletion of glutathione in cultured rat hepatocytes. *Arch. Biochem. Biophys.* **265**, 311–320.

MOORE, K.G., SCHOFIELD, B.H., HIGUCHI, K., KAJIKI, A., AU, K., PULA, P.G., BASSETT, D.B. and DANNENBERG, A.M. (1986) Two sensitive *in vitro* monitors of chemical toxicity to human and animal skin (in short term organ culture). I. Paranuclear vacuolization in glycol methacrylate tissue sections. II. Interface with 14-C-leucine incorporation. *J. Toxicol. Cutan. Ocul. Toxicol.* **5**, 285–301.

MUTASIN, D., MORRISON, L., TAKAHASHI, Y., LABIB, R., SKOUGE, J., DIAZ, L. and ANHALT, G. (1989) Definition of bullous pemphigoid antibody binding to intracellular and extracellular antigen associated with hemodesmosomes. *J. Invest. Dermatol.* **82**, 225–230.

NOVICK, M., GARD, D.H., HARDY, S.B. and SPIRA, M. (1977) Burn scar carcinoma: A review and analysis of 46 cases. *J. Trauma.* **17**, 809–817.

ORRENIUS, S. and NICOTERA, P. (1987) On the role of calcium in chemical toxicity. *Arch Toxicol.* **11**(Suppl.), 11–19.

PAPIRMEISTER, B., GROSS, C. L., PETRALI, J.P. and HIXSON, C.J. (1984) Pathology produced by sulfur mustard in human skin grafts on athymic nude mice. *J. Toxicol. Cutan. Ocul. Toxicol.* **3**, 371–408.

PAPIRMEISTER B., GROSS, C.L., MEIER, H.L., PETRALI, J.P. and JOHNSON, J.B. (1985) Molecular basis for mustard-induced vesication. *Fund Appl. Toxicol.* **5**, S134–S149.

PAPIRMEISTER, B., FEISTER, A.J., ROBINSON, S.I. and FORD, R.D. (1991) *Medical Defense Against Mustard Gas: Toxic mechanisms and pharmacological implications.* Boca Raton FL: CRC Press.

PAULET, G. (1952) Metabolisme cellulaire et action cutanee du sulfure d'ethyle dichlore (yperite). Role devolu au potentiel d'oxydation cellulaire. *CR Seances Soc. Biol.* **146**, 925–928.

PECHURA, C.M. and RALL, D.P. (1993) *Veterans at Risk. The health effects of mustard gas and lewisite.* Washington, DC: National Academy Press.

PETRALI, J.P. and OGLESBY-MEGEE, S. (1997) Toxicity of mustard gas skin lesions. *Micro. Res. Tech.* **37**(3), 221–228.

PETRALI, J.P., OGLESBY, S.B. and MILLS, K.R. (1990) Ultrastructural correlates of sulfur mustard toxicity. *J. Toxicol. Cutan. Ocular Toxicol.* **9**, 193–214.

PETRALI, J.P., OGLESBY, S.B. and JUSTUS, T.A. (1991) Morphological effects of sulfur mustard on a human skin equivalent. *J. Toxicol. Cutan. Ocular Toxicol.* **10**: 315–324.

PETRALI, J.P., OGLESBY, S. B., HAMILTON, T.A. and MILLS, K.R. (1993) Comparative morphology of sulfur mustard effects in the hairless guinea pig and a human skin equivalent. *J. Submicrosc. Cytol. Pathol.* **25**, 113–118.

PETRALI, J.P., OGLESBY, S.B. and HAMILTON, T.A. (1994) Mustard gas skin lesion and bullous pemphigoid antigen. *Proc. 52nd Annual Meeting of the Microscopy Society of America.* New Orleans, LA; pp. 254–255.

PETRALI, J.P., KAN, R.K., HAMILTON, T.A. and PLEVA, C.M. (2002) Morphological expressions of mustard gas-induced lesions: Apoptosis. Proceedings Biomedical Presentations DP21, 23rd Army Science Conference, December 2–5, Orlando, Florida.

RAY, R., LEGERE, R.H. and BROOMFIELD, C.A. (1997) Sulfur mustard-induced decrease in membrane fluidity. *J. Amer. Coll. of Toxicol.* **15**, S2-S8.

RENSHAW, B. (1946) Mechanisms in production of cutaneous injuries by sulfur and nitrogen mustards. In KIMER, W.R. (ed.) *Chemical Warfare Agents and*

Related Chemical Problems. Washington, DC; Government Printing Office, 479–520.

ROSENTHAL, D.S., SIMBULAN-ROSENTHAL, C.M.G., IYER, S., SPOONDE, A., SMITH, W.J., RAY, R. and SMULSON, M.E. (1998) Sulfur mustard induces markers of terminal differentiation and apoptosis in keratinocytes via a Ca^{2+}-calmodulin and caspase-dependent pathway. *J. Invest Dermatol.* **111**, 64–71.

RUHL, C.M., PARK, S.J., DANISA, O., MORGAN, R.F., PAPIRMEISTER, B., SIDELL, F.R., EDLICH, R.F., ANTHONY, L.S. and HIMEI, H.N. (1994) A serious skin sulfur mustard burn from an artillery shell. *J. Emergency Medicine.* **12**, 159–166.

TREVES, N. and PACK, G.T. (1930) Development of cancer in burn scars: Analysis and report of 34 cases. *Surg. Gynecol. Obst.* **51**, 749–782.

TYSON, C.A. and FRAZIER, J.M. (1993) *In vitro* biological systems. *Methods in Toxicology.* 515–524.

VEDDER, E.B. (1925) *The Medical Aspects of Chemical Warfare,* Baltimore, MD: Williams and Wilkins.

WARTHIN, A.S. (1926) Pathologic action of mustard gas (dichlorethylsulphide) In Weed, F.W. (ed.) *The Medical Department of the United States Army in the World War. Vol XIV. Medical aspects of gas warfare,* Washington, DC; Government printing office, 512–661.

WHITFIELD, D.A. (1987) A literature review upon the toxicology, mechanism of action and treatment of sulfur and nitrogen mustard poisoning. Chemical Defence Establishment, Porton, Wilts, CDE Technical Note No. 840.

WILLEMS, J.I., (1989) Clinical management of mustard gas casualties. *Ann. Med. Milit. Belg.* **3**, S1–61

WORMSER, U., SINTOV, A., BRODSKY, B. and NYSKA, A. (2000) Topical iodine preparation as therapy against sulfur mustard-induced skin lesions. *Toxicol. and Appl. Pharmacol.* **169**, 33–39.

Carcinogenesis: Current Trends in Skin Cancer Research

KAREN J AUBORN

Contents

21.1   Introduction

21.2   Susceptibility to skin cancer

21.3   Prevention

21.1   INTRODUCTION

Skin cancer is the most prevalent malignancy in fair skinned people (Diepgen and Mahler, 2002; Ley, 2002). The incidence of both the more common non-melanoma skin cancer (NMSC) and the more lethal cutaneous melanomas continue to increase, reaching epidemic numbers. NMSC accounts for up to one third of all cancers in the United States and in Australia. According to recent population based studies from Australia, the incidence rate is over 2 percent for basal cell carcinomas in males and 1 percent for squamous cell carcinomas. Mortality for NMSC is low. Surgical therapy is highly effective, but recurrence is frequent. Therefore, the associated morbidity is significant to the patient as is the burden on health care system. For melanoma, the American Cancer Society predicted there would be approximately 53,600 new cases in the US during 2002, and 7,400 deaths from melanoma during the same period. In Australia, there are over 50 new cases of melanoma per 100,000. The good news is that among cancers, skin cancer is believed to be one of the most preventable malignancies. Life style risks include ultraviolet radiation (UVR) exposure and diet. These factors can be modulated to decrease risk.

21.2   SUSCEPTIBILITY TO SKIN CANCER

Epidemiology studies and molecular data implicate exposure to ultraviolet radiation (UVR) as the most important etiological factor for risk of skin cancer. While UVR plays a central role, other agents are clearly involved. These include the immune response, certain viral infections, genetic predisposition, and diet. As shown below, these risk factors are not exclusive.

21.2.1   Ultraviolet light radiation

UVR is the carcinogenic factor in sunlight. UVR has been mainly associated as a factor for NMSC, but some role for UVR has been suggested in malignant melanoma (Grossman and Leffell, 1997). Over time, accumulation of mutations induced by UVR contributes to cancer. Most mutations are repaired or damaged cells are removed by apoptosis. However, the additive effects of mutations involved in genes involved in DNA repair, apoptosis, and control of the cell cycle can lead to tumor formation. UVR, like other agents that cause DNA damage, induces expression of the tumor suppressor gene p53, important for DNA repair, and apoptosis in response to DNA damage (Soehnge *et al.*, 1997).

■ CHAPTER 21 ■

It is, therefore, not surprising that many skin cancer cells have mutant p53. Mutations in p53 are present in about 56 percent of basal cell carcinomas (Lacour, 2002). Not only does UVR cause mutations in cellular DNA, but UVR also has profound effects on the cutaneous immune system. In an animal model of UV light-induced skin carcinogenesis, cyclooxygenase-2 was up-regulated by UVR (Fischer, 2002) which would clearly stimulate inflammatory processes (An *et al.*, 2002). Psoralen and ultraviolet A photochemotherapy (PUVA) is associated with a dose-dependent increase in the risk of non-melanoma skin cancer (Studinberg and Weller, 1993). Like ultraviolet B radiation, PUVA is both mutagenic (Nataraj *et al.*, 1997) and immunosuppressive (Ullrich, 1991) and therefore, can be considered a complete carcinogen.

21.2.2 Viruses

More and more evidence suggests that the human papillomaviruses (HPV) may have a role in promoting NMSC. These viruses can affect tumor suppressors such as p53 and retinoblastoma (zur Hausen, 2000). Epidermodysplasia verruciformis, with a papillomavirus etiology, has long been regarded as a model for nonmelonotic skin cancer (Maljewski and Jablonska, 2002). Flat warts occur in individuals with this disease, and cancers develop from lesions on sun-exposed areas. The presence (viral DNA) of a number of lesser-studied types of HPVs occur at a very high frequency in immunocompromised patients, e.g. persons with renal transplants (de Villiers, 1997). These HPVs are also being found in lesions from immunocompetent patients as well (Biliris *et al.*, 2000). Present data indicate that a primary infection occurs in the majority of individuals early in life. The virus remains latent, and prolonged UVR is needed to activate the virus or inactivate cellular genes responsible for controlled cell growth (de Villiers, 1998). Not only has UV light been shown to activate latent papillomaviruses (Amella *et al.*, 1994), but one of the viral proteins (E6) from diverse cutaneous HPV types inhibits apoptosis in response to UVR damage (Jackson and Storey, 2000). Studying HPV in skin cancer has been limited by detection methods. Currently, degenerate PCR methods are identifying many more HPV types and identifying HPV DNA in premalignant and malignant skin lesions (Biliris *et al.*, 2000, Harwood *et al.*, 1999). Consistent with the observations that HPV may be a cofactor for the development of skin cancers, several mouse strains exist with HPV transgenes and serve as models for progressive skin cancer (Arbeit *et al.*, 1994; Kang *et al.*, 2000). Other conditions add to the circumstantial evidence that HPVs are cofactors for skin cancer. The gradual loss of immunity in AIDS increases the cutaneous lesions associated with HPVs in these patients (Milburn *et al.*, 1988), and increases in skin cancers are likely with long-term survivors of AIDS. An analysis of PUVA related benign and malignant lesions found a prevalence of HPV DNA (Weinstock *et al.*, 1995).

21.2.3 Genetic disposition

The fair-skinned Caucasian population pose the greatest risk for skin cancer. Other genetic factors, such as defects in DNA repair, the immune system, or detoxifying enzymes increase risk. For example, the transmission of Epidermo-dysplasia verruciformis (described above) is autosomal recessive, and the disease has the characteristic of decreased cell-mediated immunity (Cooper *et al.*, 1990). Susceptibility loci have been identified (Ramoz *et al.*, 2000). Individuals with functional polymorphisms in the detoxifying enzymes, glutathione-S-transferases (GSTM1 and GSTT1) show enhance sensitivity to sunlight (Kerb *et al.*, 2002), and such polymorphisms occur at high frequency in Caucasians. Moreover, these GST genotypes modulated Hypericum extract (St. John's wort)—induced photosensitization.

21.2.4 Immunity

Renal transplant patients have a well documented risk of increased skin cancer. This increase is 50–100 fold (Birkeland *et al.*, 1995). The cumulative incidence of skin cancer is 27–44 percent after 10–25 years of immunosuppression (London *et al.*, 1995). This increase is concomitant with an increase in cutaneous lesions associated with HPVs; the virus is very often detected in both benign and malignant cutaneous lesions (Blessing *et al.*, 1990; Benton *et al.*, 1992).

21.2.5 Diet

A number of studies, which include animal and human studies, indicate that diet can affect skin cancer risk. A number of studies suggest that a high fat diet may directly or indirectly affect skin cancer. For example, more skin cancers occurred at an accelerated rate in mice with transgenes for HPVs when the mice were given a diet with 20 percent corn oil (Qi *et al.*, 2001). Grape skin and some other food products contain resveratrol, a phytoalexin. In a skin cancer model, it inhibited the development of preneoplastic lesions in a skin cancer model (Jang *et al.*, 1997). This phytochemical is known to act as an antioxidant, induce phase II drug-metabolizing enzymes and inhibit cylooxygenase. Low selenium (a mineral found in garlic and related foods) levels in plasma have been linked to increases risk of non-melanoma skin cancer in humans. In a study of selenium deficiency using UVR induced skin tumors in SKh:HR-hairless mice. Pence *et al.* (1994) showed the correlation between decreased risk with selenium deficiency, and that the deficiency resulted in decreases glutathione peroxidase and increases in superoxide dismutase and catalase. In another study, men with basal cell and squamous cell cancers had lower levels of beta-carotine than controls. On the other hand, high intake of cruciferous vegetables, foods with beta-carotene and vitamin C and fish were associated with a reduced risk (Lamberg, 1998). Support for antioxidants came from a cohort study in Great Britian showing a substantial protective effect for NMSC with Vitamin E (Davies *et al.*, 2002).

21.3 PREVENTION

Chemoprevention of photodamage and thus for photocarcinogenesis has been collectively referred to as photochemoprotection. Sunscreens and educational efforts may be an effective method to reduce UVR-induced photodamage. Additionally, many naturally occurring compounds such as antioxidants present in the diet have potential for human benefit. Fruits, vegetables, and certain beverages boost levels of antioxidants in the body and can serve as scavengers of sunlight-induced free radicals. For example, green tea, which is rich in polyphenolic antioxidants, has been suggested as an adjunct to sunscreen to prevent photodamage and subsequent skin cancer (Almad and Mukhtar, 2001).

A diet low in fat may reduce actinic keratosis and nomelanoma skin cancers. Expanding intervention studies support that a diet with less than 20 percent of total calories is efficacious. Patients in low-fat groups had a significant lower rate of new cancers detected at 2 years (Jaax *et al.*, 1997)

Consistent with animal studies, selenium appears to be beneficial. When a group of patients with a history of basal cell or squamous cell carcinomas were randomized into a group of persons taking 200 mg selenium per day or placebo and followed for six years, the treatment showed a trend but not significance for reducing the incidence of skin cancers. However, the study was stopped because there was a significant reduction of total cancer mortality and total cancer incidence in the selenium group (Clark *et al.*, 1996).

At a meeting of the American Academy of Dermatology (1998), Arbesman reported on the findings from more that 50 animal and human studies and suggested that the studies would support a diet of less than 20 percent calories from fat, five servings of fruit and vegetables, carotine from food equivalent to one and one-half medium carrots, vitamin E supplements, and selenium and vitamin C from food (Lamberg).

Together, studies (from basic science to intervention) support that life style change could dramatically reduce the incidence of skin cancers, particularly the NMSCs.

REFERENCES

ALMAD, N. and MUKHTAR, H. (2001) Cutaneous photochemoprotection by green tea: a brief review, *Skin Pharmacol. Applied Skin Physiol.* **14**, 69–76.

AMELLA, C.A., LOFGREN, L.A., RONN, A.M., NOURI, M., SHIKOWITZ, M.J. and STEINBERG B.M. (1994) Latent infection induced with cottontail rabbit papillomavirus. A model for human papillomavirus latency, *Am. J. Pathol.* **144**, 1167–1171.

AN, K.P., ATHAR, M., TANG, X., KATIYAR, S.K., RUSSO, J., ASZTERBAUM, M., KEPLOVICH, L., EPSTEIN, E.H. JR., MUKHTAR, H. and BICKERS, D.R. (2002) Cyclooxygenase-2 expression in murine and human nonmelanoma skin cancers: implications for therapeutic approaches, *Photochem. Photobiol.* **76**, 73–80.

ARBEIT. J.M., MUNGER, K., HOWLEY, P.M. and HANAHAN, D. (1994) Progressive squamous epithelial neoplasia in K14-human papillomavirus type 16 transgenic mice, *J. Virol.* **68**, 4358–4368.

BENTON, C., SHAHIDULLAH, H. and HUNTER, J.A.A. (1992) Human papillomavirus in the immunosuppressed, *Papillomavirus Rep.* **2**, 23–26.

BILIRIS, K.A., KOUMANTAKIN, E., DOKIANAKIN, D.N., SOURVINOS, G. and SPANDIDOS, D.A. (2000) Human papillomavirus infection of non-melanoma skin cancers in immunocompetent hosts, *Cancer Lett.* **161**, 83–88.

BIRKELAND, S.A., STORM, H.H., LAMM, L.U., BARLOW, L., BLOHME, I., FORSBERG, B., EKLUND, B., FJELDBORG, O., FRIEDBERG, M. and FRODIN, L. (1995) Cancer risk after renal transplantation in the Nordic countries, *Int. J. Cancer* **60**, 183–189.

BLESSING, K., McLAREN, K.M., MORRIS, R., BARR, B.B., BENTON, E.C., ALLOUB, M., BUNNEY, M.H., SMITH, I.W., SMART, G.E. and BIRD, C.C. (1990) Detection of human papillomavirus in skin and genital lesions of renal allograft recipients by in situ hybridization. *Histopathol.* **16**, 181–185.

CLARK, L.C., COMBS, G.F. Jr., TURNBULL, B.W., SLATE, E.H., CHALKER, D.K., CHOW, J., DAVIS, L.S., GLOVER, R.A., GRAHAM, G.F., GROSS, E.G., KRONGRAD, A., LESHER, J.L. Jr., PARK, H.K., SANDERS, B.B. Jr,. SMITH, C.L. and TAYLOR, J.R. (1996) Effects of selenium supplementation for cancer prevention in patients with carcinoma of the skin. A randomized controlled trial. Nutritional Prevention of Cancer Study Group. *J. Am. Med. Assoc.* **276**, 1957–1963.

COOPER, K.D., ANDROPHY, E.J., LOWY, D. and KATZ, S.I. (1990) Antigen presentation and T cell activation in epidermodysphasia verruciformis, *J. Invest. Dermatol.* **94**, 769–776.

DAVIES, T.W., TREASURE, F.P., Welch, A.A. and Day, N.E. (2002) Epidemiology and Health Services Research diet and basal cell cancer: results from the EPIC-Norfolk cohort, *Br. J. Dermatol.* **146**, 1017–1022.

DE VILLIERS, E.M., LAVERGNE, D., MCLAREN, K. and BENTON, E.C. (1997) Prevailing papillomavirus types in non-melanomas of the skin in renal allograft recipients, *Int. J. Cancer* **73**, 356–361.

DE VILLIERS, E.M. (1998) Human papillomavirus infections in skin cancers, *Biomed. Pharmacother.* **52**, 26–33.

DIEPGEN, T.L. and MAHLER, V. (2002) The epidemiology of skin cancer, *Br. J. Dermatol.* **146**(S61), 1–6.

FISCHER, S.M. (2002) Is cyclooxygenase-2 important in skin carcinogensis?', *J. Environ. Pathol. Toxicol. Oncol.* **21**, 183–191.

GROSSMAN, D. and LEFFELL, D.J. (1997) The molecular basis of nonmelanoma skin cancer: new understanding, *Arch. Dermatol.* **133**, 1263–1270.

HARWOOD, C.A., MCGREGOR, J.M., PROBY, C.M. and BREUER, J. (1999) Human papillomavirus and the development of non-melanoma skin cancer, *J. Clin. Pathol.*, **52**, 249–253.

JAAX, S., SCOTT, L.W., WOLF, J.E., THORNBY, J.I and BLACK, H.S. (1997) General guidelines for a low-fat diet effective in the management and prevention of nonmelanoma skin cancer, *J. Nutr. Cancer* **27**, 150–156.

JACKSON, S. and STOREY, A. (2000) E6 proteins from diverse cutaneous HPV types inhibit apoptosis in response to UV damage, *Oncogene* **19**, 592–598.

JANG, M., CAI L., UDEANI, G.O., SLOWING, K.V., THOMAS, C.F., BEECHER, C.W.W., FONG, H.H.S., FARNSWORTH, N.R., KINGHORN, A.D., RAJENDRA, R.G., MOON, R.C. and PEZZUTO, J.M. (1997) Cancer chemopreventive activity of resveratrol, a natural product derived from grapes, *Science* **275**, 218–220.

KANG, J.K., KIM, J.H., LEE, S.H., KIM, D.H., KIM, H. S., LEE, J.E. and SEO, J.S. (2000) Development of spontaneous hyperplastic skin lesions and chemically induced skin papillomas in mice expression human papillomavirus type 16 E6/E7 genes, *Cancer Lett.* **160**, 177–183.

KERB, R., BROCKMOLLER, J., SCHLAGENHAUFER, R., SPENGER, R., ROOTS, I. and BRINKMANN, U. (2002) *Am. J. Pharmacogenomics* **2**, 147–154.

LACOUR, J.P. (2002) Carcinogenesis of basal cell carcinomas: genetics and molecular mechanisms, *Br. J. Dermatol.* **146**(S61), 17–19.

LAMBERG L. (1998) Diet may affect skin cancer prevention, *J. Am. Med. Assoc.* **279**, 1427–1428.

LEY R.D. (2002) Animal models of ultraviolet radiation (UVR)-induced cutaneous melanoma, *Frontiers Bioscience* **7**, D1531–D1534.

LONDON, N.J., FARMERY, S.M., WILL, E.J., DAVISON, A.M. and LODGE, J.P. (1995) Risk of neoplasia in renal transplant patients, *Lancet* **346**, 403–406.

MAJEWSKI, S. and JABLONSKA, S. (2002) Do epidermodysplasia verruciformis human papillomaviruses contribute to malignant and benign epidermal proliferations?, *Archives Dermatol.* **138**, 649–654.

MILBURN, P.B., BRANDSMA, J.L., GOLDSMAN, C.I., TEPLITZ, E.D. and HEILMAN, E.I. (1998) Disseminated warts and evolving squamous cell carcinoma in a patient with acquired immunodeficiency syndrome, *J. Am. Acad. Dermatol.* **19**, 401–405.

NATARAJ, A.J., WOLF, P., CERRONI, L. and ANANTHASWAMY, H.N. (1997) p53 Mutation in squamous cell carcinomas from psoriasis patients treated with psoralen + PVA (PUVA), *J. Am. Acad. Dermatol.* **109**, 238–243.

PENCE, B.C., DELVER, E. and DUNN, D.M. (1994) Effects of dietary selenium on UVB-induced skin carcinogenesis and epidermal antioxidant status, *J. Invest. Dermatol.* **102**, 759–761.

QI, M., CHEN, D-Z., LIU, K. and AUBORN, K.J. (2002) N-6 polyunsaturated fatty acids increase skin but not cervical cancer in HPV 16 transgenic mice, *Cancer Res.* **62**, 433–436.

RAMOZ, N., TAIEB, A., RUEDA, L.A., MONTOYA, L.S., BOUADJAR, B., FAVRE, M. and ORTH, G. (2000) Evidence for a nonallelic heterogeneity of epidermodysplasia verruciformis with two susceptibility loc mapped to chromosome 2p21-p24 and 17q25, *J. Invest. Dermatol.* **114**, 1148–1153.

SOEHNGE, H., OUHTIT, A. and ANANTHASWAMY, O.N. (1997) Mechanisms of induction of skin cancer by UV radiation, *Frontiers Bioscience* **2**, D538–D551.

■ CHAPTER 21 ■

STUDNIBERG, H.M. and WELLER, P. (1993) PUVA, UVB, Psoriasis and non-melanoma skin cancer, *J. Am. Acad. Dermatol.* **29**, 1013–1022.

ULLRICH, S.E. (1991) Systemic immunosuppression of cell-mediated immune reactions by a monofunctional psoralen plus ultraviolet A radiation, *Photodermatol Photoimmunol Photomed.* **8**, 116–122.

WEINSTOCK, M.A., COULTER, S., BATES, J., BOGAARS, H.A., LARSON, P.L. and BURMER, G.C. (1995) Human papillomavirus and widespread cutaneous carcinoma after PUVA photochemotherapy, *Archives Dermatol.* **131**, 701–704.

ZUR HAUSEN, H. (2000) Papillomaviruses causing cancer: Evasion from host-cell control in early events of carcinogenesis, *J. Natl. Cancer Inst.* **92**, 690–698.

Retinoids and Their Mechanisms of Toxicity

WILLIAM J CUNNINGHAM AND GRAEME F BRYCE

Contents

22.1   Introduction

22.2   Retinoid classification

22.3   Basic assumptions

22.4   Variations of system, species, and route of
       delivery

22.5   Retinoid absorption, distribution, metabolism
       and excretion

22.6   Pharmacokinetics of retinoids

22.7   Metabolism of retinoids

22.8   Retinoids and their receptor interactions

22.9   Adverse effects of retinoids

22.10 Summary and conclusions

22.1   INTRODUCTION

Cloning is commonplace and the human genome is elucidated at a rapid pace. We have established a plausible pathogenesis and begun to make significant progress in design and execution of rational treatments for many diseases of the skin. Exciting progress in development of drugs that have immunomodulatory effects on psoriasis has vastly expanded our understanding of the disease itself and clarified many complex mechanisms by which the immune system can be regulated. The question of how drugs work and by what mechanisms they produce toxicity has never been more relevant or capable of solution.

About a half century after the introduction of synthetic retinoids as pharmacological agents and nearly three decades after their amazingly successful and widespread clinical usage in dermatological diseases, our understanding of how this unique class effectively clears severe nodular acne and substantially ameliorates psoriasis is developing but is not complete. The corollary question of how the pronounced side effects of retinoid therapy are ultimately mediated has been at least partially answered by discoveries relative to retinoid receptors.

The topic of toxicity of retinoids is too vast to be fully explored in all details in a single chapter but we can outline the broad and basic issues that need to be fully addressed to understand the complete mechanism of retinoid toxicity.

22.2   RETINOID CLASSIFICATION

Retinoids may be categorized by similarities of their chemical structures, by specific pharmacological effects, by the spectrum of their retinoid receptor binding and by algorithms incorporating elements of all these factors. Irrespective of method of classification, the prototypic vitamin A (retinol) and its biologically essential metabolite all-*trans*-retinoic acid, ATRA, remain the most important references.

The basic chemical structure of the first generation retinoids is similar (Figure 22.1) with a six-membered ionone ring connected to a conjugated, and thus unstable side chain capable of extensive geometric isomerization. Especially noteworthy is the facile interconversion among the trans and cis isomers (13-*cis*- and 9-*cis*-) of retinoic acid. There are however substantial differences in pharmacokinetic and metabolic behavior as well as in receptor binding properties even within this first generation.

The second generation retinoids typified by etretinate and acitretin have aromatic six-membered rings and variable side chains and terminal groups.

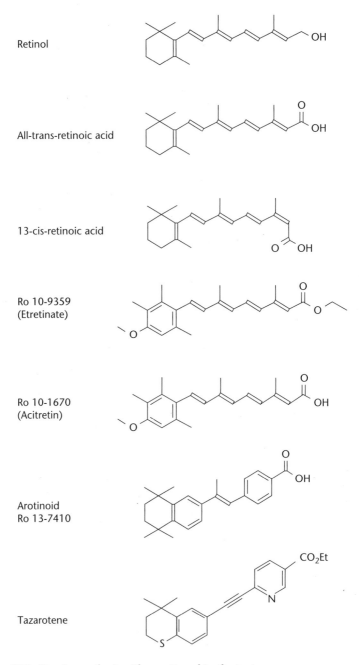

Figure 22.1: Structures of retinoids mentioned in the text.

Removal of the ethyl ester group of etretinate to give the free carboxylic acid acitretin dramatically reduces the elimination half life in humans. The reverse ethyl esterification can be induced to a significant extent by ethanol consumption leading to confusing observations regarding efficacy and side effects in patients.

Third generation retinoids have lost much of the "look" of their ancestors but not all of their "genes." Thus the arotinoids, derived through cyclization of their polyene side chain, manifest differences in receptor binding but frequently have pharmacological effects more in common with first and second generation retinoids than their structures at first glance would predict.

In this review, because of lack of complete data for most compounds, emphasis is placed upon the preponderance of data available for those retinoids whose toxicology and clinical activity have been most studied, especially all-*trans*-retinoic acid (tretinoin) and 13-*cis*-retinoic acid (isotretinoin) where clinical-toxicological correlations might be possible. Caution must be exercised, however, when extrapolating too far from the specific facts relative to any particular molecule.

22.3 BASIC ASSUMPTIONS

A useful hypothesis is that retinoids produce pharmacological effects and cause toxicity within a complicated gestalt involving a number of variously simple to highly complex mechanisms and that their varying kinetic, metabolic, enzyme, and receptor interactions all play a role in the totality or specificity of effect. There is no single and simplistic mechanism which can adequately explain the complexity of all of the potential effects of retinoids, but there are many aspects in each of these interactions which are sufficiently understood to be postulated as part of the totality of retinoid toxicity (Table 22.1). Retinoids are absorbed, bound to plasma proteins, distributed to tissues, bound to cellular receptors and to membrane and cytoplasmic binding proteins, and ultimately exert their effects through binding to specific retinoid receptors and interaction with the specific response elements of the gene to induce or repress transcription for proteins which may function as a structural component, produce a pharmacological action or further regulate other gene transcriptions. Thus several variables may at least indirectly affect overall and specific toxicity and as many aspects of regulation of retinoid ligand-gene interaction are incompletely understood, new facts are likely to require some modifications of the hypothesis.

TABLE 22.1:

Factors possibly affecting retinoid toxicity

- Inherent potential activity of the molecule
- Particulars of system, species, route of delivery
- Rate and extent of absorption
- Pharmacokinetic profile including C_{max}, AUC, time to C_{max}, elimination half life
- Plasma transport, protein carrier binding (including transcription by retinoids for induction of their own carrier proteins)
- Hepatic metabolism, storage, synthesis of metabolizing enzymes and carrier proteins
- Tissue delivery (rate, total amount), CRBP, CRABP binding
- Metabolism by P450 enzymes and P450 induction by prior retinoid administration
- Local control of P450 enzymes especially in embryological development
- RAR, RXR presence, binding affinities and total binding capacity
- Non-specific delivery to nucleus of 13-*cis* with possible intrinsic activity plus isomerization to ATRA
- Ligand-induced binding of RAR/RXR to retinoid response elements of genes with induction or repression of transcription

Furthermore, the difference between a positive and a negative action is not strictly speaking one of pharmacology alone but rather of clinical perception of the difference between pharmacological therapeutic effects and adverse "side" effects. Modification of cohesion of epithelium may thus be beneficial in a patient receiving etretinate for psoriasis of the palms and soles or for several of the epidermal dyskeratoses but appears negative in the context of mucocutaneous adverse effects in a patient receiving isotretinoin for severe acne.

22.4 VARIATIONS OF SYSTEM, SPECIES, AND ROUTE OF DELIVERY

Many observations of retinoid action from *in vitro* systems where cells are rapidly dividing, do not carry over to the *in vivo* situation where cells are growth-limited and influenced by neighboring cells and intracellular matrix. Kinetic and metabolic issues may also prevent correct extrapolation of results to the intact organism.

Retinoids may be inherently active in many species but significant differences in absorption, pharmacokinetics, metabolism and eventual pharmacological effects in the various species may be noted even in the face of similarities in receptor binding.

No more than a percent or two of retinoids applied to human skin penetrates and can access internal systems; thus, toxicity is essentially limited to local effects in most therapeutic situations. This is not at all the case in various other species where significant systemic toxicities can be produced via this route of administration because of excessive dosing and significantly higher rates of skin absorption.

Gastrointestinal absorption of retinoids is highly variable but can reach up to 90 percent absorption under appropriate conditions and thus, highly toxic amounts of retinoids may be systemically delivered by this route in humans and other species. The profound absorption, pharmacokinetic, metabolic, and species differences governing these two delivery routes mandate care in extrapolations across species or routes of delivery.

22.5   RETINOID ABSORPTION, DISTRIBUTION, METABOLISM AND EXCRETION

Retinyl palmitate is the common dietary source of vitamin A and after ingestion is hydrolyzed in the intestine by pancreatic enzymes and absorbed into intestinal cells as retinol. The absorption involves a carrier-mediated process whereby an intestinal absorption cell protein, CRBPII, binds retinol with high affinity and facilitates its uptake. In the intestinal cell, retinol is re-esterified, then incorporated into chylomicrons, and taken up in the lymphatics. A receptor-mediated internalization of chylomicrons occurs in liver hepatocytes where extensive storage of the retinol ester is possible. The entire process of intestinal absorption to hepatic storage is apparently more regulated for retinyl palmitate than for any of the synthetic retinoids.

All retinoids, once in the systemic circulation, are transported by various carrier proteins. The principal plasma protein carrier for retinol is retinol binding protein RBP, which in turn complexes with prealbumin and selectively carries the molecule to its potential sites of action. Both liver storage capacity and carrier protein capacity may be exceeded, resulting in elevations of free retinol and retinyl esters and signs and symptoms of hypervitaminosis A. RBP may be up-regulated by prior retinoid administration.

Other retinoids are carried less specifically by albumin and other serum proteins. As ATRA can be carried nonspecifically and possibly in large quantities after its administration, it may cause widespread and non-specific activity, i.e., toxicity. However, ATRA has also been demonstrated to enter retinal pigment epithelium only when bound to RBP and thus there may be an important and perhaps selective and specific method of its cellular delivery in some instances. This selectivity could also offer some protection from RA-induced retinal toxicity. 13-*cis*-RA may have non-binding protein related and therefore non-specific entry into the nucleus (Nau, 2001).

Thus we see even at the earliest points along the retinoid pathways several possible mechanisms where effect and side effect could be modulated based solely upon differences in absorption and tissue and cellular delivery mechanisms.

22.6 PHARMACOKINETICS OF RETINOIDS

All-*trans*-retinoic acid is variably absorbed and its bioavailability is enhanced with concomitant food intake. Time to maximal plasma concentrations is 1–2 hours and elimination is also rapid with a $T_{1/2}$ of 40 to 60 minutes. In several studies of doses of 45–80 mg/m²/d AUC ranged from 387 µg/L/hr to 682 µg /L/hr (Shapiro and Latriano, 1998)

Isotretinoin is absorbed best when administered with food. A single 80 mg oral dose results in mean maximum blood concentrations of 256 ng/ml with a range of 167–459 ng/ml demonstrating high inter-subject variability at a mean of 3.2 hours with a similar variable range of 1–6 hours. (Wiegand and Chou, 1998). These levels are 100–500 fold higher than mean endogenous levels. The major metabolite is 4-oxo-isotretinoin which concentrations are 87–399 ng/ml at 6–20 hours. Isomerization to the trans isomer also occurs resulting in significant levels of ATRA. The parent compound (mean steady state 160 ng/ml) and metabolites are primarily bound to albumin in the circulation. The terminal elimination of isotretinoin is 10–20 hours and that of the 4-oxo metabolite 17–50 hours. Thus in spite of roughly equivalent plasma concentrations, there is a pronounced up to 20 fold difference in elimination of ATRA or 13-*cis*-RA. This results in a large pool of non-specifically bound and potentially toxic isotretinoin and several active metabolites and isomers within the plasma, even at trough levels between daily doses.

22.7 METABOLISM OF RETINOIDS

All retinoic acids that have been used as therapeutic agents, i.e., all-*trans*-, 13-*cis*-, and 9-*cis*-retinoic acids are metabolized by similar pathways, although there are some differences in the particular set of enzymes involved. Each species is metabolized by cytochrome P450-mediated oxidative reactions first to 4-OH-derivatives and then to 4-oxo-derivatives (Figure 22.2). At both levels of metabolism there is the possibility of interconversion of the geometric isomers.

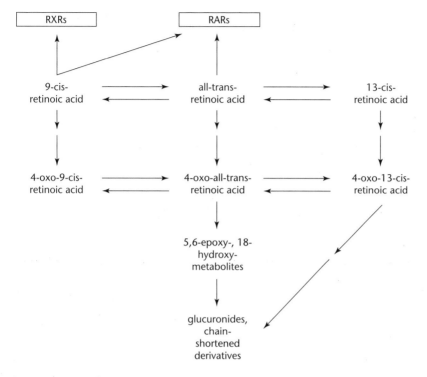

Figure 22.2: Metabolism of retinoic acid.

■

CHAPTER 22

■

The oxidations at the 4-position are, however, irreversible. Many other minor metabolites have been identified such as 5,6-epoxy-tretinoin and 18-OH-tretinoin (Napoli, 1996) but the major metabolites are the geometric isomers and the 4-oxo derivatives which may to some extent, depending on the animal species, be further transformed to water soluble glucuronides. P450 subtypes that have been shown to be significantly involved in the generation of the major metabolite (the 4-oxo derivatives) are 3A4/5, 2B6, 2C8, 2A6. The relative contributions depend on the particular retinoic acid (Marill *et al.*, 2000; Marill *et al.*, 2002). 9-*cis*-Retinoic acid has been shown in rats to be metabolized to 13,14-dihydro-9-*cis*-retinoic acid, its taurine conjugate, and also possibly to chain-shortened derivatives for excretion (Shirley *et al.*, 1996); the β-glucuronide has been identified as a urinary metabolite in humans (Sass *et al.*, 1995).

An inducible enzyme, CYP26, has recently been identified in humans (Ray *et al.*, 1997). Although all isomers of retinoic acid appear to induce its activity, only all-*trans*-retinoic acid is a substrate. The contribution of this enzyme to metabolism relative to those subtypes quoted above has not been assessed.

22.8 RETINOIDS AND THEIR RECEPTOR INTERACTIONS

Volumes have now been written about retinoid receptors, their type, structure, location, and function and it is likely that the majority of retinoid effects are genomic and mediated by the known families of receptors (Mangelsdorf *et al.*, 1995; Chambon, 1996). One long standing paradox has recently been resolved, that is the remarkable activity of 13-*cis*-retinoic acid on sebaceous cells (and hence in acne) despite the fact that, under carefully controlled conditions, it does not bind to RARs (Allenby *et al.*, 1993). However, sebocytes selectively take up 13-*cis*-retinoic acid and convert it to all-*trans*-retinoic acid within the cell where it acts as the proximal ligand (Tsukada *et al.*, 2000). Thus in this instance, 13-*cis*-retinoic acid is a prodrug for all-*trans*-retinoic acid.

Retinoid receptors are members of the large superfamily of nuclear receptors inclusive of corticoid, thyroid, vitamin D and other receptors (Evans, 1988). The two currently characterized and distinct retinoid classes of receptors are termed RAR and RXR. Each class is composed of at least three different subtypes designated alpha, beta, and gamma that are encoded by distinct genes. Retinoids bind to these nuclear receptors to form either homodimers, RXR.RXR, or heterodimers, RAR.RXR which are transcription factors that bind to specific regions of target genes termed retinoid responsive elements (RAREs). This binding causes modulation of gene transcription (Aström *et al.*, 1994). Several hundred genes have been shown to possess RAREs, which helps to explain the pleiotropic nature of retinoid action. Induction or repression of transcription may occur depending on the specifics of the retinoid, its ligand-receptor complex, and the specific RARE of the target gene. Heterodimers can also form between RXR for example and other receptor types such as the vitamin D receptor (VDR).

22.9 ADVERSE EFFECTS OF RETINOIDS

Systemic administration of pharmacologically active doses of retinoids invariably produces side effects. Skin and mucous membrane effects are nearly universal, dyslipidemias very common, bone effects seemingly less frequent and CNS effects, other than headache, uncommon. Teratogenicity is unique in that, unlike the other effects, it is preventable and effects the offspring rather than the mother. Many clinical trials have described the experience with isotretinoin with sufficient numbers of patients to realistically assess adverse event incidence and severity (Strauss *et al.*, 1984; Strauss *et al.*, 2001). The totality of side effects is qualitatively nearly identical to that of hypervitaminosis A.

As detailed above, during therapy with retinoids, levels of parent drug and metabolites are achieved which may be several hundred-fold those measured when vitamin A is administered in doses appropriate for a vitamin. Second, these levels are maintained throughout the dosing cycles by long half-lives. Third, other than retinol, other retinoids are non-specifically carried in plasma and may or may not be delivered through cells to the nucleus by specific and potentially regulating CRBP or CRABP proteins.

The reasons for this invariable toxicity are several. Can one mechanism be postulated to account for the diverse effects in all these different organ systems? We will elaborate details in several important areas of retinoid toxicity which are particularly well studied and clinically relevant i.e. mucocutaneous, dyslipidemia, teratogenicity, bone, and CNS.

22.9.1 Mucocutaneous toxicity

Mucocutaneous adverse events are nearly ubiquitous and invariable in humans receiving systemic, therapeutic doses of most retinoids and, as with other adverse events, resemble those of hypervitaminosis A. The signs and symptoms are predominantly and primarily those of "dry" skin, eyes, lips, and other external mucosal interfaces. These effects and their secondary manifestations are the result of the profound modulations of epidermal growth and differentiation produced by retinoid administration.

Some of the elucidation of retinoid effect on cellular differentiation has utilized human skin equivalents which systems correlate well with *in vivo* human epidermis (Bernard, 2002). In this study, 475 skin-related genes were analyzed comparing gene expression patterns. In the skin equivalent system, more than 40 genes were significantly modified by ATRA, 9-*cis* RA, all-*trans*-retinol, or tretinoin-containing cream with decrease in gene expression for a number of cytokeratins, cornified envelope precursors, integrins, components of desmosomes, hemi-desmosomes, and of the epidermal basement membrane. Also demonstrated was transcriptional upregulation for keratins 9 and 19, autocrine and paracrine growth factors, calmodulins, interleukin-1 alpha, other IL-1 related markers, and type II IL-1 receptor.

Extensive work with a third generation retinoid, tazarotene in psoriasis has shown that this molecule, in psoriatic lesions, skin equivalents, and keratinocyte cultures downregulates epidermal differentiation markers such as transglutaminase-K, MRP-8, SKALP, involucrin, small proline rich protein 2 (Spr-2), and keratins 6, and 16 (Duvic *et al.*, 1997). Furthermore, it upregulates markers of anti-proliferation such as TIG1, TIG2, and TIG3 and additionally down regulates markers of cell proliferation such as EGF-R, AP1 activity and ODC.

The sum of these retinoid-mediated genetically determined transcriptional effects at the morphological and functional levels of the epidermis is a profound effect on epithelial differentiation manifested by decreased cell to cell adhesion by desmosomal decrease, disruption of cell envelope formation and changes in keratin patterns. These changes produce abnormalities of barrier function and decreased stratum corneum cohesion and are the immediate cause of the major primary and secondary toxicological manifestations i.e., of signs and symptoms of dry skin, lips, eyes and other mucosae, skin irritation, slippery skin, etc.

22.9.2 Dyslipidemias

Although the true toxicity of dyslipidemias is not the elevation or decrease of specific lipids *per se* but rather the long-term consequences of the perturbation measured primarily by cardiovascular pathology, in no other of the retinoid toxicities is the undesirable effect as easily quantitated in frequency and magnitude as in that of abnormalities of lipid metabolism. Furthermore there is in these a single end point easily measured by a simple blood test, a large clinical population already studied for the perturbation and to some extent the long-term effect, and importantly a significant degree of understanding of the cellular and sub-cellular initiating activities. This may be the optimal paradigm for retinoid toxicity with potential application to the understanding of other retinoid toxic manifestations.

Dietary lipids and those synthesized in the liver, carrier proteins, enzymes and apoproteins interact in a highly complex system which is substantially perturbed by therapeutic levels of retinoids. Dyslipidemia involving serum triglyceride elevations of over 800 mg/dl (as chylomicrons and VLDL), cholesterol elevations (as LDL), and high density lipoprotein (HDL) decreases occurred in approximately 25 percent, 7 percent, and 15 percent respectively of young individuals treated for severe nodular acne with isotretinoin in standard therapeutic doses of 1 mg/kg/day. Very similar incidences and severities are observed with etretinate or acitretin therapy in spite of the pronounced differences in structure, ADME, disease indication, and age and health of the treated population. But as all regimens result in high steady state plasma drug concentrations, there is always a more than adequate level of potentially toxic drug for continuous and overwhelming interaction with all binding protein, organs, and cellular and sub-cellular systems.

Dietary lipids and endogenous lipids synthesized by the liver are carried in the blood and delivered to sites of utilization packaged in spherical structures (chylomicrons, VLDL, LDL, HDL) containing various combinations of TG, cholesterol, cholesterol esters, and phospholipids. These structures also incorporate, as an essential component, one or more hepatic-synthesized apolipoproteins that function in various ways as structural components, ligands, cofactors for enzymatic reactions, or activators or inactivators of lipoprotein lipase (LPL).

Triglycerides

Several enzymes are involved in lipid metabolism notably lipoprotein lipase, LPL, the major plasma lipolytic enzyme which hydrolyses triglycerides, TG, from chylomicrons and VLDL. Apolipoprotein C-III, apo C-III, has several functions including the inhibition of LPL and possibly also inhibition of hepatic uptake of chylomicron and VLDL remnants. Most studies in humans do not demonstrate retinoid effects on LPL but substantial evidence indicates that retinoids may induce apo C-III gene expression. Increase in apo C-III also appears to inhibit the binding of TG-rich particles to endothelial surfaces. Thus direct effects on the major catabolic enzyme of TG as well as inhibition of their uptake and thus utilization by target cells or metabolism by liver would contribute to the cause of elevations of TG.

Induction of apo C-III gene expression has been demonstrated in human hepatocytes and other cell systems and specificity for RXR agonists is demonstrated. Gene transcription of apo C-III is by a DR-1-like response element. It is further noted that several other nuclear receptors may also have a role in regulation of the apo C-III gene at the same site, thus retinoids are not the sole control of these transcriptions.

HDL

A simplistic view of HDL function is that HDL attracts and carries cholesterol from cell membranes and delivers it for hepatic metabolism and excretion into the bile. HDL incorporate many apolipoproteins but apo A-1 is particularly important in its role in "reverse cholesterol transport" e.g., in cholesterol removal from atherosclerotic lesion macrophages.

CHAPTER 22

■ 431

Although studies in many cell lines demonstrate a retinoid effect via receptor binding to the gene for apo A-I and apo A-II, in humans the levels of these apolipoproteins are not affected and other explanations for decreased HDL must be invoked. A further seeming contradiction is that retinoids have demonstrated binding and activation at the specific response element for cholesteryl ester transfer protein, CETP, transcription. This plasma protein is involved in the exchange of cholesteryl esters for TG from HDL to VLDL and LDL. The explanation for decreases in HDL with retinoid therapy requires additional information but likely involves retinoid effects on specific gene response elements affecting the lipids, enzymes or apolipoproteins involved with HDL.

22.9.3 Teratogenicity

The most significant of the toxicities of retinoids is also the most preventable. Even more so with this toxicity must all aspects of retinoid structure, ADME, and receptor binding be examined as all play a significant role in the totality of the end result.

Growth and differentiation in all tissues are complex, interrelated processes. These processes, so important in embryologic development, are highly dependent on and positively influenced by appropriate levels, timing of delivery, and local regulation of ATRA obtained from endogenous levels. The continuous and very high plasma and tissue levels of therapeutically administered retinoids natural or synthetic can substantially perturb these processes. Normal embryologic and fetal development requires meticulous, complex regulation of retinoic acid *trans*-placental concentrations, specific tissue gradients, and correct timing of RA delivery and catabolism in each developing organ system and limb and facial structure. This is normally accomplished by normal dietary intake, receptor-regulated *trans*-placental transport, and specific retinoid-retinoid receptor interaction and gene regulation.

Normal embryonic development requires highly regulated delivery and specific gene action by ATRA (McCaffery *et al.*, 1999; Thaller and Eichele, 1987). Specific tissue gradients of ATRA in proximal to distal limb buds can be demonstrated as can tissue gradients of P450RAI, its catabolic enzyme. It is reasonable to propose a mechanism by which retinoid-receptor complexes would variously induce and/or repress the gene transcription of a number of structural and functional proteins involved in growth and differentiation regulation. Normal "patterns of gene expression" would result in normal development or when perturbed result in profound abnormalities. There is little doubt that this specific retinoid-retinoid receptor interaction with the gene must be considered as the most specific, important, and penultimate of the mechanisms of retinoid production of teratogenicity.

The differences in teratogenic outcomes in rodents versus humans appears to be partly related to metabolic differences; the mouse and rat quickly glucuronidate retinoids, allowing rapid excretion and limiting *trans*-placental delivery.

22.9.4 Bone

Effects of vitamin A imbalance on skeletal development have been known for decades and need no reiteration here. Retinoid receptors have been identified in osteoprogenitor cells and given the established role of vitamin A in normal bone maturation, and previous reports of hypervitaminosis A effects at producing bony pathology, it is not unexpected to have literature reporting effects of retinoids on bone and mineral homeostasis. The limited data demonstrate that minor changes in bone structure have been observed, but that they generally lacked clinical significance. Taken together, the reports suggest that there may be a threshold exposure required to produce a clinically significant effect on bone. A typical exposure for a patient with a disorder of keratinization (DOK) might be 3 mg/kg daily for 2 years, which amounts to a total exposure of approximately 2200 mg/kg, whereas a typical acne regimen exposure, for example, is 1 mg/kg/day for 20 weeks for a total exposure of 140 mg/kg, or 15-fold less. Hyperostosis, both axial and extraspinal, was more readily documented in patients with DOKs after long-term therapy in contrast to the results in acne patients, where the radiographic observations were described variously as minimal, subtle and/or asymptomatic, and where the musculoskeletal pain was vague and did not correlate with objective physical findings or severity of the radiographic bony changes.

Biochemical studies have indicated that isotretinoin may have both a direct effect on bone tissue and on metabolism of vitamin D. However, the significance of these findings is not known, since several clinical studies have shown clearly that isotretinoin, despite inducing early elevations of markers of bone turnover, does not have a consistent effect on measured bone mineral density (Kindmark *et al.*, 1998). To date, cases of premature epiphyseal closure (PEC) related unequivocally to isotretinoin treatment for acne have not been reported in the literature. PEC seems to require higher doses for extended periods of time (Milstone *et al.*, 1982).

The effects of retinoids on bone have recently been summarized (DiGiovanna, 2001).

22.9.4 Central nervous system

Despite the level of understanding of the role of retinoic acid in the developing CNS, the question remains as to whether such retinoic acid-sensitive systems are still operative in the adult (or adolescent) brain and, if so, whether they are accessible to or modulated by exogenous isotretinoin.

Retinoic acid receptors are abundant in the brain, and whereas the retinoic acid receptor RAR-α is uniformly distributed, RAR-β and RAR-γ are restricted in their expression patterns. Likewise, the retinoic acid × receptors RXR-α and RXR-β are widely distributed but RXR-γ is localized specifically in the striatal region where dopaminergic neurons are also found (Ruberte *et al.*, 1993). The dopamine receptor D2 (D2R) has a retinoic acid response element (RARE) in the promoter region of the gene (Valdenaire *et al.*, 1994).

Whereas prenatal exposure to retinoids has been well studied and periods of particular sensitivity identified, there are few studies on the effects of postnatal administration. Exposure of rats at postnatal days 3–5 to the relatively high dose of 20 mg/kg of retinoic acid did not affect survival or produce any changes in regional brain weights (Holson *et al.*, 1997). In another study, however, a detailed histological study of rats, injected with retinoic acid when newborn, revealed the loss of a subpopulation of proliferating granule cells in the cerebellum 14 days later (Yamamoto *et al.*, 1999). It was concluded that sensitivity of cerebellar development to retinoic acid extends to the early postnatal period in rodents, which, interestingly, corresponds to the third trimester in humans.

In summary, although the role of retinoic acid in the developing CNS is well characterized, extrapolation to effects on the mature brain seem unwarranted; and absent such lines of evidence, a mechanistic association between retinoid administration and psychiatric disorders remains implausible.

22.10 SUMMARY AND CONCLUSIONS

Toxicological manifestations closely resembling hypervitaminosis A are the nearly inevitable consequence of effective systemic therapy with currently available retinoids. This is ultimately a corollary of their natural function as ligands of nuclear retinoid receptors. The specific binding of those ligand-receptor complexes to hundreds of retinoid response elements of many genes initiates transcription for functional, structural, and further regulatory proteins that are essential to cellular growth and differentiation in a wide variety of organ systems.

As with all cellular systems the complete processes must be highly regulated to result in the normal outcome. Specific and selective regulation of the timing, amount, availability and removal of the retinoid ligand from the system is in many ways bypassed by current therapeutic regimens during which there is sufficient absorption and retention of retinoids to produce sustained plasma levels of parent drug and active metabolites and isomers several hundred fold greater than endogenous levels. Excessive and continuous exposure of cells to high retinoid levels is not sufficiently prevented by non-specific plasma protein binding and tissue delivery, cellular retinoid binding protein cell delivery and local P450 metabolism. There is thus the potential for continuous interaction with hundreds of retinoid response elements that may result in incorrect, incorrectly timed, or continuous signals for gene transcription. These new patterns of gene expression may differ substantially from those ordinarily produced by endogenous retinoids and may effect profound changes in many cellular systems including important effects on expected patterns of cellular differentiation.

BIBLIOGRAPHY

ADAMSON, P.C., BALIS, F.M., SMITH, M.A., MURPHY, R.F., GODWIN, K.A. and POPLACK, D.G. (1992) Dose-dependent pharmacokinetics of all-*trans*-retinoic-acid. *Journal of the National Cancer Institute*, **84**, 1332–1335.

ALLENBY, G., BOCQUEL, M.-T., SAUNDERS, M., KAZMER, S., SPECK, J., ROSENBERGER, M., LOVEY, A., KASTNER, P., GRIPPO, J., CHAMBON, P. and LEVIN, A.A. (1993) Retinoic acid receptors and retinoid × receptors: interactions with endogenous retinoic acids. *Proceedings of the National Academy of Sciences USA,* **90**, 30–34.

ASTRÖM, A., PETTERSSON, U., CHAMBON, P. and VOORHEES, J. (1994) Retinoic acid induction of human cellular retinoic acid-binding protein-II gene transcription is mediated by retinoic acid receptor-retinoid × receptor heterodimers bound to one far upstream retinoic acid-response element with 5-base pair spacing. *Journal of Biological Chemistry*, **269**, 22334–22339.

BERNARD, F.X. (2002) Comparison of gene expression profiles in human keratinocyte mono-layer cultures, reconstituted epidermis and normal human skin; transcriptional effects of retinoid treatments in reconstituted human epidermis. *Exp. Dermatol.*, **11**(1), 59–74.

BICKERS, D.R. and SAURAT, J.H. (2001) Isotretinoin: A state-of-the-art conference. *Journal of the American Academy of Dermatology*, **45**, S125–S128.

BLANER, W.S. (2001) Cellular metabolism and actions of 13-*cis*-retinoic acid. *Journal of the American Academy of Dermatology*, **45**, S129–S135.

CHAMBON, P. (1996) A decade of molecular biology of retinoic acid receptors. *FASEB Journal*, **10**, 940–954.

CHANDRARATNA, R.A.S. (1998) Rational design of receptor-selective retinoids. *Journal of the American Academy of Dermatology*, **39**, S124–S128.

DIGIOVANNA, J.J. (2001) Isotretinoin effects on bone. *Journal of the American Academy of Dermatology*, **45**, S176–S182.

DORAN, T., SHAPIRO, S., MCLANE, J.A., BRYCE, G.F. and ECKHOFF, C. (1994) Activity and metabolism of 9-*cis* retinoic acid in models of dermatology, In: LIVREA, M., VIDALI, G. (eds) *Retinoids: From basic science to clinical applications*, Basel, Switzerland, Birkhauser, 315–328.

DUELL, E.A., ASTROM, A., GRIFFITHS, C.E., CHAMBON, P. and VOORHEES, J.J. (1992) Human skin levels of retinoic acid and cytochrome p-450-derived 4-hydroxyretinoic acid after topical application of retinoic acid *in vivo* compared to concentrations required to stimulate retinoic acid receptor-mediated transcription *in vitro*, *Journal of Clinical Investigation*, **90**, 1269–1274.

DUELL, E.A., KANG, S. and VOORHEES, J.J. (1996) Retinoic acid isomers applied to human skin *in vivo* each induce a 4-hydroxylase that inactivates only *trans* retinoic acid. *Journal of Investigative Dermatology*, **106**, 316–320.

DUVIC, M., NAGPAL, S., ASANO, A. and CHANDRARATNA, R. (1997) Molecular mechanisms of tazarotene action in psoriasis. *Journal of the American Academy of Dermatology*, **37**(2), S18–S24.

EVANS, R.M. (1988) The steroid and thyroid hormone receptor superfamily *Science*, **240**, 889–895.

FISHER, G.J., ESMANN, J., GRIFFITHS, C.E.M., TELWAR, H.S., DUELL, E.A, HAMMERBERG, C., ELDER, J.T., KARABIN, G.D., NICKOLOFF, B.J., COOPER, K.D. and VORHEES, J.J. (1991) Cellular, immunologic and biochemical characterization of topical retinoic acid-treated human skin, *Journal of Investigative Dermatology*, **96**, 699–707.

FISHER, G.J. and VOORHEES, J.J. (1996) Molecular mechanisms of retinoid actions in skin, *FASEB Journal*, **10**, 1002–1013.

GIGUERE, V. (1994) Retinoic acid receptors and cellular retinoid binding proteins: complex interplay in retinoid signaling, *Endocrine Reviews*, **15**, 61–79.

HOLSON, R.R., GAZZARA, R.A., FERGUSON, S.A., ALI, S.F., LABORDE, J.B. and ADAMS, J. (1997) Gestational retinoic acid exposure: a sensitive period for effects on neonatal mortality and cerebellar development. *Neurotoxicology and Teratology*, **19**, 335–346.

KANG, J.X., BELL, J., LEAF, A., BEARD, R.L. and CHANDRARATNA, R.A.S. (1998) Retinoic acid alters the intercellular trafficking of the mannose-6-phosphate/insulin-like growth factor II receptor and lysosomal enzymes, *Proceedings/National Academy of Science USA*, **95**, 13687–13691.

KANG, J.X., LI, Y. and LEAF, A. (1997) Mannose-6-phosphate/insulin-like growth factor-II receptor is a receptor for retinoic acid, *Proceedings/National Academy of Science USA*, **94**, 13671–13676.

KINDMARK, A., ROLLMAN, O., MALLMIN, H., PETRÉN-MALLMIN, M., LJUNGHALL, S. and MELHUS, H. (1998) Oral isotretinoin therapy in severe acne induces transient suppression of biochemical markers of bone turnover and calcium homeostasis. *Acta Dermato-Venereologica (Stockh.)*, **78**, 266–269.

MANGELSDORF, D.J., THUMMEL, C., BEATO, M., HERRLICK, P., SCHUTZ, G., UMESONO, K., BLUMBERG, B., KASTNER, P., MARK, M. and CHAMBON, P. (1995) The nuclear receptor superfamily: the second decade, *Cell*, **83**, 835–839.

MARGOLIS, D.J., ATTIE, M. and LEYDEN, J.J. (1996) Effects of isotretinoin on bone mineralization during routine therapy with isotretinoin for acne vulgaris. *Archives of Dermatology*, **132**, 769–774.

MARILL, J., CRESTEIL, T., LANOTTE, M., CHABOT, G.G. (2000) Identification of human cytochrome P450s involved in the formation of all-*trans*-retinoic acid principal metabolites. *Molecular Pharmacology*, **58**, 1341–1348.

MARILL, J., CAPRON, C.C., IDRES, N., CHABOT, G.G. (2002) Human cytochrome P450s involved in the metabolism of 9-*cis*- and 13-*cis*-retinoic acids. *Biochemical Pharmacology*, **63**, 933–943.

McCAFFERY, P., WAGNER, E., O'NEIL, J., PETKOVICH, M. and DRAGER, U.C. (1999) Dorsal and ventral retinal territories defined by retinoic acid synthesis, breakdown and nuclear receptor expression, *Mechanisms of Development*, **82**, 119–130.

MILSTONE, L.M., McGUIRE, J. and ABLOW, R.C. (1982) Premature epiphyseal closure in a child receiving oral 13-*cis*-retinoic acid. *Journal of the American Academy of Dermatology*, **7**, 663–666.

NAPOLI, J.L. (1996) Retinoic acid biosynthesis and metabolism, *FASEB Journal*, **10**, 993–1001.

CHAPTER 22

NAPOLI, J.L., BOERMAN, MH., CHAI X., ZHAI, Y. and FIORELLA, P.D. (1995) Enzymes and binding proteins affecting retinoic acid concentrations. *Journal of Steroid Biochemistry and Molecular Biology*, **53**, 497–502.

NAU, H. (2001) Teratogenicity of isotretinoin revisited: species variation and the role of all-*trans*-retinoic acid. *J. Am. Acad. Dermatol.* Nov. S183–S187.

NOY, N. (1992) The ionization behavior of retinoic acid in lipid bilayers and in membranes. *Biochimica Biophysica Acta*, **1106**, 159–164.

NOY, N. (1992a) The ionization behavior of retinoic acid in aqueous environments and bound to serum albumin, *Biochimica Biophysica Acta*, **1106**, 151–158.

PETKOVICH, P.M. (2001) Retinoic acid metabolism, *Journal of the American Academy of Dermatology*, **45**, S136–S142.

RAY, W.J., BAIN, G., YAO, M. and GOTTLEIB, D.I. (1997) CYP26, a novel mammalian cytochrome P450, is induced by retinoic acid and defines a new family, *Journal of Biological Chemistry*, **272**, 18702–18708.

ROOS, T.C., JUGERT, F., MERK, H.F. and BICKERS, D.R. (1998) Retinoid metabolism in the skin. *Pharmacological Reviews*, **50**, 315–333.

RUBERTE, E., FRIEDRICH, V., CHAMBON, P. and MORRISS-KAY, G. (1993) Retinoic acid receptors and cellular retinoid binding proteins III. Their differential transcript distribution during mouse nervous system development. *Development*, **118**, 267–282.

SASS, J.O., MASGRAU, E., SAURAT, J.H. and NAU, H. (1995) Metabolism of oral 9-*cis* retinoic acid in the human. Identification of 9-*cis* retinyl-β-glucuronide and 9-*cis*-4-oxo-retinoyl β-glucuronide as urinary metabolites, *Drug Metabolism and Disposition*, **23**, 887–891.

SEIGENTHALER, G., TOMATIS, I., CHATELLARD-GRUAZ, D., JACONI, S., ERIKSSON, U. and SAURAT, J.H. (1992) Expression of CRABP-I and –II in human epidermal cells. Alteration of relative protein amounts is linked to the state of differentiation, *Journal of Biochemistry*, **287**, 383–389.

SHAPIRO, S.S. and LATRIANO, L. (1998) Pharmacokinetic and pharmacodynamic considerations of retinoids: tretinoin. *Journal of the American Academy of Dermatology*, **39**, S13–S16.

SHIRLEY, M.A., BENNANI, Y.L., BOEHM, M.F., BREAU, A.P., PATHIRANAN, C., ULM, E.H. (1996) Oxidative and reductive metabolism of 9-*cis*-retinoic acid in the rat. Identification of 13, 14-didehydro-9-*cis*-retinoic acid and its taurine conjugate. *Drug Metabolism and Disposition*, **24**, 293–302.

STAELS, B. (2001) Regulation of lipid and lipoprotein metabolism by retinoids, *Journal of the American Academy of Dermatology*, **45**, S158–S167.

STANDEVEN, A.M., DAVIES, P.J., CHANDRARATNA, R.A.S., MADER, D.R., JOHNSON, A.T. and THOMAZY, V.A. (1996) Retinoid-induced epiphyseal plate closure in guinea pigs, *Fundamental and Applied Toxicology*, **34**, 91–98.

STRAUSS, J.S., RAPINI, R.P., SHALITA, A.R., KONECKY, E., POCHI, P.E., COMITE, H. (1984) Isotretinoin therapy for acne: results of a multicenter dose-response study. *Journal of the American Academy of Dermatology*, **10**, 490–496.

STRAUSS, J.S., LEYDEN, J.J., LUCKY, A.W., LOOKINGBILL, D.P., DRAKE, L.A., HANIFIN, J.M. *et al.* (2001) Safety of a new micronized formulation of isotretinoin in patients with severe recalcitrant nodular acne: a randomized trial comparing micronized isotretinoin with standard isotretinoin. *Journal of the American Academy of Dermatology*, **45**, 196–207.

THALLER, C. and EICHELE, G. (1987) Identification and spatial distribution of retinoids in the developing chick limb bud. *Nature*, **327**, 625–628.

TORMA, H. (2001) Interaction of isotretinoin with endogenous retinoids. *Journal of the American Academy of Dermatology*, **45**, S143–S149.

TSUKADA, M., SCHRÖDER, M., ROOS, T.C., CHANDRARATNA, R.A.S., REICHERT, U., MERK, H.F., ORFANOS, C.E. and ZOUBOULIS, C.C. (2000) 13-*cis*-retinoic acid exerts its specific activity on human sebocytes through selective intracellular isomerization to all-*trans*-retinoic acid and binding to retinoid acid receptors. *Journal of Investigational Dermatology*, **115**, 321–327.

VALDENAIRE, O., VERNIER, P., MAUS, M., DUMAS MILNE EDWARDS, J.B. and MALLET, J. (1994) Transcription of the rat dopamine-D2-receptor from 2 promoters. *European Journal Biochemistry*, **220**, 577–584.

WIEGAND, U.W. and CHOU, R.C. (1998) Pharmacokinetics of oral isotretinoin. *Journal of the American Academy of Dermatology*, **39**, S8–S12.

YAMAMOTO, M., ULLMAN, D., DRAGER, U.C. and MCCAFFREY, P. (1999) Postnatal effects of retinoic acid on cerebellar development. *Neurotoxicology and Teratology*, **21**, 141–146.

CHAPTER 22

Skin Disorders Caused by Cosmetics in China

**SHAOXI WU, NINGRU GUO, WEILI PAN
AND ZHENG MIN**

Contents

23.1 Introduction

23.2 Cosmetic contact dermatitis

23.3 Cosmetic photosensitive dermatitis

23.4 Abnormal pigmentation caused by cosmetics

23.5 Cosmetic acne

23.6 Hair injuring

23.7 Nail injuring

23.1 INTRODUCTION

Skin disorders caused by cosmetics means skin or/and its appendages damaged by cosmetics ordinarily used in daily life. They appear as macules, papules, desquamations, skin and mucous membrane dryness, hyperpigmentation, itching, and burning sensation of skin. These disorders are related to the use of cosmetics that are supposed to protect and beautify the skin.

Recently, accompanying the promotion of life level in China, as economic conditions markedly improved, cosmetic industries also developed and therefore the skin disorders caused by cosmetics markedly increased (Fu, 1983; Chen *et al.*, 1986; Xu, 1987; Cai *et al.*, 1991). The related skin disorders are more prominent in the Dermatologic clinics.

According to the "Diagnostic Standard and Treatment Principles of Skin Disorders Caused by Cosmetics" of The Ministry of Public Health and Bureau of Technology in China (GB/T17194-GB/T17194–7-1997), the skin disorders include: cosmetic contact dermatitis, cosmetic photosensitive dermatitis, cosmetic acne, cosmetic hyperpigmentation of skin, cosmetic hair injuries and cosmetic nail injuries.

23.2 COSMETIC CONTACT DERMATITIS

Cosmetic contact dermatitis is a major problem, about 70 percent of the cosmetic skin disorders. During 1992 and 1993, surveys of 10 cities organized by the Ministry of Public Health of China, detected 1493 cases of cosmetic skin disorders, of which more than 50 percent were confirmed as cosmetic contact dermatitis and allergic contact dermatitis. Primary irritant contact dermatitis is induced by deodorants, whitening agents, and epilation, etc. Allergic cosmetic contact dermatitis is mainly caused by the ordinary cosmetics and usually located over the face and neck, especially in adult women. In China, this condition resembles the data of NACDG, Netherlands, Denmark, Spain, France and United States with an incidence of 2.2 percent–12.2 percent and average of 4 percent (Adams and Maibach, 1985; Zha, 1994).

Patch testing is important for diagnosis. By patching the cosmetics which the patient uses or by using the individual chemicals, most patients would give a positive result; about 81 percent are positive in the foreign literature while 95 percent are positive in the Chinese literature (De Groot, 1987; Yue *et al.*, 1996). Positive patch test will help confirm the allergic cosmetics and further patch tests will confirm the ingredients responsible. Provocative Use Tests

CHAPTER 23

(Repeat Open Application Test) also could favor confirmation of the diagnosis (De Groot, 1987; Yue *et al.*, 1996). During testing, the suspected irritant chemicals such as in whitening agents, deodorants, and epilation cosmetics must be appropriately diluted to minimize false positive irritant responses.

23.3 COSMETIC PHOTOSENSITIVE DERMATITIS

Cosmetic photosensitive agents may cause inflammatory reactions to the skin and mucous membrane when exposed to light. In the Chinese literature, the incidence of cosmetic photosensitive dermatitis approximates 0.5 percent to 1.5 percent (Adams and Maibach, 1985; De Groot, 1987; Zha, 1994; Liu *et al.*, 1996; Wei and Huang, 1996; Yue *et al.*, 1996). In a survey of cosmetic dermatitis in 10 cities in China during 1992 and 1993, the incidence of photosensitive dermatitis was about 1.18 percent. Photoallergy testing is not available in China; thus the diagnostic criteria of cosmetic photosensitive cosmetic dermatitis is not uniform, and the above survey data may be an underestimate.

In reference to the mechanisms of photosensitive dermatitis and the pathogenesis of the photoreaction, the photosensitive dermatitis are divided into phototoxic and photoallergic, both of which are typically elicited by UVA (wavelength is between 320–420 nm) which penetrates common window glass. Phototoxic reaction is resulted by UVB (wavelength between 290–320nm) (Yang, 1992). Cosmetics allergens include antiseptics, dyes, perfumes and fluorescents of the lipsticks or the dyes, sunscreens such as the parabenzoic acid (PABA) and the steareic compoments of the lipstick, etc. (Gao and Qin, 1994).

The criteria of confirmation of the diagnosis of photosensitive dermatitis require photo patch testing.

23.4 ABNORMAL PIGMENTATION CAUSED BY COSMETICS

Hyperpigmentation or hypopigmentation of face caused by the cosmetics is common. Data in survey of cosmetic disorders during 1992 and 1993 in 10 cities in China were over 50 percent (Adams and Maibach, 1985; De Groot, 1987; Zha, 1994; Liu *et al.*, 1996; Wei and Huang, 1996; Yue *et al.*, 1996). Hyperpigmentation is more common than hypopigmentation. The former condition mostly occurred over the face and neck, which may be on one side and may be the only sign of this disorder or may be complicated with inflammation of the skin or secondary to the cosmetic contact dermatitis; photoallergic dermatitis caused abnormal pigmentation are called pigmented cosmetic dermatitis or Berloque dermatitis. As many cosmetics contained hydroquinone, it may cause the unexpected hypopigmentation or even cause the depletion of melanin of the skin. We found such complications during hair dying or after using the hair lotions which caused vitiligo-like lesions.

Disorders of pigmentation with inflammation of postinflammatory skin, hyperpigmentation could benefit from patch testing to detect the ingredients of the pathogenic portion of cosmetics; the positive reaction is about 80 percent (Wei and Huang, 1996). But when the only sign of cosmetic hyperpigmentation or as the history of pigmentation is vague and the disorder slowly developed, the patch test may be valueless for confirming the diagnosis.

23.5 COSMETIC ACNE

Cosmetic acne is not rare (Kligman and Mitts, 1972). The incidence of cosmetic acne in cosmetic skin disorders approximates 3.5 percent–10 percent (Adams and Maibach, 1985; De Groot, 1987; Zha, 1994; Liu *et al.*, 1996; Wei and Huang, 1996; Yue *et al.*, 1996). In a report of survey of 540 cases of cosmetic dermatitis, the incidence of cosmetic acne was 33 percent. The mechanism of this disorder is related to the obstruction of hair follicles with cosmetic cream, powdery coverage and other type of cosmetics, which may cause the comedones or exaggeration of the primary acne and induced inflammation of the hair follicles. In more oily cream and hair oil, it is more common.

The diagnosis of cosmetic acne must be referred to the history and clinical appearances. It is part of the differential diagnosis of acne.

In special conditions, chemical analysis of the cosmetics may define the chemicals that may induce cosmetic acne and/or performing animal experiment for confirmation. We usually use the rabbit ear as an animal model. There are two types of histological changes: follicular pores are gradually dilated and filled with dense keratotic materials; the other change is inflammation of the hair follicle but without dense keratotic materials obstruction.

23.6 HAIR INJURING

Hair injury may be caused by use of hair dyestuff, hair lotions, hair protectors, hair emollients, hair sticker, eyelash stickers, and eyelash oils, etc.

As the hair cosmetic industry gradually developed, the injuries caused by the cosmetics increased as injuries of hair shaft, fractures, splits, discoloration,

CHAPTER 23

loss of lightening and hair loss, etc. The injuries are physical or chemical, the latter being more common. The diagnosis of cosmetic hair injury depends on the history of hair cosmetics, clinical appearance, and microscopic examination of the hair shaft and hair follicle. Scanning and transmission electron microscopy may be useful. Stopping the cosmetics and therapeutic treatment may be helpful in diagnosis. Analysis of the harmful ingredient is needed, especially for detecting the overdosed ingredients. In differential diagnosis from the alopecia areata, pathological examination or even immunopathological examinations of hair follicle may be needed.

23.7 NAIL INJURING

Nail injuries caused by cosmetics include the injury of nail plate and its surrounding tissues. The injuries are not rare, because the nail cosmetics are an important portion of cosmetics. Nail cosmetics include three groups: First is the cutting and protecting cosmetics such as the nail cuticle removing cosmetics, lubricating agents, nail strengthening agents, etc. The second group includes lightening agents, etc. The third group includes cuticle removing agents, etc., organic solvents, resins, organic dying and other pigments, etc. There may be some special solvents such as acetone, potassium hydrooxide and nitrocellulose, etc. These agents could cause poisoning, irritating and allergy (Gao and Qin, 2000).

Injuries of nails caused by cosmetics includes the injury to nail plate and its surrounding tissues. Nail plate injury may produce brittle plate or onycholysis, loss of brightness of nail and deformity of nail plate. These changes may be caused by the nail cosmetics directly or indirectly by the irritation of the nail cosmetics induced the inflammation of the nail bed and its surrounding tissues. Resins in nail lacquer, and formaldhyde in nail hardening agent can induce allergic contact dermatitis of the surrounding tissues. The fluorescents in nail lacquer may cause the allergic reaction.

Diagnosis of injuries induced by the nail cosmetics depends on the history of utilizing nail lacquer, changes of the nail plates and the nail bed surrounding tissues. In the case of allergic paronychia, the diagnosis could be confirmed by patch test. As in the case of allergy to nail lacquer, besides the nail plate and its surrounding tissues, contact dermatitis may develop on the patient's face and neck. In such cases, the diagnosis must be confirmed by patch testing.

REFERENCES

ADAMS, R.M. and MAIBACH, H.I. (1985) A five year study of cosmetic reaction. *J. Am. Acad. Dermatol.*, **13**, 1062–1067.

CAI, R.K., GUY, B.Z. and LI, S.S. (1991) *Skin Health and Cosmetics*. Beijing: Light Industry Publishing Co. Ltd. (Chinese).

CHEN, M.G., FU, Z.Y. and LIU, J.C. (1986) Treatment of 89 cases of cosmetic dermatitis. *Clin. J. Dermatol.*, **6**, 295–297 (Chinese).

DE GROOT, A.C. (1987) Contact allergy to cosmetics: causative ingredients. *Contact Dermatitis*, **17**, 26–27.

FU, Z.Y. (1983) *Treatment and Prevention of Cosmetics Dermatitis in Actress*. Arts Bureau of Cultural Ministry of China, Beijing. Beijing Publisher Co. Ltd. (Chinese).

GAO, K.J. and QIN, Y.W. (1994) *Hygiene and Management of Cosmetics*. Beijing: People's Health Publisher Co. Ltd. (Chinese).

GAO, K.J. and QIN, Y.W. (2000) *Hygiene and Management of Cosmetics*. Beijing: People's Health Publisher Co. Ltd. (Chinese).

KLIGMAN, A.M. and MITTS, O.H. (1972) Acne cosmetics. *Arch. Dermatol.*, **106**, 843–844.

LIU, W., LI, H. and CAI, R.K. (1996) Clinical analysis of 87 cases of skin injuries by cosmetics. *Clin. Cosmet J.*, **2**, 75–77 (Chinese).

NAKAYAMA, H., MATSUL, S., HAYAKAWA, K., NAWAK, J. and CHHARA, A. (1984) Pigmented cosmetic dermatitis. *Int. J. Dermatol.*, **23**, 299–305.

WANG, X.S. (1992) *Handbook of Clinical Dermatology*. Shanghai: Shanghai Technology Publisher Co.Ltd. (Chinese).

WEI, C. and HUANG, T. (1996) Clinical analysis of 341 cases of cosmetic dermatitis. *Clin J. Dermatol.*, **29**, 22–25 (Chinese).

XU, H. (1987) Report of 40 cases of cosmetic dermatitis. *Wuhan M.J.*, **4**, 242–246 (Chinese).

YANG, K.L. (1992) *Dermatology*. Shanghai: Shanghai Medical University Publisher Co. Ltd. (Chinese).

YANG, K.L. and WANG, X.S. (1996) *Modern Dermatology*. Shanghai: Shanghai Medical University Publisher Co. Ltd. (Chinese).

YUE, H., ZHAU, B. and GEU, Y.S. (1996) Study of suspected cosmetics as antigen for patch test in cosmetic dermatitis. *Clin. J. Dermatol.*, **29**, 75–78 (Chinese).

CHAPTER 23

ZHA, B. (1994) Cosmetic dermatitis and control of cosmetics. *Clin. J. Dermatol.*, **23**, 38–41.

ZHAU, X.C., LIU, H. and LIU, W. (1994) Clinical analysis of 540 cases skin injuries by special series cosmetics. *J. Airforce Hosp.*, **10**, 234–236 (Chinese).

24

Drug Induced Ocular Phototoxicity

JOAN E ROBERTS

Contents

24.1 Introduction

24.2 Structure of the eye

24.3 Transmission of light through the human eye

24.4 Ocular phototoxicity induced by xenobiotics

24.5 Short screen for predicting potential phototoxicity

24.6 Additional techniques

24.7 Photochemical mechanism of phototoxicity

24.8 Biophysical studies

24.9 *In vitro* studies

24.10 Photochemical reactions in tissues

24.1 INTRODUCTION

Although the human eye is constantly subjected to both artificial and sunlight, damage rarely occurs from this light exposure unless the eye is aged (Dillon, 1991; Balasubramanian, 2000; Zigman, 2000; Andley, 2001; Roberts, 2001a) or the light is particularly intense (Sliney, 1999; 2002). However, many drugs, dietary supplements, cosmetics and diagnostic dyes have the potential to induce damage to the lens and retina in the presence of ambient light (Fraunfelder, 1982; Dayhaw-Barker, 1987; Roberts, 1996). This danger is enhanced with increased exposure to intense light because of high altitudes (Hu *et al.*, 1989), outdoor employment (Sliney, 2001), sun bed use, or phototherapy for seasonal depression (Roberts, 2000, 2001; Roberts *et al.*, 1992a).

24.2 STRUCTURE OF THE EYE

The structure of the human eye is given in Figure 24.1. The outermost layer contains the sclera, whose function is to protect the eyeball, and the cornea, which focuses incoming light onto the lens. Beneath this layer is the choroid containing the iris and ciliary body; this layer is known as the uvea. This region contains melanocytes that contain the pigment melanin, whose function is to prevent light scattering. The opening in the iris, the pupil, expands and contracts to control the amount of incoming light. Behind the iris is the lens, whose function is to focus light onto the retina. The iris and the lens are bathed in the aqueous humor, a fluid that maintains intraocular pressure; this fluid also contains various antioxidants. Transport to the lens is through the aqueous.

Behind the lens is the vitreous humor, a fluid that supports the lens and the retina and that also contains antioxidants. The retina itself contains the photoreceptor cells (rods and cones) that receive light and the neural portion (ganglion, amacrine, horizontal and bipolar cells) that transduces light signals through the retina to the optic nerve. Behind the photoreceptor cells are the retinal pigment epithelial cells, Bruch's membrane, and the posterior choroid. The photoreceptor cells are avascular; their nutrient support (ions, fluid and metabolites) is provided by the retinal pigment epithelial cells. Transport to the retinal pigment epithelial cells is carried out by the choriocapillaries across the Bruch's membrane.

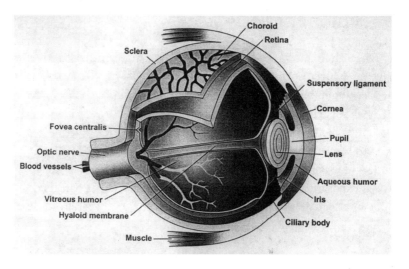

Figure 24.1: The structure of the human eye.

24.3 TRANSMISSION OF LIGHT THROUGH THE HUMAN EYE

Ambient radiation from the sun or from artificial light sources contains varying amounts of UV-C (220–290 nm), UV-B (290–320 nm), UV-A (320–400 nm), and visible light (400–700 nm). The shorter the wavelength, the greater the energy and therefore the greater the potential for biological damage. However, although the longer wavelengths are less energetic, they penetrate the eye more deeply (Roberts, 2001a)

In order for a photochemical reaction to occur in the eye, the light must be absorbed in a particular ocular tissue. The primate/human eye has unique filtering characteristics that determine in which area of the eye each wavelength of light will be absorbed (Bachem, 1956). All light of wavelengths shorter than 295 nm is cut off by the human cornea. This means that the shortest, most energetic wavelengths of light (all UV-C and some UV-B) are filtered out before they reach the human lens (Figure 24.2). Most UV light is absorbed by the lens, but the exact wavelength range depends upon age. In adults, the lens absorbs the remaining UV-B and all the UV-A (295–400 nm); therefore only visible light reaches the retina. However, the very young human lens transmits a small window of UV-B light (320 nm) to the retina, while the elderly lens filters out much of the short blue visible light (400–500 nm) (Barker *et al.*, 1991).

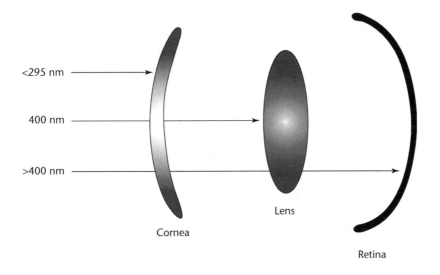

Figure 24.2: The transmission properties of the primate eye.

Transmission also differs with species; the lenses of mammals other than primates transmit ultraviolet light longer than 295 nm to the retina (Dayhaw-Barker, and Barker, 1986).

24.4   OCULAR PHOTOTOXICITY INDUCED BY XENOBIOTICS

Ultraviolet light (295–400 nm) and very short visible light (400–450 nm) are the source of most of the damage induced in the eye by direct irradiation. However, in the presence of a light activated (photosensitizing) drug (Roberts, 1984), herbal medication (Schey *et al.*, 2000) or diagnostic dye (Roberts, 1981, 1984), patients are in danger of enhanced ocular injury from both ultraviolet and all wavelengths of visible light (295–700 nm) (Roberts, 1996). The extent to which a particular dye or drug is capable of producing phototoxic side effects in the eye depends on several parameters including: 1) the chemical structure; 2) the absorption spectrum of the drug; 3) binding of the drug to ocular tissue; and 4) the ability of the drug to cross blood-ocular barriers.

24.5 SHORT SCREEN FOR PREDICTING POTENTIAL PHOTOTOXICITY

Any compound that has a tricyclic, heterocyclic or porphyrin ring structure is a potential ocular chromophore. If a drug absorbs ultraviolet light, it may damage the lens, whereas if it absorbs visible light it may also affect the retina. When exogenous sensitizers bind to ocular tissues (i.e. lens proteins (Roberts *et al.* 1991 a,b; 1990), melanin (Dayhaw-Barker and Truscott, 1988; Steiner and Buhring, 1990; Kristensen *et al.*, 1994), and DNA (Martinez and Chignell, 1998), their lifetime in the eye is extended and the hazard is enhanced. Substances that are amphiphilic or lipophilic are able to cross most blood ocular barriers (Roberts *et al.* 1991b).

In summary, there are certain chemical characteristics that allow for the prediction of potential ocular phototoxicity of a substance. These are presented in Table 24.1.

The chemical structure and absorption spectrum of a drug gives the first clear indication of potential phototoxicity. In order for a chemical compound (prescription drug, herbal medication, diagnostic dye) to induce a phototoxic response in any biological tissue, it must first absorb light. This absorption is limited by the filtering characteristics of the biological tissues involved. The human cornea absorbs all optical radiation below approximately 293 nm (Bachem, 1956). In general the lens absorbs most of the radiation between 300–400 nm, transmitting light of longer wavelengths to the retina. However, the exact filtering characteristics of the lens vary with age (Figure 24.3) and certain disease states (Barker *et al.*, 1991). Therefore a drug with an absorbance in the near UV or visible range is a potential photosensitizer of the lens and/or retina. The most potent photosensitizers usually have structures which are heterocyclic, tricyclic or porphyrin related ring systems (Figure 24.4). They

TABLE 24.1:

Short screen for predicting potential

1. Absorption spectrum	$\lambda > 295$ nm lens
	$\lambda > 400$ nm retina
2. Binding	Lens protein, DNA, melanin
3. Chemical structure	Heterocyclic, Tricyclic, Porphyrin
4. Solubility	Amphiphilic/Lipophilic
5. Skin phototoxicity	

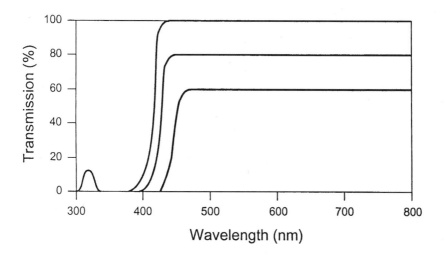

Figure 24.3: The transmission properties of the human eye as it changes with age.

should be amphiphilic or lipophilic, in order to cross blood–brain, blood–retina and aqueous–lenticular barriers.

Additional information can be obtained by measuring the absorption spectrum of the drug in the presence and absence of lens proteins, DNA and/or melanin (Dayhaw-Barker and Truscott, 1988; Steiner and Buhring, 1990; Roberts *et al. 1990,* 1991b; Kristensen *et al.*, 1994; Martinez and Chignell,1998). In the presence of any of these biomolecules, binding of the sensitizer to the biomole-cule is indicated by a red shift in the absorption spectrum of the drug. For example, the Soret band of a porphyrin is shifted to the red in the presence of cytosol lens proteins (Figure 24.5) compared to the porphyrin alone, indicating binding of the porphyrin to the lens protein. Binding of a drug to an ocular tissue would increase its retention time in the eye and therefore the drug would be more likely to induce phototoxic damage (Roberts *et al.*, 1991b).

Finally, any reports of skin phototoxicity for a particular drug should provide a clear warning of potential ocular phototoxicity. Skin phototoxicity is more readily apparent than ocular phototoxicity although it is induced by compounds with similar chemical features (Oppenlander, 1988).

24.6 ADDITIONAL TECHNIQUES

The simple screen presented above gives the first clear indication of whether or not a substance might be potentially phototoxic to ocular tissues. It is a very

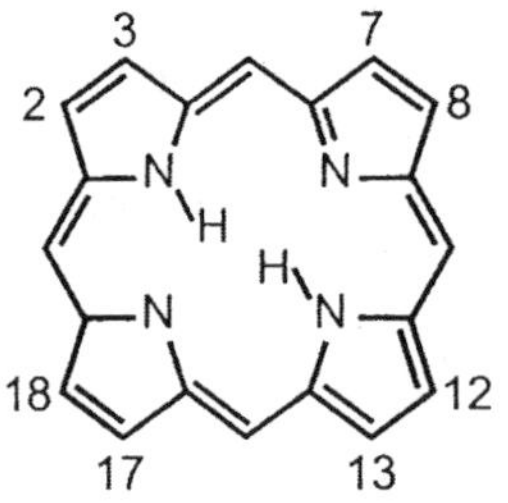

Basic Porphyrin Structure

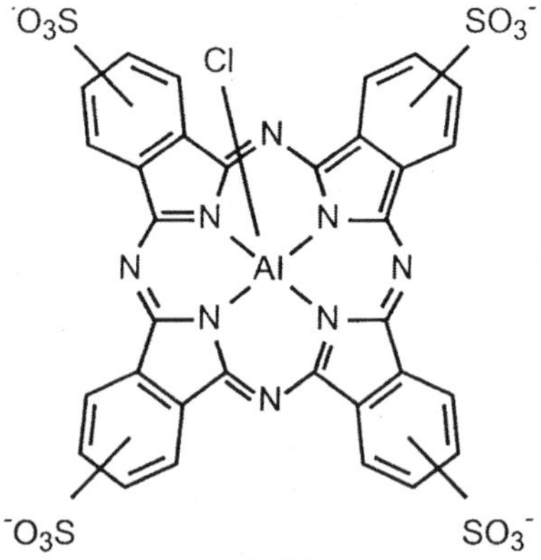

AlPCS

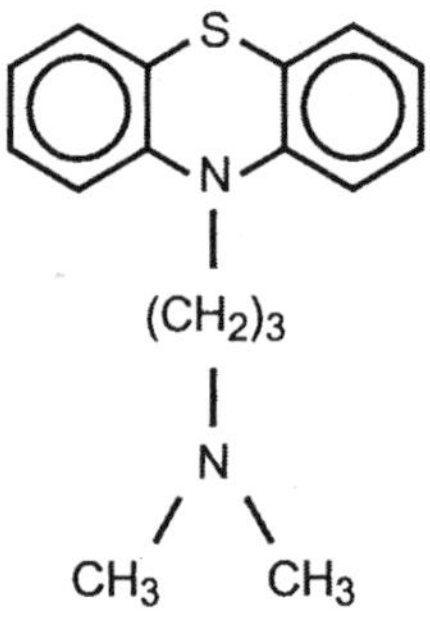

Promazine

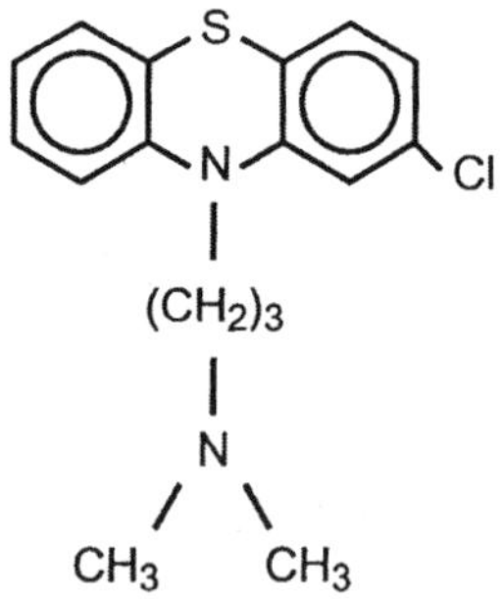

Chlorpromazine

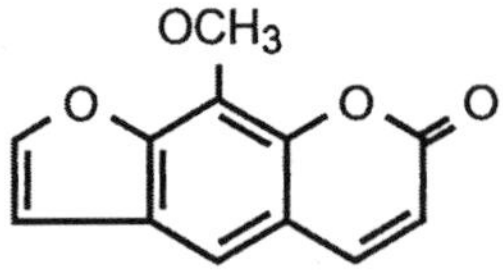

8-Methoxy Psoralen
(Xanthotoxin) (Methoxsalen)

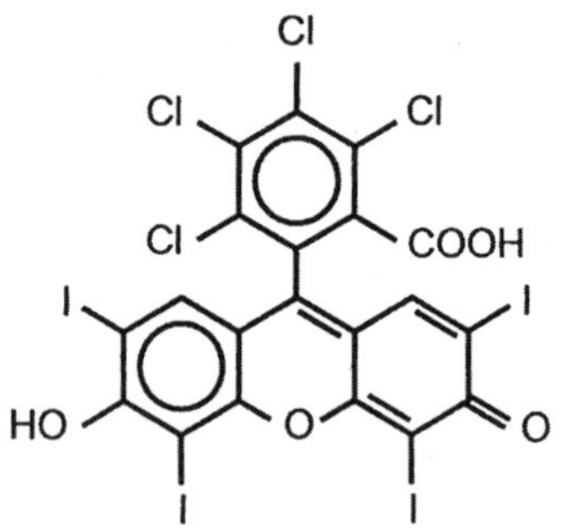

Rose Bengal

Figure 24.4: Tricyclic, heterocyclic and porphyrin ring systems of phototoxic drugs.

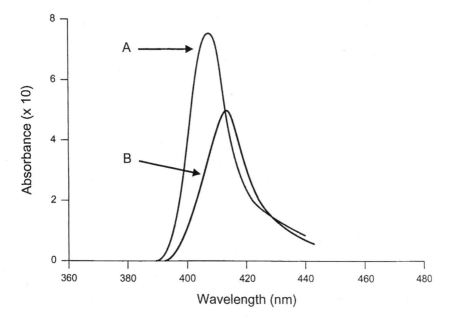

Figure 24.5: The binding of a sensitizer to lens proteins. A is the absorbance spectra of the drug and B is the absorbance spectra in the presence of lens proteins. The shift to the red is indicative of binding.

valuable tool to screen out substances that *will not* be photosensitizers in the eye. Once it has been determined that a substance is a potential photosensitizer, additional *in vitro* and biophysical assays, which take into consideration the photochemical mechanisms of phototoxicity, are useful to get a more accurate assessment of potential phototoxicity.

24.7 PHOTOCHEMICAL MECHANISM OF PHOTOTOXICITY

The molecular mechanism involved in the phototoxic damage induced in the eye is through a photooxidation reaction. This reaction begins with the absorption of light by the sensitizer (drug, dye, herbal medication), which excites the compound to the singlet state (fluorescence) and then, through intersystem crossing, goes to the triplet state. It is generally the excited triplet state of the drug/dye that then proceeds either via a Type I (free radical) or Type II (singlet oxygen) mechanism to cause the eventual biological damage (Straight and Spikes, 1985).

PHOTOOXIDATION REACTION

DRUG + light $\rightarrow$ singlet $\rightarrow$ triplet $\rightarrow$

free radicals/reactive oxygen species $\rightarrow$ Ocular damage

24.8 BIOPHYSICAL STUDIES

In complex biological systems like the eye, photooxidation can occur by either a Type I or a Type II mechanism or by both concurrently. Additional information about the precise excited state intermediates produced and the efficiency of production (quantum yield) for a phototoxic reaction in the eye can be obtained by using several photophysical techniques (flash photolysis, luminescence, pulse radiolysis, electron spin resonance) (Rodgers, 1985; Dillon and Atherton, 1990; Roberts et al., 1990, 1991a, b, 1998, 2000a, b, 2002; Dillon, 1991; Sarna et al. 1991; Reszka et al. 1992; Bilski et al. 1998; Motten et al. 1999). Determining the specific reactive intermediate(s) produced by a particular sensitizer not only defines the mechanism of toxicity but can also later be used as a tool to prevent the damage. The techniques and the reactive species that are measured are summarized in Table 24.2.

The extent of photooxidation is also influenced by the oxygen content of ocular tissues. Thus in addition to measuring excited state intermediates, the measurement of the oxygen content of a particular component of the eye is useful. The cornea is highly oxygenated and its content can be measured by the single-chamber polarographic oxygen permeability measurement method (Weissman et al., 1990). The retina is supplied with oxygen by the blood so that different portions of retinal tissues have varying but high oxygen content. This may be measured, non-invasively and *in vivo*, with a scanning laser ophthalmoscope (Ashman et al., 2001). The aqueous and the lens have low oxygen content but it is sufficient for photooxidation to occur. Measuring the excited-state

TABLE 24.2:

Biophysical studies

Technique	Reactive species
Laser flash photolysis	Triplet
Luminescence	Singlet oxygen
	Excited singlet and triplet states
Pulse radiolysis	Radicals and oxyradicals
ESR	Radicals and oxyradicals

lifetime of phosphorescent dyes in the anterior chamber provides a useful method for determining oxygen concentration *in vivo*, without penetrating the eye (Roberts *et al.*, 1992b; McLaren *et al.*, 1998).

We have confirmed that photophysical studies correlate well with *in vivo* data (Roberts *et al.*, 1991b). For instance TPPS, which binds to lens proteins, shows a long-lived triplet in the intact calf and human lens, and produces singlet oxygen efficiently, also causes photooxidative damage *in vivo* in pigmented mice.

24.9   *IN VITRO* STUDIES

24.9.1   Location/uptake of the dye/drug

For a drug, dye or herbal medication to have a toxic effect it must first be taken up into some compartment of the eye. The classical method for determining uptake into ocular tissues is *in vivo* radiolabeling. This method is time consuming and expensive, although it is effective in determining which ocular tissues have accumulated the drug in question.

An alternative method to determine uptake of a drug into ocular tissues is ocular fluorometry. After a dye or drug has absorbed light and is excited to the singlet state it can decay to the ground state, accompanied by the emission of light (fluorescence). Since most photosensitizers are fluorescent, transmitted or reflective fluorescence provides an accurate means of measuring uptake of a sensitizer into ocular tissue, a measurement that is simpler, less expensive and less arduous than using radiolabeled materials. This technique may also be used non-invasively, *in vivo*, as for instance in using a slit lamp to detect uptake of sensitizers into the human eye, or in using scanning laser ophthalmoscopes or reflective fluorometry to determine the presence of endogenous and exogenous fluorescent materials in the retina (Docchio, 1989; Docchio *et al.*, 1991; Cubeddu *et al.*, 1999; Sgarbossa *et al.*, 2001; Elsner *et al.* 2002)

24.9.2   Substrates of photooxidative damage

The targets of photooxidative reactions may be proteins, lipids, DNA, RNA, and/or cell membranes (Straight and Spikes, 1985). *In vitro* tests can be designed to determine the specific site(s) of damage to the various ocular compartments (i.e. lens and retinal epithelial cells and photoreceptor cells) and the products of those reactions.

TABLE 24.3:

In vitro studies

Technique	Substrate
Fluorescence	Sensitizer uptake
Cell culture	DNA, RNA, protein synthesis
Comet assay	DNA crosslinks
Enzyme assays	Antioxidant enzymes
Histology	Endothelial, epithelial, photoreceptor cell damage
Gel electrophoresis Amino acid analysis	Protein changes
Mass spectrometry	Lipid changes Peptide maps
TLC HPLC	Lipid oxidation Lipid peroxides DNA adducts Protein modification

Gel electrophoresis, amino acid analysis

Gel electrophoresis has been used to monitor polymerization of ocular proteins (Zigler *et al.*, 1982; Roberts 1984; Roberts *et al.*, 1985, 1992a; Kristensen *et al.*, 1995). Photopolymerization is one of the most apparent changes in ocular protein induced by photosensitizing dyes and drugs. Quantitative changes can be measured by scanning the gel and determining relative reaction rates. Specific amino acid modifications can be determined using amino acid analysis (Roberts, 1984; 1996). Zhu and Crouch (1992) have illustrated the wide variety of classical protein analysis techniques (gel electrophoresis, amino acid analysis, sequencing, isoelectric point determination, western blot, ELISA) that can be used to investigate phototoxic damage induced by dyes and drugs.

Mass spectrometry

Recent innovations in the field of mass spectrometry (Liquid secondary ion mass spectrometry (LSIMS) and electrospray ionization (ESI)) have allowed for the identification of specific amino acid modifications within large proteins through molecular weight mapping. These techniques have been applied to determine the specific sites of photooxidative damage in corneal and lenticular proteins (Schey *et al.*, 2000; Roberts *et al.*, 2001). These studies can serve as a model for defining damage from any potential phototoxic agent in the eye.

Thin layer chromatography

Thin layer chromatography is the method of choice for separating free fatty acids and phospholipids from lens (Fleschner, 1995) and retinal (Organisiak *et al.*, 1992) membranes. Thin layer chromatography/gas mass/mass spectrometry (TLC/GC/Mass Spec) may be used to measure lenticular or retinal lipid modifications (Handelman and Dratz, 1986). Specific lipids may be modified in the presence of photosensitizing agents and separated on TLC plates. The plates can then be scanned for quantitative analysis of these specific changes.

High pressure liquid chromatography

HPLC is particularly effective at separating and identifying lipid peroxides from the retina (Akasaka *et al.*, 1993). It has also been used to identify adducts formed between DNA nucleotides and phototoxic agents (Oroskar *et al.*, 1994). HPLC has been used to assess the rates of photooxidation of lens proteins in the presence of a sensitizer; with this technique it is possible to determine which amino acid modifications have been induced within the protein, where they are located, and whether sensitizing drugs may have been bound to specific lens crystallins (McDermott *et al.*, 1991).

Normalization for photons absorbed

Whatever the target tissue or extent of damage, the toxic effects of these dyes and drugs are the result of photochemical reactions. As such, their efficiency depends strongly on the number of photons absorbed by the sensitizer in the biological tissue. Therefore, in order to get an accurate comparison of the photo-sensitizing potency of various dyes and drugs with different structures and absorptive characteristics, it is essential to normalize for the number of photons absorbed by each drug in a particular system.

Normalization can be accomplished with a simple computer generated mathematical formula (Kristensen *et al.*,1995; Roberts,1996), which takes into account the absorption spectrum of the drug, the output of the lamp source used in the experiments, and the optical properties of the eye. The total relative number of photons absorbed by a drug under particular experimental conditions is the area under the product curve:

Photons Absorbed = $I \times AB \times \lambda$

Where I is the intensity of the lamp at various wavelengths, adjusted for the transmission characteristics of the cornea or lens; AB is the absorbance of the dye/drug; and λ is the number of photons per energy unit at those wavelengths. The rate of photooxidative damage is then adjusted accordingly for each sensitizer.

Cell culture/whole tissues

The first reported assay for phototoxicity in human cells (Roberts, 1981) measured changes in macromolecular synthesis in the presence and absence of a light activated drug. Other studies have assessed damage to corneal, lenticular, and retinal cells by measuring pump function, DNA crosslinks and enzyme activities both *in vitro* and *in situ* (Dayhaw-Barker, 1987; Rao and Zigler, 1992; Andley *et al.* 1994; Organisiak and Winkler, 1994; Andley, 2001, Roberts *et al.*, 2002, 1994a).

24.10 PHOTOCHEMICAL REACTIONS IN TISSUES

EXCITED STATE	→	INTERMEDIATES	→	TARGET and DAMAGE
		singlet oxygen		proteins → polymers
triplet		superoxide		lipid → peroxides
		OH·, ROO·		DNA, RNA → cross-links

In vitro techniques determine the potential damage done to an ocular substrate, which gives information about the photoefficiency of a drug should it be taken up into the various compartments of the eye. Additional information about the site of potential damage can be predicted based on which ocular substrates (proteins, DNA, lipids) are modified.

24.10.1 Site of damage

There are numerous locations subjected to phototoxic damage in the eye. The site of damage is determined by the penetration of the drug and the transmission of the appropriate wavelengths of light to that site.

Cornea

Corneal epithelial and endothelial cells may be easily damaged, leading to keratitis (Pitts *et al.*, 1976; Hull *et al.*, 1983). However, these cells have a very efficient repair mechanism and the damage is rarely permanent.

Lens

The epithelial cells of the lens, whose function is to control transport to the lens, have direct contact with the aqueous and are thus most vulnerable to photo-toxic damage. Damage to these cells would readily compromise the viability of the lens (Roberts *et al.*, 1994a; Andley, 2001). The lens fiber membrane can be photochemically harmed through damage to the lipids and /or the main intrinsic membrane protein (Roberts *et al.*, 1985). Such damage leads to changes in the refractive index resulting in a loss of transparency (opacification) (Benedek, 1971).

Phototoxic reactions can cause a modification of certain amino acids (histadine, tryptophan, cysteine) (Roberts, 1984; McDermott *et al.*, 1991) and/or a covalent attachment of sensitizer to cytosol lens proteins. In either case, the physical properties of the protein are changed, leading to aggregation and finally opacification (cataractogenesis). The covalently bound chromophore may now act as an endogenous sensitizer, producing prolonged sensitivity to light. Since there is little turnover of lens proteins this damage is cumulative.

Retina

Phototoxic damage can occur in retinal pigment epithelial tissues, the choroid and the rod outer segments which contain the photoreceptors. If the damage is not extensive, there are repair mechanisms to allow for recovery of retinal tissues. However, extensive phototoxic damage to the retina can lead to permanent blindness (Ham *et al.*, 1982; Dayhaw-Barker and Barker, 1986).

24.10.2   *In vivo* testing

The screens described above will not totally eliminate the need for accurate *in vivo* experiments. However, the function of these studies is to limit the need for *in vivo* testing of large numbers of drugs for ocular phototoxicity. Those drugs found to be highly likely to produce phototoxic side effects in the eye should be tested further in animal studies to determine the exact site and extent of damage to be expected in humans.

With simple, inexpensive *in vitro* testing, compounds can be checked for phototoxicity at the developmental stage. It may be that a portion of the molecule can be modified to reduce phototoxicity while leaving the primary drug effect intact. This may reduce the necessity of future, more costly, drug recalls.

24.10.3 Protection

Even if a drug has the potential to produce phototoxic side effects in the eye, no damage will be done if the specific wavelengths of optical radiation absorbed by the drug are blocked from transmittance to the eye. This can be easily done with wrap around eyeglasses which incorporate specific filters (Merriam, 1996; Gallas and Eisner, 2001; Sliney, 2001). Furthermore, non-toxic quenchers and scavengers could be given in conjunction with the phototoxic drug to negate its ocular side effects while still allowing for the primary effect of the drug (Roberts, 1981; Roberts *et al.*, 1991b; Roberts and Mathews-Roth, 1993; Roberts *et al.* 1994 b, c; Busch *et al.*, 1999).

ACKNOWLEDGMENT

The author wishes to thank the Hugoton Foundation for its financial support and Dr. Ann Motten, NIEHS, North Carolina for help in preparing this manuscript.

REFERENCES

AKASAKA, K., OHRUI, H. and MEGURO, H. (1993) Normal-phase high-performance liquid chromatography with a fluorimetric postcolumn detection system for lipid hydroperoxides. *J. Chromatog.* **628**, 31–35.

ANDLEY, U.P. (2001) Ocular lens photobiology. In COOHILL, T.P. and VANENZENO, D.P. (eds) *Photobiology for the 21st Century*. Kansas, Valdenmar Publishing Co., 135–142.

ANDLEY, U.P., RHIM, J.S., CHYLACK, L.T. JR. and FLEMING, T.P. (1994) Propagation and immortalization of human lens epithelial cells in culture. *Invest. Ophthalmol. Vis. Sci.* **35**, 3094–3102.

ASHMAN, R.A., REINHOLZ, F. and EIKELBOOM, R.H. (2001) Oximetry with a multiple wavelength SLO. *Int. Ophthalmol.* **23**, 343–346.

BACHEM, A., (1956) Ophthalmic action spectra. *Am. J. Ophthal.* **41**, 969–975.

BALASUBRAMANIAN, D. (2000) Ultraviolet radiation and cataract. *J. Ocul. Pharmacol. Ther.* **16**, 285–297.

BARKER, F.M., BRAINARD G.C. and DAYHAW-BARKER, P. (1991) Transmittance of the human lens as a function of age. *Invest. Ophthalmol. Vis. Sci.* **32S**, 1083.

BENEDEK, G.B. (1971) Theory of transparency of the eye. *Appl. Optics* **10**, 459–473.

BILSKI, P. KUKIELCZAK, B.M. and CHIGNELL, C.F. (1998) Photoproduction and direct spectral detection of singlet molecular oxygen in keratinocytes stained with rose bengal. *Photochem. Photobiol.* **68**, 675–678.

BUSCH, E.M., GORGELS, T.G., ROBERTS, J.E. and VAN NORREN, D. (1999) The effects of two stereoisomers of N-acetylcysteine on photochemical damage by UVA and blue light in rat retina. *Photochem. Photobiol.* **70**, 353–358.

CUBEDDU, R., TARONI, P., HU, D-N, SAKAI, N., NAKANISHI, K. and ROBERTS, J.E. (1999) Photophysical studies of A2-E, putative precursor of lipofuscin, in human retinal pigment epithelial cells. *Photochem. Photobiol.* **70**, 172–175.

DAYHAW-BARKER, P. (1987) Ocular photosensitization. *Photochem. Photobiol.* **46**, 1051–1056.

DAYHAW-BARKER, P. and TRUSCOTT, T.G. (1988) Direct detection of singlet oxygen sensitized by nalidixic acid: the effect of pH and melanin. *Photochem. Photobiol.* **47**, 765–767.

DAYHAW-BARKER, P. and BARKER, F.M. (1986) Photoeffects on the eye. In JACKSON, E.M. (ed.) *Photobiology of the Skin and the Eye*, New York, Marcel Dekker, Inc. 117–147.

DILLON, J. (1991) Photophysics and photobiology of the eye. *J. Photochem. Photobiol. B. Biol.* **10**, 23–40.

DILLON, J. and ATHERTON, S.J. (1990) Time resolved spectroscopic studies on the intact human lens. *Photochem. Photobiol.* **51**, 465–468.

DOCCHIO, F. (1989) Ocular fluorometry: principles, fluorophores, instrumentation and clinical applications. *Lasers Surg. Med.* **9**, 515–532.

DOCCHIO, F., BOULTON, M., CUBEDDU, R., RAMPONI, R. and BARKER, P.D. (1991) Age-related changes in the fluorescence of melanin and lipofuscin granules of the retinal pigment epithelium: a time resolved fluorescence spectroscopy study. *Photochem. Photobiol.* **54**, 247–253.

CHAPTER 24

ELSNER, A.E. , BURNES, S.A. and WEITER, J.J. (2002) Cone photopigment in older subjects: decreased optical density in early age-related macular degeneration. *J. Opt. Soc. Am. A* **19**, 215–221.

FLESCHNER, C.R. (1995) Fatty acid composition of triacylglycerols, free fatty acid and phospholipids from bovine lens membrane fractions. *Invest. Ophthal. Vis. Sci.* **36**, 261–264.

FRAUNFELDER, F.T. (1982) *Drug-Induced Ocular Side Effects and Drug Interactions*, 2nd ed. Philadelphia: Lea and Febiger.

GALLAS, J. and EISNER, M. (2001) Eye protection from sunlight damage. In GIACOMONI, P.U. (ed.) *Sunlight Protection in Man*, Amsterdam, Elsevier, Chapter 23, pp 437–455.

HAM, W.T., MUELLER, H.A., RUFFOLO, J.J., GUERRY, D. and GUERRY, R. K. (1982) Action spectrum for retinal injury from near ultraviolet radiation in the aphakic monkey. *Amer. J. Ophthal.* **93**, 299–305.

HANDELMAN, G.J. and DRATZ, E.A. (1986) The role of antioxidants in the retina and retinal pigment epithelium and the nature of prooxidant induced damage. *Adv. in Free Radical Biology and Medicine* **2**, 1–89.

HU, T.-S., ZHEN, Q., SPERDUTO, R.D., ZHAO, J.-L., MILTON, R.C., NAKAJIMA, A. and THE TIBET EYE STUDY GROUP (1989) Age-Related Cataract in the Tibet Eye Study. *Arch. Ophthalmol.* **107**, 666–680.

HULL, D.S., CSUKAS, S. and GREEN, K. (1983) Trifluoperazine: Corneal endothelial phototoxicity. *Photochem. Photobiol.* **38**, 425–428.

KRISTENSEN, S., ORSTEEN, A.L., SANDE, S.A. and TONNESEN, H.H. (1994) Photo-reactivity of biologically active compounds. VII. Interaction of antimalarial drugs with melanin *in vitro* as part of phototoxicity screening. *J. Photochem. Photobiol. B* **26**, 87–95.

KRISTENSEN, S., WANG, R.H., TONNESEN, H., DILLON, J. and ROBERTS, J.E. (1995) Photoreactivity of biologically active compounds. VII. Photosensitized polymerization of lens proteins by antimalarial drugs *in vitro*. *Photochem. Photobiol.* **61**, 124–130.

MARTINEZ, L. and CHIGNELL, C.F. (1998) Photocleavage of DNA by the fluoro-quinolone antibacterials. *J. Photochem. Photobiol. B.* **21**, 51–59.

MERRIAM, J.C. (1996) The concentration of light in the human lens. *Trans. Am. Ophthalmol. Soc.* **94**, 803–918.

MCDERMOTT, M., CHIESA, R., ROBERTS, J.E. and DILLON, J. (1991) Photooxidation of specific residues in alpha-crystallin polypeptides. *Biochemistry* **30**, 8653–8660.

MCLAREN, J.W., DINSLAGE, S., DILLON, J.P., ROBERTS, J.E. and BRUBAKER, R.F. (1998) Measuring oxygen tension in the anterior chamber of rabbits. *Invest. Ophthalmol. Vis. Sci.* **39**, 1899–1909.

MOTTEN A.G., MARTINEZ, L.J., HOLT, N., SIK, R. H. RESZKA, K., CHIGNELL, C.F., TONNESEN, H.H. and ROBERTS, J.E. (1999) Photophysical studies on antimalarial drugs. *Photochem. Photobiol.* **69**, 282–287.

OPPENLANDER, T. (1988) A comprehensive photochemical and photophysical assay exploring the photoreactivity of drugs. *Chimia* **42**, 331–342.

ORGANISIAK, D.T. and WINKLER, B.S. (1994) Retinal light damage: practical and theoretical considerations. *Prog. Retinal. Res.* **13**, 1–29.

ORGANISIAK, D.T., DARROW, M.A., JIANG, Y.-L., MARAK, G.E. and BLANKS, J.C. (1992) Protection by dimethylthiourea against retinal light damage in rats. *Invest. Ophthalmol. Vis. Sci.* **33**, 1187–1192.

OROSKAR, A., OLACK, G., PEAK, M.J. and GASPARRO, F.P. (1994) 4'-Aminomethyl-4,5'',8-trimethylpsoralen photochemistry: the effect of concentration and UVA fluence on photoadduct formation in poly(dA-dT) and calf thymus DNA. *Photochem. Photobiol.* **60**, 567–573.

PITTS, D.G., CULLEN, A.P. and PARR, W.H. (1976) Ocular ultraviolet effects in the rabbit eye. *DHEW (NIOSH) Publication* No. 77, 130–138.

RAO, D.M. and ZIGLER JR, J.S. (1992) Levels of reduced pyridine nucleotides and lens photodamage. *Photochem. Photobiol.* **56**, 523–528.

RESZKA, K., LOWN, J.W. and CHIGNELL, C.F. (1992) Photosensitization by anticancer agents. 10. ortho-semiquinone and superoxide radicals produced during anthapyrazole-sensitized oxidation of catechols. *Photochem. Photobiol.* **55**, 359–366.

ROBERTS, J.E. (1981) The effects of photooxidation by proflavin in HeLa cells l. The molecular mechanisms. *Photochem. Photobiol.* **33**, 55–60.

ROBERTS, J.E. (1984) The photodynamic effect of chlorpromazine, promazine and hematoporphyrin on lens protein. *Invest. Ophthalmol. Vis. Sci.* **25**, 746–750.

ROBERTS, J.E. (1996) Ocular phototoxicity. In MARZULLI, F. and MAIBACH, M. (eds) *Dermatotoxicology. 5th Edition*, Washington, DC, Taylor & Francis, Chapter 24, pp. 307–313.

ROBERTS, J.E. (2000) Light and immunomodulation. *NY Acad. Sci.* **917**, 435–445.

ROBERTS, J.E. (2001a) Ocular phototoxicity. *J. Photochem. Photobiol.* B **64**, 136–143.

CHAPTER 24

ROBERTS, J.E. (2001b) Therapeutic effects of light in humans. In COOHILL, T.P. and VALENZENO, D.P. (eds) *Photobiology for the 21st Century*, Overland Park, Kansas: Valdenmar Publishing Company, Chapter 2, pp. 17–29.

ROBERTS, J.E. and MATHEWS-ROTH, M. (1993) Cysteine ameliorates photo-sensitivity in Erythropoietic Protoporphyria. *Archives Dermatology* **129**, 1350–1351.

ROBERTS, J.E and DILLON, J. (1994c) Improvement of photodynamic therapy by selective protection of normal tissues. In JUNG, E.G. and HOLICK, M.F. (eds) *Biological Effects of Light:* Berlin, New York , Gruyter and Co., 393–399

ROBERTS, J.E., ROY, D. and DILLON, J. (1985) The photosensitized oxidation of the calf lens main intrinsic protein (MP26) with hematoporphyrin. *Curr. Eye Res.* **4**, 181-185.

ROBERTS, J.E., ATHERTON, S.J. and DILLON, J. (1990) Photophysical studies on the binding of tetrasulphonatophenylporphyrin to lens proteins. *Photochem Photobiol* 52, 845–848.

ROBERTS, J.E., ATHERTON, S.J. and DILLON , J. (1991a) Detection of porphyrin excited states in the intact bovine lens. *Photochem. Photobiol.* **54**, 855–857.

ROBERTS, J.E, KINLEY, J., YOUNG, A., JENKINS, G., ATHERTON S.J. and DILLON, J. (1991b) *In vivo* and photophysical studies on photooxidative damage to lens proteins and their protection by radioprotectors. *Photochem. Photobiol.* **53**, 33–38.

ROBERTS, J.E., REME, C., TERMAN, M. and DILLON, J. (1992a) Exposure to bright light and the concurrent use of photosensitizing drugs. *New Eng. J. Med.* **326**, 1500–1501.

ROBERTS, J.E., HARRIMAN, A., ATHERTON, S.J. and DILLON, J.E. (1992b) A non-invasive method to detect oxygen tensions and other environmental factors in the lens. *Int. Soc. Ocular Phototox.* **64** (abstract).

ROBERTS, J.E., SCHIEB, S., GARNER, W.H. and LOU, M. (1994a) Development of a new photo-oxidative induced cataract model using TPPS in an intact lens. *Invest. Ophthal. Vis. Sci.* **35**, 21–37.

ROBERTS, J.E., SELMAN, S, MORGAN, A. and DILLON, J. (1994b) Selective protection against the side effects of photodynamic therapy by radioprotectors. In JUNG, E.G. and HOLICK, M.F. (eds) *Biological Effects of Light* Berlin, New York, Gruyter and Co. , pp. 400–406.

ROBERTS, J.E., HU, D.-N. and WISHART, J.F. (1998) Pulse radiolysis studies of melatonin and chloromelatonin. *J. Photochem. Photobiol. B. Biol.* **42**, 125–132.

ROBERTS, J.E., HU, D.-N., MARTINEZ, L. and CHIGNELL, C.F. (2000a) Photophysical studies on melatonin and its receptor agonists. *J. Pineal. Res.* **29**, 94–99

ROBERTS, J.E., WISHART, J.F., MARTINEZ, L. and CHIGNELL, C.F. (2000b) Photochemical studies on xanthurenic acid. *Photochem. Photobiol.* **72**, 467–471.

ROBERTS, J.E., FINLEY, E.L., PATAT, S.A. and SCHEY, K.L. (2001) Photooxidation of lens proteins with xanthurenic acid: A putative chromophore for cataractogenesis. *Photochem. Photobiol.* **74**, 740–744.

ROBERTS, J.E., KUKIELCZAK, B.M., HU, D.-N., MILLER, D.S., BILSKI, P., SIK, R.H., MOTTEN, A.G. and CHIGNELL, C.F. (2002) The role of A2E in prevention or enhancement of light damage in human retinal pigment epithelial cells. *Photochem. Photobiol.* **75**, 184–190.

RODGERS, M.A.J. (1985) Instrumentation for the generation and detection of transient species. In BENSASSON, R.V., JORI, G., LAND, E.J. and TRUSCOTT, T.J. (eds) *Primary Photoprocesses in Biology and Medicine.* North Holland, Elsevier, 1–24.

SARNA, R., ZAJAC, J., BOWMAN, M.K. and TRUSCOTT, T.G. (1991) Photoinduced electron transfer reactions of rose bengal and selected electron donors. *J. Photochem. Photobiol. A. Chem.* **60**, 295–310.

SCHEY, K.L., PATAT, S., CHIGNELL, C.F., DATILLO, M., WANG, R.H. and ROBERTS, J.E. (2000) Photooxidation of lens proteins by hypericin (active ingredient in St. John's Wort). *Photochem. Photobiol.* **72**, 200–207.

SGARBOSSA, A., ANGELINI, N., GIOFFRE, D., YOUSSEF, T., LENCI, F. and ROBERTS, J.E. (2001) The uptake, location and fluorescence of hypericin in bovine intact lens. *Curr. Eye Res.* **21**, 597–601.

SLINEY, D.H. (2002) Geometrical gradients in the distribution of temperature and absorbed ultraviolet radiation in ocular tissues. *Dev. Ophthalmol.* **35**, 40–59.

SLINEY, D.H. (2001) Photoprotection of the eye-UV radiation and sunglasses. *J. Photochem. Photobiol. B* **64**, 166–175.

SLINEY, D.H. (1999) Geometrical assessment of ocular exposure to environmental UV radiation-implications for ophthalmic epidemiology. *J. Epidemiol.* **9**, 22–32.

STEINER, K. and BUHRING, K.U. (1990) The melanin binding of bisoprolol and its toxicological relevance. *Lens and Eye Tox. Research* **7**(3 and 4), 319–333.

STRAIGHT, R. and SPIKES, J.D. (1985) Photosensitized oxidation of biomolecules. In FRIMER, A.A. (ed.) *Singlet O, Vol IV. Polymers and Biopolymers*, Boca Raton, Fl: CRC Press, 91–143.

■ CHAPTER 24 ■

WEISSMAN, B.A., SCHWARTZ S.D., GOTTSCHALK-KATSEV N. and LEE D.A. (1990) Oxygen permeability of disposable soft contact lenses. *Am. J. Ophthalmol.* **110**, 269–273.

ZIGLER, J.S. JR, JERNIGAN, H.M. JR, PERLMUTTER, N.S. and KINOSHITA, J.H. (1982) Photodynamic cross-linking of polypeptides in intact rat lens. *Exp. Eye Res.* **35**, 239–249

ZIGMAN S. (2000) Lens UVA photobiology. *J. Ocular. Pharmacol. Ther.* **16**, 161–165.

ZHU, L. and CROUCH, R. K. (1992) Albumin in the cornea is oxidized by hydrogen peroxide. *Cornea* **11**, 567–572.

Water: Is It an Irritant?

TSEN-FANG TSAI AND HOWARD I MAIBACH

An irritant is defined as any agent, physical or chemical, capable of producing cell damage. Everything can be an irritant if applied for sufficient time and in sufficient concentration. Water, being the most abundant element of the skin, is usually regarded as banal and gentle. However, the irritancy of water is beyond doubt. All nature evolves from the water. However, as man evolved from the water and became adapted to the earthy environment, the protection from water became one of the chief functions of the skin, which is a major protective organ.

Irritant contact dermatitis is the hallmark of an irritant reaction. It has been traditionally classified into an acute and chronic type. Strong irritants will induce a clinical reaction in a single application, whereas with less potent irritants the response may be delayed and subclinical, requiring repeated or prolonged application (Hassing et al., 1982: 164). However, not all irritant reactions manifest as dermatitis. Water, being an unconventional irritant, may irritate the skin in a way other than dermatitis. Fingertip dermatitis, or wear and tear dermatitis, is the best example of cumulative irritant reaction. In this condition, hands are chronically irritated by a variety of insults, especially water. The involved skin is hardened and fissured, but typical signs of dermatitis or inflammation such as erythema, swelling or scaling are often lacking in the early stage. People who deal with wet work, such as hair dressers, hospital cleaners, cannery workers, bartenders are especially at risk (Hassing, 1990: 22). In rare conditions, water may also produce pruritus (Potasman, 1990: 26), urticaria (Medeiros, 1996: 6) or pain (Shelley and Shelley, 1998) in susceptible patients.

The occlusive patch test is a gold standard for the study of contact dermatitis. And the irritancy of water under occlusion has likewise attracted most clinical attention. Prolonged warm water immersion under occlusive shoes was considered to be the culprit of tropical-immersion-foot (Taplin and Zaias, 1966: 131). This is a condition of painful swollen feet first noticed in soldiers during the Vietnam war. Another condition is juvenile plantar dermatosis in which children, mostly atopic, present with dry, glazed and fissured forefeet. Repeated wet-to-dry process in conjunction with friction was incriminated as the main cause.

The occlusive dressing has long been used as an effective adjuvant therapy for diverse conditions such as keloid (Sawada, 1992: 45), periungual verrucae (Litt, 1978: 22) and psoriasis (Broby-Johansen, 1989: 14). Occlusion has been demonstrated to modify reactive events in Langerhans cells, and has a profound effect on cytokine production (Wood, 1994: 103). Occlusion can be achieved with either plastic dressing, silicone or by water-soaked patches. Normal skin will show typical signs of inflammation such as vasodilation, perivenular lymphocytic

CHAPTER 25

infiltration, edema, mast cells degradation and proliferation of fibroblasts after occlusion for up to two weeks (Kligman, 1996). Agner and Serup, studied skin reactions after closed patch tests and six of twenty participants had a grade 1 clinical response to water after occlusion for twenty-four hours (Agner and Serup, 1993: 28). The irritation of water under occlusion can result from the water per se or from retention of sweat, which is more irritative than the water per se (Gordon and Maibach, 1969; Hu, 1991: 182). However, a state of anhidrosis will result after prolong occlusion (Papa, 1972:59, Sulzberger and Harris, 1972: 105).

Water, as an irritant, exerts its damaging effect on the skin through different mechanisms. A normal water gradient is required for a healthy skin. The outer-most layer of stratum corneum contains 10–30 percent water, while the viable epidermis contains roughly 70 percent water. After occlusion, a change in the water gradient occurs, and an adaptation of skin physiology ensures accordingly. The normal desquamation process is highly dependent on the water gradient of the stratum corneum. Increased water content of the stratum corneum will dilute the enzymes and change the pH value important for the corneodes-molysis (Watkinson et al., 2001: 293). As a result, in macerated skin, the stratum corneum shows retentional hyperkeratosis and is shed in large sheets. Increased water content in the stratum corneum will also have a negative feedback response on the formation of natural moisturizing factors (NMFs) through the deactivation of keratohyalin granules degradation. Keratohyalin granules are the main source of NMFs. The skin surface becomes excessive dry after the removal of occlusion. This drying effect of water is best demonstrated in wet packing for management of exudative lesions.

The importance of water as a primary irritant has also been evaluated by Ramsing et al. (1997: 136). After experimental irritation by sodium lauryl sulfate in 21 healthy volunteers, one hand was exposed to water for 15 minutes twice daily for two weeks, while the other hand served as control. Water did not significantly influence transepidermal water loss, but caused a significant increase in skin blood flow, as evaluated by laser Doppler flowmetry. Clinical evaluation did not show any difference of dryness or scaling in this study. Without occlusion, the irritancy of water by itself is questionable in this model. However, it is impossible to clearly separate the effects of occlusion and water. The effect of occlusion must be conduction to the skin through water as a medium under physiologic conditions. And even though erythema alone does not equate to irritancy, temperature stimulated erythema has been observed to augment pre-existing irritation (Loffler, 2001: 81). Thus, water may also exert its irritancy through its other non-chemical nature. The temperature dependency of irritation has been well recognized (Ohlenschlaeger, 1996: 76). Besides, hydration changes the optics of the skin, and increases the penetration and absorption of the ultraviolet light. Photo-bleaching of the melanin is also more prominent in dampened hairs (Dubief, 1992: 107).

Persistent hydration of the skin surface also changes the ecological environment and supports the overgrowth of pathological organisms on skin (Aly, 1978: 71, 1981: 61; Faergemann et al., 1983: 275; Roth and James, 1989: 20). Diaper rashes and pitted keratolysis are the clear examples. Dermatophytosis complex of the toewebs is likely affected. Occlusion alone may clear the periungual verrucae, and spread the mucosal type HPV, that is condylomata acuminata, to the extragenital areas. Extraction of water soluable substances, or natural moisturizing factors (NMFs), from the skin is another mechanism. NMFs are a goup of water extractable substances, including sodium pyrrolidone carboxylic acid, sodium calcium lactate, amino acids, urea and a sugar-protein complex. These substances bind three to four times their own weight of water (Bank, 1952: 18, Jacobi, 1959: 31, Yamamura, 1989: 3). The presence of water in the stratum corneum relies on an intercellular bilayer membrane that encloses the NMFs as in an envelope (Imokawa et al., 1991: 96). Since water is the main plasticizing factor of the horny layer, the water content of the stratum corneum decreases when the NMFs are reduced, and superficial cracks might develop. The amino acid content in senile skin is decreased (Jacobson et al., 1990: 95). Frequent showering removes these water extractable substances and a delay in the replenishment of NMFs in aging skin may further aggravate this situation. It is for these reasons that frequent or prolonged bathing and showering, even without the use of soaps, is discouraged for the care of dry and senile skin (Hogstel, 1983: 9).

The importance of skin surface acidity is only unveiled recently after a long dispute (Schmid and Korting, 1995: 191). This acidic milieu is vital for both the integrity of barrier function and for the regulation of skin flora (Rippke et al., 2002: 3). The skin surface pH has also been found to be a predictor for the development of irritant contact dermatitis (Wilhelm and Maibach, 1990: 23). The irritancy of water can theoretically also result from its neutral pH of 7.0, which is alkaline compared to skin surface pH of between 4.2 to 6.0. The origin of this skin surface pH has remained enigmatic. A recent study implicates urocanic acid as a key factor in the maintenance of this acid mantle (Krien and Kermici, 2000: 115). The neutralization capacity of lesional skin in hand eczema has been shown to be defective (Schieferstein and Krich-Hlobil, 1982: 30). The change in skin surface pH has been shown in atopic dermatitis, ichthyosis, diabetes mellitis and patients on dialysis.

■ CHAPTER 25 ■

Water is a universal solvent. Trace elements in the thermal water are the corner stone of the alleged beneficial effect of crenotherapy. To the contrary, the hardness of water may sometimes contribute to the irritancy of water (Warren and Ertel, 1997: 112). Hypotonicity of pure water, and change of water pressure gradient across the stratum corneum, which may trigger the release of cytokines, may also play a role in the irritancy of water. Hydration of the stratum corneum also facilitates the penetration of foreign substances, and contributes to the development of allergic and irritant contact dermatitis. This is best exemplified in occupational contact dermatitis involving wet work (Meding and Swanbeck, 1990: 22). Occlusive dressing therapy and wet wrapping therapy involve the same principle to enhance the therapeutic effects of topical corticosteroids (Sauer, 1977: 16).

Water is the most important element in the human body. To maintain water homeostasis, a relatively dry and impermeable skin is highly desirable. Any change in this water gradient will bring about major changes in skin physiology. Water is a ubiquitous irritant, and exerts its irritancy through different mechanisms. The irritancy of water under occlusion has long been recognized. But even contact with pure water will also produce physiologic changes of the skin, and these changes might be involved in some pathological processes. Everything can be an irritant, including water.

REFERENCES

AGNER, T. and SERUP, J. (1993) Time course of occlusive effects on skin evaluated by measurement of transepidermal water loss (TEWL). *Contact Dermatitis* **28**, 6–9.

ALY, R., SHIRLEY, C., CUNICO, B. and MAIBACH, H.I. (1978) Effect of prolonged occlusion on the microbial flora, pH, carbon dioxide and transepidermal water loss on human skin. *Journal of Investigative Dermatology*, **71**, 378–381.

BANK, I.H. (1952) Factors which influence the water content of the stratum corneum. *Journal of Investigative Dermatology*, **18**, 433–440.

DUBIEF, C. (1992) Experiments with hair photodegradation. *Cosmetrics and Toiletries*, **107**, 95–102.

FAERGEMANN, J., ALY, R., WILSON, D.R. and MAIBACH, H.I. (1983) Skin occlusion: effect on Pityrosporum orbiculare, skin PCO2, pH, transepidermal water loss, and water content. *Archives of Dermatological Research*, **275**, 383–387.

GORDON, B., MAIBACH, H.I. (1969) Adhesive tape anhidrosis. *Archives of Dermatology*, **100**, 429–431.

HASSING, J.H., NATER, J.P. and BLEUMINK, E. (1982) Irritancy of low concentrations of soap and synthetic detergents as measured by skin water loss. *Dermatologica*, **164**, 314–321.

HOGSTEL, M.O. (1983) Skin care for the aged. *Journal of Gerontologic Nursing*, **9**, 431–3, 436–437.

IMOKAWA, G., KUNO, H. and KAWAI, M. (1991) Stratum corneum lipids serve as a bound-water modulator. *Journal of Investigative Dermatology*, **96**, 845–851.

JACOBI, O.K. (1959) About the mechanism of moisture regulation in the horny layer of the skin. *Proceedings of Scientific Section Toilet Goods Association*, **31**, 22–24.

JACOBSON, T.M., YÜKSEL, K.U., GEESIN, J.C., GORDON, J.S., LANE, A.T. and GRACY, R.W. (1990) Effects of aging and xerosis on the amino acid composition of human skin. *Journal of Investigative Dermatology*, **95**, 296–300.

KLIGMAN, AM. (1996) Hydration injury to the skin. In: VAN DER VALK, P.G.M. and MAIBACH, H.I. (eds) *The Irritant Contact Dermatitis Syndrome*. Boca Raton, Florida: CRC Press, 187–194.

KRIEN, P.M. and KERMICI, M. (2000) Evidence for the existence of a self-regulated enzymatic process within the human stratum corneum—an unexpected role for urocanic acid. *Journal of Investigative Dermatology*, **115**, 414–420.

LOFFLER, H.I. (2001) Skin response to thermal stimuli. *Acta Dermato-Venereologica*, **81**, 395–397.

MEDING, B. and SWANBECK, G. (1990) Occupational hand eczema in an industrial city. *Contact Dermatitis*, **22**, 13–23.

PAPA, C.M. (1972) Mechanisms of eccrine anidrosis. 3. Scanning electron microscopic study of poral occlusion. *Journal of Investigative Dermatology*, **59**, 295–298.

RAJKA, G., ALY, R., BAYLES, C., TANG, Y. and MAIBACH, H.I. (1981) The effect of short-term occlusion on the cutaneous flora in atopic dermatitis and psoriasis. *Acta Dermato-Venereologica*, **61**, 150–153.

RIPPKE, F., SCHREINER, V. and SCHWANITZ, H.J. (2002) The acidic milieu of the horny layer. *American Journal of Clinical Dermatology*, **3**, 261–272.

ROTH, R.R. and JAMES, W.D. (1989) Microbiology of the skin: resident flora, ecology, infection. *Journal of the American Academy of Dermatology*, **20**, 367–390.

SAUER, G.C. (1977) Sulzberger on ACTH, corticosteroids, and occlusive dressing therapy. *International Journal of Dermatology*, **16**, 362–364.

SCHIEFERSTEIN, G. and KRICH-HLOBIL, K. (1982) [Alkali neutralization and alkali resistance in persons with healthy skin and in eczema patients] *Dermatosen in Beruf und Umwelt*, **30**, 7–13.

SCHMID, M.H. and KORTING, H.C. (1995) The concept of the acid mantle of the skin: its relevance for the choice of skin cleansers. *Dermatology*, **191**, 276–280.

SHELLEY, W.B. and SHELLEY, E.D. (1998) Aquadynia: noradrenergic pain induced by bathing and responsive to clonidine. *Journal of the American Academy of Dermatology*, **38**, 357–358.

SULZBERGER, M.B. and HARRIS, D.R. (1972) Miliaria and anhidrosis. 3. Multiple small patches and the effects of different periods of occlusion. *Archives of Dermatology*, **105**, 845–850.

TAPLIN, D. and ZAIAS, N. (1966) Tropical immersion foot. *Military Medicine*, **131**, 814.

WARREN, R. and ERTEL, K.D. (1997) Hard water. *Cosmetics and Toiletries* **112**, 67–74.

WATKINSON, A, HARDING, C., MOORE, A. and COAN, P. (2001) Water modulation of stratum corneum chymotryptic enzyme activity and desquamation. *Archives of Dermatological Research*, **293**, 470–476.

WILHELM, K.P. and MAIBACH, H.I. (1990) Susceptibility to irritant dermatitis induced by sodium lauryl sulfate. *Journal of the American Academy of Dermatology*, **23**, 122–124.

YAMAMURA, T. and TEZUKA, T. (1989) The water-holding capacity of the stratum corneum measured by 1H-NMR. *Journal of Investigative Dermatology*, **93**, 160–164.

Sodium Lauryl Sulfate in Dermatotoxicology

CHEOL HEON LEE AND HOWARD I MAIBACH

Contents

26.1 Introduction

26.2 Application methods

26.3 Biologic endpoints

26.4 Host-related factors

26.5 Conclusion

26.1 INTRODUCTION

Sodium lauryl sulfate (SLS) is an anionic surface active agent used as an emulsifier in many pharmaceutical vehicles, cosmetics, foaming dentifrices, and foods, and it is the sodium salt of lauryl sulfate that conforms to the formula: $CH_3(CH_2)10CH_2OSO_3Na$ (Nikitakis et al., 1991). The action of SLS on surface tension is putatively the cause of its irritancy, and its great capacity for altering the stratum corneum makes it useful to enhance penetration of other substances in patch tests and in animal assays.

Kligman (1966) found no sensitization to SLS was seen in hundred volunteers in which SLS was employed in provocative or prophetic patch test procedures. There are isolated reports of contact sensitization to SLS (Sams and Smith, 1957; Prater et al; 1978; Lee et al., 2000). Some important characteristics have been proposed for irritants used experimentally: no systemic toxicity, noncarcinogenic, not a sensitizer, chemically well defined, no extreme pH value, and not a cause of cosmetic inconveniences to exposed subjects (Wahlberg and Maibach, 1980). SLS fulfills these criteria as a model irritant in the study of experimental irritant contact dermatitis.

26.2 APPLICATION METHODS

Many studies concerned with cutaneous irritation utilize a 24-h patch application. A 7-h patch (Loden and Andersson, 1996) and 4-h patch (Basketter et al., 1996) with high concentration of SLS has been developed. In real life surfactant exposure is usually of short duration, open application and cumulative. A single challenge of the skin with an irritant insult is a momentary reflection of the skin's susceptibility, which does not consider the cumulative effect of irritation or the repair mechanisms of the skin. Repetitive challenges allow for these effects. Assay methods similar to real usage situation such as repeated short duration chamber test (Frosch and Kligman, 1979a; Tupker et al., 1989a,b), repeated open application test (Lammintausta et al., 1987a; Algood et al., 1990; Wilhelm et al., 1990; Lee and Maibach, 1994), plastic occlusion stress test (POST) (van der Valk and Maibach, 1989b; Berardesca and Maibach, 1990), and soak or wash test (Lukacovic et al., 1988; Klein et al., 1992) were developed.

Tupker et al. (1997) divided the studies on SLS two categories with respect to aims. The first category, provocative testing, concerns studies in which SLS is used to induce a definite skin reaction in all individuals. The second category, susceptibility evaluation, concerns studies aimed to predict the irritant susceptibility of individuals, and investigate individual and environmental factors determining this susceptibility.

A correlation coefficient of 0.63 between a single exposure and a four-day repetitive exposure to patch testing with SLS was found (Pinnagoda *et al.*, 1989). With repeated open application of SLS for 5 days as well as a single 24-h patch test with SLS using small (8 mm) patch test chambers, only the degree of skin damage caused by the repeated open test was found associated with prior skin complaints (Lammintausta *et al.*, 1988a). Lammintausta *et al.* (1987a) observed the decrease in patch test reactivity secondary to cumulative open SLS application using small (8 mm) patch test chambers and suggested that the induced hyporeactivity might be one of false negative diagnostic patch tests. There are two contrasting responses of cumulative SLS irritation; hyporeactivity may be noted if an epidermal responses, including hyperkeratosis and dryness was a major reaction to irritant; on the other hand, if a dermal reaction, such as erythema and edema, were a major component, hyperreactivity may develop (Lee *et al.*, 1997a). Moon *et al.* (2001) suggested that repetitive mild irritation may evoke the histological changes characterized by epidermal hyperplasia with minimal inflammatory infiltration. It may depend on various factors including concentration of SLS and host related factors to be hyperreactive or hyporeactive to repeated SLS application.

There are some variations in skin responses to identical patch tests and standardization of patch test procedure is necessary to minimize the variations in patch test responses.

26.2.1 Purity and carbon length of SLS

There were significant differences in the irritant potential *in vivo* for different qualities of SLS, and there were cases in which some of the C12 chains had been substituted by longer and less irritating carbon chains (Agner *et al.*, 1989). The presence of C12 chains of SLS is known to elicit a maximum irritant reaction (Kligman and Wooding, 1967; Stillman *et al.*, 1975; Wilhelm *et al.*, 1993). Agner *et al.* (1989) suggested that only SLS qualities of high purity (>99 percent) should be used for irritant patch testing and that the quality and the purity of SLS should be stated.

26.2.2 Quantity and concentration of test solution

Quantity of test solution is important and larger quantities of test solution give more intense skin reactions, although the concentration of the irritant is kept constant (Magnusson and Hersle, 1965; Frosch and Kligman, 1979b), and Agner (1992) suggested that the Duhring chamber, the 12 mm Finn chamber, or even large chambers having bigger test areas are more effective in eliciting a response. Mikulowska and Andersson (1996) observed that the effects of 8 mm chambers could result in increased, unchanged or decreased Langerhans cells (LC) numbers, while 12 mm chambers always produced decrease in LC number. Lee *et al.* (1997b) also compared the effect of chamber size on SLS irritation on the volar forearm using three different size (8 mm, 12 mm, 18 mm) Finn chambers. The increase in skin response (visual score and transepidermal water loss (TEWL)) with the large (12 mm) Finn chamber was greater than that with the small (8 mm) Finn chamber. However, there were no significant differences between large and extra-large (18 mm) Finn chambers.

Aramaki *et al.* (2001a) studied the interrelationship between SLS concentration and duration of exposure in irritant skin reaction. The influence of SLS concentration and duration of exposure was demonstrated with a standardized coefficient value β. For TEWL, the β value of the SLS concentration was 1.5-fold higher than that found for the exposure time. For the laser Doppler flowmetry (LD), the β value of concentration was 2.5-fold higher than that of the exposure time. And they suggested that the skin reaction to SLS could be calculated by the following formulae; Δ TEWL = 14.36 × concentration + 0.82 × duration (hours) – 5.12, and LD = 30.81 × concentration + 1.09 × duration + 2.49. This estimation is only valid for a patch application of $\leq$24 h.

Brasch *et al.* (1999) have analyzed the synchronous reproducibility of patch tests with various concentrations of SLS aqueous solution (0.0625, 0.125, 0.25, 0.5, 1.0 percent) using a large Finn chamber, and they suggested that 1.0 percent SLS aqueous solution is appropriate for an irritant patch test as a positive control. Contamination with bacteria was found in the SLS solutions of lower concentrations resulting in decreased concentration of SLS and the storage of SLS solutions of very low concentrations should be at low temperature and preferably in sterile vials (Sugar *et al.*, 1999).

26.2.3   Evaporation and temperature of test solution

The penetration of SLS through the skin barrier is significantly increased by the increase of the temperature of test solution (Emilson *et al.*, 1993). Berardesca *et al.*, (1995) reported significantly different skin responses to the temperature of test solution (4°C, 20°C and 40°C). Skin damage was higher in sites treated with warmer temperatures; there was a highly significant correlation between irritation and temperature of test solution. Ohlenschlaeger *et al.* (1996) also demonstrated increased irritation on the application site of warmer solution using repeated immersions in an SLS solution at 20°C and 40°C. Transition from a packed gel state to a more fluid crystalline state in stratum corneum lipids occurs at temperatures between 38°C and 40°C and the fluidity of stratum corneum is important in the percutaneous penetration process as an explanation of increased irritancy at higher temperatures (Berardesca *et al.*, 1995). The evaporation rate of aqueous solutions from Finn chambers was reported as 1 mg/3 min (Fischer and Maibach, 1984). Evaporation from the patch before application inhibits the inflammatory response, even though the relative concentration of the irritant is increased by the process (Dahl and Roering, 1984). This inhibition of skin irritation could be the result of decreased amount or lowered temperature owing to evaporation of test solution.

26.2.4   Time of evaluation

When noninvasive measurements of the skin response are made, the interval between removal of the patch and the measurements should allow for a period of increased evaporation following occlusion. Equalization of water diffusion between the stratum corneum and the ambient air is settled after 20 min of patch removal (Stender *et al.*, 1990). For measurements of TEWL, in most papers, the interval was reported to be 30 minutes (Berardesca and Maibach, 1988b; Freeman and Maibach, 1988; Goh and Chia, 1988). The time course of TEWL after SLS patch testing demonstrated significant reduction in TEWL values from 30 to 60 min after removal of the patch, but not from 60 to 180 min (Agner and Serup, 1993), and they suggested that evaluation of irritant patch test reactions by measurement of TEWL can naturally be made at any time after removal of the patches, as long as the time period is precisely accounted for. Others have argued that a minimum waiting period of 2 or 3 hours should be allowed for evaporation of excessive water due to occlusion (Baker and Kligman, 1967; Pinnagoda *et al.*, 1989). Recently Aramaki *et al.* (2001a) suggested that TEWL measurement performed 30 min after patch removal is too early and measurement 24 hours after patch removal should be done for practical reasons.

26.2.3   Guidelines on SLS exposure methods (Tupker *et al.*, 1997)

High purity (99 percent) SLS must be used in any study, dissolved water in occlusive and open testing, while tap water may be acceptable in immersion testing. Standard sized occlusion chambers with filter paper disks corresponding to large (12 mm, 60 μl) and extra-large (18 mm, 200 μl) Finn chamber are recommended. The extra-large Finn chambers are recommended for repeated applications. For open exposures, 20 mm diameter plastic ring is advised. The volume of the solutions must be such that the total exposure area is covered (800 μl). Chambers should be applied to the skin immediately, i.e. within one minute after preparation with the test solution. TEWL measurement should be performed a minimum of 1 hour after removal of test chambers. ESCD proposed new guidelines in terms of purposes and methods of SLS exposure tests (Table 26.1).

26.3   BIOLOGIC ENDPOINTS

26.3.1   Clinical appearance of SLS reaction

Erythema, infiltration, superficial erosion can be seen during acute reaction to SLS. With higher concentrations vesicular and pustular reactions may be seen. During healing of acute reactions, scaling and fissuring will take over. The same appearance of erythema, scaling and fissuring is seen during repeated application of SLS. The soap effect consisting of fine wrinkled surface and/or chapping is not commonly seen in SLS patch test reaction (Tupker *et al.*, 1997). Most recently reported literatures have used the modified visual scoring system of Frosch and Kligman (1979a) to evaluate clinical skin reaction to SLS. Tupker *et al.* (1997) developed the guideline concerning about the visual scoring schemes for the acute and cumulative reactions to SLS (Tables 26.2 and 26.3).

26.3.2   Pathogenesis of SLS reaction

The histopathologic changes induced by SLS depend on various factors including concentration, mode of application, time of evaluation. Acute reaction to SLS application in epidermis can include hyperkeratosis, parakeratosis, spongiosis, intracellular edema, hydropic degeneration of basal cells, and necrosis (Gisslen and Magnusson, 1966; Tovell *et al.*, 1974; Mahmoud *et al.*, 1984; Willis *et al.*,

TABLE 26.1:

ESCD guidelines on SLS exposure tests with TEWL measurement[a]

	Susceptibility evaluation		Provocative testing	
	Acute	Cumulative	Acute	Cumulative
One-time occlusion test				
Application time	24 h	Not applicable	24 h	Not Applicable
Mode of application	chamber 12 mm		chamber 12 mm	
SLS w/v%	0.5%		2%	
Repeated occlusion test				
Application time	Not applicable	2 h 1×daily	Not applicable	2 h 1×daily
Application period		3 weeks[b]		3 weeks[b]
Mode of application		chamber 18 mm		chamber 18 mm
SLS w/v%		0.25%		1%
Open test				
Application time	60 min 2×daily	10 min 1×daily	Not possible[a]	10 min 1×daily
Application period	1 day	3 weeks[b]		3 weeks[b]
Mode of application	20 mm guard ring	20 mm guard ring		20 mm guard ring
SLS w/v%	10%	1%		1%
Immersion test[c]				
Immersion time	30 min 2×daily	10 min 2×daily	30 min 2×daily	10 min 1×daily
Application period	1 day	3 weeks[b]	1 day	3 weeks[b]
Mode of application	forearm immersion	forearm immersion	forearm immersion	forearm immersion
SLS w/v%	0.5%	0.5%	2%	2%

[a] Tupker, R.A., Willis, C., Berardesca, E., Lee, C.H., Fartasch, M., Agner, T. and Serup, J. (1997) 'Guidelines on sodium lauryl sulfate (SLS) exposure tests. A report from the standardization group of the European society of contact dermatitis', Contact Dermatitis, **37**: 53–69.

[b] 1 week is 5 application days.

[c] Water temperature 35°C.

TABLE 26.2:

ESCL guideline on clinical scoring of acute SLS irritant reactions[a]

Score	Qualification	Description
0	Negative	No reaction
1/2	Doubtful	Very weak erythema or minute scaling
1	Weak	Weak erythema, slight oedema, slight scaling and/or slight roughness
2	Moderate	Moderate degree of: erythema, oedema, scaling, roughness, erosions, vesicles, bullae, crusting and/or fissuring
3	Strong	Marked degree of: erythema, oedema, scaling, roughness, erosions, vesicles, bullae, crusting and/or fissuring
4	Very strong/caustic	as 3, with necrotic areas

[a] Tupker, R.A., Willis, C., Berardesca, E., Lee, C.H., Fartasch, M., Agner, T. and Serup, J. (1997) 'Guidelines on sodium lauryl sulfate (SLS) exposure tests. A report from the standardization group of the European society of contact dermatitis', *Contact Dermatitis*, **37**: 53–69.
Note. Reading 25 to 96 hours after one-time exposure.

TABLE 26.3:

ESCD guideline on clinical scoring of subacute/cumulative SLS irritant reactions[a]

Score	Qualification	Description
0	Negative	no reaction
1/2	Doubtful	Very weak erythema and/or shiny surface[b]
1	Weak	Weak erythema, diffuse or spotty, slight scaling and/or slight roughness[c]
2	Moderate	moderate degree of: erythema, scaling, roughness and/or weak oedema and/or fine fissures
3	Strong	marked degree of: erythema, scaling, roughness, oedema, fissures and/or presence of papules and/or erosions and/or vesicles
4	very strong/caustic	as 3, with necrotic areas

[a] Tupker, R.A., Willis, C., Berardesca, E., Lee, C.H., Fartasch, M., Agner, T. and Serup, J. (1997) 'Guidelines on sodium lauryl sulfate (SLS) exposure tests. A report from the standardization group of the European society of contact dermatitis', *Contact Dermatitis*, **37**: 53–69.
[b] The term 'shiny surface' is used for those minimal reactions that can only be discerned when evaluated in skimming light as a 'shiny area.'
[c] The term 'roughness' is used for reactions that can be felt as rough or dry, sometimes preceeded or followed by visible changes of the surface contour, in contrast to 'scaling,' which is accompanied by visible small flakes.

1989; Moon *et al.*, 2001). In dermis, there were variable degrees of inflammatory cell infiltration, edema, collagen degeneration. T lymphocytes are the predominant infiltrating cells and CD4(+) cells outnumbered the CD8(+) cells (Scheynius *et al.*, 1984; Ferguson *et al.*, 1985; Avnstorp *et al.*, 1987; Brasch *et al.*, 1992; Willis *et al.*, 1993). The histologic changes to cumulative SLS irritation were similar as in acute irritation, but repetitive mild irritation may evoke epidermal hyperplasia with minimal inflammatory infiltration (Moon *et al.*, 2001).

Many surfactants including SLS disrupt the skin barrier function resulting in increased TEWL (Scheuplein and Ross, 1970; Elias, 1983), and increased blood flow, clinically visible as erythema (van der Valk *et al.*, 1984). A number of hypotheses on the mechanism of SLS-induced skin irritation has been suggested. Leveque *et al.* (1993) suggested that an increase in TEWL did not necessarily imply the alteration of stratum corneum and SLS-induced dry skin could hardly be interpreted in terms of lipid removal (Froebe *et al.*, 1990). A disruption of the secondary and tertiary structure of keratin proteins may expose new water-binding sites resulting in stratum corneum hydration, and the most likely explanation of SLS-induced increase in TEWL lay in the hyperhydration of stratum corneum and a possible disorganization of lipid bilayers (Wilhelm *et al.*, 1993). Forslind (1994) proposed a domain mosaic model of skin barrier. Stratum corneum lipids are not randomly distributed, but are organized in domains. Lipids with very long chain lengths are segregated in gel, impermeable to water, and separated by grain borders populated by lipids with short chain lengths which are in fluid phase, permeable to water. Surfactants including SLS infiltrate the fluid phase permeable to water increasing the width of grain borders, and increase TEWL.

26.3.3 Noninvasive bioengineering techniques assessing SLS reaction

Several non-invasive bioengineering methods to quantify and to obtain information which is not detectable clinically have developed in recent decades (Table 26.4) (Lee and Maibach, 1995). Measurement of TEWL as a technique to evaluate skin barrier function is widely used (Berardesca and Maibach, 1988a; Wilhelm *et al.*, 1989), and a positive dose-response relationship for skin response to SLS as measured by TEWL has been demonstrated (Agner and Serup, 1990a). When attempting to quantify irritant patch test reactions by electrical conductance measurement, the intra-individual variation in the results was so high that the method was found unhelpful for this purpose (Agner and Serup, 1990b). A positive relationship was found between dose of SLS and blood flow values recorded by laser Doppler flowmetry (Nilsson *et al.*, 1982; Agner and Serup, 1990a). However, wide fluctuations in laser Doppler blood flow values in response to SLS patches were found due to spotty erythema (Freeman and

TABLE 26.4:

Noninvasive bioengineering techniques used in the evaluation of cutaneous irritation.

Technique	Measured skin function	Information obtained
Evaporimeter	Transepidermal water loss	Positive dose-response relationship for skin response to SLS Most sensitive method for SLS-induced irritation
Laser-Doppler flowmeter	Blood flow	Positive relationship between applied dose of SLS and blood flows. Wide fluctuations in response to SLS due to spotty erythema
Ultrasound	Skin thickness	No preconditioning is necessary. Good relation to SLS concentrations, but minimal correlation with erythema or epidermal damage
Impedance, conductance, capacitance	Skin hydration	Correlation with epidermal damage, but intra-individual variation is so high, this method is unhelpful
colorimeter	Skin colors	Positive correlation between changes in the a* color coordinates and doses of SLS, but not with epidermal damage

Maibach 1988). The skin color is expressed in a 3-dimensional coordinate system: a* (from green to red), b* (from blue to yellow), and L* (from black to white) values (Robertson, 1977). Color a* coordinates have been demonstrated to correlate well with visual scoring of erythema in inflammatory reactions caused by soap or SLS (Babulak *et al.*, 1986; Wilhelm *et al.*, 1989; Serup and Agner, 1990). Ultrasound examination has the advantage that no preconditioning of the subjects is necessary before measurement. Ultrasound A-scan has been found suitable for quantification of patch test reactions (Serup *et al.*, 1984; Serup and Staberg, 1987) and also a promising method for quantification of SLS-induced inflammatory response, being consistently more sensitive than measurement of skin color (Agner and Serup 1990a), and Seidenari and di Nardo (1992) demonstrated that B-scanning evaluation showed a good correlation with TEWL values in assessing superficial skin damage induced by SLS.

In a comparison among evaporimetry, laser Doppler flowmetry (LD), ultrasound A-scan and measurement of skin color, evapometry was found to be the best suited method for evaluation of SLS-induced skin damage (Wilhelm *et al.*, 1989; Agner and Serup, 1990b). Lee *et al.* (1997c) observed that measurement of erythema index using Dermaspectrometer was less sensitive than TEWL

CHAPTER 26

measurement when comparing the cutaneous irritation to two types (8 mm and 12 mm) of Finn chamber. Wilhelm *et al.* (1989) suggested that although TEWL measurements may be an accurate and sensitive method in evaluating skin irritation, color reflectance measurements may be a helpful complimentary tool for the clinician, because of its convenience. Serup (1995) suggested that transepidermal water loss is sensitive and useful in the study of corrosive irritants, such as SLS, especially in the induction phase of irritant reaction, but does not have direct clinical relevance, and the results need be backed up with other relevant measures. Fluhr *et al.* (2001) suggested that, regarding the time-dependent effect, a positive discrimination was seen for TEWL, measuring the barrier function, and the perfusion parameter LD. The discriminatory ability of TEWL was superior to that of LD. However, when evaluating SLS patch testing by bioengineering methods, TEWL measurement appears more suitable to evaluate skin reaction to SLS concentration less than 1.0 percent, whereas LD is more appropriate to evaluate pronounced skin reaction (SLS concentration ≥1 percent) (Aramaki *et al.*, 2001b).

Tupker *et al.* (1990) found that the time course of TEWL after a 24-h SLS patch test varied between different subjects. Using SLS in varying concentrations, Serup and Staberg (1987) found a delayed response only for reactions clinically scored as 1+, but not for more intense reactions, indicating that the kinetics of the response may depend on the severity of the reaction (Dahl and Trancik, 1977; Aramaki *et al.*, 2001b).

26.3.4   Recovery of SLS reaction

Wilhelm *et al.* (1994) studied the skin function during healing phase after single 24-h patch application of 0.5 percent SLS solution. Erythema was most increased directly after patch removal with a slow gradual decrease, but not completely resolved even 18 days after treatment. Stratum corneum (SC) hydration evaluated by capacitance measurements did not return to baseline values before 17 days after surfactant exposure. The repair of the SC barrier function as indicated by TEWL measurements was completed 14 days after exposure. Freeman and Maibach (1988) described augmented irritant response to repeated application of 2 percent SLS solution on the clinically improved, irritant contact dermatitis site, and suggested that although skin may appear to be morphologically normal, it may not be functionally normal. Lee *et al.* (1997a) suggested that complete recovery of skin function after acute reaction induced 1 percent SLS solution was achieved approximately 4 weeks later. Choi *et al.* (2000)

demonstrated that skin reactivity of chronically irritated sites with SLS solution showed hyperreactivity compared to normal skin even 10 weeks after chronic irritation, and suggested that chronically irritated skin required a longer recovery time than acutely irritated skin.

26.4 HOST-RELATED FACTORS

There are many host-related factors in cutaneous irritation.: those that are considered as skin disease, and those that represent variations from normal skin predisposed to irritation (Table 26.5).

26.4.1 Age

Increased susceptibility to SLS in young females compared to elderly females was reported, when assessed by visual scoring and TEWL, and the increase in TEWL values was found to be more persistent in the older group (Cua *et al.*, 1990; Elsner *et al.*, 1990). These findings imply less reaction to an irritant stimulus but a prolonged healing period in older people. There is no significant influence on skin susceptibility between the 18–50 years of age (Agner, 1991a), but significantly reduced irritant reactivity in older more than 55 years age group compared to various younger age groups (Robinson, 2002).

26.4.2 Sex

Hand eczema occurs more frequently among women than men. However, many investigators have found no sex correlation in skin susceptibility (Goh and Chia, 1988; Bjornberg, 1975; Lammintausta *et al.*, 1987b; Tupker *et al.*, 1989c). Reactivity to SLS at day 1 increased in the menstrual cycle compared to day

TABLE 26.5:

Host-related factors in cutaneous irritation

Age
Sex
Anatomic region
Race and skin color
Skin hydration
Sensitive skin
Hyperirritable skin
Skin disease (atopic dermatitis, hand eczema, seborrheic dermatitis)

■ CHAPTER 26 ■

9–11, when tested on opposite arms in healthy women (Agner *et al.*, 1991). Since no cyclical variation was found in baseline TEWL, the increased reactivity of the skin at day 1 in the menstrual cycle probably reflects an increased inflammatory reactivity, rather than changes in the barrier function. Recently Robinson (2002) reported that the male subjects responded more rapidly, and there was a significant increase in response of the male subjects compared to female subjects.

26.4.3 Anatomic region

Variation in skin responses within the same individual to identical irritant patch tests may be considerable. Van der Valk and Maibach (1989a) studied the differences in sensitivity of volar surface of the forearm to SLS and demonstrated that the potential for irritation increases from the wrist to the cubital fossa, and Panisset *et al.* (1992) showed that TEWL values next to the wrist were found greater than on the other sites of volar forearm. Cua *et al.* (1990) reported that the thigh had the highest reactivity and the palm the lowest. Henry *et al.* (1997) studied the regional variability to 1 percent SLS using corneosurfametry (OCM) bioassay and found that the dorsal hand and volar forearm were the least reactive, the neck, forehead, back and dorsal foot the most reactive sites. Dahl *et al.* (1984) found that, for simultaneous Al-patch testing with SLS, the corresponding sites on the right and the left side were scored identically in only 53 percent of cases. Using large Finn chambers (12 mm), 84 percent of SLS patches showed identical visual score when tested simultaneously on right and left arms (Agner and Serup, 1990b). Rogiers (1995) suggested that measurement of TEWL should be carried out on identical anatomic sites for all subjects involved, and the volar forearm is a good measurement site and corresponding places on the right and left forearms exhibit the same TEWL.

26.4.4 Race and skin color

Bjornberg *et al.* (1979) reported that fair skin and blue eyes showed the high intensity of the inflammatory response to a mechanical irritant. When skin color was assessed by a tri-stimulus colorimeter, an association between light reflection (L^*) from the skin surface and susceptibility to SLS was found (Agner, 1991a, b). By determination of minimal erythema dose (MED) in Caucasians, the cutaneous sensitivity to UV light and to seven different chemical irritants was found to correlate positively, while skin phototype based on complexion and history of sunburn proved less reliable (Frosch and Wissing, 1982). McFadden *et al.* (1998) found no signuficant differences in irritation thresholds to SLS between six skin phototypes. In contrast to these reports, an inclination to increased susceptibility to SLS in black and hispanic skin types as compared to white skin types was found when evaluated by measurement of TEWL (Berardesca and Maibach, 1988b, c). There were more complexing reports concerning the SLS susceptibility between Caucasian and Asian population. There was an increased cumulative irritation response in Japanese subjects versus Caucasian to various chemicals (Rapaport, 1984). Foy *et al.* (2001) demonstrated a greater acute irritant responses in Japanese women compared to Caucasian; however, cumulative irritation did not show significant increase in Japanese compared to Caucasian. Chinese displayed similar response profile in acute irritation test; however, they showed a slower and less severe response in the cumulative irritation test compared to Caucasian or Japanese subjects (Robinson, 2000). Robinson *et al.* (1998) failed to find significant differences in skin reactivity to SLS between Caucasians and Asians. However, there was a consistent trend toward increased reactivity, i.e. reduced time to respond, observed in the Asian versus Caucasian subjects (Robinson, 2002). Tanning may influence the susceptibility to irritants. A diminished reaction to SLS after UVB exposure was reported (Larmi *et al.*, 1989).

26.4.5 Skin hydration

In repetitive exposure to SLS, higher susceptibility was reported in dry skin than in clinically normal skin in eczematous subjects and controls (Tupker *et al.*, 1990). Comparing winter and summer skin, decreased skin hydration was found in winter, when a higher reactivity to SLS was also found (Agner and Serup, 1989). Low outdoor temperature and low relative humidity in the winter lead to decreased ability of the stratum corneum to retain water (Spencer *et al.*, 1975). Thus, these studies indicate that a decreased hydration state of the skin may be associated with impaired barrier function and increased skin susceptibility. In contrast, Lammintausta *et al.* (1988a) found no relationship between clinically dry skin and the response to repeated SLS exposure.

26.4.6 Sensitive skin

Frosch and Kligman (1977) reported a significant correlation between the skin response to particular irritants in healthy volunteers and patients with skin diseases. A 24-h forearm chamber exposure to 5 percent SLS solution was used for pre-selection of hyperreactors (Frosch and Kligman, 1979a). Murahata *et al.* (1986) suggested a relationship between skin susceptibility to detergents and high baseline TEWL and a highly significant correlation between baseline TEWL and TEWL after a single or repeated exposure to SLS was reported (Pinnagoda *et al.*, 1989; Tupker *et al.*, 1989c; Agner *et al.*, 1991a, b). However, other studies reported an absent or poor correlation between baseline TEWL and TEWL after SLS exposure (Berardesca and Maibach, 1988b, c; Freeman and Maibach, 1988; Wilhelm and Maibach, 1990).

Sensitive skin is a skin type having higher reactivity than normal skin and developing exaggerated reactions when exposed to external factors (Berardesca and Maibach, 1991). The stinging test using lactic acid has been widely used for the selection of sensitive skin. However, this test is based on self-perceived assessment and lacks objectivity. Seidenari *et al.* (1998) demonstrated a decrease of baseline capacitance values indicating the tendency to barrier impairment, and they suggested that dehydration can represent a basis for subjective sensations after exposure to water and soap. Lammintausta *et al.* (1988b) demonstrated a reactivity to a 24-h SLS patch test using laser Doppler velocimetry in stingers compared with non-stingers. Simion *et al.* (1995) also showed the correlations between self-perceived sensory responses to cleansing products and TEWL and colorimeter a* values. in stingers. However, other studies did not show correlation between self-assessed skin sensitivity or skin reactivity to chemosensory stimuli and skin reaction to SLS irritation (Coverly *et al.*, 1998; Robinson *et al.*, 1998; Robinson, 2002).

26.4.7 Hyperirritable skin (Excited skin syndrome)

Mitchell (1977) introduced the term "angry back" to describe the phenomenon of a single strong positive patch test reaction creating a back which is hyperreactive to other patch test applications. The excited skin syndrome was illustrated experimentally in guinea pigs and increased susceptibility to an ointment containing 1 percent SLS was observed in animals stressed by inflammatory reactions in the neck area (Andersen and Maibach, 1980). Bruynzeel *et al.* (1983) attempted to use SLS patches as markers of hyperirritability. Agner (1991b) observed no increased skin reactivity to SLS in patients with chronic or healed eczema compared to controls, while hand eczema patients with acute eczema showed an increased skin reactivity to SLS compared to controls. Shahidullah *et al.* (1969) reported increased TEWL values in the clinically normal skin of patients with eczema. But there was no significant difference in baseline TEWL values between in patients with eczema and in controls (van der Valk *et al.*, 1985; Agner, 1991b).

26.4.8 Skin diseases (atopic dermatitis, hand eczema, seborrheic dermatitis)

There is a marked abnormality in barrier function in the skin of patients with atopic dermatitis (AD), and high levels of sphingomyelin deacylase were demonstrated in the lesional and non-lesional skin of patients with AD leading to decrease of ceramide and abnormality in barrier function (Imokawa, 2001).

Di Nardo *et al.* (1996) suggested that stratum corneum ceramide content may determine a proclivity to SLS-induced irritant contact dermatitis. There are many reports of increased baseline TEWL in clinically normal skin of patients with AD (Werner and Lindberg, 1985; Agner, 1990; Tupker *et al.*, 1990; Seidenari, 1994; Nassif *et al.*, 1994; Tabata *et al.*, 1998). Agner (1990) showed that the response to SLS was statistically significantly increased in atopics compared to controls, when evaluated by visual scoring and skin thickness, but not TEWL. Nassif *et al.* (1994) suggested that atopic dermatitis patients, as well as those with a history of allergic rhinitis, had a lower irritant threshold than controls. A significantly greater intensity of response in the atopics, compared to controls, was also observed. It has also been demonstrated that a significantly greater response to SLS (Nassif *et al.*, 1994; Cowley and Farr, 1992; Agner, 1991b; Tupker *et al.*, 1990), as well as a tendency to increased skin susceptibility, is related to the degree of severeity of the dermatitis (Tupker *et al.*, 1995). There were no significant differences in TEWL between individuals who were classified as atopic but without active dermatitis, individuals with rhinoconjunctivitis or atopic asthma and healthy controls, either at the basal or at the post-SLS measurement. Enhanced skin susceptibility is only present in individuals with active dermatitis (Loeffler and Effendy, 1999). Basketter *et al.* (1998) also could not find significant differences in skin reactions to SLS in the normal skin of AD compared to control group.

Baseline TEWL values in patients with localized, inactive or healed eczema were not significantly higher than in controls (van der Valk *et al.*, 1989b; Agner, 1991b). Agner (1991b) observed no increased skin reactivity to SLS in patients with chronic or healed eczema compared to controls, while hand eczema patients with acute eczema showed an increased skin reactivity to SLS compared to controls.

CHAPTER 26

There were several reports that showed patients with seborrheic dermatitis could be easily irritated to some chemicals including SLS (Lamintausta and Maibach, 1988; Cowley and Farr, 1992). Tollesson and Frithz (1993) observed increased TEWL values and abnormality in essential fatty acids in infantile seborrheic dermatitis, and they normalized TEWL values by applying the borage oil containing gamma-linoleic acid.

26.5 CONCLUSION

It is clear that SLS data does not provide a unanimous opinion on all points. Yet, the preponderance of the observations suggest that we are beginning to understand some of the parameters, such as purity, dose, patch, anatomic site, single versus multiple application, occluded versus open application, that influence diverse response of the skin irritation.

REFERENCES

AGNER, T. (1990) Susceptibility of atopic dermatitis patients to irritant dermatitis caused by sodium lauryl sulfate, *Acta Derm. Venereol. (Stockh.)*, **71**, 296–300.

AGNER, T. (1991a) Basal transepidermal water loss, skin thickness, skin blood flow and skin colour in relation to sodium-lauryl-sulfate-induced irritation in normal skin, *Contact Dermatitis*, **25**, 108–114.

AGNER, T. (1991b) Skin susceptibility in uninvolved skin of hand eczema patients and healthy controls, *Br. J. Dermatol.*, **125**, 140–146.

AGNER, T. (1992) Noninvasive measuring methods for the investigation of irritant patch test reactions. A study of patients with hand eczema, atopic dermatitis and controls, *Acta Derm. Venereol. (Stockh.)*, suppl. **173**, 1–26.

AGNER, T. and SERUP, J. (1989) Seasonal variation of skin resistance to irritants, *Br. J. Dermatol.*, **121**, 323–328.

AGNER, T. and SERUP, J. (1990a), Sodium lauryl sulfate for irritant patch testing-A dose-response study using bioengineering methods for determination of skin irritation, *J. Invest. Dermatol.*, **95**, 543–547.

AGNER, T. and SERUP, J. (1990b) Individual and instrumental variations in irritant patch-test reactions-clinical evaluation and quantification by bioengineering methods, *Clinical Experimental Dermatol.*, **15**, 29–33.

AGNER, T. and SERUP, J. (1993) Time course of occlusive effects on skin evaluated by measurement of transepidermal water loss (TEWL): Including patch tests with sodium lauryl sulfate and water, *Contact Dermatitis*, **28**, 6–9.

AGNER, T., SERUP, J., HANDLOS, V. and BATSBERG, W. (1989) Different skin irritation abilities of different qualities of sodium lauryl sulfate, *Contact Dermatitis*, **21**, 184–188.

AGNER, T., DAMM, P. and SKOUBY, S.O. (1991) Menstrual cycle and skin reactivity, *J. Am. Acad. Dermatol.*, **24**, 566–570.

ALGOOD, G.S., ALTRINGER, L.A. and KRAUS, A.L. (1990) Development of 14 day axillary irritation test, *J. Toxicol. Cut. Ocular. Toxicol.*, **9**, 67–75.

ANDERSEN, K.E. and MAIBACH, H.I. (1980) Cumulative irritancy in the guinea pig from low grade irritant vehicles and the angry skin syndrome, *Contact Dermatitis*, **6**, 430–434.

ARAMAKI, J., LOEFFLER, C., KWANA, S., EFFENDY, I., HAPPLE, R. and LOEFFLER, H. (2001a) Irritant patch testing with sodium lauryl sulfate: interrelation between concentration and exposure time, *Brit. J. Dermatol.*, **145**, 704–708.

ARAMAKI, J., EFFENDY, I., HAPPLE, R., KWANA, S., LOEFFLER, C. and LOEFFLER, H. (2001b) Which bioengineering assay is appropriate for irritant patch testing with sodium lauryl sulfate?, *Contact Dermatitis*, **45**, 286–290.

AVNSTORP, C., RALFKIAER, E., JORGENSEN, J. and LANGE WANTZIN, G. (1987) Sequential immunophenotypic study of lymphoid infiltrate in allergic and irritant reactions, *Contact Dermatitis*, **16**, 239–245.

BABULAK. S.W., RHEIN, L.D., SCALA, D.D., SIMION. F.A. and GROVE, G.L. (1986) Quantification of erythema in a soap chamber test using the Minolta Chroma (reflectance) Meter: Comparison of instrumental results with visual assessment, *J. Soc. Cosmet. Chem.*, **37**, 475–479.

BAKER, H. and KLIGMAN, A.M. (1967) Measurement of transepidermal water loss by electrical hygrometry, *Arch. Dermatol.* **96**, 441–452.

BASKETTER, D.A., GRIFFITHS, H.A., WANG, X.M., WILHELM, K.P. and MCFADDEN, J. (1996) Individual, ethnic and seasonal variability in irritant susceptibility of skin: the implications for a predictive human patch test, *Contact Dermatitis*, **35**, 208–213.

BASKETTER, D.A., MIETTINEN, J. and LAHTI, A. (1998) Acute irritant reactivity to sodium lauryl sulfate in atopics and non-atopics, *Contact Dermatitis*, **38**, 253–257.

BERARDESCA, E. and MAIBACH, H.I. (1988a) Bioengineering and the patch test, *Contact Dermatitis*, **18**, 3–9.

BERARDESCA, E. and MAIBACH, H.I. (1988b) Racial differences in sodium lauryl sulfate induced cutaneous irritation: black and white, *Contact Dermatitis* 18, 65–70.

BERARDESCA, E and MAIBACH, H.I. (1988c) Sodium-lauryl-sulfate-induced cutaneous irritation. Comparison of white and hispanic subjects, *Contact Dermatitis,* 19, 136–140.

BERARDESCA, E. and MAIBACH, H.I. (1990) Monitoring the water-holding capacity in visually non-irritated skin by plastic occlusion stress test (POST), *Clinical Experimental Dermatol.,* 15, 107–110.

BERARDESCA, E. and MAIBACH, H.I. (1991) Sensitive skin and ethnic skin. A need for special skin-care agents. *Derm. Clin.,* 9, 89–92.

BERARDESCA, E., VIGNOLI, G.P., DISTANTE, F., BRIZZI, P. and RABBIOSI, G. (1995) Effect of water temperature on surfactant-induced skin irritation, *Contact Dermatitis,* 32, 83–87.

BJORNBERG, A. (1975) Skin reactions to primary irritants in men and women, *Acta Derm. Venereol. (Stockh.),* 55, 191–194.

BJORNBERG, A., LOWHAGEN, G. and TENGBERG, J. (1979) Relationship between intensities of skin test reactions to glass-fibres and chemical irritants, *Contact Dermatitis,* 5, 171–174.

BRASCH, J., BURGAND, J. and STERRY, W. (1992) Common pathogenetic pathways in allergic and irritant contact dermatitis, *J. Invest. Dermatol.,* 98, 364–370

BRASCH, J., BECKER, D. and EFFENDY, I. (1999) Reproducibility of irritant patch test reactions to sodium lauryl sulfate in a double-blind placebo-controlled randomized study using clinical scoring, *Contact Dermatitis,* 41, 150–155.

BRUYNZEEL, D.P., VAN KETEL, W.G., VON BLOMBERG-VAN DER FLIER, M. and SCHEPER, R.J. (1983) Angry back or the excited skin syndrome, *J. Am. Acad. Dermatol.,* 8, 392–397.

CHOI, J.M., LEE, J.Y. and CHO, B.K. (2000) Chronic irritant contact dermatitis: recovery time in man, *Contact Dermatitis,* 42, 264–269.

COVERLY, J., PETERS, L., WHITTLE, E. and BASKETTER, D.A. (1998) Susceptibility to skin stinging, non-immunologic contact urticaria and acute skin reaction; is there a relationship?, *Contact Dermatitis,* 38, 90–95.

COWLEY, N.C. and FARR, P.M. (1992) A dose-response study of irritant reactions to sodium lauryl sulfate in patients with seborrheic dermatitis and atopic eczema, *Acta Derm. Venereol. (Stockh.),* 72, 432–435.

CUA, A.B., WILHELM, K.P. and MAIBACH, H.I. (1990) Cutaneous sodium lauryl sulfate irritation potential: age and regional variability, *Br. J. Dermatol.*, **123**, 607–613.

DAHL, M.V. and ROERING, M.J. (1984) Sodium lauryl sulfate irritant patch tests. III. Evaporation of aqueous vehicle influences inflammatory response, *J. Am. Acad. Dermatol.*, **11**, 477–479.

DAHL, M.V. and TRANCIK, R.J. (1977) Sodium lauryl sulfate irritant patch tests: Degree of inflammation at various times, *Contact Dermatitis*, **3**, 263–266.

DAHL, M.V., PASS, F. and TRANCIK, R.J. (1984) Sodium lauryl sulfate irritant patch tests. II. Variation of test responses among subjects and comparison to variations of allergic responses elicited by Toxicodendron extract, *J. Am. Acad. Dermatol.*, **11**, 474–477.

DI NARDO, A., SUGINO, K., WERTZ, P., ADEMOLA, J. and MAIBACH, H.I. (1996) Sodium lauryl sulfate (SLS) induced irritant contact dermatitis: a correlation study between ceramides and *in vivo* parameters of irritation *Contact Dermatitis*, **35**, 86–91.

ELIAS, P.M. (1983) Epidermal lipids, barrier function, and desquamation *J. Invest. Dermatol.*, **80**, s44-s49.

ELSNER, P., WILHELM, D. and MAIBACH, H.I. (1990) Sodium lauryl sulfate-induced irritant contact dermatitis in vulvar and forearm skin of premenopausal and postmenopausal women, *J. Am. Acad. Dermatol.*, **23**, 648–652.

EMILSON, A., LINDBERG, M. and FORSLIND, B. (1993) The temperature effect on *in vitro* penetration of sodium lauryl sulfate and nickel chloride through human skin, *Acta Derm. Venereol. (Stockh.)*, **73**, 203–207.

FERGUSON, J., GIBBS, J.H. and SWANSON BECK, J. (1985) Lymphocyte subsets and Langerhans cells in allergic and irritant patch test reactions: histometric studies, *Contact Dermatitis*, 13, 166–174.

FISCHER, T. and MAIBACH, H.I. (1984) Finn chamber patch test technique, *Contact Dermatitis*, **11**, 137–140.

FLUHR, J.W., KUSS, O., DIEPGEN, T., LAZZERINI, S., PELOSI, A., GLOOR, M. and BERARDESCA, E. (2001) Testing for irritation with a multifactorial approach: comparison of eight non-invasive measuring techniques on five different irritation types, *Br. J. Dermatol.*, **145**, 696–703.

FORSLIND, B. (1994) A domain mosaic model of the skin barrier, *Acta Derm. Venereol. (Stockh.)*, **74**, 1–6.

CHAPTER 26

Foy, V., Weinkauf, R., Whittle, E. and Basketter, D.A. (2001) Ethnic variation in the skin irritation response, *Contact Dermatitis*, **45**, 346–349.

Freeman, S. and Maibach, H.I. (1988) Study of irritant contact dermatitis produced by repeat patch testing with sodium lauryl sulfate and assessed by visual methods, transepidermal water loss and laser Doppler velocimetry, *J. Am. Acad. Dermatol.*, **19**, 496–502.

Froebe, C.L., Simion, F.A., Rhein, L.D., Cagan, L.H. and Kligman, A.M. (1990) Stratum corneum lipid removal by surfactants: relation to *in vivo* irritation, *Dermatologica*, **181**, 277–283.

Frosch, P.J. and Kligman, A.M. (1977) Rapid blister formation in human skin with ammonium hydroxide, *Br. J. Dermatol.*, **96**, 461–473.

Frosch, P.J. and Kligman, A.M. (1979a) The soap chamber test: A new method for assessing the irritancy of soaps, *J. Am. Acad. Dermatol.*, **1**, 35–41

Frosch, P.J. and Kligman, A.M. (1979b) The Duhring chamber test, *Contact Dermatitis*, **5**, 73–81.

Frosch, P.J. and Wissing. C. (1982) Cutaneous sensitivity to ultraviolet light and chemical irritants, *Arch. Dermatol. Res.*, **272**, 269–278.

Gisslen, H. and Magnusson, B. (1966) Effects of detergents on guinea pig skin, *Acta Derm. Venereol. (Stockh.)*, **46**, 269–274.

Goh, C.L. and Chia, S.E. (1988) Skin irritability to sodium lauryl sulfate as measured by skin vapour loss by sex and race, *Clinical Experimental Dermatol.*, **13**, 16–19.

Henry, F., Goffin, V., Maibach, H.I. and Pierard, G.E. (1997) Regional differences in stratum corneum reactivity for surfactants. Quantitative assessment using the corneosurfametry bioassay, *Contact Dermatitis*, **37**, 271–275.

Imokawa, G. (2001) Lipid abnormalities in atopic dermatitis, *J. Am. Acad. Dermatol.* **45**, s29-s32.

Klein, G., Grubauer, G. and Fritsch, P. (1992) The influence of daily dish-washing with synthetic detergent on human skin, *Br. J. Dermatol.*, **127**, 131–137.

Kligman, A.M. (1966) The SLS provocative patch test in allergic contact sensitization, *J. Invest. Dermatol.*, **36**, 573–573.

Kligman, A.M. and Wooding, W.M. (1967) A method for the measurement and evaluation of irritants on human skin, *J. Invest. Dermatol.*, **49**, 78–94.

LAMINTAUSTA, K. and MAIBACH, H.I. (1988) Exogenous and endogenous factors in skin irritation, *Int. J. Dermatol.*, **27**, 213–222.

LAMMINTAUSTA, K., MAIBACH. H.I. and WILSON, D. (1987a) Human cutaneous irritation: induced hyporeactivity, *Contact Dermatitis*, **17**, 193–198.

LAMMINTAUSTA, K., MAIBACH, H.I. and WILSON, D. (1987b) Irritant reactivity in males and females, *Contact Dermatitis*, **17**, 276–280.

LAMMINTAUSTA, K., MAIBACH, H.I. and WILSON, D. (1988a) Susceptibility to cumulative and acute irritant dermatitis, *Contact Dermatitis*, **19**, 84–90.

LAMMINTAUSTA, K., MAIBACH, H.I. and WILSON, D. (1988b) Mechanisms of subjective (sensory) irritation propensity to nonimmunologic contact urticaria and objective irritation in stingers, *Derm. Beruf. Umwelt*, **36**, 45–49.

LARMI, E., LAHTI, A. and HANNUKSELA, M. (1989) Effect of ultraviolet B on nonimmunologic contact reactions induced by dimethyl sulfoxide, phenol and sodium lauryl sulfate, *Photodermatology*, **6**, 258–262.

LEE, A.Y., YOO, S.H., OH, J.G. and KIM, Y.G. (2000) 2 cases of allergic contact cheilitis from sodium lauryl sulfate in toothpaste, *Contact Dermatitis*, **42**, 111.

LEE, C.H. and MAIBACH, H.I. (1994) Study of cumulative irritant contact dermatitis in man utilizing open application on subclinically irritated skin, *Contact Dermatitis*, **30**, 271–275.

LEE, C.H. and MAIBACH, H.I. (1995) The sodium lauryl sulfate model: an overview, *Contact Dermatitis*, **33**, 1–7.

LEE, J.Y., EFFENDY, I. and MAIBACH, H.I. (1997a) Acute irritant contact dermatitis: recovery time in man, *Contact Dermatitis*, **36**, 285–290.

LEE, K.Y., PARK, C.W. and LEE, C.H. (1997b) The effect of chamber size and volume of test solution on cutaneous irritation, *Kor. J. Dermatol.*, **35**, 424–430.

LEE, K.Y., SHIN, K.Y., PARK, C.W. and LEE, C.H. (1997c) Cutaneous irritation to sodium lauryl sulfate and sodium lauroyl glutamate, *Kor. J. Dermatol.*, **35**, 491–498.

LEVEQUE, J.L., DE RIGAL,, J., SAINT-LEGER, D. and BILLY, D. (1993) How does sodium lauryl sulfate alter the skin barrier function in man? A multiparametric approach, *Skin Pharmacol.*, **6**, 111–115.

LODEN, M. and ANDERSSON, A.C. (1996) Effect of topically applied lipids on surfactant irritated skin, *Br. J. Dermatol.*, **134**, 215–220.

LOEFFLER, H. and EFFENDY, I. (1999) Skin susceptibility of atopic individuals *Contact Dermatitis*, **40**, 239–242.

LUKACOVIC, M.F., DUNLAP, F.E., MICHAELS, S.E., VISSCHER, M.O. and WATSON, D.D. (1988) Forearm wash test to evaluate the clinical mildness of cleansing products, *J. Soc. Cosmet. Chem.*, **39**, 355–366.

MAGNUSSON, B. and HERSLE, K. (1965), Patch test methods. I. A comparative study of six different types of patch tests, *Acta Derm. Venereol. (Stockh.)*, **45**, 123–128.

MAHMOUD, G., LACHAPELLE, J.M. and VAN NESTE, D. (1984) Histological assessment of skin damage by irritants: its possible use in the evaluation of a barrier cream, *Contact Dermatitis*, **11**, 179–185.

MCFADDEN, J.P., WAKELIN, S.H. and BASKETTER, D.A. (1998) Acute irritation thresholds in subjects with Type I-Type VI skin, *Contact Dermatitis*, **38**, 147–149.

MIKULOWSKA, A. and ANDERSSON, A. (1996) Sodium lauryl sulfate effect on the density of epidermal Langerhans cells: Evaluation of different test models, *Contact Dermatitis*, **34**, 397–401.

MITCHELL, J.C. (1977) Multiple concomitant positive patch test reactions, *Contact Dermatitis* **3**, 315–320.

MOON, S.H., SEO, K.I., HAN, W.S., SUH, D.H., CHO, K.H., KIM, J.J. and EUN, H.C. (2001) Pathological findings in cumulative irritation induced by SLS and croton oil in hairless mice, *Contact Dermatitis*, **44**, 240–245.

MURAHATA, R., CROVE, D.M. and ROHEIM, J.R. (1986) The use of transepidermal water loss to measure and predict the irritation response to surfactants, *Int. J. Cosmet. Science*, **8**, 225–231.

NASSIF, A., CHAN, S.C., STORRS, F.J. and HANIFIN, J.M. (1994) Abnormal skin irritancy in atopic dermatitis and in atopy without dermatitis *Arch. Dermatol.* **130**, 1402–1407.

NIKITAKIS, J.M., MCEWEN, G.N. and WENNINGER, J.A. (1991) *CTFA International Cosmetic Ingredient Dictionary* (4th edn.), Washington DC: The Cosmetic, Toiletry, and Fragrance Association Inc.

NILSSON, G.E., OTTO, U. and WAHLBERG, J.E. (1982) Assessment of skin irritancy in man by laser Doppler flowmetry, *Contact Dermatitis*, **8**, 401–406.

OHLENSCHLAEGER, J., FRIBERG, J., RAMSING, D. and AGNER, T. (1996) Temperature dependency of skin susceptibility to water and detergents, *Acta Derm. Venereol. (Stockh.)*, **76**, 274–276.

PINNAGODA, J., TUPKER, R.A., COENRAADS, P.J. and NATER, J.P. (1989) Prediction of susceptibility to an irritant response by transepidermal water loss, *Contact Dermatitis*, **20**, 341–346.

PANISSET, F., TREFFEL, P., FAIVRE, B., LECOMTE, P.B. and AGACHE, P. (1992) Trans-epidermal water loss related to volar forearm sites in humans, *Acta Derm. Venereol. (Stockh.)*, **72**, 4–5

PRATER, E., GORING, H.D. and SCHUBERT, H. (1978) Sodium lauryl sulfate—A contact allergen, *Contact Dermatitis*, **4**, 242–243.

RAPAPORT, M.J. (1984) Patch testing in Japanese subjects, *Contact Dermatitis*, **11**, 93–97.

ROBERTSON, A.R. (1977) The CIE 1976 color difference formulas, *Color Res. Appl.*, **2**, 7–11.

ROBINSON, M.K. (2000) Racial differences in acute and cumulative skin irritation responses between Caucasian and Asian populations, *Contact Dermatitis*, **42**, 134–143.

ROBINSON, M.K. (2002) Population differences in acute skin irritation responses. Race, sex, age, sensitive skin and repeat subject comparison, *Contact Dermatitis*, **46**, 86–93.

ROBINSON, M.K., PERKINS, M.A. and BASKETTER, D.A. (1998) Application of a 4-h human patch test method for comparative and investigative assessment of skin irritation, *Contact Dermatitis*, **38**, 194–202.

ROGIERS, V. (1995) Transepidermal water loss measurements in patch test assessment: The need for standardization, in: ELSNER, P. and MAIBACH, H.I. (eds) *Irritant Dermatitis. New clinical and experimental aspects*, Basel: Karger, 152–158.

SAMS, W.M. and SMITH, G. (1957) Contact dermatitis due to hydrocortisone ointment. Report of a case of sensitivity to emulsifying agents in a hydrophilic ointment base, *J.A.M.A.*, **164**, 1212–1213.

SCHEUPLEIN, R.J. and ROSS, L. (1970) Effects of surfactants and solvents on the permeability of epidermis, *J. Soc. Cosmet. Chem.*, **21**, 853–873.

SCHEYNIUS, A., FISCHER, T., FORSUM. U. and KLARESKOG, L. (1984) Phenotypic characterization in situ of inflammatory cells in allergic and irritant contact dermatitis in man, *Clinical Experimental Immunol.*, **55**, 81–90.

SEIDENARI, S. (1994) Reactivity to nickel sulfate at sodium lauryl sulfate pretreated skin sites is higher in atopics; An echographic evaluation by means of image analysis performed on 20 MHz B-scan recordings. *Acta Derm. Venereol. (Stockh.)*, **74**, 245–249.

SEIDENARI, S. and DI NARDO, A. (1992) B-scanning evaluation of irritant reactions with binary transformation and image analysis, *Acta Derm. Venereol. (Stockh.)*, (Suppl.) **175**, 9–13.

CHAPTER 26

SEIDENARI, S., FRANCOMANO, M. and MANTOVANI, L. (1998) Baseline biophysical parameters in subjects with sensitive skin, *Contact Dermatitis*, **38**, 311–315.

SERUP, J. (1995) The spectrum of irritancy and application of bioengineering techniques, in: ELSNER, P. and MAIBACH, H.I. (eds) *Irritant Dermatitis. New clinical and experimental aspects*, Basel: Karger, 131–143.

SERUP, J. and AGNER, T. (1990) Colorimetric quantification of erythema—a comparison of two colorimeters (Lange Micro Color and Minolta Chroma Meter CR-200) with a clinical scoring scheme and laser Doppler flowmetry, *Clinical Experimental Dermatol.*, **15**, 267–272.

SERUP, J. and STABERG, B. (1987) Ultrasound for assessment of allergic and irritant patch test reactions, *Contact Dermatitis*, **17**, 80–84.

SERUP, J., STABERG, B. and KLEMP, P. (1984) Quantification of cutaneous oedema in patch test reactions by measurement of skin thickness with high-frequency pulsed ultrasound, *Contact Dermatitis*, **10**, 88–93.

SHAHIDULLAH, M., RAFFLE, E.J., RIMMER, A.R. and FRAIN-BELL, W. (1969) Transepidermal water loss in patients with dermatitis, *Br. J. Dermatol.*, **81**, 722–730.

SIMION, F.A., RHEIN, L.D., MORRISON, B.M., SCALA, D.D., SALKO, D.M., KLIGMAN, A.M. and GROVE, G.L. (1995) Self-perceived sensory responses to soap and synthetic detergent bars correlate with clinical signs of irritation, *J. Am. Acad. Dermatol.*, **32**, 205–211.

SPENCER, T.S., LINAMEN, C.E., AKERS, W.A. and JONES, H.E. (1975) Temperature dependence of water content of the stratum corneum, *Br. J. Dermatol.*, **93**, 159–164.

STENDER, I.M., BLICHMANN, C. and SERUP, J. (1990) Effects of oil and water baths on the hydration state of the epidermis, *Clinical Experimental Dermatol.*, **15**, 206–209.

STILLMAN, M.A., MAIBACH, H.I. and SHALITA, A.R. (1975) Relative irritancy of free fatty acids of different chain length, *Contact Dermatitis*, **1**, 65–69.

SUGAR, M., SCHNETZ, E. and FARTASCH, M. (1999) Does sodium lauryl sulfate concentration vary with time?, *Contact Dermatitis*, **40**, 146–149.

TABATA, N., TAGAMI, H. and KLIGMAN, A.M. (1998). A 24-h occlusion exposure to 1% sodium lauryl sulfate induces a specific histopathologic inflammatory response in the xerotic skin of atopic dermatitis patients. *Acta Derm. Venereol. (Stockh.)*, **78**, 244–247.

TOLLESSON, A. and FRITHZ, A. (1993) Transepidermal water loss and water content in stratum corneum in infantile seborrheic dermatitis, *Acta Derm. Venereol. (Stockh.)*, **73**, 18–20.

TOVELL, P.W.A., WEAVER, A.C., HOPE, J. and SPROTT, W.E. (1974) The action of sodium lauryl sulfate on rat skin: an ultrastructural study, *Br. J. Dermatol.*, **90**, 501–506.

TUPKER, R.A., PINNAGODA, J., COENRAADS, P.J., KERSTHOLT, H. and NATER, J.P. (1989a) Evaluation of hand cleansers: Assessment of composition, skin compatibility by transepidermal water loss measurements, and cleansing power, *J. Soc. Cosmet. Chem.* **40**, 33–39.

TUPKER, R.A., PINNAGODA, J., COENRAADS, P.J. and NATER, J.P. (1989b) The influence of repeated exposure to surfactants on human skin as determined by transepidermal water loss and visual scoring, *Contact Dermatitis*, **20**, 108–114.

TUPKER, R.A., COENRAADS, P.J., PINNAGODA, J. and NATER, J.P. (1989c) Baseline transepidermal water loss (TEWL) as a prediction of susceptibility to sodium lauryl sulfate, *Contact Dermatitis*, **20**, 265–269.

TUPKER, R.A., PINNAGODA, J., COENRAADS, P.J. and NATER, J.P. (1990) Susceptibility to irritants: role of barrier function, skin dryness and history of atopic dermatitis, *Br. J. Dermatol.*, **123**, 199–205.

TUPKER, R.A., COENRAADS, P.J., FIDLER, V., DE JONG, M.C., VAN DER MEER, J.B., DE MONCHY, J.G. (1995) Irritant susceptibility and wheal and flare reactions to bioactive agents in atopic dermatitis (1) Influence of disease severity, *Br. J. Dermatol.*, **133**, 358–364.

TUPKER, R.A., WILLIS, C., BERARDESCA, E., LEE, C.H., FARTASCH, M., AGNER, T. and SERUP, J. (1997) Guidelines on sodium lauryl sulfate (SLS) exposure tests. A report from the standardization group of the European society of contact dermatitis, *Contact Dermatitis*, **37**, 53–69.

VAN DER VALK, P.G.M. and MAIBACH, H.I. (1989a) Potential for irritation increases from the wrist to the cubital fossa, *Br. J. Dermatol.*, **121**, 709–712.

VAN DER VALK, P.G.M. and MAIBACH, H.I. (1989b) Post-application occlusion substantially increases the irritant response of the skin to repeated short-term sodium lauryl sulfate (SLS) exposure, *Contact Dermatitis*, **21**, 335–338.

VAN DER VALK, P.G.M., NATER, J.P. and BLEUMINK, E. (1984) Skin irritancy of surfactants as assessed by water vapor loss measurements, *J. Invest. Dermatol.*, **82**, 291–293.

VAN DER VALK, P.G.M., NATER, J.P. and BLEUMINK, E. (1985) Vulnerability of the skin to surfactants in different groups of eczema patients and controls as measured by water vapour loss, *Clinical Experimental Dermatol.*, **10**, 98–103.

WAHLBERG, J.E. and MAIBACH, H.I. (1980) Nonanoic acid irritation—A positive control at routine patch testing?, *Contact Dermatitis*, **6**, 128–130.

WERNER, Y. and LINDBERG, M. (1985) Transepidermal water loss in dry and clinically normal skin in patients with atopic dermatitis *Acta Derm. Venereo. (Stockh.)*, **65**, 102–105.

WILHELM, K.P. and MAIBACH, H.I. (1990) Susceptibility to irritant dermatitis induced by sodium lauryl sulfate, *J. Am. Acad. Dermatol.*, **23**, 122–124.

WILHELM, K.P., SAUNDERS, J.C. and MAIBACH, H.I. (1989) Quantification of sodium lauryl sulfate dermatitis in man: Comparison of four techniques: skin color reflectance, transepidermal water loss, laser Doppler flow measurement and visual scores, *Arch. Dermatol. Res.*, **281**, 293–295.

WILHELM, K.P., SAUNDERS, J.C. and MAIBACH, H.I. (1990) Increased stratum corneum turnover induced by subclinical irritant dermatitis, *Br. J. Dermatol.*, **122**, 793–798.

WILHELM, K.P., CUA, A.B., WOLF, H.H. and MAIBACH, H.I. (1993) Surfactant-induced stratum corneum hydration *in vivo*: Prediction of the irritation potential of anionic surfactants, *J. Invest. Dermatol.*, **101**, 310–315.

WILHELM, KP., FREITAG, G. and WOLFF, H.H. (1994) Surfactant-induced skin irritation and skin repair. Evaluation of the acute human irritation model by noninvasive techniques, *J. Am. Acad. Dermatol.*, **30**, 944–949.

WILLIS, C.M., STEPHENS, C.J.M. and WILKINSON, J.D. (1989) Epidermal damage induced by irritants in man: a light and electron microscopic study, *J. Invest. Dermatol.*, **93**, 695–699.

WILLIS, C.M., STEPHENS, C.J.M. and WILKINSON, J.D. (1993) Differential patterns of epidermal leukocyte infiltration in patch tests reactions to structurally unrelated chemical irritants, *J. Invest. Dermatol.*, **101**, 364–370.

Barrier Creams

HONGBO ZHAI AND HOWARD I MAIBACH

Contents

27.1 Introduction

27.2 Definition and terms

27.3 Reasons to utilize BC

27.4 Mechanism of action and duration

27.5 Application methods and efficacy

27.6 US Food and Drug Administration monograph "Skin protectants"

27.7 Conclusion

27.1 INTRODUCTION

Each day skin is exposed to an infinite number of substances; some may be potentially irritants (for example, surfactants, cutting oils, acids and alkalis, etc.) or allergens (for example, poison oak/ivy, etc.). Skin barrier function may be damaged due to contact with these materials. Consequentially, irritant contact dermatitis (ICD) and allergic contact dermatitis (ACD) may develop. Minimizing exposure is recommended but often not practicable. In many occupations, such as farmers, forest firefighters, outdoor activities, hospitals, and even households such encounters are ubiquitous. Therefore, to prevent or reduce the risk of developing ICD and ACD, prophylactic measures are indicated. Application of barrier creams (BC) before or during work may play an important role in the prevention of occupational contact dermatitis and nature hand care as well.

Their efficacy in reducing the developing ICD and ACD have been documented *in vitro* and *in vivo* experimental studies (Frosch *et al.*, 1993a; Lachapelle, 1996; Zhai and Maibach, 1996a; Wigger-Alberti and Elsner, 1998; Zhai and Maibach, 1999; Wigger-Alberti and Elsner, 2000a, 2000b; Maibach and Zhai, 2000; Zhai and Maibach, 2001, 2002). Yet inappropriate BC application may induce a deleterious rather than a beneficial effect (Goh, 1991a, 1991b; Frosch *et al.*, 1993a, 1993b, 1993c, 1993d; Treffel *et al.* 1994; Zhai and Maibach, 1996b; Lachapelle 1996). This chapter emphasis BC's terms, mechanism, and other relative topics in this field.

27.2 DEFINITION AND TERMS

BC are designed to prevent or reduce the penetration and absorption of various hazardous materials into skin, preventing skin lesions and/or other toxic effects from dermal exposure (Orchard, 1984; Frosch *et al.*, 1993a; Lachapelle, 1996; Zhai and Maibach, 1996a, 1996b). BC are also called "skin protective creams (SPCs)" or "protective creams (PCs)", as well as "protective ointments," "invisible glove," "barrier," "protective" or "pre-work" creams and/or gels (lotions), "antisolvent" gels, and so on (Guillemin *et al.*, 1974; Mahmoud and Lachapelle, 1985; Loden, 1986; Goh, 1991b; Frosch *et al.*, 1993a). Frosch *et al.* (1993a) consider "skin protective creams" a more appropriate terminology since most creams do not provide a real barrier, at least not comparable to stratum corneum. We utilize BC here because this term is in general usage in industry. BC may share characteristics with moisturizers. BC's target is in the prevention of external noxious substances penetrating skin, and moisturizers are frequently used for "dry" skin conditions as well as to maintain healthy skin (Zhai and Maibach, 1998). BC and moisturizers may overlap in chemistry and function.

27.3   REASONS TO UTILIZE BC

Occupational contact dermatitis is the most common work-related injury involving millions of workers worldwide. Avoidance of these irritants or allergens may not be practical for persons whose occupation or activities mandate their working in certain environments. Certain gloves provide protective effects for corrosive agents (acids, alkalis, etc.) (Boman *et al.*, 1982; McClain and Storrs, 1992; Mellstrom *et al.*, 1996; Wigger-Alberti and Elsner, 1998). Protective clothing as well as other personal devices also plays a critical role as an important measure in industries (Mathias, 1990; Davidson, 1994). But, protective clothing may trap moisture and occlude potentially damaging substances next to the skin for prolonged periods and increase the likelihood that dermatitis will develop (Mathias, 1990; Davidson, 1994). In practice, BC are recommended only for low-grade irritants (water, detergents, organic solvents, cutting oils) (Frosch *et al.*, 1993a; Zhai and Maibach, 1996b; Wigger-Alberti and Elsner, 1998). The first line of defense against hand eczema is to wear gloves, but in many professions this is impossible because of the loss of dexterity. In some instances, an alternative would be to utilize BC. BC are also used to protect the face and neck against chemical and resinous dust and vapors (Birmingham, 1969). Many prefer to use BC rather than gloves because they do not want the hand continuously sealed inside a glove that can inhibit skin barrier function (Wigger-Alberti and Elsner, 1998). In addition, many gloves do not resist the penetration of low molecular weight chemicals. Some allergens are soluble in rubber gloves, and may penetrate the glove and produce severe dermatitis (Mathias, 1990; Estlander *et al.*, 1996; Wigger-Alberti and Elsner, 1998). Allergy to rubber latex has become a growing problem (Estlander *et al.*, 1996; Wigger-Alberti and Elsner, 1998). Furthermore, due to continuous gloves wearing, workers can develop serious symptoms (i.e., contact urticaria syndrome) including generalized urticaria, conjunctivitis, rhinitis, and asthma, etc. (Amin and Maibach, 1997; Wigger-Alberti and Elsner, 1998).

27.4   MECHANISM OF ACTION AND DURATION

Minimal information exists on the mechanisms of BC's action. The frequently quoted general rule is that water in oil (W/O) emulsions are effective against aqueous solutions of irritants and oil in water (O/W) emulsions are effective against lipophilic materials (Mathias, 1990; Frosch *et al.*, 1993a; Davidson, 1994; Lachapelle, 1996); exceptions have demonstrated (Frosch *et al.*, 1993c; Frosch and Kurte, 1994). BC may contain active ingredients presumed to work by trapping or transforming allergens or irritants (Frosch and Kurte, 1994; Lachapelle, 1996). Most believe they interfere with absorption and penetration of the allergen or irritants by physical blocking—forming a thin film that protects the skin (Orchard, 1984; Frosch and Kurte, 1994; Marks *et al.*, 1995; Lachapelle, 1996).

In order to avoid frequent interruptions for reapplication, BC are expected to remain effective for 3 or 4 hours. Most manufacturers claim that their products last ~ 4 hours. Others suggest use "as often as necessary" (Davidson, 1994). Studies document duration of action—with varying results (Reiner *et al.*, 1982; Boman *et al.*, 1982; Zhai and Maibach, 1996b; Zhai *et al.*, 1999).

27.5 APPLICATION METHODS AND EFFICACY

BC effectiveness may be influence by application methods (Packham, 1994; Wigger-Alberti *et al.*, 1997a, b). A study had been conducted to determine which areas of the hands were likely to be skipped on self-application BC by a fluorescence technique at the workplace (Wigger-Alberti *et al.*, 1997a); application of BC was incomplete, especially on the dorsal aspects of the hands. Most manufacturers suggest rubbing thoroughly onto skin; to pay special attention to cuticles and skin under nails; to let it dry approximately five minutes; to apply a thin layer of BC to all appropriate skin surfaces three to four times daily. We believe these suggestions are important for BC efficacy.

In vivo and *in vitro* methods have been developed to evaluate the efficacy of BC. Frosch *et al.* (1993a), Lachapelle (1996), Wigger-Alberti and Elsner (1998, 2000a, 2000b) and Zhai and Maibach (1996a, 1999, 2000, 2001) have extensively reviewed their efficacy.

27.6 US FOOD AND DRUG ADMINISTRATION MONOGRAPH "SKIN PROTECTANTS"

US Food and Drug Administration (FDA) identified 13 skin protectants for over-the-counter (OTC) products and regulated in Federal Register (1983). These ingredients and concentrations are listed in Table 27.1.

In addition, an OTC lotion (containing quaternium-18 bentonite) against poison ivy, oak or sumac has been approved as a New Drug Application by US FDA.

CHAPTER 27

TABLE 27.1:

US Food and Drug Administration (FDA) identified 13 skin protectants and their concentrations.

Ingredients	Concentrations
Allantoin	0.5–2%
Aluminum hydroxide gel	0.15–5%
Calamine	1–25%
Cocoa butter	50–100%
Dimethicone	1–30%
Glycerin	20–45%
Kaolin	4–20%
Petrolatum	30–100%
Shark liver oil	3 %
White petrolatum	30–100 %
Zinc acetate	0.1–2 %
Zinc carbonate	0.2–2 %
Zinc oxide	1–25 %

27.7 CONCLUSION

The efficacy of BC in preventing or reducing ICD and ACD has been well documented in many experimental environments. Obviously, BC may inhibit low-grade irritants, but should be not used as a primary protection against high-risk substances as well as corrosive agents. However, inappropriate BC application may exacerbate irritation rather than provide benefit. In particular, using BC on diseased skin may lead to increased skin irritation (Mathias, 1990; Lachapelle, 1996). People utilizing water, soaps, and detergents daily may benefit by applying BC frequently. Furthermore, BC may also shield skin from chemicals, oils and other substances and to make them easier to clean at the end of the workday (Davidson, 1994). To achieve optimal protective effects, BC should be used with careful consideration of the types of substances they are designed to protect against based on a specific exposure conditions; also, the proper use of BC should be instructed (Wigger-Alberti *et al.*, 1997a, b).

The ideal BC should be non-toxic, non-comedogenic, non-irritating, non-greasy foam, and colorless. They should keep high efficacy, but not interfere with user's manual dexterity or sensitivity. They should be easy to apply and remove, cosmetically acceptable, and economical. They may be combined with cosmetic benefits, and contain a high proportion of fatty materials (lipids) and can, therefore, also be used for skin care, especially for rough, dry or chapped skin. Furthermore, the mechanisms of BC's action should be further investigated when evaluating their efficacy. Recent investigative information will hopefully lead to controlled field trials (Berndt *et al.*, 2000; Schnetz *et al.*, 2000), so that we will have clearer insights into when and how to efficiently utilize them.

REFERENCES

AMIN, S.and MAIBACH, H.I. (1997) Immunologic contact urticaria definition. In: AMIN, S., LAHTI, A. and MAIBACH, H.I. (eds) *Contact Urticaria Syndrome,* Boca Raton: CRC Press, 11–26.

BERNDT, U., WIGGER-ALBERTI, W., GABARD, B. and ELSNER, P. (2000) Efficacy of a barrier cream and its vehicle as protective measures against occupational irritant contact dermatitis. *Contact Dermatitis,* **42**, 77–80.

BIRMINGHAM, D. (1969) Prevention of occupational skin disease. *Cutis,* **5**, 153–156.

BOMAN, A., WAHLBERG, J.E. and JOHANSSON, G. (1982) A method for the study of the effect of barrier creams and protective gloves on the percutaneous absorption of solvents. *Dermatologica,* **164**, 157–160.

DAVIDSON, C.L. (1994) Occupational contact dermatitis of the upper extremity. *Occupational Medicine,* **9**, 59–74.

ESTLANDER, T., JOLANKI, R. and KANERVA, L. (1996) Rubber glove dermatitis: a significant occupational hazard-prevention. In: ELSNER, P., LACHAPELLE, J.M., WAHLBERG, J.E. and MAIBACH, H.I. (eds) *Prevention of Contact Dermatitis. Current problem in dermatology,* Basel: Karger, 170–176.

FEDERAL REGISTER (1983) Skin protectant drug products for over-the-counter human use. *Federal Register,* **48**, 6832.

FROSCH, P.J. and KURTE, A. (1994) Efficacy of skin barrier creams. (IV). The repetitive irritation test (RIT) with a set of 4 standard irritants. *Contact Dermatitis,* **31**, 161–168.

FROSCH, P.J., KURTE, A. and PILZ, B. (1993a) Biophysical techniques for the evaluation of skin protective creams. In: FROSCH, P.J. and KLIGMAN, A.M. (eds) *Noninvasive Methods for the Quantification of Skin Functions,* Berlin: Springer-Verlag, 214–222.

FROSCH, P.J., KURTE, A. and PILZ, B. (1993b) Efficacy of skin barrier creams. (III). The repetitive irritation test (RIT) in humans. *Contact Dermatitis,* **29**, 113–118.

FROSCH, P.J., SCHULZE-DIRKS, A., HOFFMANN, M. and AXTHELM, I. (1993c) Efficacy of skin barrier creams. (II). Ineffectiveness of a popular "skin protector" against various irritants in the repetitive irritation test in the guinea pig. *Contact Dermatitis*, **29**, 74–77.

FROSCH, P.J., SCHULZE-DIRKS, A., HOFFMANN, M., AXTHELM, I. and KURTE, A. (1993d) Efficacy of skin barrier creams. (I). The repetitive irritation test (RIT) in the guinea pig. *Contact Dermatitis*, **28**, 94–100.

GOH, C.L. (1991a) Cutting oil dermatitis on guinea pig skin. (I). Cutting oil dermatitis and barrier cream. *Contact Dermatitis*, **24**, 16–21.

GOH, C.L. (1991b) Cutting oil dermatitis on guinea pig skin. (II). Emollient creams and cutting oil dermatitis. *Contact Dermatitis*, **24**, 81–85.

GUILLEMIN, M., MURSET, J.C., LOB, M. and RIQUEZ, J. (1974) Simple method to determine the efficiency of a cream used for skin protection against solvents. *British Journal of Industrial Medicine*, **31**, 310–316.

LACHAPELLE, J.M. (1996) Efficacy of protective creams and/or gels. In: ELSNER, P., LACHAPELLE, J.M., WAHLBERG, J.E. and MAIBACH, H.I. (eds) *Prevention of Contact Dermatitis. Current problem in dermatology*, Basel: Karger, 182–192.

LODEN, M. (1986) The effect of 4 barrier creams on the absorption of water, benzene, and formaldehyde into excised human skin. *Contact Dermatitis*, **14**, 292–296.

MAHMOUD, G. and LACHAPELLE, J.M. (1985) Evaluation of the protective value of an antisolvent gel by laser Doppler flowmetry and histology. *Contact Dermatitis*, **13**, 14–19.

MAIBACH, H.I. and ZHAI, H. (2000) Evaluations of barrier creams. In: WARTELL, M.A., KLEINMAN, M.T., HUEY, B.M. and DUFFY, L.M. (eds) *Strategies to Protect the Health of Deployed US Forces. Force Protection and Decontamination*, Washington DC: National Academy Press, 217–220.

MARKS, J.G. JR., FOWLER, J.F. JR., SHERETZ, E.F., RIETSCHEL, R.L. (1995) Prevention of poison ivy and poison oak allergic contact dermatitis by quaternium-18 bentonite. *Journal of the American Academy of Dermatology*, **33**, 212–216.

MATHIAS, C.G. (1990) Prevention of occupational contact dermatitis. *Journal of the American Academy of Dermatology*, **23**, 742–748.

McCLAIN, D.C. and STORRS, F. (1992) Protective effect of both a barrier cream and a polyethylene laminate glove against epoxy resin, glyceryl mono-thioglycolate, frullania, and tansy. *American Journal of Contact Dermatitis*, **13**, 201–205.

MELLSTROM, G.A., JOHANSSON, S. and NYHAMMAR, E. (1996) Barrier effect of gloves against cytostatic drugs. In: ELSNER, P., LACHAPELLE, J.M., WAHLBERG, J.E. and MAIBACH, H.I. (eds) *Prevention of Contact Dermatitis. Current problem in dermatology,* Basel: Karger, 163–169.

ORCHARD, S. (1984) Barrier creams. *Dermatologic Clinics,* 2, 619–629.

PACKHAM, C.L., PACKHAM, H.L. and RUSSELL-FELL, R. (1994) Evaluation of barrier creams: an *in vitro* technique on human skin (letter). *Acta Dermato-Venereologica,* **74**, 405–406.

REINER, R., ROSSMANN, K., VAN HOOIDONK, C., CEULEN, B.I. and BOCK, J. (1982) Ointments for the protection against organophosphate poisoning. *Arzeneimittel-Forschung,* **32**, 630–633.

SCHNETZ, E., DIEPGEN, T.L., ELSNER, P., FROSCH, P.J., KLOTZ, A.J., KRESKEN, J., KUSS, O., MERK, H., SCHWANITZ, H.J., WIGGER-ALBERTI, W. and FARTASCH, M. (2000) Multicentre study for the development of an *in vivo* model to evaluate the influence of topical formulations on irritation. *Contact Dermatitis,* **42**, 336–343.

TREFFEL, P., GABARD, B. and JUCH, R. (1994) Evaluation of barrier creams: An *in vitro* technique on human skin. *Acta Dermato-Venereologica,* **74**, 7–11.

WIGGER-ALBERTI, W. and ELSNER, P. (2000a) Barrier creams and emollients. In KANERVA, L.,ELSNER, P., WAHLBERG, J.E. and MAIBACH, H.I. (eds) *Handbook of Occupational Dermatology,* Berlin: Springer, 490–496.

WIGGER-ALBERTI, W. and ELSNER, P. (2000b) Protective creams. In: ELSNER, P. and MAIBACH, H.I. (eds) *Cosmeceuticals. Drugs vs. Cosmetics,* New York: Marcel Dekker, 189–195.

WIGGER-ALBERTI, W. and ELSNER, P. (1998) Do barrier creams and gloves prevent or provoke contact dermatitis? *American Journal of Contact Dermatitis,* **9**, 100–106.

WIGGER-ALBERTI, W., MARAFFIO, B., WERNLI, M. and ELSNER, P. (1997a) Self-application of a protective cream. Pitfalls of occupational skin protection. *Archives of Dermatology,* **133**, 861–864.

WIGGER-ALBERTI, W., MARAFFIO, B., WERNLI, M. and ELSNER, P. (1997b) Training workers at risk for occupational contact dermatitis in the application of protective creams: Efficacy of a fluorescence technique. *Dermatology,* **195**, 129–133.

ZHAI, H. and MAIBACH, H.I. (1999) Efficacy of barrier creams (skin protective creams). In: ELSNER, P., MERK, H.F. and MAIBACH, H.I. (eds) *Cosmetics. Controlled Efficacy Studies and Regulation,* Berlin: Springer, 156–166.

■ CHAPTER 27 ■

ZHAI, H. and MAIBACH, H.I. (1996a) Percutaneous penetration (Dermato-pharmacokinetics) in evaluating barrier creams. In: ELSNER, P., LACHAPELLE, J.M., WAHLBERG, J.E. and MAIBACH, H.I. (eds) *Prevention of Contact Dermatitis. Current problem in dermatology,* Basel: Karger, 193–205.

ZHAI, H. and MAIBACH, H.I. (1996b) Effect of barrier creams: human skin *in vivo. Contact Dermatitis,* **35**, 92–96.

ZHAI, H. and MAIBACH, H.I. (1998) Moisturizers in preventing irritant contact dermatitis: an overview. *Contact Dermatitis,* **38**, 241–244.

ZHAI, H. and MAIBACH, H.I. (1999) Efficacy of barrier creams (skin protective creams). In ELSNER, P., MERK, H.F. and MAIBACH, H.I. (eds) *Cosmetics. Controlled Efficacy Studies and Regulation,* Berlin: Springer, 156–166.

ZHAI, H. and MAIBACH, H.I. (2000) Models assay for evaluation of barrier formulations. In: MENNÉ, T. and MAIBACH, H.I. (eds) *Hand Eczema* (2nd edn.), Boca Raton: CRC Press, 333–337.

ZHAI, H. and MAIBACH, H.I. (2001) Tests for Skin Protection: Barrier Effect. In: BAREL, A.O., MAIBACH, H.I. and PAYE, M. (eds) *Handbook of Cosmetic Science and Technology,* New York: Marcel Dekker, Inc., 823–828.

ZHAI, H. and MAIBACH, H.I. (2002) Barrier creams—skin protectants: can you protect skin? *Journal of Cosmetic Dermatology,* **1**, 20–23.

ZHAI, H., BUDDRUS, D.J., SCHULZ, A.A., WESTER, R.C., HARTWAY, T., SERRANZANA, S. and MAIBACH, H.I. (1999) *In vitro* percutaneous absorption of sodium lauryl sulfate (SLS) in human skin decreased by Quaternium-18 bentonite gels. *In Vitro and Molecular Toxicology,* **12**, 11–15.

PART II

Methods

Methods for In Vitro Percutaneous Absorption

ROBERT L BRONAUGH

Contents

28.1 Introduction

28.2 Preliminary steps

28.3 Diffusion cells

28.4 Preparation of skin

28.5 Receptor fluid

28.6 Termination of experiment

28.7 Determination of absorption

28.8 Expression of percutaneous absorption

28.1 INTRODUCTION

In vitro percutaneous absorption methods are used for various reasons. Often it may be the only ethical way of obtaining human skin absorption data with potentially toxic chemicals. These studies also facilitate simultaneous measurement of skin metabolism which can be examined without metabolic interference from systemic organs (See Chapter 33, "Methods for *in vitro* skin metabolism studies"). The use of animals is also minimized with *in vitro* studies since many diffusion cells can be assembled from the skin of one animal.

It is important to conduct a study in a way that most closely simulates normal exposure to the chemical of interest. The length of exposure of a chemical in contact with the skin is often assumed to be 24 hours unless it is washed-off more quickly such as with a shampoo or hair color. Since the vehicle can play a major role in determining the absorption rate, the vehicle used in the absorption study should be similar to that found in normal exposure conditions.

28.2 PRELIMINARY STEPS

It is useful in the planning of studies to have knowledge of the test chemicals' solubility and partitioning properties. The log of the octanol/water partition coefficient (Log P) has been used for years as an indicator of percutaneous absorption properties. It is an indicator of the lipophilicity of a chemical which is a property necessary for it to permeate through the lipid-enriched stratum corneum layer. Water solubility is necessary for permeation through the more aqueous viable epidermal and dermal tissue. Diminished skin absorption may start to be observed with chemicals of molecular weight above 500 daltons (Bos and Meinardi, 2000).

28.3 DIFFUSION CELLS

There are two basic designs of one-chambered diffusion cells—the flow-through cell (Bronaugh and Stewart, 1985) and static cell (Franz, 1975). The one-chambered cell has a chamber (receptor) beneath the skin but is open to the environment above the skin to simulate many exposure conditions. Static diffusion cell systems are simpler in design and frequently based on the Franz diffusion cell. Receptor fluid beneath the skin is manually sampled by removing aliquots periodically for analysis. Besides the cost advantage, another important feature is their availability in a wide range of larger openings for skin that might be needed, for example, in studies with transdermal devices.

A flow-through diffusion cell (Figure 28.1) has an advantage in receptor fluid sampling, which can be done automatically using a fraction collector. The maintenance of cell viability for metabolism studies is facilitated by the continual replacement of receptor fluid. Use of a flow-through cell helps prevent high concentrations of test compound in the receptor fluid that can reduce absorption and the cell may facilitate partitioning of water insoluble chemicals from skin.

Special attention may be necessary in measuring the permeability of highly volatile compounds when the skin is not occluded to prevent evaporation. The short walls on the tops of some diffusion cells can protect the skin surface from

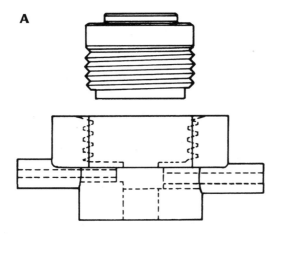

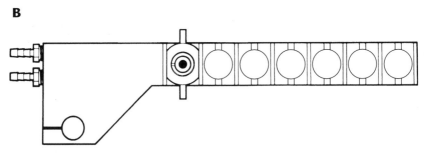

Figure 28.1: Flow-through diffusion cell and holding block. (A) Cross section of flow-through diffusion cell. (B) Aluminum holding block used to position cells over a fraction collector and to maintain the cells at a physiological temperature.

air currents and it has been suggested that this protection may be responsible for some differences observed between *in vivo* and *in vitro* results (Bronaugh and Maibach, 1985; Bronaugh *et al.*, 1985). Diffusion cells have been designed to collect evaporating material above the surface of the skin (Spencer *et al.*, 1979; Reifenrath and Robinson, 1982). These cells have proven particularly useful in studies of the effectiveness of mosquito repellents and in studies of volatile compounds that require mass balance determinations.

A two-chambered cell has two chambers of equal volume (often from 2–10 ml) that are separated by the skin membrane. Variations of the two-chambered cell have been used for years to create conditions in which the diffusion of a compound in solution can be measured from one side of the membrane to the other (Scheuplein, 1965). An infinite dose (one that is large enough to maintain constant concentration during the course of an experiment) is added to one side of the membrane and its rate of diffusion across a concentration gradient into a solution on the opposite side is determined. Usually the solutions on both sides of the membrane are stirred to ensure uniform concentrations. Studies comparing permeation through skin to Fickian diffusion through a membrane are performed in this fashion. The two-chambered cell is useful for studying mechanisms of diffusion through skin. It also is applicable to the measurement of absorption from drug delivery devices where compounds are applied to skin at an infinite dose and a steady-state rate of delivery is desired.

28.4   PREPARATION OF SKIN

Skin that is harvested from human or animal sources may need to be washed prior to further preparation for the diffusion cells. Washing should be carefully conducted with a soap and water solution followed by a water rinse.

Full-thickness skin should generally not be used for absorption studies. All or most of the dermis should be removed to simulate the *in vivo* diffusional barrier layer. Chemicals that are systemically absorbed are taken up into the blood vessels of the papillary dermis directly beneath the epidermis. A dermatome is commonly used to prepare a split-thickness preparation of skin because it can be used for all types of skin and the viability of skin can be maintained (Bronaugh and Collier, 1991). Full-thickness skin (stratum corneum side up) is fixed to a styrofoam block with hypodermic needles. The dermatome is pushed across the skin surface to prepare a layer of skin with much of the dermis removed. A dermatome section of 200 –300 μm is satisfactory since thinner preparations are difficult to make without damage to the skin.

Heat treatment is the only other practical method to remove the dermal tissue but it must be used on non-hairy skin to avoid damage to the barrier during the separation process. Full-thickness skin is submerged in 60°C water for approximately one minute and the epidermal and dermal layers can be pulled apart with forceps (Scheuplein, 1965; Bronaugh *et al.*, 1981). All but the most stable enzymes are destroyed by this process.

Chemical separation techniques (Scott *et al.*, 1986) and enzyme methods (Kitano and Okada, 1983) have only limited usage. The separation of rat skin with 2M sodium bromide can only be achieved with animals approximately 4 weeks of age. Older animals (7–8 weeks) have hair penetrating deeper into the dermis prohibiting the use of this technique. A problem with enzyme separation techniques is that degradation of the epidermal membrane can continue following assembly of the membrane in the diffusion cells (Bronaugh, unpublished observation).

The use of full thickness skin is really only justifiable when using animal skin that is already very thin, such as occurs in the mouse (400 µm) (Behl *et al.*, 1984) or rabbit. With the skin of other animals, such as the rat (800–870 µm) (Yang *et al.*, 1986), guinea pig, monkey, and pig, full thickness skin is almost 1 mm in thickness; and with human skin it can be several mm thick (Loden, 1985). Therefore, some means should be used to prepare a membrane that more accurately reflects the barrier layer in thickness. This is particularly important when examining a hydrophobic compound which diffuses slowly through the aqueous viable tissue.

After the skin is assembled in the diffusion cells, barrier integrity should be verified by measuring the absorption of a standard compound, such as tritiated water. A number of laboratories have reported permeability constant (Kp) values for tritiated water in normal skin (Dugard *et al.*, 1984; Bronaugh *et al.*, 1986), but this procedure requires dosing the skin for four–five hours for determination of the steady-state absorption of tritiated water. Bronaugh and coworkers developed a 20 minute test for tritiated water absorption to give more rapid results without hydration of skin samples (Bronaugh *et al.*, 1986).

28.5   RECEPTOR FLUID

The selection of the receptor fluid has become an increasingly important decision as investigators strive to create *in vitro* conditions that can adequately duplicate the *in vivo* situation. For measuring the absorption of water-soluble compounds, the use of normal saline or an isotonic buffer solution may be sufficient. However, some chemicals are metabolized significantly during the percutaneous absorption process (Yourick and Bronaugh, 2000). The viability of skin can be maintained for 24 h in a flow-through diffusion cell using a physiological buffer as the receptor fluid (Collier *et al.*, 1989). Metabolism and percutaneous absorption can be measured simultaneously as discussed in Chapter 33, "Methods for *in vitro* skin metabolism studies." The combined information gives a more complete picture of absorption since the actual permeating species are identified.

When fresh skin is obtained, the viability of skin can be maintained in a flow-through diffusion cell with either a tissue culture medium or a HEPES-buffered Hanks' balanced salt solution as the receptor fluid (Collier *et al.*, 1989). Bovine serum albumin (4 percent) can be added to the receptor fluid to facilitate partitioning of lipophilic compounds into the receptor fluid. Viable skin is used in studies where metabolism is of interest, but since viable skin more closely simulates the *in vivo* situation its use may also give more credibility to the penetration studies.

Sometimes surfactants (Bronaugh and Stewart, 1984) or organic solvents (Scott and Ramsey, 1987) have been added to the receptor fluid in non-viable skin studies to increase the solubility of lipophilic compounds and thereby promote free partitioning of chemicals from skin into the receptor fluid. Care must be taken to insure that damage to the skin barrier does not occur. The effectiveness of these methods will likely vary with the solubility properties of the test compound.

28.6   TERMINATION OF EXPERIMENT

At the end of a study the unabsorbed material is washed from the skin surface usually using a soap and water solution. Organic solvents have sometimes been used for more lipophilic material. For cosmetic products, removal from the skin is normally accomplished with a soap and water wash.

Barrier integrity may be rechecked with tritiated water or other standard chemical if damage to the barrier is suspected. The washing procedure itself may be damaging to the skin unless it is carefully accomplished.

28.7   DETERMINATION OF ABSORPTION

The determination of systemic percutaneous absorption is sometimes controversial in an *in vitro* diffusion cell study. Since the skin membrane can sometimes

CHAPTER 28

serve as a reservoir for absorbed material, measurement of the absorbed compound appearing in the receptor fluid alone may not be an accurate determination of systemic skin absorption. Both skin and receptor fluid levels should be measured at the end of a study. If determination of systemic absorption is desired, it is not sufficient to simply measure the receptor fluid levels. If significant amounts remain in skin, additional studies may be necessary to determine if the material in skin will eventually be systemically absorbed (see discussion below). Also, skin levels must be known in order to determine mass balance at the end of the experiment. Recoveries of at least 90 percent should be obtained unless the test compound is volatile.

Skin can be fractionated to observe localization in different layers. The stratum corneum layer can be removed from the surface of the skin by successive stripping with 10 or more pieces of cellophane tape (Kraeling and Bronaugh, 1997). Individual variation has been reported in the number of strips necessary presumably due to differences in the pressure applied to the tape and differences in the tape itself. The epidermal and dermal layers can be separated with heat as previously described in the preparation of skin.

The guidelines for skin absorption studies recommended by the European Union's Scientific Committee for Cosmetics and Non-Food Products (SCCNFP) require that material remaining in the viable skin layers (exclusive of stratum corneum) be considered as systemically absorbed (SCCNFP, 1999). The Organization for Economic and Cultural Development (OECD) draft guideline for In Vitro Skin Absorption Studies states that all material remaining in skin (including the stratum corneum) may need to be considered as systemically absorbed unless additional studies show that there is no eventual absorption (OECD, 2000).

For example, the lipophilic fragrance ingredient, musk xylol, was shown to be absorbed through hairless guinea pig and human skin (Hood *et al.*, 1996). However, substantial amounts of the fragrance were found in the skin at the end of the 24 hour studies (Table 28.1). An additional study was conducted that showed that significant amounts of the material in the skin at 24 hours diffused into the receptor fluid in the next 48 hours. These results suggest that 24-hour receptor fluid values alone do not adequately estimate systemic absorption of musk xylol.

TABLE 28.1:

Percentage of applied dose absorbed of musk xylol from oil-in-water emulsion and methanol vehicles in 24 hr

	Hairless guinea pig skin[a]		Human skin[b]	
	Oil-in-water emulsion	Methanol	Oil-in-water emulsion	Methanol
Receptor fluid	32.1 ± 1.3	25.8 ± 1.2	4.1 ± 0.7	1.0 ± 0.2
Skin	22.9 ± 2.7	18.8 ± 2.2	17.3 ± 2.3	21.3 ± 0.8
Total absorbed	55.0 ± 2.1	44.6 ± 2.4	21.5 ± 3.0	22.3 ± 0.8
24 hr skin wash	24.9 ± 1.4	5.5 ± 0.3	46.9 ± 3.2	25.9 ± 1.3
Total recovery	80.5 ± 1.9	50.4 ± 2.5	68.5 ± 2.9	45.7 ± 3.3

[a]Values are the mean ± SE of four determinations in each of three animals.
[b]Values are the mean ± SE of four or five determinations from two human subjects.

28.8 EXPRESSION OF PERCUTANEOUS ABSORPTION

Percutaneous absorption values are frequently expressed in terms of the percent of the applied dose absorbed. But these values are valid only at the concentration of the compound tested. Permeability constants are sometimes determined by dividing the steady-state absorption rate by the applied concentration of test compound. A permeability constant is therefore a normalized rate constant and is sometimes used to determine skin absorption at various doses. Errors can be introduced in these calculations if the initial lag-time in absorption is ignored and because absorption does not always increase in a linear fashion.

REFERENCES

BEHL, C.R., FLYNN, G.L., KURIHARA, T., SMITH, W.M., BELLANTONE, N.H., GATAITAN, O. and HIGUCHI, W.I. (1984) Age and anatomical site influences on alkanol permeation of skin of the male hairless mouse, *J. Soc. Cosmet. Chem.*, **35**, 237–252.

BOS, J.D. and MEINARDI, M.M.H.M. (2000) The 500 dalton rule for the skin penetration of chemical compounds and drugs, *Exp. Dermatol.* 9, 165–169.

Bronaugh, R.L. and Collier, S.W. (1991) Preparation of Human and Animal Skin, In Bronaugh, R. and Maibach, H.I. (eds) *In Vitro Percutaneous Absorption: Principles, Fundamentals, and Applications*, CRC Press Inc., Boca Raton, FL, 1–6.

Bronaugh, R.L. and Maibach, H.I. (1985) Percutaneous absorption of nitroaromatic compounds: *In vivo* and *in vitro* studies in the human and monkey, *J. Invest. Dermatol.*, **84**, 180–183.

Bronaugh R.L. and Stewart, R.F. (1984) Methods for *in vitro* percutaneous absorption studies III: Hydrophobic compounds, *J. Pharm. Sci.*, **73**, 1255–1258.

Bronaugh, R.L. and Stewart, R.F. (1985) Methods for *in vitro* percutaneous absorption studies IV: the flow-through diffusion cell, *J. Pharm. Sci.*, **74**, 64–67.

Bronaugh, R.L., Congdon, E.R. and Scheuplein, R.J., (1981) The effect of cosmetic vehicles on the penetration of N-nitrosodiethanolamine through excised human skin. *J. Invest. Dermatol.*, **76**, 94–96.

Bronaugh, R.L., Stewart, R.F., Wester, R.C., Bucks, D., Maibach, H.I. and Anderson, J. (1985) Comparison of percutaneous absorption of fragrances by humans and monkeys, *Fd. Chem. Toxicol.*, **23**, 111–114.

Bronaugh, R.L., Stewart, R.F. and Simon, M. (1986) Methods for *in vitro* percutaneous absorption studies VII: Use of excised human skin, *J. Pharm. Sci.*, **75**, 1094–1097.

Collier, S.W., Sheikh, N.M., Sakr, A., Lichtin, J.L., Stewart, R.F. and Bronaugh, R.L. (1989) Maintenance of skin viability during *in vitro* percutaneous absorption/metabolism studies, *Toxicol. Appl. Pharmacol.*, **99**, 522–533.

Dugard, P.H., Walker, M., Mawdsley, J. and Scott, R.C. (1984) Absorption of some glycol ethers through human skin *in vitro*, *Environ. Health Perspect.* **57**, 193–197.

Franz, T.J. (1975) On the relevance of *in vitro* data, *J. Invest. Dermatol.*, **64**, 190–195.

Hood, H.L., Wickett, R.R. and Bronaugh, R.L. (1996) *In vitro* percutaneous absorption of the fragrance ingredient musk xylol, *Fd. Chem. Toxicol.* **34**, 483–488.

Kitano, Y. and Okada, N. (1983) Separation of the epidermal sheet by dispase, *Brit. J. Dermatol.*, **108**, 555–560.

KRAELING, M.E.K. and BRONAUGH, R.L. (1997) *In vitro* percutaneous absorption of alpha hydroxy acids in human skin, *J. Soc. Cosmet. Chem.* **48**, 187–197.

LODEN, M. (1985) The *in vitro* hydrolysis of diisopropyl fluorophosphate during penetration through human full-thickness skin and isolated epidermis. *J. Invest. Dermatol.*, **85**, 335–339.

OECD (2000) *Environmental Health and Safety Publications: Draft Guidance Document for the Conduct of Skin Absorption Studies.* Environment Directorate. Organisation for Economic Co-operation and Development, Paris, December. www1.oecd/ehs/test/guidancewebversion.pdf/

REIFENRATH, WG. and ROBINSON, P.B. (1982) *In vitro* skin evaporation and penetration characteristics of mosquito repellents, *J. Pharm. Sci.*, **71**, 1014–1018.

SCCNFP (1999) Opinion concerning basic criteria for the *in vitro* assessment of percutaneous absorption of cosmetic ingredients—adopted by the Scientific Committee on Cosmetic Products and Non-Food Products intended for consumers during the plenary session of 23 June 1999. http:/europa.eu.int/comm/food/fs/sc/sccp/out86_en.html

SCHEUPLEIN, R.J. (1965) Mechanism of percutaneous absorption I. Routes of penetration and the influence of solubility. *J. Invest. Dermatol.*, **45**, 334–346.

SCOTT, R.C., WALKER, M. and DUGARD, P.H. (1986) *In vitro* percutaneous absorption experiments: A technique for the production of intact epidermal membranes from rat skin. *J. Soc. Cosmet. Chem.*, **37**, 35–41.

SCOTT, R.C. and RAMSEY, J.D. (1987) Comparison of the *in vivo* and *in vitro* percutaneous absorption of a lipophilic molecule (Cypermethrin, a pyrethroid insecticide). *J. Invest. Dermatol.*, **89**, 142–146.

SPENCER, T.S., HILL, J.A., FELDMANN, R.J. and MAIBACH, H.I. (1979) Evaporation of diethyltoluamide from human skin *in vivo* and *in vitro*, *J. Invest. Dermatol.*, **72**, 317–319.

YANG, J.J., ROY, T.A. and MACKERER, C.R. (1986) Percutaneous absorption of benzo(a)pyrene in the rat: Comparison of *in vivo* and *in vitro* results. *Toxicol. Ind. Health*, **2**, 409–416.

YOURICK, J.J. and BRONAUGH, R.L. (2000) Percutaneous penetration and metabolism of 2-nitro-p-phenylenediamine in human and fuzzy rat skin. *Toxicol. Appl. Pharmacol.* **166**, 13–23.

CHAPTER 28

Tape Stripping Method and Stratum Corneum

**MYEONG JUN CHOI, HONGBO ZHAI
AND HOWARD I MAIBACH**

Contents

29.1 Introduction

29.2 Stratum corneum

29.3 SC removal methods and effect of stripping

29.4 Effect of stripping factors on the tape stripping

29.5 Tape stripping versus percutaneous absorption and penetration

29.6 Tape stripping versus peptide immunization

29.7 Unanswered question and concerns to tape stripping

29.1 INTRODUCTION

Tape stripping is a useful method for removing the stratum corneum (SC) and obtaining more information about function of this thin layer as a main barrier for skin penetration. Typically an adhesive tape is pressed onto the test site and is subsequently abruptly detached. The number of tape strips need to remove the SC varies with age, sex, and possibly ethnicity (Palenske and Morhenn, 1999). Tape stripping has been used in various dermatological and pharmaceutical fields: to measure SC mass and thickness (Dreher *et al.*, 1998; Kalia *et al.*, 2001; Bashir *et al.*, 2001), to investigate percutaneous penetration and disposition of topically applied drug *in vivo* (Benfeldt and Serup, 1999; Benfeldt *et al.*, 1999; Potard *et al.*, 2000; Rougier *et al.*, 1999), and to disrupt skin barrier function (Benfeldt and Serup, 1999; Benfeldt *et al.*, 1999; Fluhr *et al.*, 2002). Also, this technique has been used to collect SC lipids samples (Weerheim and Ponec, 2001), to detect proteolytic activity associated with the SC (Beisson *et al.*, 2001), and to quantitatively estimate esterase activities in the SC (Mazereeuw-Hautier *et al.*, 2000). Stripping is a quantitative and minimally invasive assay for the detection of metal on and in the skin (Cullander *et al.*, 2000; Hostynek *et al.*, 2001). Tape stripping has been used to disrupt the skin before percutaneous peptide immunization (Seo *et al.* 2000; Takigawa *et al.*, 2001). Tape stripping is of sufficient utility to have been proposed by the FDA as part of a standard method to evaluate bioequivalence of topical dermatological dosage forms (Shah *et al.*, 1998). This method is simple, inexpensive, and minimally invasive; it has been frequently used for investigation of skin penetration, barrier function and the involvement factors in skin pathologies. Stripping is fast and easy to use in human studies.

This chapter reviews the stripping method, considering factors, analytic method of drug in the SC after stripping, and its application and summarizes recent data.

29.2 STRATUM CORNEUM

SC is a stratified squamous epithelium lining the body surface which plays an important anti-desiccating role as a barrier. SC consists of nonviable cornified cells (corneocytes) embedded in lipid-rich intercellular domains (intercorneo-cyte spaces). Intercellular domains comprise free fatty acids (FFA), cholesterol (CHOL) and ceramides (CER), together with smaller amounts of cholesteryl sulfate, sterol, triglycerides, squalene, n-alkanes, and phospholipids. SC lipids localize mainly in the intercellular space with little in the corneocytes (Moghimi *et al.*, 1999). Intercellular lipids, only if they form a continuous domain in the SC, are required for a major competent skin barrier.

In addition to lipid components, enzymes secreted in the intercorneocyte spaces are thought to be involved in barrier function and normal desquamation. Various proteases, β-glucocerebrosidase, steroid sulfatase, phospholipase A, sphinomyelinase, and lipase activities have been detected in the SC using subcellular fractionation and cytochemical techniques (Beisson *et al.*, 2001; Mazereeuw-Hautier *et al.*, 2000).

Weerheim and Ponec (2001) reported lipid analysis using Leukoflex[R] tape and ethylacetate-methanol mixture as a solvent system. With this method, levels of FFA are highest in the uppermost SC layers up to strip 4. In the following SC layers, the relative amount of FFA ranged from 15 percent to 20 percent of major SC lipid fractions. The relative amounts of CER varied from 16 to 70 percent, CHOL from 12 to 52 percent, and FFA from 12 to 64 percent. The lipid composition profile of SC varied with relation to SC depth at the tape stripping method, extraction methods and anatomical site (Bleck *et al.*, 1999; Lavrijsen *et al.*, 1994; Motta *et al.*, 1994; Weerheim and Ponec, 2001). Man-Qiang *et al.* (1993) suggested that for the formation of a competent SC barrier, the CER, CHOL, and FFA should be present in an equimolar ratio. Man *et al.* (1996) reported that three major SC lipids are required for permeability barrier homeostasis and equimolar composition of major lipids is increased up to three-fold acceleration of barrier repair.

Barrier repair creams including natural components of SC lipids have been used to treat skin disease (Chamlin *et al.*, 2001; Mortensen *et al.*, 2001). Chamlin *et al.* (2001) reported a phase I trial of a barrier repair cream in childhood atopic dermatitis.

29.3   SC REMOVAL METHODS AND EFFECT OF STRIPPING

In order to remove SC, tape stripping for mechanical removal of corneocytes and solvent extraction method to remove both polar and non-polar SC lipids are used. Tape stripping is a useful technique for selectively removing the skin's outermost layer, while solvent extraction is a delipidization process in SC.

In general, a clinical description of the barrier disruption differs depending on the disruption methods. For tape-stripped skin, the typical description was moderate erythema and a glistening surface due to total removal of the SC; for acetone-treated skin, the description was minimal or no erythema and slight superficial dryness; and for chloroform-methanol mixture the description was deep erythema and edema (Benfeldt *et al.*, 1999). Thus, an organic solvent method using chloroform-methanol mixing may be more aggressive than standard tape.

The change of skin condition after stripping differs depending on stripping (Table 29.1). Fluhr *et al.* (2002) investigated the barrier recovery pattern after tape stripping or acetone delipidization at five body sites in healthy volunteers. The fastest barrier recovery after tape stripping and acetone was observed on the forehead, followed by the back. But, there are differences in SC capacitance values following acetone and tape stripping. In the case of acetone, there are no statistically significant differences in SC capacitance between body sites. In contrast, tape stripping produces significant differences in capacitance values between body sites. The capacitance increases are related to strong barrier damage by tape stripping. However, the decrease of capacitance appears related to lipid extraction. Benfeldt and Serup (1999) reported that salicylic acid penetration greatly increased with the tape stripping, but not with acetone in the skin of hairless rats.

After barrier disruption, there are typically no adverse effects, such as infection or scarring. However, disruption of permeability barrier by tape stripping induces activiation and maturation of epidermal Langerhans cells

TABLE 29.1:

Physiological changes of the human and rat skin after stripping (from Benfeldt *et al.* 1999)

Type of skin	Barrier pertubation	None	Tape stripping[a]	Acetone[b]
Human	TEWL (g/m²/h)[c]	4.3 ± 2.2	30.6 ± 22.2	9.1 ± 7.5
	Erythema (arbitrary unit)[d]	8.7 ± 1.6	11.6 ± 2.8	9.2 ± 1.5
Rat	ΔTEWL[e]	0	69 ± 14	6 ± 3
	ΔErythema[f]	0	2.41 ± 0.87	0.95 ± 1.66

[a] Tape stripping was achieved by applying 2.5 × 5 cm (human) and 5 × 5 cm (rat) piece of Transpore tape with firm pressure and repeating the procedure 20 (human) and 10 (rat) times, respectively.

[b] Acetone was treated by gentle wiping with large cotton buds soaked in 100 percent acetone for 3 min.

[c] Fifteen minutes after barrier pertubation procedures, TEWL was measured using an Evaporimeter and recorded in triplicate.

[d] Colorimetry measures skin color by analyzing the light reflected from the skin surface according to the standization protocol for the content of green-red (a*) and yellow-blue (b*) color and skin brightness (L*). The a* redness parameter is a measure of erythema.

[e,f] TEWL and erythema from the barrier perturbed skin area minus the value from the untreated side.

(Nishijima *et al.* 1997). This process is important in inducing immune response *in vivo* and in immunizing with peptide and protein by a percutaneous method.

29.4 EFFECT OF STRIPPING FACTORS ON THE TAPE STRIPPING

When the tape stripping is employed, the following factors are important, (1) number of strips, (2) types and size of tapes, (3) the pressure applied to the strip prior to stripping and the peeling force applied for removal, (4) anatomic sites. Some parameters are summarized in Table 29.2. We summarize the effect of the type of tape and number of strips on the stripping.

Dreher *et al.* (1998) improved the method by quantifying the amount of human SC removed by each strip utilizing a colorimetric protein assay. With this method, Bashir *et al.* (2001) determined the physical and physiological effect of SC tape stripping, utilizing tapes with different physicochemical properties. Three commercial adhesive tapes utilized were D-Squame (CuDerm, Dallas, Texas, USA), Transpore (3M, St Paul, MN, USA, batch no. 2002–12 AP), and Micropore (3M, St Paul, MN, USA, batch no. 2001–08 AN). D-Squame is pre-cut into disk shape. Transpore and Micropore are provided as a standard roll. Table 29.3 shows the components of three commercial adhesive tapes and the effect of tapes on the transepidermal water loss (TEWL) depending number of strip.

Bashir *et al.* (2001) demonstrated that no significant difference was found in the kinetic parameters (mean water diffusion coefficient, SC thickness and permeability) between the tapes. However, there are differences in the mean TEWL values. Mean TEWL increases significantly as the deeper layers of the SC reached by tape stripping for the D-Squame and Transpore, but not for Micropore. Therefore, D-Squame and Transpore tapes induce a significant increase in the TEWL, while Micropore tape did not (Table 29.3). The value of TEWL was differed depending on the tape.

In order to detect and localize metals in and on the SC, a tape with low-metal adhesive tape is suitable for use with atomic absorption spectrophotometry and particle-induced X-ray emission to minimize the contamination of metal from the tape.

The number of tape strips to remove SC differs by investigator and experi-mental methods such as *in vivo* and *in vitro* assays (Table 29.2). As the number of tape strips increase, the value of TEWL is increased. The FDA guideline recommends 10 tape strips after topical application of a substance. Weerheim

TABLE 29.2:

Comparison of tape stripping methods

Type of tape	Number of stripping	Size	Applied pressure	Applied time	Study
D-Squame	40	25 mm	10 KPa	2 s	Bashir *et al.* (2001)
Transpore	40		10 KPa	2 s	Bashir *et al.* (2001)
Micropore	40		10 KPa	2 s	Bashir *et al.* (2001)
D-Squame	16	25 mm	80 g/cm^3	5 s	Potard *et al.* 2000
Leukoflex	18–20	1.5 × 5 cm	Soft pressure		Weerheim *et al.* (2001)
3M invisible	7		Controlled condition	10 s	Fernandez *et al.* (2002)
Adhesif 3M 6204	10	2 × 10 cm		2 s	Mazereeuw-Hautier *et al.* (2000)
Scotch Book tape 845	20		By rubbing six times		Alberti *et al.* (2001)
Scotch	7		1kg rubber weight was rolled over it 10 times		Wissing *et al.* (2002)
Scotch 600	2–5	4 cm	By rubbing with finger three movements		Betz *et al.* (2001)
Blenderm 3M	6	4 cm^2			Couteau *et al.* (2001)
Transpore	20	2.5 × 5 cm	Firm pressure		Benfeldt *et al.* 1999
Transpore	10	5 × 5 cm			Benfeldt and Serup (1999)
Teasfilm	20	4 cm^2			Fluhr *et al.* (2002)
D-Squame	20	3.8 cm^2	Uniform pressure	5 s	Dreher *et al.* (1998)

Tape stripping is employed with different adhesive tape, size, number of strips, and the pressure applied to the strip prior to stripping and the peeling force applied for removal.

and Ponec (2001) reported that the average number of tapes *in vivo* could be 18–20 strips. For some individuals, 40 adhesive tape strips, regardless of the type of tapes does not disrupt the SC barrier to water (Bashir *et al.* 2001). Thus, we consider the factors such as the types of tape and number of strips when applying this method.

29.4.1 Tape stripping versus SC thickness

In order to measure the SC thickness, the device for the measurement of the skin thickness can be used directly and also serial tape stripping and subsequent TEWL measurement can be used. The latter can be used not only to quantify

TABLE 29.3:

Components of three commercial tape and precise TEWL ($g/m^2/h$) data per number of strips for three common tapes at dorsal forearm site (from Bashir et al., 2001)

Number of strips	Type of tape		
	D-Squame	Transpore	Micropore
Components	Polyacrylate ester Super clear polymer	Iso-octyl acrylate, methyl acrylic acid copolymer	Iso-octyl acrylate, acrylic acid copolymer
Baseline	10.3	8.78	9.37
10	11.23	10.77	8.88
20	14.15	14.12	10.1
30	21.05	21.12	10.4
40	30.33	31.98	13.4

The tape was applied to the test site with forceps and pressed onto the skin with a standardized 10 KPa pressure for 2 s. The pressure was then removed and the tape was peeled from the skin unidirectionally.

the thickness of the SC removed by the tape stripping and but also to determine the intact membrane thickness. Some investigators have previously shown that the SC functions as a Fick's first law of water transport (Bashir et al., 2001; Kalia et al., 2001). That is, TEWL, is related to the intact membrane thickness (H) by the following equation:

$$\text{TEWL} = KD \cdot C \neq H$$

Where D is the average membrane diffusion coefficient (cm^2/s), K is the partition coefficient of water and C is the water concentration difference. From the combination of TEWL measurements, and quantification of the mass of SC removed by tape stripping, it can be used to determine the thickness of the intact SC and the diffusion coefficient of water through the SC. C has been previously defined as $1g/cm^3$ and K has been previously defined as 0.162 (Blank et al., 1984).

Schwindt et al. (1998) showed that different skin site had a difference in the SC thickness. They found that the volar forearm SC had a median thickness of 13.5 μm (utilizing Scotch Book Tape), while Bashir et al. (2001) found a median thickness of 12.6 μm with the D-Squame tape, 7.5 μm with the Transpore Tape, and 32.8 μm with Micropore. They demonstrated that the SC thickness varied depending on the tape. In fact, Micropore tape could not have simply been stripping thicker than the other two tapes—D-Squame and Transpore. As shown in Table 29.3, Micropore did not strip the components of the SC that are responsible for barrier function in the same proportions or quantity as the Squame and Transpore tapes. To calculate and compare the physical thickness of the SC, we use the same tape and the same pressure for stripping.

29.5 TAPE STRIPPING VERSUS PERCUTANEOUS ABSORPTION AND PENETRATION

Percutaneous absorption is a complicated and a complex biological process. This process initiates a series of absorption and excretion that are influenced by numerous factors. The intercellular lipid domain is a major pathway for permeation of most drugs through the SC and also acts as a major barrier for penetration into skin. As a consequence of its hydrophobic nature, the SC barrier allows the penetration of lipid soluble molecules more readily than water-soluble drugs. The hydrophilic regions in the bilayer hamper strongly lipophilic drugs. The way to overcome the properties of the corneal layer is by disrupting it, with physical methods (ultrasound, low and high-voltage electrical pulsing, and stripping) and/or chemical enhancers.

Tape stripping is mainly used to measure drug concentration and its concentration profile across the SC. SC is progressively removed by serial adhesive tape stripping and consequently, percutaneous absorption and penetration is significantly increased in pertubation skin (Table 29.4).

Benfeldt and colleagues (Benfeldt *et al.*, 1999; Befeldt and Serup, 1999) reported that salicylic acid penetration was really increased in tape stripped skin in human and hairless rats at 157 and 170-fold, respectively. Delipidization by acetone led to a doubling of the penetration in human but had no effect on penetration on hairless rats. Moon *et al.* (1990) reported that delipidization by chloroform-methanol mixture was increased by up to five-fold in hairless guinea pig (Table 29.4). Although tape stripping increased the penetration of some drugs into skin, this is not universal (Moon *et al.*, 1990; Xiong *et al.*, 1996).

Physiological and pathological factors affect drug transport across the living human skin. Bos and Meinardi (2000) suggested the 500-dalton rule for the skin penetration of chemical compounds and drugs. This size limit was changed by the skin abnormalities such as atopic dermatitis and disrupted skin.

To determine the drug concentration and profile into SC, analytical techniques are important. These techniques include skin extraction measurements, horizontal stripping and sectioning, quantitative autoradiography and spectroscopic methods. Penetration into SC is determined by tape stripping

CHAPTER 29

■ 539

TABLE 29.4:

In vivo drug penetration studies in barrier-perturbed skin

Barrier pertubation	Species	Drug	Penetration ratio*	Study
None			1	
Tape stripping	Human	Hydrocortisone	4	Feldmann and Maibach (1965)
	Hairless guinea pig	Hydrocortisone	3	Moon *et al.* (1990)
	Hairless guinea pig	Benzoic acid	2.1	Moon *et al.* (1990)
	Human	Low molecular weight Heparin	1	Xiong *et al.* (1996)
	Rat	Salicylic acid	0.8–46	Murakami *et al.* (1998)
	Human	Methylprednisolone aceponate	91.5	Gunther (1998)
	Hairless rat	Salicylic acid	170	Benfeldt and Serup (1999)
	Human	Salicylic acid	157	Benfeldt *et al.* (1999)
Delipidization	Hairless guinea pig	Hydrocortisone	5.2	Moon *et al.* (1990)
	Hairless guinea pig	Benzoic acid	2.7	Moon *et al.* (1990)
	Human	Salicylic acid	2.2	Benfeldt *et al.* (1999)
	Hairless rat	Salicylic acid	0.6	Benfeldt and Serup (1999)

* Penetration ratio varies among drugs and species investigated. Most of the studies used traditional radiolabelling techniques, where the penetration is measured as total drug absorption over 4–10 days. In case of salicylic acid, the study defined the cutaneous penetration and systemic absorption during 20-min intervals over a period of 4 h after drug administration.

followed by skin extraction and spectroscopic methods. These methods are widely used in determination of drug concentration within skin. Skin extraction is necessary to extract the drug with a suitable solvent and then an appropriate, sensitive analytical such as HPLC, GLC, and scintilation counting is used to quantify the extracted drug. The improving sensitivity of optical instrument has permitted the quantification of drugs in skin by spectroscopic methods. These methods are non-invasive and offer real time data on penetrant localization. These techniques include attenuated total reflectance Fourier transform infrared (ATR-FTIR) spectroscopy, fluorescence spectroscopy, remittance spectroscopy, and photothermal spectroscopy (Touitou *et al.*, 1998). Table 29.5 shows the characterization of the analysis method of drugs in the skin.

Tape stripping and optical spectroscopy are used as a suitable combined method to determine the horny layer profile (Weimann *et al.* 1999; 2001). The combined use of these analytical methods can test the validity of the dermato-

TABLE 29.5:

Description of the techniques available for quantifying drugs in the skin (from Touitou *et al.*, 1998)

Technique	Penetrants detected	Measuring depth	Cost	Speed	Complementary strategies
Skin extraction	Any	All strata	Inexpensive	Rapid	Separation of skin tissue Qualitative autoradiography
Horizontal sectioning	Any	All strata	Inexpensive	Rapid	Separation of foliiicles Use of follicle-free skin
Quantitative auto-radiography	Radio-labelled only	All strata	Expensive	Slow	None
ATR-FTIR spectroscopy	IR-absorbing only	SC	Expensive	Very rapid	Tape-stripping
Direct fluorescence spectroscopy	Self-fluorescent only	All strata	Medium	Rapid	Separation of follicles Quantitative fluorescent microscopy
Indirect fluorescence spectroscopy	UV-absorbing only	SC	Medium	Rapid	None
Remittance spectroscopy	UV-absorbing only	SC	Medium	Rapid	None
Photothermal spectroscopy	Strong UV-absorbing	SC	Medium	Rapid	None

■ CHAPTER 29 ■

pharmacokinetic (DPK) method to assess bioequivalence and bioavailability of topical dermatological drugs.

In addition to drug detection methods, many methods detect metal into and on the skin: inductively coupled plasma-atomic emission spectroscopy (ICP-AES), inductively coupled plasma-mass spectrometry (ICP-MS), atomic absorption spectrometry (AAS), and particle induced X-ray emission (PIXE) are widely used. ICP-AES permits detection of metals at the trace amount level, obviating the use of radioisotopes. ICP-MS is a technique applicable to µg/l (ppb) concentration of several elements in aqueous medium upon appropriate sample preparation of biological materials. AAS is the reference method accepted by the International Union of Pure and Applied Chemistry for trace element analysis. PIXE analysis with a proton microprobe allows the determination of trace elements in epidermal strata prepared by cryosection (Hostynek *et al.* 2002).

29.6 TAPE STRIPPING VERSUS PEPTIDE IMMUNIZATION

When the skin is damaged by physically, chemically, and biologically, keratino-cytes and LC become activated. In the human, disruption of permeability barrier by tape stripping induces activation of epidermal LC. Nishijima *et al.* (1997) reported that disruption of the skin barrier results in epidermal LC activation as vigorous antigen presenters for T helper cells. Takigawa *et al.* (2001) reported that acute epidermal barrier disruption by tape stripping induces LC maturation and activation in mice. The Class I and II, CD40, CD54, CD86 were expressed 24 h after tape stripping of earlobes and then the enhanced expression returned to control levels 48 h after tape stripping. Tape stripping has two potential functions for percutaneous peptide immunization. One is to increase the peptide penetration into epidermis and another is to activate the LC as an antigen presenting cells. Seo *et al.* (2000) reported that topical application of tumor-associated peptide onto the SC barrier disrupted by tape stripping in mice induces protective antitumor response *in vivo* and *in vitro*. They investigated induction of cytotoxic T lymphocytes (CTL) response on tape stripped earlobes of C57/BL6 mice by application of CTL epitope peptide onto the SC. The optimal condition of CTL response was observed 12 and 24 h after tape stripping at peptide doses of 48 and 96 μg per mouse. On the other hand, CTL induction was virtually absent when peptide was applied to intact skin.

B16 tumor cells were virtually completely rejected after epitope peptide immunization via a disrupted barrier. Also when tumor bearing mice were treated with epitope peptide on tape stripped skin, tumor cells regressed with peptide application, and 100 percent of the mice survived for 1 month and 95 percent for over 60 days. However, mice treated with peptide application to intact skin died after 34 days. Thus, percutaneous immunization provides a simple, no adjuvant system, and non-invasive means of inducing potent antitumor immunity that may be exploited for cancer immunotherapy in the human.

29.7 UNANSWERED QUESTION AND CONCERNS TO TAPE STRIPPING

Surber *et al.* (1999) reviewed the standardized tape stripping technique; many factors remain to be investigated. As shown in Table 29.2, the types and sizes of tapes utilized equally affect the method and the pressure applied to the strip prior to stripping. A preliminary FDA guideline describes a serial tape of the SC to determine the amount of drug within the skin. By the guidelines, the first tape strip is discarded, the drug is extracted from the remaining pooled strips and the quantified amount is expressed as a mass per unit area. From the guidelines, it is impossible to express the amount of drug substance per unit mass of SC and to determine the proportion of the SC that has been sampled by the tape stripping method. Recently, Bashir *et al.* (2001) attempted to improve standardization of the tape stripping method as to type of tape and pressure.

Considering the current application of tape stripping method, clinical trials for the determination of bioequivalence of topical dermatological products could be improved by standardization of tape stripping.

REFERENCES

ALBERTI, I., KALIA, Y.N., NAIK, A., BONNY, J.-D. and GUY, R.H. (2001) *In vivo* assessment of enhanced topical delivery of terbinafine to human stratum corneum, *Journal of Controlled Release*, **71**, 319–327.

BABIUK, S., BACA-ESTRADA, M., BABIUK, L.A., EWEN, C. and FOLDVARI, M. (2000) Cutaneous vaccination: the skin as an immunologically active tissue and the challenge of antigen delivery, *Journal of Controlled Release*, **66**, 199–214.

BASHIR, S.J., CHEW, A.-L., ANIGBOGU, A., DREHER, F. and MAIBACH, H.I. (2001) Physical and physiological effects of stratum corneum tape stripping. *Skin Research and Technology*, **7**, 40–48.

BEISSON, F., AOUBALA, M., MARULL, S., MOUSTACAS-GARDIES, A.-M., VOULTOURY, R., VERGER, R. and ARONDEL, V. (2001) Use of the tape stripping technique for directly quantifying esterase activities in human stratum corneum, *Analytical Biochemistry*, **290**, 179–185.

BENFELDT, E. and SERUP, J. (1999) Effect of barrier pertubation on cutaneous penetration of salicylic acid in hairless rats: *in vivo* pharmacokinetics using microdialysis and non-invasive quantification of barrier function, *Arch. Dermatology Research*, **291**, 517–526.

BENFELDT, E., SERUP, J. and MENNE, T. (1999) Effect of barrier pertubation on cutaneous salicylic acid penetration in human skin: *in vivo* pharmacokinetics using microdialysis and non-invasive quantification of barrier function, *British Journal of Dermatology*, **140**, 739–748.

BETZ, G., NOWBAKHT, P., IMBODEN, R. and IMANIDIS, G. (2001) Heparin penetration into and permeation through human skin from aqueous and liposomal formulations *in vitro*, *International Journal of Phamaceutics*, **228**, 147–159.

BLANK, I.H., MOLONEY, J., EMSLIE, A.G., SIMEN, I. and APT, C. (1984) The diffusion of water across the stratum corneum as a function of its water content, *Journal of Investigative Dermatology*, **82**, 188–194.

BLECK, O., ABECK, D., RING, J., HOPPE, U., VIETZKE, J.P., WOLBER, R., BRANDT, O. and SCHREINER, V. (1999) Two ceramide subfractions detectable in CER (AS) position by HPTLC in skin surface lipids of non-lesional skin of atopic eczema, *Journal of Investigative Dermatology*, **37**, 911–917.

BOS, J.D. and MEINARDI, M.M.H.M. (2000) The 500 dalton rule for the skin penetration of chemical compounds and drugs, *Experimental Dermatology*, **9**, 165–169.

CHAMLIN, S.L., FRIEDEN, I.J., FEWLER, A., WILLIAMS, M., KAO, J., SHEN, M. and ELIAS, P.M. (2001) Ceramide-dominant, barrier-repair lipids improve chilhood atopic dermatitis, *Arch. Dermatology*, **137**, 1110–1112.

COUTEAU, C., PEREZ-CULLEL, N., CONNAN, A.E. and COIFFARD, L.J.M. (2001) Stripping method to quantify absorption of two sunscreens in human, *International Journal of Phamaceutic*, **222**, 153–157.

CULLANDER, C., JESKE, S., IMBERT, D., GRANT, P.G. and BENCH, G. (2000) A quantitative minimally invasive assay for the detection of metals in the stratum corneum, *Journal of Phamaceutical and Biomedical Analysis*, **22**, 265–279.

DARY, C.C., BAANCATO, J.N. and SALEH, M.A. (2001) Chemomorphic analysis of melathion in skin layers of the rat: Implications for the use of dermatopharmacokinetic tape stripping in exposure assessment to pesticides, *Regulatory Toxicology and Pharmacology*, **34**, 234–248.

DREHER, F., ARENS, A., HOSTYNEK, J.J., MUDUMBA, S., ADEMOLA, J. and MAIBACH, H.I. (1998) Colorimetric method for quantifying human stratum corneum removed by adhesive tape stripping, *Acta Derma. Venerel.*, **78**, 186–189.

FELDMANN, R.J. and MAIBACH, H.I. (1965) Penetration of 14-hydrocortisone through normal skin, *Arch. Dermatol.*, **91**, 661–666.

FERNANDEZ, C., NIELLOUD, F., FORTUNE, R., VIAN, L. and MARTI-MESTRES, G. (2002) Benzophenone-3: rapid prediction and evaluation using non-invasive methods of *in vivo* human penetration, *Journal of Pharmaceutical and Biomedical Analysis*, **28**, 57–63.

FLUHR, J.W., DICKEL, H., KUSS, O., WEYHER, I., DIEPGEN, T.L. and BERARDESCA, E. (2002) Impact of anatomical location on barrier recovery, surface pH and stratum corneum hydration after acute barrier disruption, *British Journal of Dermatology*, **146**, 770–776.

GUNTHER, C., KECSKES, A., STAKS, T. and TAUBER, U. (1998) Percutaneous absorption of methyprednisolone aceponate following topical application of Advantan lotion on intact, inflamed and stripped skin of male volunteers, *Skin Pharmacol. Appl. Skin Physiology*, **11**, 35–42.

HOSTYNEK, J.J., DREHER, F., NAKADA, T, SCHWINDT, D., ANIGBOGU, A. and MAIBACH, H.I. (2001) Human stratum corneum absorption of nickel salts. Investigation of depth profiles by tape stripping *in vivo*, *Acta Derm. Venereol.*, **212**, 11–18.

HOSTYNEK, J.J., REAGAN, K.E. and MAIBACH, H.I. (2002) Release of nickel ion from the metal and its alloys as cause of nickel allergy. In HOSTYNEK, J.J. and MAIBACH, H.I. (eds) *Nickel and the Skin. Absorption, Immunology, Epidemiology, and Metallurgy*, Boca Raton: CRC Press, 99–145.

KALIA, Y.N., ALBERT, I., NAIK, A. and GUY, R.H. (2001) Assessment of topical bioavailability *in vivo*: The importance of stratum corneum thickness, *Skin Pharmacol. Appl. Skin Physiology*, **14**, 82–86.

LAVRIJSEN, A.P.M., HIGOUNENC, I.M., WEERHEIM, A., OESTMANN, E., TUINEENBURG, E.E., BODDE, H.E. and PONEC, M. (1994) Validation of an *in vivo* extraction method for human stratum corneum ceramides, *Arch. Dermatology Research*, **286**, 495–503.

MAN, M.M., FEINGOLD, K.R., THORNFELDT, C.R. and ELIAS, P.M. (1996) Optimization of physiological lipid mixtures for barrier repair, *Journal of Investigative Dermatology*, **106**, 1096–1101.

MAN-QIANG, M., FEINGOLD, K.B. and ELIAS, P.M. (1993) Exogenous lipids influence permeability barrier recovery in acetone treated murine skin, *Arch. Dermatology*, **129**, 728–738.

■ CHAPTER 29 ■

MAZEREEUW-HAUTIER, J., REDOULES, D., TARROUX, R., CHARVERON, M., SALLES, J.P., SIMON, M.F., CERUTTI, I., ASSALIT, M.F., GALL, Y., BONAFE, J.L. and CHAP, H. (2000) Identification of pancreatic type I secreted phospholipase A2 in human epidermis and its determination by tape stripping, *British Journal of Dermatology*, **142**, 424–431.

MOGHIMI, H.R., BARRY, B.W. and WILLIAMS, A.C. (1999) Stratum corneum and barrier performance. A model lamellar structural approach. In: BRONAUGH, R.L. and MAIBACH, H.I. (eds) *Percutaneous Absorption. Drug-Cosmetics-Mechanism-Methodology*, New York: Marcel Dekker, 515–553.

MOON, K.C., WESTER, R.C. and MAIBACH, H.I. (1990) Diseased skin models in the hairless guinea pig: *in vivo* percutaneous absorption, *Dermatologica*, **180**, 8–12.

MORTENSEN, J.T., BJERRING, P. and CRAMERS, M. (2001) Locobase repair cream following CO_2 laser skin resurfacing reduces interstitial fluid oozing, *Journal of Cosmetic Laser Therapy*, **3**, 155–158.

MOTTA, S., SESAN, S., MONTI, M., GIULIANI, A. and CAPUTO, R. (1994) Inter-lamellar lipid differences in human stratum corneum, *Acta Derma. Venereol.*, **186**, 131–132.

MURAKAMI, T., YOSHIOKA, M., OKAMOTO, I., YUMOTO, R., HIGASHI, Y., OKAHARA, K. and YATA, N. (1998) Effect of ointment bases on topical and transdermal delivery of sallicylic acid in rats: evaluation by skin microdialysis, *Journal of Pharmaceutical Pharmacology*, **50**, 55–61.

NISHIJIMA, T., TOKURA, Y., IMOKAWA, G., SEO, N., FURUKAWA, F. and TAKIGAWA, M. (1997) Altered permeability and disordered cutaneous immunoregulatory function in mice with acute barrier disruption, *Journal of Investigative Dermatology*, **109**, 175–182.

PALENSKE, J. and MORHENN, V.B. (1999) Changes in the skin's capacitance after damage to the stratum corneum in humans, *Journal of Cutan. Medical Surgery*, **3**, 127–131.

POTARD, G., LAUGEL, C., SCHAEFER, H. and MARTY, J.-P. (2000) The stripping technique: *In vitro* absorption and penetration of five UV filter on excised fresh human skin, *Skin Pharmacol. Appl Skin Physiology*, **13**, 336–344.

ROUGIER, A., DUPUIS, D., LOTTE, C., MAIBACH, H.I. (1999) Stripping method for measuring percutaneous absorption *in vivo*. In BRONAUGH, R.L. and MAIBACH, H.I. (eds) *Percutaneous Absorption. Drug-Cosmetics-Mechanism-Methodology*, New York: Marcel Dekker, 375–394.

SCHWINDT, D.A., WILHELM, K.P. and MAIBACH, H.I. (1998) Water diffusion characteristics of human stratum corneum at different anatomical sites *in vivo*, *Journal of Investigative Dermatology*, **111**, 385–389.

SEO, N., TOKURA, Y., NISHIJIMA, T., HASHIZUME, H., FURUKAWA, F. and TAKIGAWA, M. (2000) Percutaneous peptide immunization via corneum barrier-disrupted murine for experimental tumor immunoprophylaxis, *Proceeding National Academic Science USA*, **97**, 371–376.

SHAH, V.P., FLYNN, G.L., YACOBI, A., MAIBACH, H.I., BON, C., FLEISCHER, N.M., FRANZ, T.J., KAPLAN, L.J., KAWAMOTO, J., LESKO, L.J., MARTY, J.-P., PERSHING, L.K., SHAEFER, H., SEQUEIRA, J.A., SHRIVASTAVA, S.P., WILKINS, J. and WILLIAMS, R.L. (1998) Bioequivalence of topical dermatological dosage forms—methods of evaluation of bioequivalence. *Pharmaceutical Research* **15**, 167–171.

SURBER, C., SCHWARB, F.P. and SMITH, E.W. (1999) Tape-stripping technique. In BRONAUGH, R.L. and MAIBACH, H.I. (eds) *Percutaneous Absorption. Drug-Cosmetics-Mechanism-Methodology*, New York: Marcel Dekker, 395–409.

TAKIGAWA, M., TOKURA, Y., HASHIZUME, H., YAGI, H. and SEO, N. (2001) Percutaneous peptide immunization via corneum barrier-disrupted murine for experimental tumor immunoprophylaxis, *Annals of the New York Academy of Science*, **941**, 139–146.

TOUITOU, E., MEIDAN, V.M. and HORWIWITZ, E. (1998) Methods for quantitative determination of drug localized in the skin, *Journal of Controlled Release*, **56**, 7–21.

XIONG, G.L., QUAN, D. and MAIBACH, H.I. (1996) Effect of penetration enhancers on *in vitro* percutaneous absorption of low molecular weight heparin through human skin, *Journal of Controlled Release*, **42**, 289–296.

WEERHEIM, A. and PONEC, M. (2001) Determination of stratum corneum lipid profile by tape stripping in combination with high-performance thin-layer chromatography. *Arch. Dermatol. Research*, **293**, 191–199.

WEIGMANN, H., LADEMANN, J., MEFFERT, H., SCHAEFER, H. and SRERRY, W. (1999) Determination of the horny layer profile by tape stripping in combination with optical spectroscopy in the visible range as a prerequisite to quantify percutaneous absorption, *Skin Pharmacol. Appl. Skin Physiology*, **12**, 34–45.

WEIGMANN, H.J., LADEMANN, J., SCHANZER, S., LINEMANN, U., VON PELCHRZIM, R., SCHAEFER, H., STERRY, W. and SHAH, V. (2001) Correlation of the local distribution of topically applied substances inside the stratum corneum determined by tape stripping to differences in bioavailability, *Skin Pharmacol. Appl Skin Physiology*, **14**, 98–102.

WISSING, S.A. and MULLER, R.H. (2002) Solid lipid nanoparticles as carrier for sunscreens: *in vitro* release and *in vivo* skin penetration, *Journal of Controlled Release*, **81**, 225–233.

Percutaneous Absorption of Hazardous Substances from Soil and Water

RONALD C WESTER AND HOWARD I MAIBACH

Contents

30.1   Introduction

30.2   Percutaneous absorption

30.3   *In vitro* diffusion versus *in vivo*

30.4   Soil load

30.5   Discussion

30.1 INTRODUCTION

Contamination of soil and water (ground and surface water) and the transfer of hazardous chemical is a major concern. When the large surface area of skin is exposed to contaminated soil and water (work, play, swim, daily bath), skin absorption may be significant. Brown *et al.* (1984) suggested that skin absorption of contaminants in water has been underestimated and that ingestion may not constitute the sole, or even the primary route of expense. Soil has become an environmental depository for potentially hazardous chemicals. Exposure through work in pesticide-sprayed areas on chemical dump sites seems obvious. However, there may be hidden dangers in weekend gardening or in the child's play area.

This chapter demonstrates potential risk from contaminated soil and water, and discusses potential error in dependence on model systems without validation.

30.2 PERCUTANEOUS ABSORPTION

30.2.1 Solvents

Numerous sites have significant levels of organic contaminants in soil, which are either slowly released or degraded, providing a potential long-term source for chemical exposures. Remediation clean-up cost vary dramatically with the level to which soil must be decontaminated. However, a difficulty in establishing soil clean-up level stems, in part, from our lack of knowledge of the dermal bioavailability of chemicals following exposure to environmental mediums. Compared to dermal exposures with neat or aqueous compound, little is understood about the dermal bioavailability of solvents in soil, dust, sludge, or sediment matrices. A method has been developed to determine dermal uptake of solvents under nonsteady state conditions using real-time breath analysis in rats, monkeys, and human volunteers. The exhaled breath was analyzed using an ion trap mass spectrometer, which can continually quantitate chemicals in the exhaled breath stream in the 1–5 ppb range. The resulting exhaled breath data were evaluated using physiologically based pharmacokinetic (PBPK) models to estimate dermal permeability constants (K_p), under various exposure conditions. Exposures have been conducted comparing the impact of exposure matrix (soil versus water), occlusion versus non-occlusion, and species-differences on the percutaneous absorption of methyl chloroform, trichloroethylene, and pentachloroethylene. Studies have demonstrated that rat skin is roughly 40× more permeable than human skin, that bioavailability is decreased when exposures are in a soil versus aqueous matrix, and that under non-occluded exposure conditions the majority of the compound is lost to volatilization and unavailable for absorption. These results have clearly illustrated that the methodology was sufficiently sensitive to enable the conduct of animal and human dermal studies at low exposure concentrations over small body surface areas, for short periods of time.

Table 30.1 summarizes PBPK estimates for solvent human *in vivo* dermal absorption. Hand immersion is a volunteer sitting comfortably with his/her hand immersed in a bucket of water or soil containing one of the solvents. The volunteer wears a facemask. The volunteer inhales fresh air from an air tank. The mask has a special device that switches between inhalation and exhalation. Thus the volunteer exhales through a different pathway such that the exhaled breath goes to a tandem ion-trap mass spectrometer (MS/MS) coupled to a computer which records and can display real-time (every few second if wanted) the solvent concentration in the exhaled breath (Poet *et al.*, 2000a, 2000b, 2002).

Table 30.2 gives PBPK model estimates for the dermal absorption of TCE in rats. Estimated permeability constants are listed. Generally, solvent dermal absorption is less for humans than for rats. In both species solvent absorption is less from soil than from water. This may be due to water's ability to retain solvent within a matrix on the skin better than with soil.

The combination of real-time breath analysis and PBPK modeling provides an opportunity to effectively follow the changing kinetics of uptake, distribution, and elimination phases of a compound throughout a dermal exposure. The

TABLE 30.1:

PBPK model estimates for human *in vivo* dermal absorption

Solvent	Treatment	K_p (cm/hr)
Methylchloroform (TCA)	Water hand immersion	0.0063 ± 0.0006
Trichloroethylene (TCE)	Soil hand immersion	0.0015 ± 0.0005
	Water patch	0.019 ± 0.001
	Soil hand immersion	0.0074 ± 0.000
	Soil patch	0.0043 ± 0.002
Perchlorolthylene (PCE)	Soil hand immersion	0.0009 ± 0.0003

TABLE 30.2:
PBPK model estimates for the dermal absorption of TCE in rats

Exposure concentration	$K_p{}^a$ (cm/hr)			Amount absorbed (mg)			Total TCE recovered[b] (%)		
Occluded water[c] (mg/l)									
1,600	0.31	±	0.018	7.5	±	1.4	100	±	5.2
600	0.30	±	0.006	2.7	±	0.4	103	±	5.1
Average	0.31	±	0.014				102	±	5.6
Nonoccluded soil[c] (mg/kg)									
40,600	0.087	±	0.002	1.5	±	1.4	98	±	8.8
20,300	0.085	±	0.003	7.3	±	2.7	97	±	5.7
5,000	0.085	±	0.003	1.7	±	0.8	101	±	1.4
Average	0.086	±	0.003				99	±	6.0
Occluded soil[c] (mg/kg)									
15,600	0.090	±	0.003	40	±	15	99	±	2.2
5,300	0.089	±	0.002	14	±	3.7	99	±	2.4
Average	0.090	±	0.002				99	±	1.0

[a] Water K_p values are significantly from soil (p<0.01) for both occluded and nonoccluded studies. There is no significant difference in K_p between occluded and nonoccluded soil exposures.
[b] The total TCE recovered was calculated from percent absorbed (estimated from PBPK model), percent remaining in media (soil or water), and percent in charcoal path, where appropriate (as measured using GC headspace analysis), ± SD. The amount absorbed by the body for nonoccluded soil exposure is for a 3 h exposure (n = 3), ± SD.

sensitivity of the ASGDI-MS/MS system for exhaled-breath analysis is pivotal in enabling studies wherein human volunteers are exposed to low levels of compounds for short periods of time. This real-time, *in vivo* method is suitable for studying the percutaneous absorption of volatile chemicals, and allows exposures to be conducted under a variety of exposure conditions, including occluded versus non-occluded, rat versus monkey versus human, and soil versus water matrices (Thrall *et al.*, 2000).

30.2.2 Organic chemicals

DDT, Benzo[a]pyrene, Chlordane, Pentachlorophenol, 2, 4-D

Table 30.3 gives the *in vitro* (human skin) and *in vivo* (Rhesus monkey) percutaneous absorption of organic chemicals from soil and a comparative vehicle (water or solvent, depending on vehicle). The soil is the same source (Yolo County) for all chemicals. For each chemical the concentration of mass (µg) per unit skin area (cm²) is the same for each vehicle. It should be pointed out that chemical selection was done according to chemical interest, as

TABLE 30.3:

In vitro and *in vivo* percutaneous absorption of organic chemicals

Compound	Vehicle	Skin			Percent dose *In vitro* Receptor fluid			*In vivo*		
DDT	acetone	18.1	±	13.4	0.08	±	0.02	18.9	±	9.4
	soil	1.0	±	0.7	0.04	±	0.01	3.3	±	0.5
Ben[a]pyrene	acetone	23.7	±	9.7	0.09	±	0.06	51.0	±	22.0
	soil	1.4	±	0.9	0.01	±	0.06	13.2	±	3.4
Chlordane	acetone	10.8	±	8.2	0.07	±	0.06	6.0	±	2.8
	soil	0.3	±	0.3	0.04	±	0.05	4.2	±	1.8
Pentachlorophenol	acetone	3.7	±	1.7	0.6	±	0.09	29.2	±	5.8
	soil	0.11	±	0.04	0.01	±	0.00	24.4	±	6.4

expressed by Cal EPA and US EPA. Thus the chemicals exhibit high logP octanol/water partition coefficients, rather than a range of logPs (Table 30.4). The *in vivo* human skin percutaneous absorption is expressed as chemical percent dose in receptor fluid accumulation and skin content. Chemicals with higher logPs are lipophilic and therefore are not soluble in biological fluid receptor fluid (plasma, buffered saline) (Wester *et al.*, 1990a, 1990b, 1992a).

Receptor fluid (human plasma) accumulation of DDT was negligible in the *in vitro* study due to solubility restriction. Human skin content was 18.1 percent dose from acetone vehicle. *In vivo* absorption in the Rhesus monkey was 18.9 percent dose from acetone vehicle. These values are comparable to the published 10 percent dose absorbed *in vivo* in man from acetone vehicle. Percutaneous absorption from soil was predicted to be 1.0 percent dose in human skin *in vitro* and a comparative 3.3 percent dose *in vivo* in rhesus monkey.

TABLE 30.4:

Octanol / water partition coefficients of compounds

Compounds	LogP
DDT	6.91
Benzo[a]pyrene	5.97
Chlordane	5.58
Pentachlorophenol	5.12
2,4-D	2.81
PCBs	mixture
Aroclor 1242	(high logP)
Aroclor 1254	(high logP)

In vivo percutaneous absorption of benzo[a]pyrene is high –51.0 percent reported here for rhesus monkey and 48.3 percent (Bronaugh *et al.*, 1986) and 35.3 percent (Yang *et al.*, 1989) for the rat. Benzo[a]pyrene absorption from soil was approximately one-fourth that of solvent vehicle (Wester *et al.*, 1990a).

For chlordane, pentachlorophenol, and 2,4-D, the *in vivo* percutaneous absorption in rhesus monkey from soil was equal to or slightly less than that obtained from solvent vehicle (Table 30.3). Validation to man *in vivo* is available for 2,4-D where the percutaneous absorption is the same for rhesus monkey and man. *In vitro* percutaneous absorption is variable, probably due to solubility problems relative to high lipophilicity.

30.2.3 PCBs

Table 30.5 gives the *in vitro* and *in vivo* percutaneous absorption of PCBs (Wester *et al.*, 1993a). As with the other organic chemicals with high logP, receptor fluid accumulation *in vitro* was essentially nil. Skin accumulation *in vitro* did exhibit some PCB accumulation. *In vivo*, PCB percutaneous absorption for both Aroclor 1242 and 1254 was (a) high, ranging from 14 to 21 percent, and (b) generally independent of formulation vehicle. Thus, PCBs have a strong affinity for skin and are relatively easily absorbed into and through skin. Figure 30.1 summarizes absorption from solvent and soil.

TABLE 30.5:

In vitro and *in vivo* percutaneous absorption of PCBs

Compound	Vehicle	Skin	Percent dose *In vitro* Receptor fluid	*In vivo*
PCBs (1242)	acetone	—	—	21.4 ± 8.5
	TCB	—	—	18.0 ± 8.3
	mineral oil	6.4 ± 6.3	0.3 ± 0.6	20.8 ± 8.3
	soil	1.6 ± 1.1	0.04 ± 0.05	14.1 ± 1.0
PCB (1254)	acetone	—	—	14.6 ± 3.6
	TCB	—	—	20.8 ± 8.3
	mineral oil	10.0 ± 16.5	0.1 ± 0.07	20.4 ± 8.5
	soil	2.8 ± 2.8	0.04 ± 0.05	13.8 ± 2.7

CHAPTER 30

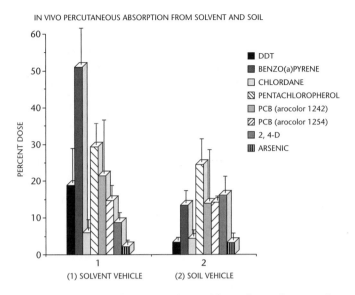

IN VIVO PERCUTANEOUS ABSORPTION FROM SOLVENT AND SOIL

Figure 30.1: In percutaneous absorption of several hazardous substances from soil and solvent (either acetone or water). Overall, soil reduced absorption to about 60 percent, compared to solvent. This is caution, however, because the absorption of some compounds is the same for soil and solvent.

30.2.4 Metals

Arsenic, cadmium, mercury

Selected salts of arsenic, cadmium, and mercury are soluble in water, and thus are amenable to *in vitro* percutaneous absorption with human skin. Arsenic absorption *in vitro* was 2.0 percent (1.0 percent skin plus 0.9 percent receptor fluid), and the same *in vivo* in rhesus monkey. Absorption from soil was equal to (*in vivo*) or approximately one-third (*in vitro*). Cadmium and mercury both accumulate in human skin, and are slowly absorbed into the body. (It should be noted that *in vivo* studies with cadmium and mercury are difficult to perform; cadmium accumulates in the body and mercury is not excreted via urine.) Note the high skin content with cadmium and mercury (Table 30.6) (Wester *et al.*, 1992a, 1993b).

TABLE 30.6:

In vitro and *in vivo* percutaneous absorption of metals

Compound	Vehicle	Skin		Percent dose *In vitro* Receptor fluid		*In vivo*	
Arsenic	water	1.0	± 1.0	0.9	± 1.1	2.0	± 1.2
	soil	0.3	± 0.2	0.4	± 0.5	3.2	± 1.9
Cadmium	water	6.7	± 4.8	0.4	± 0.2	—	
	soil	0.09	± 0.03	0.03	± 0.02	—	
Mercury	water	28.5	± 6.3	0.07	± 0.01	—	
	soil	7.9	± 2.2	0.06	± 0.01	—	

30.3 *IN VITRO* DIFFUSION VERSUS *IN VIVO*

Regulatory agencies have developed an affinity for a calculated permeability coefficient (K_p) for risk assessment. Permeability coefficients are easiest determined from the time course of chemical diffusion from a vehicle (water, soil) across the skin barrier into a receptor fluid. Table 30.7 compares *in vitro* diffusion receptor fluid absorption with *in vivo* percutaneous absorption. Receptor fluid accumulation for the higher logP chemicals (Table 30.4) is negligible. This is due to basic chemistry—the compounds are not soluble in the water based receptor fluid. Based on these receptor fluid accumulations these chemicals are not absorbed by skin. Risk assessment would contain an extreme false negative component. That point where the diffusion system and receptor fluid accumulation gives a true K_p or manufactures a false K_p has not been determined. Regulatory agents should have some *in vivo* validation before blindly accepting an *in vitro* K_p.

30.4 SOIL LOAD

A popular assumption is that only the fine particles of soil which stick to the skin transfer contaminants from the soil to the skin. This is the monolayer theory. If it was only the fine soil particles, then all of the data shown in this chapter could not exist, because the fine particles were not used (sieved out for laboratory personnel safety reasons). Besides, contaminants will transfer between large surfaces (table, couch, etc.) and skin, even between people. And, certainly, the first soil monolayer to contact the skin during planting of the first rose bush will not be the same monolayer after planting the twentieth bush.

■ CHAPTER 30 ■

TABLE 30.7:

In vitro receptor fluid versus *in vivo* percutaneous absorption

Compound	Vehicle	Percent dose *In vitro* Receptor fluid	*In vivo*
DDT	Acetone	0.08 ± 0.02	18.9 ± 9.4
	Soil	0.04 ± 0.01	3.3 ± 0.5
Benzo[a]pyrene	Acetone	0.09 ± 0.06	51.0 ± 22.0
	Soil	0.01 ± 0.06	13.2 ± 3.4
Chlordane	Acetone	0.07 ± 0.06	6.0 ± 2.8
	Soil	0.04 ± 0.05	4.2 ± 1.8
Pentachlorophenol	Acetone	0.6 ± 0.09	29.2 ± 5.8
	Soil	0.01 ± 0.00	24.4 ± 6.4
PCBs (1242)	Acetone	—	21.4 ± 8.5
	TCB	—	18.0 ± 8.3
	Mineral oil	0.3 ± 0.6	20.8 ± 8.3
	Soil	0.04 ± 0.05	14.1 ± 1.0
PCBs (1254)	Acetone	—	14.6 ± 3.6
	TCB	—	20.8 ± 8.3
	Mineral oil	0.1 ± 0.07	20.4 ± 8.5
	Soil	0.04 ± 0.05	13.8 ± 2.7
2,4-D	Acetone	—	2.6 ± 2.1
	Soil	0.02 ± 0.01	15.9 ± 4.7
Arsenic	Water	0.9 ± 1.1	2.0 ± 1.2
	Soil	0.03 ± 0.5	3.2 ± 1.9
Cadmium	Water	0.4 ± 0.2	—
	Soil	0.03 ± 0.02	—
Mercury	Water	0.07 ± 0.01	—
	Soil	0.06 ± 0.01	—

However, the computer model needs the monolayer therefore it has to exist. Table 30.8 shows the effect of soil load. Note the chemical concentration was kept constant while soil load was varied.

30.5 DISCUSSION

The evolution of skin resulted in a tissue that protects precious body fluids and constituents from excessive uptake of water and contaminants in the external environment. The outermost surface of the skin that emerged for human is the stratum corneum, which restricts but does not prevent penetration of water and other molecules. This is a complex lipid-protein structure that is exposed to contaminants during bathing, swimming, and exposure to the environment. Industrial growth has resulted in the production of organic chemical and toxic metals whose disposal resulted in contamination. As a man or woman settles

TABLE 30.8:

Effect of Soil Load on 2,4-D Percutaneous Absorption

System	Soil load[a] (mg/cm²)	Percent dose absorbed[b]
In vivo, rhesus monkey	1	9.8 ± 4.0
	40	15.9 ± 4.7
In vitro, human skin	5	1.8 ± 1.7
	10	1.7 ± 1.3
	40	1.4 ± 1.2

[a] Concentration of 2,4-D chemical per cm² skin area was kept constant, while soil load per cm² skin area was varied.
[b] In vivo percutaneous absorption measured by urinary ^{14}C accumulation; *in vitro* absorption determined by ^{14}C skin content.
[c] Mean ± SD (n=4).

into a tub or a child sits in the dirt for a day of play, the skin (the largest organ of the body), acts as a lipid sink (stratum corneum) for the lipid-soluble contaminants. Skin also serves as transfer membrane for water and whatever contaminants may be dissolved in it. It is most important to note that (a) water transfers through skin and can carry chemicals, and (b) the outer layer of skin is lipid in nature. Thus, highly lipophilic chemicals such as DDT, PCBs, and chlordane residing in soil will quickly transfer to skin. Percutaneous absorption can be linear, orderly, and predictive (a measured flux from water). However, evidence exists that chemicals may transfer to skin with short-term exposure.

Regulators should be cautious as *in vitro* and computer models are developed for risk assessment. Validation is needed to avoid false negative assessment.

REFERENCES

BRONAUGH, R.L. and STEWARD, R.F. (1986) Methods for *in vitro* percutaneous absorption studies. VI. Preparation of the barrier layer. *J. Pharm. Sci.* **75**, 487–491.

BRONAUGH, R.L., STEWARD, R.F. and STORM, J.E. (1989) Extent of cutaneous metabolism during percutaneous absorption xenobiotics. *Toxicol. Appl. Pharmacol.* **99**, 534–543.

BROWN, H.S., BISHOP, D.R. and ROWAN, C.A. (1984) The role of skin absorption as a route of exposure for volatile organic compounds (VOCs) in drinking water. *Am. J. Public Health* **74**, 479:484.

CHAPTER 30

POET, T.S., THRALL, K.D., CORLEY, R.A., HUI, X., EDWARDS, J.A., WEITZ, K.K., MAIBACH, H.I. and WESTER, R.C. (2000a) Utility of real time breath analysis and physiologically based pharmacokinetic modeling to determine the percutaneous absorption of methyl chloroform in rats and humans. *Toxicol. Sci.* **54**, 42–51.

POET, T.S., CORLEY, R.A., THRALL, K.D., EDWARDS, J.A., TANOJO, H., WEITZ, K.K., HUI, X., MAIBACH, H.I. and WESTER, R.C. (2000b) Assessment of the percutaneous absorption of trichloroethylene in rats and humans using MS/MS real-time breath analysis and physiologically based pharmacokinetic modeling. *Toxicol. Sci.* **56**, 61–72.

POET, T.S., WEITZ, K.K., GIES, R.A., EDWARDS, J.A., THRALL, K.D., CORLEY, R.A., TANOJO, H., HUI, X., MAIBACH, H.I. and WESTER, R.C. (2002) PBPK modeling of the percutaneous absorption of perchlorolthylene from a soil matrix in rats and humans. *Toxicol. Sci.* **67**, 17–31.

REIGNER, B.G., GUNGON, R.A., HOAG M.K. and TOZER, T.N. (1991) Pentachlorophenol toxicokinetics after intravenous and oral administration to rat. *Zenobiotica* **21**, 1547–1558.

SHU, H., TEITEBAUM, P., WEBB, A.S., MARPLE, L., BRUNCK, B., DEL ROSSI, D., MURRAY, F.J. and PAUSTENBACH, D. (1988) Bioavailability of soil-bound TCDD. Dermal bioavailability in the rat. *Fund. Appl. Toxicol.* **10**, 335–343.

THRALL, K.D., POET, T.S., CORLEY, R.A., TANOJO, H., EDWARDS, J.A., WEITZ, K.K., HUI, X., MAIBACH, H.I. and WESTER, R.C. (2000) A real-time *in vivo* method for studying the percutaneous absorption of volatile chemicals. *Int. J. Occup. Environ. Health* **6**, 96–103.

WESTER, R.C., MAIBACH, H.I., BUCKS, D.A.W., SEDIK, L., MELENDRES, J., LIAO, C. and DIZIO, S. (1990a) Percutaneous absorption of [^{14}C] DDT and benzo[a]pyrene from soil. *Fundam. Appl. Toxicol.* **15**, 510–516.

WESTER, R.C., MAIBACH, H.I., SEDIK, L., MELENDRES, J., WADE, M. and DIZIO, S. (1990b) *In vitro* percutaneous absorption of pentachlorophenol from soil. *Fundam. Appl. Toxicol.* **19**, 68–71.

WESTER, R.C., MAIBACH, H.I., SEDIK, L., MELENDRES, J., LIAO, C.L. and DIZIO, S. (1992a) Percutaneous absorption of cadmium from water and soil. *J. Toxicol. Environ. Health* **35**, 269–277.

WESTER, R.C., MAIBACH, H.I., SEDIK, L., MELENDRES, J. and J., WADE, M. (1993a) *In vivo* and *in vitro* percutaneous absorption and skin decontamination of arsenic from water and soil. *Fundam. Appl. Toxicol.* **20**, 336–340.

WESTER, R.C., MAIBACH, H.I., SEDIK, L., MELENDRES, J. and J., WADE, M. (1993b) Percutaneous absorption of PCBs from soil: *In vivo* rhesus monkey, *in vitro* human skin, and binding to powdered human stratum corneum. *J. Toxicol. Environ. Health* **39**, 375–382.

YANG, J.J., ROY, T.A. KRUEGER, A.J., NEIL, W. and MACKERER, C.R. (1989) *In vitro* and *in vivo* percutaneous absorption of benzo[a]pyrene from petroleum crude-fortified soil in the rat. *Bull. Environ. Contam. Toxicol.* **43**, 207–214.

Isolated Perfused Porcine Skin Flap

JIM E RIVIERE

Contents

31.1 Introduction

31.2 Overview of method

31.3 Applications

31.4 Discussion

31.1   INTRODUCTION

There are numerous methods which have been employed to assess the percutaneous absorption of toxic chemicals using both *in vitro* and *in vivo* animal models. There is little debate that *in vivo* human studies are optimal for predicting the absorption of topically applied chemicals in man. However, for highly toxic or carcinogenic chemicals, ethics preclude conducting such studies when a risk analysis is to be conducted. Similar considerations apply to the humane use of animal surrogates. For chemicals which pose little direct adverse risk to man or animals, experimental design and sampling limitations often apply to any *in vivo* study. An important limitation is the inability to noninvasively sample the venous drainage of a topical application site to determine the true cutaneous flux for use as an input into systemic risk assessment models. Similarly, extensive biopsies may not be taken to quantitate subtle, pre-clinical morphological or biochemical manifestations of dermatotoxicity.

The next alternative in the hierarchy of model systems would be *in vitro* diffusion cell studies using human skin. Although in most cases these methods may appear to be preferred, there are limitations that may seriously detract from their usefulness. These include studies where vasoactive compounds are being used or where the magnitude or distribution of cutaneous blood flow would affect the subsequent rate and extent of compound absorption or pattern of cutaneous distribution. Vascular changes could result from compound-induced cutaneous irritation where released inflammatory mediators could directly modulate vascular physiology. Some *in vitro* models are not optimal for studying the kinetics of cutaneous metabolism. Another problem is availability of disease-free, fresh human skin from the same individual and body region. Variability in tissue sources may introduce an unacceptably high degree of intersample variation. If the effects of chemical or physical pre-treatment on subsequent chemical absorption are to be studied, ethical considerations may preclude these studies being done in man. These limitations also apply to recently developed living skin equivalent (LSE) models and *in vitro* animal studies.

Isolated perfused skin studies, such as the isolated perfused porcine skin flap (IPPSF) developed in our laboratory and described in this chapter, may be the "missing link" in the hierarchy of classic *in vitro* and *in vivo* models. The primary advantages of isolated perfused systems relate to:

1   the presence of a functional cutaneous vascular system;
2   the ease of continuously sampling venous perfusate;

3   the ability to conduct mass-balance and metabolism studies;

4   the availability of a large dosing surface area;

5   the capability of simultaneously assessing transdermal chemical flux and biomarkers of cutaneous toxicity;

6   the ability to conduct morphological evaluations at the end of a study in the samepreparation that an absorption study was conducted; and

7   the ease with which experimental conditions (temperature, humidity, perfusate flow and composition) can be manipulated and controlled without being concerned with interference from systemic feedback processes as is usually seen *in vivo*.

Isolated kidney, liver and lung perfusions have been recognized as mainstay models for toxicology and pharmacology for many decades. Part of their acceptance relates to the ease of harvest since these organs are all characterized by having "closed" vascular systems with anatomically identifiable arterial inputs and venous outputs, both amenable to catheterizations with minimal expertise in surgery. In contrast, outside of the possible exception of ears, skin does not possess such a closed vascular system.

Rabbit and pig ears have been used as perfused skin systems to assess percutaneous absorption of topically applied compounds (Behrendt and Kampffmeyer, 1989; de Lange *et al.*, 1992; Celesti *et al.*, 1993). We feel that a fundamental problem with these systems is that the skin of the pinna is different (hair density, adnexial structures) than other body sites and has a much greater degree of blood perfusion (Monteiro-Riviere *et al.*, 1990; Monteiro-Riviere *et al.*, 1993a). Additionally, the vasculature is specialized because of the unique thermoregulatory demands placed on this appendage. Auricular arteries perfuse a complex tissue bed consisting of skin, subcutaneous tissue, muscle and cartilage. We believe that these additional factors outweigh the obvious economic benefits of obtaining ears from laboratory animals or abattoirs. Also, reports have appeared sporadically in the literature on perfused pieces of animal and human skin being used in various studies (Feldberg and Paton, 1951; Kjaersgaard, 1954; Hiernickel, 1985; Kietzmann *et al.*, 1991), however none have ever been optimized or validated for percutaneous absorption studies.

31.2 OVERVIEW OF METHOD

31.2.1 Surgical preparation and perfusion

The IPPSF is a single pedicle axial pattern tubed skin flap created from the abdominal skin of weanling pigs. This area was selected because it is perfused by direct cutaneous arteries (superficial epigastric artery) and drained by the associated paired venous commitantes. This allows a tube of skin to be created whose sole vascular supply may be cannulated and perfused *ex vivo*. The formation of a tubed flap allows the wound edges to be apposed and after a short healing period of two days the preparation only drains via the venous system. This area of skin has also been used to created the *in situ* rat/human skin flap system (Krueger *et al.*, 1985) and recently an isolated perfused human non-tubed skin flap model (Kreidstein *et al.*, 1991). The IPPSF is fully described in the original publications describing its use (Riviere *et al.*, 1986; Monteiro-Riviere *et al.*, 1987; Riviere and Monteiro-Riviere, 1991). In addition, our group has developed an isolated perfused equine skin flap for use in assessing percutaneous absorption of chemicals across horse skin (Bristol *et al.*, 1991) and a perfused human tumor bearing flap for use in anticancer drug targeting investigations (Vaden *et al.*, 1993).

The IPPSF is created in a two-stage surgical procedure (Figure 31.1) (Bowman *et al.*, 1991). Two flaps are created on each pig using the right and left caudal superficial epigastric arteries. Depending on the experimental design, this allows one flap to serve as a control for the other during perfusion studies so as to minimize inter-flap variability. In Stage I surgery, conducted aseptically and under inhalational anesthesia, a 4×12 cm area of skin previously shown to be perfused by this artery is demarcated, excised, tubed and allowed to remain on the pig. Two days later, a time found to be optimal based on morphological criteria (Monteiro-Riviere *et al.*, 1987), the flap is excised and the artery cannulated in a simpler Stage II procedure. Both flaps are then removed and placed in the isolated perfusion chambers described below. The small incision remaining on the pig is allowed to heal and then the pig can be returned to its prior disposition (sale, other uses).

The isolated perfusion apparatus depicted in Figure 31.2 is a custom Plexiglas chamber designed to maintain the skin flap in a temperature and humidity regulated environment. Perfusion pressure, flow, pH and temperature are set for desired conditions dictated by the experimental design and continuously monitored. The perfusion media is a modified Krebs-Ringer bicarbonate buffer

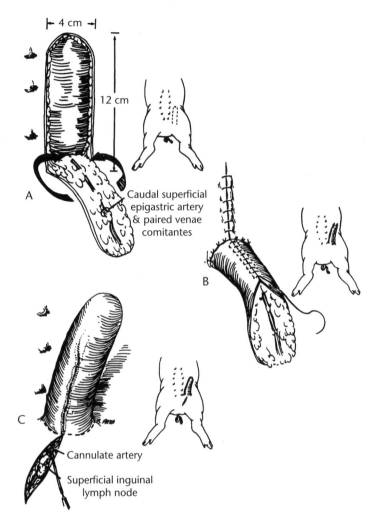

Figure 31.1: Two stage surgical procedure used to create isolated perfused porcine skin flaps. A single pedicle axial pattern tubed skin flap is created in Stage One (A) and harvested two days later in the Stage Two (B) procedure.

(pH 7.4, 350 mOsm/kg) containing albumin (45g/L) and supplied with glucose (80–120 mg/dl) as the primary energy source. Albumin is added to provide the oncotic pressure required to maintain capillary patency as dictated by Starling's laws, and to facilitate the absorption of lipophilic penetrants that otherwise would not be soluble in a pure aqueous buffer system. Normal perfusate flow

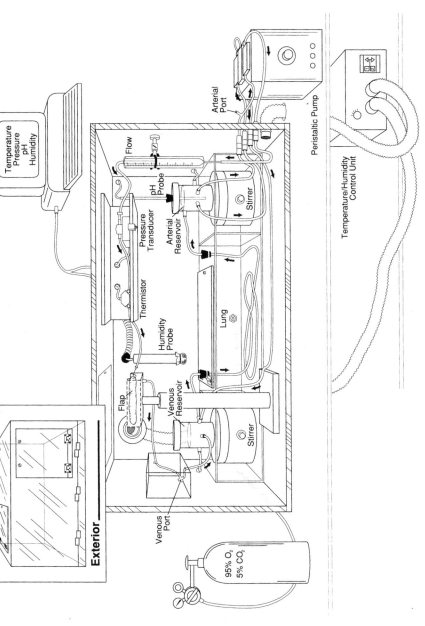

Figure 31.2: Temperature and humidity controlled chamber used to maintain IPPSF viability and environmental conditions throughout an experiment.

through the skin is maintained at 1 ml/min/flap (3–7 ml/min/100 g) with a mean arterial cannula pressure ranging from 30 to 70 mmHG. With this system, flaps may be maintained biochemically and morphologically viable for up to 24 hours. Two experimental configurations are possible for flap perfusion: recirculating and non-recirculating. For most studies, the single pass non-recirculating system is used. Our laboratory has perfused over 2200 IPPSFs and several hundred more have also been independently perfused in non-academic laboratories to which the technique has been transferred.

31.3   APPLICATIONS

There have been three general types of studies conducted in the IPPSF: toxicology, percutaneous absorption (including biotransformation and pharma-cokinetic modeling) and cutaneous drug distribution (drug administered by intra-arterial infusion) studies. The first two of these will be addressed in this chapter.

31.3.1   Assessment of flap viability and development of biomarkers for toxicity assessment

Viability of the preparations are monitored real-time by assessing perfusate pressure and glucose utilization. We have found that during perfusion of a normal IPPSF, the most sensitive indicator of vascular function, and thus of vascular toxicity in dermatotoxicology experiments, is the parameter of vascular resistance calculated as perfusate pressure divided by flow. This parameter has also been used as an endpoint in pharmacological experiments when autonomic drug activity has been studied (Rogers and Riviere, 1994). Glucose utilization, calculated from the arterial–venous extraction ratio and perfusate flow, has been used as a marker of direct cutaneous toxicity of chemicals (King and Monteiro-Riviere, 1990; King et al., 1992; Monteiro-Riviere, 1992; Srikrishna et al., 1992) with decreases in cumulative glucose utilization being suggestive of direct chemical toxicity. However, glucose utilization may also be dependent upon the extent of capillary perfusion, since only cells which are being perfused are capable of extracting glucose from the arterial perfusate (Rogers and Riviere, 1994). A decrease in glucose utilization is definitely a manifestation of chemical activity, however a chemical-induced decrease in epidermal glucose utilization may be blunted by increased capillary perfusion. Independent markers of capillary perfusion (e.g. microspheres) are being assessed for utility in this area.

Depending on the experimental design, a number of more specialized markers of viability, or loss thereof, may be assessed. Previously, we have assessed lactate production as a marker of epidermal glucose utilization and have observed decreased lactate production coexistent with decreased glucose utilization. Also, we have monitored the release of inflammatory mediators into the perfusate as biomarkers for physical or chemical-induced toxicity. These have included PGE_2, $PGF_{2\alpha}$, and interleukins 1 and 8 as indicators of cutaneous inflammation (Monteiro-Riviere, 1992; Zhang et al., 1995a, b). Prostaglandin fluxes changed with compounds which altered vascular resistance. We have used these prostaglandin fluxes as endpoints in pharmacologic intervention studies designed to block a cutaneous toxicant's effect by pre-exposure infusion of a specific antagonist. For example, in order to dissect out the role of prostaglandins in sulfur mustard (HD)-induced cutaneous vesication, we demonstrated that perfusion with the non-steroidal anti-inflammatory drug (NSAID) indomethacin blunted both PGE_2 release and altered vascular resistance, but did not completely prevent blister formation (Zhang et al., 1995b). Similarly, infusion of pyridostigmine bromide modulated interleukin 8 and PGE_2 release seen after exposure to topical irritants (Monteiro-Riviere et al., 2003).

The final markers of dermatotoxicity are the myriad of morphological endpoints which may be assessed easily at the termination of an experiment. Specimens are routinely collected for light microscopy to evaluate skin viability and integrity (Monteiro-Riviere et al., 1987). These studies are pivotal in assessing the nature of cutaneous toxicity produced (Monteiro-Riviere, 1992; Monteiro-Riviere et al., 2001). For a more specific insight into the mechanism of an observed effect, transmission electron microscopy may also be performed (Monteiro-Riviere et al., 1987, Monteiro-Riviere, 1990). These studies give a better indication of what is actually occurring within the epidermal cells at a level before light microscopy or gross observation indicate an adverse effect. For even more specific details, specialized morphological procedures may be conducted. These have included enzyme histochemistry to probe biochemical pathways affected by cutaneous toxicants (King et al., 1992; Srikrishna et al., 1992), immunohistochemistry and immunoelectron microscopy to study the specific molecular targets involved in vesication secondary to chemical alkylation (King et al., 1994; Monteiro-Riviere and Inman, 1995; Zhang et al., 1995c) or topical jet-fuel exposure (Rhyne et al., 2002), and X-ray diffraction microscopy to probe pathways of metal penetration (Monteiro-Riviere et al., 1994a).

Although every one of the aforementioned biomarkers may be assessed in other skin models, the unique strength of the IPPSF is that all may be simultaneously evaluated in the same preparation. For example, we have recently demonstrated the utility of the IPPSF to serve as a humane *in vitro* model for UVB phototoxicity (Monteiro-Riviere *et al.*, 1994b). In these studies, physiological parameters such as vascular resistance, glucose utilization and prostaglandin (PGE$_2$) efflux could be simultaneously evaluated in the same preparation as morphometric quantitation of pyknotic "sunburn" cells and estimation of epidermal growth fraction using histochemical staining for the proliferating cell nuclear antigen (PCNA). In chemical-induced dermatotoxicity, compound flux through the skin can simultaneously be determined in the same preparation that physiological and morphological endpoints are being evaluated. Such studies have been conducted with paraquat (Srikrishna *et al.*, 1992), lewisite (King *et al.*, 1992), 2-chloroethyl methyl sulfide (King and Monteiro-Riviere, 1990), lidocaine iontophoresis (Monteiro-Riviere, 1990) and electroporation (Riviere *et al.*, 1995), and very recently with complex chemical mixtures. Chapter 4 in the present text on chemical mixtures should be consulted for details on some of these studies.

This approach offers many unique advantages. First it guarantees that cutaneous exposure to a penetrating molecule actually occurred. Second, it allows quantitation of this exposure and subsequent correlation to severity of toxicity observed. Finally, it would allow the development of linked toxico-kinetic-toxicodynamic models to be developed which should shed insight into the mechanisms of cutaneous toxicity.

31.3.2 Absorption studies

The IPPSF has also been extensively utilized to quantitate the cutaneous penetration and absorption of topically applied compounds for which systemic exposure could result in toxicity. There are a number of levels of sophistication which can be employed depending upon the nature of the penetrant and the precision desired. The simplest approach is to measure compound flux into the venous perfusate and express this as the percent of applied dose absorbed (Figure 31.3). The compound remaining on the skin surface and within the skin can be easily assessed, especially if radiolabeled chemical was employed. This method is accurate if most of the absorption is complete at the end of an experiment (e.g. venous fluxes are approaching background). The amount of penetrated chemical in the venous effluent may then be determined as the area under the curve (AUC) of the venous efflux profile.

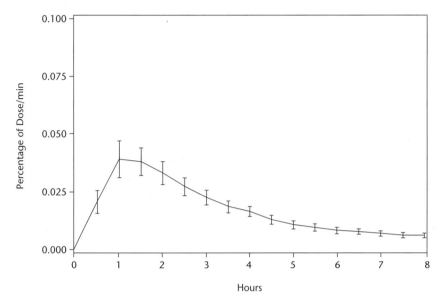

Figure 31.3: Typical IPPSF venous flux profile for a percutaneous absorption experiment (mean ± SD).

At the end of a topical treatment, additional studies may be conducted to determine the amount and distribution of penetrated compound within local tissues. The most precise technique available for this purpose is to take a core biopsy through the dosing site, snap freeze it in liquid nitrogen, and then cut serial sections in order to precisely localize chemical distribution within the skin as a function of penetration depth. In these studies which are fully described in the literature (Riviere *et al.*, 1992a; Monteiro-Riviere *et al.*, 1993b), the surface of the application site is first gently washed with a mild soap solution and then dried with gauze. Cellophane tape is then applied to "strip" the stratum corneum. A biopsy punch is used to take the core of tissue which is then embedded in OCT compound, quenched in an isopentane well cooled by liquid nitrogen and immediately stored at –80°C until it is sectioned in a cryostat. Each tissue section (representing a disk of skin containing radiolabeled compound), along with the washes and tape strips, are then combusted and radioactivity determined using liquid scintillation spectroscopy. The resulting data is a depth penetration profile for the compound under study (Figure 31.4). Although similar studies may be conducted *in vivo*, the advantage of the IPPSF is that this data is obtained in the same preparation that venous flux of the

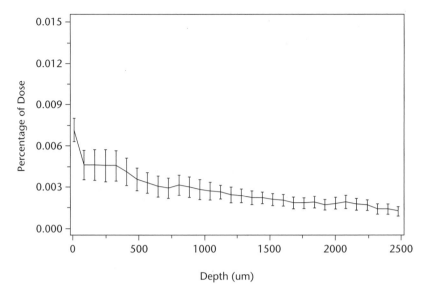

Figure 31.4: Typical IPPSF tissue distribution profile seen after topical administration (mean ± SD).

compound is determined, allowing the investigator to assess factors which modulate tissue penetration from absorption into the vasculature. This approach was utilized to assess the effect of various environmental exposure variables on the absorption of TCB (Qiao and Riviere, 2000). Finally, a technique was recently developed to assess the absorption of volatile compounds in this model (Riviere *et al.*, 2000).

Percutaneous absorption in the IPPSF was correlated ($r^2 \approx 0.8$) to *in vivo* human absorption for five diverse compounds (Wester *et al.*, 1998). The IPPSF estimate for absorption used was the amount absorbed into the perfusate plus the amounts penetrated into the skin. Comparative absorption values (% Dose; Mean + SD) were:

Compound	Human			IPPSF		
salicylic acid	6.5	±	5	7.5	±	2.6
theophylline	16.9	±	11.3	11.8	±	3.8
2,4-dimethylamine	1.1	±	0.3	3.8	±	0.6
diethyl hexyl phthalic acid	1.8	±	0.5	3.9	±	2.4
ρ-amino benzoic acid	11.5	±	6.3	5.9	±	3.7

31.3.3 Dermatopharmacokinetic studies

The greatest level of precision which may be achieved with this system is to apply pharmacokinetic models to either extrapolate to the *in vivo* situation or quantitate the fate of drug within the skin. These are especially adaptable to a system such as the IPPSF because venous drug efflux can be readily determined, which is the starting point for the analysis. These strategies are outlined in Figure 31.5. If the goal of the study is to predict *in vivo* disposition, then one should view the IPPSF as a "living" infusion pump whose output flux (venous efflux) is actually the input into the systemic circulation. First, this approach allows one to use porcine skin data to model human skin penetration with human systemic pharmacokinetic data to avoid interspecies differences in drug distribution, metabolism or elimination. Second, this strategy allows one to predict the actual serum drug concentration-time profile that may be seen *in*

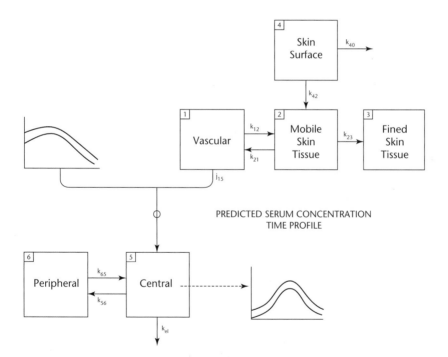

Figure 31.5: Conceptual approach to using IPPSF absorption profile (upper left) or dermatopharmacokinetic model (upper right) as input into a systemic pharmacokinetic model (lower left) to predict an *in vivo* serum concentration-time profile.

vivo. This approach has been used to predict the *in vivo* disposition of a number of drugs, including arbutamine and LHRH (Riviere *et al.*, 1992b; Heit *et al.*, 1993; Williams and Riviere, 1994). The systemic input may either be the observed IPPSF venous efflux profile or the pharmacokinetic simulation of this profile.

This brings us to the second use of pharmacokinetic modeling which is to predict the shape of the cutaneous efflux profile based on factors governing the absorption and distribution of the drug. Our group initiated these studies using drug infused into the arterial cannula whereby arterial and venous extraction of the drug could be determined. This approach allowed the basic structure of our IPPSF model to be determined (Williams and Riviere, 1989a). The specific volumes of the extracellular and intracellular spaces were then validated using dual radiolabeled albumin and inulin infusions (Williams and Riviere, 1989b). The next step was to add a percutaneous absorption component (Williams *et al.*, 1990; Carver *et al.*, 1989) which is the basic model depicted in Figure 31.5. This approach allows one to conduct an experiment over an eight hour period and use the venous efflux profile to determine the parameters of the pharmaco-kinetic model. If the venous efflux profiles demonstrated a peak or beginning of a plateau phase, then using the model parameters, the eight hour data may be extrapolated to extended time points. Such correlations ($r^2 \approx 0.9$) were deter-mined between extrapolated IPPSF profiles and observed six day absorptions for a number of diverse compounds, further demonstrating both the utility of the IPPSF to predict percutaneous absorption in humans as well as the underlying similarity between pig and human skin (Riviere and Monteiro-Riviere, 1991). Since only the total fraction of a topically applied dose absorbed was predicted in these situations, *in vivo* pharmacokinetic data was not needed since a blood concentration-time profile was not available.

The only data used in the models presented above are actual venous efflux profiles and residual compound recovered at the end of an experiment (e.g. unabsorbed chemical bound to dosing device, skin surface wipes and drug in the flap). The precision of such models may be greatly improved if the tissue penetration data described above (stratum corneum residues by tape strips, serial sections of biopsy cores) are also included in the data analysis. Additionally, if other *in vitro* data such as stratum corneum partition coefficients and rates of evaporation are independently determined in porcine skin (Williams *et al.*, 1994), more sophisticated models may be developed which can shed much greater insight into the mechanisms governing chemical absorption and penetration. Figure 31.6 depicts such a model which incorporates the fate of the vehicle used to apply the drug, since it is widely acknowledged (but seldomly

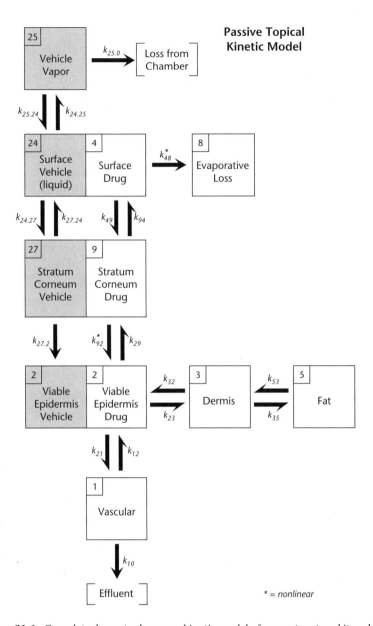

Figure 31.6: Complete dermatopharmacokinetic model of a penetrant and its vehicle (shaded) utilizing multiple data points obtained from IPPSF experiments (venous effluent profiles and tissue samples as seen in Figures 31.3 and 31.4) and parameters from parallel *in vitro* studies.

modeled) that vehicle effects the rate and extent of penetration of many compounds (Williams and Riviere, 1995). This approach allows one to take into account penetrating chemical or vehicle interactions with stratum corneum lipids (e.g. enhancers such as Azone®) which could alter permeability, to be directly incorporated into the analysis. The work has been extended to study the simultaneous absorption of multiple (>2) penetrants so that a mechanistic approach to assessing exposure to chemical mixtures may be developed (Riviere et al., 1995). This approach is now being applied to the complex absorption patterns seen in topical jet fuel exposure (Riviere et al., 1999). Finally, absorption of toxic compounds which may alter their own absorption secondary to cutaneous toxicity of the penetrant has been studied using the chemical vesicant sulfur mustard (Riviere et al., 1995). In this model, absorption profiles could only be precisely described if the vascular compartment was modulated as a function of sulfur mustard in the skin. This was independently correlated to vascular volume/permeability using inulin infusions to measure vascular space.

The major limitation to all pharmacokinetic approaches such as these relate to the large data requirements needed to solve model parameters. A full solution for a model such as presented in Figure 31.6 requires a series of replicated experiments using a single chemical applied at different doses and experiments terminated at various time points.

As mentioned above, in vitro studies would be conducted to obtain specific biophysical parameter estimates. All data is simultaneously analyzed. For many compounds, specific components of the full model may not be required and thus in reality, the actual model fitted is simpler. Statistical algorithms are presently being developed to select the optimum model for the specific compound being studied and collapse the remainder of the model structure into a matrix from which individual rate parameters cannot be extracted (Smith et al., 1995). This work has now resulted in the collapse of an equation that describes an IPPSF efflux profile to a three parameter equation: $Y(t) = A (e^{-bt} - e^{-dt})$ which adequately describes most IPPSF flux profiles (Riviere et al., 2001). This approach allows emphasis to be placed only on those compartments or processes which are important for the chemical being studied, yet retains the general structure of the model for all compounds so that future extrapolations are facilitated.

31.3.4 Cutaneous biotransformation

The final aspect of assessing percutaneous absorption which has not been considered up to this point is cutaneous biotransformation. The IPPSF is ideally suited for this purpose and has been used to study metabolism of pesticides, drugs and endogenous compounds (Bikle *et al.*, 1994; Carver *et al.*, 1990; Chang *et al.*, 1994; Riviere *et al.*, 1994, 1996). Specific pharmacokinetic models which incorporate IPPSF data and *in vivo* disposition have been constructed (Qiao *et al.*, 1994; Qiao and Riviere, 1995). These studies demonstrate a number of important features of percutaneous absorption of chemicals which are bio-transformed during passage through the skin. The method of dose application significantly affects the metabolic profile observed in the venous efflux. Occlusion enhances the fraction of parathion metabolized to para-nitrophenol both in the IPPSF and the *in vivo* pig. The mechanism of this effect has not been determined, although it illustrates the inherent complexity of skin relative to assessing the fate of chemicals applied on its surface. By constructing dermato-pharmacokinetic models to address these phenomena, quantitative parameters describing absorption and cutaneous distribution independent of biotrans-formation may be used as experimental endpoints.

The primary implication of biotransformation to risk assessment is that the *in vitro* to *in vivo* extrapolation strategy outlined in Figure 31.6 is actually oversimplified since it assumes all inputs from the skin to the general circulation are in the form of parent chemical. In reality, multiple inputs from the skin to systemic circulation are required making the extrapolation process more complex. *In vivo* work requires that studies be done both intravenously and topically so that systemic and cutaneous metabolism may be separated. Dosing methods must also be assessed if effects such as occlusion are to be quantitated.

31.3.5 Percutaneous absorption of vasoactive chemicals

One of the major advantages of using an isolated perfused tissue preparation is the presence of an intact vascular system with dermal microcirculation. This is important from the perspective of assessing the effect of altered blood flow on compound disposition as well as determining how a penetrating chemical's inherent vasoactivity affects its own fate. Unlike other organ systems, the range of blood flow possible through mammalian skin is tremendous because of its role in thermoregulation. The primary impact of altered dermal perfusion on the disposition of penetrated chemical may be on the surface area of the exchanging capillaries being perfused which determines the actual volume of dermis which is perfused and thus is available for systemic absorption (Riviere and Williams, 1992; Williams and Riviere, 1995). Alternatively, changes in dermal perfusion resulting from modulation of arterial-venous shunt activity may completely bypass areas of skin or result in deeper dermal penetration, a phenomenon observed *in vivo* with piroxicam (Monteiro-Riviere *et al.*, 1993b). Changes in dermal perfusion may be initiated by physiological homeostatic mechanisms, by exposure to vasoactive drugs or secondarily by chemical-induced irritation with concomitant release of vasoactive inflammatory mediators (e.g. prostaglandins). Using glucose utilization as a measurement of exchanging capillary perfusion, we have recently begun to map out the IPPSF vascular response to the infusion of vasoactive drugs in an attempt to experimentally define the pharmacodynamics of vasoactive drugs in this system for future integration into a comprehensive pharmacokinetic-pharmacodynamic model (Rogers and Riviere, 1994).

The impact of a drug's vasoactivity on its rate and extent of percutaneous absorption and distribution within skin can best be illustrated with IPPSF studies on the iontophoretic transdermal delivery of lidocaine co-administered with the vasodilator tolazoline or the vasoconstrictor norepinephrine (Riviere *et al.*, 1991; Riviere *et al.*, 1992a). Co-iontophoresis of both these compounds using *in vitro* diffusion cell systems resulted in essentially no effect on lidocaine flux. However, identical *in vivo* dosing conditions resulted in increased blood concentrations when tolazoline was present. As can be seen in Figure 31.7, tolazoline enhanced and norepinephrine decreased lidocaine flux in IPPSF studies. When one examined the concentrations in the skin underlying these electrodes, the opposite pattern was seen. These vascular effects have now been incorporated into our dermatopharmacokinetic model (Williams and Riviere, 1993). These studies clearly demonstrate the importance of the microcirculation on determining the non-steady state profile of drug delivery and dermal disposition.

31.4 DISCUSSION

The above presentation should have provided the reader with an overview of the uses of a perfused skin model such as the IPPSF in percutaneous absorption and dermatotoxicokinetic studies. One of its major advantages is that both absorption and toxicity may be assessed in the same preparation. The pharmacokinetic models developed are experimentally verifiable. The major limitations are centered on the cost of the preparation and the technical expertise required to successfully conduct the studies. The overall cost is significantly greater than *in vitro* diffusion cell studies or *in vivo* rodent experiments, comparable to human skin equivalent and larger mammal (dog, pig, primate) *in vivo* work and much less expensive than human trials. However, cost alone is not a sufficient

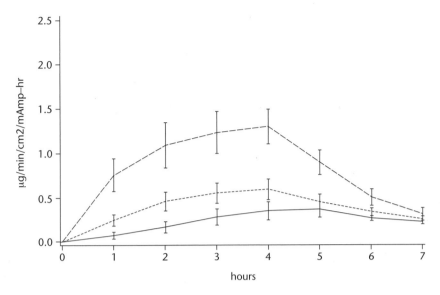

Figure 31.7: IPPSF venous efflux profile of iontophoretically delivered lidocaine (---) demonstrating vascular effect with enhanced delivery after tolazoline (——) and reduced delivery after norepinephrine (—) coadministration.

criterion. These studies are humane; and more information may be gathered than is obtainable with either *in vitro* or *in vivo* work. Optimal benefit may be achieved if these studies serve as a bridge between *in vitro* human/animal and *in vivo* animal work and the ultimate *in vivo* human exposure scenario.

31.4.1 Integrated approach to dermal risk assessment using a dermatopharmacokinetic template

The optimal method to assess all of the aforementioned complex events is to use a hierarchy of experimental model systems ranging from *in vitro* diffusion cells for animals and humans to perfused skin studies such as the IPPSF to *in vivo* animal and human studies. By designing such experiments using a comprehensive dermatopharmacokinetic model as a template, the limitations of each system may be delineated and a complete understanding of the rate limiting steps in the process defined. For example, there is general consensus that the major biological differences between humans and other species in regard to a chemical's percutaneous absorption is the nature of the stratum corneum lipids and patterns of biotransformation. As others have documented, the lipids of the stratum corneum of the pig are very similar to man and may be the primary reason that with *in vivo* comparisons, pigs and humans are often very similar. Such data is often not available relative to biotransformation. However, patterns of biotransformation may be determined from *in vitro* human diffusion cell or skin-equivalent studies and can be directly compared to *in vitro* pig data collected under identical conditions. Any differences observed may then be incorporated into the dermatopharmacokinetic model. The limitations to solely rely on the *in vitro* human data relate to the lack of proper anatomical orientation and lack of microcirculation which could alter the rate of parent chemical and metabolite penetration and thus pattern of biotransformation.

Any prediction errors purely inherent to the *in vitro* to *in vivo* extrapolation may be studied directly in the pig and a correction vector incorporated into the kinetic template. With these limitations defined, reasonable extrapolations to humans may then be made. Importantly, physiological or pathological processes which have been theoretically or experimentally shown to be important in either *in vitro* human or *in vivo* animal studies may be simulated. Using this approach, these hypotheses may then be tested in a reduced number of human clinical studies. More importantly, for many extremely toxic chemicals, human studies are never possible due to ethical limitations. This makes the pharmacokinetic approach, capable of synthesizing and integrating data from many levels of experimentation, an optimal strategy for human risk assessment. The same holds for drugs in very early stages of preclinical development.

In conclusion, the IPPSF appears to be a useful humane experimental model system for assessing both a chemical's percutaneous absorption profile and dermatotoxic potential. The IPPSF's greatest strength is the ability to experimentally characterize both phenomena simultaneously. By utilizing a fixed template to guide experimental design, one is assured that maximum information may be obtained from each individual study while maintaining the ability to extrapolate across chemicals.

REFERENCES

BEHRENDT, H. and KAMPFFMEYER, H.G. (1989) Absorption and ester cleavage or methyl salicylate by skin of single-pass perfused rabbit ears. *Xenobiotica* **19**, 131–141.

BIKLE, D.D., HALLORAN, B.P. and RIVIERE, J.E. (1994) Production of 1,25 dihydroxyvitamine D$_3$ by perfused pig skin. *J. Invest. Dermatol.* **102**, 796–798.

BOWMAN, K.F., MONTEIRO-RIVIERE, N.A. and RIVIERE, J.E. (1991) Development of surgical techniques for preparation of *in vitro* isolated perfused porcine skin flaps for percutaneous absorption studies. *Am. J. Vet. Res.* **25**, 75–82.

BRISTOL, D.G., RIVIERE, J.E., MONTEIRO-RIVIERE, N.A., BOWMAN, K.F. and ROGERS, R.A. (1991) The isolated perfused equine skin flap: Preparation and metabolic parameters. *Vet. Surg.* **20**, 424–433.

CARVER, M.P., WILLIAMS, P.L. and RIVIERE, J.E. (1989) The isolated perfused porcine skin flap (IPPSF). III. Percutaneous absorption pharmacokinetics of organophosphates, steroids, benzoic acid and caffeine. *Toxicol. Appl. Pharmacol.* **97**, 324–337.

CARVER, M.P., LEVI, P.E. and RIVIERE, J.E. (1990) Parathion metabolism during percutaneous absorption in perfused porcine skin. *Pest. Biochem. Physiol.* **38**, 245–254.

CELESTI, L., MURRATZU, C., VALOTI, M., SGARAGLI, G. and CORTI, P. (1993) The single-pass perfused rabbit ear as a model for studying percutaneous absorption of clonazepam, *Meth. Find. Exp. Vlin. Pharmacol.* **15**, 49–56.

CHANG, S.K., WILLIAMS, P.L., DAUTERMAN, W.C. and RIVIERE, J.E. (1994) Percutaneous absorption, dermatopharmacokinetics, and related biotransformation studies of carbaryl, lindane, malathion and parathion in isolated perfused porcine skin. *Toxicology* **91**, 269–280.

FELDBERG, W. and PATON, W.D.M. (1951) Release of histamine from skin and muscle in the cat by opium alkaloids and other histamine liberators. *J. Physiol.* **114**, 490–509.

HEIT, M., WILLIAMS, P., JAYES, F.L., CHANG, S.K. and RIVIERE, J.E. (1993) Transdermal iontophoretic peptide delivery. *In vitro* and *In vivo* studies with luteinizing hormone releasing hormone (LHRH). *J. Pharm. Sci.* **82**, 240–243.

HIERNICKEL, H. (1985) An improved method for *in vitro* perfusion of human skin. *Br. J. Dermatol.* **112**, 299–305.

KIETZMANN, M., ARENS, D., LOSCHER, W. and LUBACH, D. (1991) Studies on the percutaneous absorption of dexamethasone using a new *in vitro* model, the isolated perfused bovine udder, In: SCOTT, R.C., GUY, R.H., HADGRAFT, J. and BODEE, H.E. (eds) *Prediction of Percutaneous Penetration*, London: IBC Technical Services, Ltd, 519–526.

KING, J.R. and MONTEIRO-RIVIERE, N.A. (1990) Cutaneous toxicity of 2-chloroethyl methyl sulfide in isolated perfused porcine skin. *Toxicol. Appl. Pharmacol.* **104**, 167–179.

CHAPTER 31

KING, J.R., RIVIERE, J.E. and MONTEIRO-RIVIERE, N.A. (1992) Characterization of lewisite toxicity in isolated perfused skin. *Toxicol. Appl. Pharmacol.* **116**, 189–201.

KING, J.R., PETERS, B.P. and MONTEIRO-RIVIERE, N.A. (1994) Matrix molecules of the epidermal basement membrane as targets for chemical vesication with lewisite. *Toxicol. Appl. Pharmacol.* **126**, 164–173.

KJAERSGAARD, A.R. (1954) Perfusion of isolated dog skin. *J. Invest. Dermatol.* **22**, 135–141.

KREUGER, G.G., WOJCIECHOWSKI, Z.J., BURTON, S.A., GILHAR, A., HUETHER, S.E., LEONARD, L.G., ROHR, U.D., PETELENZ, T.J., HIGUCHI, W.I. and PERSHING, L.K. (1985) The development of a rat/human skin flap served by a defined and accessible vasculature on a congenitally athymic (Nude) rat. *Fundam. Appl. Toxicol.* **5**, S112-S121.

KREIDSTEIN, M.L., PANG, C.Y., LEVINE, R.H. and KNOWLTON, R.J. (1991) The isolated perfused human skin flap: Design, perfusion technique, metabolism and vascular reactivity. *Plas. Reconstr. Surg.* **87**, 741–749.

DE LANGE, J., VAN ECK, P., ELLIOTT, G.R., DE KORT, W.L.A.M. and WOLTHIUS, O.L. (1992) The isolated blood-perfused pig ear: An inexpensive and animal saving model for skin penetration studies. *J. Pharmacol. Toxicol. Meth.* **27**, 71–77.

MONTEIRO-RIVIERE, N.A. (1990) Altered epidermal morphology secondary to lidocaine iontophoresis: *In vivo* and *In Vitro* studies in porcine skin. *Fundam. Appl. Toxicol.* **15**, 174–185.

MONTEIRO-RIVIERE, N.A. (1992) Use of isolated perfused skin model in dermatotoxicology. *In Vitro Toxicol.* **5**, 219–233.

MONTEIRO-RIVIERE, N.A. and INMAN, A.O. (1995) Indirect immunohisto-chemistry and immunoelectron microscopy distribution of eight epidermal-dermal junction epitopes in the pig and in isolated perfused skin treated with bis (2-chloroethyl) sulfide. *Toxicol. Pathol.* **23**, 313–325.

MONTEIRO-RIVIERE, N.A., BOWMAN, K.F., SCHEIDT, V.J. and RIVIERE, J.E. (1987) The isolated perfused porcine skin flap (IPPSF): II. Ultrastructural and histological characterization of epidermal viability. *In Vitro Toxicol.* **1**, 241–252.

MONTEIRO-RIVIERE, N.A., BRISTOL, D.G., MANNING, T.O., ROGERS, R.A. and RIVIERE, J.E. (1990) Interspecies and interregional analysis of the comparative histological thickness and laser Doppler blood flow measurements at five cutaneous sites in nine species. *J. Invest. Dermatol.* **95**, 582–586.

MONTEIRO-RIVIERE, N.A., STINSON, A.W. and CALHOUN, H.L. (1993a) Integument. In: DELLMANN, H.D. (ed) *Textbook of Veterinary Histology*, 4th Ed., Philadelphia: Lea and Febiger, 285–312.

MONTEIRO-RIVIERE, N.A., INMAN, A.O., RIVIERE, J.E., MCNEILL, and FRANCOEUR, M.L. (1993b) Topical penetration of piroxicam is dependent on the distribution of the local cutaneous vasculature. *Pharm. Res.* 10, 1326–1331.

MONTEIRO-RIVIERE, N.A., INMAN, A.O. and RIVIERE, J.E. (1994a) Identification of the pathway of iontophoretic drug delivery: Light and ultrastructural studies using mercuric chloride in pigs. *Pharm. Res.* 11, 251–256.

MONTEIRO-RIVIERE, N.A., INMAN, A.O. and RIVIERE, J.E. (1994b) Development and characterization of a novel skin model for phototoxicology. *Photodermatol, Photoimmunol. Photomed,* 10, 235–243.

MONTEIRO-RIVIERE, N.A., INMAN, A.O. and RIVIERE, J.E. (2001) The effects of short term high dose and low dose dermal exposure to jet A, JP-8, and JP-8 +100 jet fuels. *J. Appl. Toxicol.* 21, 485–494.

MONTEIRO-RIVIERE, N.A., BAYNES, R.E. and RIVIERE, J.E. (2003) Pyridostigmine bromide modulates topical irritant-induced cytokine release from human epidermal keratinocytes and isolated perfused porcine skin. *Toxicology* 183, 15–28.

QIAO, G.L. and RIVIERE, J.E. (1995) Significant effects of application site and occlusion on the pharmacokinetics of cutaneous penetration and biotransformation of parathion In Vivo in swine. *J. Pharm. Sci.* 84, 425–432.

QIAO, G.L. and RIVIERE, J.E. (2000) Dermal absorption and tissue disposition of 3,3',4,4'-tetrachlorobiphenyl (TCB) in an *ex vivo* pig model: Assessing the impact of dermal exposure variables. *Int. J. Occup. Environ. Health* 6, 127–137.

QIAO, G.L., WILLIAMS, P.L. and RIVIERE, J.E. (1994) Percutaneous absorption, biotransformation and systemic disposition of parathion *in vivo* in swine. I. Comprehensive pharmacokinetic model. *Drug Metab. Dispos.* 22, 459–471.

RHYNE, B.N., PIRONE, J.P., RIVIERE, J.E. and MONTEIRO-RIVIERE, N.A. (2002) The use of enzyme histochemistry in detecting cutaneous toxicity of three topically applied jet fuel mixtures. *Toxicol. Mechanisms Methods* 12, 17–34.

RIVIERE, J.E. and MONTEIRO-RIVIERE, N.A. (1991) The isolated perfused porcine skin flap as an *in vitro* model for percutaneous absorption and cutaneous toxicology. *Critical Reviews in Toxicol.* 21, 329–344.

RIVIERE, J.E. and WILLIAMS, P.L. (1992) Pharmacokinetic implications of changing blood flow in skin. *J. Pharm. Sci.* 81, 601–602.

CHAPTER 31

RIVIERE, J.E., BOWMAN, K.F., MONTEIRO-RIVIERE, N.A., CARVER, M.P. and DIX, L.P. (1986) The isolated perfused porcine skin flap (IPPSF). I. A novel *in vitro* model for percutaneous absorption and cutaneous toxicology studies. *Fundam. Appl. Toxicol.* **7**, 444–453.

RIVIERE, J.E., SAGE, B.S. and WILLIAMS, P.L. (1991) The effects of vasoactive drugs on transdermal lidocaine iontophoresis. *J. Pharm. Sci.* **80**, 615–620.

RIVIERE, J.E., MONTEIRO-RIVIERE, N.A. and INMAN, A.O. (1992a) Determination of lidocaine concentration in skin after transdermal iontophoresis: Effects of vasoactive drugs. *Pharm. Res.* **9**, 211–214.

RIVIERE, J.E., WILLIAMS, P.L., HILLMAN, R. and MISHKY, L. (1992b) Quantitative prediction of transdermal iontophoretic delivery of arbutamine in humans using the *in vitro* isolated perfused porcine skin flap (IPPSF). *J. Pharm. Sci.* **81**, 504–507.

RIVIERE, J.E., BROOKS, J.D., WILLIAMS, P.L. and MONTEIRO-RIVIERE, N.A. (1995a) Toxicokinetics of topical sulfur-mustard penetration, disposition and vascular toxicity in isolated perfused porcine skin. *Toxicol. Appl. Pharmacol.* **135**, 25–34.

RIVIERE, J.E., MONTEIRO-RIVIERE, N.A., ROGERS, R.A., BOMMANNAN, D., TAMADA, J.A. and POTTS, R.O. (1995b) Pulsatile transdermal delivery of LHRH using electroporation. Drug delivery and skin toxicology. *J. Contr. Release* **36**, 229–233.

RIVIERE, J.E., WILLIAMS, P.L. and MONTEIRO-RIVIERE, N.A. (1995c) Mechanistically defined chemical mixtures (MDCM): A new experimental paradigm for risk assessment applied to skin. *Toxicologist* **15**, 323–324.

RIVIERE, J.E., BROOKS, J.D., WILLIAMS, P.L., McGOWAN, E. and FRANCOEUR, M.L. (1996) Cutaneous metabolism of isosorbide dinitrate after transdermal administration in isolated perfused porcine skin. *Int. J. Pharm.* **127**, 213–217.

RIVIERE, J.E., MONTEIRO-RIVIERE, N.A., BROOKS, J.D., BUDSABA, K. and SMITH, C.E. (1999) Dermal absorption and distribution of topically dosed jet fuels Jet A, JP-8, and JP-8(100). *Toxicol. Appl. Pharmacol.* **160**, 60–75.

RIVIERE, J.E., BROOKS, J.D. and QIAO, G.L. (2000) Methods for assessing the percutaneous absorption of volatile chemicals in isolated perfused skin: Studies with chloropentafluorobenzene (CPFB) and dichlorobenzene (DCB). *Toxicol. Methods* **10**, 265–281.

RIVIERE, J.E., SMITH, C.E., BUDSABA, K., BROOKS, J.D., OLAJOS, E.J., SALEM, H. and MONTEIRO-RIVIERE, N.A. (2001) Use of methyl salicylate as a simulant to predict the percutaneous absorption of sulfur mustard. *J. Applied Toxicology* **21**, 91–99.

ROGERS, R.A. and RIVIERE, J.E. (1994) Pharmacologic modulation of cutaneous vascular resistance in the isolated perfused porcine skin flap (IPPSF). *J. Pharm. Sci.* **83**, 1682–1689.

SMITH, C.E., WILLIAMS, P.L. and RIVIERE, J.E. (1995) Compartment model of skin transport. A dominant eigenvalue approach. *Proc. Biometrics Sec. Am. Stat. Assoc.* Washington DC, 449–454.

SRIKRISHNA,V., RIVIERE, J.E. and MONTEIRO-RIVIERE, N.A. (1992) Cutaneous toxicity and absorption of paraquat in porcine skin. *Toxicol. Appl. Pharmacol.* **115**, 89–97.

VADEN, S.L., PAGE, R.L., PETERS, B.P., CLINE, J.M. and RIVIERE, J.E. (1993) Development and characterization of an isolated and perfused tumor and skin preparation for evaluation of drug disposition. *Cancer Research* **53**, 101–105.

WESTER, R.C., MELENDRES, J., SEDIK, L., MAIBACH, H.I. and RIVIERE, J.E. (1998) Percutaneous absorption of salicylic acid, theophylline, 2,4-dimethylamine, diethyl hexylphthalic acid and ρ-aminobenzoic acid in the isolated perfused porcine skin flap compared to man. *Toxicol. Appl. Pharmacol.* **151**, 159–165.

WILLIAMS, P.L. and RIVIERE, J.E. (1989a) Definition of a physiologic pharmacokinetic model of cutaneous drug distribution using the isolated perfused porcine skin flap (IPPSF). *J. Pharm. Sci.* **78**, 550–555.

WILLIAMS, P.L. and RIVIERE, J.E. (1989b) Estimation of physiological volumes in the isolated perfused porcine skin flap. *Res. Commun. Chem. Pathol. Pharmacol.* **66**, 145–158.

WILLIAMS, P.L. and RIVIERE, J.E. (1993) A model describing transdermal iontophoretic delivery of lidocaine incorporating consideration of cutaneous microvascular state. *J. Pharm. Sci.* **82**, 1080–1084.

WILLIAMS, P.L. and RIVIERE, J.E. (1994) A "full-space" method for predicting *in vivo* transdermal plasma drug profiles reflecting both cutaneous and systemic variability. *J. Pharm. Sci.* **83**, 1062–1064.

WILLIAMS, P.L. and RIVIERE, J.E. (1995) A biophysically-based dermatopharmacokinetic compartment model for quantifying percutaneous penetration and absorption of topically applied agents. I. Theory. *J. Pharm. Sci.* **84**, 599–608.

WILLIAMS, P.L., CARVER, M.P. and RIVIERE, J.E. (1990) A physiologically relevant pharmacokinetic model of xenobiotic percutaneous absorption utilizing the isolated perfused porcine skin flap (IPPSF). *J. Pharm. Sci.* **79**, 305–311.

CHAPTER 31

WILLIAMS, P.L., BROOKS, J.D., INMAN, A.I., MONTEIRO-RIVIERE, N.A. and RIVIERE, J.E. (1994) Determination of physiochemical properties of phenol, par anitrophenol, acetone and ethanol relevant to quantitating their percutaneous absorption in porcine skin. *Res. Commun. Chem. Pathol. Pharmacol.* **83**, 61–75.

ZHANG, A., RIVIERE, J.E. and MONTEIRO-RIVIERE, N.A. (1995a) Evaluation of protective effects of sodium thiosulfate, cysteine, niacinamide and indomethacin on sulfur mustard-treated isolated perfused porcine skin. *Chem.-Biol. Interact.* **96**, 249–262.

ZHANG, A., RIVIERE, J.E. and MONTEIRO-RIVIERE, N.A. (1995b) Topical sulfur mustard induces changes in prostaglandins and interleukin 1α in isolated perfused porcine skin. *In Vitro Toxicol.* **8**, 149–157.

ZHANG, A., PETERS B.P. and MONTEIRO-RIVIERE, N.A. (1995c) Assessment of sulfur mustard interaction with basement membrane components. *Cell Biol. Toxicol.* **11**, 89–101.

Physiologically Based Pharmacokinetic Modeling

32

JAMES N MCDOUGAL*

Contents

32.1   Introduction

32.2   Why use PB-PK models?

32.3   When can PB-PK models be used?

32.4   What are the components of a PB-PK model?

32.5   How do you develop PB-PK models?

32.6   Conclusion

32.7   Nomenclature

* The author gratefully acknowledges the support of the Air Force Office of Scientific Research and the National Institute of Occupational Safety and Health.

32.1   INTRODUCTION

Understanding and quantifying the penetration of chemicals into and through the skin is important in both pharmacology and toxicology. In nearly every case, the species of interest is the human species, although laboratory animals are often used as surrogates, particularly in the case of toxicological studies. Appropriate use of laboratory animals necessitates understanding differences between species so that the process of extrapolation to humans is meaningful. This is vital for *in vivo* animal studies, which are often more complex than *in vitro* animal studies. *In vivo* studies have the advantage of intact skin that has blood flow, is alive and is responsive. Metabolism, nervous and humoral responses are also present and therefore living skin more accurately reflects human exposure scenarios. Traditionally, the analysis of *in vivo* skin penetration in laboratory animals has involved estimation of the amount of chemical that has penetrated using either blood concentrations or the amount of chemical excreted after a dermal exposure. These methods are descriptive; applicability of the results is limited by the appropriateness of the specific experimental design and the similarities between the laboratory species chosen and humans.

Due to the increase in the availability of computer hardware and software over the last two decades, methods that are based on physiological and pharmacokinetic principles are now feasible alternatives for analysis of *in vivo* skin penetration. These physiologically-based pharmacokinetic (PB-PK) approaches mathematically describe the dynamics of chemicals in the body in terms of rates of blood flow, permeability of membranes and partitioning of chemicals into tissues. Characterizing absorption in terms of parameters, which are measurable and species specific, facilitates extrapolations to the real species of interest, providing these parameters are known or can be determined for humans. This chapter describes physiologically-based pharmacokinetic models, their use as a tool to quantify and understand the process of dermal absorption and penetration, and their suitability for dose, route and species extrapolation.

32.2   WHY USE PB-PK MODELS?

One of the big advantages of dermal PB-PK models over traditional *in vivo* methods is the ability to accurately describe non-linear biochemical and physical processes. Describing skin penetration based on blood concentrations or excretion rates, as "percent absorbed," assumes all processes have a simple linear relationship with the exposure concentration. When non-linear processes occur in the absorption, distribution, metabolism or elimination of a chemical, describing penetration as "percent absorbed" does not provide information that can be applied to situations other than the experimental situation. Skin penetration may not be linear when there is binding or metabolism in the skin or when skin blood flow is a limiting factor. Many biochemical processes in the body are non-linear, for example the percent of chemical metabolized per hour at a low liver concentration may be much greater than the percent metabolized per hour at a high liver concentration. A quantitative description of saturable kinetics in the model may allow it to be predictive of blood or tissue concentrations from various doses. A complete mathematical description of dermal pharmacokinetics takes mass balance throughout the animal into account, and makes it possible to estimate fluxes (amount/time) and permeability constants (distance/time). These expressions of the penetration process are required to accurately predict penetration in other situations (that is, different exposure area, time or concentration) when nonlinear processes are present.

A properly validated PB-PK description of the skin will provide more information from each experiment than is possible without it. For example, if it is the chemical concentration in an organ or tissue that is important, by understanding the quantitative relationship between blood concentrations and tissue concentrations, serial blood sampling may provide the estimate of the tissue dose that is required without the need for an invasive procedure to sample tissue concentrations. Another good example would be the estimation of rate of metabolism in the skin. Proper comparison of a PB-PK description of metabolite production after an intravenous infusion with the rates of metabolite production after application to the skin at several concentrations allows the metabolic parameters in the skin to be estimated.

In this age of increased concern over the use of animals in research, it is important to try to reduce animal use and get the most information from each animal that must be used. Before any experimentation, PB-PK models can often be used to form predictions that will help in designing experimental doses and sampling times, thus avoiding "range finding" experiments. During the experiment, PB-PK descriptions may allow the use of fewer animals because it may not be necessary to sacrifice animals at various time points to get tissue concentrations. After the study is complete, PB-PK models allow one to extrapolate results to other exposure areas, times or concentrations, possibly eliminating the need to repeat an experiment under different conditions.

Another important reason for using physiologically-based pharmacokinetic modeling of skin penetration is to acquire the experience necessary to extrapolate to other species. Classical pharmacokinetic modeling assumes that the body can be adequately described by one to three compartments based on the shape of the semilogarithmic plot of plasma concentration versus time (Gibaldi and Perrier, 1982). The most common classical description is a two compartment linear system where one compartment is the plasma and the other all remaining body water and tissues. Using this type of model, the plasma concentration curve can be fit by a distributive phase (a) and a post-distributive phase (b). This type of model is useful in clinical situations for determining dose or dose regimen. Classical modeling has occasionally been used in skin penetration studies (Cooper, 1976; Wallace and Barnett, 1978; Peck *et al.*, 1981; Chandrasekaran *et al.*, 1978; Birmingham *et al.*, 1979; Guy *et al.*, 1982; Kubota and Ishizake, 1986).

Figure 32.1 is a schematic representation of the classical two compartment pharmacokinetic model having a body compartment connected with the plasma. The first order transfer rates (K_{12}, K_{21}, K_{10}) are descriptive of a particular situation (Gibaldi and Perrier, 1982) but do not allow extrapolation to other exposure conditions or species because their physiological basis is obscure. PB-PK models are better suited for extrapolation because their physiological basis is well defined. It has been shown that a PB-PK model for the inhalation of styrene in rats can be predictive of blood and exhaled air concentrations of styrene in humans after scaling-up the physiological and metabolic constants (Ramsey and Andersen, 1984). Extrapolation with a PB-PK model is only limited by the ability of the modeler to quantitatively describe the species differences in the pharmacokinetic and physiological processes involved.

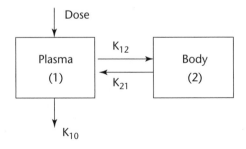

Figure 32.1: Classical pharmacokinetic model with two compartments and first order transfer and elimination rates.

32.3   WHEN CAN PB-PK MODELS BE USED?

PB-PK models can be used in nearly any *in vivo* experimental situation in which the physiological and pharmacokinetic processes can be described adequately for the purposes of the scientific question to be answered. It is often not necessary to have an exhaustive description of the animal to be studied—only the simplest description that "works." It is possible to imagine a PB-PK model that describes blood flow, partition coefficients and metabolic characteristics for each organ in a specific mammal, but a single scientific question that would require such an exaustive description could not be imagined! Normally it is sufficient to combine many organs into several lumped compartments that have similar blood flows and partition coefficients. The requirement for quantitative understanding of these conceptual processes is both the strong point and the Achilles heel of PB-PK modeling. Quantitative descriptions are the strong point because of their basis in underlying principles, but they are the weak point because of the level of understanding required is not easy to achieve. Often the initial description of a particular process is not adequate but through experimentation and more careful description, based on sound pharmacokinetic and physiological principles, the fundamental understanding of the processes involved can be increased.

32.4   WHAT ARE THE COMPONENTS OF A PB-PK MODEL?

Simply speaking, a mammalian organism is comprised of diverse, sometimes metabolically active, pools of fluid separated by membranes which prohibit, permit or promote passage of the fluids and/or their dissolved contents. These fluids and membranes obey and can therefore be described by the physical laws of fluid dynamics, transport and diffusion. Skin is one of the most important membranes because it separates and protects animals from their environment. The major fluids, which contribute 60 percent of body weight, are blood plasma, interstitial fluids and intracellular fluids. Plasma, the most important fluid because of its continuous motion, transports the red cells, white cells, platelets and soluble components in the blood. Interstitial fluid, which bathes cells with three times the volume of the plasma, is diffuse and separated from the plasma only by capillary walls. The comparatively static intracellular fluid is separated from the extracellular fluids by specialized cell membranes with sophisticated transport systems. The membranes in the tissues that keep these fluids organized are protein-lipid structures of varying thicknesses, which may contain alterable apertures and carry metabolic enzymes. With this uncomplicated description as a basis, most pharmacokinetic processes can be simplified and described in terms of flows, volumes, solubilities, diffusion and metabolic rates. When these physiological and biochemical processes can be quantified, a mathematical description can be constructed and compared with experiments to accurately describe the processes involved (see reviews by Himmelstein and Lutz, 1979; Lutz *et al.*, 1980; Gerlowski and Jain, 1983; Clewell and Andersen, 1989).

32.4.1 Tissue compartments

The building block of a PB-PK model is the compartment. A compartment is a collection of fluids or tissues and/or organs that are grouped together because of similar physiological and pharmacokinetic characteristics rather than anatomical considerations (Lutz *et al.*, 1980). Each lumped compartment receives inward flux of chemical in the blood flow, has a volume and may incorporate binding or loss of chemical through outward flux or metabolism. Subcompartments may be necessary to accurately describe barriers to movement or sequestration of chemical. Figure 32.2 illustrates a lumped compartment.

Even this level of complexity is not always necessary to adequately describe the processes that are occurring. The transport of chemical across the thin capillary wall may be so rapid that the plasma and interstitial fluid have equivalent concentrations and therefore it may be possible to combine the plasma and interstitial fluid subcompartments into one extracellular fluid subcompartment. Diffusion across cellular membranes into the intracellular

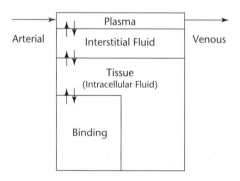

Figure 32.2: Diagrammatic description of a lumped compartment with three subcompartments and binding in the tissue subcompartment.

fluid may be so rapid that flow of the blood to the compartment is the rate limiting factor affecting uptake of a chemical and therefore it may be possible to avoid subcompartments completely. The free concentration of chemical in the plasma, interstitial fluid or intracellular fluid subcompartments will depend on whether binding or metabolism occurs in the subcompartment.

Penetration of the skin is a process that lends itself to PB-PK modeling. Compartments are chosen based on an understanding of the pharmacokinetics of the chemical and the purpose for the model. Figure 32.3 shows a model with five simple compartments that was designed for predicting blood concentrations from different exposure times and concentrations on the skin. Each compartment is assumed to be well-stirred, flow limited and has no subcompartments. Potential losses of chemical are evaporation from the skin, hepatic metabolism, and exhalation. The description is of the venous equilibration type, without blood volume being specified.

The skin compartment is discussed in detail in the next subsection. The rapidly perfused compartment lumps tissues with high blood flow, and high affinity for the chemical. It represents kidney, viscera, brain and other richly perfused organs. The slowly perfused compartment has low blood flow, low affinity for the chemical and represents muscle and other poorly perfused tissues and organs. The fat compartment has low blood flow, high affinity for the chemical and represents various types of fat. These characteristics are important

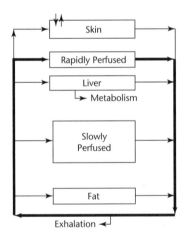

Figure 32.3: Diagrammatic representation of a PB-PK model with five simple compartments connected by blood flow. Compartment volumes and blood flows are approximately to scale.

criteria in choosing the compartments. According to this description, the sole route of entry for the chemical is the skin and elimination is by way of diffusion out of the skin followed by metabolism in the liver, and exhalation (if the chemical is volatile). Additional compartments would be required for a chemical which was eliminated in the kidney, or if concentration in a target organ (e.g. testis) is of particular interest.

32.4.2 Skin compartment

A skin compartment is just a special subset of tissue compartments that, because it is the defined portal of entry and has definable anatomy and physiology, needs to be further elaborated. Figure 32.4 illustrates a skin compartment that contains most of the anatomical detail that may be important in skin penetration (Bookout *et al.*, 1996, 1997). Most of this detail will not be necessary for any particular chemical, but is described here for completeness. Each subcompartment communicates in both directions with adjacent compartments and each has a concentration, volume and affinity for the chemical of interest. The surface subcompartment, although not strictly part of the skin, is crucial to making the PB-PK model functional. The surface area exposed, exposure concentration, amount applied to skin, and affinity of the chemical for the vehicle (if any) are all incorporated into this subcompartment. If evaporation is occurring or if the chemical is applied in a vehicle and the vehicle has a penetration rate of its own, terms characterizing these events must be incorporated into the description so the concentration in the surface subcompartment, which is the driving force for penetration, is accurately described.

The stratum corneum subcompartment represents the thin, densely packed, fully differentiated keratinocytes. This layer is the principal barrier to penetration for most chemicals due to the compactness of its lipid-protein matrix (Marzulli

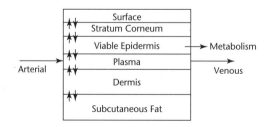

Figure 32.4: Diagrammatic representation of a skin compartment with six subcompartments and metabolism occurring in the viable epidermis.

■ CHAPTER 32 ■

and Tregear, 1961; Scheuplein, 1967; Mershon, 1975; Elias and Friend, 1975; Dugard and Scott, 1984). The stratum corneum has the potential to act as a reservoir for lipophilic chemicals and may provide binding sites. There is little, if any, metabolic activity and no active transport processes (Scheuplein, 1967) associated with this lifeless layer. In this description, the stratum corneum is treated as if it were homogeneous and well-stirred. This gross over-simplification will not apply for all chemicals. For other types of chemicals, it may be necessary to model the stratum corneum as the multilayered structure that it actually is (Blank and Scheuplein, 1964; Odland, 1983). Partial differential equations can be written to describe the skin if the concentration gradient within the skin is significant.

The viable epidermis subcompartment contains cells formed in the basal layer which become keratinized and more compact as they migrate toward the surface to form the stratum corneum. The majority of the metabolic activity of the skin is found in this layer and it may provide binding sites (Marzulli *et al.*, 1969; Pannatier *et al.*, 1978; Finnin and Schuster, 1985).

The plasma subcompartment in the skin provides blood flow to the dermis. Its vasculature is neurally regulated, provides nutrients and other essential chemicals to the skin and affords a means for dissipation of body heat from the extremities. Pharmacokinetically, the plasma subcompartment receives chemicals that penetrate the skin but it also receives chemicals from arterial blood. Chemicals leave the skin via the venous blood or by metabolism. In this simplified description, the plasma subcompartment is between the viable epidermis and the dermis when, in fact, it is imbedded in the papillary dermis (Braverman and Keh-Yen, 1983; Odland, 1983).

The dermis subcompartment provides structural support for the epidermal layers above. It consists of a thick fibrous matrix of elastin and collagen and is more porous than the other compartments. Chemicals may bind to these structural components as they transit through the skin. The collagen in the dermis constitutes approximately 77 percent of the dry mass of the skin (Odland, 1983). The upper part of the dermis contains capillaries that provide nutrients to the viable epidermis.

The subcutaneous fat subcompartment represents a layer of variable thickness, which is poorly perfused but may provide a reservoir for lipophilic chemicals. Because it is perfused, it could be an important compartment in its own right, even though it is below the level of the capillary beds.

Although the subcompartments make this skin compartment fairly complex for modeling purposes, it is still an obvious oversimplification of the actual intricacy of mammalian skin. Notably missing are appendages (sweat glands, hair follicles, and sebaceous glands) which have been suggested to be contributing pathways for absorption at early times with slowly diffusing electrically charged chemicals (Scheuplein, 1967; Mershon, 1975). Bookout and collaborators (1997) have described physiologically based modeling of appendages.

32.4.3 Flux equations

Flux equations are the key to an appropriate model (see Flynn *et al.*, 1974, for an excellent review of mass transport). The rate of change of amount (expressed as a product of volume and concentration) in a subcompartment at any time is a balance between inward flux and outward flux:

$$V \frac{dC}{dt} = Influx_{total} - Efflux_{total} \tag{32.1}$$

where V is the volume, C is the free concentration (mass/volume), and *Influx* and *Efflux* are sums of the fluxes (mass/time) in each direction (equations (32.2)–(32.4)). The general form for the equation describing unidirectional flux where transportation of a chemical is occurring because of bulk flow of the medium is:

$$Flux = QC \tag{32.2}$$

where Q is flow (volume/time) of the medium.

When the membrane between subcompartments (e.g. capillary or cell membrane) acts as a barrier to simple diffusion or when adjacent compartments such as the viable epidermis and dermis in Figure 32.4 act like there is a membrane between them, the flux from outside to inside is described by the permeability-area product and the concentration difference across the membrane:

$$Flux = PA(C_{out} - C_{in}) \tag{32.3}$$

where P is permeability (distance/time), A is area (distance^2), and C_{out}, C_{in} are the free concentrations at the outer and inner surfaces of the membrane. The thermodynamic activity differential actually drives the transport process and, if the chemicals across the barrier are in different media, it is the effective concentration at the interface that must be used in the calculation. Therefore, the concentration must be adjusted for partitioning between the media.

In some cases, movement across a barrier between subcompartments may not be by simple diffusion. If there is a saturable, active process involved, the description for flux is often represented by:

$$Flux = \frac{kVC}{K_T + C} \tag{32.4}$$

where k is the maximum transport rate (mass/volume $\times$ time), and K_T is the Michaelis-like constant (mass/volume).

32.4.3 Binding, metabolism and excretion

The free concentration of chemical in a subcompartment can also be reduced by binding to proteins or cellular macromolecules, by several types of metabolic processes and by excretion (Lutz et al., 1980; Gerlowski and Jain, 1983). Normally, these processes are either first-order, saturable or some combination of the two. If the process is first-order, the general equation is:

$$Loss = rCV \tag{32.5}$$

where Loss has the same units as Flux (mass/time) and r is a proportionality constant (time^{-1}). This description of loss will have the same form regardless of whether the first-order loss is due to irreversible binding, metabolism or excretion.

When the binding, metabolism or excretion is saturable, the loss can be described by an equation of the same form as equation (32.4) (Lutz et al., 1980; Gerlowski and Jain, 1983). The equation for saturable metabolism is:

$$Loss = \frac{V_{max}C}{K_m + C} \tag{32.6}$$

where V_{max} is the maximum reaction velocity (mass/time) and K_m is the Michaelis Constant.

32.4.4 Mass balance equations

Each lumped compartment

In general, for each subcompartment in Figure 32.2 a differential equation in the form of equation (32.1) can be constructed. Equations (32.7)–(32.9) are for plasma, interstitial fluid and intercellular fluid in tissues, respectively:

$$V_p \frac{dC_p}{dt} = Q_t(C_a - C_v) + P_{is}A_{is}\left(\frac{C_{is}}{R_{is/p}} - C_p\right)$$ (32.7)

$$V_{is}\frac{dC_{is}}{dt} = P_{is}A_{is}\left(C_p - \frac{C_{is}}{R_{is/p}}\right) + P_tA_t\left(\frac{C_t}{R_{t/is}} - C_{is}\right)$$ (32.8)

$$V_t\frac{dC_t}{dt} = P_tA_t\left(C_{is} - \frac{C_t}{R_{t/is}}\right) - rC_tV_t$$ (32.9)

where subscripts p, is and t refer to the plasma, interstitial and tissue (intercellular fluid) subcompartments, respectively (see Nomenclature). C_a is concentration in the arterial blood, C_v is the concentration in venous blood, and R is the partition coefficient between the media indicated by its subscripts. The concentration in the lumped compartment is the volume average of the concentration of the subcompartments:

$$C_i = \frac{C_pV_p + C_{is}V_{is} + C_tV_t}{V_p + V_{is} + V_t}$$ (32.10)

Each of the compartments in the general model shown in Figure 32.3 could require treatment as a diffusion limited lumped compartment as described above; however, the simplification shown in equation (32.18) will adequately describe the pharmacokinetic behavior of many lipid soluble organic chemicals.

Skin compartment

For skin subcompartments in Figure 32.4, equations (32.11)–(32.17) account for mass fluxes within each subcompartment:

$$V_{sfc}\frac{dC_{sfc}}{dt} = P_{sc}A_{sc}\left(\frac{C_{sc}}{R_{sc/sfc}} - C_{sfc}\right)$$ (32.11)

$$V_{sc}\frac{dC_{sc}}{dt} = P_{sc}A_{sc}\left(C_{sfc} - \frac{C_{sc}}{R_{sc/sfc}}\right) + P_{ve}A_{ve}\left(\frac{C_{ve}}{R_{ve/sc}} - C_{sc}\right)$$ (32.12)

$$V_{ve}\frac{dC_{ve}}{dt} = P_{ve}A_{ve}\left(C_{sc} - \frac{C_{ve}}{R_{ve/sc}}\right) + P_pA_p\left(\frac{C_p}{R_{p/ve}} - C_{ve}\right) - \frac{V_{max}C_{ve}}{K_m + C_{ve}}$$ (32.13)

$$V_d \frac{dC_p}{dt} = Q_{sk}\left(C_a - C_v\right) + P_p A_p \left(C_{ve} - \frac{C_p}{R_{p/ve}}\right) + P_d A_d \left(\frac{C_d}{R_{d/p}} - C_p\right) \tag{32.14}$$

$$V_p \frac{dC_d}{dt} = P_d A_d \left(C_p - \frac{C_d}{R_{d/p}}\right) + P_{sf} A_{sf} \left(\frac{C_{sf}}{R_{sf/p}} - C_d\right) \tag{32.15}$$

$$V_{sf} \frac{dC_{sf}}{dt} = P_{sf} A_{sf} \left(C_d - \frac{C_{sf}}{R_{sf/d}}\right) \tag{32.16}$$

where the subscripts *sfc, sc, ve, d, p, sf* and *sk* stand for surface, stratum corneum, viable epidermis, dermis, plasma, subcutaneous fat and skin, respectively. The concentration in the skin as a whole is the volume average of the concentration of the subcompartments:

$$C_{sk} = \frac{C_{sc} V_{sc} + C_{ve} V_{ve} + C_p V_p + C_d V_d + C_{sf} V_{sf}}{V_{sc} + V_{ve} + V_p + V_d + V_{sf}} \tag{32.17}$$

It must be emphasized that these are theoretical descriptions of the process of skin penetration. These compartments have been chosen based on the current understanding of what may be the most important structural components involved. Exploration and understanding of these concepts will determine which are important subcompartments for each specific chemical to be studied.

Simplifying assumptions

For completeness, the hypothetical compartments in Figures 32.3 and 32.4 have been relatively rigorously described using the PB-PK approach to diffusion limitation in each subcompartment; however, until methods are developed to measure the permeability-area products (*PA*) for the subcompartment interfaces, many simplifications must be made to make the description useful for extrapolation. One simplifying approach has been to lump *P* and *A* together into a single term which has units of volume/time and is estimated or fit (Lutz *et al.*, 1980; Miller *et al.*, 1981; Angelo *et al.*, 1984; Gabrielsson *et al.*, 1985). A problem with the combined term is lack of knowledge about how to scale this term so that it can be applied to another species. It has been assumed that the permeability term is related to a constant physical process across species and the area can be scaled according to body weight (Gabrielsson *et al.*, 1985).

There are several assumptions that have been used to collapse the subcompartments shown in Figures 32.2, 32.3 and 32.4 and therefore reduce the complexity of the problem. When transfer across the cell membrane is the rate limiting step, the plasma and interstitial subcompartments can be combined into a single extracellular compartment (Lutz *et al.*, 1980; Gerlowski and Jain, 1983). When blood flow to the tissue is the rate limiting step (i.e. delivery of the chemical in the blood flow is much less than diffusion into the tissue), all subcompartments can be collapsed into a single well-stirred compartment where the rate of change in amount of chemical in the compartment as a whole is related to blood flow and the difference between arterial blood and venous blood concentrations (Lutz *et al.*, 1977; Mintun *et al.*, 1980; Andersen, 1981; Lutz *et al.*, 1984; Matthews and Dedrick, 1984; Clewell and Andersen, 1985; Andersen *et al.* 1987; Leung *et al.*, 1988; Fisher *et al.*, 1989) which is a consolidation of equations (32.1) and (32.2):

$$V_i \frac{dC_i}{dt} = Q_i \left(C_a - \frac{C_i}{R_{i/b}} \right) \tag{32.18}$$

where the *i* subscript refers to any compartment and $R_{i/b}$ is the partition coefficient between the tissue and blood. It has also been assumed that the concentration of chemical in tissue is in equilibrium with mixed venous blood. The second concentration term, tissue concentration (C_i) divided by the tissue to blood partition coefficient, is substituted for the concentration in venous blood, assuming the equilibrium condition:

$$R_{i/b} = \frac{C_i}{C_v} \tag{32.19}$$

where C_v is the concentration in venous blood leaving the tissue.

Full PB-PK model

When differential equations are written for the skin and body compartments, they need to be connected in a way that total mass in the whole organism is conserved. The mass balance in the liver compartment is the same as equation (32.18) except for the addition of saturable metabolism (equation (32.6)).

$$V_l \frac{dC_l}{dt} = Q_l \left(C_a - \frac{C_l}{R_{l/b}} \right) - \frac{V_{max} \frac{C_l}{R_{l/b}}}{K_m + \frac{C_l}{R_{l/B}}} \tag{32.20}$$

where C_l is the concentration in the liver. The simple skin compartment in Figure 32.3 can be described as a single well-stirred compartment with simple diffusion:

$$V_{sk}\frac{dC_{sk}}{dt} = Q_{sk}\left(C_a - \frac{C_{sk}}{R_{sk/b}}\right) + P_{sk}A_{sk}\left(C_{sfc} - \frac{C_{sk}}{R_{sk/sfc}}\right)$$

(32.21)

The first term on the right side of the equation describes the effect of blood flow, the second term is the net flux of chemical into the skin from the skin surface.

The concentration of chemical in mixed venous blood is the flow weighted average of all the concentrations leaving a compartment:

$$C_v = \frac{\Sigma_i(Q_iC_i)}{Q_c}$$

(32.22)

where Q_c is cardiac output (total blood flow).

32.4.5 Parameters of a model

The parameters required for the model will depend on the compartments that have been chosen based on pharmacokinetics. It is important to know which parameters are available, or can be determined, because they may be the limiting factors in the structure of the model. Physiological parameters for rats with a model for volatile lipophilic chemicals (McDougal et al., 1986) is shown in Table 32.1.

It is important that the sum of the individual blood flows equals the total cardiac output. The sum of the volumes of the compartments only accounts for 91 percent of the body weight. The other 9 percent that is not accounted for is nonperfused tissue such as fur, crystalline bone, cartilage, and teeth.

Chemical-specific parameters of a model are partition coefficients, binding coefficients and metabolic rates. Partition coefficients describe the ratio of chemical concentrations in different materials at equilibrium. They reflect the solubility of a chemical in biological fluids and tissues and are essential components of physiologically based models. Some of the partition coefficients determined by Gargas et al. (1989) that have been used for a PB-PK model of dermal absorption of organic vapors (McDougal et al., 1990) are shown in Table 32.2. These partition coefficients for volatile chemicals were measured by determining, at equilibrium, the ratio of concentrations in the blood or tissue

TABLE 32.1:

Physiological parameters from a PB-PK model for rats.

Lumped compartment	Blood flow (cardiac output) %	Volume (body weight) %
Rapidly perfused	56	5
Liver	20	4
Slowly perfused	10	65
Fat	9	7
Skin	5	10

TABLE 32.2:

Partition coefficients for some organic chemicals

Chemical	Muscle/air	Fat/air	Liver/air	Blood/air
Styrene	46.7	3476	140.7	40.2
m-Xylene	41.9	1859	92.0	46.0
Toluene	27.7	1021	82.8	18.0
Perchloroethylene	20.0	1638	69.9	19.9
Benzene	10.3	499	17.8	17.8
Halothane	4.5	182	7.6	5.3
Hexane	2.9	159	12.0	2.3

to the concentration in air. Tissue/blood partition coefficients can be estimated by dividing the tissue/air partition coefficient by the blood/air partition coefficient. Jepson *et al.* (1994) developed a method to measure blood/saline and tissue/saline partition coefficients for nonvolatile chemicals (<1 mm Hg at 20°C) using filtration under pressure. In this case, tissue/blood partition coefficients can be estimated by dividing the tissue/saline partition coefficient by the blood/saline partition coefficient.

Metabolic constants describe the rate of loss of chemical from a lumped compartment. Table 32.3 shows saturable (V_{max} and K_m) and first-order (K_{fo}) metabolic constants for several volatile organics from McDougal *et al.* (1990). Most of these metabolic constants for rats were determined *in vivo* by gas uptake techniques (Gargas *et al.*, 1986), but they can also be determined *in vitro* (Dedrick *et al.*, 1972; Sato and Nakajima, 1979; Reitz *et al.*, 1988). Kedderis (1997) has evaluated the extrapolation of *in vitro* enzyme induction to humans.

TABLE 32.3:

Metabolic constants for some organic chemicals

Chemical	V_{max} (mg/kg/hr)	K_m (mg/liter)	K_{fo} (kg^{-1}hr^{-1})
Styrene	8.4	0.4	0.0
m-Xylene	4.2	0.4	2.0
Toluene	4.7	1.0	0.0
Perchloroethylene	0.0	0.0	0.3
Benzene	3.3	0.6	0.0
Halothane	7.0	0.2	0.0
Hexane	6.0	0.4	3.4

32.4.6   Computer simulations

PB-PK models are sets of time dependent, non-linear simultaneous differential equations such as those described above. Most common computer programming languages, such as FORTRAN, BASIC and C could be used to solve these differential equations simultaneously although the ease at which it could be done would be greatly improved with add-on integration routines and plotting packages. Continuous system simulation languages such as Advanced Continuous Simulation Language (ACSL) (AEgis Technology Group Inc., Huntsville AL) and MATLAB® (The Math Works Inc., Natick, MA), Berkley Madona™ (Kagi, Emeryville, CA), ModelMaker (Borland®, Scotts Valley, CA), which were designed for engineering simulations, make the process of coding, debugging, modifying and running a PB-PK model much easier. Simulation languages are interactive and allow easy data entry, on-line changes of model parameters, and plotting of the results. These simulation languages have been the most important factor influencing the increased use of PB-PK models.

32.5   HOW DO YOU DEVELOP PB-PK MODELS?

PB-PK models are unlike "canned" computer programs that can be used for various purposes once they are written. They are radically different from such multipurpose programs as statistical routines, spreadsheets and databases because the structure of a PB-PK model is dependent on the interaction of a specific chemical with a specific species. The result of using a PB-PK model for a chemical other than that for which it was intended would be like using an Ohio state tax preparation package to prepare a California state tax return. Each unique chemical-species interaction requires that the salient physiological and pharmacokinetic principles be understood and quantitatively described. Development of a PB-PK model is an iterative process that requires insight, trial and error, and careful laboratory investigation. PB-PK models can and should be developed before the first laboratory experiment. As knowledge is gained in the laboratory, each new understanding should be quantitatively described in the model. Simulation and experimentation should be accomplished concurrently. Simulation prior to experimentation will allow appropriate data to be collected. Experimentation will confirm or increase the understanding that is quantified in the model. The key is understanding at the appropriate level as opposed to description on a superficial level.

32.5.1   Choose compartments

Decisions about the form of the skin compartment are related to the behavior of the chemical in the skin. Lag time (the time before steady state penetration rate is achieved) is the single most important determining factor. If lag time prior to achieving steady state absorption is short i.e. 15 minutes, a simple well-stirred homogeneous skin compartment (Figure 32.3) may be an adequate description. If the lag time is longer, which is more common, it will be necessary to include part or all of the skin subcompartments shown in Figure 32.4. Distribution of the chemical in the skin will determine which compartments are important to describe explicitly. Many of the methods that have been developed to study the skin will be useful for increasing the understanding required for an appropriate mathematical description. These include *in vitro* methods for metabolism and penetration, laser Doppler velocimetry, tape stripping, and ultrastructural analysis by light or electron microscopy.

Deciding which compartments, in addition to a skin, to include in a model requires knowledge of the pharmacokinetics of the chemical of interest. Depending on the chemical, pharmacokinetic information may be available from the literature or it may need to be determined in the laboratory before determining the structure of the model. Compartments must be included in a model to represent the major organs of metabolism and excretion. For example, a chemical that is primarily eliminated in the urine by an active process would require a kidney compartment, but a chemical that is eliminated primarily by exhalation would require a lung compartment. Metabolism studies with radio-labeled chemicals or other analytical methods, such as gas chromatography or high-performance liquid chromatography, will provide the kinetic data required to choose the important compartments for loss of parent chemical. Additional lumped compartments must be included to account for distribution of the chemical in the animal. A lipophilic chemical would require a fat compartment or compartments while a chemical that does not distribute to the fat would not. Distribution studies with radiolabeled or non-labeled chemicals provide the details necessary for appropriate choices of compartments. New analytical methods such as positron emission tomography or nuclear magnetic residence imaging appear promising and may provide valuable distribution information in the whole animal. Organs in which the chemical has similar distribution may be lumped together if the organs have similar blood flow per weight of tissue. Blood flow to organs can be determined from the literature or from microsphere techniques. Other compartments that may be desired in the model would be representative of target organs for toxicity or therapeutic effect.

Decisions about the form of a lumped compartment and the requirement for subcompartments depend on the relationship between blood flow to the compartment, volume of the compartment and solubility of the chemical in the compartment. Deciding whether the limiting factor in transfer of chemical from blood to the compartment is flow or diffusion is not always simple experimentally (Riggs, 1963). It is probably best to assume blood flow is the limiting factor unless there is evidence otherwise or flow-limitation does not adequately describe the behavior of a compartment. The most important principle in PB-PK modeling is to use the simplest description that adequately describes the behavior of the chemical.

32.5.2 Determine physiological parameters

Species-specific physiological parameters, i.e. blood flow and volumes of organs, are often available in the physiology handbooks or reviews (Snyder *et al.*, 1974; Fiserova-Bergerova *et al.*, 1983; Gerlowski and Jain, 1983; USEPA, 1987) or from published PB-PK models (Adolf, 1949; Dedrick, 1973; Lutz *et al.*, 1980; Ramsey and Andersen, 1984; Corley *et al.*, 1990, 2000; Bouchard *et al.*, 2001; Timchalk *et al.*, 2002). It is necessary to make decisions about which physiological parameters to use from the literature because there will undoubtedly be a range of values available. One must avoid the temptation to change the physiological parameters to fall outside this normal range in order to obtain agreement between prediction and observation. If this temptation is not resisted, the result will be the loss of the ability to extrapolate. The physiological parameters in a PB-PK model for any species should be robust and not change when a different chemical is modeled, unless there is sound evidence that the chemical specifically causes changes, e.g. blood flow. When prediction and observation do not agree there are two explanations: either the results of the experiment are not accurate or the model assumptions are inadequate. Once experimental calculations have been checked, the best approach is to determine if the structure of the model is adequate. In some cases, an important compartment has been overlooked or a diffusion limitation has been described as a flow limitation.

32.5.3 Determine chemical parameters

Metabolic constants, partition coefficients and binding coefficients are much less available in the literature than the physiological parameters and they must often be determined experimentally. Metabolic constants can be determined in many ways, both *in vitro* and *in vivo*. Methods used specifically for PB-PK modeling are the tissue homogenate methods of Dedrick *et al.* (1972) and *in vivo* gas uptake methods for measuring metabolism of volatile chemicals (Gargas *et al.*, 1986). Partition coefficients for volatile chemicals in blood and tissue homogenates can be determined by the vial equilibration technique (Gargas *et al.*, 1989). Partition coefficients for nonvolatile chemicals can be determined by measuring tissue and blood concentrations after continuous dosing to achieve equilibrium. Binding, which is distinguished from partitioning because it is not linearly related to concentration, can be determined by various methods (Dedrick and Bischoff, 1968; Lin *et al.*, 1982). The same caveat about changing physiological parameters to fit the data applies to the chemical parameters. Halving the blood/air partition coefficient because it fits the experimental results better may solve an immediate problem at the expense of the general applicability of the model.

32.5.4 Validate model where absorption is absent

Before a PB-PK model can be used to describe the process of absorption through the skin, it is necessary to gain some confidence in the quantitative description of pharmacokinetics when absorption is absent. The model should successfully simulate blood concentrations, tissue concentrations or expired breath after intravenous exposures at several concentrations. Urinary or fecal excretion could also be used for validation, but they are not optimum because sampling times are critical. Ideally, prolonged intravenous infusions at several concentrations and intravenous boluses at several concentrations should be used to make sure that the physiological and pharmacokinetic parameters chosen will adequately describe the processes of distribution, metabolism and excretion for a wide range of concentrations. An alternative approach would be to achieve the same confidence with subcutaneous infusions using minipumps.

32.5.5 Validate model with dermal absorption

Once the parameters not involved in absorption are fixed, then the model can be used to understand the process of absorption through the skin. Parent chemical distribution in the body after absorption through the skin and hepatic metabolism will follow the same principles independent of the absorption process. When these processes are understood and quantified, the rate of absorption through the skin can be determined based on blood, tissue, breath or excreta concentrations. Permeability constants can be determined by using the model to determine total chemical absorbed as long as the concentration on the skin and the surface area are known (McDougal *et al.*, 1986). Figure 32.5 shows predicted blood concentrations for several organic chemicals when rats were exposed dermally to carefully controlled vapor concentrations during whole-body exposures with respiratory protection (McDougal *et al.*, 1986).

32.5.6 Extrapolation to humans

The ability to extrapolate from laboratory species to man is one of the most important reasons for using PB-PK models. Ramsey and Andersen (1984) have shown that a physiologically-based pharmacokinetic model for inhalation of styrene vapors in rodents can predict the pharmacokinetic behavior of inhaled styrene in humans by changing the blood flows, organ volumes and partition coefficients to those of humans. The same principles could be used to extrapolate dermal absorption studies to humans if differences in skin structure are taken into account. It will be possible to quantify the species differences in blood flow, differences in stratum corneum, epidermal and subcutaneous fat thickness and composition, as well as the effect of the type and number of appendages on skin penetration in various species.

It has been shown that organic vapor penetration rates determined in rats using a PB-PK model are two to four times greater than penetration rates in humans calculated from the literature based on the total absorbed after whole-body exposures (McDougal *et al.*, 1990). The consistency of these comparisons suggests that differences in permeability may be due to physical differences in the skin. Using this as an example, it is important to understand some of the approaches and limitations involved in extrapolation to humans. It is not possible to directly extrapolate, with any confidence, the published PB-PK model for organic vapors in rats to the published human studies. This is because the human studies were based on urinary output and/or exhaled breath and the rat studies were based on blood concentrations. It would be fairly easy to make the rat model capable of predicting exhaled breath and urinary output by adding urinary output and validating the rat model for these routes of excretion.

Once the rat model accurately predicted experimental results for urinary output and exhaled breath, the rat model could be used to address the human data by changing the physiological, pharmacokinetic and biochemical parameters in the model to those of the human. For example, alveolar ventilation rates, blood flows, organ volumes, and urine volumes would need to be changed to those of the human. Partition coefficients, metabolic rates, and urinary excretion rates would need to be found or determined for each chemical of interest and changed in the model. With the published rat description, permeability constants were determined with confidence because the model was validated with a route where complex absorption was absent, i.e. inhalation. If the scaled-up rat model did not predict the dermal exposures in humans, it could be because the permeability constant in humans is different (as suspected) or because the physiological, or pharmacokinetic parameters used for humans were incorrect. It would be necessary to make sure that these parameters were correct in humans with a route of absorption other than dermal.

Providing the rest of the description was correct, any inaccuracy in the prediction would be due to differences in permeability constant in the skin, and the permeability constant could be estimated by determining the constant required to fit the data. If the simple skin compartment (equation (32.21)) were descriptive for this chemical in the rat it would most likely be descriptive of the same chemical in the human. Other types of chemicals, which penetrate more slowly than organic vapors, may require that the skin be broken into some or all of the subcompartments described in equations (32.11)–(32.16). In such a case, the subcompartments would also require that the structural differences in the skin between species be understood and quantified.

Other types of skin models that use first order rate constants to describe the transfer of chemicals between subcompartments have been developed. They are excellent descriptive models but do not extrapolate to other species well, because the first order rate constant is a composite of the permeability, area exposed and the partition coefficient. These models have been reviewed and compared with PB-PK models by Roberts *et al.* (1999) and McCarley and Bunge (2001).

32.5.7 When the model fails

Paradoxically, models are often most useful when they fail to adequately describe the experimental data. During the process of developing a more adequate description of the pharmacokinetic processes involved, insight can be gained which will apply to other situations and increase the understanding of the skin, specifically, and pharmacokinetics, in general. It is the physiological foundation of the description that forces an investigator to design experiments to determine where the description is inaccurate. When frustration occurs, it is important to remember that the behavior of chemicals in living systems is not arbitrary. Chemicals and biological systems interact in accordance with physicochemical principles, which once understood are very reasonable and reliable. PB-PK modeling is an iterative process that requires theory and observation to come closer together until the final result is achieved.

32.5.8 Value of PB-PK skin models

PB-PK modeling can increase the understanding of the effect of vehicles on penetration rates and penetration enhancement. Jepson and McDougal (1999) showed the importance of the skin/vehicle partition coefficient by demonstrating that permeability, measured *in vivo*, could be extrapolated between different vehicles (water, corn oil and mineral oil) with a reasonable degree of accuracy. Traditionally, flux measurements must be made on a system that is at or near steady state. Jepson and McDougal (1997) demonstrated that a PB-PK model could be used as a tool to estimate *in vivo* permeability in a situation such as an organic chemical in a small volume of water where steady state is never achieved. These models have also been shown to accurately describe *in vitro* skin and receptor solution concentrations in the first 20 minutes of organic chemical in aqueous vehicle (McDougal and Jurgens, 2001). Real time breath analysis has been linked with PB-PK modeling as a tool to investigate human dermal absorption of volatile chemicals from water (Poet *et al.*, 2000; Thrall *et al.*, 2000) and soil (Thrall *et al.*, 2000; Poet *et al.*, 2002). This noninvasive approach wouldn't be available without a PB-PK model to estimate body burden.

32.5.9   Future of PB-PK skin models

Improved skin compartments can be developed and validated which include some of the subcompartments shown in Figure 32.4 to be predictive of penetration rates of chemicals that have more complicated absorption profiles. Pharmacodynamic models that quantitatively describe the molecular events that occur in the skin with local toxicity (for example, psoriasis, contact dermatitis or skin cancer) can be developed. These models might describe tissue levels, production and turnover rates of important proteins, signaling molecules and/or mRNA levels that are responsible for deleterious changes in skin function. With appropriate biologically based models, it is possible to make the connection between amount of chemical on the surface and the therapeutic or toxic effect. When validated, these validated models could be applied to the development of biomarkers and prophylaxis.

32.6   CONCLUSION

Physiologically-based pharmacokinetic models provide tremendous capacity to increase the understanding of skin absorption and the effects of chemicals in the skin. The ability to extrapolate between *in vivo* exposure conditions, doses and species allows laboratory animal studies to provide a wealth of information applicable to human exposure situations. The ability to apply quantitative descriptions to processes occurring in the skin is limited only by our ability to understand the processes involved.

32.7   NOMENCLATURE

C	Concentration (mass/volume)
V	Volume
A	Area (distance^2)
Q	Flow (volume/time)
P	Permeability (distance/time)
K_m	Michaelis metabolic constant (mass/volume)
K_T	Michaelis-like transport constant (mass/volume)
k	Maximum transport rate (mass/volume × time)
r	Proportionality constant (time^{-1})
R	Partition coefficient (unitless, ratio of concentrations)
V_{max}	Maximum velocity (mass/time)

■ CHAPTER 32 ■

32.7.1 Subscripts

a	arterial
b	blood
c	cardiac output
d	dermis
e	extracellular
i	*i*th tissue
is	interstitial
p	plasma
sc	stratum corneum
sf	subcutaneous fat
sfc	surface
sk	skin
t	tissue
v	venous
ve	viable epidermis

REFERENCES

ADOLF, E.F. (1949) Quantitative relations in the physiological constitutions of mammals. *Science* **109**, 579–585.

ANDERSEN, M.E. (1981) A physiologically-based toxicokinetic description of the metabolism of inhaled gases and vapors: Analysis at steady state. *Toxicol. Appl. Pharmacol.* **60**, 509–526.

ANDERSEN, M.E., CLEWELL III, H.J., GARGAS, M.L., SMITH, F.A. and REITZ, R.H. (1987) Physiologically based pharmacokinetics and the risk assessment process for methylene chloride. *Toxicol. Appl. Pharmacol.* **87**, 185–205.

ANGELO, M.J., BISCHOFF, K.B., PRITCHARD, A.B. and PRESSER, M.A. (1984) *J. Pharmacokin. Biopharm.* **12**, 413–436.

BIRMINGHAM, B.K., GREENE, D.S. and RHODES, C.T. (1979) Systemic absorption of topical salicylic acid. *Int. J. Dermatol.* **18**, 228–231.

BLANK, I.H. and SHEUPLEIN, R.J. (1964) The epidermal barrier. In ROOK, A. and CHAMPION, R.H. (eds) *Progress in Biological Sciences in Relation to Dermatology.* Cambridge University Press, Cambridge Mass. p. 246–261.

BOOKOUT, JR., R.L., MCDANIEL, C.R., QUINN, D.W. and MCDOUGAL, J.N. (1996) Multilayered dermal subcompartments for modeling chemical absorption. *SAR and QSAR in Environmental Research.* **5**, 133–150.

BOOKOUT, JR., R.L., QUINN, D.W. and McDOUGAL, J.N. (1997) Parallel dermal subcompartments for modeling chemical absorption. *SAR and QSAR in Environmental Research.* **7**, 259–279.

BOUCHARD M., BRUNET R.C., DROZ P.O. and CARRIER, G. (2001) A biologically based dynamic model for predicting the disposition of methanol and its metabolites in animals and humans. *Toxicol. Sci.* **64**, 169–184.

BRAVERMAN, I.M. and KEH-YEN, A. (1983) Ultrastructure of the human dermal microcirculation. IV. Valve-containing collecting veins at the dermal-subcutaneous junction. *J. Invest. Dermatol.* **81**, 438–442.

CHANDRASEKARAN, S.K., BAYNE, W. and SHAW J.E. (1978) Pharmacokinetics of drug permeation through human skin. *J. Pharmaceut. Sci.* **67**, 1370–1374.

CLEWELL III, H.J. and ANDERSEN, M.E. (1985) Risk assessment extrapolations and physiological modeling. *Toxicol. Indust. Health* **1**, 111–131.

CLEWELL III, H.J. and ANDERSEN, M.E. (1989) Improving toxicology testing protocols using computer simulations. *Toxicol. Letters* **49**, 139–158.

COOPER, E.R. (1976) Pharmacokinetics of skin penetration. *J. Pharmaceut. Sci.* **65**, 1396–1397.

CORLEY R.A., MENDRALA, A.L., SMITH, F.A., STAATS, D.A., GARGAS, M.L., CONOLLY, R.B., ANDERSEN, M.E. and REITZ, R.H. (1990) Development of a physiologically based pharmacokinetic model for chloroform. *Toxicol. Appl. Pharmacol.* **103**, 512–527.

CORLEY, R.A., ENGLISH, J.C., HILL, T.S., FIORICA, L.A. and MORGOTT, D.A. (2000) Development of a physiologically based pharmacokinetic model for hydroquinone. *Toxicol. Appl. Pharmacol.* **165**, 163–74.

DEDRICK, R.L. (1973) Animal scale-up. *J. Pharmacokin. Biopharm.* **1**, 435–461.

DEDRICK, R.L. and BISCHOFF, K.B. (1968) Pharmacokinetics in applications of the artificial kidney. *Chem. Engr. Prog. Symp. Ser.* No. 84. **64**, 32–44.

DEDRICK, R.L., FORRESTER, D.D. and HO, D.H.W. (1972) *In vitro–in vivo* correlation of drug metabolism-deamination of 1-b-D arabinofuranosylcytosine. *Biochem. Pharmacol.* **21**, 1–16.

DUGARD, P.H. and SCOTT, R.C. (1984) Absorption through skin. In BADEN, H.P. (ed.) *Chemotherapy of Psoriasis*, Oxford: Pergamon Press, 125–144.

ELIAS, P.M. and FRIEND, D.S. (1975) The permeability barrier in mammalian epidermis. *J. Cell Biol.* **65**, 180–191.

FINNIN, M.J. and SCHUSTER, S. (1985) Phase 1 and phase 2 drug metabolism in isolated epidermal cells from adult hairless mice and in whole human hair follicles. *Biochem. Pharmacol.* **34**, 3571–3575.

CHAPTER 32

FISEROVA-BERGEROVA, V. and HUGHES, H.C. (1983) Species differences on bioavailability of inhaled vapors and gases. In FISERVOA-BERGEROVA, V. (ed.) *Modeling of Inhalation Exposure to Vapors: Uptake, Distribution and Elimination,* Vol 2. CRC Press, Boca Raton, Florida, 97–106.

FISHER, J.W., WHITTAKER, T.A., TAYLOR, D.H., CLEWELL III, H.J. and ANDERSEN, M.E. (1989) Physiologically based pharmacokinetic modeling of the pregnant rat: A multiroute exposure model for trichloroethylene and its metabolite, trichloroacetic acid. *Toxicol. Appl. Pharmacol.* **99**, 395–414.

FLYNN, G.L., YALKOWSKY, S.H. and ROSEMAN, T.J. (1974) Mass transport phenomenon and models: Theoretical concepts. *J. Pharm. Sci.* **63**, 479–509.

GARGAS, M.L., ANDERSEN, M.E. and CLEWELL III, H.J. (1986) A physiologically based simulation approach for determining metabolic constants from gas uptake data. *Toxicol. Appl. Pharmacol.* **86**, 341–352.

GARGAS, M.L., BURGESS, R.J., VOISARD, D.E., CASON, G.H. and ANDERSEN, M.E. (1989) Partition coefficients of low-molecular-weight volatile chemicals in various liquids and tissues. *Toxicol. Appl. Pharmacol.* **98**, 87–99.

GABRIELSSON, J.L., JOHANSSON, P., BONDESSON, U. and PAALZOW, L.K. (1985) Analysis of methadone disposition in the pregnant rat by means of a physiological flow model. *J. Pharmacokin. Biopharm.* **13**, 355–372.

GERLOWSKI, L.E. and JAIN, R.K. (1983) Physiologically based pharmacokinetic modeling: Principles and applications. *J. Pharm. Sci.* **72**, 1103–1127.

GIBALDI, M. and PERRIER, D. (1982) *Pharmacokinetics.* New York: Marcel Dekker, Inc.

GUY, R.H., HADGRAFT, J. and MAIBACH, H.I. (1982) A pharmacokinetic model for percutaneous absorption. *Int. J. Pharm.* **11**, 119–129.

HIMMELSTEIN, K.J. and LUTZ, R.J. (1979) A review of the application of physiologically-based pharmacokinetic modeling. *J. Pharmacokin. Biopharm.* **7**, 127–137.

JEPSON, G.W., HOOVER, D.K., BLACK, R.K., McCAFFERTY, J.D., MAHLE, D.A. and GEARHART, J.M. (1994) A partition coefficient determination method for nonvolatile chemicals in biological tissues. *Fundam. Appl. Toxicol.* **22**, 519–524.

JEPSON, G.W. and McDOUGAL, J.N. (1997) Physiologically based modeling of nonsteady state dermal absorption of halogenated methanes from an aqueous solution. *Toxicol. Appl. Pharmacol.* **144**, 315–324.

JEPSON, G.W. and MCDOUGAL, J.N. (1999) Predicting vehicle effects on the dermal absorption of halogenated methanes using physiologically based modeling. *Toxicol. Sci.* **48**, 180–188.

KEDDERIS, G.L. (1997) Extrapolation of *in vitro* enzyme induction data to humans *in vivo*. *Chemico-Biological Interact.* **107**, 109–121.

KUBOTA, K. and ISHIZAKI. T. (1986) A calculation of percutaneous drug absorption—I. Theoretical. *Comput. Biol. Med.* **16**, 17–19.

LEUNG, H-W, KU, R.H., PAUSTENBACH, D.J. and ANDERSEN, M.E. (1988) A physiologically based pharmacokinetic model for 2,3,7,8-tetrachlorodibenzo-*p*-dioxin in C57BL/6J and DBA/2J mice. *Toxicol. Letters* **42**, 15–28.

LIN, J.H., SUGIYAMA, Y., AWAZY, S. and HANANO, M. (1982) *In vitro* and *in vivo* evaluation of the tissue-to blood partition coefficient for phyusiological pharmacokinetic models. *J. Pharmacokin. Biopharm.* **10**, 637–647.

LUTZ, R.J., DEDRICK, R.L. and ZAHARKO, D.S. (1980) Physiological pharmaco-kinetics: An *in vivo* approach to membrane transport. *Pharmacol. Ther.* **11**, 559–592.

LUTZ, R.J., DEDRICK, R.L., MATTHEWS, H.B., ELING, T.E. and ANDERSON, M.W. (1977) A preliminary pharmacokinetic model for several chlorinated biphenyls in the rat. *Drug Metab. Dispos.* **5**, 386–395.

LUTZ, R.J., DEDRICK, R.L., TUEY, D., SIPES, I.G., ANDERSON, M.W. and MATTHEWS, H.B. (1984) Comparison of the pharmacokinetics of several polychlorinated biphenyls in mouse, rat, dog, and monkey by means of a physiological pharmacokinetic model. *Drug Metab. Dispos.* **12**, 527–535.

MARZULLI, F.N. and TREGEAR, R.T. (1961) Identification of a barrier layer in the skin. *J. Physiol.* **157**, 52–53.

MARZULLI, F.N., BROWN, D.W.C and MAIBACH, H.I. (1969) Techniques for studying skin penetration. *Toxicol. Appl. Pharmacol.* **sup. 3**, 76–83.

MATTHEWS, H.B. and DEDRICK, R.L. (1984) Pharmacokinetics of PCBs. *Ann. Rev. Pharmacol. Toxicol.* **24**, 85–103.

MERSHON, M.M. (1975) Barrier surfaces of skin. In Advances in Chemistry Series, No. 145, *Applied Chemistry at Protein Interfaces*, American Chemical Society, 41–73.

McCARLEY, K.D. and BUNGE, A.L. (2001) Pharmacokinetic models of dermal absorption. *J. Pharmaceut. Sci.* **90**, 1699–1719.

McDOUGAL, J.N. and JURGENS J.M. (2001) Short term dermal absorption and penetration of chemicals from aqueous solutions: Theory and experiment. *Risk Analysis,* **21**, 719–726.

■ CHAPTER 32 ■

McDOUGAL, J.N., JEPSON, G.W., CLEWELL III, H.J., MacNAUGHTON, M.G. and ANDERSEN, M.E. (1986) A physiological pharmacokinetic model for dermal absorption of vapors in the rat. *Toxicol. Appl. Pharmacol.* **85**, 286–294.

McDOUGAL, J.N., JEPSON, G.W., CLEWELL III, H.J., GARGAS, M.L. and ANDERSEN, M.E. (1990) Dermal absorption of organic chemical vapors in rats and humans. *Fundam. Appl. Toxicol.* **14**, 299–308.

MILLER, S.C., HIMMELSTEIN, K.J. and PATTON, T.F. (1981) A physiologically based pharmacokinetic model for the intraocular distribution of pilocarpine in rabbits. *J. Pharmacokin. Biopharm.* **9**, 653–677.

MINTUN, M., HIMMELSTEIN, K.J., SCHRODER, R.L., GIBALDI, M. and SHEN, D.D. (1980) Tissue distribution kinetics of tetraethylammonium ion in the rat. *J. Pharmacokin. Biopharm.* **8**, 373–409.

ODLAND, G.F. (1983) Structure of skin. In GOLDSMITH, L.A. (ed.) *Biochemistry and Physiology of the Skin* V. 1. Oxford: Oxford University Press, 3–63.

PANNATIER, A., JENNER, P., TESTA, B. and ETTER, J.C. (1978) The skin as a drug-metabolizing organ. *Drug Metab. Rev.* **8**, 319–343.

PECK, C.C., LEE, K. and BECKER, C.E. (1981) Continuous transepidermal drug collection: Basis for use in assessing drug intake and pharmacokinetics. *J. Pharmacokin. Biopharm.* **9**, 41–57.

POET, T.S., THRALL, K.D., CORLEY, R.A., HUI, X., EDWARDS, J.A., WEITZ, K.K., MAIBACH, H.I. and WESTER, R.C. (2000) Utility of real time breath analysis and physiologically based pharmacokinetic modeling to determine the percutaneous absorption of methyl chloroform in rats and humans. *Toxicol. Sci.* **54**, 42–51.

POET, T.S., WEITZ, K.K., GIES, R.A., EDWARDS, J.A., THRALL, K.D., CORLEY, R.A., TANOJO, H., HUI, X., MAIBACH, H.I. and WESTER, R.C. (2002) PBPK modeling of the percutaneous absorption of perchloroethylene from a soil matrix in rats and humans. *Toxicol. Sci.* **67**, 17–31.

RAMSEY, J.C. and ANDERSEN, M.E. (1984) A physiologically based description of the inhalation pharmacokinetics of styrene in rats and humans. *Toxicol. Appl. Pharmacol.* **73**, 159–175.

REITZ, R.H., MENDRALA, A.L., PARK, C.N., ANDERSEN, M.E. and GUENGERICH, F.P. (1988) Incorporation of *in vitro* enzyme data into the physiologically-based pharmacokinetic (PB-PK) model for methylene chloride: implications for risk assessment. *Tox. Letters* **43**, 97–116.

RIGGS, D.S. (1963) *The Mathematical Approach to Physiological Problems: A critical primer*. Cambridge, Mass: MIT Press.

ROBERTS, M.S., ANISSIMOV, Y.G. and GONSALVEZ, R.A. (1999) Mathematical models in percutaneous absorption. In BRONAUGH, R.L. and MAIBACH, H.I. (eds) *Percutaneous Absorption: Drugs–Cosmetics–Mechanisms–Methodology*. New York, NY: Marcel Dekker, Inc. 3–55.

SATO, A. and NAKAJIMA, T. (1979) A vial-equilibration method to evaluate the drug-metabolizing enzyme activity for volatile hydrocarbons. *Toxicol. Appl. Pharmacol.* **47**, 41–46.

SCHEUPLEIN, R.J. (1967) Mechanism of percutaneous absorption. II. Transient diffusion and relative importance of various routes of skin penetration. *J. Invest. Dermatol.* **48**, 79–88.

SNYDER, W.S., COOK, M.J., NASSET, E.S., KARHHAUSEN, L.R., HOWELLS, G.P. and TIPTON, I.H. (1974, *Report of the Task Group on Reference Man*, Oxford, UK: Pergamon Press.

THRALL K.D., POET T.S., CORLEY R.A., TANOJO H., EDWARDS J.A., WEITZ K.K., HUI X., MAIBACH H.I. and WESTER R.C. (2000) A real-time *in vivo* method for studying the percutaneous absorption of volatile chemicals. *Int. J. Occup. Environ. Health* **6**, 96–103.

TIMCHALK, C., NOLAN, R.J., MENDRALA, A.L., DITTENBER, D.A., BRZAK, K.A. and MATTSSON, J.L. (2002) A physiologically based pharmacokinetic and pharma-codynamic (PBPK/PD) model for the organophosphate insecticide chlorpyrifos in rats and humans. *Toxicol. Sci.* **66**, 34–53.

UNITED STATES ENVIRONMENTAL PROTECTION AGENCY (EPA) (1988) *Reference Physiological Parameters in Pharmacokinetic Modeling*. US Environmental Protection Agency, Office of Health and Environmental Assessment, Office of Research and Development, Washington, DC, EPA/600/6–88/004.

WALLACE, S.M. and BARNETT, G. (1978) Pharmacokinetic analysis of percutaneous absorption: Evidence of parallel pathways for methotrexate. *J. Pharmacokin. Biopharm.* 6, 315–325.

■ CHAPTER 32 ■

Methods for In Vitro Skin Metabolism Studies

33

ROBERT L BRONAUGH

Contents

33.1 Introduction

33.2 Reasons for doing *in vitro* studies

33.3 Maintenance of skin viability in diffusion cells

33.4 Skin viability assays

33.5 Skin metabolism during *in vitro* absorption studies

33.1 INTRODUCTION

It has been known for years that enzymes in skin catalyze a wide variety of metabolic reactions (Pannatier *et al.*, 1978; Bickers, 1980; Kappus, 1989). All of the major enzymes important for systemic metabolism in the liver and other tissues have been identified in skin (Pannatier *et al.*, 1978). Often enzyme activity has been found to be lower in skin (on a per mg tissue basis) when compared to the liver (Bronaugh *et al.*, 1989; Muckhtar and Bickers, 1981). However, the skin is the largest organ in the body with a surface area of 2 m^2 and total weight estimated at 4 kg—about three times that of the liver (Pannatier *et al.*, 1978). Therefore, the skin can play an important role as a portal of entry of chemicals into the body.

Some chemical groups such as esters, primary amines, alcohols and acids are particularly susceptible to metabolism in skin. Many esters are hydrolyzed by esterase to their parent alcohol and acid molecules (Boehnlein *et al.*, 1994; Kenney *et al.*, 1995). Primary amines are frequently acetylated during percutaneous absorption through skin (Nathan *et al.*, 1990; Kraeling *et al.*, 1996; Yourick and Bronaugh, 2000). Oxidation/reduction and conjugation of alcohols and acids are commonly observed in skin (Nathan *et al.*,1990; Boehnlein *et al.*, 1994).

Chemicals that undergo significant metabolism in skin may exhibit greater or lesser biological activity than predicted simply from skin penetration studies. A more thorough examination of the safety or efficacy of these compounds can be determined by evaluating skin absorption and metabolism simultaneously using *in vitro* techniques.

33.2 REASONS FOR DOING *IN VITRO* STUDIES

Skin metabolism studies are difficult to accurately conduct *in vivo* because of systemic metabolism that takes place before samples are collected in the blood, urine or other site. *In vitro* studies isolate the skin from the metabolic activity in the rest of the body. When studies are conducted using viable skin in diffusion cells, metabolites can be measured in skin homogenates or in the receptor fluid directly beneath the skin. Also, *in vitro* studies may be the only ethical way to obtain human skin metabolism data for chemicals with safety concerns.

33.3   MAINTENANCE OF SKIN VIABILITY IN DIFFUSION CELLS

The assembly of skin in diffusion cells is described in general terms in Chapter 28, "Methods for *in vitro* percutaneous absorption." This chapter will discuss methods for maintaining viable skin in metabolism studies.

Human or animal skin should be freshly obtained. Skin previously frozen for shipping or storage is unsuitable for metabolism studies. Enzyme activity with some stable enzymes can sometimes still be observed in non-viable skin but the activity may be at a reduced level as observed for esterase activity (Boehnlein *et al.*, 1994; Kenney *et al.*, 1995).

The viability of rat skin was maintained for at least 24 hours in flow through diffusion cells using several physiological buffers as the receptor fluid (Collier *et al.*, 1989). For 24-hr studies the use of flow-through cells is likely required so that nutrients are continually provided to the skin.

Although a tissue culture media (minimal essential media, MEM) was satisfactory in maintaining skin viability, it was not required. Simpler balanced salt solutions such as HEPES-buffered Hanks' balanced salt solution (HHBSS) or Dulbecco modified phosphate-buffered saline worked just as well and are potentially less problematic for analytical reasons. Some of the vitamins, cofactors and amino acids contained in MEM absorb in UV light and can interfere with UV detection during HPLC analysis. Bovine serum albumin (BSA) has been added to the receptor fluid to enhance the partitioning of lipophilic test compounds from skin into the receptor fluid.

33.4   SKIN VIABILITY ASSAYS

Viability of skin was primarily assessed in our initial studies by measuring aerobic and anaerobic glucose utilization (Collier *et al.*, 1989). Anaerobic metabolism of glucose to lactic acid predominates in skin and so this assay has been commonly used. Glucose is the primary energy source for skin cells and has been monitored by tissue banks to assess skin viability for transplants (May and DeClement, 1981). We used electron and light microscopy techniques to assess viability by demonstrating that the cellular organelles were still intact at the end of 24 hour studies. Skin metabolism of estradiol and testosterone was also maintained for 24 hours.

We have observed that the addition of 4 percent BSA to HHBSS results in a low-ering of lactate levels measured in the skin viability assay (Hood and Bronaugh,

1999). Therefore, the 3-[4,5-dimethylthiazol-2yl]-2,5-diphenyltetrazolium bromide (MTT) assay was adapted to assess skin viability when BSA was required in the receptor fluid. The MTT assay of skin viability was not affected by addition of BSA to the receptor fluid. The viability of human, fuzzy rat and hairless guinea pig skin was found to be maintained for 24 hours. However, the assay can only be conducted at the end of a study when skin can be removed from the diffusion cell. The lactate measurement of glucose utilization can be conducted during the course of an experiment.

33.5 SKIN METABOLISM DURING *IN VITRO* ABSORPTION STUDIES

Early studies from our laboratory used intact viable dermatome skin sections from mice, rats, hairless guinea pigs, and humans in flow through diffusion cells to study the penetration and metabolism of estradiol and testosterone (Collier *et al.*, 1989), AETT and BHT (Bronaugh *et al.*, 1989), benzo[a]pyrene and 7-ethoxycoumarin (Storm *et al.*, 1990), and azo colors (Collier *et al.*, 1993).

The percutaneous absorption and metabolism of three structurally related compounds, benzoic acid, p-aminobenzoic acid (PABA), and ethyl amino-benzoate (benzocaine) were determined *in vitro* with hairless guinea pig and human skin (Nathan *et al.*, 1990). Approximately 7 percent of the absorbed benzoic acid was conjugated with glycine to form hippuric acid. Acetylation of primary amines was found to be an important metabolic step in skin. For benzocaine, a molecule susceptible to both N-acetylation and ester hydrolysis, 80 percent of the absorbed material was acetylated, while less than 10 percent of the absorbed ester was hydrolyzed. PABA was much more slowly absorbed than benzocaine and was also less extensively N-acetylated. Acetyl-PABA was found primarily in the receptor fluid at the end of the experiments but the receptor fluid contained only 20 percent of the absorbed dose. Much of the absorbed PABA remained unmetabolized and in the skin as might be expected for an effective sunscreen agent. The compound in skin would probably not have been exposed to N-acetylating enzymes if it was localized primarily in the stratum corneum. A similar pattern of benzocaine metabolism was observed in human and hairless guinea pig skin, however there appeared to be less enzyme activity in human skin.

The effect of benzocaine dose on its absorption and metabolism was determined in the hairless guinea pig (Kraeling *et al.*, 1996). It was of interest to determine if metabolism of absorbed benzocaine remained extensive when the

■ CHAPTER 33 ■

radiotracer doses used in our earlier studies were increased to doses simulating human use conditions as a local anesthetic. Percutaneous penetration of benzocaine increased 50-fold when the applied dose increased from 2 to 200 µg/cm². Metabolism of benzocaine to acetylbenzocaine was reduced at the higher dose but still approximately one-third of the absorbed dose was metabolized (Table 33.1). The metabolism of benzocaine in skin may not effect the local anesthetic activity of a topical commercial product since benzocaine and acetylbenzocaine were found to have similar potencies in reducing conductance in the isolated squid giant axon (Kraeling et al., 1996).

Esterase activity and alcohol dehydrogenase activity were characterized in hairless guinea pig skin with the model compounds methyl salicylate and benzyl alcohol (Boehnlein et al., 1994). Subsequently, the absorption and metabolism of the cosmetic ingredient retinyl palmitate was determined in human and hairless guinea pig skin.

The metabolism of methyl salicylate was determined in viable and non-viable hairless guinea pig skin. In viable skin over 50 percent of the absorbed compound was hydrolyzed by esterases in skin to salicylic acid. Twenty-one percent of the

TABLE 33.1:

Effect of benzocaine dose on its metabolism; percentage distribution of benzocaine and metabolites in receptor fluid and skin in 24 h.

Location and compound	Dose level								
	2 µg/cm²			40 µg/cm²			200 µg/cm²		
Receptor fluid									
Benzocaine	9.6	±	4.2	50.7	±	6.6	54.0	±	5.2
AcBenz	83.8	±	4.4	43.8	±	5.7	37.9	±	3.6
PABA	1.0	±	0.3	0.1	±	0.1	0.9	±	0.5
AcPABA	5.1	±	1.0	5.8	±	0.9	7.2	±	1.7
Skin									
Benzocaine	26.7	±	14.2	2.4	±	2.4	62.7	±	12.2
AcBenz	6.9	±	6.9	34.4	±	20.3	20.9	±	11.7
PABA	4.3	±	4.3	3.2	±	3.2	1.5	±	1.3
AcPABA	24.7	±	14.9	15.2	±	16.0	14.9	±	1.2
Total									
Benzocaine	10.7	±	3.3	49.9	±	6.5	57.3	±	3.7
AcBenz	80.5	±	3.8	43.6	±	5.6	34.3	±	3.4
PABA	1.4	±	0.2	0.1	±	0.1	0.9	±	0.5
AcPABA	6.5	±	1.0	5.9	±	1.0	7.6	±	2.0

Values are the mean ± S.E. for 1–6 determinations in each of three animals. The 40 µg/cm² dose level values are the mean ± S.E. of 2–3 determinations in each of four animals. The dosing vehicle was acetone. AcBenz = acetylbenzocaine; PABA = p-aminobenzoic acid; AcPABA = acetylPABA absorbed compound was further conjugated with glycine to form salicyluric acid. Greater esterase activity was observed in male skin. Esterase is a stable enzyme and hydrolysis of methyl salicylate also occurred in non-viable skin. However no conjugation of salicylic acid was observed in non-viable skin.

Oxidation of benzyl alcohol was also observed in hairless guinea pig skin. Approximately 50 percent of the absorbed benzyl alcohol was oxidized to benzoic acid in viable skin with a small portion of this compound being further metabolized to the glycine conjugate—hippuric acid. As with the ester, significant activity was also observed in non-viable skin and greater oxidation of the alcohol was obtained with male skin.

The absorption and metabolism of retinyl palmitate was measured to see if ester hydrolysis and alcohol oxidation occurred with this cosmetic ingredient. Most of the absorbed radioactivity remained in the skin. A substantial amount of the absorbed compound was hydrolyzed to retinol but no oxidation of the alcohol to retinoic acid was observed. Any effects of retinyl palmitate on the structure of skin may be due to the formation of retinol during percutaneous absorption.

Absorption values from *in vitro* studies with viable hairless guinea pig skin have been found to compare closely with *in vivo* results for phenanthrene (Ng *et al.*, 1991) and for pyrene, benzo[a]pyrene, and di(2-ethylhexyl) phthalate (Ng *et al.*, 1992). Also, significant metabolism was observed *in vitro* during the absorption of all four compounds.

Phenanthrene was metabolized *in vitro* to 9,10-dihydrodiol, 3,4-dihydrodiol, 1,2-dihydrodiol and traces of hydroxy phenanthrenes (Ng *et al.*, 1991). Following topical administration of phenanthrene, approximately 7 percent of the percutaneously absorbed material was converted to the dihydrodiol metabolites.

Numerous metabolites of benzo[a]pyrene were formed during percutaneous absorption through hairless guinea pig skin (Ng *et al.*, 1992). Of particular interest was the identification of benzo[a]pyrene 7,8,9,10 tetrahydrotetrol in the diffusion cell receptor fluid. This metabolite is the hydrolysis product of the ultimate carcinogen, 7,8-dihydroxy, 9,10-epoxy-7,8,9,10-tetrahydro-benzo[a]pyrene. This study demonstrates that skin metabolism is likely responsible for skin tumors formed following topical benzo[a]pyrene administration. In the earlier phenanthrene study (Ng *et al.*, 1991), no known carcinogenic metabolites were formed during skin permeation. This finding is consistent with the lack of tumorigenicity of phenanthrene in rodents.

Since the systemic toxicity of topically applied compounds is sometimes evaluated by the oral route of administration, the effect of route of administration

CHAPTER 33

on metabolism of (^{14}C) 2 nitro-p-phenylenediamine (2NPPD) was examined *in vitro* in the fuzzy rat (Yourick and Bronaugh, 2000). Rat skin dermatomed to approximately 250 µm and full thickness rat intestinal tissue (from the jejunum) were assembled into flow-through diffusion cells perfused with HHBSS to maintain viability. 2NPPD was applied for 30 minutes to skin in a semi-permanent hair dye formulation and to intestine in HHBSS (pH 6.5). Similar amounts of radioactivity penetrated into the receptor fluid from each tissue during the 24 h studies.

The metabolism of 2NPPD was determined in receptor fluid fractions using an HPLC method. More than 50 percent of the 2NPPD applied to skin remained unmetabolized while only 40 percent of 2NPPD was unmetabolized by intestine (Figure 33.1). Substantially more acetylation of 2NPPD to N4-acetyl-2NPPD occurred during absorption through skin. However triaminobenzene was formed to a greater extent in intestine. The amount of sulfated 2NPPD and/or metabolites (actual compound or compounds not determined) was also greater in effluent from intestinal tissue. The extent of metabolism of 2NPPD in human

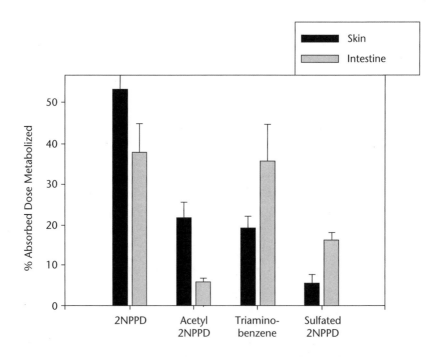

Figure 33.1: Metabolism of 2NPPD during absorption through rat skin and intestinal tissue. Values are the mean ± S.E. of three individual rat studies (n=3).

skin (semipermanent hair dye vehicle) was also determined. Approximately 60 percent of the absorbed radioactivity was metabolized to equal amounts of triaminobenzene and N4-acetyl-2NPPD. No sulfated compounds were found in effluents from human skin. These studies showed significant differences in metabolism during penetration through human and rat skin as well as differences in metabolism through rat skin and intestinal tissue.

REFERENCES

BICKERS, D.R. (1980) The skin as a site of drug and chemical metabolism. In DRILL, V.A. and LAZAR, P. (eds) *Current Concepts in Cutaneous Toxicity.* New York: Academic Press, 95–126.

BOEHNLEIN, J., SAKR, A., LICHTIN, J.L. and BRONAUGH, R.L. (1994) Characterization of esterase and alcohol dehydrogenase activity in skin. Metabolism of retinyl palmitate to retinol (Vitamin A) during percutaneous absorption, *Pharm. Res.,* **11,** 1155–1159.

BRONAUGH, R.L., STEWART, R.F. and STORM, J.E. (1989) Extent of cutaneous metabolism during percutaneous absorption of xenobiotics, *Toxicol. Appl. Pharmacol.,* **99,** 534–543.

COLLIER, S.W., SHEIKH, N.M., SAKR, A., LICHTIN, J.L., STEWART, R.F. and BRONAUGH, R.L. (1989) Maintenance of skin viability during *in vitro* percutaneous absorption /metabolism studies, *Toxicol. Appl. Pharmacol.,* **99,** 522–533.

COLLIER, S.W., STORM, J.E. and BRONAUGH, R.L. (1993) Reduction of azo dyes during *in vitro* percutaneous absorption, *Toxicol. Appl. Pharmacol.,* **118,** 73–79.

HOOD, H.L. and BRONAUGH, R.L., (1999) A comparison of skin viability assays for *in vitro* skin absorption/metabolism studies, *In Vitro and Mol. Toxicol.,* **12,** 3–9.

KAPPUS, H. (1989) Drug metabolism in the skin. In GREAVES, M.W. and SCHUSTER, S. (eds) *Pharmacology of the Skin II.* New York: Springer-Verlag, 123–163.

KENNEY, G.E., SAKR, A., LICHTIN, J.L., CHOU, H. and BRONAUGH, R.L. (1995) *In vitro* absorption and metabolism of Padimate-O and a nitrosamine formed in Padimate-O containing cosmetic products, *J. Soc. Cosmet. Chem.,* **46,** 117–127.

KRAELING, M.E.K., LIPICKY, R.J. and BRONAUGH, R.L. (1996) Metabolism of benzocaine during percutaneous absorption in the hairless guinea pig: Acetylbenzocaine formation and activity, *Skin Pharmacol.*, **9**, 221–230.

MAY, S.R. and DECLEMENT, F.A. (1981) Skin banking. Part III Cadaveric allograft skin viability, *J. Burn Care Rehab.*, **2**, 128–141.

MUKHTAR, H. and BICKERS, D.R. (1981) Drug Metabolism in Skin, *Drug Metab. Dispos.* **9**, 311–314.

NATHAN, D., SAKR, A., LICHTIN, J.L. and BRONAUGH, R.L. (1990) *In vitro* skin absorption and metabolism of benzoic acid, p-aminobenzoic acid, and benzocaine in the hairless guinea pig, *Pharm. Res.*, **7**, 1147–1151.

NG, K.M.E., CHU, I., BRONAUGH, R.L., FRANKLIN, C.A. and SOMERS, D.A. (1991) Percutaneous absorption/metabolism of phenanthrene in the hairless guinea pig: Comparison of *in vitro* and *in vivo* results, *Fund. Appl. Toxicol.*, **16**, 517–524.

NG, K.M.E., CHU, I., BRONAUGH, R.L., FRANKLIN, C.A. and SOMERS, D.A. (1992) Percutaneous absorption and metabolism of pyrene, benzo[a]pyrene, and di(2-ethylhexyl) phthalate: Comparison of *in vitro* and *in vivo* results in the hairless guinea pig, *Toxicol. Appl. Pharmacol.*, **115**, 216–223.

PANNATIER, A., JENNER, P., TESTA, B. and ETTER, J.C. (1978) The skin as a drug-metabolizing organ, *Drug Metab. Rev.* **8**, 319–343.

STORM, J.E., COLLIER, S.W., STEWART, R.F. and BRONAUGH, R.L. (1990) Metabolism of xenobiotics during percutaneous penetration: Role of absorption rate and cutaneous enzyme activity, *Fund. Appl. Toxicol.*, **15**, 132–141.

YOURICK, J.J. and BRONAUGH, R.L. (2000) Percutaneous penetration and metabolism of 2-nitro-p-phenylenediamine in human and fuzzy rat skin, *Toxicol. Appl. Pharmacol.*, **166**, 13–23.

Transdermal Drug Delivery Systems: Dermatologic and Other Adverse Reactions

CHERYL LEVIN AND HOWARD I MAIBACH

Contents

34.1 Introduction

34.2 Scopolamine

34.3 Clonidine

34.4 Nitroglycerin

34.5 Nicotine

34.6 Estradiol

34.7 Estrogen/progesterone

34.8 Testosterone

34.9 Fentanyl

34.10 Future

34.1 INTRODUCTION

Transdermal therapeutic systems (TTS) provide an effective method to deliver certain drugs through skin. Lipophilic drugs with relatively high potency and high volume of distribution are promising candidates for transcutaneous delivery. Currently, eight TTS are marketed (scopolamine, clonidine, nitroglycerin, nicotine, estradiol, estradiol/progesterone, and fentanyl) (Hogan and Cottam, 1991). Transdermal delivery provides a constant, controlled amount of drug, and eliminates the gastrointestinal and hepatic "first-pass" metabolism experienced with oral medication. Other advantages include the avoidance of high peak levels in achieving a steady state concentration and increased patient compliance. Although beneficial, these devices have adverse effects. One major limitation in transdermal delivery is allergic contact dermatitis. This delayed hypersensitivity reaction may result from various components of the TTS, namely the drug, its vehicle, or the adhesive used to secure the TTS to the skin (Ademola and Maibach, 1997). Other skin-related side effects from transdermal systems include irritant dermatitis, hypo- or hyperpigmentation, erythema, pruritis and excoriation.

34.2 SCOPOLAMINE

Scopolamine, the first drug to be delivered transdermally, is currently used to treat motion sickness and postoperative nausea (Brown and Langer, 1988; Stromberg, 1991). As opposed to other transdermal systems which are applied to the thick-skinned trunk, scopolamine is applied to the thin-skinned postauricular area.

There have been few reported cases of allergic contact dermatitis with this TTS (Fisher, 1984) (Trozak, 1985) (Van der Willigen *et al.*, 1988). Gordon *et al.* reported delayed type hypersensitivity reactions in an unexpectedly high rate (10 percent) of users (Gordon *et al.*, 1989). However, the report's high results may reflect the subjects wearing the patch for a prolonged period. Patch tests have confirmed that scopolamine is the sensitizing agent in most cases. No reported systemic contact dermatitis cross reactions to atropine have occurred (Trozak, 1985). Allergic contact dermatitis may be confirmed by patch testing 1 percent scopolamine in petrolatum or water (Fisher, 1984).

Irritant contact dermatitis (ICD) has been reported with both placebo and active scopolamine patches (Homick *et al.*, 1983). Atopic dermatitis or other active dermatitis patients are particularly susceptible to scopolamine-induced

ICD. The incidence of ICD is directly proportional to the period of occlusion. Repetitive patch application to the same site also contributes to an increased incidence of ICD.

There are also many non-dermatologic side effects associated with transdermal scopolamine, mostly associated with scopolamine's anticholinergic effects. The most common scopolamine-induced adverse events are visual disturbances and dry mouth, which occurs in 18 percent and 8 percent of patients taking the TTS, respectively (Kranke *et al.*, 2002). Anisocoria, due to the transfer of medication from the medication disk to the patient's eye (i.e. by rubbing the patch and then one's eyes), has been reported in several cases (Carlston, 1982; Rodor *et al.*, 1989). Scopolamine has also precipitated glaucoma in a few instances; therefore, it is recommended to avoid its usage in patients predisposed to glaucoma.

Children and the elderly should also avoid usage of scopolamine patches due to the associated delirium in these patients (Anon, 2001). Delirious patients may fail to remember that the patches contain medicine and may not follow guidelines as to their usage. Patients with acetylcholine deficiency should exert particular caution in using scopolamine patches as this may lead to an overdose of the anticholinergic effect and may produce a delirious state (MacEwan *et al.*, 1985).

Finally, application of scopolamine patch for longer than three days may result in scopolamine withdrawal syndrome. Symptoms include nausea, vomiting, paresthesias of extremities and intermittent sweating (Saxena and Saxena, 1990). Withdrawal symptoms often resolve within hours of removal of the scopolamine patch. Severe cases of physiological chemical dependency may require hospitalization. Tapered reduction is necessary to prevent severe withdrawal symptoms in these patients.

34.3 CLONIDINE

Clonidine is a centrally acting alpha-adrenoreceptor agonist used for the treatment of hypertension. It also has efficacy in smoking cessation, reduction of post-orchiectomy hot flashes, alcohol withdrawal, and reduction of spinal spasticity. Although early allergencity tests in guinea pigs failed to identify clonidine as a sensitizer, once accessible many users developed allergic contact dermatitis (Shaw *et al.*, 1987). Therefore, some claim that weak allergens occluding the skin may not be identified with routine guinea pig models (Scheper *et al.*, 1990). Others suggest that the immunosuppressive effects of clonidine on the induction of sensitization in unrelated allergens may account for the inability to detect clonidine sensitization with acute exposure (Robinson, 1990). Kalish *et al.* has developed another predictive model of clonidine sensitization (among other weak allergens) using CBA/J mice (Kalish, 1996).

Compliance with transdermal clonidine therapy is high and patients commonly prefer it to oral therapy. However, local severe skin reactions commonly occur and are the most frequent reason for discontinuing transdermal clonidine treatment (Prisant, 2002). Erythema, pruritis, scaling, excoriation, vesiculation, induration and allergic contact dermatitis have been associated with transdermal clonidine utilization in up to 50 percent of cases (Boekhorst, 1983; Grattan and Kennedy, 1985; Groth *et al.*, 1985; Maibach, 1987; Horning *et al.*, 1988; Fillingim *et al.*, 1989; Corazza *et al.*, 1995; Polster *et al.*, 1999). Hyper- and hypopigmentation have also occurred. The incidence of skin reactions increased with the dose and duration of use. Only 2 to 3 percent of topically sensitized patients experience systemic reactions when challenged with oral clonidine (Maibach, 1985; Corazza *et al.*, 1995). Therefore, the current recommendation is to continue oral treatment when topical application is no longer feasible. Clinical studies suggest that the incidence of sensitization to allergic contact dermatitis is higher in females and lower in blacks (Holdiness, 1989).

A majority of studies record sensitization from clonidine itself. However, Corazza *et al.* reported a patient with allergy to the TTS *in toto* and not to the recommended concentrations of the drug itself (Corazza *et al.*, 1995). This hypersensitivity reaction may be due to an impure compound formation resulting from the interaction of clonidine and acetaldehyde, a component of the TTS (Holdiness, 1989). Dermatitis from other components of the transdermal patch has rarely been reported. One patient with concomitant mycosis fungiosis developed allergic contact dermatitis from a clonidine patch (Polster *et al.*, 1999). The etiology of the ACD could not be determined as patch testing was not performed. The current recommendation for patch testing is 9 percent clonidine in petrolatum (Hogan and Cottam, 1991). The dermatotoxicologic experience with clonidine led to the observation that predictive assays (Draize Repeat Insult Patch test) for transdermals may need to be twelve weeks rather than the typical 6 weeks (unpublished data).

Unsubstantiated reports suggest that skin pretreatment with hydrocortisone, an aluminum-magnesia suspension, or the anti-inflammatory beclomethasone dipropionate reduces the clonidine-induced contact dermatitis in sensitized patients (McChesney, 1991). A study by Silva *et al.* tested a 0.1 ml maalox suspension (of alumina, magnesia and simethicone). Thin application of the

CHAPTER 34

pretreatment solution to back skin prior to application of the clonidine TTS reduced dermatitis in one patient and prevented the type IV hypersensitivity reaction in the other two patients. Clonidine's hypertensive effect was maintained (Silva and Berman, 1992). Hydrocortisone pre-application has been found to increase the absorption of clonidine, although the exact mechanism has yet to be elucidated (Ito and O'Conner, 1991). Further studies must be performed to investigate the effects of various skin pretreatment drugs on the development of ACD from clonidine TTS.

Side effects not directly skin-related include dry mouth, sedation, dizziness, lethargy and constipation. Systemic side effects have been reported in children who chew or ingest the clonidine patch (Caravati and Bennett, 1988; Corneli et al., 1989; Harris, 1990; Yablon and Sipiski, 1993). There have also been two case reports of children developing systemic toxicity following dermal clonidine exposure (Reed and Hamburg, 1986).

34.4 NITROGLYCERIN

The topically applied prophylactic anti-anginal drug nitroglycerin has rarely caused allergic contact dermatitis (Vaillant et al., 1990; de la Fuente et al., 1994). Irritant reactions have been observed in about 15 percent of cases, though erythema has often been attributed to nitroglycerin's vasodilatory effect and not to allergy or irritation (Vaillant et al., 1990).

None of the 3273 patients participating in a large cohort study presented with a nitroglycerin-induced hypersensitivity reaction (Harari et al., 1987; Carmichael and Foulds, 1989). Similarly, a prospective study of 33 patients found that none experienced ACD (Vaillant et al., 1990). Kounis et al. reported four of 320 (1.2 percent) patients with an allergic reaction from a nitroglycerin patch, including one generalized anaphylactic response (Kounis et al., 1996).

In the past decade, only four isolated cases of ACD from nitroglycerin TTS have been reported (Carmichael and Foulds, 1989; Di Landro et al., 1989; Torres et al., 1992; Machet et al., 1999). Nitroglycerin was responsible for the dermatitis in two of these cases (Carmichael and Foulds, 1989; Torres et al., 1992) while one case reported allergy to the TTS in toto but not to a placebo patch or nitroglycerin (Di Landro et al., 1989). Patch testing was not performed in the final case report, though the dermatitis was observed in two transdermal systems (Machet et al., 1999).

Reaction to the TTS system but not to nitroglycerin is rare (Carmichael and Foulds, 1989; Torres et al., 1992; Wainright et al., 1993). It has been hypothesized that the complex composition of the patch could be responsible for the dermatitis. The nitroglycerin patch consists of nitroglycerin adsorbed on lactose and bathed in a medical silicone fluid. The rate controlling membrane is made of an ethylene vinyl acetate copolymer. Individual components of the TTS should be tested to determine the etiology of the hypersensitivity reaction. Finnish occupational ACD reports suggest patch testing with 0.5–2 percent nitroglycerin in petrolatum (Kanerva *et al.*, 1991).

Patients who experience ACD to transdermal nitroglycerin generally do not develop ACD when given oral glycerlyl trinitrate. Nevertheless, it is recommended that patients allergic to the nitroglycerin patches are patch tested before oral glyceryl trinitrate is given.

It is important to remove transdermal nitroglycerin patches before defibrillating a patient because of the potential for explosions. There was one case report of a first-degree burn in a man who was defibrillated without removing the patch (Panacek *et al.*, 1992). Another case report describes the development of second-degree burns in a man who wore a transdermal nitroglycerin patch and stood too close to a leaky microwave oven (Murray, 1984). It was originally assumed that the explosion occurred when the microwave radiation heated the metallic element in the disk; a subsequent study found that this was unlikely to be the cause (Mosley *et al.*, 1990).

34.5 NICOTINE

The nicotine patch has been implicated in adverse skin reactions, including allergic contact dermatitis. Up to 50 percent of patients have experienced localized skin reactions such as erythema, burning, or itching upon application of the patch (Abelin *et al.*, 1989; Transdermal Nicotine Study Group, 1991). Generally, the skin irriation is minor and may be treated with topical 1 percent hydrocortisone. The cutaneous pharmacologic effects of nicotine are extensively reviewed by E. Smith *et al.* (1992).

In a majority of hypersensitivity reactions from this TTS, the active drug nicotine has been responsible. One study involving 183 heavy smokers reported a 2.6 percent incidence of ACD from nicotine among patients using transdermal patches (Eichelberg *et al.*, 1989). Similar results in a JAMA study found 16 of 664 patients (2.4 percent) with nicotine allergy to the TTS, 11 of whom were confirmed by rechallenge (Abelin *et al.*, 1989). Finally, Jordan *et al.* reported three of 186 subjects exhibiting evidence of delayed contact sensititzation to ACD (Jordan, 1992). However, in each of these studies, patch testing was not performed, and therefore allergy to other components of the TTS cannot be ruled out. In contrast, 5 of 14 volunteers with a history of adverse skin reactions to TTS experienced sensitization to nicotine, as confirmed by patch testing. One individual reacted to the patch itself (Bircher *et al.*, 1991).

There have also been several case reports of ACD from nicotine patches (Farm, 1993; Fiore and Hartman, 1993; Vincenzi *et al.*, 1993; Dwyer and Forsyth, 1994; von Bahr and Wahlberg, 1997). Patch testing confirmed nicotine as the responsible agent in a majority of these cases (Farm, 1993; Vincenzi, Tosti *et al.*, 1993). One report involved systemic reactions, including papulovesicular rashes in places of high pressure from underwear. The switch to nicotine gum induced further systemic spread to the legs and feet (Farm, 1993).

Two reports suggest that components of the patch itself are cause for the allergic response. However, patch testing was performed only in one of these cases, which found methacrylates to be the causative agent (Dwyer and Forsyth, 1994).

Patients displaying symptoms of ACD should be patch tested to confirm the source of the allergy. The observed erythema may not be an allergic reaction at all, but may result from the vasodilatory effect of nicotine, as was reported in one case (von Bahr and Wahlberg, 1997). The recommended test agent and concentration for patch testing is an aqueous solution of 10 percent nicotine base (Bircher *et al.*, 1991; Vincenzi *et al.*, 1993). Patients who are confirmed allergic to the nicotine patch should be advised against smoking cigarettes to avoid a potentially serious systemic response.

Patients with severe angina pectoris, serious arrhythmias and those immediately post-myocardial infarction should be advised against using the nicotine patches. Nicotine excess and nicotine withdrawal produce similar side effects, including insomnia, dizziness, anxiety, irritability, fatigue and stomach upset (Hogan and Cottam, 1991).

34.6 ESTRADIOL

Useful in suppressing hot flashes among postmenopausal women, estradiol patches are a source of skin irritation among 2–>25 percent of users (Utian, 1987; McCarthy *et al.*, 1992; The transdermal HRT investigators group, 1993; de Cetina and Reyes, 1999). Adverse skin reactions are more prevalent in tropical climates (Bhathena *et al.*, 1998; de Cetina and Reyes, 1999), probably due to the increased occlusive effects of the warm, humid environment. Erythema and cutaneous irritation may be responsible for the discontinuance of transdermal estradiol in 2–7 percent of women. Prolonged local hyperpigmentation in estradiol users has been reported in two patients. One patient experienced UVB-induced hyperpigmentation (to treat an unrelated skin disorder) while wearing an estradiol patch.

Two types of estradiol TTS are currently marketed. The drug reservoir system is composed of a reservoir containing the drug, a rate-limiting membrane and an adhesive. The newer matrix system eliminates the alcohol-based reservoir and incorporates the estrogen into the adhesive. Matrix patches may cause fewer skin reactions than reservoir patches according to both unsubstantiated and published reports (The transdermal HRT investigators group, 1993; Howie and Heimer, 1995; Ross et al., 1997).

There have been several reported cases of allergic contact dermatitis from transdermally applied estradiol. Most studies implicate a component of the TTS and not estradiol as the sensitizing agent. Several reports of allergic contact dermatitis from the receptacle constituents (McBurney et al., 1989), ethanol (Pecquet et al., 1992; Grebe et al., 1993), or a component of the drug reservoir (Torres et al., 1992) such as hydroxypropyl cellulose (Schwartz and Clendenning, 1988), have been recorded. In one patient, there was a putative cross-reactivity between the propylene glycol vehicle used in acyclovir cream 5 percent used to treat herpes simplex labialis infection and the hydroxypropyl cellulose in an estradiol patch (Corazza et al., 1993). The two compounds share a chemical similarity and propylene glycol has been indicated in inducing sensitization by other allergens (Hannuksela, 1987).

ACD from estradiol TTS has been confirmed by patch testing in only four reported cases (Boehnicke and Gall, 1996; El-Sayed et al., 1996; Goncalo et al., 1999), with two reporting systemic effects as well (Goncalo et al., 1999; Corazza et al., 2002). However, estradiol was the probable sensitizing agent in other unsubstantiated reports (McBurney et al., 1989; Carmichael and Foulds, 1992; Quince et al., 1996). Thus far there is no declared vehicle and concentration for patch testing, though two studies have found testing in 96 percent ethanol to be appropriate (Boehnicke and Gall, 1996; Goncalo et al., 1999).

As with other estrogen replacement therapies, the most commonly reported side effects include breast tenderness, headache, nausea and abdominal pain. Recent studies indicate that hormone replacement therapy, including transdermal estradiol, may not provide benefit to all post-menopausal patients (Women's Health Initiative randomized controlled trial, 2002).

■ CHAPTER 34 ■

34.7 ESTROGEN/PROGESTERONE

Most recently, a combination estrogen/progesterone patch was developed for use as a transdermal contraceptive. Side effects are typical of hormonal contraception. They include irritant reactions, nausea, emotional lability, headache and breast discomfort. To date, there have been no reported cases of allergic contact dermatitis to the estrogen/progesterone contaceptive patch.

34.8 TESTOSTERONE

The testosterone transdermal patch may be applied to scrotal or glabrous skin. Scrotal skin allows the highest rate of percutaneous absorption for steroids and thus can be utilized to deliver higher levels of drug (Bals-Pratch et al., 1986). In order to improve adhesion to the scrotal skin, the area must be shaved before applying the patch. This may lead to skin irritation at the application site.

There is only one confirmed case of allergic contact dermatits from TTS testosterone, a system utilized to treat hypogonadal men (Buckley et al., 1997). A man with Kleinefelter's syndrome became allergic to the testosterone within the nonscrotal TTS (Andropatch), as validated by patch testing. A mild allergic reaction to one of the patch excipients also occurred in one patient. The reaction involved a mild transient erythema. A large cohort study by Jordan compared irritation and allergy associated with nonscrotal and scrotal transdermal systems in 60 healthy adult males (Jordan, 1997). The incidence of irritation and allergy were significantly higher ($p<0.0001$) in the nonscrotal system, although patch testing was not performed. Further studies are necessary to understand the adverse effects of various components of both scrotal and nonscrotal TTS on skin.

Some men may experience fluid retention, acne, and temporary gynecosmastia resulting from the testosterone patch (Kohn et al., 2000).

34.9 FENTANYL

The opioid fentanyl is used as a pre-anesthetic analgesic and to relieve patients in chronic pain (Calis, 1992). There are currently no reported cases of ACD from fentanyl. Adverse skin reactions include pruritis, erythema and a diffuse, nonpruritic papular rash. Though these reactions are due to irritation and not an allergic response, they may persist for several days due to the drug depository left in the skin (Calis, 1992). Similar skin reactions have occurred in other transdermal systems, and are most likely due to a component of the patch and not the drug itself. Bacterial or fungal overgrowth may also be responsible for the irritant reaction. Pretreatment with chlorhexidine may reduce irritation by preventing bacterial overgrowth.

Respiratory depression is the most serious adverse event associated with transdermal fentanyl. Hypoventilation has been described in approximately 2 percent of cancer patients using the fentanyl patch. Death occurred in one fentanyl user who slept on a heated waterbed (Press, 1993). The cutaneous hyperthermia resulted in increased fentanyl uptake and systemic toxicity. Systemic toxicity leading to respiratory depression also occurred in one patient who abused the opioid by scraping the contents of a fentanyl patch and smoking it (Marquardt and Tharratt, 1993). Twenty-eight to 84 percent of the original drug amount may be present following therapeutic use (Marquardt et al., 1995). Patches must be disposed of properly to prevent potential abuse. Direct body contact leading to secondary systemic toxicity has been reported. A child experienced respiratory depression when a fentanyl patch worn by his grandmother was transferred to him during the night (Hardwick et al., 1997). Naloxone should immediately be given to patients experiencing fentanyl toxicity.

34.10 FUTURE

The advantages associated with TTS, including avoidance of the first-pass metabolism, elimination of "peaks and valleys" and improved patient compliance, have led to continual interest in the development of new transdermal systems. Some transdermal systems that may be available in the US in the near future include insulin (Sen et al., 2002) and asthma (Kato et al., 2002) medication.

The current transdermal delivery systems are useful for delivering small, lipophilic molecules through the skin. However, there are many compounds that do not meet these requirements. New techniques are being developed to allow the transfer of hydrophilic, charged drugs through the skin. "Active" transdermal drug delivery involves utilizing external driving forces on the stratum corneum in order to allow penetration of the molecule of interest (Barry, 2001).

Electrically-assisted methods include iontophoresis, phonophoresis, electroporation, magnetophoresis, and photochemical waves. Iontophoresis passes an electric current through the skin and thereby provides the driving force to enable penetration of ions into the skin (Singh *et al.*, 1995). The development of transdermal insulin may require the use of iontophoresis (Rastogi and Singh, 2002). Phonophoresis utilizes ultrasound energy to enhance drug penetration. Higher frequency energy enables greater penetration but also is associated with greater adverse events. Electroporation uses strong, brief pulses of electric current to punch holes in the stratum corneum. These holes close 1 to 30 minutes following the electrical stimulus (Banga and Prausntiz, 1998). Electroporation coupled with iontophoresis may be helpful in the delivery of some drugs (Badkar *et al.*, 1999). The application of high gradient magnetic fields and vibrational forces to biological systems is termed magnetophoresis. Magnetophoresis may be effective in the delivery of terbutaline sulfate (TS), a drug widely used for the treatment of acute and chronic bronchitis patients (Narasimha and Shobha Rani, 1999). Laser-induced stress waves, known as photochemical waves, may also be of benefit in drug delivery.

Hydrating agents and chemical enhancers also increase pore size to enhance drug delivery. Moisturizers are the primary hydrating agents. There are numerous chemical enhancers, including benzalkonium chloride, oleyl alcohol and alphaterpineol (Monti *et al.*, 2001). Transdermal delivery may be most improved utilizing a combination of chemical enhancers and electically-assisted devices (Terahara *et al.*, 2002).

The stratum corneum may also be removed or bypassed utilizing ablation, microneedles or follicular delivery. Pulsed CO_2 lasers are used in tissue ablation to damage the skin. Microneedle enhanced transdermal drug delivery also damages the skin by creating channels for drug diffusion across the stratum corneum. The existing needles are 150 microns long and leave holes about one micron in diameter when removed from the skin. Originally developed for the microelectronics industry, the tiny needles can avoid causing pain because they penetrate only the outermost layer of skin that contains no nerve endings (Henry *et al.*, 1998). Follicular media include liposomes, ethosomes, transfersomes and niosomes. While passive transdermal systems have been on the market for more than twenty years, active transdermal systems are still not available for clinical use. Further clinical trials are needed to evaluate the safety and efficacy of the active transdermal products.

REFERENCES

ANON (2001) Scopolamine: new preparations. Reference treatment for death rattle. *Prescrire Int.* **10**(54), 99–101.

ABELIN, T., BUEHLER, A., *et al.* (1989) Controlled trial of transdermal nicotine patch in tobacco withdrawal. *Lancet.* **1**(8628), 7–10.

ADEMOLA, J. and MAIBACH, H. (1997) Safety assessment of transdermal and topical dermatological products. In GHOSH, T., PFISTER, W. and YUM, S. (eds) *Transdermal and Topical Drug Delivery Systems.* Buffalo Grove: Interpharm Press.

BADKAR, A., BETAGERI, G., *et al.* (1999) Enhancement of transdermal iontophoretic delivery of a liposomal formulation of colchicine by electroporation. *Drug Delivery.* **6**, 111–115.

BALS-PRATCH, M., YOON, Y., *et al.* (1986) Transdermal testosterone substitution therapy for male hypogonadism. *Lancet.* **2**, 943–946.

BANGA, A. and PRAUSNTIZ, M. (1998) Assessing the potential of skin electroporation for the delivery of protein- and gene-based drugs. *Trends Biotechnol.* **16**, 408–412.

BARRY, B. (2001) Novel mechanisms and devices to enable successful transdermal drug delivery. *Eur. J. Pharm. Sci.* **14**(2), 101–114.

BHATHENA, R., ANKLESARIA, B., *et al.* (1998) The influence of transdermal oestradiol replacement therapy and medroxyprogesterone acetate on serum lipids and lipoproteins. *Br. J. Pharmacol.* **45**(2), 170–172.

BIRCHER, A., HOWALD, H., *et al.* (1991) Adverse skin reactions to nicotine in a transdermal therapeutic system. *Contact Derm.* **25**(4), 230–236.

BOEHNICKE, W.-H. and GALL, H. (1996) Type IV hypersensitivity to topical estradiol in a patient tolerant to it orally. *Contact Derm.* **35**, 187–188.

BOEKHORST, J. (1983) Allergic contact dermatitis with transdermal clonidine. *Lancet.* **2**, 1031–1032.

BROWN, L. and LANGER, R. (1988) Transdermal delivery of drugs. *Annual Review of Medicine* **39**, 221–229.

BUCKLEY, D., WILKINSON, S., *et al.* (1997) Contact allergy to a testosterone patch. *Contact Dermatitis.* **39**, 91–92.

CALIS, K. (1992) Transdermally administered fentanyl for pain management. *Clin. Pharmacokinet.* **11**(1), 22–36.

CARAVATI, E. and BENNETT, D. (1988) Clonidine transdermal patch poisoning. *Ann. Emerg. Med.* **17**(2), 175–176.

CARLSTON, J. (1982) Unilateral dilated pupil from scopolamine disk. *J. Am. Med Assoc.* **248**, 31.

CARMICHAEL, A. and FOULDS, I. (1989) Allergic contact dermatitis from transdermal nitroglycerin. *Contact Dermatitis.* **21**, 113–114.

■ CHAPTER 34 ■

CARMICHAEL, A. and FOULDS, I. (1992) Allergic contact dermatitis from estradiol in oestrogen patches. *Contact Derm.* **26**, 194–195.

CORAZZA, M., MANTOVANI, L., *et al.* (1995) Allergic contact dermatitis from a clonidine transdermal delivery system. *Contact Derm.* **32**(4), 246.

CORAZZA, M., MANTOVANI, L., *et al.* (2002) Allergic contact dermatitis from transdermal estradiol and systemic contact dermatitis from oral estradiol. A case report. *J. Reprod. Med.* **47**(6), 507–509.

CORAZZA, M., VIRGILI, A., *et al.* (1993) Propylene glycol allergy from acyclovir cream with cross-reactivity to hydroxypropyl cellulose in a transdermal estradiol system. *Contact Derm.* **29**, 283–284.

CORNELI, H.M., BANNER, W. W., VERNON, D.D. and SWENSON, P.H. (1989) Toddler eats clonidine patch and nearly quits smoking for life. *JAMA.* **261**(1), 42.

DE CETINA, T. and REYES, L. (1999) Skin reactions to transdermal estrogen replacement therapy in a tropical climate. *Int. J. Gynaecol. Obstet.* **64**(1), 71–72.

DE LA FUENTE, P. R., MEDINA, A., *et al.* (1994) Contact dermatitis from nitroglycerin. *Annals of Allergy* **72**, 344–346.

DI LANDRO, A., VALSECCHI, R., *et al.* (1989) Contact dermatitis from Nitroderm. *Contact Derm.* **21**(2), 115–116.

DWYER, C. and FORSYTH, A. (1994) Allergic contact dermatitis from methacrylates in a nicotine transdermal patch. *Contact Derm.* **30**, 309–310.

EICHELBERG, D., STOLZE, P., *et al.* (1989) Contact allergies induced by TTS-treatment. *Methods Find. Exp. Clin. Pharmacol.* **11**(3), 223–225.

EL-SAYED, F., BAYLE-LEBEY, P., *et al.* (1996) Sensibilisation systemique au 17-B-oestradiol induite par voie transcutanee. *Ann Dermatol. Venereol.* **123**, 26–28.

FARM, G. (1993) Contact allergy to nicotine from a nicotine patch. *Contact Derm.* **29**(4), 214–215.

FILLINGIM, J.M, MATZEK, K.M., HUGHES, E.M., JOHNSON, P.A., SHARON, G.S. (1989) Long-term treatment with transdermal clonidine in mild hypertension. *Clin. Ther.* **11**(3), 398–408.

FIORE, M. and HARTMAN, M. (1993) Side effects of nicotine patches. *JAMA.* **270**, 2735.

FISHER, A. (1984) Dermatitis due to therapeutic systems. *Cutis.* **34**, 526–531.

GONCALO, M., OLIVEIRA, H., *et al.* (1999) Allergic and systemic contact dermatitis from estradiol. *Contact Derm.* **40**, 58–59.

GORDON, D., SHUPAK, A., *et al.* (1989) Allergic contact dermatitis caused by transdermal hyoscine. *Br. J. Dermatol.* **298**, 1220–1226.

GRATTAN, C. and KENNEDY, C. (1985) Allergic contact dermatitis to transdermal clonidine. *Contact Derm.* **19**, 225–226.

GREBE, S., ADAMS, J., *et al.* (1993) Systemic sensitization ot ethanol by transdermal estrogen patches. *Arch. Dermatol.* **129**, 379–380.

GROTH, H., VETTER, H., *et al.* (1985) Transdermal clonidine in essential hypertension: Problems during long-term treatment. In WEBER, M., DRAYER, I. and KOLLOCH, R. (eds) *Low Dose Oral and Transdermal Therapy of Hypertension.* Darmstadt: Steinkopff Verlag, 60–65.

HANNUKSELA, M. (1987) Propylene glycol promotes allergic patch test reactions. *Bollettino di Dermatologia Allergologica e Professionale.* **2**, 40–44.

HARARI, Z., SOMMER, I., *et al.* (1987) Multifocal contact dermatitis to Nitroderm TTS 5 with extensive postinflammatory hypermelanosis. *Dermatologica.* **174**, 249–252.

HARDWICK, W., KING, W., *et al.* (1997) Respiratory depression in a child unintentionally exposed to transdermal fentanyl patch. *South. Med. J.* **90**(9), 962–964.

HARRIS, J. (1990) Clonidine patch toxicity. *DICP.* **24**(12), 1191–1194.

HENRY, S., MCALLISTER, D., *et al.* (1998) Microfabricated microneedles: a novel approach to transdermal drug delivery. *J Pharm. Sci.* **87**(8), 922–925.

HOGAN, D. and COTTAM, J. (1991) Dermatological aspects of transdermal drug delivery systems. In MARZULLI, F. and MAIBACH, H. (eds) *Dermatotoxicology.* Washington DC: Taylor and Francis, 75–86.

HOLDINESS, M. (1989) A review of contact dermatitis associated with transdermal therapeutic systems. *Contact Derm.* **20**(1), 3–9.

HOMICK, J., KOHL, R., *et al.* (1983) Transdermal scopolamine in the prevention of motion sickness: Evaluation of the time course and efficacy. *Aviat. Space Environ. Med.* **54**, 994–1000.

HORNING, J., ZAWADA JR, E., *et al.* (1988) Efficacy and safety of two-year therapy with transdermal clonidine for essential hypertension. *Chest.* **93**, 941–945.

HOWIE, H. and HEIMER, G. (1995) A multicenter randomized parallel group study comparing a new estradiol matrix patch and a registered reservoir patch. *Menopause.* **2**, 43–48.

ITO, M. and O'CONNER, D. (1991) Skin pretreatment and the use of transdermal clonidine. *Am. J. Med.* **91**(1A), 42S–49S.

■ CHAPTER 34 ■

JORDAN, W. J. (1997) Allergy and topical irritation associated with transdermal testosterone administration: a comparison of scrotal and nonscrotal transdermal systems. *Am. J. Cont Derm.* **8**(2), 108–113.

JORDAN, W. P. (1992) Clinical evaluation of the contact sensitization potential of a transdermal nicotine system (Nicoderm). *J. Fam. Pract.* **34**(6), 709–712.

KALISH, R., WOOD, J.A., WILLE, J.J., KYDONIEUS, A. (1996) Sensitization of mice to topically applied drugs: albuterol, chlorpheniramine, clonidine and nadolol. *Contact Derm.* **35**(2), 76–82.

KANERVA, L., LAINE, R., *et al.* (1991) Occupational allergic contact dermatitis caused by nitroglycerin. *Contact Dermatitis.* **24**(5), 356–362.

KATO, H., NAGATA, O., *et al.* (2002) [Development of transdermal formulation of tulobuterol for the treatment of bronchial asthma]. *Yakugaku Zasshi.* **122**(1), 57–69.

KOHN, F., RING, J., *et al.* (2000) [Dermatologic aspects of male hypogonadism] [Article in German]. *Hautarzt.* **51**(4), 223–230.

KOUNIS, N., ZAVRAS, G., *et al.* (1996) Allergic reactions to local glyceryl trinitrate administration. *Br. J. Clin. Pract.* **50**(8), 437–439.

KRANKE, P., MORIN, A., *et al.* (2002) The efficacy and safety of transdermal scopolamine for the prevention of postoperative nausea and vomiting: a quantitative systematic review. *Anesth. Analg.* **95**, 133–143.

MACEWAN, G., WILLIAM, R., *et al.* (1985) Psychosis due to transdermally administered scopolamine. *Can. Med. Assoc.* **133**, 4331–4332.

MACHET, L., MARTIN, L., *et al.* (1999) Allergic contact dermatitis from nitroglycerin contained in 2 transdermal systems. *Dermatology.* **198**(1), 106–107.

MAIBACH, H. (1985) Clonidine: irritant and allergic contact dermatitis assays. *Contact Derm.* **12**(4), 192–195.

MAIBACH, H. (1987) Oral substitution in patients sensitized by transdermal clonidine treatment. *Contact Derm.* **16**, 1–8.

MARQUARDT, K. and THARRATT, R. (1993) Fentanyl smokes. *Vet. Hum. Toxicol.* **35**, 362.

MARQUARDT, K., THARRATT, R., *et al.* (1995) Fentanyl remaining in a transdermal system following 3 days of continuous use. *Ann. Pharmacother.* **29**, 969–971.

MCBURNEY, E., NOEL, S., *et al.* (1989) Contact dermatitis to transdermal estradiol system. *J. Am. Acad. Dematol.* **20**, 508–510.

McCarthy, T., Dramusic, V., *et al.* (1992) Use of two types of estradiol-releasing skin patches for menopausal patients in a tropical climate. *Am. J. Obstet. Gynecol.* **166**, 2005–2010.

McChesney, J. (1991) Preventing the contact dermatitis caused by a transdermal clonidine patch [letter]. *West. J. Med.* **154**(6), 736.

Monti, D., Giannelli, R., *et al.* (2001) Comparison of the effect of ultrasound and of chemical enhancers on transdermal permeation of caffeine and morphine through hairless mouse skin *in vitro*. *Int. J. Pharm.* **229**(1–2), 131–137.

Mosley, H., Johnston, S., *et al.* (1990) The influence of microwave radiation on transdermal delivery systems. *Br. J. Dermatol.* **122**, 361–363.

Murray, K. (1984) Hazards of microwave ovens to transdermal delivery systems. *N. Engl. J. Med.* **310**, 721.

Narasimha, M.S. and Shobha Rani, R. (1999) Effect of magnetic field on the permeation of salbutamol sulfate and terbutaline sulfate. *Indian Drugs.* **36**, 663–664.

Panacek, E., Munger, M., *et al.* (1992) Report of nitropatch explosions complicating defibrillation. *Am. J. Emerg. Med.* **10**(2), 128–129.

Pecquet, C., Pradalier, A., *et al.* (1992) Allergic contact dermatitis from ethanol in a transdermal estradiol patch. *Contact Derm.* **27**(4), 275–276.

Polster, A., Warner, M.R., Camisa, C. (1999) Allergic contact dermatitis from transdermal clonidine in a patient with mycosis fungoides. *Cutis.* **63**(3), 154–155.

Press, A. (1993). Mother sues over painkiller patch. *Pensacola Times*, November 15: 4B.

Prisant, L. (2002) Transdermal clonidine skin reactions. *J. Clin. Hypertens.* **4**(2), 136–138.

Quince, S., Garde, A., *et al.* (1996) Allergic contact dermatitis from estradiol in a transdermal therapeutic system. *Allergy* **51**, 62–63.

Rastogi, S. and Singh, J. (2002) Transepidermal transport enhancement of insulin by lipid extraction and iontophoresis. *Pharm. Res.* **19**(4), 427–433.

Reed, M. and Hamburg, E. (1986) Person-to-person transfer of transdermal drug delivery systems: A case report. *N. Engl. J. Med.* **314**, 1120–1121.

Robinson MK, S.T. (1990) Immunosuppressive effects of clonidine on the induction of contact sensitization in the balb/c mouse. *J. Invest. Dermatol.* **95**(5), 587–591.

CHAPTER 34

RODOR, F., COTTIN, C., *et al.* (1989) [Transdermal scopolamine and mydriasis]. *Therapie.* **44**, 447–448.

ROSS, D., REES, M., *et al.* (1997) Randomised crossover comparison of skin irritation with two transdermal oestradiol patches. *Br. Med. J.* **315**(7103), 288.

SAXENA, K. and SAXENA, S. (1990) Scopolamine withdrawal syndrome. *Postgrad. Med. J.* **87**(1), 63–66.

SCHEPER, R.J., VON BLOMBERG, B.M.E., DE GROOT, J., GOEPTAR, A.R., LANG, M., OOSTENDORP, R.A., BRUYNZEEL, D.P. and VAN TOL, R.G. (1990) Low allergenicity of clonidine impedes studies of sensitization mechanisms in guinea pig models. *Contact Derm.* **23**(2), 81–89.

SCHWARTZ, B. and CLENDENNING, W. (1988) Allergic contact dermatitis from hydroxypropyl cellulose in a transdermal estradiol patch. *Contact Derm.* **18**, 106–107.

SEN, A., DALY, M., *et al.* (2002) Transdermal insulin delivery using lipid enhanced electroporation. *Biochim. Biophys. Acta.* **1564**(1), 5–8.

SHAW, J., CRAMER, M., *et al.* (1987a) Rate-controlled transdermal therapy utilizing polymeric membranes. *Transderm. Deliv. Drugs.* **1**, 102–116.

SILVA, S. and BERMAN, B. (1992) The effect of topical maalox on transdermal clonidine-induced contact dermatitis. *American Journal of Contact Dermatitis* **3**, 79–82.

Singh, P., Anliker, M., *et al.* (1995) Facilitated drug delivery during transdermal iontophoresis. *Curr. Prob. Dermatol.* **22**, 184–188.

SMITH, E., SMITH, K., *et al.* (1992) The local side effects of transdermally absorbed nicotine. *Skin Pharmacol.* **5**(2), 69–76.

STROMBERG, B. (1991) Transdermal scopolamine for the control of postoperative nausea. *American Surgeon* **57**(11), 712–715.

TERAHARA, T., MITRAGOTRI, S., *et al.* (2002) Porous resins as a cavitation enhancer for low-frequency sonophoresis. *J. Pharm. Sci. Technol.* **91**(3), 753–759.

THE TRANSDERMAL HRT INVESTIGATORS GROUP (1993) A randomized study to compare the effectiveness, tolerability and acceptability of two different transdermal estradiol replacement therapies. *Int. J. Fertil.* **38**, 5–11.

TORRES, V., LOPES, J., *et al.* (1992) Allergic contact dermatitis from nitroglycerin and estradiol transdermal therapeutic systems. *Contact Derm.* **26**(1), 53–54.

TRANSDERMAL NICOTINE STUDY GROUP (1991) *J. Am. Med. Assoc.* **266**, 3133–3138.

TROZAK, D. (1985) Delayed hypersensitivity to scopolamine delivered by a transdermal device. *J. Am. Acad. Dematol.* **13**, 247–251.

UTIAN, W. (1987) Transdermal estradiol overall safety profile. *Am. J. Obstet. Gynecol.* **156**, 1336–1338.

VAILLANT, L., BIETTE, S., *et al.* (1990) Skin acceptance of transcutaneous nitro-glycerin patches: a prospective study of 33 patients. *Contact Dermatitis.* **23**(3), 142–145.

VAN DER WILLIGEN, A., ORANJE, A., *et al.* (1988) Delayed hypersensitivity to scopolamine in transdermal therapuetic systems. *J. Am. Acad. Dematol.* **18**, 146–147.

VINCENZI, C., TOSTI, A., *et al.* (1993) Allergic contact dermatitis from transdermal nicotine systems. *Contact Derm.* **29**(2), 104–105.

VON BAHR, B. and WAHLBERG, J. (1997) Reactivity to nicotine patches wrongly blamed on contact allergy. *Contact Derm.* **37**(1), 44–45.

WAINRIGHT, R., FORAN, J., *et al.* (1993) The long-term safety and tolerability of transdermal glyceryl trinitrate, when used with a patch-free interval in patients with stable angina. *British Journal of Clinical Practice* **47**, 178–182.

WOMEN'S HEALTH INITIATIVE RANDOMIZED CONTROLLED TRIAL (2002) Risks and benefits of estrogen plus progestin in healthy post-menopausal women: principal results. *JAMA.* **288**(3), 321–333.

YABLON, S. and SIPISKI, M. (1993) Effect of transdermal clonidine on spinal spasticity. A case series. *Am. J. Phys. Med. Rehabil.* **72**(3), 154–157.

■ CHAPTER 34 ■

ANNEX

TABLE 34.1:
Allergic contact dermatitis from transdermal systems

Drug	Incidence of allergic contact dermatitis	Specific etiology	Reference
Scopolamine	Rare	The active drug in most cases	Fisher (1984); Trozak (1985); Van der Willigen et al. (1988); Gordon et al. (1989)
Clonidine	Relatively common Reported in up to 50% of cases	The active drug in most cases	Grattan et al. (1985); Groth et al. (1985); Weber et al. (1984); Boekhorst (1983); Horning et al. (1988); Maibach (1987); Fillingim et al. (1989); Corazza et al. (1995); Polster et al. (1999), 26
Nitroglycerin	Rare	The active drug in most cases	Harari et al. (1987); Carmichael (1994); Carmichael et al. (1989); Torres et al. (1992); Landro et al. (1989); Machet et al. (1999); Kounis et al. (1996); Torres et al. (1992); Wainright et al. (1993)
Nicotine	Somewhat common	The active drug in most cases	Eichelberg et al. (1989); Abelin et al. (1989); Jordan (1992); Bircher et al. (1991);Vincenzi et al. (1993); Farm (1993); Von Bahr et al. (1997); Dwyer et al. (1994); Fiore et al. (1993).
Estradiol	Relatively common	A component of the TTS other than the active drug in most cases	McBurney et al. (1989); Grebe et al., (1993); Pecquet et al. (1992); Torres et al. (1992); Schwartz et al. (1988); Corazza et al. (1993); Boehnicke et al. (1996); El-Sayed et al. (1996); Goncalo et al. (1999); Corraza et al. (2002)
Testosterone	Rare	The active drug	Buckley et al. (1997)
Fentanyl	No reported cases		

TABLE 34.2:

Overview of Adverse Reactions from Transdermal Systems

Drug	Major adverse reactions
Scopolamine	• visual disturbances and dry mouth • anisocoria • glaucoma • delirium in children and elderly • withdrawal syndrome
Clonidine	• skin reactions, including allergic contact dermatitis, erythema, pruritis, scaling, excoriation, vesiculation and induration • dry mouth • sedation • dizziness • lethargy • constipation
Nitroglycerin	• erythema • irritant contact dermatitis • potential for burns ("arc explosions")
Nicotine	• skin reactions, including allergic contact dermatitis, erythema, burning, or itching • withdrawal and excess syndrome
Nstradiol	• breast tenderness • headache • nausea • abdominal pain • erythema • irritant contact dermatitis
Estrogen/Progesterone	• irritant reactions • nausea • emotional lability • headache • breast discomfort
Testosterone	• fluid retention • acne • temporary gynecosmastia • irritant contact dermatitis
Fentanyl	• pruritis • erythema • diffuse, nonpruritic papular rash • respiratory depression

Predictive Toxicology Methods for Transdermal Delivery Systems

ANNE CHESTER, WEI-QI LIN, MARY PREVO,
MICHEL CORMIER AND JAMES MATRIANO

Contents

35.1   Introduction

35.2   Toxicology evaluation plan

35.3   Irritation

35.4   Sensitization

35.5   Summary

35.1 INTRODUCTION

Predicting potential toxicologic responses to transdermal delivery is a complex procedure, involving both traditional toxicology protocols for evaluating results of systemic exposure and topical studies assessing skin–drug interactions and reactions. Evaluation of individual drug and system components is followed by final system testing to assess possible interactions. Risk is estimated by analyzing toxicologic data quantitatively, with estimation of human exposure based on dose-response extrapolations. Formulation or system changes designed to minimize risk are evaluated. In some instances local intolerance to a compound—due either to irritation or sensitization—may preclude development of a transdermal product despite efficacious plasma levels. For viable projects with acceptable toxicologic profiles, a strategy is implemented to manage risk of irritation and sensitization. In addition to the usual drug-specific systemic toxicology and regulatory issues, a toxicology evaluation plan for transdermal dosage forms must include primary and cumulative irritation and sensitization testing. The plan must also take into account FDA's categorization of new transdermal systems as new chemical entities (NCEs) subject to standard nonclinical testing procedures.

35.2 TOXICOLOGY EVALUATION PLAN

Development of a toxicology evaluation plan for a transdermal system involves two major stages: assessment of previous experience with both the drug(s) and system components, and selection of necessary and appropriate tests. Assessment of previous experience includes review of data in the literature and in regulatory submissions available through the Freedom of Information Act. Substantial published knowledge of the drug allows analysis of the effects of various doses and regimens and generally reduces testing requirements. Information about oral, intravenous, and especially subcutaneous administration may be used for comparison or to support the safety and efficacy of transdermal delivery when equivalent plasma levels are achieved and no significant biotransformation occurs. Literature and other available data about compounds previously cleared by the US Food and Drug Administration (FDA) may be useful in determining areas for additional study. Similarly, evaluations of proposed system materials in the literature and previous FDA submissions may provide valuable information about individual system components or possible interactions of materials.

■ CHAPTER 35 ■

An additional factor in the evaluation plan is the categorization by FDA of new transdermal systems as new chemical entities (NCEs) subject to standard non-clinical testing procedures. A complete toxicology profile-including subchronic, chronic, carcinogenic, and genotoxic assays-is required for all compounds delivered transdermally. The requirement may be reduced when systems incorporate a compound already marketed in another dosage form. Transdermal systems that achieve lower plasma drug levels than other marketed forms of the drug and systems that incorporate drugs and/or components previously evaluated for irritation or topical sensitization may require few nonclinical studies.

Structure-activity relationship (SAR) and quantitative structure-activity relationship (QSAR) analyses in toxicology reveal interactions between chemicals and biological systems. These analyses help to determine whether a chemical poses a potential risk to biological systems, discover its potential cross-reactions, and evaluate the reliability of the published data. Several reports describe efforts to use structure-activity analysis predictively (Hostynek *et al.*, 1996; Basketter, 1998; Barratt and Langowski, 1999; Barratt, 2000; Barratt *et al.*, 2000; Gerberick and Robinson, 2000; McKinney *et al.*, 2000; Kodithala *et al.*, 2002). One approach is to use an expert system based on rules defining structural alerts to determine SARs in contact sensitization (Ashby *et al.*, 1995). Another is to discern the major subgroups associated with sensitization (alkylating agents, benzoylating agents, and so on) and derive QSARs for each grouping. Data for incorporation in QSAR databases can be generated by different tests, including the mouse ear sensitivity test (MEST), murine local lymph node assay (LLNA) (see Murine Models), guinea pig maximization test (GPMT), and Freund's complete adjuvant test (FCA). A systematic analysis of these data can help determine features that make a chemical a sensitizer and identify minimal structural requirements for the recognition of an allergen.

For example, an SAR model developed by Enslein and colleagues (1988) predicts probable ($p = 0.3$–0.7) severity of eye irritation for the Draize test or equivalent tests. A program incorporating modeling data allows evaluation of cyclic and noncyclic compounds and produces a composite judgment of probable eye irritation (negative, mild, moderate, and severe) with 91 to 95 percent overall accuracy, according to the product literature.

An effort to develop a comprehensive allergic contact dermatitis model involved development of a biologically based QSAR model (Hostynek *et al.*, 1996; Roberts and Basketter, 2000). The model was developed through tabulation of descriptors from structural analyses of 35 compounds known to be moderate to severe allergens, and 36 non-allergens selected from molecules of diverse structure and functionality, from formaldehyde to steroids. The method used two-value multiple regression analysis, through progressive elimination of descriptors with low statistical strength, to produce a predictive model based on five indicator variables and four continuous variables from an initial set of 22. This model successfully classified 34 of the 35 allergens (97 percent sensitivity) and 33 of the 36 non-allergens (92 percent sensitivity). *In vivo* validation of the classification model against murine LLNA data confirmed all predicted allergens and two of the three non-allergens at all concentrations tested. Limitations to the model included the use of data generated from a variety of different animal models and clinical experience, and the small pool of available data, which in most cases prevented the use of a single animal model. In addition, although classification was successful, efforts to predict allergic potency were limited by the quality of the data, the limited predictability of metabolism in the skin, and the reactivity of certain structures. Despite these limitations, QSAR classification allows an early estimation of the risk/benefit ratio-and consequently some prioritization and streamlining of the drug development process-before resources are committed to laboratory studies.

Studies of skin metabolism may also be required. Although transdermal administration bypasses hepatic circulation, molecules absorbed through the skin will come into contact with the skin's metabolic system. (For a comprehensive review of the skin's enzymatic activity, see Noonan and Wester, 1985; Steinstrasser and Merkle, 1995; Baron and Merk, 2001.) Skin metabolism may alter the delivery profile and pharmacological effects of some percutaneously absorbed compounds (Guy and Hadgraft, 1982; Boehnlein *et al.*, 1994, Hashiguchi *et al.*, 1998, Tang-Liu *et al.*, 1999; see also Chapter 10 of this book). The effects of first-pass skin metabolism of transdermally delivered compounds can be predicted by *in vitro* biotransformation studies (Cormier *et al.*, 1991; Friedberg, 1998; Brand *et al.*, 2000; Smith *et al.*, 2000; Sintov, *et al.*, 2002). The toxicology profile of compounds may be altered by the quantitative modification of metabolic pathways caused by skin metabolism (Bucks, 1984; Cleary *et al.*, 1984). These changes, which are sometimes measured by comparison with oral or intravenous data, may result in local irritation, sensitization, or adverse systemic effects. Changes resulting from skin metabolism may also transform inactive prodrugs with favorable permeation characteristics into metabolically active parent drugs (Tauber, 1989; Imoto *et al.*, 1996; Sintov *et al.*, 2002). In addition, genetic variations in the skin's enzymatic activity may account for differences in therapeutic efficacy among patients. Generally, however, the effect of the skin's first-pass metabolism is slight since skin cells have lower intrinsic metabolic activity than hepatocytes, and only a few cell layers within a limited area are perfused by a transdermally delivered compound. For example, skin metabolism of propranolol, which is metabolized extensively by the liver, was almost negligible (Cormier *et al.*, 1991).

Toxicokinetic analysis—pharmacokinetic analysis applied to dose-ranging and definitive toxicity testing—is increasingly important to determine drug exposure in nonclinical toxicology protocols for transdermal and other dosage forms, and is included in guidelines drafted by the International Conference on Harmonization (Federal Register, 1995). Toxicokinetic studies describe the relationship between systemic exposure, dose administered, and time, providing data to support safety claims at various doses. Results of these studies contribute to the design of subsequent nonclinical studies. (For protocol details for toxicokinetic studies, see Kantrowitz and Yacobi, 1994.) Because transdermal delivery of drugs bypasses the first-pass effect, the drug to metabolite ratio changes.

Phototoxicity issues may also need to be addressed with transdermal drug delivery. Although phototoxicity testing is conducted primarily in humans, both the FDA and OECD have draft guidelines for photosafety testing (including phototoxicity, photoallergy, photogenotoxicity, photocarcinogenicity) and provide decision trees to assist in the evaluation. According to the OECD, photosafety testing is indicated if the drug absorbs light between 270 and 700 nm on the UV-visible light absorption spectrum, and if the drug is topically applied or accumulates in light exposed areas. The OECD considers the *in vitro* 3T3 NRU phototoxicity assay validated and provides a test guideline. This assay can be used to evaluate the drug substance, but other testing may be required on the finished drug product. If additional *in vivo* testing is warranted, a controlled clinical trial is suggested. The FDA has stated that testing only the drug substance may be acceptable, but that the drug product (final formulation) should be tested if the product absorbs light between 290 and 700 nm as well as if the product is ". . . applied to the skin or eyes, or persist or accumulate in one of these areas, or 2) are known to affect the skin or eyes." The FDA does not specify how to test for photosafety, but acknowledges the use of *in vitro* studies, *in vivo* nonclinical studies, and human clinical studies, and encourages ". . . the submission of specific data that may help in evaluating the regulatory acceptance of such assays." The Interagency Coordinating Committee on the Validation of Alternative Methods (ICCVAM) is expected to evaluate the 3T3 *in vitro* assay, but no information is available as of this writing. The communication of risk is key; factors to consider include the half-life, acute or chronic use, pharmacologic class, and persistence in the skin (especially in areas exposed to sunlight). If the risk is sufficient, additional tests may evaluate photoallergy, photogenotoxicity, and/or photocarcinogenicity.

Polymers used in transdermal systems need to be evaluated for potential adverse effects before testing the drug delivery system in humans. Polymers used in transdermal drug delivery systems may not penetrate the skin themselves, but components of the polymer, such as residual monomers, reactive agents, or processing additives, may migrate. The effects of polymers or extracts will depend on unique chemical characteristics and the amount (or dose) of polymer/extract administered. To assist in the selection of materials, literature from the manufacturer and data from published studies should be reviewed for clinical and nonclinical safety information (Venkatraman *et al.*, 2000).

The polymer and extracts should be biocompatible since they are in contact with components that do penetrate the skin. If necessary, *in vitro* and *in vivo* tests are conducted to evaluate the biocompatibility of the polymer and/or extract and of the drug delivery system and thus to assess the safety of the system. *In vitro* studies should be conducted before initiating *in vivo* studies. The tests listed in ISO/ANSI/AAMI Standard 10993, Biological Evaluation of Medical Devices, are intended to provide testing strategies for medical devices. There are similar guidelines in the United States Pharmacopeia 23 for plastics used as drug containers. These tests may also be used to test biocompatibility of polymers used in transdermal drug delivery systems.

Extracts may also be tested for the potential to cause topical sensitization. Preparation of polymer extracts is defined by guidelines, but the choice of conditions should come close to the conditions of manufacture of the drug delivery system. Extracts are evaluated in *in vitro* cytotoxicity tests as well as in *in vivo* irritation, intracutaneous injection, systemic injection, and implantation studies. A sample of the polymer may also be evaluated in these *in vivo* tests. The final transdermal drug delivery system must also be evaluated in standard nonclinical toxicology studies to evaluate safety of the system.

If there is systemic absorption of a polymer or a permeation enhancer that is not a new chemical entity (NCE), manufacturer information and published scientific literature should be reviewed. If data indicate that blood levels are acceptable based on historical exposure or existing toxicology data, then conducting irritation and sensitization studies with the final formulation and providing a written review and justification of the use of the polymer or permeation enhancer may be all that is necessary.

■ CHAPTER 35 ■

If the polymer or permeation enhancer is released systemically and *is* an NCE, a series of *in vitro* and *in vivo* genotoxicity studies should be conducted. If the assays reveal a genotoxic result in multiple assays, development of the polymer or permeation enhancer should be halted. If no genotoxic activity is present, a full toxicology program consisting of acute, chronic, reproduction, and carcinogenicity testing is likely to be required. Additional toxicology studies (irritation and sensitization) would need to be conducted with the final formulation.

New adhesives should also be tested for biocompatibility. Extracts may be evaluated in *in vitro* cytotoxicity tests and *in vivo* irritation, intracutaneous injection, systemic injection, and implantation studies. Placebo transdermal systems may be tested in irritation studies to evaluate the contribution of the adhesive to irritation. Sensitization studies should always include placebos to differentiate reactions between the drug and the excipients.

Beyond these general toxicology considerations, irritation and sensitization tests are a primary focus for evaluating a transdermal dosage form. Laboratory procedures used to predict the potential for irritation and sensitization associated with transdermal system use are discussed in the following sections.

35.3 IRRITATION

35.3.1 *In vivo* irritation testing

Primary irritation is most often tested by modifications of the original Draize test. Draize-type tests have been used by several government bodies, including the Department of Transportation, the Consumer Product Safety Commission, the Environmental Protection Agency, and the Organization for Economic Cooperation and Development (Patrick and Maibach, 1994). Despite adoption of these tests in the Federal Hazardous Substance Act, reproducibility and applicability to human experience have been questioned (York and Steiling, 1998). The test has the following limitations:

- It tends to over predict irritation, although its intended use is to identify severe hazards.
- Critics note its inability to differentiate mild and moderate irritants.
- Choice of animals may be critical to the outcome of irritation assays.
- The rabbit model predicts severe irritants, but may over predict responses or fail to identify substances that produce minimal irritation in humans

(Phillips *et al.*, 1972). Tests of mild to moderate irritants in albino or hairless guinea pigs may help clarify the irritation potential of these compounds in humans.

- It yields little information about the mechanism(s) of irritation.
- It is unsatisfactory for mild irritants or colored preparations and in situations where the adhesiveness of materials masks or exaggerates responses.

Raw materials, intermediates, and final products are routinely tested in acute (single application) primary skin irritation studies, which allow applications of powders, liquids, gels, films, and transdermal systems (Chapter 33). Transdermal systems should be applied for the intended dosing interval in humans (e.g., for a 7-day transdermal system, apply for 7 days).

Additional tests on the components of a transdermal system as well as on the final formulation and placebo may include a subchronic irritation and dermal toxicity study (Steinberg *et al.*, 1975; Robinson and Perkins, 2002). Plasma concentrations are determined on the first and last day to substantiate systemic exposure during these studies (28 to 90 days). Release of drug from the transdermal system may also be determined by measuring residual drug in used systems. For both active and placebo systems, erythema and edema of the skin sites are also monitored, and clinical pathology and histology observations are made to establish dose-related drug effects. Here again, the system should be applied for the intended dosing interval in humans. Typically, transdermal systems are not applied to the same skin site on people, and therefore, applications should be rotated among two to four skin sites on the toxicology animal model (guinea pigs, rabbits, pigs).

35.3.2 *In vitro* irritation testing

Increasingly, the pharmaceutical and cosmetic industries rely on methods that employ cell culture techniques as scientifically and economically preferable to animal testing for screening xenobiotics (Gad, 1990; Robinson *et al.*, 2002). These techniques offer the following advantages:

- Organ and cell cultures can predict acute damage by agents to keratinocytes or other cell types and can reveal factors contributing to tissue damage.
- *In vitro* tests have measurable endpoints.
- They are quick, sensitive, reproducible, and adaptive to various cell types.

- Endpoints used to assess cytotoxicity involve objective evaluation and give few false negative results. Other assays, notably those that evaluate cell morphology, can result in false negatives—for example, formalin preserves membrane structures.

Conducting the experiment on cells derived from skin is recommended; normal human fibroblasts and keratinocytes are the best choices. Reconstituted human skin models allow testing of complex formulations and xenobiotics with poor water solubility characteristics (Roguet, 1999; Robinson *et al.*, 2002; Zuang *et al.*, 2002). These models have a stratum corneum that, like normal human skin, provides a barrier to permeation. Permeability constants for several tested compounds are at least one order of magnitude higher through reconstituted skin than through normal human skin, however (Zghoul *et al.*, 2001). The primary disadvantages to this model are cost and poor adaptability to large-scale cytotoxicity screening.

Two assays—the Neutral Red Assay and the mitchondrial toxicity test (MTT)—are drawing increasing interest despite some limitations, and offer ease of application, objectivity, and the opportunity for automation. The Neutral Red Uptake Assay assesses the integrity of the lysosomal compartment (Bulychev *et al.*, 1978). One drawback of this assay is the potential interference with lysosomotropic agents and ionophores (Reijngoud and Tager, 1976; Cramb, 1986). The modified MTT is used to screen for *in vitro* cytotoxicity of agents on human keratinocytes (Swisher *et al.*, 1989). The assay is unsuitable for the following materials: (1) substances that spontaneously reduce MTT, including glutathione and other sulfhydryl-containing molecules, and (2) those that inhibit the mitochondrial dehydrogenases responsible for metabolizing MTT. XTT, a recently introduced tetrazolium salt, does not require formazan solubilization prior to absorbance measurements (Roehm *et al.*, 1991).

Many other indicators of cell viability have been used as well. Assays that monitor cell membrane integrity have been widely recognized as indicators of irreversible cell damage. Such assays include nuclear and cellular staining by membrane impermeant dyes (e.g., trypan blue, propidium iodide), release of trapped cytoplasmic probes (fluorescein and derivatives), and leakage of intracellular enzymes such as lactate dehydrogenase and acid phosphatase (Roguet, 1999; Eun and Suh, 2000). Other methods assess the release of inflammation markers such as prostaglandin E_2 or interleukin-1 alpha (Roguet 1999). Unfortunately, most of these assays are not readily adaptable to large-scale cytotoxicity screening.

Since test materials may potentially interfere with the assay, the use of several *in vitro* tests that target different cellular endpoints maximizes the degree of confidence in cytotoxicity results (Osborne and Perkins, 1994; Sina *et al.*, 1995, Husøy *et al.*, 1993). For example, the Neutral Red assay measures lysosomal uptake and the MTT evaluates enzymatic cleavage; it is very unlikely that a given agent could interfere with both assays. Nevertheless, when complex mixtures are studied, a third assay—performed in parallel—should be considered.

While individual components or combinations of chemicals can be evaluated for cytotoxicity in classic isolated cell culture models, the testing of water insoluble compounds or final formulations presents another degree of complexity. Here also, reconstituted skin models are particularly well suited. The Minimal Essential Medium (MEM) Assay and Agar Diffusion Method are used to evaluate polymers and potentially leachable substances to ensure that they are nontoxic and biocompatible with *in vivo* reference points (Eagle, 1959; Guess *et al.*, 1965). For the MEM assay, the polymer (amount based on US Pharmacopeia guidelines; USP NF 2002) is extracted in MEM for 24 hours. The culture medium is replaced with extract-containing medium, and cytotoxicity is measured by microscopic examination of morphological alterations (presence or absence of a confluent monolayer, intracellular granulation, cellular swelling and crenation, and the percentage of cell lysis) at 24, 48, and 72 hours. Exclusion of dye can confirm cell viability. In the Agar Diffusion Method, a layer of agar is present between the target cell and the material being tested. The zone where cytotoxicity is observed beyond the initial application site constitutes the endpoint of the assay.

35.3.3   *In vitro/in vivo* correlation

In vitro models do not allow adequate study of the effect local vasculature has on removal of compounds from the skin or the reversibility of the inflammatory response following removal. The absence of vasculature and the incomplete inflammatory response and repair mechanisms thus limit the accuracy of *in vitro* systems in predicting skin irritation. Nevertheless, reasonably good rank correlations have been observed between relative toxicity produced *in vitro* and skin irritation produced *in vivo* in animals or in humans (Swisher *et al.*, 1988; Dickson *et al.*, 1994; Osborne and Perkins, 1994; Sina *et al.*, 1995; Eun and Suh, 2000; Zuang *et al.*, 2002). The correlation seems to improve markedly when the *in vitro* data are compared with eye irritation produced *in vivo* in the Draize test (Marinovich *et al.*, 1990). This finding probably indicates that the lack of a permeation barrier produces the discrepancy between *in vivo* and *in vitro* results and that, for many compounds, cellular damage is the initial event that triggers skin irritation.

35.4 SENSITIZATION

Skin sensitization, or contact sensitization, is a delayed-type immune response mediated by T-cells. The induction period varies from days to months depending on the sensitizer, the administration regimen, the presence of adjuvant, and the species. Typically, if sensitization has occurred, inflammation develops within 24 h after re-exposure to the sensitizing compound.

Numerous tests and strategies, including both *in vivo* and *in vitro*, are available, developed, and have been adopted by several regulatory agencies to identify potential skin sensitizers (Maurer *et al.*, 1994; Basketter *et al.*, 1995; Gerberick *et al.*, 2000; Ryan *et al.*, 2000, 2001; Kimber *et al.*, 2001a, b). The EEC suggests the guinea pig maximization test as the first test, based on the original literature and its validation with moderate or weak allergens. Other validated protocols using guinea pigs are acceptable under certain circumstances. In addition, the OECD accepts the MEST and various LLNA screening tests (see Murine Models), which may be useful to screen therapeutic compounds or excipients of transdermal systems. *In vitro* methods include lymphocyte proliferation assays and the assay of lymphokines (e.g., macrophage inhibitor factor) released by sensitized lymphocytes on exposure to antigen (Kimber *et al.*, 2001, a, b; Ryan *et al.*, 2001). The final transdermal system formulation should be tested in the guinea pig model.

35.4.1   Guinea pig model

The guinea pig is the animal most frequently used to evaluate the potential for compounds to produce contact sensitization. Kimber and colleagues (2001a) reviewed the guinea pig assays that are predictive for contact sensitization (for other reviews, see Kligman and Basketter, 1995; Frankild *et al.*, 1996; Basketter and Kimber, 2001). In most study designs, albino guinea pigs are used. These animals weigh 250 to 500 g and are divided into test and control groups containing 10 to 20 animals. Testing lasts approximately 5 weeks and includes an induction phase, a rest period, and a topical challenge. Skin sites are evaluated at 2, 24, and 48 h after the test compound is removed. Red and swollen sites on test animals indicate sensitization. Sensitization potential is characterized based on the number of animals exhibiting reactions (0–8 percent—weak to 81–100 percent—extreme).

The hairless guinea pig is also used as a predictive model to study irritation and sensitization. Hairless guinea pigs are derived from a natural mutation, are euthymic, and are hairless except for continuous growth of hair at the nose and feet. The hairless guinea pig strain offers a cost-effective alternative to the Hartley guinea pig strain, since depilation or shaving is not required. In addition, undue irritation during removal of bandages is reduced, and application sites are not obscured by hair growth during scoring. Hairless guinea pigs have been evaluated in primary skin irritation and sensitization studies (Chester *et al.*, 1988; Buehler and Kreuzman, 1990).

Delayed contact hypersensitivity testing of transdermal delivery systems must not under-predict potential toxic effects. Protocols designed to test products that wash off the skin may not be optimal for systems that deliver drugs through the skin. The sensitization potential of the drug is assessed early in the development program, before the development of the transdermal product. In one modified FCA protocol for evaluation of a compound's sensitization potential, five intradermal injections of drug emulsified in FCA are administered in a 10-day period and augmented with occlusive topical application. Other modifications or combined FCA and topical applications have been reported as well (Klecak, 1985; Sato, 1985; Kimber *et al.*, 2001a). After the usual waiting period, challenges are made either by intradermal injection or occlusive application of the compound. For evaluation of compounds with good transdermal flux, intermediate formulations, or final formulations, a modified Buehler protocol may be used (Tsuchiya *et al.*, 1982). This modified protocol may use five or more 24-h occlusive applications of materials over a 3-week period (Chester *et al.*, 1988). Topical applications can be augmented by FCA injections, with or without drug, to the shoulder region. Treatment sites for the first and last inductions are scored for erythema/edema at 2 and 24 hours after removal of the test article. Approximately 2 weeks after the last topical application of the induction period, all groups are challenged with 24-h occlusive topical application of appropriate test and control formulations.

Modifications of these standard methods have been adopted to test transdermal systems. For example, transdermal systems are applied three times a week for 3 weeks. The protocol should include at least three groups: one group of at least 10 guinea pigs induced with the placebo formulation (final formulation with permeation enhancers if appropriate, but no drug), one group of 10 guinea pigs induced with the final formulation with drug, and a positive

■ CHAPTER 35 ■

control group. The positive control group animals are typically induced with a topical application, not a transdermal system, of a known moderate to severe sensitizer to demonstrate that the animals can mount a sensitization response. This group may only require five animals. As with topical applications, transdermal applications can be augmented by FCA injections, with or without drug, to the shoulder region. After a rest period of 2 weeks, each animal in the transdermal group is challenged with both the placebo and active systems. This will differentiate any sensitization reactions to drug from those to excipient(s). If the intended dosing interval of the transdermal system is greater than 24 h, the design of sensitization studies may be modified, e.g., each induction application may be 48 h instead of 24 h. If a second challenge is needed to confirm responses, the transdermal animals can be rechallenged 2 weeks after the first challenge. Challenges may include intradermal injections of the drug and/or each excipient/permeation enhancer to differentiate the causative compound. For each additional challenge, the challenge materials should be applied in the same manner to an additional group of 5 naïve guinea pigs to act as an irritation control group. For all challenges, skin sites are evaluated at 2, 24, and 48 hours (or longer if indicated) after the test compound or the transdermal system is removed. The scoring system remains the same, and a reaction is generally considered positive when a combined erythema and edema score of 2 or greater is still present 48 h after removal of the system. Sensitization potential is characterized based on the number of animals exhibiting reactions (0–8 percent—weak to 81–100 percent—extreme).

35.4.2 Murine models

When testing a component and not the transdermal system, murine models such as the MEST and LLNAs have objective endpoints and allow evaluation of pigmented materials. Murine assays also reduce cost, time of test duration, number of animals used, and required care space.

Procedures to evaluate the potential for human sensitization include *in vitro* methods such as the assay of lymphokines (e.g., macrophage inhibitor factor) released by sensitized lymphocytes upon exposure to antigen and lymphocyte proliferation assays (Ryan *et al.*, 2001). *In vivo* methods include the MEST and LLNA noted above.

The MEST (Gad *et al.*, 1986) is a thoroughly investigated assay that evaluates compounds for their potential to sensitize mice by quantitatively measuring mouse ear thickness following re-exposure to a sensitizing agent. The presence or absence of sensitization is judged by percent difference between test and control ears. Sensitization has occurred if the ear of one or more animals is at least 20 percent thicker than the control ear. Incidence of false positives is less than one in a thousand. One or more unequivocal responses in a group of 10 animals are considered a positive result. A single response or more indicate that the compound is a moderate or strong sensitizer.

Using the highest possible test material concentration (mildly irritating for induction) is thought to guarantee the maximal sensitization response. However, some studies indicate that multiple dose studies will increase sensitivity (Gad 1994).

The MEST was developed to overcome the subjective grading of guinea pig erythema in response to allergens. In addition, it reduces cost, time (duration of test is shorter), the number of animals, and the required care space. Finally the assay allows for evaluation of pigmented materials.

The murine LLNA focuses on the central events during contact sensitization: activation and clonal expansion of allergen-reactive T lymphocytes (Kimber et al., 1986). Increases in lymph node weight and lymphocyte proliferative responses were measured following exposure to various sensitizing agents (Kimber et al., 1990; Gerberick et al., 2000). Chemicals are classified as "strong" or "not strong" sensitizers according to the level of [3H] thymidine incorporation recorded. A positive response is when one or more concentrations elicit a threefold or greater increase in isotope incorporation over vehicle control. The LLNA has been validated by the Interagency Coordinating Committee on the Validation of Alternative methods (ICCVAM) and peer reviewed (Dean et al., 2001; Sailstad et al., 2001). The Center for Drug Evaluation and Research and the Center for Biologics Evaluation and Research of the FDA have accepted the LLNA as an acceptable alternative to the guinea pig studies for hazard identification when appropriate.

A major advantage of the LLNA is the objective endpoint. In the guinea pig methods, there are difficulties in interpreting the challenge-induced skin reactions. In contrast to MEST, this test does not rely on the use of adjuvants, and irritant and nonsensitizing compounds appear not to interfere with the immunological status of the draining lymph node. The test may be made more sensitive by the careful use of interleukin 2 (Kimber and Weisenberger, 1989).

In 1992, both the OECD and EEC reduced the number of primary recommended tests and accepted primarily the Buehler and the maximization tests; the EEC favors the maximization test as the first test (Maurer et al., 1994). It was recommended that tests be based on the original literature; in addition,

CHAPTER 35

validation occurs with moderate/or weak allergens, other validated protocols are acceptable in certain cases, and the OECD accepts MEST and LLNA as screening tests. Positive results in these *in vitro* tests are sufficient, but negative results in mouse tests have to be confirmed in guinea pig tests.

The results of animal sensitization studies must be related to potential human hazards. Unfortunately, human populations show greater variability than do animal test systems. This is particularly problematic because a negative sensitizer in the test does not guarantee that the compound will not sensitize humans. For example, standard predictive tests in guinea pigs indicated that clonidine was not a sensitizer. This observation was confirmed in clinical trials. Following introduction in the marketplace a large number of users (19 percent) became sensitized to transdermal clonidine after prolonged use. Conversely, a weak sensitizer with good potential utility for therapy may not need to be abandoned, but may need to be patch tested in humans.

35.5 SUMMARY

This chapter describes toxicity tests used for establishing the safety of a transdermal delivery system. In addition to sensitization and irritation potentials, standard preclinical testing procedures for any new drug to be approved for marketing are required. In the United States, the FDA treats all new transdermal dosage forms as NCEs; however a transdermal system incorporating a drug or compound already approved in a different dosage form may have a swifter approval process. Systemic safety may not be an issue if the dosage for drugs to be delivered transdermally produces plasma levels far lower than those produced by marketed forms of the same drug. If systemic safety has already been adequately demonstrated, nonclinical studies may be minimal or not required.

REFERENCES

ASHBY, J., BASKETTER, D.A., PATON, D. and KIMBER, I. (1995) Structure activity relationships in skin sensitization using the murine local lymph node assay, *Toxicology*, **103**, 177–194.

BARON, J.M. and MERK, H.F. (2001) Drug metabolism in the skin, *Curr. Opin. Allergy Clin. Immunol.*, **1**, 287–291.

BARRATT, M.D. (2000) Prediction of toxicity from chemical structure, *Cell. Biol. Toxicol.*, **16**, 1–13.

BARRATT, M.D. and LANGOWSKI, J.J. (1999) Validation and subsequent development of the DEREK skin sensitization rulebase by analysis of the BgVV list of contact allergens, *J. Chem. Inf. Comput. Sci.*, **39**, 294–298.

BARRATT, M.D., CASTELL, J.V., MIRANDA, M.A. and LANGOWSKI, J.J. (2000) Development of an expert system rulebase for the prospective identification of photoallergens, *J. Photochem. Photobiol.*, **58**, 54–61.

BASKETTER, D.A. (1998) Chemistry of contact allergens and irritants, *Am. J. Contact. Dermat.*, **9**, 119–124.

BASKETTER, D.A. and KIMBER, I. (2001) Predictive testing in contact allergy: Facts and future, *Allergy*, **56**, 937–943.

BASKETTER, D.A., SCHOLES, E.W., CHAMBERLAIN, M. and BARRATT, M.D. (1995) An alternative strategy to the use of guinea pigs for the identification of skin sensitization hazard, *Food Chem. Toxicol.*, **33**, 1051–1056.

BOEHNLEIN, J., SAKR, A., LICHTIN, J.L. and BRONAUGH, R.L. (1994) Characterization of esterase and alcohol dehydrogenase activity in skin: metabolism of retinyl palmitate to retinal (vitamin A) during percutaneous absorption, *Pharm. Res.*, **11**, 1155–1159.

BRAND, R.M., HANNAH, T.L., MUELLER, C., CETIN, Y. and HAMEL, F.G. (2000) A novel system to study the impact of epithelial barriers on cellular metabolism, *Ann. Biomed. Eng.*, **28**, 1210–1217.

BUCKS, D.A.W. (1984) Skin structure and metabolism relevance to the design of cutaneous therapeutics, *Pharm. Res.*, **1**, 148–153.

BUEHLER, E.V. and KREUZMAN, J.J. (1990) Comparable sensitivity of hairless and Hartley strain guinea pigs to a primary irritant and a sensitizer, *J. Toxicol. Cutan. Ocular Toxicol.*, **9**, 163–168.

BULYCHEV, A., TROUET, A. and TULKENS, P. (1978) Uptake and intracellular distribution of neutral red in cultured fibroblasts, *Exp. Cell. Res.*, **115**, 343–355.

CHESTER, A.E., TERRELL, T.G., NAVE, E., DORR, A.E. and DE PASS, L.R. (1988) Dermal sensitization study in hairless guinea pigs with dinitrochlorobenzene and ethyl aminobenzoate, *J. Toxicol. Cutan. Ocular Toxicol.*, **7**, 273–281.

CLEARY, G.W. (1984) Transdermal controlled release systems, in LANGER, R.S. and WISE, D.L., (eds) *Medical Applications Of Controlled Release*, Boca Raton, FL: CRC Press, 203–251.

COMMITTEE FOR PROPRIETARY MEDICINAL PRODUCTS (CPMP) (2001) Note for Guidance on Photosafety Testing. Online. Available HTTP: <http://www.cpmp/swp/398/01.draft> (accessed March 2001).

■ CHAPTER 35 ■

CORMIER, M., LEDGER, P., MARTY, J.P. and AMKRAUT, A. (1991) *In vitro* cutaneous biotransformation of propronolol, *J. Invest. Dermatol.*, **97**, 447–453.

CRAMB, G. (1986) Selective lysosomal uptake and accumulation of the beta-adrenergic antagonist propranolol in cultured and isolated cell systems, *Biochem. Pharmacol.*, **35**, 1365–1372.

DEAN, J.H., TWERDOK, L.E., TICE, R.R., SAILSTAD, D.M., HATTAN, D.G. and STOKES, W.S. (2001) ICCVAM evaluation of the murine local lymph node assay II. Conclusions and recommendations of an independent scientific peer review panel, *Reg. Tox. Pharm.*, **34**, 258–273.

DICKSON, F.M., LAWRENCE, J.N. and BENFORD, D.J. (1994) Cytotoxicity of 12 chemicals of known human and animal skin irritation potential in human keratinocyte cultures, *Toxicol. In Vitro*, **8**, 661–663.

EAGLE, H. (1959) Amino acid metabolism in mammalian cell cultures, *Science*, **130**, 432–437.

ENSLEIN, K., BORGSTEDT, H.H., BLAKE, B.W. and HART, J.B. (1988) Prediction of rabbit skin irritation severity by structure–activity relationships, *Toxicol. In Vitro*, **1**, 129–147.

EUN, H.C. and SUH, D.H. (2000) Comprehensive outlook of *in vitro* tests for assessing skin irritancy as alternatives to Draize tests, *J. Dermatol. Sci.*, **24**, 77–91.

Federal Register (1995) *Federal Register* **60**(40) March 1: 11264–11268.

FOOD and DRUG ADMINISTRATION (2000) Guidance to the Industry: Photosafety Testing. Online. Available HTTP: <http://www.fda.gov.draft> (accessed January 2000).

FRANKILD, S., BASKETTER, D.A. and ANDERSEN, K.E. (1996) The value and limitations of rechallenge in the guinea pig maximization test, *Contact Dermatitis*, **35**, 135–140.

FRIEDBERG, T. (1998) Molecular biological methods for characterizing drug-metabolizing enzymes in hepatic and extrahepatic tissues, *Skin Pharmacol. Appl. Skin Physiol.*, **11**, 61–69.

GAD, S.C. (1994) The Mouse Ear Swelling Test (MEST) in the 1990s, *Toxicology*, **93**, 33–46.

GAD, S.C. (1990) Recent development in replacing, reducing, and refining animal use in toxicologic research and testing, *Fundam. Appl. Toxicol.*, **15**, 8–16.

GAD, S.C., DUNN, B.H., DOBBS, D.N., REILLY, C. and WALSH, R.D. (1986) Development and validation of an alternative dermal sensitization test: The Mouse Ear Swelling Test (MEST), *Toxicol. Appl. Pharmacol.*, **84**, 93–114.

GERBERICK, G.F. and ROBINSON, M.K. (2000) A skin sensitization risk assessment approach for evaluation of new ingredients and products, *Am. J. Contact Dermat.*, **11**, 65–73.

GERBERICK, G.F., RYAN, C.A., KIMBER, I., DEARMAN, R.J., LEA, L.J. and BASKETTER, D.A. (2000) Local lymph node assay: validation assessment for regulatory purposes, *Am. J. Contact Dermat.*, **11**, 3–18.

GUESS, W.L., ROSENKLUTH, S.A., SCHMIDT, B. and AUTAIN, J. (1965) Agar diffusion method for toxicity screening of plastics on cultural cell monolayers, *J. Pharm. Sci.*, **54**, 1545–1547.

GUY, R.H. and HADGRAFT, J. (1982) Percutaneous absorption with saturable metabolism, *Int. J. Pharm.*, **11**, 187–197.

HASHIGUCHI, T., TAKADA, A., IKESUE, A., OHTA, J., YAMAGUCHI, T., YASUTAKE, T. and OTAGIRI, M. (1998) Evaluation of the topical delivery of a prednisolone derivative based upon percutaneous penetration kinetic analysis, *Biol. Pharm. Bull.*, **21**, 882–885.

HOSTYNEK, J.J., MAGEE, P.S. and MAIBACH, H.I. (1996) QSAR predictive of contact allergy: Scope and limitations, *Curr. Probl. Dermatol.*, **25**, 18–27.

HUSØY, T., SYVERSEN, T. and JENSSEN, J. (1993) Comparisons of four *in vitro* cytotoxicity tests: The MTT assay, NR assay, uridine incorporation and protein measurements, *Toxicol. In Vitro*, **7**, 149–154.

IMOTO, H., ZHOU, Z., STINCHCOMB, A.L. and FLYNN, G.L. (1996) Transdermal prodrug concepts: Permeation of buprenorphine and its alkyl esters through hairless mouse skin and influence of vehicles, *Biol. Pharm. Bull.*, **19**, 263–267.

INTERAGENCY COODINATING COMMITTEE ON THE VALIDATION OF ALTERNATIVE METHODS. PHOTOTOXICITY WORKING GROUP (2000) Draft Proposal for a New Guideline: 432. *In Vitro* 3T3 NRU Phototoxicity Test. Online. Available HTTP: <http://iccvam.niehs.nih.gov/groups/pwg.htm> (accessed 31 May 2002).

KANTROWITZ, J. and YACOBI, A. (1994) Toxicokinetics, in STARK, K.(ed.) *Handbook of Experimental Pharmacology*, Berlin: Springer-Verlag, **10**, 383–403.

KIMBER, I. and WEISENBERGER, C. (1989) A murine local lymph node assay for the identification of contact allergens. Assay development and results of an initial validation study, *Arch. Toxicol.*, **63**, 274–282.

CHAPTER 35

KIMBER, I., MITCHELL, J.A. and GRIFFIN, A.C. (1986) Development of a murine local lymph node assay for the determination of sensitizing potential, *Food Chem. Toxicol.*, **24**, 585–586.

KIMBER, I, HILTON, J. and BOTHAM, P.A. (1990) Identification of contact allergens using the murine local lymph node assay: Comparisons with the Buehler Occluded Patch Test in guinea pigs, *J. Appl. Toxicol.*, **10**, 173–180.

KIMBER, I., BASKETTER, D.A., BERTHOLD, K., BUTLER, M., GARRIGUE, J.L., LEA, L., NEWSOME, C., ROGGEBAND, R., STEILING, W., STROPP, G., WATERMAN, S. and WIEMANN, C. (2001a) Skin sensitization testing in potency and risk assessment, *Toxicol. Sci.*, **59**, 198–208.

KIMBER, I., PICHOWSKI, J.S., BETTS, C.J., CUMBERBATCH, M., BASKETTER, D.A. and DEARMAN, R.J. (2001b) Alternative approaches to the identification and characterization of chemical allergens, *Toxicol. In Vitro*, **15**, 307–312.

KLECAK, G. (1985) The Freund's complete adjuvant test and the open epicutaneous test: A complementary test procedure for realistic assessment of allergenic potential, *Curr. Probl. Dematol.*, **14**, 152–171.

KLIGMAN, A.M. and BASKETTER, D.A. (1995) A critical commentary and updating of the guinea pig maximization test, *Contact Dermatitis*, **32**, 129–134.

KODITHALA, K., HOPFINGER, A.J., THOMPSON, E.D. and ROBINSON, M.K. (2002) Prediction of skin irritation from organic chemicals using membrane-interaction QSAR analysis, *Toxicol. Sci.*, **66**, 336–346.

MARINOVICH, M., TRAGNI, E., CORSINI, A. and GALLI, C.L. (1990) Quantification of *in vitro* cytotoxicity of surfactants: Correlation with their eye irritation potential, *J. Toxicol. Cutan. Ocular Toxicol.*, **9**, 169–178.

MAURER, T. ARTHUR, A. and BENTLEY, P. (1994) Guinea-pig contact sensitization assays, *Toxicology*, **93**, 47–54.

McKINNEY, J.D., WALLER, R.A., NEWMAN, M.C. and GERBERICK, F. (2000) The practice of structure activity relationships (SAR) in toxicology, *Toxicol. Sci.*, **56**, 8–17.

NOONAN, P.K. and WESTER, R.C. (1985) Cutaneous metabolism of xenobiotics, in BRONAUGH, R.L. and MAIBACH, H.I. (eds) *Percutaneous Absorption,* New York: Marcel Dekker, 65–85.

OSBORNE, R. and PERKINS, M.A. (1994) An approach for development of alternative test methods based on mechanisms of skin irritation, *Food Chem. Toxicol.*, **32**, 133–142.

PATRICK, E. and MAIBACH, H.I. (1994) Dermatotoxicology, in Hayes, A.W. (ed) *Principles and Methods of Toxicology*, New York: Raven Press, 767–803.

PHILLIPS, L., STEINBERG, M., MAIBACH, H.I. and AKERS, W.A. (1972) A comparison of rabbit and human skin responses to certain irritants, *Toxicol. Appl. Pharmacol.*, 21, 369–382.

REIJNGOUD, D.J. and TAGER, J.M. (1976) Chloroquine accumulation in isolated rat liver lysosomes, *FEBS Lett.*, 64, 231–235.

ROBERTS, D.W. and BASKETTER, D.A. (2000) Quantitative structure-activity relationships: Sulfonate esters in the local lymph node assay, *Contact Dermatitis*, 42, 154–161.

ROBINSON, M.K., COHEN, C., DE FRAISSINETTE ADE, B., PONEC, M., WHITTLE, E. and FENTEM, J.H. (2002) Non-animal testing strategies for assessment of the skin corrosion and skin irritation potential of ingredients and finished products, *Food Chem. Toxicol.*, 40, 573–592.

ROBINSON, M.K. and PERKINS, M.A. (2002) A strategy for skin irritation testing, *Am. J. Contact Dermat.*, 13, 21–29.

ROEHM, N.W., RODGERS, G.H., HATFIELD, S.M. and GLASEBROOK, A.L. (1991) An improved colorimetric assay for cell proliferation and viability utilizing the tetrazolium salt XTT, *J. Immunol. Methods*, 142, 257–265.

ROGUET, R. (1999) Use of skin cell cultures for *in vitro* assessment of corrosion and cutaneous irritancy, *Cell. Biol. Toxicol.*, 15, 63–75.

RYAN, C.A., GERBERICK, G.F., CRUSE, L.W., BASKETTER, D.A., LEA, L., BLAIKIE, L., DEARMAN, R.J., WARBRICK, E.V. and KIMBER, I. (2000) Activity of human contact allergens in the murine local lymph node assay, *Contact Dermatitis*, 43, 95–102.

RYAN, C.A., HULETTE, B.C. and GERBERICK, G.F. (2001) Approaches for the development of cell-based *in vitro* methods for contact sensitization, *Toxicol. In Vitro*, 15, 43–55.

SAILSTAD, D., HATTAN, D., HILL, R.N. and STOKES, W.S. (2001) ICCVAM evaluation of the murine local lymph node assay. The ICCVAM review process, *Reg. Tox. Pharm.*, 34, 249–257.

SATO, Y. (1985) Modified guinea pig maximization test, *Curr. Probl. Dermatol.*, 14, 193–200.

SINA, J.F., GALER, D.M., SUSSMAN, R.G., GAUTHERON, P.D., SARGENT, E.V., LEONG, B., SHAH, P.V., CURREN, R.D. and MILLER, K. (1995) A collaborative evaluation of seven alternatives to the Draize eye irritation test using pharmaceutical intermediates, *Fundam. Appl. Toxicol.*, 26, 20–31.

CHAPTER 35

SINTOV, A.C., BEHAR-CANETTI, C., FRIEDMAN, Y. and TAMARKIN, D. (2002) Percutaneous penetration and skin metabolism of ethylsalicylate-containing agent, TU-2100: *In-vitro* and *in-vivo* evaluation in guinea pigs, *J. Control. Release*, **79**, 113–122.

SMITH, C.K., MOORE, C.A., ELAHI, E.N., SMART, A.T. and HOTCHKISS, S.A. (2000) Human skin absorption and metabolism of the contact allergens, cinnamic aldehyde, and cinnamic alcohol, *Toxicol. Appl. Pharmacol.*, **168**, 189–199.

STEINBERG, M., AKERS, W.A., WEEKS, M.H., MCCREESH, A.H. and MAIBACH, H.I. (1975) A comparison of test techniques based on rabbit and human skin responses to irritants with recommendation regarding the evaluation of mildly or moderately irritating compounds, in MAIBACH, H.I. (ed.) *Animal Models In Dermatology*, New York: Churchill Livingstone, 1–11.

STEINSTRASSER, I. and MERKLE, H.P. (1995) Dermal metabolism of topically applied drugs: Pathways and models reconsidered, *Pharm. Acta Helv.*, **70**, 3–24.

SWISHER, D.A., CORMIER, M., JOHNSON, J. and LEDGER, P.W. (1989) A cytotoxicity assay using normal human keratinocytes: Characterization and applications, in MAIBACH, H.I. and LOWE, N.H. (eds) *Models in Dermatology*, vol. 4, Basel: Karger, 131–137.

SWISHER, D.A., PREVO, M.E. and LEDGER, P.W. (1988) The MTT *in vitro* cytotoxicity test: Correlation with cutaneous irritancy in two animal models, in GOLDBERG, A.M. (ed.) *Progress in In Vitro Toxicology. Alternative Methods in Toxicology Series*, New York: Mary Ann Liebert, 265–269.

TANG-LIU, D.D., MATSUMOTO, R.M. and USANSKY, J.I. (1999) Clinical pharmacokinetics and drug metabolism of tazarotene: A novel topical treatment for acne and psoriasis, *Clin. Pharmacokinet.*, **37**, 273–287.

TAUBER, U. (1989) Drug metabolism in the skin: Advantages and disadvantages, in HADGRAFT, J. and GUY, R.H. (eds) *Transdermal Drug Delivery: Developmental Issues and Research Initiatives*, New York: Marcel Dekker, 99–111.

TSUCHIYA, S., KONDO, M., OKAMOTO, K. and TAKASE, Y. (1982) Studies on contact hypersensitivity in the guinea pig, *Contact Dermatitis*, **8**, 246–255.

US PHARMACOPEIAL CONVENTION (1995) *United States Pharmacopeia (USP 23), National Formulary (NF 18)*, Rockville MD: US Pharmacopeial Convention 1995, 1697–1699.

VENKATRAMAN, S., DAVAR, N., CHESTER, A. and KLEINER, L. (2000) An overview of controlled-release systems, in WISE, D. (ed.) *Handbook of Pharmaceutical Controlled Release Technology*, New York: Marcel Dekker, 431–463.

YORK, M. and STEILING, W. (1998) A critical review of the assessment of eye irritation potential using the Draize rabbit eye test, *J. Appl. Toxicol.*, **18**, 233–240.

ZGHOUL, N., FUCHS, R., LEHR, C.M. and SCHAEFER, U.F. (2001) Reconstructed skin equivalents for assessing percutaneous drug absorption from pharmaceutical formulations, *ALTEX* **18**, 103–106.

ZUANG, V., BALLS, M., BOTHAM, P.A., COQUETTE, S.A., CORSINI, E., CURREN, R.D., ELLIOTT, G.R., FENTEM, J.H., HEYLINGS, J.R., LIEBSCH, M., MEDINA, J., ROGUET, R., VAN DE SANDT, J.J., WIEMANN, C. and WORTH, A.P. (2002) Follow-up to the ECVAM prevalidation study on *in vitro* tests for acute skin irritation. The European Center for the Validation of Alternative Methods Skin Irritation Task Force Report 2, *Altern. Lab. Anim.*, **30**, 109–129.

CHAPTER 35

Animal, Human and In Vitro Test Methods for Predicting Skin Irritation

CHERYL LEVIN AND HOWARD I MAIBACH

Contents

36.1 Introduction

36.2 Animal models

36.3 *In-vitro* assays

36.4 Human models

36.1 INTRODUCTION

Contact with external irritating agents, such as dishwashing liquid, enzymes, or raw meat can result in irritant contact dermatitis (ICD), a localized nonimmunologic condition. ICD ensues when irritant stimuli overpower the defense and repair capacities of the skin (Goldner and Jackson, 1994; Walle, 2000). Exposure to potent irritants or exposure to mild irritants for an extended period of time will increase the likelihood of developing ICD.

Preventive measures, including the utilization of proper skin care, the avoidance of harsh soaps and the use of protective garments such as gloves, will decrease the risk of irritant dermatitis occurring. In addition, it is of crucial importance to test the irritant potential of any substance that will be applied to human skin, so that its likelihood of inducing irritant dermatitis is known. Federal regulatory agencies require toxicity testing to determine the safety or hazard of various chemicals and products prior to human exposure. This information is used to properly classify and label products according to their potential hazard (Bashir and Maibach, 2000).

No one assay is able to accurately portray irritation in its entirety. This is because irritant dermatitis may result from either acute or cumulative injury, and may involve inflammation or skin necrosis (corrosive). A number of animal, human and *in vitro* test methods have been developed, each portraying some but not all aspects of irritation. Each model has its unique benefits and limitations.

36.2 ANIMAL MODELS

36.2.1 Draize rabbit assay

In order to evaluate primary irritation and corrosion, the Draize animal model or one of its modifications is utilized. The Draize rabbit test was developed in 1944, and has since been adopted in the US Federal Hazardous Substance Act (FHSA) (code of FR) (Patrick and Maibach, 1989). The test involves two (1 square inch) test sites on the dorsal skin of six albino rabbits. One site is abraded (through use of a hypodermic needle across the rabbit skin) and the other site remains intact. The stratum corneum is broken on the abraded site, without loss of blood. The undiluted "irritant" materials (0.5 g for solids or 0.5 ml for liquids) are placed on a patch and applied to the test sites. They are secured with two layers of surgical gauze (1 inch (2.5 cm) squared) and tape. The animal is

CHAPTER 36

wrapped in cloth so that the patches are secure for a 24-h period. Assessment of erythema and edema, utilizing the scale noted in Table 36.1, takes place 24 h and 72 h following patch application. Severe reactions are again assessed on days 7 or 14. Radiolabeled tracers or biochemical techniques to monitor skin healing is also utilized by some investigators. Other investigators supplement with histological evaluation of skin tissue (Mezei *et al.*, 1966; Murphy *et al.*, 1979).

The Draize test ultimately quantifies irritation with the primary irritation index (PII), which averages the erythema and edema scores of each test site and then adds the averages together. Materials producing a PII of <2 are considered nonirritating, 2–5 mildly irritating, >5 severely irritating and require precautionary labeling. Subsequent studies have demonstrated that the PII is somewhat subjective because the scoring of erythema and edema require clinical judgment (Patil *et al.*, 1998).

Main critics of the Draize test oppose the harsh treatment of animals. They argue that the Draize test is unreliable at distinguishing between mild and moderate irritants. Furthermore, they believe the Draize is not an accurate predictor of skin irritancy as it does not include vesiculation, severe eschar formation or ulceration in evaluating the PII. Finally, they argue that the Draize procedure is not reproducible (Weil and Scala, 1971) and they question its relevance with regard to human experience (Edwards, 1972; Nixon *et al.*, 1975; Shillaker *et al.*, 1989). Proponents of the Draize test point out that the test is somewhat inaccurate but it generally overpredicts the severity of skin damage produced by chemicals, and thereby errs on the side of safety for the consumer

TABLE 36.1:

Draize scoring system

Erythema	
No erythema	0
Slight erythema	1
Well-defined erythema	2
Moderate or severe erythema	3
Severe erythema or slight eschar formation (injuries in depth)	4
Edema	
No edema	0
Very slight edema	1
Slight edema (well-defined edges)	2
Moderate edema (raised >1 mm)	3
Severe edema (raised >1 mm and extending beyond the area of exposure)	4

Adapted from Patrick and Maibach (1989).

(Patil *et al.*, 1996). This topic is hotly debated. In the meantime, the Draize assays are recommended by regulatory bodies.

36.2.2 Modified Draize models

The Draize test has been modified in response to harsh criticisms over the past years. Alterations include changing the preferred species, use of fewer animals, testing on only intact skin and reduction of the exposure period to irritants. Please note Table 36.2 for a comparison of the modified Draize tests

36.2.3 Cumulative irritation assays

Frequently, irritant contact dermatitis is produced through cumulative exposure to a weak irritant. While the Draize assay assesses acute exposure to a strong irritant, there have been many assays developed to measure repetitive, cumulative irritation. One such assay was developed by Justice *et al.* (1961). They measured epidermal erosion through a repeat animal patch (RAP) test for comparing irritant potential of surfactants. In their study, solutions were occlusively applied to the clipped dorsum of albino mice for a 10-minute interval. The process was repeated seven times and the skin was subsequently examined microscopically for epidermal erosion.

The repetitive irritation test (RIT), as described by Frosch *et al.* (1993), utilizes guinea pigs as the animal model in determining the protective efficacy of creams

■ CHAPTER 36 ■

TABLE 36.2:

Modified Draize irritation method

	Draize	FHSA[1]	FIFRA[2]	DOT[3]	OECD[4]
No. of animals	3	6	6	6	6
Abrasion	yes	yes	2 of each	no	no
Exposure period (h)	24	24	4	4	4
Examination (h)	24, 72	24, 72	0.5, 1, 24, 48, 72	4, 48	0.5, 1, 24, 48, 72
Excluded from testing	—	—	toxic materials ph 2 or 11.5	—	toxic materials ph 2 or 11.5

Notes:
[1] FHSA, Federal Hazardous Substance Act
[2] FIFRA, Federal Insecticide, Fungicide and Rodenticide Act
[3] DOT, Department of Transportation
[4] OECD, Organization for Economic Cooperation and Development

Adapted from Bashir and Maibach (2000).

against various chemical irritants. In one study, the irritants sodium hydroxide (NaOH), sodium lauryl sulfate (SLS) and toluene were administered daily for 2 weeks to shaved dorsal skin of guinea pigs. Barrier creams were applied two hours prior to and immediately following irritant exposure. Visual scoring, laser Doppler flowmetry (LDF) and transepidermal water loss (TEWL) quantified resultant erythema. The study found one barrier cream effective against SLS and toluene injury, while another barrier cream studied did not show any efficacy. In general, the RIT is most useful in evaluating the efficacy of barrier creams in preventing cumulative irritation.

To rank products for their irritant potential, repeat application patch tests have been developed. Diluted potential irritants are occlusively applied to the same site for 15 to 21 days. The sensitivity of the test is influenced by both the duration of occlusion and the type of patch used to apply the irritants. In general, a longer occlusive period will result in enhanced percutaneous penetration. Similarly, the Draize-type gauze dressing will produce less percutaneous penetration as compared to the Duhring metal chambers. In order to facilitate interpretation of test results, a reference material that is of similar use or that produces a known effect is incorporated into the test. Rabbits and guinea pigs are the most commonly used animal species in the repeat application test (Phillips et al., 1972; Wahlberg, 1993). In a recent study, Kobayashi et al. (1999) studied the effects of propranolol as an irritant utilizing both primary and cumulative irritation assays. In both assays, skin irritation and histopathological changes were observed in all guinea pigs treated with propranolol, and those tended to increase with the increase of propranolol dosage. The skin reactions increased with the application times of propranolol up to 7 days in the cumulative skin irritation study. Scoring of the test sites were made in accordance with the following scale: 0 = No reaction, 1+ = Mild erythema covering the entire patch area, 2+ = Erythema and edema, 3+ = Erythema, edema, vesicles, 4+ = Erythema, edema, and bullae.

One variation of the repeat application patch test involves measuring the edema-producing capacity of irritants utilizing a guinea pig model. Visual inspection and Harpenden calipers measure skin thickness following application of irritants for 3–21 days. This model demonstrates clear dose-response relationships and discriminating power for all irritants, excluding acids and alkalis (Wahlberg, 1993).

Open application assays, developed by Marzulli and Maibach (1975), involve application of irritants onto the backs of rabbits 16 times over a 3-week period. Visual scoring of erythema and skin thickness measurements are utilized to quantify results. A high degree of correlation has been observed when comparing erythema and skin thickness data. In addition, the results of 60 test substances in rabbits strongly correlated with the results of cumulative irritation studies in man, suggesting that the rabbit assay is a useful model.

A modified open application assay was performed by Anderson *et al.* (1986). In his assay, irritants are applied once a day for 3 days to a 1-cm^2 test site on the backs of guinea pigs. Sites are evaluated visually for erythema and edema. In addition, biopsies are taken and skin samples are stained with May-Grunward-Giemsa under oil immersion, to evaluate epidermal thickness and dermal infiltration. Irritants are compared to the standard irritant, 2 percent SLS and their potency is ranked. Extensive processing involved in properly performing this assay may limit its usefulness.

36.2.4 Immersion assay

Aqueous detergent solutions and other surfactant-based products are evaluated for irritancy using the guinea pig immersion assay (Calandra, 1971; MacMillan *et al.*, 1975; Gupta *et al.*, 1992). This assay involves placing 10 guinea pigs in a restraining device that is immersed in a 40°C test solution for 4 h daily for a total of 3 days (Kooyman and Snyder, 1942). The restraining apparatus allows the guinea pig's head to be above the solution. Twenty-four hours following the final immersion, the animals' flanks are shaved and evaluated for erythema, edema and fissures. In one study, the dermatotoxic effects of detergents in guinea pigs and humans were concomitantly tested (Gupta *et al.*, 1992). The immersion assay was utilized to test guinea pigs, while the patch assay tested humans. Irritation of guinea pig skin led to epidermal erosion and a 40–60 percent increase in histamine content. Seven of eight human subjects had a positive patch test to the same irritants, indicating a strong correlation between the guinea pig and human models.

36.2.5 Mouse ear model

The mouse ear model is used to evaluate the degree of inflammation associated with shampoos or surfactant-based products. Uttley and Van Abbe (1973) first described the mouse model when they applied undiluted shampoos to one ear of mice daily for 4 days. They visually assessed the erythema, vessel dilation and edema. However, the anesthetic used to anesthetize the mice in this study may have altered the development of inflammation and confounded results.

More recently, Patrick and Maibach (1987) applied surfactants to measure mouse ear thickness at various time points following irritant application. Pretreating the ear with croton oil or 12-O-tetradecanoylphorbol 13-acetate 72 h prior to irritant application increased the sensitivity of the assay. This assay was most useful in testing surfactant-based products and had little efficacy with oily or highly perfumed materials.

36.2.6   Recent assays

Recent animal assays have been developed to quantify irritant response. Humphrey *et al.* (1993) measured Evans blue dye recovered from rat skin after exposing the skin to inflammatory agents. Trush *et al.* (1994) assessed the dermal inflammatory response to numerous irritants by measuring the level of myelo-peroxidase enzyme in polymorphonuclear leukocytes in young CD-1 mice.

36.2.7   Conclusion

Animal assays must be interpreted with caution. Dose-response measurements must be followed. Draize scores are most accurate when compared to related compounds with a record of human exposure. It is important to note that occlusive application does not enhance percutaneous penetration for all materials.

Responses in animal models, particularly the guinea pig and the rabbit, have a high degree of correlation to those of humans, but some inconsistencies have occurred. Major discrepancies in irritant response between different animal species tested under identical conditions have occurred (Llewellyn *et al.*, 1972; Gilman *et al.*, 1978), particularly with regard to weak irritants and colored materials. Subjective visual scoring techniques have accounted for some of these discrepancies. It is prudent to utilize other methodologies in addition to the animal model when evaluating a putative irritant.

36.3   *IN-VITRO* ASSAYS

In vitro skin irritation assays are of potential benefit in addressing humane concerns associated with animal testing. These "alternative" methods may potentially reduce the number of animals needed in irritation testing, or in some cases may fully replace the need to use animals. In recent years, a number of *in vitro* skin irritation assays have been developed. However, most of these have not been evaluated in validation studies to determine their usefulness, limitations and compliance with regulatory testing requirements. Furthermore, dose-response relationships have not been established for *in vitro* methods.

Studies evaluating *in vitro* testing thus far indicate usefulness in predicting starting doses for *in vivo* studies, potentially reducing the number of animals used for such determinations. Additionally, other studies suggest an association between *in vitro* cytotoxicity and human lethal blood concentrations. The US Interagency Coordinating Committee on the Validation of Alternative Methods (ICCVAM) and the US National Toxicology Program Center for the Evaluation of Alternative Toxicological Methods (NICEATM), were established to evaluate *in vitro* irritant testing. To date, there are four approved irritation assays, namely Corrositex®, Epiderm™, Episkin™ and Rat Skin Transcutaneous Electrical Resistance (TER) Assays.

Corrositex® is a collagen matrix acting as synthetic skin, and is used to assess the dermal corrosivity potential of chemicals. Should a chemical pass through the biobarrier by diffusion and/or destruction, Corrositex® elicits a color change in the underlying liquid Chemical Detection System (CDS). Corrositex® is currently used by the US Department of Transportation (US DOT) to assign categories of corrosivity for labeling purposes according to United Nations (UN) guidelines. However, its use is limited to specific chemical classes, including acids, acid derivatives, acylhalides, alkylamines and polyalkyamines, bases, cholorosilanes, metal halides, and oxyhalides.

A peer review panel of NICEATM and ICCVAM elucidated some of the advantages to Corrositex®, including its possible usefulness in replacing or reducing the number of animals required. Positive test results often eliminate the need for animal testing. When further animal testing is necessary, often only one animal is required to confirm a corrosive chemical. The panel also concluded that most of the chemicals identified as negative by Corrositex® or nonqualifying in the detection system are unlikely to be corrosive when tested on animals for irritation potential.

EpiDerm™ (EPI-200) is a three-dimensional human skin model that uses cell viability as a measure of corrosivity. It has been utilized with several common tests of cytotoxicity and irritancy, including MTT, IL-la, PGE_2, LDH, and sodium fluorescein permeability.

EPISKIN™ is a three-dimensional human skin model comprised of a reconstructed epidermis and a functional stratum corneum. In a study supported by the European Centre for the Validation of Alternative Methods (ECVAM), EPISKIN™ was useful in testing all types of potential irritants, including organic

TABLE 36.3:

In vitro assays

Assay	Description	Methodology
Corrositex®	Collagen matrix acting as synthetic skin	A color change in the underlying liquid Chemical Detection System when irritant passes through matrix
Epiderm™	Three dimensional matrix acting as synthetic skin	Cell viability as a measure of corrosivity
Episkin™	Three dimensional matrix acting as synthetic skin	Cell viability as a measure of corrosivity
TER	Skin disks taken from the pelts of humanely killed young rats	Significantly lower inherent transcutaneous electrical resistance when skin barrier is compromised

acids, organic bases, neutral organics, inorganic acids, inorganic bases, inorganic salts, electrophiles, phenols and soaps/surfactants. With both EPISKIN™ and EpiDerm™, the test material is topically applied to the skin for up to four hours with subsequent assessment of the effects on cell viability.

In the TER Assay, irritants will portray a loss of normal stratum corneum integrity and barrier function. A reduced barrier function will exhibit a significantly lower inherent transcutaneous electrical resistance. TER involves up to 24 h application of test material to the epidermal surfaces of skin disks taken from the pelts of humanely killed young rats. Comparing Epiderm, Episkin and TER, only EPISKIN was able to significantly distinguish between two particular types of chemicals. Currently, the ICCVAM recommends that EPIDERM, EPISKIN and TER are used to assess the dermal corrosivity potential of chemicals in a "weight-of-evidence" approach. In general, positive corrosivity tests will not require further testing, while negative corrosivity will.

In-vitro assays are promising and have significant interest to toxicologists. The future promises a greater use for *in vitro* irritancy testing.

36.4 HUMAN MODELS

Following the development of the patch test, Draize *et al.* suggested a 24 h single application patch test in humans. Human testing facilitates extrapolation of data to the clinical setting. Many variations of the single-application test have been developed. Testing is often performed on undiseased skin (Skog, 1960) of the dorsal upper arm or back. The required test area is small and up to ten materials may be tested simultaneously and compared. A reference irritant substance is often included to account for variability in test responses. In general, screening of new materials involves open application on the back or dorsal upper arm for a short amount of time (30 min to 1 h) to minimize potential adverse events in subjects.

36.4.1 Single-application patch testing

The National Academy of Sciences (National Academy of Sciences and Committee for the Revision of NAS Publication 1138, 1977) recommended a 4-h single-application patch test protocol for routine testing of skin irritation in humans. In general, patches are occluded onto the dorsal upper arm or back skin of patients. The degree of occlusion varies according to the type of occlusive device; the Hilltop or Duhring chambers or an occlusive tape will enhance percutaneous penetration as compared to a non-occlusive tape or cotton bandage (Patil *et al.*, 1996). Potentially volatile materials should always be tested with a non-occlusive tape.

Exposure time to the putative irritant varies greatly, and is often customized by the investigator. Volatile chemicals are generally applied for 30 min to 1 h while some chemicals have been applied for more than 24 h.

Following patch removal, skin is rinsed with water to remove residue. Skin responses are evaluated 30 min to 1 h following patch removal in order to allow hydration and pressure effects of the patch to subside. Another evaluation is performed 24 h following patch removal. The animal Draize scale is used to analyze test results (see Table 36.1). The Draize scale does not include papular, vesicular, or bullous responses; other scales have been developed to address these needs.

Single-application patch tests generally heal within one week. Depigmentation at the test site results in some subjects.

36.4.2 Cumulative irritation test

Utilizing statistical analysis of test data, Kligman and Woodling (1967) calculated the IT50 (time to produce irritation in 50 percent of subjects) and ID50 (dose required to produce irritation in 50 percent of subjects following a 24 h exposure). Their work formed the basis for the 21-day cumulative irritation assay. The "21 day assay" is used to screen new formulas prior to marketing. The original assay involved application of a 1-in (2.5 cm) square of Webril saturated with the test material (either liquid or 0.5 g of viscous substance) to the skin of the undamaged upper back. Occlusive tape secured the patch. Twenty-four hours after patch application, the test site is examined and the patch is reapplied. The test is repeated for 21 days.

Two modifications of the cumulative irritation test were studied by Wigger-Alberti *et al.* (1997a). One assay involved Finn chamber application of metal-working fluids onto the midback of volunteers for one day. The sites were evaluated and the fluids were then reapplied for an additional two days. In the other assay, a 2-week, 6-h per day repetitive irritation test (excluding weekends) was utilized. Better discrimination of irritancy and shorter duration was observed with the 3-day model.

36.4.3 Chamber scarification test

The chamber scarification test assesses the irritancy potential of materials on damaged skin (Frosch and Kligman, 1976; 1977). Subjects included in this assay are highly sensitive to 24 h exposure to 5 percent SLS (they form vesicles, severe erythema and edema post application). Six to eight 10 mm² areas on the volar forearms are scratched eight times with a 30-gauge needle. Scarification damages the epidermal layer without drawing blood. Four scratches are parallel and the other four are perpendicular to the test site. 0.1 g of test material (or 0.1 mL of liquid) is then applied to the scarified area for 24 h via Duhring chambers. Non-occlusive tape is used to secure the chambers in place. With fresh specimens, patches are applied daily for 3 days. A visual scoring scale is used to quantify test results thirty minutes following patch removal. An analogous area of intact skin must be scored as well, so that evaluation is based upon comparison between compromised and intact skin. The visual score of scarified test sites divided by the score of intact test sites, known as the scaarification index, allows this comparison to be made. The relationship of this assay to prediction of irritant response from routine use has yet to be established.

36.4.4 Immersion tests

Patch tests often overpredict the irritant potential of some materials. Immersion tests were established to improve irritancy prediction by mimicking consumer use. Kooyman and Snyder developed the arm immersion technique to compare the relative irritancy of two soap or detergent products (Kooyman and Snyder, 1942). Soap solutions of up to 3 percent are prepared in troughs and subjects immersed one hand and forearm in each trough, comparing different products or concentrations. Temperature is maintained at 41°C (105°F). The exposure period varies between 10 and 15 min a day for a total of 5 days or until observable irritation is produced on both arms. The antecubital fossa is generally the first area to experience irritation, followed by the hands (Justice *et al.*, 1961) (Kooyman and Snyder, 1942).

More recently, variations on the arm immersion technique have developed so that the antecubital fossa and the hands are separately tested. Variations incorporate different dosing regimens or measuring different endpoints. Clarys *et al.* (1997) (Clarys and Barel, 1997) investigated the effects of temperature and anionic character on the degree of irritation caused by detergents. Transepidermal water loss (TEWL), erythema (colorimetry, a* parameter), and skin dryness (capacitance) were used to quantify test results. The irritant response was increased by higher temperature and higher anionic content. Utilizing a modified arm immersion technique, Allenby *et al.* (1993) noticed that once skin had been compromised (erythema of 1+ on a visual scale), irritants applied to the forearm and back caused an exaggerated response.

36.4.5 Soap chamber technique

The "chapping" potential of bar soaps is evaluated with the soap chamber technique, developed by Frosch and Kligman (1979). While patch testing is useful in predicting erythema, it does not address the dryness, flaking and fissuring observed with bar soap use. Using this method, 0.1 ml of an 8 percent soap solution is applied to the forearm via Duhring chambers fitted with Webril pads. Non-occlusive tape is used to secure the chambers. Patches are applied for 24 h on day 1 and 6 h on days 2–5. If severe erythema at the test site occurs, the investigator must discontinue the study. Skin responses are evaluated with visual scoring of erythema, scaling and fissures. This test correlates well with skin-washing procedures but tends to overpredict irritant response of some materials.

36.4.6 Protective barrier assessment

The skin barrier function assays test the efficacy of protective creams in preventing an irritant response. Zhai *et al.* (1998) studied the effect of barrier creams in reducing erythema, edema, vesiculation and maceration. Subjects were given creams and then irritated with either SLS or ammonium hydroxide. Paraffin wax in cetyl alcohol was the most effective in preventing irritation.

CHAPTER 36

In another study by Wigger-Alberti and Elsner (1997a), petrolatum was applied to the backs of 20 subjects. Subjects were then exposed to SLS, NaOH, toluene and lactic acid. Irritation was assessed by visual scoring, TEWL and colorimetry. Petrolatum was found to be an effective barrier cream against SLS, NaOH and lactic acid and moderately effective against toluene.

Frosch *et al.* (1993) revised the RIT (see animal model section) to evaluate the effect of two barrier creams in preventing SLS-induced irritation. The irritant was applied to the ventral forearms of human subjects for 30 min daily for 2 weeks. Visual scoring, laser Doppler flowmetry (LDF), colorimetry and TEWL were utilized to assess resultant erythema. TEWL was found most useful in quantifying results, while colorimetry was the least beneficial.

36.4.7 Bioengineering methods

Modern bioengineering methods utilized to quantify test results include transepidermal water loss (TEWL), capacitance, ultrasound, laser Doppler flowmetry, spectroscopy and chromametry (colorimetry). Most of the assays described were developed before the introduction of these bioengineering methods. These methods allow a more precise quantification of test results. These techniques are described in detail by Patil *et al.* (1998).

REFERENCES

ALLENBY, C., BASKETTER, D., *et al.* (1993) An arm immersion model of compromised skin. (I) Influence on irritant reactions. *Contact Derm.* 28(2), 84–88.

ANDERSON, C., SUNDBERG, K., *et al.* (1986) Animal model for assessment of skin irritancy. *Contact Derm* 15, 143–151.

BASHIR, S. and MAIBACH, H. (2000) Methods for testing irritant potential. In MENNE, T. and MAIBACH, H. (eds) *Hand Eczema*. New York: CRC Press, 367–376.

CALANDRA, J. (1971) Comments on the guinea pig immersion test. *CFTA Cosmet. J.* 3(3), 47.

CLARYS, P. and BAREL, A.O. (1997) Comparison of three detergents using the patch test and the hand/forearm immersion test as measurements of irritancy. *J. Soc. Cosmet. Chem.* 48, 141–149.

CLARYS, P., MANOU, I., *et al.* (1997) Influence of temperature on irritation in the hand/forearm immersion test. *Contact Derm.* 36(5), 240–243.

EDWARDS, C. (1972) Hazardous substances. Proposed revision of test for primary skin irritants. *Federal Register* **37**(27), 625–627, 636.

FROSCH, P. and KLIGMAN, A. (1976) The chamber scarification test for irritancy. *Contact Derm.* **2**, 314–324.

FROSCH, P. and KLIGMAN, A. (1977) The chamber scarification test for testing the irritancy of topically applied substances. In DRILL, V. and LAZAR, P. (eds) *Cutaneous Toxicity.* New York: Academic Press, 150.

FROSCH, P.J. and KLIGMAN, A.M. (1979) The soap chamber test. A new method for assessing the irritancy of soaps. *J. Am. Acad. Dermatol.* **1**, 35–41.

FROSCH, P., SCHULZE-DIRKS, A., *et al.* (1993) Efficacy of skin barrier creams. The repetitive irritation test (RIT) in the guinea pig. *Contact Dermatitis* **28**, 94–100.

GILMAN, M., EVANS, R., *et al.* (1978) The influence of concentration, exposure duration, and patch occlusivity upon rabbit primary dermal irritation indices. *Drug and Chemical Toxicology* **1**(4), 391–400.

GOLDNER, R. and JACKSON, E. (1994) Irritant contact dermatitis. In HOGAN, D. (ed.) *Occupational Skin Disorders.* New York: Igaku-Shoin Medical Publishers, 23.

GUPTA, B., MATHUR, A., *et al.* (1992) Dermal exposure to irritants. *Vet. Hum. Toxicol.* **34**(5), 405–407.

HUMPHREY, D. (1993) Measurement of cutaneous microvascular exudates using Evans blue. *Biotechnic and Histochemistry* **68**(6), 342–349.

JUSTICE, J., TRAVERS, J., *et al.* (1961) The correlation between animal tests and human tests in assessing product mildness. *Proc. Sci. Section Toilet Goods Assoc.* **35**, 12–17.

KLIGMAN, A. and WOODING, W. (1967) A method for the measurement and evaluation of irritants on human skin. *Journal of Investigative Dermatology* **49**, 78–94.

Kobayashi, I., Hosaka, K., *et al.* (1999) Skin toxicity of propranolol in guinea pigs. *J. Toxicol. Sci.* **24**(2), 103–112.

KOOYMAN, D. and SNYDER, F. (1942) Tests for the mildness of soaps. *Arch. Dermatol. Syphilol.* **46**, 846–855.

LLEWELLYN, P., MARSHALL, S., *et al.* (1972) A comparison of rabbit and human skin response to certain irritants. *Toxicology and Applied Pharmacology* **21**, 369–382.

MACMILLAN, F., RAM, R., *et al.* (1975) A comparison of the skin irritation produced by cosmetic ingredients and formulations in the rabbit, guinea pig and beagle dog to that observed in the human. In MAIBACH, H. (ed.) *Animal Models in Dermatology.* Edinburgh: Churchill Livingstone, 399–402.

MARZULLI, F. and MAIBACH, H. (1975) The rabbit as a model for evaluating skin irritants: A comparison of results obtained on animals and man using repeated skin exposure. *Food and Cosmetics Toxicology* **13**, 533–540.

MEZEI, M. *et al.* (1966) Dermatitic effect of nonionic surfactants. I. Gross, microscopic, and metabolic changes in rabbit skin treated with nonionic surface-active agents. *Journal of Pharmaceutical Science and Technology* **55**, 584–590.

MURPHY, J., WATSON, E., *et al.* (1979) Cutaneous irritation in the topical application of 30 antineoplastic agents to New Zealand white rabbits. *Toxicology* **14**, 117–130.

NATIONAL ACADEMY OF SCIENCES and COMMITTEE FOR THE REVISION OF NAS PUBLICATION 1138 (1977) Principles and procedures for evaluating the toxicity of household substances, pp. 23–59. Washington DC, National Academy of Sciences.

NIXON, G., TYSON, C., *et al.* (1975) Interspecies comparison of skin irritancy. *Toxicology and Applied Pharmacology* **31**, 481–490.

PATIL, S., PATRICK, E., *et al.* (1996) Animal, human and *in vitro* test methods for predicting skin irritation. In MARZULLI, F. and MAIBACH, H. (eds) *Dermatotoxicology.* Fifth Edition. Washington DC: Taylor and Francis.

PATIL, S., PATRICK, E., *et al.* (1998) Animal, human and *in vitro* test methods for predicting skin irritation. In MARZULLI, F. and MAIBACH, H. (eds) *Dermatotoxicology methods: the laboratory worker's vade mecum.* Washington DC: Taylor and Francis, 89–104.

PATRICK, E. and MAIBACH, H. (1987) A novel predictive assay in mice. *Toxicologist* **7**, 84.

PATRICK, E. and MAIBACH, H. (1989) Comparison of the time course, dose response and mediators of chemicially induced skin irritation in three species. In FROSCH, P., DOOMS-GOOSSENS, A., LACHAPELLE, J.-M., RYCROFT, R.J.G. and SCHEPER, R.J. (eds) *Current Topics in Contact Dermatitis.* New York: Springer-Verlag.

PHILLIPS, L., STEINBERG, M., *et al.* (1972) A comparison of rabbit and human skin responses to certain irritants. *Toxicology and Applied Pharmacology* **21**, 369–382.

SHILLAKER, R., BELL, G., *et al.* (1989) Guinea pig maximization test for skin sensitisation: The use of fewer test animals. *Archives of Toxicology* **63**(4), 283–288.

SKOG, E. (1960) Primary irritant and allergic eczematous reactions in patients with different dermatoses. *Acta Derm. Venereol.* **40**, 307–312.

TRUSH, M., ENGER, P., *et al.* (1994) Myeloperoxidase as a biomarker of skin irritation and inflammation. *Food and Chemical Toxicology* **32**(2), 143–147.

UTTLEY, M. and VAN ABBE, N. (1973) Primary irritation of the skin: mouse ear test and human patch test procedures. *J. Soc. Cosmet. Chem.* **24**, 217–227.

WAHLBERG, J. (1993) Measurement of skin fold thickness in the guinea pig. Assessment of edema-inducing capacity of cutting fluids in responses to certain irritants. *Contact Derm.* **28**, 141–145.

WALLE, H.V.D. (2000) Irritant contact dermatitis. In MENNE, T. and MAIBACH, H. (eds) *Hand Eczema*. New York: CRC Press, 133–139.

WEIL, C. and SCALA, R. (1971) Study of intra- and inter-laboratory variability in the results of rabbit eye and skin irritation tests. *Toxicology and Applied Pharmacology* **19**, 276–360.

WIGGER-ALBERTI, W. and ELSNER, P. (1997a) Petrolatum prevents irritation in a human cumulative exposure model *in vivo*. *Dermatology* **194**(3), 247–250.

WIGGER-ALBERTI, W., HINNEN, U., *et al.* (1997b) Predictive testing of metal-working fluids: a comparison of 2 cumulative human irritation models and correlation human irritation models and correlation with epidemiological data. *Contact Derm.* **36**(1), 14–20.

ZHAI, H., WILLARD, P., *et al.* (1998) Evaluating skin-protective materials against contact irritants and allergens. An *in vivo* screening human model. *Contact Derm.* **38**(3), 155–158.

CHAPTER 36

Analysis of Structural Change in Intercellular Lipids of Human Stratum Corneum Induced by Surfactants

Electron Paramagnetic Resonance (EPR) Study

YOSHIAKI KAWASAKI, JUN-ICHI MIZUSHIMA
AND HOWARD I MAIBACH

Contents

37.1 Introduction

37.2 What is Electron Paramagnetic Resonance (EPR) spectroscopy?

37.3 Experimental design

37.4 Results and discussion

37.5 Conclusion

37.1 INTRODUCTION

The human skin is the largest organ in the body and serves the major function of protecting the underlying tissues from external elements. The skin offers a formidable barrier in the form of a multilayered stratum corneum that is renewed continuously by the underlying epidermis. With increasing use of cosmetics and cleansing products, the human skin is brought into contact with the variety of excipients used in these topical formulations. Many of these contain surfactants which can have toxic and irritating effects on skin. In addition, these amphiphillic molecules can partition into the stratum corneum and compromise the epidermal barrier function.

The intercellular lipid lamellae in the stratum corneum constitute the main epidermal barrier to the diffusion of water and other solutes (Elias and Friend, 1975; Elias, 1981; Wertz and Downing, 1982; Elias, 1983; Landman, 1986). These lipids, arranged in multiple layers between the corneocytes (Swartzendruber *et al.*, 1989; Wertz *et al.*, 1989), consist of ceramides (40–50 percent), free fatty acids (15–25 percent), cholesterol (15–25 percent) and cholesterol sulfate (5–10 percent) (Swartzendruber *et al.*, 1987; Gray *et al.*, 1982; Long *et al.*, 1985). Information on the molecular structure of these lipids is important in elaborating a rational design for effective penetration enhancers in transdermal drug delivery (Woodford and Barry, 1986) and to understand the mechanism of irritant dermatitis and other stratum corneum diseases. This information has been obtained by thermal analysis (Van Duzee, 1975; Golden *et al.*, 1987; Bouwstra *et al.*, 1992), X-ray diffraction study (Vilkes *et al.*, 1973; White *et al.*, 1988; Bouwstra *et al.*, 1991a, b; Garson *et al.*, 1991; Bouwstra *et al.*, 1994), FT-IR spectroscopy (Bommannann *et al.*, 1990; Krill *et al.*, 1992) and electron paramagnetic resonance spectroscopy (EPR) (Rehfeld *et al.*, 1988; 1990).

Several investigators (Imokawa *et al.*, 1975; Faucher and Goddard, 1978; Imokawa, 1980; Fulmer and Kramer, 1986; Rhein *et al.*, 1986; Froebe *et al.*, 1990; Rhein *et al.*, 1990; Barker *et al.*, 1991; Giridhar and Acosta, 1993; Wilmer *et al.*, 1994) have demonstrated that stratum corneum swelling, protein denaturation, lipid removal, inhibition of cellular proliferation and chemical mediator release contribute to irritation reactions. However, the mechanism of irritant dermatitis has not yet been understood and defined completely.

On the other hand, permeability is increased by an increase in fluidity both in biological and artificial membranes, suggesting a correlation between flux and fluidity (Knutson *et al.*, 1985; Golden *et al.*, 1987). The dynamic properties of intercellular lipids in the stratum corneum are incompletely characterized; the effect of surfactants has not been studied in detail.

CHAPTER 37

Electron paramagnetic resonance (EPR) employing nitroxide spin probes, known as the spin labeling method, has been utilized as a valuable spectroscopic method for providing information about the dynamic structure of membranes (Sauerheber *et al.*, 1977; Curtain and Gorden, 1984). Spin probes are specifically incorporated into the lipid or lipid part of biological membranes. Thus, each label reflects the properties of different membrane regions. EPR spectra of membrane incorporated spin probes are sensitive to the rotational mobility and orientation of the probes, and to the polarity of the environment surrounding the probes.

In this chapter, the influence of surfactants on the intercellular lipid structure of cadaver stratum corneum and the stripped stratum corneum will be discussed, based on Spin-Label Electron Paramagnetic Resonance (EPR) spectroscopy. Techniques used to investigate fluidity of intercellular lipid layers of human stratum corneum will also be reviewed. In the meantime, we will also show the correlation between EPR spectral data and human clinical data such as trans-epidermal water loss (TEWL).

37.2 WHAT IS ELECTRON PARAMAGNETIC RESONANCE (EPR) SPECTROSCOPY?

Electron paramagnetic resonance (EPR), also known as electron spin resonance (ESR), is the name given to the process of resonant absorption of microwave radiation by paramagnetic ions or molecules, with at least one unpaired electron spin in the presence of a static magnetic field. EPR was discovered by Zavoisky in 1944. It has a wide range of applications in chemistry, physics, biology, and medicine: it may be used to probe the "static" structure of solid and liquid systems, and is also very useful in investigating dynamic processes.

Most biological systems give no intrinsic EPR signal because they have no unpaired electrons. Therefore, if EPR is to be used in studying these systems such as lipid membranes or macromolecules, one or more radicals known as spin labels must be coupled to the system under investigation. The spin label thus is an extrinsic probe or reporter group providing information that reflects the state of the biological system.

37.2.1 Principles

The detailed principles of EPR are explained in the book written by Wertz and Bolton (1972) Here, EPR principles are introduced in brief.

The principles of EPR are similar to those of NMR (Nuclear Magnetic Resonance). The magnetic moment of an unpaired electron is given by

$$m = -g_e \, (eh \, / \, 4\pi m_e) \, m_s \; (\text{SI})$$

in which g_e is the electronic g-factor (a number very nearly equal to 2). $-e$ and m_e are respectively the electronic charge and mass, and m_s is the spin quantum number (equal to $\pm 1/2$). The quantity in parentheses in the first equation is called the *Bohr magneton*, and has the value of 9.2732×10^{-24} J T^{-1} in SI units (9.2732×10^{-21} erg G^{-1}). In an applied magnetic field of strength B, the transition of an electron from ground to the excited state requires energy

$$\Delta E = g_e \, (eh \, / \, 4\pi m_e) \, B \; (\text{SI})$$

In a magnetic field of 2T (20 kG), this energy corresponds to the absorption of radiation of the frequency

$$\upsilon = \Delta E \, / h = 2 \times (9.273 \times 10^{-24} \, \text{JT}^{-1})(2 \text{ T}) \, / \, 6.62 \times 10^{-34} \, \text{Js} = 5.6 \times 10^{10} \, \text{Hz}$$

which is in the microwave region of the spectrum.

Paramagnetic substances are detected readily by EPR. About 10^{-13} mole of a substance gives an observable signal, so this technique is one of the most sensitive of all spectroscopic tools (Eisenberg and Crothers, 1979).

The effect of a neighboring nuclear spin on the resonance of an unpaired electron is called hyperfine coupling. For an electron in a magnetic field, there are two orientations and two quantum states (Figure 37.1(a)), giving a possible combination of four quantum states for the electron-nucleus pair. Nuclear spin "splits" each electron quantum state into two states. Because the selection rules for transitions in hyperfine coupling are $\Delta m_s = \pm 1$ and $\Delta m_I = 0$, there can only be two transitions among these four states for which electromagnetic radiation can be absorbed. Vertical arrows in Figure 37.1(b) show these two transitions.

For the ^{14}N nucleus, for example, $I = 1$, so there are three nuclear spin quantum states. Thus, a nearby ^{14}N nucleus splits the electronic levels into six levels. Three transitions are allowed among the six levels; consequently, the spectrum consists of three absorption bands.

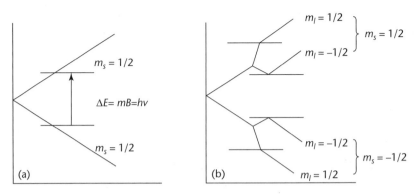

Figure 37.1: Energy levels of an unpaired electron with spin quantum states $m_s = 1/2$: (a) in magnetic field; and (b) in a magnetic field and coupled to a nuclear spin of $I = 1/2$, with nuclear spin quantum.

37.2.2 Electron spin resonance spectrometer

A modern ESR instrument consists of three basic units: (a) a microwave bridge and resonator, (b) a variable field magnet and (c) signal amplification circuitry (Figure 37.2).

Microwaves of the desired frequency are generated by either a klystron or Gunn diode. Their intensity is adjusted by an attenuator and transmitted via a waveguide to the sample chamber/resonator. During resonance, a small amount of microwaves is reflected from the resonator and detected by a Shottky diode.

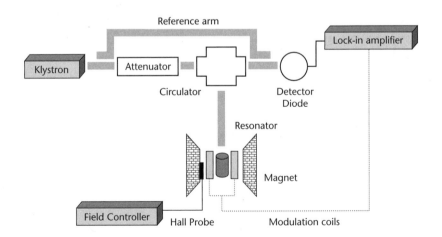

Figure 37.2: Block diagram of a typical EPR spectrometer.

To separate the reflected and incident microwaves, a circulator is placed between the attenuator and resonator. The circulator channels the microwaves in a forward direction: incident microwaves to the resonator and reflected microwaves to the detector. The bridge often contains an additional pathway—a reference arm which taps off a small fraction of the microwaves from the source—which bypasses the resonator and falls onto the detector to ensure its bias for the optimal detection of small intensity changes during resonance.

A static magnetic field is provided by an electromagnet stabilized by a Hall probe. The field is slowly swept by varying the amount of current passing through the electromagnet.

37.2.3 Spin labeling method; paramagnetic nitroxide molecules that serve as probes in membranes

McConnell *et al.* (1972) showed that significant information could be derived about macromolecules and membranes from the EPR spectra of bound nitroxide molecules. These are stable molecules that possess an unpaired $2p$ electron. The unpaired electron endows the molecules with strong EPR spectra. 5-Doxyl Stearic Acid (5-DSA) is one of the most commonly used spin probes and its structure is shown in Figure 37.3. A nitroxide molecule bound to a macromolecule is called a spin label.

Because the ^{14}N nucleus in a nitroxide molecule is near the unpaired electron, there is an interaction between them, thereby producing hyperfine splitting in the EPR spectrum. The ^{14}N nucleus has a spin of one, and consequently three absorption bands appear in the EPR spectra. The EPR spectra are usually recorded as the first derivative of the absorption spectrum, so instead of three bands there are three rise-and-dip spikes, which are the derivatives of the three bands. Triplet signals, which are sharp, can be observed when the spin-probe moves freely, as shown in Figure 37.4. However, the spectrum becomes broader when spin probe mobility is restricted by interaction with other components. When the spin

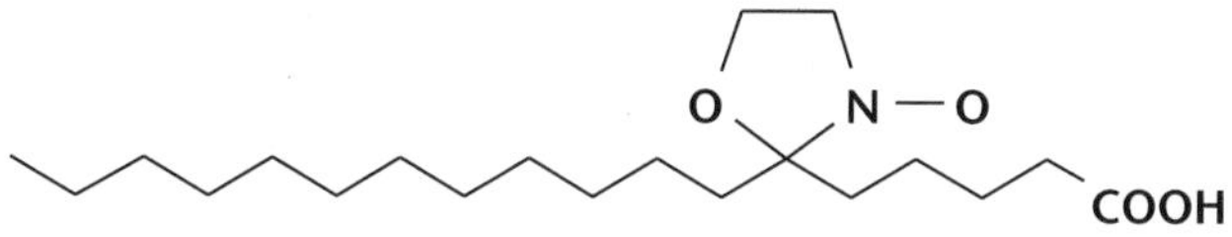

Figure 37.3: Chemical structure of spin probe; 5-Doxyl Stearic Acid (-DSA).

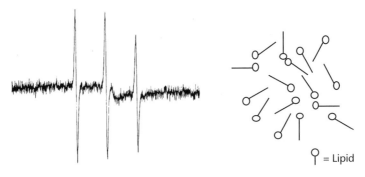

Figure 37.4: EPR spectrum of 5-DSA in aqueous solution.

probe is incorporated into the highly-oriented intercellular lipid structure of normal skin, the probe cannot move freely due to the rigidity of the lipid structure, and its EPR spectrum represents the broad profile as seen in Figure 37.5(a). Once the normal structure is completely destroyed by chemical and/or physical stress, there is nothing to inhibit probe mobility, and the EPR spectrum profiles become sharp, as in Figure 37.5(b). The EPR spectral profile represents the rigidity of the environment of the spin probe. To express the rigidity quantitatively, an order parameter S is calculated from the EPR spectrum.

Spin labels provide information about the molecules to which they are bound. They can report the rate of motion of the molecule to which they have been covalently bound, or the amount of thermal motion in a membrane into which they have been inserted. The principle is that the bands of the EPR spectrum are broadened when the spin label is immobilized and narrowed when it is tumbling rapidly. The narrowing comes from the more rapid relaxation of the spin when neighboring groups are moving rapidly with respect to the spin label.

A second type of information is the polarity of the local environment surrounding the spin probe. The extent of splitting of the side bands from the central band depends on the dielectric constant of the medium in which the spin label is dissolved. Solvents of high dielectric constant augment the polarity of the N-O bond and increase the splitting. By measuring the splitting, an estimate can be made of the polarity of the surroundings of the spin label. This is of interest, for example, when a spin label is bound to a membrane, since it allows one to determine if the label is bound near the polar head groups or near the non-polar hydrocarbon chains (Mehlhorn and Keith, 1972).

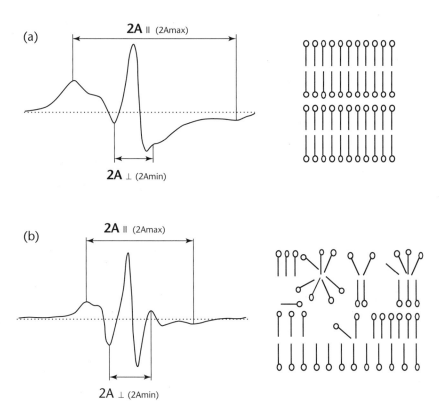

Figure 37.5: EPR spectrum of 5-DSA labeled stratum corneum from cadaver, (a) non-treatment (control), (b) treated with 1%wt SLS (sodium lauryl sulfate) for 24 hours.

37.2.4   How to read the EPR spectrum; calculation of order parameter S

Order parameters were calculated according to Griffith and Jost (1976), Hubbell and McConnell (1971), and Marsh (1981):

$$S = (A\| - A\perp) / [A_{ZZ} - 1/2 (A_{XX} + A_{YY})](a_0/a_0')$$

where 2 A$\|$ is identified with the outer maximum hyperfine splitting A_{max}, and A$\perp$ is obtained from the inner minimum hyperfine splitting A_{min} (Figure 37.5).

a$_0$ is the isotropic hyperfine splitting constant for nitroxide molecules in the crystal state.

$$a_0 = (A_{XX} + A_{YY} + A_{ZZ}) / 3$$

■ CHAPTER 37 ■

The values used to describe the rapid anisotropic motion of membrane-incorporated probes of the fatty acid type are:

$$(A_{XX}, A_{YY}, A_{ZZ}) = (6.1, 6.1, 32.4) \text{ Gauss}$$

Similarly the isotropic hyperfine coupling constant for the spin label in the membrane (a_0') is given by:

$$a_0' = (A\| + 2\, A\bot) / 3$$

a_0' values are sensitive to the polarity in the environment of the spin labels since increases in a_0' value reflect an increase in the polarity of the medium.

The order parameter provides a measure of the flexibility of the spin labels in the membrane. It follows that $S = 1$ for highly oriented (rigid) states and $S = 0$ for completely isotropic motion (liquid). Increases of order parameter reflect decreases in the segmental flexibility of the spin label, and conversely decreases in the order parameter S reflect increases in the flexibility (Curtain and Gorden, 1984).

37.3 EXPERIMENTAL DESIGN

37.3.1 EPR measurement of stratum corneum from cadaver; spin labeling and surfactant treatment procedure

Human abdominal skin was obtained from a fresh cadaver with a dermatome. Epidermis was separated from dermis by immersing the skin in a 60°C water bath set for 2 min. followed by mechanical removal. Then, the epidermis was placed, stratum corneum side up, on the filter paper and floated on 0.5%wt trypsin (type II; Sigma) in a Tris-HCl buffer solution (pH 7.4) for two hours at 37°C. After incubation, any softened epidermis was removed by mild agitation of the stratum corneum sheet. Stratum corneum was dried and stored in a desiccator at −70°C for 3–4 days. Details are described by Quan (Quan and Maibach, 1994; Quan et al., 1995).

One slice of dry stratum corneum sheet (approximately 0.5 cm²; ~0.7 cm × ~0.7 cm) was incubated in a 1.0 mg/dl 5-DSA aqueous solution (2.6×10^{-5} M; FW = 384.6) for two hours at 37°C and washed gently with deionized water to remove the excess spin label.

Surfactant treatment was as follows: a spin-labeled section of stratum corneum was immersed in surfactant aqueous solution and incubated at 37°C for one hour. The stratum corneum was taken out of the surfactant solution at indicated times. After rinsing with deionized water and removing the excess water, the stratum corneum was mounted on a flat surface EPR cell and EPR spectra were recorded.

The control EPR spectrum was recorded for the spin-labeled section of stratum corneum kept in the deionized water at 37°C instead of that kept in the surfactant solution.

37.3.2 EPR measurement of stripped human stratum corneum; spin labeling and surfactant treatment procedure

Two hundred μl of aqueous solution of 1.00%wt surfactants were applied to the mid-volar forearm using occlusive polypropylene chambers (1.8 cm diameter; Hilltop Laboratory, Cincinnati, OH, USA) for 24 h. Deionized water served as vehicle controls. Application sites for the different treatments were rotated to avoid an anatomical selection bias (Van der Valk and Maibach, 1989; Cua *et al.*, 1990; Lee *et al.*, 1994). Each site was examined visually by the same investigator and using following instrumental methods; transdermal water loss (TEWL), electrical conductance and chromametry.

After these non-invasive measurements, patch site stratum corneum was removed from the volar side of the forearm skin by a single stripping with one drop of cyanoacrylate resin onto a quartz glass in accordance with the method of Imokawa *et al.* (1991). Stripped stratum corneum attached to a quartz glass was spin labeled with a drop (approximately 30 μl) of 1.0 mg/dl 5-DSA solution for 30 minutes at 37°C, then washed with deionized water to remove excess spin probe on the stripped skin surface.

Stripped stratum corneum was attached to a quartz cell and EPR measurement was similarly conducted for cadaver stratum corneum.

37.4 RESULTS AND DISCUSSION

37.4.1 Effect of surfactants on the intercellular lipid fluidity of cadaver stratum corneum

Kawasaki *et al.* (1995; 1997; 1999) and Mizushima *et al.* (2000) have examined the influence of surfactants on human stratum corneum obtained from cadaver (Table 37.1).

■ CHAPTER 37 ■

TABLE 37.1:

Order parameters of stratum corneum treated with surfactants and clinical observations

Category	Sample name	Concentration (%wt)	Order parameter S	Visual scores (average ± SD)	Visual scores (average ± SD) g/m²/h
Control	Water		0.89 ± 0.04	0.00 ± 0.00	5.0 ± 1.1
Anionic	SLS (Sodium lauryl sulfate)	1.0	0.47 ± 0.05	0.79 ± 0.30	13.6 ± 3.1
	SL (Sodium laurate)	1.0	0.65 ± 0.06	0.08 ± 0.20	7.1 ± 3.9
		5.0	0.52 ± 0.04	0.67 ± 0.30	13.3 ± 3.7
	SLES (Sodium lauryl POE (3) ether sulfate)	1.0	0.62 ± 0.06	0.42 ± 0.30	7.6 ± 2.8
	SLEC (Sodium lauryl POE (3) ether carboxylate)	1.0	0.62 ± 0.05	0.08 ± 0.20	7.4 ± 2.9
	SLG (Monosodium lauryl glutamate)	1.0	0.73 ± 0.07	0.04 ± 0.10	6.7 ± 3.5
		5.0	0.77 ± 0.08	0.13 ± 0.20	5.5 ± 2.3
Cationic	MSAC (Monostearylammonium chloride)	1.0	0.68 ± 0.02	NA	10.2 ± 1.9
Amphoteric	HEA	1.0	0.75 ± 0.02	NA	9.2 ± 0.8

NA: Visual grading is different from that of anionics.

The surfactant molecule, which is amphiphillic to water and lipid, may be incorporated into structured lipids (lamellar structure). The order parameter calculated from 1.00%wt SLS treated stratum corneum was 0.47, indicating a disordering of the lipid structure. On the contrary, the high order parameter value (0.73) for 1.00%wt SLG meant less of an effect on the structured lipid compared to the control order parameter value (0.89). Treatment with 1.00%wt solution of SL, SLES and SLEC revealed intermediate levels between SLG and SLS. Lipid disorder induced by MSAC and HEA, which are classified into a category different from anionic surfactants, also revealed intermediate levels between SLS and SLG. Note that 1.00%wt MSAC and 1.00%wt HEA, which are quaternary and amphoteric compounds respectively, lead to less disorder in lipid structure than 1.00%wt SLS, although the irritation potential of surfactants is widely assumed to follow the pattern below in which quaternaries are the most irritating; quaternaries > amphoterics > anionics > nonionics (Rieger, 1997). These two compounds (1.00%wt MSAC and 1.00%wt HEA) have plus charges. Their interaction with stratum corneum may be different from that of anionics such as SLS. A plus charge might have more attractive interaction with proteins electrically because proteins are generally thought to be negatively charged.

The change of order parameter corresponds to the structural changes in lipid layers. We can speculate that there are two phases in the increase of fluidity in lipid structure (decreasing the order parameter). The first phase is an effect of surfactants incorporated into the lamellar structures. If the surfactant interferes with or decreases lateral interactions between lipids, mobility increases in a way similar to the phase conversion from liquid crystal to gel in the lamellar layers. The second phase is the destruction of lamellar structure by micellization or solubilization of lipids by the surfactant. In this case, lipids no longer have dimensional restrictions and gain much higher mobility.

The results shown in Table 37.2 indicate that mobility increase induced by SLG can be attributed to phase-one structural changes in the lipid layers and that SLS might cause further disruption of the structures of lipid layers. The role of water in the stratum corneum must be also considered in an examination of the effects of surfactants on lipid layers. Treatment with anionic surfactants might influence water penetration and/or skin swelling (Takino *et al.*, 1996). Rhein *et al.* (1986; 1990) examined the swelling of stratum corneum caused by surfactants and reported that the swelling effect of surfactants suggests a mechanism of action as the basis for *in vivo* irritation potential.

Figure 37.6 shows the correlation between the order parameter obtained from an EPR spectrum and the clinical readings. The correlation coefficients

■ CHAPTER 37 ■

TABLE 37.2:

EPR spectral data and clinical data of SLS/SLG mixtures

Sample name	Averaged order parameter (mean ± SD; n=3)	Human patch (mean ± SD)	
		Visual score	TEWL (g H₂O/m²/h)
Control	0.86 ± 0.03	0.53 ± 0.08	13.0 ± 1.0
0.25%wt SLS	0.70 ± 0.02	0.73 ± 0.08	22.3 ± 1.7
0.50%wt SLS	0.66 ± 0.04	0.70 ± 0.10	22.3 ± 1.7
0.75%wt SLS	0.64 ± 0.03	0.87 ± 0.14	22.7 ± 1.5
1.00%wt SLS	0.56 ± 0.03	1.03 ± 0.15	25.4 ± 2.6
0.25%wt SLS + 0.75%wt SLG	0.81 ± 0.07	0.42 ± 0.30	20.0 ± 1.7
0.50%wt SLS + 0.50%wt SLG	0.71 ± 0.00	0.08 ± 0.20	20.7 ± 1.9
0.75%wt SLS + 0.25%wt SLG	0.66 ± 0.04	0.04 ± 0.10	21.2 ± 2.6
0.25%wt SLS + 1.00%wt SLG	0.81 ± 0.05	NA	NA
0.50%wt SLS + 1.00%wt SLG	0.79 ± 0.05	NA	NA
0.75%wt SLS + 1.00%wt SLG	0.74 ± 0.04	NA	NA
1.00%wt SLS + 1.00%wt SLG	0.66 ± 0.05	NA	NA
1.00%wt SLG	0.82 ± 0.02	0.67 ± 0.08	15.8 ± 1.1

Note: Error bars: Mean ± SD, n=3 for order parameters, Mean ± SD, n=15 for clinical data
NA : Not available in Imokawa *et al.* (1991).

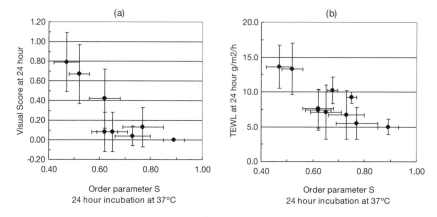

Figure 37.6: Correlation between clinical data of 24 hour patch and order parameter S of 5-DSA labeled cadaver stratum corneum incubated in surfactant solution for 1 hour at 37°C: (a) Correlation between order parameters and visual scores; (b) Correlation between order parameters and TEWL.

(*Note:* Error bars : Mean ± SD, n=3 for order parameter ; Mean ± SD, n=14 for clinical data.)

(r^2) of visual score and TEWL values were 0.76 and 0.83, respectively. The order parameter correlates to TEWL values better than to visual scores. This difference may be explainable in that TEWL is a direct measure of water barrier function, while visual scores represent total skin reactions including physical or structural changes of skin tissue due to physiological or biological reactions with surfactants. The visual score and colorimetry, showed similar correlation coefficients, which mainly reflect reactions of the skin including edema of the epidermis and upper dermis, perivascular infiltrates and vasodilation. The order parameter might not predict subsequent skin reactions after a disorder of the lipid structure caused by the denaturation of proteins or mucosaccarides in the dermis.

Order parameter measurement of stratum corneum may predict the minimal difference in irritation potential among a range of surfactants.

37.4.2 Effect of surfactant mixtures (SLS/SLG) on intercellular lipid fluidity of cadaver stratum corneum

As discussed previously, SLS was the most severely irritating and SLG the mildest amongst the anionic surfactants tested. Kawasaki *et al.* (1999) examined the influence of surfactant mixtures (SLS/SLG) on the intercellular lipid fluidity of stratum corneum obtained from cadaver skin.

The order parameter of water-treated stratum corneum (vehicle control) was 0.86 ± 0.03. Anionic surfactants as amphiphilic molecules may be incorporated into structured lipids (the lamellar structure). The order parameter calculated from 1.00%wt SLS treated stratum corneum was 0.56 ± 0.03, indicating disorder in the lipid structure. On the contrary, the high order parameter value (0.82 ± 0.02) for 1.00%wt SLG meant that less lipid structure was disordered; 1.00%wt SLG was almost equal to water. Treatment with 0.25%wt, 0.50%wt and 0.75%wt SLS solutions revealed intermediate levels between 1.00%wt SLG and 1.00%wt SLS.

Each order parameter of 5-DSA labeled stratum corneum treated with SLS/SLG mixtures (the total concentration was constant at 1.00%wt) showed higher values than those of 0.25%wt, 0.50%wt, 0.75%wt SLS, respectively. There were no statistically significant differences between 0.50%wt SLS and 0.50%wt SLS / 0.50%wt SLG, and between 0.75%wt SLS and 0.75%wt SLS / 0.25%wt SLG ($p>0.05$). These profiles are also supported by the results of Kanari *et al.* (1993).

These results suggest that SLG inhibited SLS-induced lipid fluidization. To confirm the anti-fluidization of SLG, SLS/SLG mixture solutions were prepared with the SLG concentration constant at 1.00%wt, and 5-DSA labeled stratum

CHAPTER 37

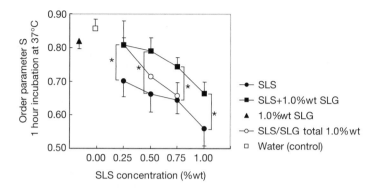

Figure 37.7: Order parameter of 5-DSA labeled cadaver stratum corneum treated with water, SLS, SLG, and LSL/SLG mixtures (total concentration 1.00wt%, 1.00wt% SLG addition to the SLS solutions.
Error bars : Mean ± SD, $n=3$;
* indicates that $p < 0.05$)

corneum was treated with them. Then the EPR spectra were measured. The calculated order parameters are plotted in Figure 37.7.

Order parameters at each SLS concentration (0.25, 0.50, 0.75 and 1.00%wt SLS) with 1.00%wt SLG, showed higher values than those of SLS-only solutions. There were statistically significant differences between solutions with and without 1.00%wt SLG ($P<0.05$), suggesting that the addition of 1.00%wt SLG inhibits the fluidization of intercellular lipids induced by SLS. It may be hypothesized that the direct interactions between SLS and intercellular lipids were interrupted by SLG and the log P (partition coefficient; log {[SLS] $_{lipid}$ / [SLS] $_{bulk}$}) of SLS into the intercellular lipid may be decreased.

The role of water in the stratum corneum must also be considered in analyzing the effects of surfactants on lipid layers. Alonso *et al.* (1995; 1996) reported that water increases the fluidity of the intercellular lipids of rat stratum corneum in the region closer to the hydrophilic area but not in the lipophillic area, deep inside the intercellular lipid layer.

The order parameter correlated to the clinical readings (Figure 37.8). The correlation coefficients (r^2) of visual score and TEWL values were 0.73 and 0.83, respectively. The order parameter correlates to TEWL values better than to visual scores, which are same result as shown in the previous section.

The order parameters represent the disorder of stratum corneum induced by short-term surfactant contact. However, the clinical data represent skin irritation

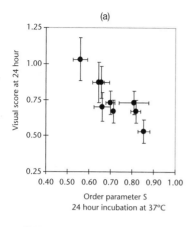 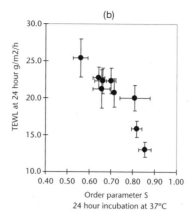

Figure 37.8: Correlation between clinical data of 24 hour patch and order parameter S of 5-DSA labeled cadaver stratum corneum incubated in surfactant solution for 1 hour at 37°C: (a) Correlation between order parameters and visual scores; (b) Correlation between order parameters and TEWL.

(*Note:* Error bars : Mean ± SD, $n=3$ for order parameter ; Mean ± SD, $n=15$ for clinical data.)

---

reactions induced by 24-hour occlusive contact with surfactants. Order parameter measurement of stratum corneum may predict the minimal difference in irritation potential among a range of surfactants.

37.4.3 Correlation between CMC and intercellular lipid fluidization for SLS

1.00 wt% SLS causes more fluidization than other anionic surfactants. We still must ask: how long must there be contact with severe anionic surfactant SLS before fluidization happens in lipids? How much alteration is induced by how much concentration of SLS?

Figure 37.9 (unpublished data) shows the incubation time dependence of an EPR spectrum with different SLS concentrations. With increasing incubation time, the order parameter was decreased. However, each profile of incubation time dependence had a plateau at the region of 6 hours and thereafter. The skin lipid alteration induced by SLS was typically completed within 6 hours at a given concentration. However, each alteration level in intercellular lipids depended on its SLS concentration.

As the concentration of SLS increases, the order parameter at 24-hour incubation decreases drastically in the range of 0 to 0.25%wt of SLS (Figure

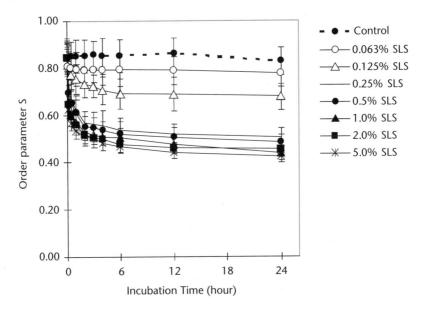

Figure 37.9: Time dependence of order parameters of 5-DSA labeled stratum corneum in SLS solution at various concentrations.

(*Note:* Error bars : Mean ± SD, *n*=5.)

37.10) However, the order parameters calculated from the stratum corneum treated with SLS at more than 0.5%wt had no significant difference, showing around 0.45 ~0.49. This critical point between 0.25 and 0.5%wt (8.7~17.3 mM) may correspond to the CMC (Critical Micelle Concentration) for SLS at 37°C. Rosen (1978) reported that the CMC of SLS is 8.6 mM at 40°C and 8.2 mM at 25°C.

This behavior is consistent with the following general concerns among experts: monomeric surfactants can penetrate the skin. Monomeric molecules are also the species that are initially adsorbed into the various surfaces within the skin; we cannot ignore secondary bonding due to hydrophobic effects. Thus, the concentration of monomeric species probably plays a major role in skin and surfactant interactions (Rieger, 1995).

37.4.4 EPR study utilizing human stripped stratum corneum

All the previous data are based on human stratum corneum obtained from cadaver skin. In order to define the structural changes in intercellular lipids

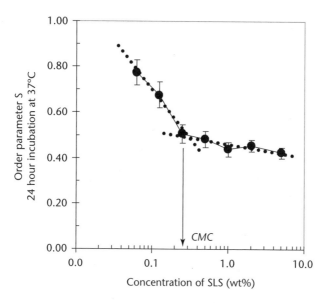

Figure 37.10: Correlation between SLS concentration and order parameters of 5-DSA labeled cadaver stratum corneum incubated at 37°C for 24 hours

(*Note:* Error bars ; Mean ± SD for *n*=5.)

induced by the topical application of surfactants and to discuss the correlation between lipid alteration and skin irritation reactions, choosing human stratum corneum from cadavers for a substrate as a model site of skin irritation is much better than using animal skins such as those of guinea pigs and rats, or using lecithin liposomes. But stratum corneum is not sufficient for discussing the mechanism of irritant dermatitis. Cadaver stratum corneum is just a substrate, not a living system which has a recovery system induced by signals such as chemical mediators. With the new procedure for measuring EPR spectra on human stripped stratum corneum, information on the dynamics of living skin may be provided.

Mizushima *et al.* (2000) examined EPR spectral data on stratum corneum from cadaver skin and stripped skin treated with three types of surfactants.

The correlation between order parameters of 5-DSA labeled cadaver stratum corneum treated with surfactants and those of 5-DSA labeled stripped stratum corneum was summarized in Figure 37.11.

It was possible for EPR spectra having sufficient signal intensity to read, to be obtained from stripped stratum corneum. The order parameters obtained from

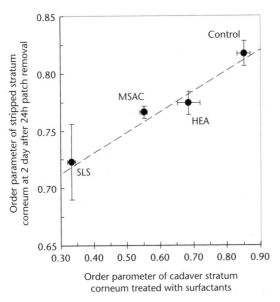

Figure 37.11: Correlation of order parameters between *cadaver stratum corneum* and *stripped stratum corneum*.

(*Note:* Error bars ; Mean ± SD for *n*=5.)
Cadaver stratum corneum = −3.883 + 5.833*Stripped stratum corneum

stripped stratum corneum are larger than those of cadaver stratum corneum. However, a high correlation between them was observed. Hence, the order parameters of cadaver stratum corneum reflect the fluidity of the intercellular lipids in the irritated skin.

The order parameter of SLS treated cadaver stratum corneum is smaller than that of stripped stratum corneum. This difference may be due to the barrier-reconstruction property of skin itself. The epidermis can synthesize lipid immediately after barrier disruption (Grubauer *et al.*, 1989). Skin barrier function was 80 percent repaired by 6 to 8 h, when skin was treated with acetone (Elias and Feingold, 1992).

The correlation between the order parameter of stripped stratum corneum and clinical readings are follows; the correlation coefficient between order parameter and visual score, TEWL values on the second day after patch removal, were 0.526, 0.708, respectively. The correlation with TEWL is high, as shown in Figure 37.12. This result consists of *in vitro* data based on cadaver stratum corneum.

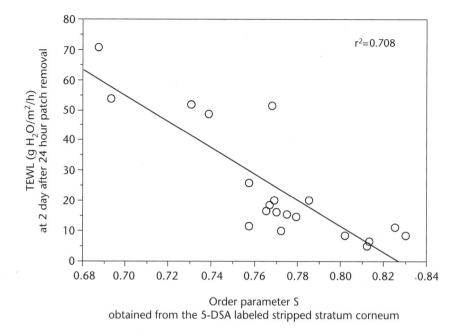

Figure 37.12: The correlation between TEWL and order parameters at 2nd day after 24 hour patch removal.

37.4.5 Water may affect the Order Parameter S

The role of water in the stratum corneum must be also considered for an understanding of the effects of surfactants on lipid layers. Alonso *et al.* (1995; 1996) reported that water increases the fluidity of intercellular lipids of rat stratum corneum at the region close to the hydrophilic area, but not in the lipophilic area, deep inside the intercellular lipid layer. Treatment with anionic surfactants may influence water penetration into stratum corneum. In case that the stratum corneum from a cadaver is treated with SLS and SLG for one hour, the order parameter decreases with the dose dependency of the surfactants. When order parameter is followed over time under dry conditions, those values increase. After 24 hours, the order parameter becomes higher than in the control (Kawasaki *et al.*, 1997). It is suggested that the altering of water content in cadaver stratum corneum affects the order parameter. This does not simply mean loss of water, because after the untreated control stratum corneum dries, the order parameter still shows a minimal order parameter change.

To investigate such effects of surfactants, Mizushima *et al.* (2001) measured the EPR spectra on cadaver stratum corneum treated with four concentrations of SLS under wet conditions just after incubation. The EPR spectra were measured again on the same samples after they were dried at room temperature for one hour. They also weighed each cadaver stratum corneum sample three times as follows; 1. before labeling (initial weight of each stratum corneum), 2. just after the treatment/ EPR measurement of stratum corneum under wet conditions, and 3. after the second EPR measurement of stratum corneum under dry conditions.

As shown in Table 37.3, under wet conditions, the order parameter S decreased and the weight of each cadaver stratum corneum increased with SLS dose dependency. On the contrary, under dry conditions, the order parameter increased with the dose dependency of SLS compared to the untreated control, which meant that the fluidity of the stratum corneum increased greatly before surfactant treatment. The weight of each cadaver stratum corneum sheet decreased with SLS dose dependency. So we can say that the effect of SLS on stratum corneum is not only to alter the fluidity of the lipid bilayer, but also to change the water-holding capacity of the lipid bilayer. This might be due to depletion of and/or change in the intercellular lipid lamellae such as fatty acids, cholesterol derivatives, and/or materials which cooperate with the keratin protein and amino acids as natural moisturizing factors.

Two phases can be hypothesized in the increase of fluidity in lipid structures. The first phase is in the effect of surfactants incorporated into the lamellar structures. If the surfactant interferes with or decreases lateral interactions

TABLE 37.3:

The order parameters S obtained from SLS treated cadaver stratum corneum ($n=3$) and its weight, measured under wet and dry conditions

SLS concentration (%wt)	Order parameter		Weight increase (%)	
	Wet condition	Dry condition	Wet condition	Dry condition
0.00	0.81 ± 0.01	0.82 ± 0.01	155.2 ± 4.3	95.2 ± 4.9
0.13	0.79 ± 0.01	0.83 ± 0.01	195.0 ± 9.8	87.1 ± 11.5
0.25	0.71 ± 0.01	0.84 ± 0.01	289.5 ± 47.7	82.5 ± 6.4
0.50	0.63 ± 0.02	0.84 ± 0.01	337.7 ± 28.8	81.6 ± 5.3
1.00	0.59 ± 0.01	0.84 ± 0.01	351.9 ± 21.3	80.3 ± 14.2

Note: The weight of the stratum corneum sheet is defined as 100 (%) just before labeling with 5-DSA aqueous solution.

between lipids, mobility increases in a way similar to the phase conversion from liquid crystal to gel in the lamellar layers. The second phase is the destruction of the lamellar structure by means of micellization or solubilization of the lipid layer by the surfactant. In this case, lipids no longer have dimensional restrictions and gain much higher mobility. The surfactant might have changed the water-holding capacity of the stratum corneum, and the water content may change the fluidity of stratum corneum lipids. We have to consider the water content of stratum corneum because it will alter the fluidity of intercellular lipids. To evaluate the effects of chemicals such as surfactants on stratum corneum lipids which may change the water holding capacity, we have to consider the existing water content of stratum corneum in measuring the EPR spectra.

37.5 CONCLUSION

The toxic manifestations of topically applied substances may induce immediate phenomena (such as corrosion or primary irritation), delayed phenomena (such as sensitization), phenomena which require an additional vector (such as phototoxicity), and systemic phenomena (paraquat toxicity). Such reactions cannot occur unless the toxic agent reaches a viable part of the skin by going through the stratum corneum with accompanying intercellular lipid structure disruption. If the toxicant can be stored in or absorbed by a skin layer without any alteration in lipid structure, it may not reach the viable tissues at all or may be released relatively slowly, thus effectively prolonging the symptoms

EPR spin labeling is a robust method for monitoring the structural change in intercellular lipids induced by topically applied surfactants. We have shown that order parameter is an easy to use and quantifiable method for predicting irritation reactions in the skin. In particular, EPR measurement on stripped stratum corneum may reflect the actual skin condition with regard to lipid structure. It may also aid in investigating the irritation potential of general chemicals, effects of topical penetration enhancers, drug delivery systems and skin diseases such as xerosis and atopic dermatitis.

REFERENCES

ALONSO, A., MEIRELLES, N.C. and TABAK, M. (1995) Effect of hydration upon the fluidity of intercellular membranes of stratum corneum: an EPR study, *Biochimica et Biophysica Acta* **1237**, 6–115.

CHAPTER 37

ALONSO, A., MEIRELLES, N.C., YUSHMANOV, V.E. and TABAK, M. (1996) Water increases the fluidity of intercellular membranes of stratum corneum: correlation with water permeability, elasticity and electrical resistance properties, *J. Invest. Dermatol.* **106**, 1058–1063.

BARKER, J., MITRA, R., GRIFFITHS, C., DIXIT, V. and NICKOLOFF, B. (1991) Keratinocytes as initiators of inflammation, *Lancet* **337**, 211–214.

Bommannann, D., Potts, R.O. and Guy, R.H. (1990) Examination of stratum corneum barrier function in vivo by infrared spectroscopy, *J. Invest. Dermatol.* **95**, 403–408.

BOUWSTRA, J.A., DE VRIES, M.A., DORIS, G.S., BRAS, W., BRUSSEE, J. and PONEC, M. (1991a) Thermodynamic and structural aspects of the skin barrier, *J. Controlled Release* **15**, 209–220.

BOUWSTRA, J.A., GOORIS, G.S., VAN DER SPEK, J.A. and BRAS, W. (1991b) Structural investigations of human stratum corneum by small-angle X-ray scattering, *J. Invest. Dermatol.* **97**, 1005–1012.

BOUWSTRA, J.A., GOORIS, G.S., DE VRIES, M.A., VAN DER SPEK, J.A. and BRAS, W. (1992) Structure of human stratum corneum as a function of temperature and hydration : A wide-angle X-ray diffraction study, *Intl. J. Phram.* **84**, 205–216.

BOUWSTRA, J.A., GOORIS, G.D., VAN DER SPEK, J.A., LAVRIJSEN, S. and BRAS, W. (1994) The lipid and protein structure of mouse stratum corneum: a wide and small angle diffraction study, *Biochim. Biophys. Acta* **1212**, 183–192.

CUA, A., WILHELM, K. and MAIBACH, H.I. (1990) Cutaneous sodium lauryl sulfate irritation potential: age and regional variability, *Br. J. Dermatol.* **123**, 607–163.

CURTAIN, C.C. and GORDEN, L.M. (1984) ESR spectroscopy of membranes, in VENTER, J.C. and HARRISON, L.C. (ed.) *Membranes, Detergents and Receptor Solubilization*, New York: Alan R. Liss, 177–213.

EISENBERG, D. and CROTHERS, D. (1979) *Physical Chemistry with Application to the Life Science*, Menlo Park: The Benjamin/Cummings Publishing Company, Inc.

ELIAS, P.M. (1981) Epidermal lipids, membrane, and keratinization, *Int. J. Dermtol.* **20**, 1–19.

ELIAS, P.M. (1983) Epidermal lipids, barrier function, and desquamation, *J. Invest. Dermatol.* **80**, 44–49.

ELIAS, P.M. and FEINGOLD, K. (1992) Lipids and the epidermal water barrier: metabolism, regulation, and pathophysiology, *Semin. Dermatol.* **11**, 176–178.

ELIAS, P.M. and FRIEND, D.S. (1975) The permeability barrier in mammalian epidermis, *J. Cell. Biol.* **65**, 180–191.

FAUCHER, J.A. and GODDARD, E.D. (1978) Interaction of keratinous substrates with sodium lauryl sulfate: I. Sorption, *J. Soc. Cosmet. Chem.* **29**, 323–337.

FROEBE, C.L., SIMON, F.A., RHEIN, L.D., CAGAN, R.H. and KLIGMAN, A. (1990) Stratum corneum lipid removal by surfactants: relation to in vivo irritation, *Dermatologica* **181**, 277–283.

FULMER, A.W. and KRAMER, G.J. (1986) Stratum corneum lipid abnormalities in surfactant-induced dry scaly skin, *J. Invest. Dermatol.* **86**, 598–602.

GARSON, J.C., DOUCET, J., LEVEUQUE, J.L. and TSOUCARIS, G. (1991) Oriented structure in human stratum corneum revealed by X-ray diffraction, *J. Invest. Dermatol.* **96**, 43–49.

GIRIDHAR, J. and ACOSTA, D. (1993) Evaluation of cytotoxicity potential of surfactants using primary rat keratinocyte culture as an *in vitro* cutaneous model, *In Vitro Toxicol. A Journal of Molecular and Cellular Toxicology* **6**, 33–46.

GOLDEN, G.M., GUZEK, D.B., KENNEDY, A.H., MCKIE, J.E. and POTTS, R.O. (1987) Stratum corneum lipid phase transitions and water barrier properties, *Biochemistry* **26**, 2382–2388.

GOLDEN, G.M., MCKIE, J.E. and POTTS, R.O. (1987) Role of stratum corneum lipid fluidity in transdermal drug flux, *J. Pharm. Sci.* **76**, 25–28.

GRAY, G.M., WHITE, R.J. and YARDLEY, H.J. (1982) Lipid composition of the superficial stratum corneum cells of pig epidermis, *Br. J. Dermatol.* **106**, 59–63.

GRIFFITH, O.H. and JOST, P.C. (1976) Lipid spin labels in biological membrane, in BERLINER, L.J. (ed.) *Spin Labeling Theory and Applications*, New York: Academic Press, 453–523.

GRUBAUER, G., FEINGOLD, K. and ELIAS, P.M. (1989) Transepidermal water loss: The signal for recovery of barrier structure and function, *J. Lipid Res.* **30**, 232–333.

HUBBEL, W.L. and MCCONNELL, H.M. (1971) Molecular motion in spin-labeled phospholipids and membranes, *J. Am. Chem. Soc.* **93**, 314–326.

IMOKAWA, G. (1980) Comparative study on the mechanism of irritation by sulfate and phosphate type anionic surfactants, *J. Soc. Cosmet. Chem.* **31**, 45–66.

IMOKAWA, G., ABE, A., JIN, K., HIGAKI, Y., KAWASHIMA, M. and HIDANO, A. (1991) Decreased level of ceramides in stratum corneum of atopic dermatitis: An etiologic factor in atopic dry skin, *J. Invest. Dermatol.* **96**, 523–526.

CHAPTER 37

IMOKAWA, G., SUMURA, K. and KATSUMI, M. (1975) Study on skin roughness by surfactants: II. Correlation between protein denaturation and skin roughness, *J. Am. Oil Chem. Soc.* **52**, 484–489.

KANARI, M., KAWASAKI, Y. and SAKAMOTO, K. (1993) Acylglutamate as an anti-irritant for mild detergent system, *J. Soc. Cosmet. Chem. Jpn.* **27**, 498–505.

KAWASAKI, Y., QUAN, D., SAKAMOTO, K. and MAIBACH, H.I. (1997) Electron resonance study on the influence of anionic surfactants on human skin, *Dermatology* **194**, 238–242.

KAWASAKI, Y., QUAN, D., SAKAMOTO, K., COOKE, R. and MAIBACH, H.I. (1999) Influence of surfactant mixtures on intercellular lipid fluidity and skin barrier function, *Skin Research Technology*, **5**, 96–101.

KAWASAKI, Y., TAKINO, Y., OHNUMA, M., SAKAMOTO, K., and MAIBACH, H.I. (1995) Correlation between *in vivo* skin irritation and intercellular lipid fluidity; ESR spin-labeling method, Abstract of 9th Japan Society of Animal Test Alternatives, Kyoto Japan.

KNUTSON, K., POTTS, R.O., GUZEK, D.B., GOLDEN, G.M., LAMBERT, W.J., MCKIE, J.E. and HIGUCHI, W.I. (1985) Macro- and molecular physical-chemical considerations in understanding drug transport in the stratum corneum, *J. Controlled Release* **2**, 67–87.

KRILL, S.L., KNUTSON, K. and HIGUCHI, W.I. (1992) The stratum corneum lipid thermotropic phase behavior, *Biochim. Biophys. Acta* **1112**, 281–286.

LANDMAN, L. (1986) Epidermal permeability barrier: transformation of lamellar granule-disks into intercellular sheets by a membrane-fusion process, a freeze-fracture study, *J. Invest. Dermatol.* **87**, 202–209.

LEE, C.H., KAWASAKI, Y. and MAIBACH, H.I. (1994) Effect of surfactant mixtures on irritant contact dermatitis potential in man : sodium lauroyl glutamate and sodium lauryl sulfate, *Contact Dermatitis* **30**, 205–209.

LONG, S.A., WERTZ, P.W., STRAUSS, J.S. and DOWNING, D.T. (1985) Human stratum corneum polar lipids and desquamation, *Arch. Dermatol. Res.* **277**, 284–287.

MARSH, D. (1981) Electron paramagnetic resonance: spin labels, in GRELL, E. (ed.), *Membrane Spectroscopy*, Berlin: Springer, 51–142.

MCCONNELL, H.M., DEVAUX, P., SCANDELLA, C.J. (1972) Electron spin resonance. In FOX, C.F. (ed.) *Membrane Fusion*. New York: Academic Press, 27–37.

MEHLHORN, R.J. and KEITH, A.D. (1972) Spin labeling of biological membranes. In FOX, C.F. and KEITH, A.D. (eds.) *Membrane Molecular Biology*. Stamford: Sinauer Associates, 192.

MIZUSHIMA, J., KAWASAKI, Y., INO, M., SAKAMOTO, K., KAWASHIMA, M. and MAIBACH, H.I. (2001) Effect of surfactants on human stratum corneum utilizing electron paramagnetic resonance spectroscopy—from the point of view of water content, *J. Japanese Cosmetic Science Society* **25**, 130–135.

MIZUSHIMA, J., KAWASAKI, Y., TABOHASHI, T., KITANO, T., SAKAMOTO, K., KAWASHIMA, M., COOKE, R., and MAIBACH, H.I. (2000a) Effect of surfactants on human stratum corneum: Electron paramagnetic resonance study, *Intl. J. Pharm.* **197**, 193–202.

MIZUSHIMA, J., KAWASAKI, Y., TABOHASHI, T., KITANO, T., SAKAMOTO, K., KAWASHIMA, M., COOKE, R., and MAIBACH, H.I. (2000b) Effect of surfactants on human stratum corneum: Electron Paramagnetic Resonance study, *Intl. J. Pharm.* **197**, 193–202.

QUAN, D. and MAIBACH, H.I. (1994) An electron paramagnetic resonance study: I. Effect of Azone on 5-doxyl stearic acid-labeled human stratum corneum, *Int. J. Pharm.* **104**, 61–72.

QUAN, D., COOKE, R.A. and MAIBACH, H.I. (1995) An electron paramagnetic resonance study of human epidermal lipids using 5-doxyl stearic acid. *J. Controlled Release* **36**, 235–241.

REHFELD, S.J., PLACHY, W.Z., HOU, S.Y.E. and ELIAS, P.M. (1990) Localization of lipid microdomains and thermal phenomena in murine stratum corneum and isolated membrane complexes: an electron spin resonance study. *J. Invest. Dermatol.* **95**, 217–223.

REHFELD, S.J., PLACHY, W.Z., WILLIAM, W.I. and ELIAS, P.M. (1988) Calorimetric and electron spin resonance examination of lipid phase transitions in human stratum corneum: molecular basis for normal cohesion and abnormal desquamation in recessive X-linked ichthyosis, *J. Invest. Dermatol.* **91**, 499–505.

RHEIN, L.D., ROBBINS, C.R., FERNEE, K. and CANTORE, R. (1986) Surfactant structure effects on swelling of isolated human stratum corneum, *J. Soc. Cosmet. Chem.* **37**, 125–139.

RHEIN, L.D., SIMION, F.A., HILL, R.L., CAGAN, R.H., MATTAI, J., MAIBACH, H.I. (1990) Human cutaneous response to a mixed surfactant system: role of solution phenomena in controlling surfactant irritation, *Dermatologica* **180**, 18–23.

RIEGER, M.M. (1995) Surfactant interactions with skin, *Cosmetics & Toiletries* **110**, 31–50.

■ CHAPTER 37 ■

RIEGER, M.M. (1997) The skin irritation potential of quaternaries, *J. Soc. Cosmet. Chem.* **48**, 307–317.

ROSEN, M.J. (1978) *Micelle Formation by Surfactants in "Surfactants and Interfacial Phenomena"*, New York: John Wiley & Sons, 83–122.

SAUERHEBER, R.D., GORDEN, L.M., CROSLAND, R.D. and KUWAHARA, M.D. (1977) Spin-label studies on rat liver and heart plasma membranes; Do probe interactions interfere with the measurement of membrane properties?, *J. Membr. Biol.* **31**, 131–139.

SWARTZENDRUBER, D.C., WERTZ, P.W., KITKO, D.J., MADISON, K.C. and DOWNING, D.T. (1989) Molecular models of the intercellular lipid lamellae in mammalian stratum corneum, *J. Invest. Dermatol.* **92**, 251–257.

SWARTZENDRUBER, D.C., WERTZ, P.W., MADISON, K.C. and DOWNING, D.T. (1987) Evidence that the corneocyte has a chemically bound lipid envelope, *J. Invest. Dermtol.* **88**, 709–713.

TAKINO, Y., KAWASAKI, Y., SAKAMOTO, K. and HIGUCHI, W.I. (1996) Influence of anionic surfactants to skin: the change of the water permeability and electric resistance, Abstract of 19th IFSCC International Congress, Sydney.

VAN DER VALK, P.G.M. and MAIBACH, H.I. (1989) Potential for irritation increases from the wrist to the cubital fossa, *Br. J. Dermatol.* **121**, 709–712.

VAN DUZEE, B.F. (1975) Thermal analysis of human stratum corneum, *J. Invest. Dermatol.* **65**, 404–408.

VILKES, G.L., NGUYEN, A.L. and WILDHAUER, R. (1973) Structure-property relations of human and neonatal rat stratum corneum: I. Thermal stability of the crystalline lipid structure as studied by X-ray diffraction and differential thermal analysis. *Biochim. Biophys. Acta* **304**, 267–275.

WERTZ, J.E. and BOLTON, J.R. (1972) *Electron Spin Resonance: Elementary Theory and Applications*, New York: McGraw-Hill.

WERTZ, P.W. and DOWNING, D.T. (1982) Glycolipids in mammalian epidermis: structure and function in the water barrier. *Science*, **217**, 1261–1262.

WERTZ, P.W., SWARTZENDRUBER, D.C., KITKO, D.J., MADISON, K.C. and DOWNING, D.T. (1989) The role of the corneocyte lipid envelopes in cohesion of the stratum corneum, *J. Invest. Dermtol.*, **93**, 169–172.

WHITE, S.H., MIREJOVSKI, D. and KING, G.I. (1988) Structure of lamellar lipid domains and corneocyte envelopes of murine stratum corneum. An X-ray diffraction study, *Biochemistry*, **27**, 3725–3732.

WILMER, J., BURLESON, F., KAYAM, F., KANNO, J. and LUSTER, M. (1994) Cytokine induction in human epidermal keratinocytes exposed to contact irritants and its relation to chemical-induced inflammation in mouse skin. *J. Invest. Dermatol.* **102**, 915–922.

WOODFORD, R. and BARRY, B.W. (1986) Penetration enhancers and the percutaneous absorption of drugs: an update, *J. Toxicol. Cutaneous Ocul. Toxicol.* **5**, 167–177.

38

Test Methods for Allergic Contact Dermatitis in Animals

GEORG KLECAK

Contents

38.1 Introduction

38.2 General principles

38.3 The guinea pig maximization test

38.4 Split adjuvant technique

38.5 The optimization test

38.6 Freund's complete adjuvant test

38.7 The modified Draize test

38.8 The Buehler test

38.9 The open epicutaneous test

38.10 Modified guinea pig maximization test

38.11 The cumulative contact enhancement test

38.12 The epicutaneous maximization test

38.13 Single-injection adjuvant test

38.14 The Tierexperimenteller Nachweis (TINA) test

38.15 The footpad test

38.16 The guinea pig allergy test adapted to cosmetic ingredients

38.17 The ear/flank test (Stevens test)

38.18 Conclusions

38.1 INTRODUCTION

Among the dermatotoxicologic community working on immune skin effects manifested as *allergic contact dermatitis*, the proven effective strategy has been to develop and apply animal assays for identification of chemical xenobiotics with allergenic potential and to assess the sensitization hazard potential of these environmental contactants for human beings. Since 1935 (Landsteiner and Jacobs, 1935) the guinea pig has represented the reference animal model.

Besides the official regulatory guinea pig methods listed in Appendix 3 of the OECD Test Guidelines (No. 406; OECD, 1992), another category of "nonregulatory"/investigative testing strategies is represented by various modifications of the Draize test, the guinea pig maximization test, and the split adjuvant test (Figure 38.1).

The main purpose of this chapter is to convey to the reader a general understanding of the rationale, the design, and predictive value of each particular testing strategy, reviewed here.

The common principle of all these methods is to initiate exposure(s) of a test article or its test samples to the same skin site or area (*induction phase*), which after a rest period of at least 7 d is followed by a *challenge exposure* of the article or of its test sample(s) to a virgin skin site or area.

Animal bioassay data currently are generated from experimental designs, outlined in various testing guidelines issued by OECD (1981, 1992), EEC (1983), U.S. Environmental Protection Agency/TSCA (1985), U.S. Environmental Protection Agency/FIFRA (1984), OSHA (1987), CTFA (1981), and Japan/MAFF (1985) for allergenicity assessment of single chemicals and "end-use" products. Generally, guinea pig assays vary with respect to administration route and mode, exposed skin surface conditions, frequency, number and duration of exposures, and dosing of a test article (Table 38.1). Variations among testing protocols give rise to differences in their sensitivity and predictivity (Marzulli and Maguire, 1982). The key factors influencing the outcome of a skin sensitization assay in guinea pigs are of biological (genetic), chemical, and operative origin.

The main biological factor is the choice of a suitable guinea pig strain. Guinea pigs of Hartley, Pirbright, or Himalayan white strains, weighing 350–400 g, are known to be "good responders" in spite of differences in response to some human contact allergens (Chase, 1941; Polak *et al.*, 1968; Parker *et al.*, 1975; Rockwell, 1955; Stampf and Benezra, 1982). Only with exposure to moderate or weak contact allergens do the operative factors have an effect on the

CHAPTER 38

"REGULATORY" PROCEDURES

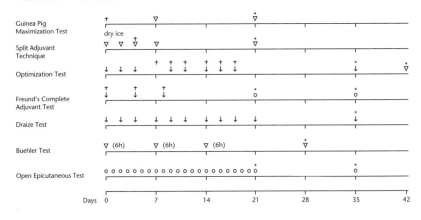

"NON-REGULATORY" PROCEDURES

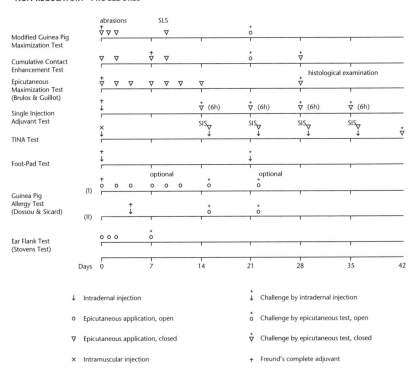

↓   Intradernal injection

o   Epicutaneous application, open

▽   Epicutaneous application, closed

×   Intramuscular injection

↓   Challenge by intradernal injection

o   Challenge by epicutaneous test, open

▽   Challenge by epicutaneous test, closed

+   Freund's complete adjuvant

Figure 38.1: Guinea pig contact allergy tests: procedure for induction and challenge.

sensitization rate of test animals (Goodfrey and Baer, 1991). Of these, the following should be considered:

1 Mode and manner of exposure—Repeated, intradermal or occlusive applications onto the same skin site or area are more efficient for induction of contact allergy than the open application (Kligman, 1966b).

2 Skin conditions—Application over slightly inflamed, scarified, or sodium lauryl sulfate (SLS) pretreated skin site improves the sensitizing rate of weak sensitizers (Vinson *et al.*, 1965; Baker, 1968; Kligman, 1966a).

3 Use of "adjuvants"—Employment of Freund's complete adjuvant (FCA) for induction has maximal stimulating effect on the immune mechanism and may convert chemicals with poor allergenic properties into moderate or strong sensitizers (Goodfrey and Baer, 1971; Andersen, 1985).

4 Dosing—The use of higher concentrations and higher dosing increases the sensitization rate (Magnusson and Kligman, 1970; Marzulli and Maibach, 1974; Christensen *et al.*, 1984).

5 Vehicle choice—Marked differences in the intensity and frequency of skin reactions were found when different vehicles were used (van der Walle *et al.*, 1982; Björkner and Niklasson, 1984).

6 Occlusion—An occlusion time of 24 h or longer results in uniform immune responses, reduces the vehicle effect, and yields a lower response level than that found by open exposure (Magnusson and Hersle, 1965; Pirilä, 1974).

7 Area of sensitizing exposure—The size of skin surface patches used for induction should be >4 cm^2, while the appropriate size for challenge patches would be 2–4 cm^2 (White *et al.*, 1986).

8 Dose-response effect—Graded skin response is induced and elicited by using graded concentrations in sensitization protocol, enabling determination of end points as minimal sensitizing eliciting and maximal nonsensitizing/ noneliciting concentration level (Bronaugh *et al.*, 1994).

9 Animal—Care and housing conditions (Andersen, 1993; US Department of Health, Education, and Welfare, 1978).

38.2 GENERAL PRINCIPLES

The following points belong to the obligatory (elementary) parts of every study protocol for allergenicity assessment involving experimental animals.

CHAPTER 38

38.2.1 Preliminary irritation test

A special group of four to six animals is used to establish a suitable (moderate irritant) concentration for intradermal or epicutaneous induction treatment and the highest nonirritant one for challenging. In addition care has to be taken that FCA treatment may lower the threshold for the primary non-irritant concentration in test animals (Magnusson, 1980).

38.2.2 Controls

It is necessary to include negative or vehicle control animals in the test strategy to ensure that the challenge reactions, seen in test animals, are of allergic origin and not due to skin irritancy. Controls have to be treated in exactly the same manner as the test animals, except that during the induction phase the use of a test article is omitted.

For rechallenge or crosstest it is essential to incorporate a new set of four to six naive control animals. The use of positive controls is required in order to validate the test procedure and system (guinea pig colony), twice a year using one of the moderate and weak contact sensitizers (hydroxcitronellal, neomycine sulfate, benzocaine).

38.2.3 Evaluation

Evaluation of skin reactions is usually performed by visual scoring of erythema, edema, and other clinical changes of skin using various grading scales. Magnusson and Kligman (1969, 1970) prefer to use an ordinal scale:

−	=	no visible change
+	=	patchy erythema
+ +	=	confluent erythema
+ + +	=	confluent erythema and edema

It is possible to assign numerical values to these gradings. An exceptional case is the optimization test, in which "reaction volume" in microliters serves as the parameter for evaluation of skin reactions.

The scoring system is of relative value, but comparison of frequency, intensity, and duration of reactions elicited on test and control animals generally permits an unequivocal decision as to whether sensitization has occurred or not.

38.2.4 Classification

A potential contact sensitizer is classified as any article that produces in a nonadjuvant assay at least 15 percent of test animals with allergic contact dermatitis. A negative result is one in which no skin reaction was elicited in any of the experimental animals. All other results would be classified as questionable and indicate the need of rechallenging or study repetition.

Based on the results of an adjuvant test, each test article that sensitizes at least 8 percent of test animals is classified as sensitizer. In case of a lower percentage of sensitized animals, a rechallenge is recommended for confirmation of challenge results (Figure 38.1).

38.3 THE GUINEA PIG MAXIMIZATION TEST

In the guinea pig maximization test (GPMT), as described by Magnusson and Kligman (1969, 1970), 20 test and 10–20 control guinea pigs are used (Figure 38.2.).

The induction, consisting of two phases, is initiated (d 0) by paired intradermal injections (0.1 ml each) into the clipped and shaved shoulder region of the test animals of

1   Complete Freund's adjuvant (FCA).

GUINEA PIG MAXIMIZATION TEST (GPMT)

	INDUCTION			CHALLENGE
	Day	0	7	21
2 groups 20 animals each	A – 0.1ml test material i.d. B – 0.1ml......................FCA i.d. C – 0.1ml test material+ FCA i.d.		occlusive 48 h test material	occlusive 24 h test mat. + vehicle
a. TEST				
b. VEHICLE CONTROL		Treated in the same way and manner except that use of test sample is omitted during induction phase		

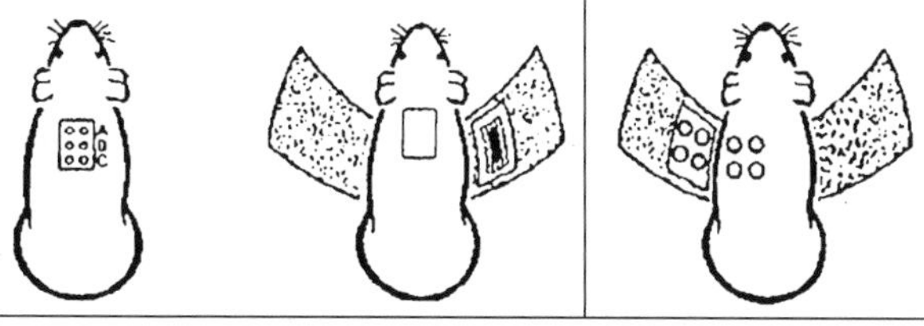

Figure 38.2: Guinea pig maximization test (GPMT).

2   Test article in suitable vehicle (water, paraffin oil, propylene glycol).

3   Mixture of dissolved or suspended test article with FCA (1:1).

On d 7, for boosting, a topical occlusive patch is applied for 48 h on the shoulder region, which has been clipped 24 h before.

For induction of sensitization, the use of a mildly or moderately irritating test concentration is recommended. When nonirritating test articles are involved, pretreatment of the freshly clipped shoulder region with 10 percent SLS is indicated on d 6.

Challenge is performed on d 21. On the left flank of all animals a skin site of 4 cm^2 is shaved, to which the test article is applied in suitable vehicle at primary nonirritating concentration(s) using a 24-h occlusive "patch unit" with Finn chambers, for example. The vehicle may be simultaneously tested, if indicated. The challenge reactions are examined 24 and 48 h after removal of the patch, scored according to a standard rating scale, and the classification of allergenic potential is graded from none to extreme. Rechallenge or cross-test may follow at weekly intervals, always on contralateral flanks.

Control animals are treated similar to test animals, except that during the induction phase the test article is omitted.

The GPMT is a very sensitive procedure for allergenicity screening of test articles (Maurer *et al.*, 1978; Kero and Hannuksela, 1980; Stampf and Benezra, 1982; Andersen, 1985, 1993; Anderson *et al.*, 1984, 1985; Andersen and Maibach, 1985a, 1985b; Wahlberg and Boman, 1985) with a tendency to overestimate the potency of many weak, mild, and moderate human sensitizers. Even if its experimental data are less suitable for sensitization hazard calculation related to intended, accidental, or occasional exposure of human skin to various environmental allergens, the GPMT is strongly recommended as a legislative method.

Due to limits and deficiencies of this testing strategy, various modifications of the GPMT are utilized to improve its predictivity (Rochas *et al.*, 1977; Kozuka *et al.*, 1981; Sato *et al.*, 1981; Guillot and Gonnet, 1985; Maurer and Hess, 1989). The use of fewer test animals was recommended by Hofman *et al.* (1987) and Shillaker *et al.* (1989).

38.4   SPLIT ADJUVANT TECHNIQUE

In this assay (Figure 38.3) the test article and FCA are administered separately (Maguire, 1973, 1975, 1985; Maguire and Cipriano, 1985), and two groups of 10–20 guinea pigs each are involved.

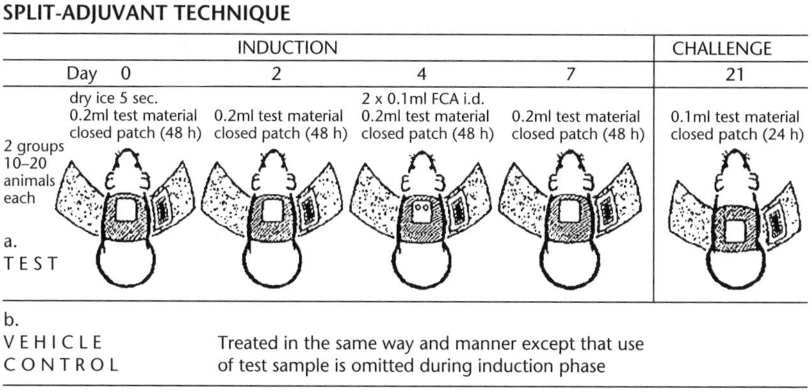

SPLIT-ADJUVANT TECHNIQUE

	INDUCTION				CHALLENGE
Day 0	2	4	7		21
dry ice 5 sec. 0.2ml test material closed patch (48 h)	0.2ml test material closed patch (48 h)	2 x 0.1ml FCA i.d. 0.2ml test material closed patch (48 h)	0.2ml test material closed patch (48 h)		0.1ml test material closed patch (24 h)

2 groups 10–20 animals each

a. T E S T

b. V E H I C L E C O N T R O L — Treated in the same way and manner except that use of test sample is omitted during induction phase

Figure 38.3: Split-adjuvant technique.

38.4.1 Induction

On d 0 the skin of the suprascapular region is shaved to remove hair and loose keratin. Thereafter, a window dressing is fixed over this skin site. The induction site of 2 cm^2 is exposed to "dry ice" for at minimum 5 s prior to application of 0.2 ml semisolid or 0.1 ml liquid test sample, covered with filter paper, fixed with adhesive tape, and kept under occlusion for 48 h. This procedure is repeated every other day up to a total of four induction treatments On d 4, prior to topical application of the test sample, 2 intradermal injections of 0.1 ml FCA are administered symmetrical into the induction site. On d 9 the dressing is removed.

38.4.2 Challenge

On d 21 challenge is performed by 24 h occlusive or open patch test application of 0.5 ml semisolid test article, or 0.1 ml if liquids are tested, to a virgin clipped skin site on the dorsal back measuring 2 cm^2. Controls are treated similarly, except that test article administration is omitted during induction phase. Reading and scoring of elicited skin reactions is done on d 22, 23, and 24. Rechallenge or cross-tests can follow at in intervals of 10 d.

This test protocol is designed for testing of chemicals as well as "end use" products. It is somewhat less sensitive than the GPMT. Its performance is rather complicated, and is stressful for animals due to the use of window dressing during the induction phase.

CHAPTER 38

MODIFIED SPLIT ADJUVANT TEST

	INDUCTION				CHALLENGE
Day	0	2	4	7	21
2 groups 10–20 animals each	0.2ml test mat. e.c.*	0.2ml test mat. e.c.*	2 x 0.1ml FCA i.d. 0.2ml test mat. e.c.*	0.2ml test mat. e.c.*	0.1ml test material closed patch (24 h)

a.
T E S T

b.
V E H I C L E
C O N T R O L

Treated in the same way and manner except that use of test sample is omitted during induction phase

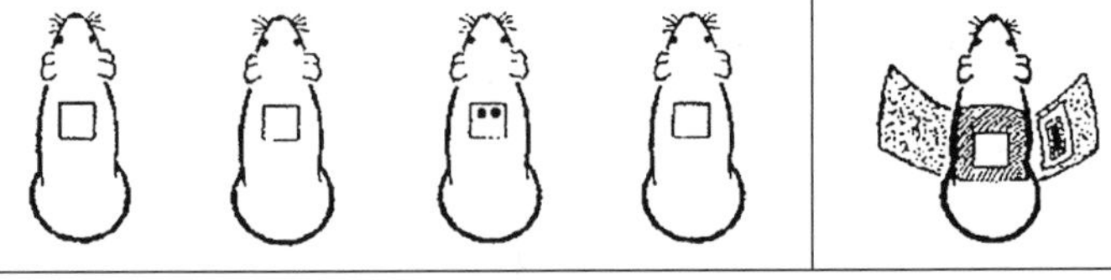

* application on reexcoriated skin

Figure 38.4: Modified split adjuvant test.

In the modified Maguire Test (MM) (Figure 38.4) by Prince and Prince (1977) or Rao *et al.* (1981) the use of occluded patches is replaced by open application of 0.2 ml of the test sample onto the reexcoriated (with sandpaper or tape) skin site in the suprascapular region. The MM is carried out under test conditions that are closer to the "in-use" situation, due to separate and open application of allergens. The database is relatively new.

38.5 THE OPTIMIZATION TEST

As described by Maurer (1974, 1985) and Maurer *et al.* (1978, 1980), the optimization test (OPT) protocol involves two groups of 20 test and control animals (Figure 38.5).

38.5.1 Sequence of induction

On d 0 two intradermal injections of the test article, dissolved or suspended (0.1 percent) in suitable vehicle, are administered into a shaved flank (0.05 ml) and dorsal area (0.1 ml) of the test animals.

On d 2 and 4, injections (0.1 ml) of a 0.1 percent test sample are given into the back area. Approximately 24 h after each of the four initial intradermal injections during the first week of induction the reaction sites are depilated, and the skin reactions are examined, by measuring and multiplying the two

OPTIMIZATION TEST

	INDUCTION		CHALLENGE	
Week	1	2–3	5–7	6
2 groups 20 animals each	0.1ml: 0.1% solution in NaCl i.d.	0.1ml: 0.1% solution in FCA i.d.	0.1ml: 0.1% solution in NaCl i.d.	occlusive 24 h sub-irritant concentration in petrolatum
a. T E S T	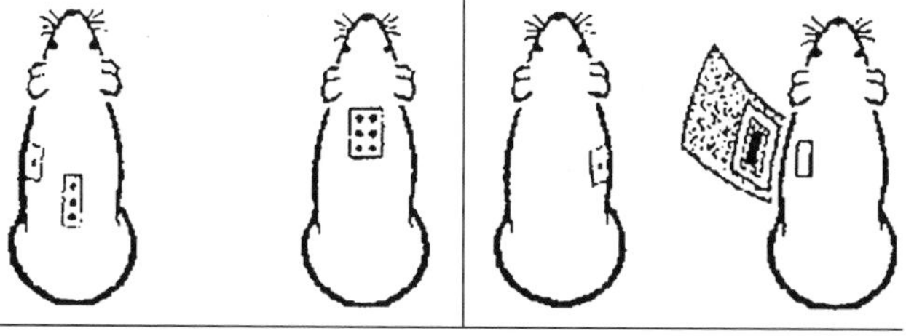			
b. V E H I C L E C O N T R O L	Treated in the same way and manner except that use of test sample is omitted during induction phase			

Figure 38.5: Optimization test.

largest perpendicular diameters and the skin-fold thickness to obtain the "reaction volume" and calculate skin irritation threshold for each animal.

On d 6, an intracutaneous dose (0.1 ml) of a 1:1 emulsion or mixture of a dissolved or suspended test article in vehicle with FCA is administered into the clipped nuchal region. This intracutaneous administration is repeated on d 8, 10, 12, 14, and 16.

38.5.2 First challenge

About 2 wk after the last induction, the 0.1 percent test sample is injected with 0.05 ml into a virgin skin area on the contralateral flank, and the 24-h skin reactions are measured.

38.5.3 Assessment

If the reaction volume of the challenge injection is greater than the skin irritation threshold, the animal is termed as sensitized (positive). The second parameter represents skin reactions, which were induced and elicited in control animals. For final evaluation the number of "positive" test animals is compared with the number of control animals that show nonspecific reactions of comparable intensity, using the exact Fisher test.

A second challenge can be performed 1 wk later if the results of the first challenge are negative or marginal, using a maximum nonirritant concentration of the test article in suitable vehicle for open or occlusive exposure. Skin reactions are examined 24, 48, or 72 h after challenge and classified according to a standard rating scale.

Control animals are treated in the same manner as test animals, except that during induction the administration of test article is omitted.

Variation in reactions to epidermal challenge is taken into account by means of statistical group comparison and the Fisher test.

The optimization test and the maximization method are almost equally efficient (Maurer et al., 1980; Stampf et al., 1982; Stampf and Benezra, 1982). Both test protocols may overclassify some chemicals in terms of their sensitizing potential for humans and share similar merits and deficiencies.

The OPT has a database of industrial chemicals, warranting more flexible objective assessment of skin responses.

38.6 FREUND'S COMPLETE ADJUVANT TEST

Freund's complete adjuvant test (FCAT; Figure 38.6) uses a test and a control group of 10–20 guinea pigs each (Klecak et al., 1977; Klecak, 1982, 1985).

Induction is performed in the suprascapular region. A skin site of approximately 6×2 cm is shaved and an intradermal injection of 0.1 ml of a 1:1 mixture or emulsion of FCA and the dissolved test article at a concentration of 5 percent or less is administered on d 0, 4, and 8.

Challenge is performed on d 21 on clipped flank skin using open application. Up to 6 concentrations (the minimal irritating one and its 1:3 nonirritating dilutions) of the test article in suitable vehicle may be used and are applied to a test site of 2 cm^2 at a dose of 0.025 ml (liquids) or 0.01 ml (semisolids), which had been marked with a circular stamp.

Control animals are treated similarly, except that the use of test article during induction phase is omitted.

Challenge reactions are examined 24, 48, and 72 h after challenging and graded according to a standard rating scale. Rechallenge and cross-test may be performed in intervals of 10–14 d on the contralateral flank. For each rechallenge or cross-test at least four new control animals need to be used.

FCA TEST

	INDUCTION	CHALLENGE
	Day 0, 4, 8	21.35
2 groups 10–20 animals each a. T E S T	every second day 0.1ml 5% sol. in FCA i.d. 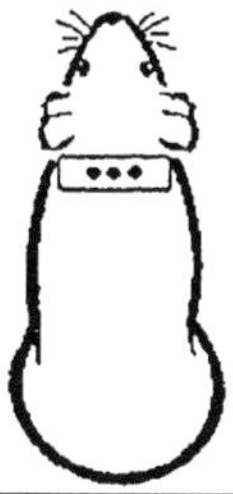 	0.025ml/2cm^2 e.c. A = min. irritating conc. B = A:3 max. non irritating conc. C = B:3 D = C:3 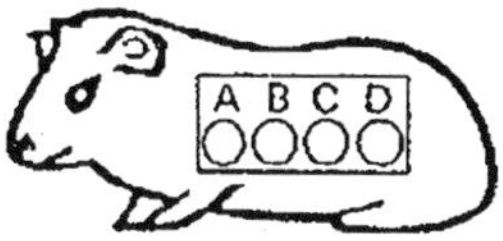

b. V E H I C L E C O N T R O L	Treated in the same way and manner except that use of test sample is omitted during induction phase

Figure 38.6: FCA test.

The FCAT is easy to perform, economical, and as sensitive as the GPMT. It is not suitable for testing insoluble test articles or "end-use" products, and tends to overestimate the allergenic potential of weak and moderate human contact allergens. Nevertheless, it yields quantitative data in the form of a threshold concentration for elicitation of allergic contact dermatitis, based on the endpoint determination (Stampf *et al.*, 1982; van der Walle and Bensink, 1982; van der Walle *et al.*, 1982; Klecak, 1985; J. Avalos *et al.*, 1989; Gäfvert, 1994).

The FCA test in sequential combination with the open epicutaneous test represents an adequate program for detection of strong and moderate, as well as weak, allergenic potential of single chemicals and injectible "end-use" products. Both animal assays (FCAT and OET) yield data of predictive value regarding actual risk estimate of contact sensitization in humans under anticipated use conditions and occasional or accidental exposure.

38.7 THE MODIFIED DRAIZE TEST

The aim of all modifications of the Draize test (Draize, 1955, 1959) is to enhance the sensitivity of this animal assay for detecting weaker skin sensitizers by increasing the test concentration as high as to cause moderate irritant skin responses at maximum (Voss, 1958), including control animals for challenging (Maurer *et al.*, 1978), replacement of intradermal administration by open application (Prince and Prince, 1977), increased frequency of exposures by rechallenge and or repetition of the whole study course in the same test animal group (double Draize test), or shortening the duration of the induction to 1-d treatment by administration of four intradermal injections at sites overlying the axillary and inguinal lymph nodes (Sharp, 1978).

The procedure of the modified Draize test (MDT), according to Johnson and Goodwin (1985), consists of two parts, and involves two groups of 10 guinea pigs each (Figure 38.7).

38.7.1 Part I

Induction phase

Ten test animals are used. On d 0, 4 intradermal administrations of the test article at a dose of 0.1 ml and at a concentration corresponding to 2.5 times the intradermal challenge concentration (ICC, may cause slight but perceptible irritation on guinea pig skin) on the clipped skin site overlying both axillary and inguinal lymph nodes are employed.

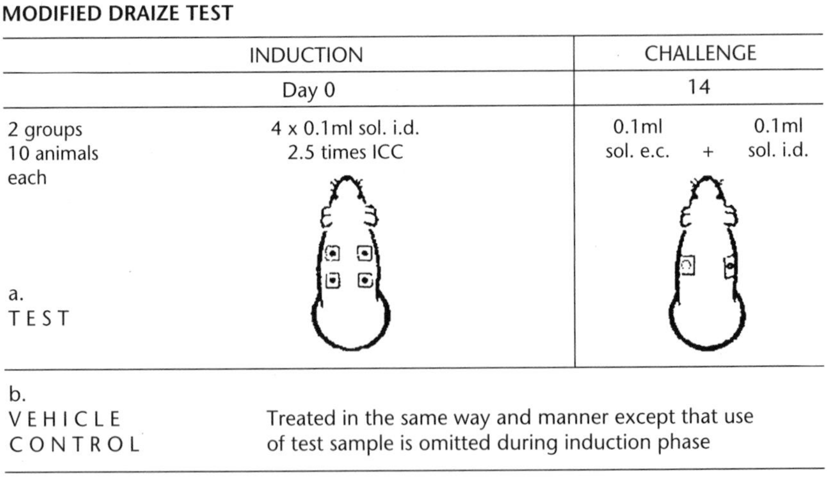

MODIFIED DRAIZE TEST

	INDUCTION	CHALLENGE
	Day 0	14
2 groups 10 animals each	4 x 0.1ml sol. i.d. 2.5 times ICC	0.1ml 0.1ml sol. e.c. + sol. i.d.

a.
TEST

b.
VEHICLE
CONTROL
    Treated in the same way and manner except that use of test sample is omitted during induction phase

Figure 38.7: Modified Draize test.

Resulting 24-h skin reactions are examined, their intensity graded (erythema and edema), and the average reaction size evaluated based on the measurement of the longitudinal and lateral axes diameters of each of the four skin reactions.

Challenge phase

On d 14 each of the experimental animals is challenged, using intradermal administration of 0.1 ml of the test articles in suitable solvents at a nonirritant or slightly irritant concentration at maximum on one clipped flank, and open epicutaneously on the opposite clipped flank with 0.1 ml of the test samples at primary nonirritant concentration to a circular test site of about 8 cm^2. The 24-h reactions are examined, graded, and their size evaluated. Confirmation rechallenge may follow on d 21 and 28. For each rechallenge 10 control animals, which had been treated with FCA for induction solely, are challenged similarly to the test animals.

38.7.2   Part II

If both challenge tests of Part I are negative (no evidence that skin sensitization occurred in test animals), a second set of intradermal injections is administered on d 35. The challenge procedure is similar to the one described for Part I, but confirmation rechallenge is done intradermally and epicutaneously in weekly intervals. New control animals have to be involved.

This technique is suitable for testing of soluble or suspensible chemicals exclusively, and is significantly more sensitive than the Draize guinea pig test, though still less sensitive than the GPMT and the FCAT.

38.8   THE BUEHLER TEST

The standardized protocol (Figure 38.8) involves a group of 20 tests and one or more groups of 10 control animals each (Bühler, 1965, 1982, 1985; Bühler and Griffith, 1975; Griffith and Bühler, 1969; Ritz and Bühler, 1980).

The induction phase is performed by 1 or 3 weekly occlusive application(s) of the test sample at a slight to moderately irritating concentration for at minimum 3 or at maximum 9 wk. The induction skin site of approximately 8 cm^2 on the animal's left shoulder is clipped 24 h before the guinea pigs are placed into restrainers and, using 4-cm^2 occlusive patches for 6 hours, Webril pads with 0.4 ml test sample or Hill-Top chambers with 0.2 ml test sample at

BUEHLER TEST

	INDUCTION			CHALLENGE	
	Day 0	7	14	28	
3 groups 10-20 animals each	occlusive 6 h 0.5ml sol.	occlusive 6 h 0.5ml sol.	occlusive 6 h 0.5ml sol.	occlusive 24 h 0.5ml sol. Test site	occlusive 24 h 0.5ml sol. Control site
a. TEST					
b. VEHICLE CONTROL	Treated in the same way and manner except that use of test sample is omitted during induction phase				
c. NEGATIVE CONTROL	Challenged only				

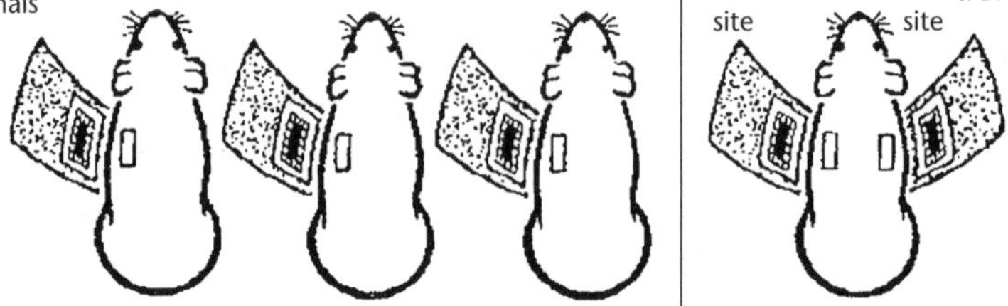

Figure 38.8: Buehler test.

the highest possible (moderate irritating) or anticipated use concentration, are fixed to the skin.

For the challenge phase, when a rest period of 14 d has passed after the last induction exposure, test animals and 10 controls are challenged by application of 0.2–0.5 ml of the test sample at primary nonirritating concentration(s) to a naive clipped back skin site under an occlusive patch for 6 h.

During the induction and challenge procedure the animals are kept in a specially designed restrainer, which prevents their movement and enables attachment of the occlusive patch with a rubber dental dam, slightly pulled and fastened to the restrainer.

The observations and gradings of elicited skin reactions on previously depilated test sites are done 24 and 48 h after challenge.

Single or multiple rechallenge(s) or cross-test(s) may follow at intervals of 1 or 2 wk, always to a virgin skin site on the animal's back. If indicated, a vehicle may be used additionally.

Control animals are treated in the same manner, except that the use of test article for induction is omitted.

For evaluation, two parameters are used: The *incidence index* is an expression of the number of responding animals out of the total test animals, while the severity index is calculated from the total sum of 24-h and/or 48-h reaction grades divided by the number of animals exposed.

The Buehler test is suitable for testing single chemicals as well as "end-use" products. This assay is uneconomical, time-consuming, and the validity of results is usually limited to use concentration.

Nevertheless, the Buehler test is often recommended as a legislative method, especially in the United States.

38.9   THE OPEN EPICUTANEOUS TEST

In the open epicutaneous test (OET) a test article and/or its sample(s) are applied epicutaneously uncovered to the test site with intact skin surface (Figure 38.9). Constant volumes per square centimeter of each test sample are applied to standard areas of the clipped flank skin during the induction and elicitation phase of the assay. For OET at least six guinea pigs are utilized for every test concentration group, while "end-use" products are tested in 20 animals. Ten guinea pigs constitute a control group (Klecak *et al.*, 1977).

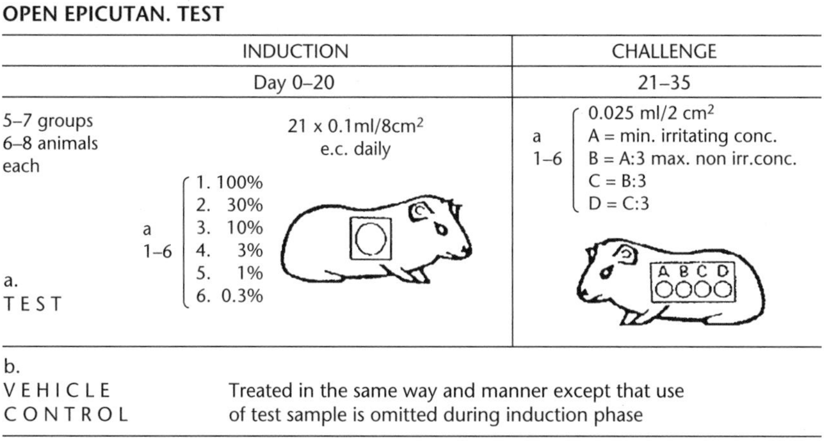

■ CHAPTER 38 ■

OPEN EPICUTAN. TEST

	INDUCTION	CHALLENGE
	Day 0–20	21–35

5–7 groups
6–8 animals
each
 	
a.
T E S T
	21 x 0.1ml/8cm²
	e.c. daily
	
	a 1. 100%
	1–6 2. 30%
	  3. 10%
	  4. 3%
	  5. 1%
	  6. 0.3%
		0.025 ml/2 cm²
		a A = min. irritating conc.
		1–6 B = A:3 max. non irr.conc.
		  C = B:3
		  D = C:3

b. V E H I C L E C O N T R O L	Treated in the same way and manner except that use of test sample is omitted during induction phase	

Figure 38.9: Open epicutaneous test.

Induction requires daily applications on 5 or 7 consecutive days per week of 0.1 ml of the neat test article or its progressively diluted (3:1) solutions, emulsions, or suspensions, usually to the same skin area of 8 cm² on a clipped flank, with 20 exposures in total. In cases where moderate to strong skin reactions are induced on test animals, the application sites are changed.

For challenge, on d 21 or 29 all experimental animals are treated on the contra-lateral clipped flank with the test article and/or its dilutions at the minimal irritating and some lower primary nonirritant concentrations at a dose of 0.025 ml (solutions) or 0.01 ml (semisolids) per circular test site of about 2 cm² in size. Vehicle may be involved at challenge, if indicated.

Control animals are treated similarly, except that the use of test article is omitted during induction.

The reactions are read and recorded 24, 48, and/or 72 h after challenging. Rechallenge(s) or cross-tests can follow at intervals of 10–14 days, always on the contralateral flank.

This technique shows no limitations in terms of physicochemical properties of test articles, has high flexibility, and enables prediction of health risk calculation related to intended, occasional, or accidental exposure of human skin to various types of potential contact allergens, since dose-related experimental data are obtained (Klecak, 1982).

The OET fails when borderline sensitizers are tested or test articles with limited skin penetration capability are involved. A complementary testing program, combining either the FCAT or GPMT with the OET, is adequate to define conditions under which a contact allergen can act as a skin sensitizer in humans or not, a crucial point in predictive testing (Stampf et al., 1982; van der Walle et al., 1982; van der Walle and Bensink, 1982; Kero and Hannuksela, 1980). A good correlation exists between HRIPT and OET results (Klecak, 1985).

38.10 MODIFIED GUINEA PIG MAXIMIZATION TEST

There are several drawbacks to the modified guinea pig maximization text (GPMT). For example, intradermal administration is an unnatural exposure route for a contact allergen, often resulting in overestimation of allergenicity of test articles. It is not suitable for testing poorly soluble or insoluble test articles and "end-use" products, since these are not injectible.

The modified protocol (Sato et al., 1981, 1984; Sato, 1985) differs from the GPMT shown in Figure 38.10 in that for the first induction phase on 10 test

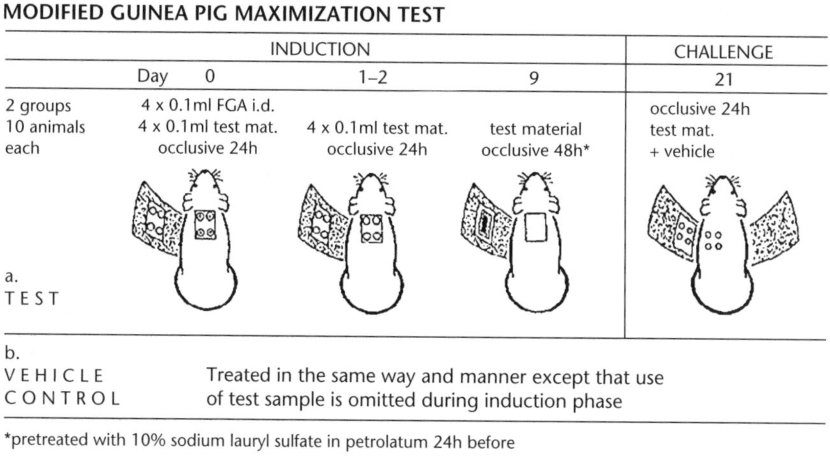

MODIFIED GUINEA PIG MAXIMIZATION TEST

	INDUCTION			CHALLENGE
Day 0	1–2	9		21
2 groups 10 animals each	4 x 0.1ml FGA i.d. 4 x 0.1ml test mat. occlusive 24h	4 x 0.1ml test mat. occlusive 24h	test material occlusive 48h*	occlusive 24h test mat. + vehicle

a.
T E S T

b.
V E H I C L E   Treated in the same way and manner except that use
C O N T R O L   of test sample is omitted during induction phase

*pretreated with 10% sodium lauryl sulfate in petrolatum 24h before

Figure 38.10: Modified guinea pig maximization test.

animals, four injections of 0.1 ml FCA emulsified with bidistilled water (1:1) are administered intradermally into the comers of a 4×2 cm skin site on the clipped nuchal skin area. Thereafter the sites of injection are abraded by superficial incisions and each of them is covered with a circular lint patch of 1.5 cm in diameter with 0.1 ml (0.1 g) of the test sample, occlusively fixed in place for 24 h. Skin abrasion and application of the four patches under occlusion are repeated on the next 2 d.

Approximately 24 h prior to the second induction treatment by a 48-h occlusive patch test of 2.5×4 cm with the test sample on d 9, the nuchal area of animals is clipped, shaved, and the skin treated with 10 percent SLS in petrolatum if indicated.

Another variant of the first induction phase, as proposed by Maurer and Hess (1989), consists of four intradermal injections of a 1:1 FCA/saline emulsion, followed by a 24-h occlusive application of the test article in white petrolatum or of a neat "end-use" product.

The challenge is performed on d 21, using occlusive patch or open (uncovered) application, on the clipped flank skin. For the 24-h occlusive patch the test sample is incorporated into petrolatum or other suitable vehicle and applied at a dose of 50 mg to the lint patch of 2.5×4.0 cm, or a Finn chamber "patch unit" can be involved, which is occlusively fixed to the test site. For the open challenge 0.01 ml (10mg) of the test sample is applied directly to a circular test site 1.5 cm in diameter.

The challenge sites are evaluated and scored 24 and 48 h after initiation of the challenge exposure. If appropriate, rechallenge and cross-tests are done in weekly intervals on contralateral flanks. The 10 control animals are treated in the same way as the test animals, except that during induction, application of the test article is omitted. This testing strategy is suitable for allergenicity assessment of neat chemicals and "end-use" products. It is sensitive enough to identify weak contact allergens, and yields quantitative data in the form of threshold concentrations, which improves its predictive value.

38.11 THE CUMULATIVE CONTACT ENHANCEMENT TEST

The test protocol for this animal bioassay (Figure 38.11) involves separate application of Freund's complete adjuvant and the test articles (Tsuchiya *et al.*, 1982). The epidermal application of the test sample for induction simulates more accurately common exposure conditions to a potential environmental contact allergen. Two groups of 10 guinea pigs are used at minimum.

For induction the test animals are exposed to the test sample on d 0, 2, 7, and 9, at a dose of 0.2 ml of liquids or 0.1 ml of semisolids, applied to a linen patch of 2 × 4 cm and fixed under a 24-h occlusive patch to the clipped suprascapular area. On d 7, prior to the patch application, 2 × 0.1 ml of Freund's

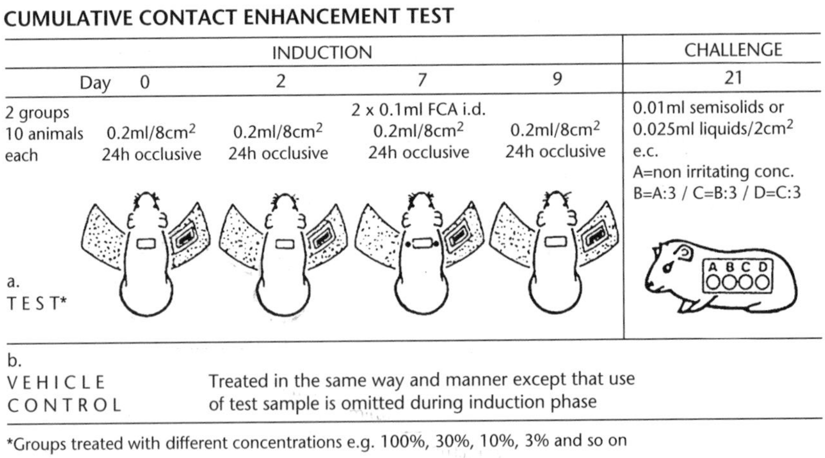

CUMULATIVE CONTACT ENHANCEMENT TEST

	INDUCTION				CHALLENGE
Day	0	2	7	9	21
2 groups 10 animals each	0.2ml/8cm² 24h occlusive	0.2ml/8cm² 24h occlusive	2 × 0.1ml FCA i.d. 0.2ml/8cm² 24h occlusive	0.2ml/8cm² 24h occlusive	0.01ml semisolids or 0.025ml liquids/2cm² e.c. A=non irritating conc. B=A:3 / C=B:3 / D=C:3

a.
TEST*

b.
VEHICLE
CONTROL   Treated in the same way and manner except that use
                 of test sample is omitted during induction phase

*Groups treated with different concentrations e.g. 100%, 30%, 10%, 3% and so on

Figure 38.11: Cumulative contact enhancement test.

complete adjuvant is administered intradermally parallel on each side of the application area.

For the challenge test, on d 21 one animal flank is shaved and 0.01 ml (semi-solids) or 0.025 ml (liquids) of the test sample, at nonirritating concentrations, is applied to circular skin area(s) of 2 cm in diameter using open application or 24-h occlusive patches. Rechallenge(s) may be performed to the contralateral flank in 7–10 d of sequence. The 24-, 48-, and 72-h skin reactions are scored according to a standard rating scale. Controls are treated in the same manner, except that the use of test article is omitted during the induction phase.

The cumulative contact enhancement test (CCET) is specified as a suitable tool to categorize contact allergens as weak or moderate and/or severe skin sensitizers (Tsuchiya *et al.*, 1985; Scheper *et al.*, 1990; Gäfvert, 1994).

This test strategy is recommended to screen allergenicity of poorly soluble or insoluble chemicals as well as "end-use" products. The database is relatively new.

Two short period or abbreviated variants of the CCET were reported by Kashima *et al.* (1993a, 1993b), which are designated as the AP 2 test (FCA intradermally and 24-h occlusive patch on d 0 and 4 for induction), and the CAP 2 test (cyclophosphamide i.p. on d 0 and FCA intradermally with occlusive patch on d 3 and 7). In both variants the challenge test is performed on d 14 followed by scoring of elicited skin reactions as described by the CCET.

Both methods shorten the test, and in the CAP 2 test the cyclophosphamide effectively enhances the skin reaction of the guinea pig to weak allergens.

38.12   THE EPICUTANEOUS MAXIMIZATION TEST

This test protocol is designed to assess the allergenic potential of "end-use" products and their single compounds (Brulos *et al.*, 1977a). It includes epicutaneous application of a test article, using occlusive patch and intradermal administration of complete Freund's adjuvant. Macroscopic readings of doubtful challenge skin reactions are evaluated microscopically; 20 guinea pigs are involved (Figure 38.12).

The preliminary test, initiated prior to the main study, is performed as follows: On d 0 the test article is applied as such or diluted at a dose of 0.5 ml (liquids, semisolids) or 0.5 g (moistened solids), using the 48-h occlusive patch on a shaved skin area of 2 cm^2 behind the left shoulder blade. Readings of the treated skin sites are performed 1, 6, 24, and 48 h after removal of the patch, and skin reactions are scored. Animals showing moderate to severe skin responses (strong reactors) must be replaced.

■ CHAPTER 38 ■

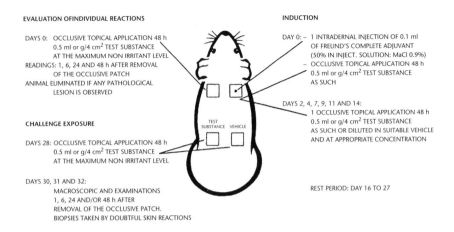

EVALUATION OFINDIVIDUAL REACTIONS

DAYS 0: OCCLUSIVE TOPICAL APPLICATION 48 h
0.5 ml or g/4 cm² TEST SUBSTANCE
AT THE MAXIMUM NON IRRITANT LEVEL
READINGS: 1, 6, 24 AND 48 h AFTER REMOVAL
OF THE OCCLUSIVE PATCH
ANIMAL ELIMINATED IF ANY PATHOLOGICAL
LESION IS OBSERVED

CHALLENGE EXPOSURE

DAYS 28: OCCLUSIVE TOPICAL APPLICATION 48 h
0.5 ml or g/4 cm² TEST SUBSTANCE
AT THE MAXIMUM NON IRRITANT LEVEL

DAYS 30, 31 AND 32:
MACROSCOPIC AND EXAMINATIONS
1, 6, 24 AND/OR 48 h AFTER
REMOVAL OF THE OCCLUSIVE PATCH.
BIOPSIES TAKEN BY DOUBTFUL SKIN REACTIONS

TEST SUBSTANCE   VEHICLE

INDUCTION

DAY 0: – 1 INTRADERNAL INJECTION OF 0.1 ml
OF FREUND'S COMPLETE ADJUVANT
(50% IN INJECT. SOLUTION: MaCl 0.9%)
– OCCLUSIVE TOPICAL APPLICATION 48 h
0.5 ml or g/4 cm² TEST SUBSTANCE
AS SUCH

DAYS 2, 4, 7, 9, 11 AND 14:
1 OCCLUSIVE TOPICAL APPLICATION 48 h
0.5 ml or g/4 cm² TEST SUBSTANCE
AS SUCH OR DILUTED IN SUITABLE VEHICLE
AND AT APPROPRIATE CONCENTRATION

REST PERIOD: DAY 16 TO 27

Figure 38.12: Epicutaneous maximization test. From Guillot and Gonnet (1985). Reprinted with permission.

For the main study, details concerning the induction as well as the challenge phase of this experimental design are best reproduced in Figure 38.12, as completed by Guillot -and Gonnet (1985).

Skin responses to challenge test are scored according to a standard grading scale. Histological examinations are performed in cases where skin lesions occur or reactions are doubtful.

Biopsies are carried out about 6 h after the first reading or immediately after subsequent readings. Excised skin specimens are fixed and embedded in paraffin, and sections are stained with hematoxylin and eosin. No control animals are involved in this assay.

Authors reported (Rochas *et al.*, 1977; Guillot and Gonnet, 1985) that in their hands the test is sufficiently sensitive to identify "end-use" products or their components that show even a slight allergenic potential.

38.13 SINGLE-INJECTION ADJUVANT TEST

In the eyes of the originators (Goodwin *et al.*, 1981) the single-injection adjuvant test (SIAT) procedure is simple to perform, and represents a suitable alternative to the GPMT of Magnusson and Kligman (1970). This technique is a modification of the methodology used by Connor *et al.* (1975) for allergenicity studies with sultone sensitizers in alkyl ether sulfates. Two groups of 10 guinea pigs each are used (Figure 38.13).

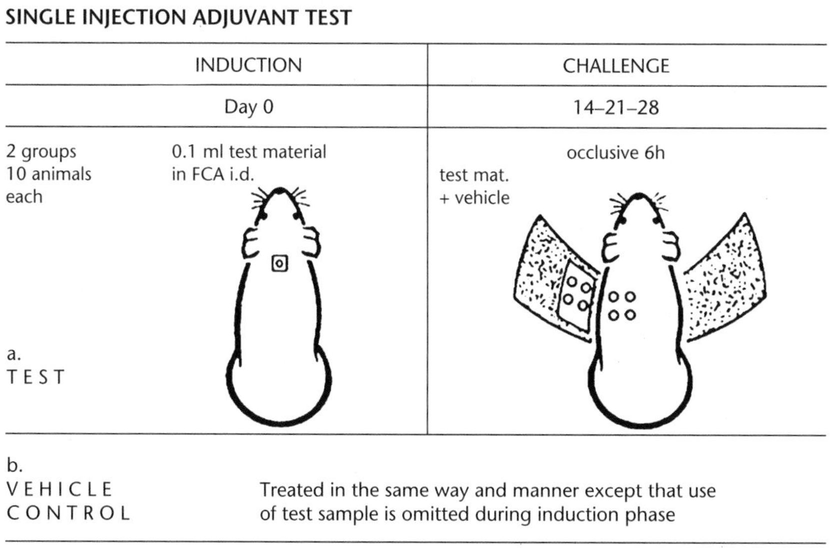

SINGLE INJECTION ADJUVANT TEST

	INDUCTION	CHALLENGE
	Day 0	14–21–28

a.
TEST

b. VEHICLE CONTROL	Treated in the same way and manner except that use of test sample is omitted during induction phase

Figure 38.13: Single-injection adjuvant test.

For the induction phase, the dissolved or suspended test article in a minimal quantity of suitable solvent is mixed with FCA to the chosen "final" induction concentration, determined in a preliminary irritation test, causing not more than moderate skin irritation. This mixture is injected intradermally at a dose of 0.1 ml between the animal's shoulders.

The challenge test is performed on d 14. Filter paper in aluminum patch test cups or Finn chambers or other type of "patch unit" is saturated with primary nonirritating concentration(s) of the test article and applied occlusively for 6 h to a shaved skin site on one animal flank. Subsequent rechallenge(s) may be performed at weekly intervals, necessitating the use of four new control animals. Controls are treated similar to test animals, except that during induction the test article is omitted.

The skin test sites are examined approximately 22 and 46 h after removal of the patch, and the elicited skin reactions are estimated according to a standard scoring system.

The sensitivity of the SIAT can be improved by increasing the number of intradermal exposures during the induction phase (DIAT and/or TIAT, i.e., double and/or triple induction injection), and/or by rechallenging (booster effect).

Even if less sensitive than the GPMT of Magnusson, the SLAT is easy to perform, more flexible, and not as time-consuming. Other merits and deficiencies are discussed by Goodwin *et al.* (1983), Goodwin and Johnson (1985), and Basketter and Allenby (1991). SIAT is not suitable for testing nonsoluble or suspensible chemicals and "end-use" products.

38.14 THE TIEREXPERIMENTELLER NACHWEIS (TINA) TEST

This test protocol involves 25 test and 10 control guinea pigs (Figure 38.14). The induction procedure requires intramuscular and intradermal administration, as well as a cloth patch test to apply the test sample to the animal (Ziegler, 1976, 1977; Ziegler and Süss, 1985).

At d 0 a mixture of FCA and the test article at a dose of 0.2 ml and at a slightly irritant concentration is administered intramuscularly into all four extremities and into the clipped neck region of the test animal. On d 14 the neck region and one flank of the animals are shaved. Then 10 percent SLS in Vaseline or 70 percent dimethyl sulfoxide (DMSO) is applied to the flank skin. At 24 h later, 0.1 ml of the test sample, at a minimal irritant concentration, is administered

TINA TEST

	INDUCTION		CHALLENGE
	Day 0	15–22–29–36	42
2 groups of animals	5 x 0.2 ml test mat. in FCA i.m.	0.1 ml test mat. i.d. + test material closed patch (24h)*	0.1 ml test material closed patch (24h)

a.
TEST*

b.
VEHICLE
CONTROL — Treated in the same way and manner except that use of test sample is omitted during induction phase

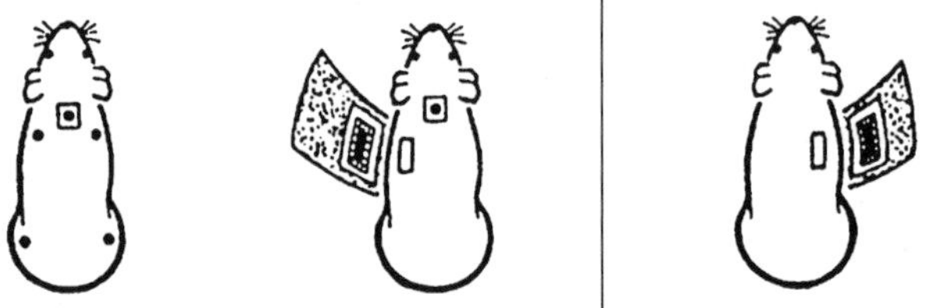

*pretreated with 10% sodium lauryl sulfate in petrolatum or DMSO 24h before

Figure 38.14: TINA test.

intradermally into the neck region. Simultaneously the flank skin is exposed to the test sample at a slightly irritant concentration, using a 24-h occlusive patch. On d 17 the patch is removed. This double exposure to the corresponding skin sites is repeated four times at weekly intervals.

On d 42 the right flank of all experimental animals is shaved for challenging. The challenge test is performed on the shaved contralateral flank on d 42 using a 24-h occlusive patch test with the test article at a nonirritant concentration in suitable vehicle. Readings of skin responses and their grading are performed on four subsequent days. Skin reactions with a duration of 48 h and more are considered positive.

Control animals are treated similarly to test animals, except that the use of the test article is omitted during the induction phase. Rechallenge or cross-test may follow at intervals of 7–14 d.

The TINA test is a sensitive but time-consuming procedure and is not suitable for testing poorly soluble or insoluble test articles, semisolids, or "end-use" products. The database is new.

38.15 THE FOOTPAD TEST

Two groups of 10 guinea pigs each are used (OECD, 1992) for this test (Figure 38.15).

For induction, on d 0 a 1 percent mixture or suspension (w/v) of the test article in complete Freund's adjuvant is administered at a dose of 0.05 ml into the front footpad of the test animals. The challenge test is performed on d 7. The test article usually is dissolved at a concentration of 1 percent (primary nonirritating one) or less in a vehicle formulated from guinea pig fat:dioxone: acetone (1:2:7) and applied open epicutaneously to the clipped flank skin at a dose of 0.3 ml to a circular test site of 8 cm^2. About 24 h after challenge, the test area is depilated and washed off with lukewarm water (37°C). Approximately 3 h after depilation, examination and grading of the elicited skin response are done according to a standard rating scale. Rating of these skin reactions is repeated 24 h later.

Control animals are treated in the same way as test animals, except that the use of the test article during induction is omitted.

The footpad test may be modified by using intradermal administration of the test article at primary nonirritating concentration in bidistilled water or in saline for challenging. Limits and deficiencies of this animal assay are similar to those of the Draize test. The database of this animal assay is poor.

FOOT-PAD TEST

	INDUCTION	CHALLENGE
	Day 0	21
2 groups 10 animals each	footpad injection: 0.05 ml 1% sol. in FCA 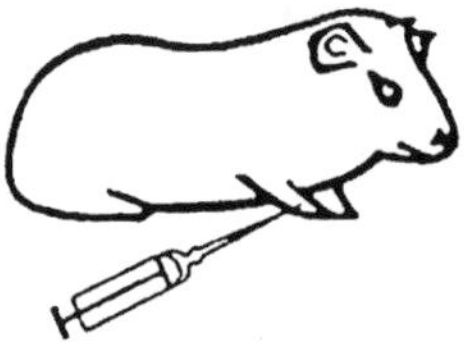	0.3 ml e.c. 1% solution in solvent system of guinea pig fat: dioxan: aceton, 1: 2: 7. 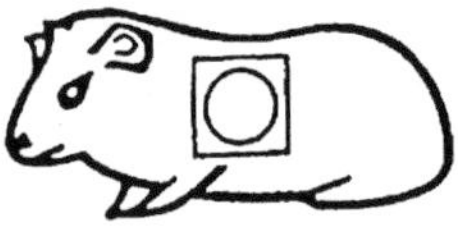
a. TEST		
b. VEHICLE CONTROL	Treated in the same way and manner except that use of test sample is omitted during induction phase	

Figure 38.15: Footpad test.

38.16 THE GUINEA PIG ALLERGY TEST ADAPTED TO COSMETIC INGREDIENTS

To evaluate the safety of different types of cosmetic formulations, toiletries, and their individual components, the authors developed a testing methodology based on the combination of two protocols (Dossou *et al.*, 1985).

Three groups of 12 or 24 guinea pigs each are used: one group for topical application, one for intradermal administration of a test article, and one control group. If indicated, additional vehicle groups can be added. After each epicutaneous application, animals are placed into individual restrainers for 2–4 h, allowing no movement and licking.

38.16.1 Protocol I—Induction by topical route

On d 0 all animals are treated with 0.2 ml Freund's complete adjuvant, administered into the footpad of one of the animal's hind legs, which has been cleaned with ethanol. An area of 3×5 cm on the scapular region is shaved (hair product testing) and depilated (skin product testing) on d 0, 2, and 4, about 6 h prior to open application of a dose of 0.5 ml of the neat test article or its dilutions or suspensions in suitable vehicle to this test site. If appropriate (weaker contact allergen), the total number of induction exposures can be increased up to nine (Figure 38.16).

38.16.2 Protocol II—Induction by injection

The test animal group is treated by administration of a 1:1 mixture of FCA/ dissolved test article or 1:1 emulsion of (FCA + unsoluble test article)/bidistilled water into the footpad of one of the animal's hind legs (Figure 38.17).

For the challenge, after a rest period of 11 d all experimental animals are challenged by open application of 10 µl of one or more test samples, which are not skin irritating, to the clipped and depilated back and lumbar region. The elicited reactions are read 24 and 48 h after challenging and the intensity is scored. Both protocols can be modified by rinsing the test article, increasing the frequency of exposure during induction, and involving cross-tests or

GUINEA PIG ALLERGY TEST (1)

	INDUCTION		CHALLENGE
	Day 0	2–4	15
3 groups 8 animals each	0.2 ml FCA footpad test material 0.5 ml/15 cm² e.c.	test material 0.5 ml/15 cm² e.c.	test material 0.01 ml e.c.

a. TEST

b. VEHICLE CONTROL — Treated in the same way and manner except that use of test sample is omitted during induction phase

c. FCA CONTROL — During induction treated with FCA i.d. exclusively and challenged

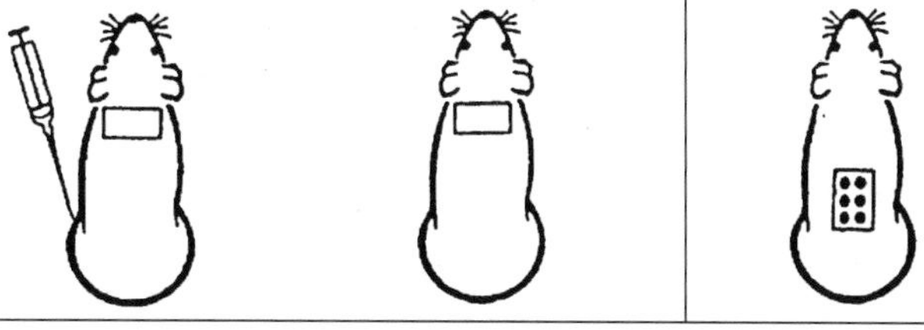

Figure 38.16: Guinea pig allergy test (1).

GUINEA PIG ALLERGY TEST (2)

INDUCTION			CHALLENGE
Day 0–3		4	15
2 groups 8 animals each	no treatment	0.2 ml FCA + test material footpad inject.	test material 0.01 ml e.c.

a.
TEST

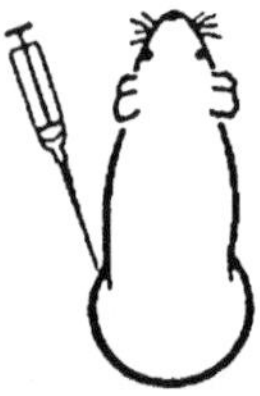

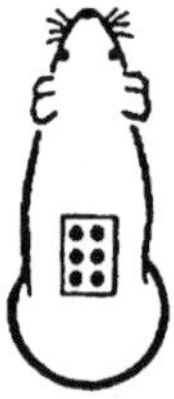

b.
VEHICLE
CONTROL — Treated in the same way and manner except that use of test sample is omitted during induction phase

Figure 38.17: Guinea pig allergy test (2).

rechallenge tests. The control group is challenged in the same way as the test group, except that use of the test article is omitted during induction.

The two protocols are complementary and linked. The topical route protocol simulates the conditions of anticipated exposure to "end-use" products, while the intradermal route is as exaggerated and sensitive as the GPMT. This assay is simple to perform, variable, sensitive, and suitable for testing of dermatologics, cosmetics, and toiletries as well as single chemicals, but during immobilization is stressing for the animals. The database is new.

38.17 THE EAR/FLANK TEST (STEVENS TEST)

This animal assay (Figure 38.18) is recommended as useful for rapid sensitization potential screening of a wide range of industrial chemicals by Stevens (1967). The use of the ears for induction of sensitization has been described by Davies (1964). Two groups of 10 guinea pigs each are used.

For the induction phase the test article, diluted in suitable vehicle and at an appropriate concentration, is applied once daily on 3 consecutive days to the outer surface of the ears at a dose of 0.1 ml per ear.

EAR FLANK TEST (STEVENS TEST)

	INDUCTION	CHALLENGE
	Day 0–1–2	7
2 groups 10 animals each	0.1 ml per ear e.c. 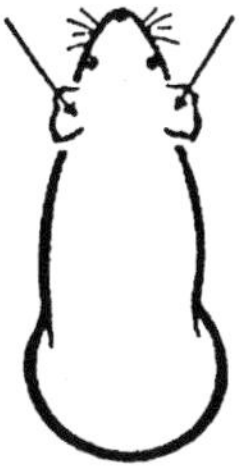	0.2 ml/cm² e.c.
a. TEST		
b. VEHICLE CONTROL	Treated in the same way and manner except that use of test sample is omitted during induction phase	

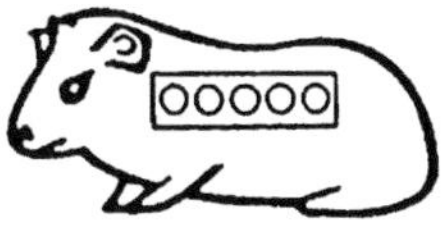

Figure 38.18: Ear flank test (Stevens test).

For challenging, on d 7 a range of primary nonirritant concentrations of test article in suitable vehicle and at a dose of 0.2 ml are applied to a clipped flank of 10 test animals on a marked circular area with a diameter of 1.0 cm. Control animals are challenged. Elicited skin reactions are graded 24 h later according to a standard rating scale. Rechallenge or cross test may follow at intervals of 1–2 wk on contralateral flanks.

There are four advantages of the ear/flank test:

1 No clipping or shaving of the outer surface of the ears is required before treatment.
2 The flanks are virgin skin test sites.
3 Test material applied to the ear appears not to be interfered with by the guinea pig, and thus the use of occlusive dosing can be avoided.
4 It is suitable for testing of final or end-use products.

The classification system is not intended to imply that this animal assay fails to detect weak sensitizers. However, even a negative result in the ear/flank test may be utilizable in predicting that an industrial product is not a strong contact sensitizer. The database is relatively slim.

38.18 CONCLUSIONS

The most promising preventive measure for reducing the incidence of allergic contact dermatitis in a population is to limit the contamination of our environment with potential contact allergens (Dept. of Health, Education, and Welfare, 1975).

A skilled, selected, and properly performed animal assay on guinea pigs offers a useful tool to assess the sensitizing potential of individual chemicals as well as "end-use" products (Andersen and Maibach, 1985a, 1985b). This becomes increasingly important as more predictive animal data become available for which a good correlation exists with epidemiological findings. It is of paramount importance in safety assessment that the difference between animal skin sensitizing risk and human health hazard is clearly stated. Thus, for the purpose of hazard evaluation, a positive result originating from animal sensitization assay does not necessarily mean that a hazard for humans exists, taking assumed exposure conditions to environmental contactants into consideration.

REFERENCES

ANDERSEN, K.E. (1985) Guinea pig maximization test: Effect of type of Freund's complete adjuvant emulsion and of challenge site location. *Derm. Beruf. Umwelt* **33**, 132–136.

ANDERSEN, K.E. (1993) Potency evaluation of contact allergens—Dose-response studies using the guinea pig maximization test. *Nordiske Seminar og Arbejdsrapporter*, Copenhagen.

ANDERSEN, K.E. and MAIBACH, H.I. (1985a) Contact allergy predictive tests in guinea pigs. *Curr. Probl. Dermatol.* **4**, 59–61.

ANDERSEN, K.E. and MAIBACH, H.I. (1985b; Guinea pig sensitization assays an overview. *Curr. Probl. Dermatol.* **14**, 263–290.

ANDERSEN, K.E., BOMAN, A., HAMANN, K. and WAHLBERG, J.E. (1984) Guinea pig maximization tests with formaldehyde releasers. Results from two laboratories. *Contact Dermatitis* **10**, 257–266.

ANDERSEN, K.E., BOMAN, A., VOLUND, A.A. and WAHLBERG, J.E. (1985) Induction of formaldehyde contact sensitivity: Dose-response relationship in the guinea pig maximization test. *Acta Dermato-Venereol. (Stockh.)* **65**, 472–478.

AVALOS, J., MOORE, H.W., REED, M.W. and RODRIGUEZ, E. (1989) Sensitizing potential of cyclobutene diones. *Contact Dermatitis* **21**, 341.

BAKER, H. (1968) The effects of dimethylsulfoxide, dimethylformamide and dimethylacetamide on the cutaneous barrier to water in human skin. *J. Invest. Dermatol.* **50**, 282–288.

BASKETTER, D.A. and ALLENBY, C.F. (1991) Studies on the phenomena in delayed contact hypersensitivity reactions. *Contact Dermatitis* **25**, 160–171.

BJÖRKNER, B. and NIKLASSON, B. (1984) Influence of the vehicle on elicitation of contact allergic reactions to acrylic compounds in the guinea pig. *Contact Dermatitis* **11**, 268–278.

BRONAUGH, R.L., ROBERTS, C.D. and McCAY, J.L. (1994) Dose-response relationship in skin sensitization. *Food Chem. Toxicol.* **32**, 113–117.

BRULOS, M.F., GUILLOT, J.P., MARTINI, M.C. and COTTE, J. (1977) The influence of perfumes on the sensitizing potential of cosmetic bases. I. A technique for evaluating sensitizing potential. *J. Soc. Cosmet. Chem.* **28**, 357–365.

BÜHLER, E.V. (1965) Delayed contact hypersensitivity in the guinea pig. *Arch. Dermatol.* **91**, 171–177.

BÜHLER, E.V. (1982) Comment on guinea pig test methods. *Food Chem. Toxicol.* **20**, 494–495.

BÜHLER, E.V. (1985) A rationale for the selection of occlusion to induce and elicit delayed contact hypersensitivity in the guinea pig. A prospective test. *Curr. Problems Dermatol.* **14**, 39–58.

BÜHLER, E..V. and GRIFFITH, F. (1975) Experimental skin sensitization in the guinea pig and man. In MAIBACH, H. (ed.) *Animal Models in Dermatology*, Edinburgh: Churchill Livingstone, 56–66.

CHASE, M.W. (1941) Inheritance in guinea pigs of the susceptibility to skin sensitization with simple chemical compounds. *J. Exp. Med.* **73**, 711–726.

CHRISTENSEN, O.B., CHRISTENSEN M.B. and MAIBACH, H.I. (1984) Effect of vehicle on elicitation of DNCB contact allergy in guinea pig. *Contact Dermatitis* **10**, 166–169.

CONNOR, D.S., RITZ, H.L., AMPULSKI, R.S., KOWOLLIK, H.G., LIM, P., THOMAS, D.W. and PARKHURST, R. (1975) Identification of certain sultones as the sensitizers in an alkyl ethoxy sulfate. *Fette Seifen Anstrichm.* **77**, 25–29.

CTFA SAFETY TESTING GUIDELINES. (1981) Adjunct to the CTFA Safety Substantiation Guidelines (1976). In *The CTFA Technical Guidelines*. Washington, DC: Cosmetic, Toiletry and Fragrance Association.

DAVIES, G. E. (1964) *Proc. European Society for the Study of Drug Toxicity* 4. Excerpta Medica Foundation Int. Congr. Serv. No. 81.

CHAPTER 38

DEPARTMENT of HEALTH, EDUCATION and WELFARE. (1975) Investigation of Consumer's Perception of Adverse Reactions to Consumer Products. Contracted to Westat, Inc., Rockville, Md., contract 223738052, June. Rockville, MD: Consumer Safety Statistic Staff, Office of Planning and Evaluation, Office of the Commissioner, Food and Drug Administration.

DOSSOU, K. G., SICARD, C., KALOPISSIS, O., REYMOND, D. and SCHAEFER, H. (1985) Guinea pig allergy test adapted to cosmetic ingredients. *Curr. Problems Dermatol.* **14**, 248–262.

DRAIZE, J. H. (1955) Dermal toxicity. *Food Drug Cosmet. Law J.* **10**, 722–732.

DRAIZE, J. H. (1959) Intracutaneous sensitization test in guinea pig. In Appraisal of the safety of chemicals in food, drugs and cosmetics. In *Dermal Toxicity*, p. 46. Austin, TX: Association of Food and Drug Officials of the United States, Texas State Department of Health.

EUROPEAN ECONOMIC COMMISSION (1983) Commission Directive of 29 July 1983 adapting to technical progress for the 5th time. Council Directive 67/648/EEC on the approximation of laws, regulations, and administration provisions relating to the classification packaging and labelling of dangerous substances. *J. Eur. Communities* **L251**, 27–1.

GÄFVERT, E. (1994) Allergenic components in modified and unmodified rosin. *Acta Dermato-Venereol. (Stockh.) Suppl.* **184**, 1–36.

GOODFREY, H. P. and BAER, H. (1971) The effect of physical and chemical properties of the sensitizing substance on the induction and elicitation of delayed contact sensitivity. *J. Immunol* **105**, 431–441.

GOODWIN, B. F. J. and JOHNSON, A. W. (1985) Single injection adjuvant test. In ANDERSON, K.E. and MAIBACH, H.I. (eds), *Current Problems in Dermatology*, Basel: Karger, Vol. 14, 201–207.

GOODWIN, B. F. I., CREVEL, R. W. R. and JOHNSON, A. W. (1981) A comparison of three guinea pig sensitization procedures for the detection of 19 reported human contact sensitizers. *Contact Dermatitis* **7**, 248–258.

GOODWIN, B. F. J., ROBERTS, D. W., WILLIAMS, D. L. and JOHNSON, A. W. (1983) Skin sensitization potential of saturated and unsaturated sultones. In GIBSON, G., HUBBARD, R. and PARKE, C. V. (eds), *Immunotoxicology*, London: Academic Press, 443–448.

GRIFFITH, J. F. and BÜHLER, E. V. (1969) Experimental Skin Sensitization in the Guinea Pig and Man. Cincinnati, OH: Procter and Gamble Co. Presented at the 26th Annual Meeting, American Academy of Dermatologists, Bar Harbor, ME.

GUILLOT, J. P. and GONNET, J. F. (1985) The epiculaneous maximization test. *Curr. Problems Dermatol.* **14**, 220–247.

HOFMANN, T., DIEHL, K. -H., LEIST, K. -H. and WEIGAND, W. (1987) The feasibility of sensitization studies using fewer test animals. *Arch. Toxicol.* **60**, 470–471.

JAPAN/MAFF (1985) *Testing Guidelines for the Evaluation of Safety of Agricultural Chemicals.* Tokyo: The Ministry of Agriculture, Forestry and Fisheries.

JOHNSON, A. W. and GOODWIN, B. F. J. (1985) The Draize test and modifications. *Curr. Problems Dermatol.* **14**, 31–38.

KASHIMA, R., OYAKE, Y., OKADA, J. and IKEDA, Y. (1993a) Studies of new short-period method for delayed contact hypersensitivity assay in the guinea pig. (I.) Development and comparison with other methods. *Contact Dermatitis* **28**, 235–242.

KASHIMA, R., OYAKE, Y., OKADA, J. and IKEDA, Y. (1993b) Studies of new short-period method for delayed contact hypersensitivity assay in the guinea pig (2.) Studies of the enhancement effect of cyclophosphamide. *Contact Dermatitis* **29**, 26–32.

KERO, M. and HANNUKSELA, M. (1980) Guinea pig maximization test, open epicutaneous test and chamber test in induction of delayed contact hypersensitivity. *Contact Dermatitis* **6**, 341–344.

KLECAK, G. (1982) Identification of contact allergens: Predictive tests in animals. In MARZILLI, F. and MAIBACH, H.I. (eds) *Dermatotoxicology*, 2nd ed., New York: Hemisphere, 200–219.

KLECAK, G. (1985) The Freund's complete adjuvant test and open epicutaneous test. A complementary test procedure for realistic assessment of allergenic potential. *Curr. Problems Dermatol.* **14**, 152–171.

KLECAK, G., GELEICK, H. and FREY, I. R. (1977) Screening of fragrance materials for allergenicity in the guinea pig. I. Comparison of four testing methods. *J. Soc. Cosmet. Chem.* **28**, 53–64.

KLIGMAN, A. M. (1966a) The SLS provocative patch test. *J. Invest. Dermatol.* **46**, 573–589.

KLIGMAN, A. M. (1966b) The identification of contact allergens by human assay II. Factors influencing the induction and measurement of allergic contact dermatitis. *J. Invest. Dermatol.* **47**, 375–392.

KOZUKA, T., MORIKAVA F. and OHTA, S. (1981) A modified technique of guinea pig testing to identify delayed hypersensitivity allergens. *Contact Dermatitis* **7**, 225–237.

LANDSTEINER, K. and JACOBS, J. (1935) Studies on sensitization of animals with simple chemical compounds. *J. Exp. Med.* **61**, 643–656.

MAGNUSSON, B. and HERSLE, K. (1965) Patch test methods: I. A comparative study of six different types of patch tests. *Acta Dermato-Venereol. (Stockh.)* **45**, 123–128.

MAGNUSSON, B. and KLIGMAN, A. M. (1969) The identification of contact allergens by animal assay. The guinea pig maximization test. *J. Invest. Dermatol.* **52**, 268–276.

MAGNUSSON, B. and KLIGMAN, A. M. (1970) *Allergic Contact Dermatitis in the Guinea Pig. Identification of contact allergens.* Springfield, IL: Charles C. Thomas.

MAGUIRE, H. C. (1973) The bioassay of contact allergens in the guinea pig. *J. Soc. Cosmet. Chem.* **24**, 151–162.

MAGUIRE, H. C. (1975) Estimation of the allergenicity of prospective contact sensitizers in the guinea pig. In MAIBACH, H. (eds), *Animal Models in Dermatology*, Edinburgh: Churchill Livingstone, 67–75.

MAGUIRE, H. C., Jr. (1985) Estimation of the allergenicity of prospective human contact sensitizers in the guinea pig. In MAIBACH, H. and LOWE, N.J. (eds) *Models in Dermatology*, Vol. 2, Basel: Karger, 234–239.

MAGUIRE, H. C., Jr. and Cipriano, D. (1985) Split adjuvant test. *Curr. Problems Dermatol.* **14**, 107–113.

MARZULLI, F. and MAGUIRE, H. C., Jr. (1982) Usefulness and limitations of various guinea pig test methods in detecting human skin sensitizers— Validation of guinea pig tests for skin hypersensitivity. *Food Cosmet. Toxicol.* **20**, 67–74.

MARZULLI, F. N. and MAIBACH, H. I. (1974) The use of graded concentrations in studying skin sensitizers: Experimental contact sensitization in man. *Food Cosmet. Toxicol.* **12**, 219–227.

MAURER, T. (1974) Tierexperimentelle Methoden zur prädiktiven Erfassung sensibilisierender Eigenschaften von Kontaktallergenen. Inauguraldissertation, Universität Basel.

MAURER, T. (1985) The optimization test. *Curr. Problems Dermatol.* **14**, 114–151.

MAURER, T. and HESS, R. (1989) The Maximization Test for skin sensitization potential—Updating the standard protocol and validation of a modified protocol. *Fd. Chem. Toxic.* **27**, 807–811.

MAURER, T., THOMANN, P. WEIRICH, E. G. and HESS, R. (1978) Predictive evaluation in animals of the contact allergenic potential of medically important substances. I. Comparison of different methods of inducing and measuring cutaneous sensitization. *Contact Dermatitis* **4**, 321–333.

MAURER, T., WEIRICH, E. C. and HESS, R. (1980) The optimlzation test in guinea pigs in relation to other prediction sensitization methods. *Toxicology* **15**, 163–171.

OCCUPATIONAL SAFETY and HEALTH ADMINISTRATION (1987) *Toxic and Hazardous Hazard Communication Standard.* CFR Title 29, Chapter XVII, Part 1910, Subpart Z, Section 1910. 1200, p. 91.

ORGANIZATION for ECONOMIC COOPERATION and DEVELOPMENT (1992) *Guidelines for Testing of Chemicals.* Director of Information, OECD, Paris, France, 1981, revised 1992.

PARKER, D., SOMMER, G. and TURK, J. L. (1975) Variation in guinea pig responsiveness. *Cell. Immunol.* **18**, 233–238.

PIRILÄ, V. (1974) Chamber test versus lapptest. Förhandlingar vid Nordisk Dermatologisk Forening 20 Möte, 43.

Polak, L., BARNES, J. M. and TURK, J. L. (1968) The genetic control of contact sensitization to inorganic metal compounds in guinea-pigs. *Immunology* **14**, 707–711.

PRINCE, H. N. and PRINCE, T. G. (1977) Comparative guinea pig assays for contact hypersensitivity. *Cosmet. Toiletries* **92**, 53–58.

RAO, K. S., BETSO, J. E. and OLSON, K. J. (1981) A collection of guinea pig sensitization. The results grouped by chemical class. *Drug Chem. Toxicol.* **4**, 331–351.

RITZ, H. L. and BÜHLER, E. V. (1980) Planning conduct, and interpretation of guinea pig sensitization patch tests. In DRILL, V.A. and LAZAR, P. (eds) *Current Concepts in Cutaneous Toxicity* New York: Academic Press, 25–40.

ROCHAS, H., GUILLOT, J. P., MARTINI, M. C. and COTTE, J. (1977), Contribution à l'etude de l'influence des parfums sur le pouvoir sensibilisant de bases cosmetique. 2ème partie: Role du parfum sur le pouvoir sensibilisant de bases cosmetique. *J. Soc. Cosmet. Chem.* **28**, 367–375.

ROCKWELL, E. M. (1955) Study of several factors influencing contact irritation and sensitization. *J. Invest. Dermatol.* **24**, 35–49.

SATO, Y. (1985) Modified guinea pig maximization test. *Curr Probl. Dermatol.* **14**, 193–200.

■ CHAPTER 38 ■

SATO, Y., KATSUMURA, Y., ICHIKAWA, H. KOBAYASHI, T., KOZUKA, T., MORIKAWA, F. and OHTA, S. (1981) A modified technique of guinea pig testing to identify delayed hypersensitivity allergens. *Contact Dermatitis* **7**, 225–237.

SATO, Y., KUTSUNA, H., KOBAYASHI, T. and MITSUI, T. (1984) D&C Nos. 10 and 11. Chemical composition analysis and delayed contact hypersensitivity testing in the guinea pig. *Contact Dermatitis* **10**, 30–38.

SHARP, D. W. (1978) The sensitization potential of some perfume ingredients tested, using a modified Draize procedure. *Toxicology* **9**, 261–271.

SCHEPER, R. J., VON BLOMBERG, B. M. E., DE GROOT, J., GOEPTAR, A. R., LANG, M., OSTENDORP, R. A. J., BRUYNZEEL, D. P. and VAN TOL, R. G. L. (1990) Low allergenicity of clonidine impedes studies of sensitization mechanisms in guinea pig models. *Contact Dermatitis* **23**, 81–89.

SHILLAKER, R. O., GRAHAM, M. B., HODGSON, I. T. and PADGHAM, M. D. (1989) Guinea pig maximisation test for skin sensitisation: The use of fewer test animals. *Arch. Toxicol.* **63**, 281.

STAMPF, J.-L. and BENEZRA, C. (1982) The sensitizing capacity of helenin and of two of its main constituents, the sesquiterpene lactones alantolactone and isoalantolactone: A comparison of epicutaneous and intradermal sensitizing methods and of different strains of guinea pigs. *Contact Dermatitis* **8**, 16–24.

STAMPF, J.-L., BENEZRA, C. and ASAKAWA, Y. (1982) Stereospecificity of allergic contact dermatitis (ACD) to enantiomers. Part III. Experimentally induced ACD to natural sesquiterpene dialdehyde polygodial in guinea pigs. *Arch. Dermatol. Res.* **274**, 277–281.

STEVENS, M. A. (1967) Use of the albino guinea-pig to detect the skin-sensitizing ability of chemicals. *Br. J. Ind. Med.* **24**, 189.

TSUCHIYA, S., KONDO. M., OKAMOTO, K. and Takase, Y. (1982) Studies on contact hypersensitivity in the guinea pig. The cumulative contact enhancement test. *Contact Dermatitis* **8**, 246–255.

TSUCHIYA, S., KONDO, M., OKAMOTO, K. and TAKASE, Y. (1985) The cumulative contact enhancement test. *Curr. Problems Dermatol.* **14**, 208–219.

US DEPARTMENT OF HEALTH, EDUCATION and WELFARE (1978) Guide for the care and use of laboratory animals. U.S. Department of Health, Education and Welfare. Public Health Service, National Institute of Health. Revised Publication No. (NIH) 78-23.

US ENVIRONMENTAL PROTECTION AGENCY/FIFRA (1984) Environmental Protection Agency Pesticide Assessment Guidelines; Subdivision F—Hazard

Evaluation: Human and Domestic Animals. Office of Pesticide Programs. PB86–108958. Series 81-6.

US ENVIRONMENTAL PROTECTION AGENCY/TSCA (1985) Environmental Protection Agency—Toxic Substances Control Act Test Guidelines; Final Rules—Subpart E—Specific Organ/Tissue Toxicity, 796.4100. Dermal sensitisation. *Fed. Reg.* **50**(188), 39425.

VAN DER WALLE, H. B. and BENSINK, T. (1982) Cross reaction pattern of 26 acrylic monomers on guinea pig skin. *Contact Dermatitis* **8**, 376–382.

VAN DER WALLE, H. B., KLECAK, G., GELEICK, H. and BENSINK, T. (1982) Sensitizing potentials of 14 mono(meth)acrylates in the guinea pig. *Contact Dermatitis* **8**, 223–235.

VINSON, L. J., SINGER, E. J., KOEHLER, W. R., LEHMAN, M. D. and MAUSRAT, T. (1965) The nature of the epidermal barrier and some factors influencing skin permeability. *Toxicol. Appl. Pharmacol.* **7**, 7–19.

VOSS, J. G. (1958) Skin sensitisation by mercaptans of low molecular weight. *J. Invest. Dermatol.* **31**, 273–279.

WAHLBERG, J. E. and BOMAN, A. (1985) Guinea pig maximization test. *Curr. Problems Dermatol.* **14**, 59–106.

WAHLBERG, J. E. and FREGERT, S. (1985) Guinea pig maximization test. In MAIBACH, H. and LOWE, N.J. (eds) *Models in Dermatology*, Vol. 2, Basel: Karger, 225–233.

WHITE, S. I., FRIEDMANN, P. S., MOSS, C. and SIMPSON, J. M. (1986) The effect of altering area of application and dose per unit area on sensitization by DNCB. *Br. J. Dermatol.* **115**, 663–668.

ZESCH, A. (1974) Wechselbeziehungen zwischen Haut, Vehikel und Arzneimittel bei der Penetration in die menschliche Haut. II. Vehikel und Penetration. *Fette Seiten Anstrichm.* **76**, 312–318.

ZIEGLER, V. (1976) Tierexperimenteller Nachweis stark allergener Eigenschaften von Industrieprodukten. Dissert. Promot. B, Karl-Marx-Univ., Leipzig.

ZIEGLER, V. (1977) Der tierexperimentelle Nachweis allergener Eigenschaften von Industrieprodukten. *Dermatol. Monatsschr.* **163**, 387–391.

ZIEGLER, V., REINICKE, A., Andreas, V. and Süss, E. (1984) Empfehlungen zum Einsatz von Dimethylsulfoxid (DMSO) anstelle des Natriumlaurilsulfates bei der tierexperimentellen Prüfung neuer Allergene nach der TGL 32591. *Dermatol. Monatsschr.* **170**, 186.

CHAPTER 38

ZIEGLER, V. and SÜSS, E. (1985) The TINA test. *Curr. Problems Dermatol.* **14**, 172–192.

ZIEGLER, V., SÜSS, E., STANDAU, H. and HASERT, K. (1972) Der Meerschweinchen-Maximizatioptest zum Nachweis der sensibilisierenden Wirkung wichtiger Industrieprodukte. *Allerg. Immunol.* **18**, 203–208.

Test Methods for Allergic Contact Dermatitis in Humans

FRANCIS N MARZULLI AND HOWARD I MAIBACH

Contents

39.1   Introduction

39.2   Predictive tests

39.3   Diagnostic tests

39.4   Excited skin syndrome

39.1   INTRODUCTION

Allergic contact dermatitis (ACD) is a commonly occurring inflammatory skin disease that appears as a delayed skin response following skin contact with an allergenic chemical. It is characterized by erythema, edema, and vesiculation. Regulatory agencies such as the Food and Drug Administration (FDA), US Environmental Protection Agency (EPA), and Consumer Product Safety Commission (CPSC) often require that chemicals and untested substances that are intended to be newly introduced into the marketplace be evaluated for this hazard potential.

ACD has widespread occurrence, in part because of the annual introduction of large numbers of new chemicals into the marketplace, some of which are ultimately found to be allergenic under use conditions. In addition, older allergenic chemicals employed in occupational settings provide a continuing source of skin disease and are difficult to eliminate from the environment.

Medicaments and cosmetics contain preservatives and fragrances that may be allergenic (Bandmann *et al.*, 1972; Marzulli and Maibach, 1980; Opdyke, 1974). A more detailed list of allergenic substances would include rubber, plastics, metals, epoxy resins, wood products, metal-working fluids, printing chemicals, and others (Maibach, 1987). Culinary and nonedible plants constitute another sizable source of allergenic chemicals (Fisher, 1986).

The *American Journal of Contact Allergy*, started in 1989, was introduced as the official journal of the American Contact Dermatitis Society. It and the older nondomestic journal *Contact Dermatitis* are the current principal sources of information about ACD. *Dermatosen's* articles in German and English provide many scholarly presentations.

Although ACD closely resembles irritant contact dermatitis on gross inspection of the skin, ACD has an immunologic etiology that is lacking in irritant dermatitis. Accordingly, tests for ACD potential must demonstrate that the chemical is capable of producing a more severe subsequent skin effect than was encountered on initial contact, signifying an allergic (altered) response rather than an irritant response. Conversely, skin irritation as a cause for skin effects must be excluded. That is, a positive skin response at challenge must be produced by a clearly nonirritant concentration of the test substance.

Animal tests are often preferred as compared with human tests for predicting human ACD potential. This is a precautionary measure that is undertaken to avoid sensitizing a significant segment of the human population to the test

■ CHAPTER 39 ■

chemical and to a vast array of closely related (cross-reacting) chemicals that will be encountered by the test subject at a later time.

Nonanimal *in vitro* alternative tests are currently under investigation but none has been validated to date.

Human tests for ACD potential are often needed as followup to animal tests, since the correlation between animal and human test results is not exact (Marzulli and Maguire, 1982). Human tests are employed both for forecasting ACD potential of new chemicals and for diagnosing ACD in clinical patients that present themselves to investigative dermatologists for evaluation and treatment of contact dermatitis.

Allergenic chemicals are sometimes purposefully introduced into the marketplace if there is some medical benefit to be achieved, and the therapeutic index suggests that the concentration required for efficacy is below that likely to result in sensitization of large numbers of users. Benzoyl peroxide is allergenic and falls into this category. It is marketed as a drug for treating acne vulgaris, with a warning label to discontinue use if ACD occurs. Others, like formaldehyde, have a potential for sensitizing, but may be well tolerated at low concentrations and appropriate use concentrations.

39.2 PREDICTIVE TESTS

A large database exists involving animals and humans that have been tested with a wide variety of chemicals for skin sensitization potential. These data are available for study of the relationship of chemical structure and potency as skin sensitizers. Dupuis and Benezra (1983) and Benezra *et al.* (1989) summarized chemical properties that appeared to be associated with a propensity for skin sensitization. More recently, structure—activity relationships were investigated by Ferguson *et al.* (1994). This group has targeted electrophilicity as an important factor in a chemical's capacity to sensitize. Accordingly, they have employed measures of electrophilicity to predict sensitization potential.

Human test methods for forecasting skin sensitization potential were largely developed and refined during the period 1941–1975 and are summarized in Table 39.1. Currently, the modified maximization technique of Kligman and Epstein (1975) and the modified Draize procedure (Table 39.1) are methods of choice.

In these human studies, the test chemical is applied to the skin under an occlusive patch. This chemical trauma is repeated 7–10 times over a three week period in order to induce sensitization of the test chemical. This is followed by a rest period of 10 days to 2 weeks. The skin is then challenged (to see if an immune-based altered response has taken place) using a new skin site and application of a nonirritant concentration of the test material under occlusion. Induction may be accomplished by employing enhancing techniques such as repetition of the chemical insult (Shelanski, 1951), using a high concentration of test material at induction (Marzulli and Maibach, 1973, 1974), treating the skin with sodium lauryl sulfate (SLS) (Kligman, 1966b), skin stripping (Spier and Sixt, 1955), or freezing (Epstein *et al.*, 1963). Freund's adjuvant (Freund, 1951) was among the earliest techniques to improve the sensitization response in animal tests.

The size of the test population is important with regard to interpretation of findings. Henderson and Riley (1945) discussed how the total number of test participants employed may affect the predictive accuracy of the data obtained, when analyzed statistically. Careful consideration must be given to two aspects:

1 The sample size of test subjects must be large enough so that results are valid for the population at large, yet small enough to be logistically feasible in the laboratory.
2 The laboratory test must have the capacity to predict likelihood of occurrence under use conditions.

39.3 DIAGNOSTIC TESTS

In diagnostic tests, a preparation is applied to a clinical patient's skin under an occlusive patch for 48 h and the skin is evaluated for evidence of erythema, edema, or more severe skin changes occurring 24, 48, or 72 h after removal of the patch. Allergenic materials are thereby identified by producing skin disease on a small scale with offending chemicals.

The American Academy of Dermatology has worked collaboratively with Hermal Pharmaceutical Laboratories, Inc., Route 145, Oak Hill, New York, NY 12460. This organization can provide further details regarding diagnostic test methods and types and sources of test allergens. A booklet by James G. Marks and Vincent A. DeLeo (1992) entitled Patch Testing for Contact and Occupational Dermatology is available from Hermal Laboratories.

The North American Contact Dermatitis Group, a task force of the American Academy of Dermatology, consisting of a dozen or so dermatologist specialists, focuses attention on allergic contact dermatitis. They review test methods,

■ CHAPTER 39 ■

TABLE 39.1:
Predictive tests for skin sensitization of humans

Test	Test: Number of subjects	Test substance amount or concentration	Vehicle	Skin site	Type patch	Induction: Number of patches	Duration	Rest	Challenge	Reference
Schwartz	200	Fabric			Fabric	1	5 d	10 d	48 h patch; observe 10 d	Schwartz (1941)
Schwartz	200	1 in. fabric, liquid or powder		Arm, thigh, or back	Cellophane covered with 2 × 2 in. Elastoplast	1	72 h	7–10 d	72 h; same site; observe 3 d	Schwartz (1960)
"Prophetic" Schwartz-Peck	200	¼ in. square 4-ply gauze, liquid saturated[a]	Petrolatum or corn oil	Arm or back	1 in. square nonwaterproof cellophane covered with 2 in. square adhesive plaster	1	24 h or 3 or 4 d	10–14 d	48 h; any site especially thin keratin; observe 3 d; compare new and old formulas	Schwartz and Peck (1944); Schwartz (1951)
"Repeated insult" Shelanski	200	Proportional to area of ultimate use	Mineral oil		Occlusion; follows Schwartz test	10–15	24 h every other day; same site	2–3 wk	48 h patch	Shelanski (1951); Shelanski and Shelanski (1953)
"Repeated insult" Draize	100 males 100 females	0.5 ml or 0.5 g		Arm or back	1 in. square	10	24 h alternate days	10–14 d	Repeat patch on new site	Draize et al. (1944). Shehinski (1951); Draize (1959)

Modified Draize	200	0.5 ml or 0.5 g (high concentration)	Petrolatum	Arm	Square BandAid, no perforations	10	48 h	2 wk	Patch on new site 72 h with nonirritant concentration	Marzulli and Maibach (1973, 1974)
"Maximization" Kligman	25	1 ml 5% SLS[b] followed by 1 ml 25% test material	Petrolatum	Forearm or calf	1.5 in. square Webril occluded with Blenderm; held in place with perforated plastic tape	5 (same site)	24 h SLS followed by 48 h test material for each of 5 inducing applications	10 d	1 in. square patch on lower back or forearm; 0.4 ml of 10% SLS for 1 h followed in 24 h by 0.4 ml of 10% test material for 48 h	Kligman (1966a)
Modified "maximization"	25	Same as maximization	Petrolatum			7	24 h SLS followed by 48 h test material for each of 7 inducing applications; no patch for 24 h between each of 7 inducing applications	10 d	2% SLS for ½ h followed by 48 h patch with test material	Kligman and Epstein (1975)

[a] Modified for solids, powders, ointments, and cosmetics. Concentration, amount, area, and site of application are considered important in evaluating results. Authors recommended that cosmetics be tested uncovered.

[b] Sodium lauryl sulfate (SLS) pretreatment is used to produce moderate inflammation of the skin. SLS is mixed with test material when compatible. SLS is eliminated when the test material is a strong irritant.

TABLE 39.2:

Results of tests on 1119 patients with suspected allergic contact dermatitis, using 32 "standard allergens"

Allergens[a]	Total tallied	Interpretation			Relevance		
		Allergic	Doubtful	Irritant	Present	Past	Relevance (%)
Balsam of Peru 25% petrolatum	1122	37	13	2	10	3	35
Benzocaine 5% petrolatum	1135	40	3	0	18	6	60
Benzoyl peroxide 1% petrolatum	1115	20	6	3	6	2	40
Black rubber paraphenylenediamine mix (PPD mix 0.6% petrolatum)[b]	1140	16	1	3	10	1	69
Caine mix less benzocaine 3% petrolatum[c]	1117	22	7	8	7	4	50
Carba mix 3% petrolatum (carba rubber mix)[d]	1135	38	14	6	23	4	71
Cinnamic alcohol 5% petrolatum	1046	28	4	4	13	2	54
Cinnamic aldehyde 2% petrolatum	1048	62	21	60	22	5	44
Dibucaine 1% petrolatum	1009	8	1	2	2	1	38
Cyclomethycaine sulfate 1% petrolatum	1012	8	1	4	2	0	25
Epoxy resin 1% petrolatum	1129	21	3	0	9	3	57
Ethylenediamine dihydrochloride 1% petrolatum	1120	66	2	0	28	18	70
Eugenol 4% petrolatum	1016	14	3	5	3	3	43
Formaldehyde 2% water	1144	70	9	13	27	5	46
Hydroxycitronellal 4% petrolatum	1049	16	2	2	6	2	50
Imidazolidinyl urea 2% water	1134	17	5	2	5	0	29
Isoeugenol 4% petrolatum	1012	24	5	1	5	3	34
Lanolin alcohol (wool wax alcohol) 30% petrolatum	1135	14	5	1	10	1	79
Mercapto mix 1% petrolatum (mercapto rubber mix)[e]	1132	30	3	0	21	3	80
Mercaptobenzothiazole 1% petrolatum	1141	33	4	2	21	4	76
Neomycin sulfate 20% petrolatum	1131	75	5	2	25	19	59
Nickel sulfate 2.5% petrolatum	1123	109	7	8	40	43	76
Oak moss 5% petrolatum	1038	20	3	0	7	4	55

para-Tertiary-butylphenol formaldehyde resin 1% petrolatum	1129	9	0	3	5	2	78
Potassium dichromate 0.5% petrolatum	1138	59	15	34	19	7	44
p-Phenylenediamine 1% petrolatum	1138	79	6	2	33	14	59
Quaternium-15 2% petrolatum	1129	76	1	0	37	6	57
Quaternium-15 2% water	1103	43	12	0	25	0	58
Rosin (colophony) 20% petrolatum	1132	22	4	0	8	1	41
Tetracaine 1% petrolatum	1014	8	1	2	1	3	50
Thimerosal 0.1% petrolatum	1137	70	10	4	15	20	50
Thiuram mix 1% petrolatum (thiuram rubber mix)[f]	1137	44	8	0	25	5	68

[a] Not every patient was tested with every allergen.

[b] *N*-Pheny-*N'*-cyctohexyl-*p*-phenylenediamine 0.25 per cent, *N*-isopropyl-*N'*-phenyl-*p*-phenylenediamine 0.10 per cent *N,N'*-diphenyl-*p*~phenylenediamine 0.25 per cent.

[c] Dibucaine 1 per cent, tetracaine 1 per cent, cyclomethycaine sulfate 1 per cent.

[d] Diphenylguanidine 1.0 per cent, zinc diethyldithiocarbamate 1.0 per cent, zinc diethyldithiocarbamate 1.0 per cent.

[e] *N*-Cyclohexyl-2-benzothiazolesulfenamide 0.333 per cent, 2,2'-benzothiazyl disulfide 0.333 per cent, 4-morpholinyl-2-benzothiazyl disulfide 0.333 per cent.

[f] Tetramethylthiuram disulfide 0.25 per cent, tetramethylthiuram monosulfide 0.25 per cent, tetramethylthiuram disulfide 0.25 per cent, dipentamethylenethiuram disulfide 0.25 per cent.

standardize techniques, collect information relating to the ACD potential of marketplace products and chemicals, and publish their findings.

One of the more recent refinements in interpretation of diagnostic test results consists of an assessment of the relevance of positive patch-test findings to the diagnosis. The investigator must first establish that positive patch-test results are consistent with a history of exposure to a particular chemical in a product and must exclude other possible environmental exposure conditions. Next, the location of the present dermatitis must correspond to the site of contact with the putative offending chemical. Finally, the patch-test concentration must be nonirritating, as can be demonstrated by a dose-response effect when dilution of the putative allergen is employed. An operational definition of ACD has been suggested (Ale and Maibach, 1995) using the following algorithm to establish the relation between a positive patch test and the likelihood of clinical ACD: 1) history of exposure, 2) appropriate morphology, 3) positive patch test to a non-irritating concentration of the putative allergen, 4) repeat patch test if excited skin syndrome is operative (more than one positive patch test), 5) employ serial dilution patch testing to distinguish allergen from marginal irritant, 6) employ use test or open patch test, 7) resolution of dermatitis.

An example of test results obtained by the North American Contact Dermatitis Group was reported by Storrs *et al.* (1989) and is given in Table 39.2. The most common sensitizers identified were nickel, *p*-phenylenediamine, quaternium-15, neomycin, thimerosol, formaldehyde, cinnamic aldehyde, ethylenediamine, potassium dichromate, and thiuram mix. Ten participating investigation centers were involved, including five university clinics, two large multispecialty clinics, and three private offices.

39.4 EXCITED SKIN SYNDROME

"Angry back" and "excited skin" are terms used to describe a hyperirritable skin condition that occurs when multiple concomitant inflammatory skin conditions prevail. When this hypersensitive skin condition exists, false positive test results may occur. Details and strategies for dealing with the situation are discussed by Bruynzeel and Maibach (1991).

REFERENCES

ALE, S. I. and MAIBACH, H. I. (1995) Clinical relevance in allergic contact dermatitis: An algorithmic approach. *Dermatosen* **43**, 119–121.

BANDMANN, H. J., CALNAN, C. D., CRONIN, E., FREGERT, S., HJORTH, N., MAGNUSSON, B., MAIBACH, H., MALTEN, K. F., MENEGHINI, C. L., PIRILA, V. and WILKINSON, D. W. (1972) Dermatitis from applied medicaments. *Arch. Dermatol.* **106**, 335–337.

BENEZRA, C., SIGMAN, C. and MAIBACH, H. (1989) A systematic search for structure-activity relationships of skin contact sensitization: II. para-phenylenediamines. *Semin. Dermatol.* **8**, 88–93.

BRUYNZEEL D. and MAIBACH, H. I. (1991) Excited skin syndrome and the hypo-reactive state: Current status. In MENNE, T. and MAIBACH, H. I. (eds) *Exogenous Dermatoses: Environmental dermatitis*, Boca Raton, FL: CRC Press, 141–150.

DE GROOT, A. and WEYLAND, J. (1988) Kathon CG: A review. *J. Am Acad. Dermatol.* **18**, 350–358.

DRAIZE, J. H. (1959) Dermal toxicity. In *Appraisal of the Safety of Chemicals in Foods, Drugs and Cosmetics*. Austin, TX: Assoctatton of Food and Drug Officials of the United States, Texas State Department of Health.

DRAIZE, J. H., WOODARD, G. and CALVERY, H. D. (1944) Methods for the study of irritation and toxicity of substances applied topically to the skin and mucous membranes. *J. Pharmacol. Exp. Ther.* **83**, 377–390.

DUPUIS, A. and BENEZRA, C. (1983) *Allergic contact dermatitis to simplc chemicals. A molecular approach.* New York: Marcel Dekker.

EPSTEIN, W. L., KLIGMAN. A. and SENECAL, I. P. (1963) Role of regionally mph nodes in contact sensitization *Arch. Dermatol.* **88**, 789–792.

FERGUSON, J., ROSENKRANZ, H. S., KLOPMAN, C. and KAROL, M. (1994) Structural determinants of dermal and respiratory sensitization determined using a computer-assisted structure-activity expert system (multicase). Abstracts of the 33rd annual meeting. *Toxicologist* **14** (1).

FISHER, A. A. (1986) *Contact Dermatitis*, 3rd ed. Philadelphia: Lea and Febiger.

FREUND, J. (1951) Effect of paraffin oil and mycobacteria on antibody formation and sensitization: Review. *Am. J. Clin. Pathol.* **21**, 645.

HENDERSON, C. R., and RILEY, E. C. (1945) Certain statistical considerations in patch testing. *J. Invest. Dermatol.* **6**, 227–232.

KLIGMAN, A. M. (1966a) The identification of human allergens by human assay. III. The maximization test. A procedure for screening and rating contact sensitizers. *J. Invest. Dermatol.* **43**, 393-409.

KLIGMAN, A. M. (1966b) The SLS provocative patch test in allergic contact sensitization. *J. Invest. Dermatol.* **46**, 573–585.

■ CHAPTER 39 ■

KLIGMAN, A. M. and Epstein, W. L. (1975) Updating the maximization test for identifying contact allergens. *Contact Dermatitis* **1**, 231 –239.

MARKS, J. C. and DeLED, V. A. (1992) *Patch Testing for Contact and Occupational Dermatology.* St. Louis, MO: Mosby.

MAIBACH, H. (1987) *Occupational and Industrial Dermatology.* 2nd ed. Chicago: Year Book Medical.

MARZULLI, F. and MAGUIRE, H. (1982) Usefulness and limitations of various guinea-pig test methods in detecting human skin sensitizers—validation of guinea-pig tests for skin hypersensitivity. *Food Chem. Toxicol.* **20**, 67–74.

MARZULLI, F. and MAIBACH, H. (1973) Antimicrobials: Experimental contact sensitization in man. *J. Soc. Cosmet. Chem.* **24**, 399–421.

MARZULLI, F. and MAIBACH, H. (1974) The use of graded concentrations in studying skin sensitizers: Experimental contact sensitization in man. *Food Cosmet. Toxicol.* **12**, 219–227.

MARZULLI, F. and MAIBACH, H. (1980) Contact allergy: Predictive testing of fragrance ingredients in humans by Draize and maximization methods. *Environ. Pathol. Toxicol.* **3**, 235–245.

OPDYKE, D. L. (1974) Monographs on fragrance raw materials. *Food. Cosmet. Toxicol.* **12**, 807–1016.

SHELANSKI, H. A. (1951) Experience with and considerations of the human patch test method. *J. Soc. Cosmet. Chem.* **2**, 324–331.

SHELANSKI, H. A. and SHELANSKI, M.V. (1953) A new technique of human patch tests. *Proc. Sci. Sect. Toilet Goods Assoc.* **19**, 46–49.

SCHWARTZ, L. (1941) Dermatitis from new synthetic resin fabric finishes. *J. Invest. Dermatol.* **4**, 459–470.

SCHWARTZ, L . (1951) The skin testing of new cosmetics. *J. Soc. Cosmet. Chem.* **2**, 321–324.

SCHWARTZ, L. (1960) Twenty-two years experience in the performiance of 200,000 prophetic patch tests. *South. Med. J.* **53**, 478–483.

SCHWARTZ, L. and PECK, S. M. (1944) The patch test in contact dermatitis. *Public Health Rep.* **59**, 546–557.

SPIER, H. W. and SIXT, I. (1955) Untersuchungen uber die Abhangigkeit des Ausfalles der exzem Lappchenpraben von der Hornschichtdicke. *Hautarzt* **6**, 152–159.

STORRS, F., ROSENTHAL, L. E., ADAMS, R. M., *et al.* (1989) Prevalence and relevance of allergic reactions in patients patch-tested in North America—1984 to 1985. *J. Am. Acad. Dermatol.* **20**, 1038–1045.

Immunoadjuvants in Prospective Testing for Contact Allergens

40

HENRY C MAGUIRE, JR

Contents

40.1 Introduction

40.2 Complete Freund's adjuvant

40.3 P. acnes

40.4 Cyclophosphamide

40.5 Local anticancer drugs

40.6 Cytokines

40.7 Miscellany

40.1 INTRODUCTION

In this chapter we deal with predictive tests that are intended to identify the ability of substances to induce allergic contact dermatitis (ACD) in man. Such predictive or prospective testing was initially performed in groups of 100–200 volunteers (Draize *et al.*, 1944; Schwartz, 1960). Conditions were arranged in one or more ways so that the likelihood of sensitization was increased. 1. The concentration of the test substance at induction was increased. 2. The material was repeatedly applied to the sensitization site. 3. The barrier layer was damaged (scraping, stripping or detergent) or rendered more permeable by occlusion or DMSO. 4. Inflammation in the sensitization site was induced by SLS (sodium lauryl sulfate), freezing or scraping (Kligman, 1966a and 1966b; Marzulli and Maibach, 1983, Kligman and Epstein, 1975). Immunoadjuvants were not used. Challenge was by patch test, often under occlusion, where the test material was usually presented at a high non-irritating concentration, not necessarily representing use exposure. All of these maneuvers were designed to increase the sensitizing rate so that reasonable extrapolation could be made to very large groups. Of course, appropriate extrapolation from the harsh sensitization conditions of the prospective tests to the real world of allergen exposure requires experience and much common sense.

Immunological adjuvants are substances that up-regulate the induction of the immune response to an allergen or antigens. In the case of contact allergens, the incidence and/or intensity of the delayed type hypersensitivity (DTH) skin sensitization is increased. With prospective testing of materials for their ability to induce ACD we deal with adjuvants that heighten the T cell response. There is a substantial argument about whether the specific effector T-cell of ACD is of the CD4 or CD8 phenotype. The dominant opinion now is that the specific cell is a CD8+ T cell, two decades ago the CD4+ T cells were considered the key specific T cell. It is likely that the specific effector T-cell can be either (or both), perhaps depending on the allergen or mode of sensitization. (Cher and Mosmann, 1987; Wang *et al.*, 2001; Akiba *et al.*, 2002)

The prospective testing of substances for their allergenicity in experimental animals can be done without the use of immunoadjuvants. For instance, the guinea pig non-adjuvant testing methods such as those of Draize (a modification of Landsteiner's technique) or of Buehler rely on multiple injections or applications (with occlusion) of the test material to the sensitization site to enhance the acquisition of DTH to the allergen (Landsteiner and Jacobs, 1935; Draize *et al.*, 1944; Draize, 1959; Buehler 1965; Buehler and Griffith, 1975).

CHAPTER 40

These non-adjuvant testing methods are excellent for the identification of strong, moderate and sometimes of weak sensitizers; however, very weak sensitizers are likely to be missed (Magnusson and Kligman, 1969, 1970; Klecak, 1983; Marzulli and Maguire, 1982). For the purpose of non-specifically magnifying the allergenicity of test materials so as to render very weak allergens sensitizing in at least some test animals, immunoadjuvants are required. It is our intention to discuss immunoadjuvants that have been or might be used to enhance the acquisition of allergic contact dermatitis and photoallergic contact dermatitis in laboratory animals for prospective testing.

A number of immunoadjuvants that increase the acquisition of ACD or delayed type hypersensitivity reactions in experimental animals are given in Table 40.1. It is remarkable that the mechanisms of immunoadjuvant activity of all of these substances are poorly understood, even in the case of the widely used complete Freund's adjuvant. Much immunoadjuvant research is trial and error, and the justification for the specifics of particular laboratory protocols is largely based on empirical findings.

TABLE 40.1:

Immunoadjuvants for prospective testing

Complete Freund's adjuvant
Propionibacterium acnes (C. parvum)
Cyclophosphamide
Local cancer chemotherapeutic drugs
Recombinant cytokines
Miscellany

Immunoadjuvants can enhance either the B-cell or the T-cell response or both responses. Immunoadjuvants such as alum and incomplete Freund's adjuvant (paraffin oil plus emulsifier), which are primarily B-cell stimulants, are not of practical value for upregulating ACD; these adjuvants are not discussed here.

The guinea pig is the classical experimental animal for DTH to contact allergens and for prospective testing of possible sensitizers. The mouse model of Kimber et al., which is gaining currency, in its present form does not use immunoadjuvants (Chapter 41 this volume). Other possible experimental animals such as the rat and rabbit are not used for prospective testing of possible contact allergens. Viable Bacillus Calmette-Guerin (BCG) injected into the sensitization site has been reported to increase the acquisition of allergic contact dermatitis to dinitrochlorobenzene in patients with advanced cancer (Berd *et al.*, 1982). However, it is unlikely, for ethical and regulatory reasons, that BCG or other injectable immunoadjuvants will be used for prospective testing in man. Therefore, our discussion here of immunoadjuvants for prospective testing of contact allergens is necessarily focused on the guinea pig.

There are two underlying, substantially proven, assumptions of prospective testing of materials for their allergenicity in the guinea pig. 1. that the allergenicity scores of test materials in the guinea pig and in man are the same (strong and weak sensitizers of the guinea pig, in parallel, are strong and weak sensitizers of man) and 2. that the rank order of sensitization rates is not changed by the use of immunoadjuvants, i.e., there is roughly equal magnification by immunoadjuvants of the immune response to different contact allergens.

40.2   COMPLETE FREUND'S ADJUVANT

Incomplete Freund's adjuvant is paraffin oil with the addition, usually, of a water-in-oil emulsifier. Complete Freund's adjuvant (CFA) is incomplete Freund's adjuvant plus heat-killed tubercle bacilli. CFA very strongly and consistently increases T-cell responses. It derives from the observation in the guinea pig more than sixty years ago that the injection of viable tubercle bacilli into the skin rendered that skin much more efficient for the induction of delayed-type hypersensitivity (DTH) to proteins that were later injected into the same site (Dienes and Schoenheit, 1926; Dienes and Mallory, 1932). Later, it was found that DTH to tuberculin and to other proteins could very efficiently be induced utilizing killed tubercle bacilli in paraffin oil; unsaturated oils were unsatisfactory vehicles (Couland, 1935; Saenz, 1939; Freund and McDermott, 1942). The finding that haptenized (picrylated) spleen cells emulsified in Freund's complete adjuvant induced very strong ACD to picryl chloride (Landsteiner and Chase, 1941; Chase, 1954) extended the applicability of complete Freund's adjuvant to contact allergens. Later it was discovered that sensitization to contact allergens could be intensified by the intradermal injection of Freund's complete adjuvant and the application of the sensitizer to the injected skin site. This finding allowed complete Freund's adjuvant to be used as an immunopotentiator for essentially all possible contact allergens and photocontact allergens and it is an important element in the construction of the Magnusson-Kligman guinea pig maximization test (Magnusson and Kligman, 1970). Immunopotentiation by separate administration of allergen and adjuvant requires that the sites of CFA and of contact allergen drain into

CHAPTER 40

the same regional lymph nodes; for an immunoadjuvant effect, contact in the skin of CFA and allergen is not necessary (Maguire 1972, 1974).

Complete Freund's adjuvant is currently used in a number of prospective tests in the guinea pig (Klecak, Chapter 38 this volume). An important consideration is that CFA does not perturb the relative ranking of the contact allergens (Magnusson and Kligman, 1970; Marzulli and Maguire, 1982); weak allergens (remain relatively weak vis-à-vis strong allergens, as assessed by the incidence and intensity of the challenge reactions). CFA techniques in the various prospective tests that use them are easily learned and performed, a major advantage. Drawbacks of CFA are its induction of chronic cutaneous ulcers at CFA injection sites and the production of migratory granulomas and of "adjuvant arthritis" (Chase, 1959; Pearson, 1959). These side effects are the major reasons why CFA is not used in humans.

40.3 P. ACNES

Killed Propionibacterium acnes (P. acnes or C. parvum) in a saline vehicle was at one time widely used in the immunotherapy of human tumors and of tumors in experimental animals (Woodruff, 1980). It has been shown to regularly heighten the acquisition of DTH to contact allergens in mice, rats and guinea pigs, as well as to facilitate the induction of photoallergy (Maguire, 1981; Maguire and Cipriano, 1983; Maguire and Kaidbey, 1982). In mice, 30 µg of heat-killed P. acnes in saline is injected intradermally into the skin and the contact allergen is pipetted onto that site. As with CFA, the contact allergen and P. acnes do not have to come into contact with one another in the skin, nor do they have to be administered at the same time; however, an absolute requirement is that they share common draining lymph nodes. A substantial advantage of P. acnes is its relative lack of toxicity in the doses needed for immunopotentiation. Its potential as an immunoadjuvant for prospective testing in experimental animals of allergens and photoallergens has not been explored yet. Preparations of killed P. acnes (or one or more fractions of the bacterium) could well be a substitute for complete Freund's adjuvant.

In recent studies we have found that heat-killed P. acnes is also a very effective immunoadjuvant for the induction of delayed type hypersensitivity by plasmids that express proteins (to be published). In model pre-clinical and clinical studies, vaccines using recombinant plasmids that express different proteins have been found to be safe and are likely to be effective (Lowrie and Whalen, 2000).

40.4 CYCLOPHOSPHAMIDE

Cyclophosphamide is a substantial immunosuppressant, as are most of the cancer chemotherapeutic drugs. However, it was observed by Maguire and Ettore in 1967 and confirmed by Hunziger (1968) that treatment of guinea pigs with cyclophosphamide prior to application of sensitizer resulted in a marked increase in the intensity of the acquired ACD as well as a prolongation of the challenge reactions. Numerous laboratories have confirmed this observation and extended it to other species including chickens, rats, mice, hamsters and humans, and to DTH to protein antigens (Katz *et al.*, 1974; Maguire *et al.*, 1976, 1979; Maguire, 1980; Jaffee and Maguire, 1981; Berd *et al.*, 1982). The mechanism of immuno-potentiation with cyclophosphamide pretreatment seems to rely on the selective inhibition of a precursor population of cells with specific suppressor activity, although the exact way in which this is accomplished remains to be defined. While particular experiments have suggested that cyclophosphamide (Cy) pretreatment would be useful in prospective testing, at least one large-scale study comparing guinea pig tests utilizing CFA with and without cyclophospha-mide pretreatment concluded that Cy pretreatment was not an advantage (Marzulli and Maguire, 1982). Whether Cy would be a benefit in other protocols, such as the lymph node assay of Kimber in mice remains to be examined.

Melphalan is another cancer chemotherapeutic drug with immunosup-pressive and immunoadjuvant properties similar to cyclophosphamide. As taught us by Mocyr and co-workers in a long series of papers, immunologically these cancer chemotherapeutic drugs have similar immunomodulatory properties (Dray and Mocyr, 1989).

40.5 LOCAL ANTICANCER DRUGS

Some years ago, Scheper and co-workers made the startling finding that local cancer chemotherapeutic drugs injected into the sensitization site could upregulate the acquisition of contact sensitivity (Boerrigter and Scheper, 1984). The phenomenon, originally described in guinea pigs, also was demonstrated by that group in mice. Not all cancer chemotherapeutic drugs work equally well; some do not work at all (Limpens *et al.*, 1990). The timing of drug in relation to allergen differs from that of immunopotentiation with systemic cyclophosphamide in that the local drug is typically given after the allergen. The phenomenon can be seen with complete antigens as well as with contact allergens (haptens); however, it is sensitive to dose of drug: very high doses can be inhibitory and very low doses are ineffective. An important issue is whether a general protocol can be worked out, particularly with respect to dose and time of drug that would be applicable to all potential contact allergens. An evaluation of local anticancer drugs as immunoadjuvants for prospective testing remains to be done. A large data base would be required.

40.6 CYTOKINES

Studies of the regulation of the immune response have identified an array of interleukins (numbering 27 at this writing) as well as other cytokines (chemokines) that modulate the activity of T cells and B cells. The genes for many of the cytokines have been cloned and the recombinant protein products are available for mice and humans. Indeed, future protocols of immunopotentiation for the purpose of prospective testing of substances for their allergenicity and photoallergenicity are likely to include one or more of these recombinant molecules. It is important to remember that nearly all of the cytokines structurally have species specificity. For many, the structural specificity is reflected in specificity of function e.g. human GM-CSF and human IL-12 are inactive in the mouse or guinea pig. Inhibitory interleukins such as interleukin 4 (IL-4) and interleukin 10 (IL-10), which suppress contact allergy, clearly are not of interest as immunopotentiators for ACD (Enk *et al.*, 1994). However, a number of cytokines have been demonstrated to heighten the acquisition of DTH; we discuss two here.

40.6.1 Gamma-interferon

Gamma-interferon (IFN-gamma) is a homodimeric molecule consisting of two 18-kD polypeptides; it is variably glycosylated but its biological activity does not require glycosylation. Activated T cells are the predominant source of IFN-gamma. IFN-gamma has many different activities on cells, all of which appear to be mediated by specific gamma-interferon receptors; these receptors are different from the receptors of the alpha- and beta-(type I) interferons. Gamma-interferon activates macrophages as well as certain other cell types, especially natural killer (NK) cells, and it induces the expression of tumor necrosis factor (TNF) alpha as well as certain other cytokines. TNF-alpha is required for the expression of ACD; well-sensitized mice treated with antibody to TNF-alpha at the time of ACD challenge fail to show positive allergic contact reactions (Bromberg *et al.*, 1992).

Gamma-interferon favors the generation of TH-1 cells (the T cells that mediate delayed type hypersensitivity) and suppresses the development of and cytokine secretion by TH-2 cells. TH-2 cells and their products (especially IL-4 and IL-10) are generally suppressive of TH-1 cells. Further, a prominent effect of IFN-gamma is to induce a marked increase in expression of class II major histocompatibility complex molecules (which present antigen for delayed type hypersensitivity reactions) on the cell surface of antigen presenting cells (Skoskiewicz *et al.*, 1985).

Playfair and his group have conducted important studies of mouse IFN-gamma as an immunological adjuvant using as antigen the malarial parasite Palasmodium yoellii (Playfair and DeSouza, 1987; Heath *et al.*, 1989). They found that IFN-gamma was an effective immunoadjuvant when given with the antigen, particularly as relates to cell-mediated responses and the capacity to heighten the activity of a vaccine based on killed parasites.

Our laboratory has studied the immunopotentiation of ACD in the mouse utilizing recombinant murine gamma-interferon (Maguire *et al.*, 1987, 1989). Gamma-interferon injected into the sensitization site heightens the acquisition of DTH to the contact allergens DNFB (1-fluoro-2,4-dinitrobenzene) and oxazolone (4-ethoxymethylene-2-phenyl-oxazolone). In a typical experiment, groups of BALB/c mice were injected intradermally with murine recombinant gamma-interferon or with vehicle, and were sensitized by the application of oxazolone to the skin site. They were ear challenged 6 days later; measurements of ear thickness were taken at baseline and at 24 hours and 48 hours. (This is a standard way to assess DTH to contact allergens in mice and other rodents (Asherson and Ptak, 1968). The results are shown in Figure 40.1. Clearly, IFN-gamma substantially increased the induced sensitivity.

Immunopotentiation of ACD by IFN-gamma was also demonstrated in the experiments with the contact allergen oxazolone. Further, we found that a significant immunoadjuvant effect could be realized when IFN-gamma was given as late as 2 days after the administration of allergen. This latter finding suggests that immunopotentiation with IFN-gamma is not simply the result of the increased expression of class II major histocompatability surface antigens on the antigen-presenting cells but other mechanisms such as stimulation by IFN-gamma of the clonalization of antigen-selected T cells in the regional lymph nodes and/or TH-1 polarization of the immune response, might be involved.

Immunopotentiation of DTH to contact allergens in the mouse with IFN-gamma appears to be a local rather than systemic event. Thus, if the sites of

■ CHAPTER 40 ■

GROUP	DAY 0	DAY 7	DAY 8
(6) I	Gamma-IFN, Oxaz.	Oxaz. Ear Challenge	10.2
(6) II	Vehicle Oxaz.	DITTO	6.5
(6) III	——	DITTO	1.5

Figure 40.1: Mice were injected intradermally in a clipped site on the right rear flank with 0.1 ml of 1 percent normal mouse serum in saline containing 500u murine recombinant IFN-gamma (Group I) or with vehicle (Group II). Immediately following the intradermal injections mice of both groups were sensitized by the application of 20 µl of 5 percent oxazolone in acetone: corn oil (9:1). Seven days later, mice of both groups, as well as mice of a toxicity control group (Group III), were tested on the right ear with 7 µl of 0.1 percent oxazolone after baseline ear thickness measurements. Ear thicknesses were again measured at 24 hours. The average increases in ear thicknesses (mm $\times$ 10^{-2}) of each group of mice are shown. Group 1>2,3, p<.01.

administration of allergen and of IFN-gamma are distant, the immunopotentiation by IFN-gamma is lost. As far as we are aware, comparable experiments focused on the immunoadjuvant effect of local IFN-gamma have not been done in humans; however, their feasibility (and the possible utility of IFN-gamma in vaccines) is suggested by the lack of toxicity of intradermal recombinant gamma-interferon when given to patients (Kaplan et al., 1989).

40.6.2 Interleukin-12

Interleukin 12 (IL-12) is a heterodimeric molecule consisting of 35-kD and 40-kD chains. It is secreted by macrophages and dendritic cells, and was initially identified as a factor that stimulated NK cells and, as a separate observation, cytotoxic T cells (Kobayashi et al., 1989; Stern et al., 1992; Trinchieri, 1994). The human and the murine cDNAs have been cloned, sequenced, and expressed. IL-12, like gamma-IFN, is relatively species specific. In vitro studies indicate that it directs the induction of a TH-1 response and that some of its activities are inhibited by interleukin-10 (D'Andrea et al., 1993). In vivo studies have shown that treatment of mice with intraperitoneal IL-12 inhibits the growth of several syngeneic tumors. The peritumoral administration of IL-12 to a transplanted renal-cell carcinoma (RENCA) in syngeneic mice led to tumor inhibition and regression (Brunda et al., 1993). This inhibition of growth by IL-12 has been shown with a number of other transplantable tumors.

We have studied murine recombinant interleukin-12 as an immunoadjuvant for ACD in the mouse (Maguire, 1995). We have observed that the administration of IL-12 (as opposed to saline) immediately before contact sensitization markedly heightened the induced allergic contact dermatitis as measured by an increase in ear thickness. In a typical experiment, one group of five Balb/c albino female mice were injected intraperitoneally with 1.6 ug murine recombinant interleukin-12. A second group were given vehicle (saline) intraperitoneally. Both groups of mice were contact sensitized by the application of 10 μl 1 percent DNFB to a clipped area on the rear flank. Fourteen days later both groups were ear challenged with 0.1 percent of DNFB and measurements were taken of ear thickness at baseline, at 24 hours and at 48 hours (Figure 40.2).

IL-12 administration does not up-regulate the expression of DTH when given at the time of challenge. As opposed to IFN-gamma, administration of IL-12 at a distant site, as well as locally, enhances the acquisition of contact allergy to DNFB and to oxazolone. Intraperitoneal IL-12 in well-tolerated doses is a consistently effective Th-1 immunoadjuvant. This gives a considerable advantage to IL-12 over interferon-gamma, since immunopotentiation with systemic gamma interferon fails. Cyclophosphamide pretreatment and IL-12 intraperitoneally synergistically immunopotentiate the acquisition of ACD. The field of IL-12 immunobiology is still evolving, and further interesting findings can be expected that will provide the basis for including IL-12 in prospective testing protocols.

Other cytokines that are potential candidates for immunopotentiation in prospective testing include interleukin-1 (IL-1), granulocyte macrophage colony-stimulating factor (GM-CSF), and interleukin-2 (IL-2). In particular contexts these molecules have been shown to increase the induction of specific T-cell immunity.

GROUP	DAY 0	DAY 0	DAY 14	DAY 15	DAY 16
(5) I	IL-12 IP	DNFB 1%	DNFB 0.1%	5.6	8.7
(6) II	Saline IP	Rear Flank	Ear Test	2.2	2.8

Figure 40.2: Mice were injected intraperitoneally with 1.6 μg of murine recombinant interleukin-12 on Day 0. Immediately following the interleukin-12, these mice (group 1) and a control group of mice (group 2) were sensitized by the application of 10 μl of 1 percent DNFB in an acetone: olive oil (9:1) vehicle. Fourteen days later, mice of both groups, were tested on the ear with 0.1 percent DNFB after baseline thickness measurements were made. Ear thicknesses were measured again at 24 hours and at 48 hours. The average increase in ear thickness (mm.X10(-2)) of each group of mice is shown: Group 1>2 p<.01.

■ CHAPTER 40 ■

To my knowledge, they have not been examined as possible immunoadjuvants in the prospective testing of materials for contact allergenicity.

40.7 MISCELLANY

40.7.1 Anti-interleukin 10 antibody

A key player in the regulation of the immune response by cytokines is interleukin 10 (Il-10). It down-regulates both immune and non-immune inflammatory reactions. Thus, the primary irritant reaction to croton oil and the DNFB challenge reaction, in DNFB sensitized mice, as well as the induction of allergic contact dermatitis to DNFB is reduced when the mice are treated systemically with Il-10 (Ferguson et al., 1994). Contrariwise, monoclonal antibody that specifically neutralizes Il-10 up-regulates both the acquisition and the expression of allergic contact dermatitis (Maguire et al., 1997). As expected, Il-10 knockout mice had increased type 1 (Th-1) reactivity to immunogens (Halak et al., 1999). Anti-Il-10 antibody could be a useful immunoadjuvant for the prospective testing of contact allergens, particularly in mice.

40.7.2 Plasmids expressing cytokines and chemokines

In mice, a number of cytokines expressed by plasmids have been shown to up-regulated the Th-1 response when given with a plasmid expressing the immunogen. These plasmids with immunoadjuvant activity include plasmids expressing IL-12, GM-CSF, gamma-interferon, Il-8 and RANTES (Kim et al., 2000). In general, the endpoints have been the result of *in vitro* studies. We have examined a number of plasmids expressing cytokines for their ability to up-regulate the induction of DTH to contact allergens in the mouse. The basic design of the experiments was as follows: plamid was injected intradermally in a clipped site on the back of the mouse and, one or two days later, the particular sensitizer was applied topically to the same site (Kim et al. 1999) A typical experiment is shown with plasmid expressing murine recombinant Il-12 (pcIl-12) and the contact sensitizer, oxazolone in Figure 40.3. Other cytokines that behaved as immunoadjuvants in similar experiments included pcGM-CSF, and, curiously, pcIl-10. The use of plasmids expressing various cytokines and co-stimulatory molecules is an active area of investigation, particularly as relates to the design of effective human and veterinary vaccines. The technology has not yet been applied to the prospective testing of contact allergens.

GROUP	DAY 0	DAY 1	DAY 13	DAY 14	DAY 15
(5) I	pcIl-12	Oxaz.	Oxaz.	11.2	8.9
(5) II	pcDNA3	Sens.	Ear	6.3	6.4
(5) III	—	—	Chall.	2.0	2.4

Figure 40.3: Up-regulating the induction of ACD with plasmid expressing Il-12. Mice were injected intradermally in a clipped site on the back with pcIl-12 (Group I) or with the plasmid backbone, pcDNA3 (Group II) on Day 0. Next day, 20 µl of 5 percent oxazolone was applied to the sites. Day 13, these mice and mice of a toxicity control group were ear challenged with 10 µl of 0.2 percent oxazolone. The increases in ear thickness at 24 hours and at 48 hours are shown (mm.X10(-2)). (GROUP I>II,III at 24 hours and at 48 hours, p<.05.)

40.7.3 Immunostimulatory DNA

Bacterial DNA expressing particular unmethylated CpG sequences can behave as immunological adjuvants and up-regulate the TH-1 immune response associated with DTH (van Uden and Raz, 2000). The active DNA has been shown to stimulate innate immunity by reaction with a particular toll-like receptor (TLR9). As a result, there is secretion of a number of proinflamatory cytokines that can up-regulate the immune response (Aderem and Ulevitch, 2000; Akira *et al.*, 2001). For example, imiquimod (Aldara®), a compound with immunoadjuvant qualities that is utilized in dermatology for the treatment of viral warts, acts through TLR7 (Hemmi *et al.*, 2002). Materials that activate innate immunity are potentially useful as immunoadjuvants for prospective tests designed to identify contact allergens.

REFERENCES

ADEREM A. and ULEVITCH R.J. (2000) Toll-like receptors in the induction of the innate immune response. *Nature* **406**, 782–787.

AKIBA H., KEHREN J., DUCLUZEAU M.-T., KRASTEVA M., HERAND F., KAISERLAIN D., KANEKO F. and NICOLAS J.-F. (2002) Skin inflammation during contact hypersensitivity is mediated by early recruitment of CD8+ T cytotoxic 1 cells inducing keratinocyte apoptosis. *J. Immunol.* **168**, 3079–3087.

AKIRA S., TAKEDA K. and KAISHO T. (2001) Toll-like receptors: critical proteins linking innate and acquired immunity. *Nature Immunology* **2**, 675–680.

ASHERSON, G.L. and PTAK, W. (1969) Contact and delayed hypersensitivity in the mouse 1. Active sensitization and passive transfer. *Immunology* **15**, 405–416.

CHAPTER 40

BERD, D., MASTRANGELO, M., ENGSTROM, P., PAUL, A. and MAGUIRE, H. (1982) Augmentation of the human immune response by cyclophosphamide. *Cancer Res.* **42**, 4862–4866.

BOERRIGTER, G.H. and SCHEPER, R.J. (1984) Local administration of the cytostatic drug 4-hydroperoxy-cyclophosphamide (4-HPCY) facilitates cell-mediated immune reactions. *Clin. Exp. Immunol.* **58**, 161–166.

BROMBERG, J.S., CHAVIN, K.D. and KUNKEL, S.L. (1992) Anti-tumor necrosis factor antibodies suppress cell-mediated immunity *in vivo. J. Immunol.* **148**, 3412–3417.

BRUNDA, M.J., LINSTRO, L., WARTIER, R.R., WRIGHT, R.B., HUBBARD, B.R., MURPHY, M., WOLF, S.F. and GATELY, M.K. (1993) Anti-tumor and anti-metastatic activity of interleukin 12 against murine tumors. *J. Exp. Med.* **178**, 1223–1230.

BUEHLER, E.V. (1965) Delayed contact hypersensitivity in the guinea pig. *Arch. Dermatol.* **91**, 171–177.

BUEHLER, E.V. and GRIFFITH, F. (1975) Experimental skin sensitization in the guinea pig and man. In MAIBACH, H. (ed.) *Animal Models in Dermatology*, Edinburgh: Churchill Livingstone, 56–66.

CHASE, M.W. (1954) Experimental sensitization with particular reference to picryl chloride. *Int. Arch. Allergy* **5**, 163.

CHASE, M.W. (1959) Disseminated granulomata in the guinea pig. In SHAFFER, J.H., LoGRIPPO, G.A. and CHASE, M.W. (eds) *Mechanisms of Hypersensitivity*, Boston: Little, Brown, 673–678.

CHER, D.J. and MOSMANN, T.R. (1987) Two types of murine helper T cell clone. II. Delayed-type hypersensitivity is mediated by Th-1 clones. *J. Immunol.* **138**, 3688–3694.

COULAND, E. (1935) Caracteres de l'etat allergique observe chez les animaux de laboratoire apres injections de bacilles de Koch enrobes dans la paraffine. *C. R. Soc. Biol.* **119**, 368.

D'ANDREA, A., ASTE-AMEZAGA, M., VATIANTE, N.M., XIAOJING, M., KUBIN, M. and TRINCHIERI, G. (1993) Interleukin 10 (IL-l0) inhibits human lymphocyte interferon gamma production by suppressing natural-killer cell stimulatory factor/IL-l2 synthesis in accessory cells. *J. Exp. Med.* **178**, 1041–1048.

DIENES, L. and MALLORY, T.B. (1932) Histological studies of hypersensitive reaction. Part I. The contrast between the histological responses in the tuberculin (allergic) type and the anaphylactic type of skin reactions. *Am. J. Path.* **8**, 689.

DIENES, L. and SCHOENHEIT, E.W. (1926) Local hypersensitiveness in tuberculous guinea pigs. *Proc. Soc. Exp. Biol. Med.* **24**, 132.

DRAIZE, J.H. (1959) Appraisal of the safety of chemicals in foods, drugs and cosmetics. In *Dermal Toxicity*, Austin, TX: Association of Food and Drug Officials of the United States, Texas State Department of Health, 46.

DRAIZE, J.H., WOODGARD, G. and CALVERY, H.O. (1944) Methods for the study of irritation and toxicity of substances applied topically to the skin and mucous membranes. *J. Pharmacol. Exp. Ther.* **82**, 377–390.

DRAY S. and MOKYR M.B. (1989) Cyclophosphamide and melphalan as immunopotentiating agents in cancer therapy. *Med. Oncology and Tumor Pharmacotherapy* **6**, 77–85.

ENK, A.H., SALOGA, J. BECKER, D., MOHAMADZADEH, M. and KNOP, J. (1994) Induction of hapten-specific tolerance by interleukin-10 *in vivo*. *J. Exp. Med.* **179**, 1397–1402.

FERGUSON T.A., DUBE P. and GRIFFITH T.S. (1994) Regulation of contact hypersensitivity by Il-10. *J. Exp. Med.* **179**, 1597–1604.

FREUND, J. and MCDERMOTT, K. (1942) Sensitization to horse serum by means of adjuvants. *Proc. Soc. Exp. Bio. Med.* **49**, 548.

HALAK, B.K., MAGUIRE, H.C. JR. and LATTIME, E.C. (1999) Tumor-induced interleukin-10 inhibits type 1 immune responses directed at a tumor antigen as well as a non-tumor antigen present at the tumor site. *Cancer Res.* **59**, 911–917.

HEATH, A.W., DEVEY, M.E., BROWN, I.N., RICHARDS, C.E. and PLAYFAIR, H.J.L. (1989) Interferon gamma as an adjuvant in immunocompromised mice. *Immunology* **67**, 520–524.

HEMMI, H., KAISHO, T., TAKEUCHI, O., SATO, S., SANJO, H., HOSHINO, K., HORIUCHI, T., TOMIZAWA, H., TAKEDA, K. and AKIRA, S. (2002) Small antiviral compounds activate immune cells via the TLR7 MYD88-dependent signaling pathways. *Nature Immunology* **3**, 196–200.

HUNZIGER, N. (1968) Effect of cyclophosphamide on the contact eczema in guinea pigs. *Dermatologica.* **136**, 187–191.

JAFFEE, B.D. and MAGUIRE, H.C., JR. (1981) Delayed-type hypersensitivity and immunological tolerance to contact allergens in the rat. *Fed. Proc.* **40**, 4312.

KAPLAN, G., MATHUR, N.K., JOB, C.K., NATHAN, I. and COHN, 2. A. (1989) Effect of multiple interferon injections on the disposal of mycobacterium leprae. *Proc. Nati. Acad. Sci. USA* **86**, 8073–8077.

KATZ, S.I., PARKER, D., SOMMER, G. and TURK J.L. (1974) Suppressor cells in normal immunization as a basic homeostatic phenomenon. *Nature (Land.)* **248**, 612–614.

KIM, J.J., MAGUIRE, H.C. JR., NOTTINGHAM, L.K., MORRISON, L.D., TSAI, A., SIN, J.J., CHALIAN, A.A. and WEINER, D.B. (1998) Coadministration of IL-12 or Il-10 expression cassettes drives immune responses toward a Th-1 phenotype. *J. Interferon, Cytokine Res.* **18**, 537–547.

KIM, J.J. YANG, J.-S., DENTCHEV, T., DANG, K. and WEINER, D.B. (2000) Chemokine gene adjuvants can modulate immune responses induced by DNA vaccines. *J. Interferon and Cytokine Research* **20**, 487–498.

KLECAK, G. (1983) Identification of contact allergens: Predictive tests in animals. In MARZULLI, F.N. and MAIBACH, H.I. (eds.) *Dermatotoxicology*, 2nd ed. Washington, DC: Hemisphere.

KLIGMAN, A.M. (1966a) The identification of contact allergens by human assay, III the maximization test. A procedure for screening and rating contact sensitizers. *J. Invest. Derm.* **47**, 393–409.

KLIGMAN, A.M. (1966b) The SLS-provocative patch test in allergic contact sensitization. *J. Invest. Derm.* **46**, 573–583.

KLIGMAN, A.M. and EPSTEIN, W. (1975) Updating the maximization test for identifying contact allergens. *Contact Dermatitis* **1**, 23 1–239.

KOBAYASHI, M., FITZ, L., RYAN, M., HEWICK, R.M., CLARK, S.C., CHART, S., LOUDON, R., SHERMAN, F., PERUSSIA, B. and TRINCHIERI, G. (1989) Identification and purification of natural killer cell stimulatory factor (NKSF), a cytokine with multiple biological effects on human lymphocytes. *J. Exp. Med.* 170, 827–845.

LANDSTEINER, K. and CHASE, M.W. (1941) Studies in the sensitization of animals with simple chemical compounds. IX. Skin sensitization induced by injection of conjugates. *J. Exp. Med.* **73**, 431–438.

LANDSTEINER, K. and JACOBS, J. (1935) Studies on sensitization of animals with simple chemical compounds. *J. Exp. Med.* **61**, 643–656.

LIMPENS, J., GARSSEN, J., GENNERAAD, W.T.V. and SCHEPER, R.J. (1990) Enhancing effects of locally administered cytostatic drugs on T-effector cell functions in mice. *Int. J. Immunopharmacol.* **12**, 77–88.

LOWRIE, D.R. and WHALEN, R.G. (eds) (2000) *DNA Vaccine*, Totowa, NJ: Humana Press.

MAGNUSSON, B. and KLIGMAN, A.M. (1969) The identification of contact allergens by animal assay. The guinea pig maximization test. *J. Invest. Dermatol.* **52**, 268–276.

MAGNUSSON, B. and KLIGMAN, A.M. (1970) *Allergic Contact Dermatitis in the Guinea Pig. Identification of Contact Allergens*. Springfield, IL: Charles C. Thomas.

MAGUIRE, H.C. Jr. (1996) Cyclophosphamide in interleukin-12 synergistically upregulate the acquisition of allergic contact dermatitis in the mouse. *Acta Derm. Venereol.* **76**, 277–279.

MAGUIRE, H.C., Jr. (1972) Mechanism of intensification by complete Freund's adjuvant of the acquisition of delayed hypersensitivity in the guinea pig. *Immunol. Commun.* **1**, 239–246.

MAGUIRE, H.C., Jr. (1974) Alteration in the acquisition of delayed hypersensitivity in the guinea pig. *Allergy* **8**, 13–26.

MAGUIRE, H.C., Jr. (1980) Allergic contact dermatitis in the hamster. *J. Invest. Dermatol.* **75**, 166–169.

MAGUIRE, H.C., Jr. (1981) Immunopotentiation of allergic contact dermatitis in the guinea pig with C. parvum (P. acnes). *Acta Dermato-Venereal, (Stockh.)* **615**, 65–67.

MAGUIRE, H.C., Jr. (1995) Murine recombinant interleukin-12 increases the acquisition of allergic contact dermatitis in the mouse. *Int. Arch. Allergy Immunol.* **106**, 166–168.

MAGUIRE H.C., JR. and CIPRIANO, D. (1983) Immunopotentiation of cell-mediated hypersensitivity by C. parvum (P. acnes). *Int. Arch. Allergy Appl. Immunol.* **701**, 34–39.

MAGUIRE H.C., JR. and ETTORE, V.L. (1967) Enhancement of Dinitrochlorobenzene (DNCB) contact sensitization of cyclophosphamide in the guinea pig. *J. Invest. Dermatol.* **48**, 39–43.

MAGUIRE, H.C., JR. and KAIDBEY, K. (1982) Experimental photoallergic contact dermatitis: A mouse model. *J. Invest. Dermatol.* **79**, 147–152.

MAGUIRE H.C. JR., KETCHA K.A. and LATTIME, E.C. (1997) Neutralizing anti-Il-10 antibody upregulates the induction and elicitation of contact hypersensitivity. *J. Interferon and Cytokine Res.* **17**, 763–768.

MAGUIRE H.C., JR., RANK, R.G. and WEIDANZ, W.P. (1976) Allergic contact dermatitis to low molecular weight allergens in the chicken. *Int. Arch. Allergy Appl. Immunol.* **50**, 737–744.

MAGUIRE H.C., JR., FARIS, L. and WEIDANZ, W. (1979) Cyclophosphamide intensifies the acquisition of allergic contact dermatitis in mice rendered B-cell deficient by heterologous anti-IgM antisera. *Immunology* **37**, 367–372.

MAGUIRE H.C., JR., GUIDOTTI, M. and WEIDANZ, W. (1987) Immunopotentiation of allergic contact dermatitis (ACD) in the mouse by local injection of gamma interferon. *Clin. Res.* **35**, 8–11 (abstr.).

MAGUIRE, H.C., JR., GUIDOTTI, M.B. and WEIDANZ, W.P. (1989) Local murine recombinant interferon heightens the acquisition of allergic contact dermatitis in the mouse. *Int. Arch. Allergy* **88**, 345–347.

MARZULLI, F. and MAGUIRE, H.C., JR. (1982) Usefulness and limitation of various guinea pig tests for skin hypersensitivity. *Food Cosmet. Toxicol.* **201**, 61–74.

CHAPTER 40

MARZULLI, F.N. and MAIBACH, H.I. (1983) Contact allergy: Predictive testing in humans. In Marzulli, F.N. and Maibach, H.I. (eds) *Dermatotoxicology*, New York: Hemisphere, 279–299.

PEARSON, C.M. (1959) Development of arthritis in the rat following injection with adjuvant. In SHAFFER, J.H., LoGRIPPO, G.A. and CHASE, M.W. (eds) *Mechanisms of Hypersensitivity*, Boston: Little, Brown, 647–671.

PLAYFAIR, J.H.L. and DESOUZA, J.B. (1987) Recombinant gamma interferon is a potent adjuvant for a murine malaria vaccine in mice. *Clin. Exp. Immunol.* **67**, 5–10.

SAENZ, A. (1939) Influence de la desensibilisation sur la dispersion des germes de surinfection chew des cobayes rendus hyperallergiques au moyen de bacilles tuberculeux morts enrobes dan l'huile de Vaseline. *C. R. Soc. Biol.* **130**, 219.

SCHWARTZ, L. (1960) Twenty-two years experience in the performance of 200,000 prosthetic-patch tests, *South. Med. J.* **53**, 478–483.

SKOSKIEWICZ, M.J., COLVIN, R.B., SCHNEEBERGER, E.E. and RUSSELL, P.S. (1985) Widespread and selected induction of major histocompatibility complex-determined antigens *in vivo* by interferon. *J. Exp. Med.* **162**, 1645–1664.

STEM, A.S., PODLASKI, F.J., HULMES, J.D., PAN, Y.-C.E., QUINN, P.M., WOLITZHY, A.G., FAMILLETTI, P.C., STREMLO, D.L., TRUITT, T., CHIZZOHITE, R. and GATELY, M.K. (1990) Purification to homogeneity and partial characterization of cytotoxic lymphocyte maturation factor from human B-lymphoblastoid cells. *Proc. Natl. Acad. Sci.* **87**, 6808–6812.

TRINCHIERI, G. (1994) Interleukin-12 and its role in the generation of Th-1 cells. *Immunol. Today* **14**, 335–337.

VAN UDEN, J.H. and RAZ, E. (2000) Immunostimulatory DNA sequences, in LOWRIE, D.B. and WHALEN, R.G. (eds) *DNA Vaccines*, Totowa, New Jersey: Humana Press, 145–168.

WANG, B., FELICIANI, C., FREED, I., CAI, C. AND SAUDER, D.N. (2001) Insights into molecular mechanisms of contact hypersensitivity gained from gene knockout studies. *J. Leukocyte Biol.* **70**, 185–190.

WOODRUFF, M.F.A. (1980) *The Interaction of Cancer and Host*. New York: Grune and Stratton.

The Local Lymph Node Assay

IAN KIMBER, DAVID A BASKETTER,
G FRANK GERBERICK AND REBECCA J DEARMAN

Contents

41.1 Introduction

41.2 Development of the LLNA

41.3 Evaluation and validation

41.4 Current international regulatory status of the LLNA

41.5 The LLNA and assessment of relative potency

41.6 Integration of LLNA data into risk assessment

41.7 Conclusions

41.1 INTRODUCTION

The acquisition of skin sensitization is dependent upon the initiation of a cell-mediated immune response. The relevant events can be summarized briefly as follows. Sensitization is induced when an individual (an inherently susceptible individual) is exposed topically to a sufficient amount of contact allergen. The chemical allergen either directly or indirectly associates with protein and is recognized and internalized by cutaneous dendritic cells, the most important of which in this context are epidermal Langerhans cells (LC). It is now clear that LC play a number of pivotal roles in the generation of cutaneous immune responses and the induction of skin sensitization; their most important responsibility being the transport of antigen, via the afferent lymphatics, to draining lymph nodes. During this migration from the skin, LC are subject to a functional maturation with the result that by the time of their arrival in lymph nodes they have acquired the characteristics of immunostimulatory antigen presenting cells (Cumberbatch *et al.*, 2000; Kimber *et al.*, 1998a; 2000). In the lymph nodes antigen is presented to responsive T lymphocytes and these cells become activated and are induced to divide and differentiate. Cell division results in a selective clonal expansion of allergen-responsive T lymphocytes; this quantitative increase in specific T lymphocytes being the cellular basis for sensitization and immunological memory. If the now sensitized subject is exposed again to the same chemical, at the same or a different site, then this expanded population of specific T lymphocytes will recognize and respond to allergen in the skin and trigger an accelerated and more aggressive secondary immune response, that in turn causes the cutaneous inflammation that is recognized clinically as allergic contact dermatitis. The molecular and cellular mechanisms that result in the induction and elicitation of contact allergy have been reviewed extensively elsewhere (Grabbe and Schwarz, 1998; Kimber *et al.*, 2002; Kimber and Dearman, 2002). For the purposes of this chapter it is sufficient to say that the ability of chemical allergens to induce the activation of skin draining lymph nodes and to stimulate lymph node cell (LNC) proliferative responses are the events upon which the local lymph node assay (LLNA) is founded.

There are several review articles that consider various aspects of the LLNA (Kimber *et al.*, 1994; Dearman *et al.*, 1999; Gerberick *et al.*, 1999; 2000; Basketter and Kimber, 2001; Basketter *et al.*, 2001a; 2002). The purposes here are to review the development and subsequent evaluation and validation of the LLNA and to examine the use of this method for hazard identification, potency evaluation and risk assessment.

41.2 DEVELOPMENT OF THE LLNA

Based upon an appreciation of the events induced during skin sensitization, the objective was to determine whether a method for hazard identification could be developed in mice that might be used as a viable alternative to the then favored guinea pig assays. In contrast to those guinea pig methods (in which activity is measured as a function of challenge-induced cutaneous reactions in previously sensitized animals), the strategy adopted was to focus on events during the induction phase of skin sensitization, and in particular on changes provoked in lymph nodes draining the site of exposure. Several parameters of lymph node activation could be viewed as legitimate potential correlates of skin sensitization, including increases in lymph node weight and cellularity, the appearance of pyroninophilic cells and the stimulation of LNC turnover (Kimber *et al.*, 1986; Kimber and Weisenberger, 1989). Preliminary investigations revealed, however, that of these the induction of LNC proliferation represented to most sensitive and most selective marker of skin sensitizing activity. In initial studies proliferative activity had been measured *in vitro* during culture of draining LNC with [^{3}H] thymidine (^{3}H-TdR) (Kimber *et al.*, 1986; Kimber and Weisenberger, 1989). One important development, however, was to measure instead lymph node hyperplastic responses *in situ* (Kimber, 1989; Kimber *et al.*, 1989). This adaptation not only provided a more holistic and more sensitive assessment of LNC proliferative activity, it also served to obviate the need for tissue culture. It is this form of the LLNA that has been the subject of extensive evaluations and that was subsequently validated.

The basic protocol for the LLNA has been described in detail elsewhere (Gerberick *et al.*, 1992; Kimber and Basketter, 1992; Hilton and Kimber, 1995; Kimber, 1998), but can be summarized briefly as follows. Mice of CBA strain are used. Groups of mice receive topical applications of various concentrations of the test chemical (or of the relevant vehicle control) daily for three consecutive days. Recommendations regarding suitable test concentrations are available elsewhere (Kimber and Basketter, 1992). For the purposes of hazard identification it may be considered desirable to select the highest recommended test concentrations. In practice, however, this is not always possible. Concerns regarding local or systemic toxicity, and/or poor solubility, may dictate a more conservative approach.

Several vehicles may be used, and again those usually favored are considered elsewhere (Kimber and Basketter, 1992; Basketter and Kimber, 1996; Dearman *et al.*, 1999). Decisions regarding the choice of vehicle (in the context of hazard identification at least) are reached usually on the basis of suitability for topical application and the solubility of the test material. It is relevant to mention here that the vehicle in which a chemical allergen is encountered at skin surfaces can have a significant impact on the extent to which skin sensitization is acquired, and on the vigor of responses in the LLNA (Cumberbatch *et al.*, 1993; Dearman *et al.*, 1996; Heylings *et al.*, 1996; Warbrick *et al.*, 1999a; Basketter *et al.*, 2001b; Wright *et al.*, 2001). There is no doubt that the vehicle matrix also influences the elicitation of responses in other methods for the identification of contact allergens. Although vehicle effects have, in practice, little or no impact on the performance of the LLNA in the context of hazard identification, they are (quite rightly) of more significance when considering LLNA dose responses for the purposes of potency and risk assessment. This issue will be addressed again later.

Five days following the initiation of exposure, mice receive an intravenous injection of ^{3}H-TdR. Animals are sacrificed 5 hours later and draining auricular lymph nodes excised. These are either pooled for each experimental group, or alternatively are pooled on a per animal basis. Single cell suspensions of LNC are prepared and the cells washed and suspended in trichloroacetic acid (TCA) for at least 12 hours at 4°C. Precipitates are suspended in TCA and transferred to an appropriate scintillation fluid. The incorporation by draining LNC of ^{3}H-TdR is measured by scintillation counting and recorded as mean disintegrations per minute (dpm) for each experimental group, or for each animal. In those instances where it is deemed appropriate to include within the test protocol a positive control it is recommended that hexyl cinnamic aldehyde (HCA) is used for this purpose (Dearman *et al.*, 1998; 2001).

For each concentration of test material a stimulation index (SI) is calculated using as the comparator the value derived from the concurrent vehicle control. Skin sensitizers are defined as those chemicals, that at one or more test concentrations, are able to induce an SI of 3 or greater. It is important to recognize that the original decision to use an SI value of 3 as the criterion for a positive response in the LLNA was arbitrary; the choice being made on the basis of experience with a range of chemical allergens and non-sensitizing chemicals. However, it would appear that the decision was correct, since continued experience has revealed that in practice an SI of 3 appears to provide an accurate identification of skin sensitizing chemicals. Moreover, a retrospective analysis of results obtained with some 134 chemicals in the LLNA was reported in 1999 (Basketter *et al.*, 1999a). The data were subjected to a rigorous mathematical assessment using Receiver Operator Characteristic (ROC) curves. The conclusion drawn from these analyses was that an SI value of 3 provides an appropriate criterion for the identification of contact allergens (Basketter *et al.*, 1999a). Despite the proven value of an SI of 3 for hazard identification, some flexibility is appropriate when interpreting LLNA data. It has been recommended previously (Kimber and Basketter, 1992) that the characteristics of dose-response relationships and other factors should be taken into account. Thus for instance, if a test chemical were to display a dose-related increase in LNC proliferative activity that just failed at the highest concentration to achieve an SI of 3 then it would probably be inappropriate to conclude that the material lacked any potential to cause skin sensitization. In such cases it would be prudent to conduct a repeat analysis using, if possible, higher concentrations of the test chemical and/or a different vehicle.

A summary of the conduct of the standard LLNA is illustrated in Figure 41.1.

Before leaving the conduct of the LLNA and considering its performance, it is appropriate to acknowledge that some other investigators have proposed modifications to the basic protocol. Such vary in their scope and complexity. Some suggested changes are relatively modest, such as for instance the use of an alternative isotope, or non-isotopic methods, for measurement of LNC proliferation (Ladics *et al.*, 1995; Takeyoshi *et al.*, 2001), or the consideration of the use of mouse strains other than CBA (Woolhiser *et al.*, 2000). However, other proposals call for much more substantial changes to the standard protocol (Ikarashi *et al.*, 1993; 1994; 1996; Homey *et al.*, 1998; Ulrich *et al.*, 1998; van Och *et al.*, 2000; De Jong *et al.*, 2002; 2001). Such modifications of the standard method in mice have not been evaluated thoroughly, or validated formally, and will not be considered here. Neither do we consider here the merits or otherwise of conduct of the LLNA in species other than the mouse (Maurer and Kimber, 1991; Ikarashi *et al.*, 1992; Arts *et al.*, 1996: Clottens *et al.*, 1996; Kashima *et al.*, 1996).

41.3 EVALUATION AND VALIDATION

The LLNA was developed initially as a method for hazard identification. Although it is now clear that the LLNA is also of considerable utility in determination of relative potency and in the risk assessment process, it is for the purposes of hazard identification that the assay has been formally validated. That process of evaluation and validation is described here. Use of the LLNA for potency and risk assessment is considered later.

The LLNA has been evaluated extensively in both national and international inter-laboratory collaborative trials (Basketter *et al.*, 1991; 1996; Kimber *et al.*,

TEST MATERIAL / VEHICLE

DAYS 0,1,2

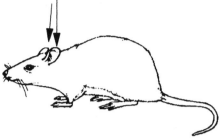

Three consecutive daily 25 μl applications of
various concentrations of the test material to the
dorsum of both ears. Control mice receive identical
treatment with the same volume of vehicle alone.

DAY 5

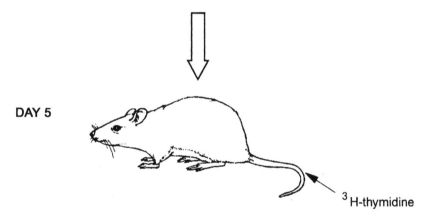

^{3}H-thymidine

All mice (test and control) are injected
intravenously via the tail vein with 20 μCi of
^{3}H-thymidine in 250 μl of phosphate buffered saline

5 HOURS

Draining auricular lymph nodes are excised and
pooled for each experimental group and processed
for β-scintillation counting

Figure 41.1: Conduct of the standard local lymph node assay.

1991; 1995; 1998b; Kimber and Basketter, 1992; Scholes *et al.*, 1992; Loveless *et al.*, 1996), and has been the subject of searching comparisons with guinea pig predictive test methods and human sensitization data (Kimber *et al.*, 1990a; 1994; Basketter and Scholes, 1992; Basketter *et al.*, 1991; 1992; 1993; 1994; Ryan *et al.*, 2000). Collectively, these investigations comprised analyses of a wide variety of chemicals. In addition, however, more discrete investigations of specific groups of materials have been conducted using either the standard LLNA, or modifications of it. Among these are studies of biocides (Botham *et al.*, 1991; Hilton *et al.*, 1998; Basketter *et al.*, 1999b; Warbrick *et al.*, 1999a), fragrance materials and materials used in personal care products (Hilton *et al.*, 1996; Wright *et al.*, 2001), metal salts (Basketter *et al.*, 1999c), rubber chemicals (De Jong *et al.*, 2002), petrochemicals (Edwards *et al.*, 1994), dyes (Sailstad *et al.*, 1994) and chemical mutagens and rodent carcinogens (Ashby *et al.*, 1993; Warbrick *et al.*, 2001). On the basis of these investigations and additional practical experience gained from the use of the method, the conclusion drawn was that the LLNA represented a viable alternative to guinea pig tests for the identification of contact allergens (Basketter *et al.*, 1996; Chamberlain and Basketter, 1996; Gerberick *et al.*, 2000).

Against this background the LLNA was submitted in 1998 for consideration by the Interagency Coordinating Committee on the Validation of Alternative Methods (ICCVAM), an organization established in the USA by 14 Federal regulatory and research agencies to harmonize the development, validation and acceptance of new toxicological test methods (NIH, 1999). A peer review panel was appointed by ICCVAM and after intensive scrutiny of the method it concluded that, compared with other predictive tests, the LLNA offers advantages with respect to animal welfare (specifically in terms of refinement and reduction). The panel also recommended that the LLNA could be used as a stand-alone alternative for the purposes of hazard identification, subject to the implementation of certain protocol modifications. These proposed modifications included considerations of selection of mouse strain, the individual identification of mice, analysis of body weight changes, the use of statistical analyses and the incorporation of a concurrent positive control (NIH, 1999; Dean *et al.*, 2001; Haneke *et al.*, 2001; Sailstad *et al.*, 2001). The utility and application of these modifications have been the subject recently of a detailed commentary (Basketter *et al.*, 2002), and a similar analysis here would be beyond the scope of this chapter. The important point is, however, that the LLNA was subjected to rigorous independent scrutiny and validated by ICCVAM as an appropriate method for hazard identification. There soon followed a similar endorsement by the European Centre for the Validation of Alternative Methods (ECVAM) (Balls and Hellsten, 2000). In the light of these developments the current regulatory status of the LLNA is outlined briefly in the next section.

Although the LLNA has been shown in the context of the validation exercises summarized above to have levels of sensitivity, selectivity and overall accuracy comparable with, or better than, the commonly used guinea pig tests, questions are nevertheless raised about specific issues relating to test performance. Among these are the ability of the assay to detect metal allergens (and in particular nickel), and the prevalence of false positive responses.

Nickel is a common human allergen. Although modest responses to nickel chloride and nickel sulfate can be elicited in mice (Kimber *et al.*, 1990b; Gerberick *et al.*, 1992), the consensus is that nickel salts usually fail to test positive in the LLNA (Kimber *et al.*, 1994). However, it has also often proven difficult to elicit responses to nickel salts in guinea pig tests (Buehler, 1965; Goodwin *et al.*, 1981). The likelihood is that nickel is probably only a very weak allergen and that the high prevalence of sensitization in some societies is due to the ubiquitous distribution of this substance and the extensive opportunities for exposure. The ability of the LLNA to detect metal salts that are known to be implicated in allergic contact dermatitis has now been examined systematically. Thirteen metal salts were studied, of which eight were considered to be contact allergens. The remaining five were considered not to cause skin sensitization. With the exception of nickel chloride, all known allergens (tin chloride, cobalt chloride, mercuric chloride, ammonium tetrachloroplatinate, potassium dichromate, beryllium sulfate, and gold chloride) were found to elicit positive responses in the LLNA (Basketter *et al.*, 1999c). Of the five non-sensitizers, four (zinc sulfate, lead acetate, manganese chloride, and aluminum chloride) failed to induce positive LLNA responses, and only one (copper chloride) tested positive (Basketter *et al.*, 1999c). Taken together, these data indicate that, in the majority of instances, the LLNA provides an accurate assessment of the likely skin sensitizing potential of metal salts. The argument is, however, rather academic given new metal allergens are very unlikely to be discovered.

The other issue is the possibility of false positive results. One apparent anomaly in the performance of the LLNA is the fact that sodium lauryl sulfate, a non-sensitizing skin irritant, has been shown by some investigators to elicit positive, albeit weak, responses (Basketter *et al.*, 1994; Kimber *et al.*, 1994; Montelius *et al.*, 1994; Loveless *et al.*, 1996). It is possible that SLS may represent something of a special case, insofar as it is known that this chemical is able to cause the migration of epidermal LC to the skin draining lymph nodes

■ CHAPTER 41 ■

(Cumberbatch *et al.*, 1993), although the relevance of this for the initiation of LNC proliferative activity is not clear. Even if certain skin irritants are able in some instances to provoke comparatively low level activity in draining lymph nodes, this does not necessarily compromise the correct interpretation of test data, or prevent the accurate identification of chemicals that have the potential to cause skin sensitization (Basketter *et al.*, 1998). Moreover, it is important to appreciate that the majority of non-sensitizing skin irritants fail to elicit positive responses in the LLNA (Kimber *et al.*, 1991; Gerberick *et al.*, 1992; 1995; Basketter *et al.*, 1998).

41.4 CURRENT INTERNATIONAL REGULATORY STATUS OF THE LLNA

The adoption of a new test method into regulatory guidelines represents a substantial challenge, demanding a general scientific consensus on its suitability, as well as acceptance via the formal processes prescribed for validation. As described above, this latter step was undertaken for the LLNA via ICCVAM. The report of this independent review has been published (NIH, 1999). ICCVAM concluded that the method was fully valid as a standalone alternative to, or replacement for, existing guinea pig tests. As a result, the LLNA was adopted by several federal regulatory agencies in the USA as an accepted method for skin sensitization testing. In addition, the LLNA has been incorporated into a new Test Guideline (No. 429) by the Organization for Economic Cooperation and Development (OECD) and it was expected that this would be published late in 2002. In parallel, the European Union (EU) has prepared a new test method on the LLNA (B42); the text closely following that prepared by the OECD. The LLNA has been approved at the technical level and is also expected to appear in the Official Journal of the European Union later in 2002. Anticipating these changes, at least one Competent Authority in the EU (the UK Health and Safety Executive) has formally changed its policy, confirming that the LLNA is now its test method of choice for the identification of chemicals possessing skin sensitization hazard.

41.5 THE LLNA AND ASSESSMENT OF RELATIVE POTENCY

Although accurate identification of hazard is a required first step in any toxicological evaluation, it does not of itself necessarily inform the risk assessment process. What is really needed, in concert with an appreciation of likely conditions of exposure, is information regarding toxicological potency. With respect to the induction of skin sensitization, potency should be defined as a function of the amount of chemical that is necessary to induce sensitization in a previously naïve subject. In fact, the most compelling illustration of this in humans derives from volunteer studies conducted by Friedmann and colleagues. They were able to demonstrate that, in most circumstances at least, the acquisition of skin sensitization is critically dependent upon the amount of chemical experienced per unit area of skin (Friedmann, 1990). Recently, a major focus of attention has been on defining how the LLNA can be used to assess experimentally the relative sensitizing potency of contact allergens (Kimber and Basketter, 1997; Basketter *et al.*, 2001a; Kimber *et al.*, 2001)

The induction by chemical allergens of proliferative responses in draining lymph nodes provides not only a marker of skin sensitizing activity, but also a quantitative correlate of the extent of sensitization (Kimber *et al.*, 1999; Kimber and Dearman, 1991). It is reasonable, therefore, to speculate that it should be possible to determine the relative potency of chemicals on the basis of the vigor of responses induced in the LLNA. For this purpose an EC3 value is derived from dose-related activity in the LLNA; an EC3 value being defined as the amount of chemical (absolute amount of chemical or chemical per unit area, or percentage or molar concentration) that is required to induce in the assay a response of the magnitude that in practice defines skin sensitizing potential (an SI of 3).

Careful thought was given to the most suitable method for deriving EC3 values from LLNA dose-responses. Investigations were conducted in which three possible approaches were compared: quadratic regression analysis, Richard's model and simple linear interpolation. The conclusion drawn was that linear interpolation between values either side of the threefold SI on an LLNA dose-response curve provides the most robust and most convenient method for calculation of EC3 values (Basketter *et al.*, 1999d). This approach can be expressed mathematically as:

$$EC3 = c + [(3 - d)/(b\text{-}d)] \times (a - c)$$

where (a,b) and (c,d) are the coordinates, respectively, of data points lying immediately above and immediately below the SI value of 3.

It could be argued that there are available more sophisticated approaches for interrogation of dose-response relationships and that the application of these might provide for greater accuracy. Although it might appear scientifically

■ CHAPTER 41 ■

heretical to reject such methods in favor of the much more straightforward approach of linear extrapolation, as will become apparent, it is neither necessary nor helpful for classification purposes to measure with great accuracy small, and probably biologically insignificant, differences between chemical allergens in terms of EC3 values.

Experience to date reveals that EC3 values are very robust parameters of LLNA responses, both with time within a single laboratory, and also between laboratories. Thus, for instance, it was found in studies of HCA conducted by a single laboratory over a 10 month period that EC3 values were very consistent, ranging from 6.9 percent to 9.6 percent (Dearman *et al.*, 1998). Similar consistency was found when EC3 values for *p*-phenylenediamine (PPD) were measured each month over a 4 month period (Warbrick *et al.*, 1999b). The results of inter-laboratory collaborative trials of the LLNA demonstrated that very similar EC3 values were derived when the same chemical was analyzed in several independent laboratories (Kimber *et al.*, 1995; 1998b; Loveless *et al.*, 1996; Warbrick *et al.*, 1999b).

In practice, EC3 values have been used successfully to determine the relative skin sensitizing potency of several series of chemicals, including isothiazolinone biocides (Basketter *et al.*, 1999b), dinitrohalobenzenes (Basketter *et al.*, 1997) and various aldehydes (Basketter *et al.*, 2001c).

The real test of the utility of relative potency measurements based on EC3 values is the extent to which they are congruent with what is known of the activity of sensitizing chemicals among human populations. To address this issue analyses were undertaken in partnership with clinical dermatologists who provided a view of the relative skin sensitizing potency of two series of known human contact allergens. Chemicals were classified according to relative potency based on clinical judgment and experience. These classifications were then compared with EC3 values derived for the same chemicals. In each of two investigations there was a very close correlation between clinical potency and EC3 values (Basketter *et al.*, 2000; Gerberick *et al.*, 2001b). Based on these analyses, and other investigations, the view is that the most appropriate potency classifications would use the following descriptors: *strong, moderate, weak, extremely weak and non-sensitizer.* One recommendation for equating these classifications to EC3 values used as the unit for the latter exposure per unit area of skin (μg of chemical/cm^2 of skin surface). The proposed classification was: *strong* (EC3 <100 μg/cm^2); *moderate* (100–1000 μg/cm^2); *weak* (1000–10,000 μg/cm^2) and *extremely weak* (>10,000 μg/cm^2). Non-sensitizing chemicals would not have a measurable EC3 value because, by definition, they fail at all test concentrations to provoke a three-fold or greater increase in LNC proliferation compared with vehicle controls (Gerberick *et al.*, 2001b). It must be emphasized that this is only one possible classification scheme for grading contact allergens as a function of EC3 values. Nevertheless, it does have the merit of providing a rank order that correlates well with human experience of sensitizing potential.

Before considering how in practice the relative potency of contact allergens based on EC3 values can be integrated into the risk assessment process, it is necessary to address one point that was alluded to earlier; the relevance of vehicle matrix for relative potency. It is clear that the form in which a chemical is encountered at skin surfaces can impact upon the effectiveness with which contact sensitization is acquired, and this is of potential importance in establishing likely risks to human health. There is good evidence that the vehicle in which a chemical allergen is applied to the skin can have a significant influence on LLNA responses and EC3 values; the implication being that the vehicle may affect overall sensitizing potency (Basketter *et al.*, 2001b; Lea *et al.*, 1999; Warbrick *et al.*, 1999a; 1999b; Wright *et al.*, 2001). It is not possible currently to draw any conclusions regarding which vehicles may potentiate skin sensitization. Indeed, such generalizations may not be possible as experience to date suggests that the impact of vehicle upon the effectiveness of sensitization will vary significantly according to the physicochemical characteristics and dose of the chemical allergen. Notwithstanding these uncertainties there is every reason to conclude that the vehicle formulation can influence the induction of skin sensitization and that this is an important consideration when developing risk assessments.

41.6   INTEGRATION OF LLNA DATA INTO RISK ASSESSMENT

Skin sensitization risk assessment of new chemicals is a critical step before their introduction into the workplace and/or marketplace. The basic process used for evaluating the skin sensitization risk of a new product ingredient is to consider a no effect/safety factor approach. This is a stepwise approach that may involve analytical assessments, preclinical skin sensitization testing, clinical evaluation, and benchmarking of resulting data against similar ingredients or product types (Robinson *et al.*, 1989; Gerberick *et al.*, 1993; Kimber and Basketter, 1997; Basketter, 1998; Gerberick and Robinson, 2000). It is the potential for an adverse effect to occur in humans exposed during manufacturing or product use that is being determined. This approach incorporates assessment of both inherent

■ CHAPTER 41 ■

toxicity and exposure to the new ingredient. Specifically, it involves determination of the likely extent of exposure to the test material (exposure assessment), and its sensitization potency (dose-response assessment). It is the ability of the LLNA to assess skin sensitization potency that makes it an invaluable tool for conducting sound, quantitative exposure-based risk assessments (Robinson *et al.*, 2000; Gerberick *et al.*, 2001a).

Despite the importance of potency estimation in the development of accurate risk assessments, there has been only relatively modest progress in the definition of appropriate experimental models. The standard guinea pig tests, such as the maximization test, were successful at hazard identification (Andersen and Maibach, 1985; Botham *et al.*, 1991), and there has been some interest in the use of a modified guinea pig maximization test for consideration of relative potency. Of note has been the work of Andersen and co-workers, who manipulated the guinea pig maximization test in order to obtain dose-response data (Andersen *et al.*, 1995). However, the LLNA provides new opportunities for the objective and quantitative estimation of skin sensitization potency (Kimber and Basketter, 1997; Dearman *et al.*, 1999).

Experience to date with this approach has been encouraging; clear differences between skin sensitizing chemicals can be discerned and such differences appear to correlate closely with the ability of the materials to induce contact allergy in experimental models and with what is known of their sensitizing activity in humans (Hilton *et al.*, 1998; Basketter *et al.*, 1999; Basketter *et al.*, 2000; Gerberick *et al.*, 2001b). As discussed previously, the LLNA can be useful in developing classification schemes for ranking the potency of chemical allergens tested in the LLNA. Therefore, the LLNA as a preclinical tool provides critical skin sensitization potency information (EC3 values) that allows assessors to estimate the potential risk to workers or consumers. Moreover, the ability of the LLNA to measure relative potency may provide a basis for regulators to use such data to guide them in when and how to inform individuals of potential risks.

41.7 CONCLUSIONS

The local lymph node assay has proven value for the purposes of skin sensitization hazard identification. It has been formally validated in this respect and has been accepted broadly in regulatory guidelines. It has also been acknowledged that the assay also offers important animal benefits. Fewer animals are needed and animals are subject to reduced trauma and discomfort. Moreover, the LLNA provides a coherent approach to defining relative potency as an important contribution to the risk assessment process.

REFERENCES

ANDERSEN, K.E. and MAIBACH, HI. (1985) Guinea pig sensitisation assays: An overview. In ANDERSEN, K.E. and MAIBACH, H.I. (eds) *Contact Allergy Predictive Tests in Guinea Pigs, Current Problems in Dermatology.* Vol.14, New York: Karger, 59–106.

ANDERSEN, K.E., VOLUND, A. and FRANKILD, S. (1995) The guinea pig maximization test with a multiple dose design. *Acta Derm. Venereol.* **75**, 463–469.

ARTS, J.H.E., DROGE, S.C.M., BLOKSMA, N. and KUPER, C.F. (1996) Local lymph node activation in rats after dermal application of the sensitizers 2,4-dinitrochlorobenzene and trimellitic anhydride. *Fd. Chem. Toxic.* **34**, 55–62.

ASHBY, J., HILTON, J., DEARMAN, R.J., CALLANDER, R.D. and KIMBER, I. (1993) Mechanistic relationship among mutagenicity, skin sensitisation and skin carcinogenicity. *Environ. Health Perspect.* **101**, 62–67.

BALLS, M. and HELLSTEN, E. (2000) Statement on the validity of the local lymph node assay for skin sensitisation testing. ECVAM Joint Research Centre, European Commission, Ispra. *Altern. Lab. Animals* 28, 366–367.

BASKETTER, D.A. (1998) Skin sensitization: risk assessment. *Int. J. Cosmet. Sci.* 20, 141–150.

BASKETTER, D.A., BLAIKIE, L., DEARMAN, R.J., KIMBER, I., RYAN, C.A., GERBERICK, G.F., HARVEY, P., EVANS, P., WHITE, I.R. and RYCROFT, R.J.G. (2000) Use of the local lymph node assay for the estimation of relative contact allergenic potency. *Contact Derm.* **42**, 344–348.

BASKETTER, D.A., DEARMAN, R.J., HILTON, J. and KIMBER, I. (1997) Dinitrohalobenzenes: evaluation of relative skin sensitization potential using the local lymph node assay. *Contact Derm.* **36**, 97–100.

BASKETTER, D.A., GERBERICK, G.F. and KIMBER, I. (2001a) Measurement of allergenic potency using the local lymph node assay. *Trends Pharmacol. Sci.* **22**, 264–265.

BASKETTER, D.A., GERBERICK, G.F. and KIMBER, I. (2001b) Skin sensitization, vehicle effects and the local lymph node assay. *Fd. Chem. Toxic.* **39**, 621–627.

BASKETTER, D.A., EVANS, P., FIELDER, R.J., GERBERICK, G.F., DEARMAN, R.J. and KIMBER, I. (2002) Local lymph node assay—validation, conduct and use in practice. *Fd. Chem. Toxic.* **40**, 593–598.

■ CHAPTER 41 ■

BASKETTER, D.A., GERBERICK, G.F. and KIMBER, I. (1998) Strategies for identifying false positive responses in predictive skin sensitization tests. *Fd. Chem. Toxic.* **36**, 327–333.

BASKETTER, D.A., GERBERICK, G.F., KIMBER, I. and LOVELESS, S.E. (1996) The local lymph node assay: a viable alternative to currently accepted skin sensitisation tests. *Fd. Chem. Toxic.* **34**, 985–997.

BASKETTER, D.A. and KIMBER, I. (1996) Olive oil: suitability for use as a vehicle in the local lymph node assay. *Contact Derm.* 35, 190–191.

BASKETTER, D.A. and KIMBER, I. (2001) Predictive testing in contact allergy: facts and future. *Allergy* 56, 937–943.

BASKETTER, D.A. and SCHOLES, E.W. (1992) Comparison of the local lymph node assay with the guinea-pig maximization test for the detection of a range of contact allergens. *Fd. Chem. Toxic.* **60**, 65–69.

BASKETTER, D.A., LEA, L.J., COOPER, K.J., RYAN, C.A., GERBERICK, G.F., DEARMAN, R.J. and KIMBER, I. (1999c) Identification of metal allergens in the local lymph node assay. *Am. J. Contact Derm.* **10**, 297–212.

BASKETTER, D.A., LEA, L.J., COOPER, K., STOCKS, J., DICKENS, A., PATE, I., DEARMAN, R.J. and KIMBER, I. (1999a) Threshold for classification as a skin sensitizer in the local lymph node assay: a statistical evaluation. *Fd. Chem. Toxic.* **37**, 1167–1174.

BASKETTER, D.A., LEA, L.J., DICKENS, A., BRIGGS, D., PATE, I., DEARMAN, R.J. and KIMBER, I. (1999d) A comparison of statistical approaches to the derivation of EC3 values from local lymph node assay dose responses. *J. Appl. Toxicol.* **19**, 261–266.

BASKETTER, D.A., RODFORD, R., KIMBER, I., SMITH, I. and WAHLBERG, J.E. (1999b) Skin sensitization risk assessment: a comparative evaluation of 3 isothiazolinone biocides. *Contact Derm.* **40**, 150–154.

BASKETTER, D.A., SCHOLES, E.W., CUMBERBATCH, M., EVANS, C.D. and KIMBER, I. (1992) Sulphanilic acid: divergent results in the guinea pig maximization test and the local lymph node assay. *Contact Derm.* **27**, 209–213.

BASKETTER, D.A., SCHOLES, E.W. and KIMBER, I. (1994) The performance of the local lymph node assay with chemicals identified as contact allergens in the human maximization test. *Fd. Chem. Toxic.* **32**, 543–547.

BASKETTER, D.A., SCHOLES, E.W., KIMBER, I., BOTHAM, P.A., HILTON, J., MILLER, K., ROBBINS, M.C., HARRISON, P.T.C. and WAITE, S.J. (1991) Interlaboratory evaluation of the local lymph node assay with 25 chemicals and comparison with guinea pig test data. *Toxicol. Meth.* **1**, 30–43.

BASKETTER, D.A., SELBIE, E., SCHOLES, E.W., LEES, D., KIMBER, I. and BOTHAM, P.A. (1993) Results with OECD recommended positive control sensitisers in the maximization, Buehler and local lymph node assays. *Fd. Chem. Toxic.* **31**, 63–67.

BASKETTER, D.A., WRIGHT, Z.M., WARBRICK, E.V., DEARMAN, R.J., KIMBER, I., RYAN, C.A., GERBERICK, G.F. and WHITE, I.R. (2001c) Human potency predictions for aldehydes using the local lymph node assay. *Contact Derm.* **45**, 89–94.

BOTHAM, P.A., BASKETTER, D.A., MAURER, TH., MUELLER, D., POTOKAR, M. and BONTINCK, W.J. (1991a) Skin sensitization—a critical review of predictive test methods in animal and man. *Fd. Chem. Toxic.* **29**, 275–286.

BOTHAM, P.A., HILTON, J., EVANS, C.D., LEES, D. and HALL, T.J. (1991b) Assessment of the relative skin sensitising potency of 3 biocides using the local lymph node assay. *Contact Derm.* **25**, 172–177.

BUEHLER, E.V. (1965) Delayed contact hypersensitivity in the guinea pig. *Arch. Dermatol.* **91**, 171–177.

CHAMBERLAIN, M. and BASKETTER, D.A. (1996) The local lymph node assay: status of validation. *Fd. Chem. Toxic.* **34**, 999–1002.

CLOTTENS, F.L., BREYSSENS, A., DE RAEVE, H., DEMEDTS, M. and NEMERY, B. (1996) Assessment of the ear swelling test and local lymph node assay in hamsters. *Toxicol. Meth.* **35**, 167–172.

CUMBERBATCH, M., DEARMAN, R.J., GRIFFITHS, C.E.M. and KIMBER, I. (2000) Langerhans cell migration. *Clin. Exp. Dermatol.* **25**, 413–418.

CUMBERBATCH, M., SCOTT, R.C., BASKETTER, D.A., SCHOLES, E.W., HILTON, J. DEARMAN, R.J. and KIMBER, I. (1993) Influence of sodium lauryl sulfate on 2,4-dinitrochlorobenzene induced lymph node activation. *Toxicology* **77**, 181–191.

DEAN, J.H., TWERDOK, L.E., TICE, R.R., SAILSTAD, D.M., HATTAN, D.G. and STOKES, W.S. (2001) ICCVAM evaluation of the murine local lymph node assay. II Conclusions and recommendations of an independent scientific peer review panel. *Reg. Toxicol. Pharmacol.* **34**, 258–273.

DEARMAN, R.J., BASKETTER, D.A. and KIMBER, I. (1999) Local lymph node assay: use in hazard and risk assessment. *J. Appl. Toxicol.* **19**, 299–306.

DEARMAN, R.J., CUMBERBATCH, M. HILTON, J., CLOWES, H.M., FIELDING, I., HEYLINGS, J.R. and KIMBER, I. (1996) Influence of dibutyl phthalate on dermal sensitization to fluorescein isothiocyanate. *Fundam. Appl. Toxicol.* **33**, 24–30.

DEARMAN, R.J., HILTON, J., EVANS P., HARVEY, P., BASKETTER, D.A. and KIMBER, I. (1998) Temporal stability of local lymph node assay responses to hexyl cinnamic aldehyde. *J. Appl. Toxicol.* **18**, 281–284.

DEARMAN, R.J., WRIGHT, Z.M., BASKETTER, D.A., RYAN, C.A., GERBERICK, G.F. and KIMBER, I. (2001) The suitability of hexyl cinnamic aldehyde as a calibrant for the murine local lymph node assay. *Contact Derm.* **44**, 357–361.

DE JONG, W.H., VAN OCH, F.M.M., DEN HARTOG, C.F., SPIEKSTRA, S.W., SLOB, W., VANDEBRIEL, R.J. and VAN LOVEREN, H. (2002) Ranking of allergenic potency of rubber chemicals in a modified local lymph node assay. *Toxicol. Sci.* **66**, 226–232.

EDWARDS, D.A., SORRANO, T.M., AMORUSO, M.A., HOUSE, R.V., TUMMEY, A.C., TRIMMER, G.W., THOMAS, P.T. and RIBEIRO, P.L. (1994) Screening petrochemicals for contact hypersensitivity potential: a comparison of the murine local lymph node assay with guinea pig and human test data. *Fundam. Appl. Toxicol.* **23**, 179–187.

FRIEDMANN, P.S. (1990) The immunology of allergic contact dermatitis: the DNCB story. *Adv. Dermatol.* **5**, 175–196.

GERBERICK, G.F. and ROBINSON M.K. (2000) A skin sensitization risk assessment approach for evaluation of new ingredients and products. *Am. J. Contact Derm.* **11**, 65–73.

GERBERICK, G.F., BASKETTER, D.A. and KIMBER, I. (1999) Contact sensitization hazard identification. *Comments on Toxicol.* **7**, 31–41.

GERBERICK, G.F., HOUSE, R.V., FLETCHER, E.R. and RYAN, C.A. (1992) Examination of the local lymph node assay for use in contact sensitization risk assessment. *Fundam. Appl. Toxicol.* **19**, 438–445.

GERBERICK, G.F., ROBINSON, M.K., FELTER, S.P., WHITE, I.R. and BASKETTER, D.A. (2001a) Understanding fragrance allergy using an exposure-based risk assessment approach. *Contact Derm.* **45**, 333–340.

GERBERICK, G.F., ROBINSON, M.K., RYAN, C.A., DEARMAN, R.J., KIMBER, I., BASKETTER, D.A., WRIGHT, Z and MARKS, J.G. (2001b) Contact allergenic potency: correlation of human and local lymph node assay data. *Am. J. Contact Derm.* **12**, 156–161.

GERBERICK, G.F., ROBINSON, M.K. and STOTTS, J. (1993) An approach to allergic contact sensitization risk assessment of new chemicals and product ingredients. *Am. J. Contact Derm.* **4**, 205–211.

GERBERICK, G.F., RYAN, C.A., KIMBER, I, DEARMAN, R.J., LEA, L.J. and BASKETTER, D.A. (2000) Local lymph node assay: validation assessment for regulatory purposes. *Am. J.Contact Derm.* **11**, 3–18.

GOODWIN, B.F.J., CREVEL, R.W.R. and JOHNSON, A.W. (1981) A comparison of three guinea pig sensitization procedures for the detection of 19 human contact sensitizers. *Contact Derm.* **7**, 248–258.

GRABBE, S. and SCHWARZ, T. (1998) Immunoregulatory mechanisms involved in the elicitation of allergic contact dermatitis. *Immunol. Today* **19**, 37–44.

HANEKE, K.E., TICE, R.R., CARSON, B.L., MARGOLIN, B. and STOKES, W.S. (2001) ICCVAM evaluation of the murine local lymph node assay. III. Data analyses completed by the National Toxicology Program Interagency Center for the Evaluation of Alternative Toxicological Methods. *Reg. Toxicol. Pharmacol.* **34**, 274–286.

HEYLINGS, J.R., CLOWES, H.M., CUMBERBATCH, M., DEARMAN, R.J., FIELDING, I., HILTON, J. and KIMBER, I. (1996) Sensitization to 2,4-dinitrochlorobenzene: influence of vehicle on absorption and lymph node activation. *Toxicology* **109**, 57–65.

HILTON, J. and KIMBER, I. (1995) The murine local lymph node assay. In O'HARE, S. and ATTERWILL, C.K. (eds) *Methods in Molecular Biology, Vol. 43: In Vitro Toxicity Testing Protocols.* Totawa NJ, Humana Press, 227–235.

HILTON, J., DEARMAN, R.J., FIELDING, I., BASKETTER, D.A. and KIMBER, I. (1996) Evaluation of the sensitising potential of eugenol and isoeugenol in mice and guinea pigs. *J. Appl. Toxicol.* **16**, 459–464.

HILTON, J., DEARMAN, R.J., HARVEY, P., EVANS, P., BASKETTER, D.A. and KIMBER, I. (1998) Estimation of relative skin sensitizing potency using the local lymph node assay: a comparison of formaldehyde with glutaraldehyde. *Am. J. Contact Derm.* **9**, 29–33.

HOMEY, B., VON SCHILLING, C., BLUMEL J., SCHUPPE, H.-C., RUZICKA, T., AHR, H.J., LEHMANN, P. and VOHR, H.-W. (1998) An integrated model for the differentiation of chemical-induced allergic and irritant skin reactions. *Toxicol. Appl. Pharmacol.* **153**, 83–94.

IKARASHI, Y., OHNO, K., MOMMA, J., TSUCHIYA, T. and NAKAMURA, A. (1994) Assessment of contact sensitivity of four thiourea rubber accelerators: comparison of two mouse lymph node assays with the guinea pig maximization test. *Fd. Chem. Toxic.* **32**, 1067–1072.

IKARASHI, Y., OHNO, K., TSUCHIYA, T. and NAKAMURA, A. (1992) Differences in draining lymph node cell proliferation among mice, rats and guinea pigs following exposure to metal allergens. *Toxicology* **76**, 283–292.

IKARASHI, Y., TSUCHIYA, T. and NAKAMURA, A. (1993). A sensitive mouse lymph node assay with two application phases for detection of contact allergens. *Arch. Toxicol.* **67**, 629–636.

IKARASHI, Y., TSUCHIYA, T. and NAKAMURA, A. (1996) Application of a sensitive mouse lymph node assay for detection of contact sensitization capacity of dyes. *J Appl. Toxicol.* **16**, 349–354.

KASHIMA, R., OYAKE, Y., OKADA, J. and IKEDA, Y. (1996) Improved *ex vivo/in vitro* lymph node cell proliferation assay in guinea pigs for a screening test of contact hypersensitivity to chemical compounds. *Toxicology* **114**, 47–55.

KIMBER, I. (1989) Aspects of the immune response to contact allergens: opportunities for the development and modification of predictive test methods. *Fd. Chem. Toxic.* **27**, 755–762.

KIMBER, I. (1998) The local lymph node assay. In MARZULLI, F.N. and MAIBACH, H.I. (eds) *Dermatotoxicology Methods: The Laboratory Worker's Vade Mecum.* Washington DC, Taylor and Francis, 145–152.

KIMBER, I. and BASKETTER, D.A. (1992) The murine local lymph node assay: a commentary on collaborative trials and new directions. *Fd. Chem. Toxic.* **30**, 165–169.

KIMBER, I. and BASKETTER, D.A. (1997) Contact sensitization: a new approach to risk assessment. *Human Ecol. Risk Assess.* **3**, 385–395.

KIMBER, I. and DEARMAN, R.J. (1991) Investigation of lymph node cell proliferation as a possible immunological correlate of contact sensitising potential. *Fd. Chem. Toxic.* **29**, 125–129.

KIMBER, I. and DEARMAN, R.J. (2002) Allergic contact dermatitis: the cellular effectors. *Contact Derm.* **46**, 1–5.

KIMBER, I. and WEISENBERGER, C. (1989) A murine local lymph node assay for the identification of contact allergens. Assay development and results of an initial validation study. *Arch. Toxicol.* **63**, 274–282.

KIMBER, I., BASKETTER, D.A., BERTHOLD, K., BUTLER, M., GARRIGUE, J-L., LEA, L., NEWSOME, C., ROGGEBAND, R., STEILING, W., STROPP, G., WATERMAN, S. and WIEMANN, C. (2001) Skin sensitization testing in potency and risk assessment. *Toxicol. Sci.* **59**, 198–208.

KIMBER, I., BASKETTER, D.A., GERBERICK, G.F. and DEARMAN, R.J. (2002) Allergic contact dermatitis. *Int. Immunopharmacol.* **2**, 201–211.

KIMBER, I., BENTLEY, A. and HILTON, J. (1990b) Contact sensitization of mice to nickel sulfate and potassium dichromate. *Contact Derm.* **23**, 325–330.

KIMBER, I., CUMBERBATCH, M., DEARMAN, R.J., BHUSHAN, M. and GRIFFITHS, C.E.M. (2000) Cytokines and chemokines in the initiation and regulation of epidermal Langerhans cell mobilization. *Br. J. Dermatol.* **142**, 401–412.

KIMBER, I., DEARMAN, R.J., CUMBERBATCH, M. and HUBY R.J.D. (1998a) Langerhans cells and chemical allergy. *Curr. Opinion Immunol.* **10**, 614–619.

KIMBER, I., DEARMAN, R.J., SCHOLES, E.W. and BASKETTER, D.A. (1994) The local lymph node assay: developments and applications. *Toxicology* **93**, 13–31.

KIMBER, I., GERBERICK, G.F. and BASKETTER, D.A. (1999) Thresholds in contact sensitization: theoretical and practical considerations. *Fd. Chem. Toxic.* **37**, 553–560.

KIMBER, I., HILTON, J. and BOTHAM, P.A. (1990a) Identification of contact allergens using murine local lymph node assay: comparisons with the Buehler occluded patch test in guinea pigs. *J. Appl. Toxicol.* **10**, 173–180.

KIMBER, I., HILTON, J., BOTHAM, P.A., BASKETTER, D.A., SCHOLES, E.W., MILLER, K., ROBBINS, M.C., HARRISON, P.T.C., GRAY, T.J.B. and WAITE, S.J. (1991) The murine local lymph node assay: results of an interlaboratory trial. *Toxicol. Lett.* **55**, 203–213.

KIMBER, I., HILTON, J., DEARMAN, R.J., GERBERICK, G.F., RYAN, C.A., BASKETTER, D.A., LEA, L., HOUSE, R.V., LADICS, G.S., LOVELESS, S.E. and HASTINGS, K. (1998b) Assessment of the skin sensitizing potential of topical medicaments using the local lymph node assay: an inter-laboratory evaluation. *J. Toxicol. Environ. Health* **53**, 563–579.

KIMBER, I., HILTON, J., DEARMAN, R.J., GERBERICK, G.F., RYAN, C.A., BASKETTER, D.A., SCHOLES, E.W., LOVELESS, S.E., LADICS, G.S., HOUSE, R.V. and GUY, A. (1995) An international evaluation of the murine local lymph node assay and comparison of modified procedures. *Toxicology* **103**, 63–73.

KIMBER, I., HILTON, J. and WEISENBERGER, C. (1989) The murine local lymph node assay for identification of contact allergens: a preliminary evaluation of in situ measurement of lymphocyte proliferation. *Contact Derm.* **21**, 215–220.

KIMBER, I., MITCHELL, J.A. and GRIFFIN, A.C. (1986) Development of a murine local lymph node assay for the determination of sensitizing potential. *Fd. Chem. Toxic.* **24**, 585–586.

CHAPTER 41

KLINGMAN, A.M. (1966a) The identification of contact allergens by human assay: III The maximization test. A procedure for screening and rating contact sensitizers. *J. Invest. Derm.* **47**, 393–409.

KLINGMAN, A.M. (1966b) The SLS provocative patch in allergic contact sensitization. *J. Invest. Derm.* **46**, 573–585.

LADICS, G.S., SMITH, C., HEAPS, K.L. and LOVELESS, S.E. (1995) Comparison of I^{125}-iododeoxyuridine (^{125}IUdR) and [^{3}H] thymidine ([^{3}H]TdR) for assessing cell proliferation in the murine local lymph node assay. *Toxicol. Meth.* **5**, 143–152.

LEA, L.J., WARBRICK, E.V., DEARMAN, R.J., KIMBER, I. and BASKETTER, D.A. (1999) The impact of vehicle on assessment of relative skin sensitization potency of 1,4-dihydroquinone in the local lymph node assay. *Am. J. Contact Derm.* **10**, 213–218.

LOVELESS, S.E., LADICS, G.S., GERBERICK, G.F., RYAN, C.A., BASKETTER, D.A., SCHOLES, E.W., HOUSE, R.V., HILTON, J., DEARMAN, R.J. and KIMBER, I. (1996) Further evaluation of the local lymph node assay in the final phase of an international collaborative trial. *Toxicology* **108**, 141–152.

MAURER, T. and KIMBER, I. (1991) Draining lymph node cell activation in guinea pigs: comparisons with the murine local lymph node assay. *Toxicology* **69**, 209–218.

MONTELIUS, J., WAHLKVIST, H., BOMAN, A., FERNSTROM, P., GRABERGS, L. and WAHLBERG, J.E. (1994) Experience with the murine local lymph node assay: inability to discriminate between allergens and irritants. *Acta. Dermatol. Venereol.* **74**, 22–27.

NIH (1999) The Murine Local Lymph Node Assay: A Test Method for Assessing the Allergic Contact Dermatitis Potential of Chemicals/Compounds. NIH No. 99–4494.

OECD (2002) Local Lymph Node Assay. Test Guideline no 429, Organisation for Economic Cooperation and Development, Paris.

ROBINSON, M.K., GERBERICK, G.F., RYAN, C.A., MCNAMEE, P., WHITE, I.R. and BASKETTER, D.A. (2000). The importance of exposure estimation in the assessment of skin sensitisation risk. *Contact Derm.* **42**, 251–259.

ROBINSON, M.K., STOTTS, J., DANNEMAN, P.J., NUSAIR, T.L. and BAY, P.H. (1989) A risk assessment process for allergic contact sensitization. *Fd. Chem. Toxic.* **27**, 479–489.

RYAN, C.A., GERBERICK, G.F., CRUSE, L.W., BASKETTER, D.A., LEA, L., BLAIKIE, L., DEARMAN, R.J., WARBRICK, E.V. and KIMBER, I. (2000) Activity of human contact allergens in the murine local lymph node assay. *Contact Derm.* **43**, 95–102.

SAILSTAD, D.M., HATTAN, D., HILL, R.N. and STOKES, W.S. (2001) ICCVAM evaluation of the murine local lymph node assay. I. The ICCVAM review process. *Reg. Toxicol. Pharmacol.* **34**, 249–257.

SAILSTAD, D., TEPPER, J.S., DOERFLER, D.L., QASIM, M. and SELGRADE, M.K. (1994) Evaluation of an azo and two anthraquinone dyes for allergic potential. *Fundam. Appl. Toxicol.* **23**, 569–577.

SCHOLES, E.W., BASKETTER, D.A., SARLL, A.E., KIMBER, I., EVANS, C.D., MILLER, K., ROBBINS, M.C., HARRISON, P.T.C. and WAITE, S.J. (1992) The local lymph node assay: results of a final inter-laboratory validation under field conditions. *J. Appl. Toxicol.* **12**, 217–222.

SCHWARTZ, L. (1960) Twenty-two years experience on the performance 200,000 prophetic-patch tests. *South. Med. J.* **53**, 478–483.

TAKEYOSHI, M., YAMASAKI, K., YAKABE, Y., TAKATSUKI, M. and KIMBER, I. (2001) Development of a non-radio isotopic endpoint of murine local lymph node assay based on 5-bromo-2'-deoxyuridine (BrdU) incorporation. *Toxicol. Lett.* **119**, 203–208.

ULRICH, P., HOMEY, B. and VOHR, H.-W. (1998) A modified local lymph node assay for the differentiation of contact photoallergy from phototoxicity by analysis of cytokine expression in skin-draining lymph node cells. *Toxicology* **125**, 149–168.

ULRICH, P., STREICH, J. and SUTER, W. (2001) Intralaboratory validation of alternative endpoints in the murine local lymph node assay for the identification of contact allergic potential: primary ear skin irritation and ear-draining lymph node hyperplasia induced by topical chemicals. *Arch. Toxicol.* **74**, 733–744.

VAN OCH, F.M.M., SLOB, W., DE JONG, W.H., VANDEBRIEL, R.J. and VAN LOVEREN, H. (2000) A quantitative method for assessing the sensitizing potency of low molecular weight chemicals using a local lymph node assay: employment of regression method that includes determination of the uncertainty margins. *Toxicology* **146**, 49–59.

WARBRICK, E.V., DEARMAN, R.J., ASHBY, J., SCHMEZER, P. and KIMBER, I. (2001) Preliminary assessment of the skin sensitizing activity of selected rodent carcinogens using the local lymph node assay. *Toxicology* **163**, 63–69.

WARBRICK, E.V., DEARMAN, R.J., BASKETTER, D.A. and KIMBER, I. (1999a) Influence of application vehicle on skin sensitization to methylchloroisothiazolinone/

■ CHAPTER 41 ■

methylisothiazolinone: an analysis using the local lymph node assay. *Contact Derm.* **41**, 325–329.

WARBRICK, E.V., DEARMAN, R.J., LEA, L.J., BASKETTER, D.A. and KIMBER, I. (1999b) Local lymph node assay responses to paraphenylenediamine: intra- and inter-laboratory studies. *J. Appl. Toxicol.* **19**, 255–260.

WOOLHISER, M.R., MUNSON, A.E. and MEADE, B.J. (2000) Comparison of mouse strains using the local lymph node assay. *Toxicology* **146**, 221–227.

WRIGHT, Z.M., BASKETTER, D.A., BLAIKIE, L., COOPER, K.J., WARBRICK, E.V., DEARMAN, R.J. and KIMBER, I. (2001) Vehicle effects on skin sensitizing potency of four chemicals: assessment using the local lymph node assay. *Int. J. Cosmet. Sci.* **23**, 75–83.

Contact Urticaria and the Contact Urticaria Syndrome (Immediate Contact Reactions)

SMITA AMIN, ARTO LAHTI
AND HOWARD I MAIBACH

Contents

42.1 Introduction

42.2 Symptoms

42.3 Etiology and mechanisms

42.4 Diagnostic tests

42.5 Summary

42.1 INTRODUCTION

The contact urticaria syndrome (CUS) (immediate contact reactions) comprises a heterogeneous group of inflammatory reactions that appear. usually within minutes, after contact with the eliciting substance. They include not only wheal and flare but also transient erythema and may lead to eczema.

The epidemiology of these reactions is inadequately documented. The first such studies were performed in Hawaii (Elpern, 1985a, 1985b, 1986), Poland (Rudzki *et al.*, 1985), Sweden (Nilsson, 1985), Denmark (Veien *et al.*, 1987), Finland (Turjanmaa, 1987), and Switzerland (Weissenbach *et al.*, 1988). These studies suggested that immediate contact reactions are common in dermatologic practice. Some substances cause immediate reactions in almost everyone at the first contact (methyl nicotinate), but others need a period of sensitization (latex rubber).

Since the original description of the contact urticaria syndrome in 1975 (Maibach and Johnson), new cases are published with increasing frequency.

42.2 SYMPTOMS

Immediate contact reactions appear on normal or eczematous skin within minutes to an hour or so after agents capable of producing this type of reaction have been in contact with the skin. They disappear within 24 h, usually within a few hours. The symptoms can be classified according to morphology and severity: Itching, tingling or burning accompanied by erythema are the weakest type of immediate contact reaction and are often produced by cosmetics (Emmons and Marks, 1985) and fruits and vegetables. Local wheal-and-flare is the prototype reaction of contact urticaria. Generalized urticaria after a local contact is uncommon. Tiny vesicles may rapidly appear on the fingers in protein contact dermatitis. Apart from the skin, effects may also appear in other organs in cases of strong hypersensitivity, thus leading us to neologize the term called contact urticaria syndrome. In some cases, immediate contact reactions can be demonstrated only on slightly or previously affected skin, and it can be part of the mechanism responsible for maintenance of chronic eczemas (Hannuksela, 1980; Maibach, 1976; Veien *et al.*, 1987).

There has been confusion in using terms such as contact urticaria, immediate contact reactions, atopic contact dermatitis, and protein contact dermatitis (Table 42.1). Immediate contact urticaria includes both urticaria and other reactions, whereas protein contact dermatitis means allergic or nonallergic eczematous dermatitis caused by proteins or proteinaceous materials.

■ CHAPTER 42 ■

TABLE 42.1:

Terminology of contact urticaria syndrome

Term	Remarks
Immediate contact reaction	Includes urticarial, eczematous, and other immediate reactions
Contact urticaria	Allergic (type I) and nonallergic (type II) contact urticaria reactions
Protein contact dermatitis	Allergic or nonallergic eczematous reactions caused by proteins or proteinaceous material

42.3 ETIOLOGY AND MECHANISMS

The mechanisms underlying contact reactions are divided into two main types, namely, immunologic [immunoglobin E (IgE) mediated] and nonimmunologic immediate contact reactions (Lahti and Maibach, 1987). However, there are substances causing immediate contact reactions whose mechanism (immunologic or not) remains unknown.

Tables 42.2–42.4 present agents that have been reported to cause immediate contact reactions. They include chemicals in medications, industrial contactants, components of cosmetic products and of foods and drinks, and chemically undefined environmental agents. The pathogenetic classification (nonimmunologic versus immunologic) is also given but in many instances it is arbitrary,

TABLE 42.2:

Substances that have caused local reactions and anaphylactic symptoms in skin tests

Aminophenazone
Ampicillin
Balsam of Peru
Bacitracin
Chloramphenicol
Diethyltoluamide
Egg
Epoxy resin
Latex protein (rubber products)
Mechlorethamine
Neomycin
Penicillin
Streptomycin

TABLE 42.3:

Agents producing immunologic contact urticaria (ICU)

Animal products
    Amnion fluid
    Blood
    Brucella aborrus (Trunnel *et al.*, 1985)
    Cercariae
    Cheylerus malaccensis (Yoshikawa, 1985)
    Chironomidae, *Chironomus thummi thummi* (Mittelbach, 1983)
    Cockroaches
    Dander (Agrup and Sjostedt, 1985; Weissenbach *et al.*, 1988)
    Dermestes macularus Degeer (Lewis-Jones, 1985)
    Gelatine (Wahi and Kleinhans, 1989)
    Gut
    Hair
    Listrophorus gibbus (Burns, 1987)
    Liver
    Locust (Monk, 1988: Tee *et al.*, 1988)
    Mealworm, *Tenibrio molitor* (Bernstein *et al.*, 1983)
    Placenta
    Saliva (Valsecchi and Cainelli, 1989)
    Serum
    Silk
    Spider mite, *Terranychus urticae* (Reunala *et al.*, 1983)
    Wool
Food
    Dairy
        Cheese
        Egg
        Milk (Boso and Brestel, 1987; Salo *et al.*, 1986)
    Fruits
        Apple (Halmepuro and Løwenstein, 1985; Pigatto *et al.*, 1983)
        Apricot
        Banana
        Kiwi
        Mango
        Orange
        Peach
        Plum
    Grains
        Buckwheat (Valdivieso *et al.*, 1989)
        Maize
        Malt
        Rice (Lezaun *et al.*, 1994)
        Wheat
        Wheat bran
    Honey
    Nuts/seeds
        Peanut
        Sesame seed
        Sunflower seed

■ CHAPTER 42 ■

TABLE 42.3:

(*Continued*)

Meats
    Beef
    Chicken
    Lamb
    Liver
    Turkey
    Seafood
        Fish (Kavli and Moseng, 1987: Melino *et al.*, 1987: Díaz-Sánchez *et al.*, 1994)
        Prawns
        Shrimp (Nagano *et al.*, 1984)
    Vegetables
        Beans
        Cabbage
        Carrot (Muñoz *et al.*, 1985)
        Celery (Krernser and Lindemayr, 1983; Wuthrich and Dietschi, 1985)
        Chives
        Cucumber
        Endive
        Lettuce
        Onion
        Parsley
        Parsnip
        Potato (Larkö *et al.*, 1983)
        Rutabaga (swede)
        Tomato
        Soybean
    Fragrances and flavorings
        Balsam of Peru
        Menthol
        Vanillin
Medicaments
    Acetylsalicylic acid
    Antibiotics
        Ampicillin
        Bacitracin
        Cephalosporins
            Cefotiam dihydrochloride (Mizutani *et al.*, 1994)
        Chloramphenicol (Schewach-Millet and Shpiro, 1985)
        Gentamicin
        Iodochlorhydroxyquin
        Mezlocillin (Keller and Schwanitz, 1993)
        Neomycin
        Nifuroxime (Aaronson, 1969)
        Penicillin (Rudzki and Rebandel, 1985)
        Rifamycin (Grob *et al.*, 1987)
        Streptomycin
        Virginiamycin (Baes, 1974)
    Benzocaine (Kleinhans and Zwissler, 1980)
    Benzoyl peroxide
    Clobetasol 17-propionate (Gottmann-Lückerath, 1982)

Dinitrochlorobenzene (Valsecchi et al., 1986: van Hecke and Santosa, 1985)
Etophenamate (Pinol and Carapeto, 1984)
Fumaric acid derivatives (de Haan et al., 1994)
Mechlorethamine
Phenothiazines
    Chlorpromazine (Lovell et al., 1986)
    Levomepromazine (Johansson, 1988)
    Promethazine
Pyrazolones
    Aminophenazone (Lombardi et al., 1983)
    Methamizole
    Propylphenazone
Tocopherol (Kassen and Mitchell, 1974)
Metals
    Copper (Shelley et al., 1983)
    Nickel (Valsecchi and Cainelli, 1987)
    Platinum
    Rhodium
Plant products (Lahti, 1986b)
    Algae
    Birch
    Camomile
    Castor bean
    Chrysanthemum (Tanaka et al., 1987)
    Cinchona (Dooms-Goossens et al., 1986a)
    Colophony (Rivers and Rycroft, 1987)
    Corn starch Assalve et al., 1988: Fisher, 1987)
    Cotoneaster
    Emetin
    Fennel (La Rosa et al., 1986)
    Garlic
    Grevillea juniperina (Apted, 1988a)
    Hakea suaveolens (Apted, 1988b)
    Hawthorn, Crataegus monogyna (Steinman et al., 1984)
    Henna
    Latex rubber (Axelsson et al., 1987; Frosh et al., 1986: Morales et al., 1989;
        Spaner et al., 1989: van der Meeren and van Erp, 1986; Wrangsjö et al., 1988)
    Lichens
    Lily (Lahti, 1986a)
    Lime (Picardo et al., 1988)
    Limonium tataricum (Quirce et al., 1993)
    Mahogany
    Mustard (Kavli and Moseng, 1987)
    Papain (Santucci et al., 1985)
    Perfumes
    Pickles (Edwards and Edwards, 1984a)
    Rose (Kleinhans, 1985)
    Rouge
    Spices (Niinimäki. 1987)
    Strawberry (Grattan and Harman, 1985)
    Teak
    Tobacco (Tosti et al., 1987)
    Tulip (Lahti, 1986a)
    Winged bean (Lovell and Rycroft, 1984)

■ CHAPTER 42 ■

TABLE 42.3:

(Continued)

Preservatives and disinfectants
    Benzoic acid (Nethercott *et al.*, 1984)
Benzyl alcohol
    Chlorhexidine (Bergqvist-Karlsson, 1988; Fisher, 1989; Nishioka *et al.*, 1984)
    Chloramine
    Chiorocresol (Goncalo *et al.*, 1987)
    1,3-Diiodo-2-hydroxypropane (Löwenfeld, 1928)
    Formaldehyde (Andersen and Maibach, 1984: Lindskov, 1982)
    Gentian violet (Francois *et al.*, 1970)
    Hexantriol (Tachibana *et al.*, 1977)
    para-Hydroxybenzoic acid (Bottger *et al.*, 1981)
    Parabens (Henry *et al.*, 1979)
    Phenylmercuric propionate
    orrho-Phenylphenate (Tuer *et al.*, 1986)
    Polysorbates
    Sodium hypochlorite
Sorbitan monolaurate
Tropicamide (Guilt *et al.*, 1979)
Enzymes
    alpha-Amylasc (Moren *et al.*, 1993)
    Cellulases (Tarvainen *et al.*, 1991)
    Xylanases (Tarvainen *et al.*, 1991)
Miscellaneous
    Acetyl acetone (Sterry and Schmoll, 1985)
    Acrylic monomer
    Alcohols (amyl, butyl, ethyl, isopropyl) (Rilliet *et al.*, 1980)
    Aliphatic polyamide
    Ammonia
    Ammonium persulfate
    Aminothiazole
    Benzophenone
    Butylated hydroxytoluene
    Carbonless copy paper
    Chlorothanil (Dannaker *et al.*, 1993)
    Cu(II) acetyl acetonate (Sterry and Schmoll, 1985)
    Denatonium benzoate
    Diethyltoluamide
    Epoxy resin (Jolanki *et al.*, 1987)
    Formaldehyde resin
    Lanolin alcohols
    Lindane
    Methyl ethyl ketone (Varigos and Nurse, 1986)
    Monoamvlamine
    Naphtha (Goodfield and Saihan, 1988)
    Naphihylacetic acid (Camarasa, 1986)
    Nylon (Dooms-Goossens *et al.*, 1986b; Hatch and Maibach, 1985)
    Oleylamide
    Paraphenylenediamine (Edwards and Edwards, 1984b; Temesvari, 1984)
    Patent blue dye
    Perlon

Phosphorus sesquisulfide (Payero et al., 1985)
Plastic
Polypropylene (Tosti et al., 1986)
Polyethylene glycol
Potassium ferricyanide
Seminal fluid (Blair and Parish. 1985
Sodium silicate
Sodium sulfide
Sulfur dioxide
Terpinyl acetate
Textile finish (de Groot and Gerkens, 1989)
Vinyl pyridine
Zinc diethyldithiocarbamate

TABLE 42.4:

Agents producing nonimmunologic contact urticaria (NICU)

Animals
    Arthropods
    Caterpillars (Ducombs et al., 1983: Edwards et al., 1986)
    Corals
    Jellyfish
    Moths
    Sea anemones
Foods
    Cayenne pepper
    Cows milk (Oranje et al., 1992, 1994)
    Fish
    Mustard
    Thyme
Fragrances and flavorings
    Balsam of Peru
    Benzaldehyde
    Cassia (cinnamon oil)
    Cinnamic acid
    Cinnamic aldehyde (Emmons and Marks, 1985; Gum et al., 1984: Larsen, 1985;
        Helton and Storrs, 1994)
Medicaments
    Alcohols (Wilkin and Fortner, 1985)
    Benzocaine
    Camphor
    Cantharides
    Capsaicin
    Chlorophorm
    Dimethyl sulfoxide
    Friar's balsam
    Iodine
    Methyl salicylate
    Methylene green
    Myrrh

■ CHAPTER 42 ■

TABLE 42.4:

(*Continued*)

    Nicotinic acid esters
    Resorcinol
    Tar extracts
    Tincture of benzoin
    Witch hazel
Metals
    Cobalt
Plants
    Nettles (Kulze and Greaves, 1988; Oliver *et al.*, 1991)
    Seaweed
Preservatives and disinfectants
    Acetic acid (Burral *et al.*, 1990)
    Benzoid acid
    Chlorocresol (Freitas and Brandão, 1986)
    Formaldehyde
    Sodium benzoate
    Sorbic acid (Soschin and Leyden, 1986)
Miscellaneous
    Butyric acid
    Diethyl fumarate (Lahti and Maibach, 1985a; White and Cronin, 1984)
    Histamine
    Pine oil
    Propylene glycol (Funk and Maibach, 1994)
    Pyridine carboxaldehyde Archer and Cronin. 1986: Hannuksela *et al.*, 1989)
    Sulfur (Böttger *et al.*, 1981)
    Turpentine

---

because the mechanisms of various contact reactions are unclear or mainly because a pathogenic evaluation was not performed.

Increasing awareness of immediate contact reactions will expand the list of etiologic agents, and more thorough understanding of pathophysiologic mechanisms will lead to a better and more rational classification of these reactions than at present. The international epidemic of latex protein contact urticaria has led to an awareness of the syndrome among surgeons, anesthesiologists, pediatricians, and gynecologists.

42.3.1 Immediate contact urticaria (ICU), IgE-mediated contact reactions (Type I)

Immunologic contact urticaria reactions are immediate reactions in people who have previously become sensitized to the causative agent. In some cases of immunologic contact reaction, the respiratory, gastrointestinal, and genital tracts may have been the routes of sensitization. However, natural latex and some foods can sensitize people through the skin.

In skin challenge, the molecules of a contact reactant penetrate the epidermis and react with specific IgE molecules attached to mast-cell membranes. Cutaneous symptoms (erythema and edema) are elicited by vasoactive substances, mainly histamine released from mast cells. The role of histamine is important, but other mediators of inflammation, such as prostaglandins, leukotrienes, and kinins, may also influence the intensity of response. However, little is known regarding the dynamics of their interplay in clinical situations. More is known about the mediators of nonimmunologic contact urticaria (NICU).

Not only do mast cells and circulating basophils have Fc receptors for IgE molecules, but also eosinophils (Capron et at., 1981), peripheral B and T lymphocytes (Yodoi and Iskizaka, 1979), platelets (Joseph et at., 1983), monocytes (Melewicz and Spiegelberg, 1980), and alveolar macrophages (Joseph et al., 1980) can bind IgE. These findings make the issue of immunologic contact urticaria (ICU) more complicated than was believed earlier.

Patients with atopic dermatitis, but not other atopics or normal controls, have IgE on their epidermal Langerhans cells (Barker et al., 1988; Bruynzeel-Koomen, 1986; Bruynzeel-Koomen et al., 1986). This finding may provide an explanation for the high frequency of positive patch-test reactions to inhalant allergens, such as house dust mites, birch and grass pollen, and animal danders, in these patients (Adinoff et al., 1988; Leung et al., 1987; Mitchell et al., 1986; Reitamo et al., 1986; Tigalonowa et al., 1988). An important function of epidermal Langerhans cells is antigen presentation in delayed-type contact allergic reaction, but it can be hypothesized that protein allergens (inhalant, food, etc.) for type I immediate contact reactions bind to specific IgE molecules present on epidermal Langerhans cells, which become apposed to mononuclear cells (Najem and Hull, 1989) and induce a delayed-type hypersensitivity reaction resulting in eczematous skin lesions. This may be the mechanism whereby repeated immediate contact reactions lead to more persistent eczematous skin lesions.

Contact urticaria to rubber latex is a typical example of immediate immuno-logic contact reaction and is common (Estlander et al., 1987; Pecquet and Leynadier, 1993; Turjanmaa, 1987; Turjanmaa and Reunala, 1988; Wrangsjo et al., 1986). Anaphylactic symptoms and generalized urticaria have occurred after contact with surgical (Axelsson et al., 1987; Carrillo et al., 1986; Spaner et al., 1989; Turjanmaa et al., 1988a) and household rubber gloves (Seifert et al.,

1987). These reactions have been shown to be immediate, allergic, and IgE-mediated (Frosch *et al.*, 1986; Seifert *et al.*, 1987; Turjanmaa and Reunala, 1989; Turjanmaa *et al.*, 1989). The allergens are among the proteins that constitute 1–2 per cent of natural latex. Allergy to latex can be established by open application, skin prick tests (Turjanmaa *et al.*, 1988c), and the latex radioallergo-sorbent test (RAST) (Turjanmaa *et al.*, 1988b).

Veterinary surgeons can contract contact urticaria on the hand after contact with cow amnion fluid, but they do not acquire reactions to cow dander in clinical provocation tests or in skin prick tests with cow epithelium extracts. RAST investigations have shown that antibodies to cow amnion fluid and serum, but not to epithelia, can be found in the sera of veterinary surgeons. The allergen causing contact urticaria in these cases is a compound of amnion fluid and serum but not of the epithelium of cows (Kalveram *et al.*, 1986).

Foods are the most common causes of immediate allergic contact reactions (Table 42.3). The orolaryngeal area is a site where immediate reactions are provoked by food allergens, frequently among atopic individuals. Of 230 patients allergic to birch pollen, 152 (66 per cent) gave a history of itching, tingling, or edema of the lips and tongue and hoarseness or irritation of the throat when eating raw fruits and vegetables such as apple, potato, carrot, and tomato (Hannuksela and Lahti, 1977). Plum, peach, cherry, kiwi, celery, and parsnip can also elicit immediate contact reactions in birch pollen-allergic people. Positive results ("scratch-chamber" test) with suspected raw fruits and vegetables were noted in 36 per cent of 230 patients. Apple, carrot, parsnip, and potato elicited reactions more often than swede (rutabaga), tomato, onion, celery, and parsley. The clinical relevance of the skin test results with apple. potato, and carrot was 80–90 per cent. Only 7 of 158 (4 per cent) atopic patients who were not allergic to birch pollen had positive skin test reactions to any of the fruits and vegetables.

RAST and RAST inhibition studies have confirmed the cross-allergy between birch pollen and fruits and vegetables. All immunological determinants in apple, carrot, and celery tuber appeared to be present also in birch pollen but not vice versa (Halmepuro and Løvenstein, 1985; Halmepuro *et al.*, 1984).

42.3.2 Protein contact dermatitis

The term "protein contact dermatitis" was introduced (Hjorth and Roed-Petersen, 1976) for people with hand eczema demonstrating immediate symptoms when the skin was exposed to certain food proteins. Most of these individuals handled job-related food products for a protracted period before the symptoms appeared. Itching, erythema, urticarial swelling, or small vesicles appear on fingers or dorsa of hands within 30 min of contact with fish or shellfish. Wheat flour (causing baker's dermatitis) and natural rubber proteins are other examples of immediate contact reactions. Protein contact dermatitis may appear without previous urticarial rashes, but it may also be a result of repeated contact urticaria (Hannuksela, 1986). It is probable that both immuno-logic and nonimmunologic (irritant) types of protein contact reactions exist. Eczematous reactions are indistinguishable from primary irritant or allergic dermatitis, and careful study of the patient's history and the performance of skin tests ensure correct diagnosis. Awareness of these reactions provides profound relief for some hand eczema patients (Menné and Maibach, 1994; Turanmaa, 1994).

42.3.3 Nonimmunologic contact urticaria

Nonimmunologic contact urticaria (NICU) occurs without previous sensitization and is the most common type of immediate contact reaction. The reaction remains localized and does not spread to become generalized urticaria, nor does it cause systemic symptoms. Typically, the strength of the reaction varies from erythema to an urticarial response. depending on the concentration, the skin area exposed, the mode of exposure, and the substance itself (Lahti, 1980).

Potent and well-studied substances producing nonimmunologic immediate contact reactions (Table 42.4) include benzoic acid, sorbic acid, cinnamic acid, cinnamic aldehyde, and nicotinic acid esters. Under optimal conditions more than half of the individuals react with local erythema and edema to these substances within 45 min of application if the concentration is high enough. Benzoic acid, sorbic acid, and sodium benzoate, preservatives for cosmetics and other topical preparations, are capable of producing immediate contact reactions at concentrations from 0.1 to 0.2 per cent (Lahti, 1980; Soschin and Leyden, 1986).

Cinnamic aldehyde at a concentration of 0.01 per cent may elicit erythema with a burning or stinging feeling in the skin. Some mouthwashes and chewing gums contain cinnamic aldehyde at concentrations that produce a pleasant tingling or "lively" sensation in the mouth and enhance the sale of the product. Higher concentrations produce lip swelling or contact urticaria.

The skin of the face, neck, back, and extensor sides of the upper extremities react more readily than other parts of the body; the soles and palms are the least sensitive areas (Gollhausen and Kligman, 1985; Lahti, 1980). Scratching does not enhance the reactivity, nor does occlusion, for benzoic acid.

The mechanism of nonimmunologic contact urticaria has not been established, but possible mechanisms are a direct influence upon dermal vessel walls or a non-antibody-mediated release of histamine, prostaglandins, leukotrienes, substance P, or other inflammatory mediators (Lahti and Maibach, 1987). No specific antibodies against the causative agent are in the serum.

It was earlier presumed that substances eliciting nonimmunologic contact urticaria also result in nonspecific histamine release from mast cells. However, antihistamines, hydroxyzine, and terfenadine did not inhibit reactions to benzoic acid, cinnamic acid, cinnamic aldehyde. methyl nicotinate, or dimethyl sulfoxide but they did inhibit reactions to histamine in the prick test (Lahti, 1980, 1987). The results suggest that histamine is not the main mediator in NICU.

Effect of Nonsteroidal Anti-inflammatory Drugs

Nonimmunologic contact reactions to benzoic acid, cinnamic acid, cinnamic aldehyde, methyl nicotinate, and diethyl fumarate can be inhibited by peroral acetylsalicylic acid and indomethacin (Lahti et al., 1983. 1987) and by topical application of diclofenac or naproxene gels (Johansson and Lahti, 1988). Inhibition by acetylsalicylic acid can last up to 4 days (Kujala and Lahti, 1989). The mechanism by which nonsteroidal anti-inflammatory drugs (NSAIDs) inhibit contact reactions in human skin has not been defined, but it may be ascribed to a common pharmacological action, that is, inhibition of prostaglandin bioformation.

Role of sensory nerves

Capsaicin (trans-8-methyl-N-vanillyl-6-nonenamide), the most abundant of the pungent principles of the red pepper (Capsicum), is known to induce vasodilatation and protein extravasation by specific release of bioactive peptides, for example, substance P, from axons of unmyelinated C-fibers of the sensory nerves. Pretreatment with capsaicin inhibits erythema reactions in histamine skin tests (Bernstein et al., 1981; Wallengren and Moller. 1986). However, pretreatment with capsaicin inhibited neither erythema nor edema elicited by benzoic acid or methyl nicotinate (Larmi et al., 1989). The result suggests that pathways sensitive to capsaicin are not substantially involved.

Topical anesthesia (lidocaine plus prilocaine) can inhibit erythema and edema reactions to histamine and also to benzoic acid and methyl nicotinate, but it is not known whether the inhibitory effect is due to the influence on the sensory nerves of the skin only, or if the anesthetic affects other cell types or regulatory mechanisms of immediate type skin inflammation (Larmi *et al.*, 1989).

Effect of ultraviolet irradiation

Immediate contact reactions to benzoic acid and methyl nicotinate can also be inhibited by ultraviolet (UV) B and A light exposure, an effect that lasts for at least 2 wk (Larmi *et al.*, 1988). An interesting observation was the fact that UV irradiation had systemic effects; it inhibited reactions on nonirradiated skin sites, too (Larmi. 1989). The mechanism of UV inhibition is not known, but it does not seem to be due to thickening of the stratum corneum (Larmi, 1989).

Little is known about the histology of immediate contact reactions. In studies with nicotinates, the accumulation of mononuclear cell perivascular infiltrate was seen from 15 min and that of neutrophils from 2 h onward, persisting up to 48 h in normal subjects. Leukocytoclasis was also observed. The cell infiltrate was seen to a lesser degree in 1 of 6 atopic eczema patients but not in normal subjects treated with 600 mg acetylsalicylic acid before the nicotinate application (Daroczy and Temesvari, 1988; English *et al.*, 1987).

Animal model for nonimmunologic contact urticarial reactions

Animal models permit identification of agents capable of immediate contact reactions and mechanistic studies (Lahti, 1988). Guinea pig body skin reacts with rapidly appearing erythema to cinnamic aldehyde, methyl nicotinate, and dimethyl sulfoxide but not to benzoic acid, sorbic acid, or cinnamic acid. Any of these substances applied to the guinea pig ear lobe causes erythema and edema to appear. Quantification of edema by measuring changes in the ear thickness with a micrometer caliper is an accurate, reproducible. and rapid method (Lahti and Maibach, 1984).

Analogous reactions can be elicited in the ear lobes of other laboratory animals. Cinnamic aldehyde and dimethyl sulfoxide produce ear swelling in the rat and mouse, but benzoic acid, sorbic acid, cinnamic acid, diethyl fumarate, and methyl nicotinate produce no response. This suggests that either several

CHAPTER 42

■ 831

mechanisms are involved in immediate contact reactions from different substances or there are differences in the activation of mediators of inflammation between guinea pig, rat, and mouse (Lahti and Maibach, 1985a, 1985b).

The swelling response in the guinea pig ear lobe is dependent on the concentrations of the eliciting substance. The maximal response is a roughly 100 per cent increase in ear thickness, which appears within 50 mm of application.

Biopsies taken from the guinea pig ear lobe 40 mm after application of test substances show marked dermal edema and intra- and perivascular infiltrates of heterophilic (neutrophilic in humans) granulocytes: they appear to be characteristic of nonimmunologic contact urticaria in the guinea pig ear (Anderson, 1988; Lahti and Maibach, 1984; Lahti *et al.*, 1986).

A decrease in response to contact urticaria is noticed after reapplication of the test substances to the guinea pig ear on the following day (Lahti and Maibach, 1985c). The tachyphylaxis is not specific to the substance that produces it, and the reactivity to other agents decreases as well. The length of the refractory period varies with the compound used. It is 4 d for methyl nicotinate, 8 d for diethyl fumarate and cinnamic aldehyde, and up to 16 d for benzoic acid, cinnamic acid, and dimethyl sulfoxide.

The reaction of guinea pig ear lobe to nonimmunologic contact urticaria seems to be similar to that of human skin. The similarities include the morphology, the time course of maximal response, the concentrations of the eliciting substances, the tachyphylaxis phenomenon (Lahti, 1980), and the lack of an inhibitory effect of antihistamines on contact reactions (Labti, 1987; Lahti *et al.*, 1986).

Specificity of the reaction

Pyridine carboxaldehyde (PCA) is one of the many substances that can produce nonimmunologic immediate contact reactions (Archer and Cronin, 1986). It has three isomers: 2-, 3-, and 4-PCA. according to the position of the aldehyde group on the pyridine ring. 3-PCA is the strongest and 2-PCA the weakest contact reactant in both the human skin and guinea pig ear swelling test (Hannuksela *et al.*, 1989; Lahti and Maibach, 1984). Only a slight change in the molecular structure of a chemical can greatly alter its capacity to produce nonimmunologic immediate contact reactions.

42.4 DIAGNOSTIC TESTS

The diagnosis of immediate contact reactions is based on a full medical history and on skin tests with suspected substances.

42.4.1 Tests for both immunologic (ICU) and nonimmunologic contact urticaria (NICU)

The simplest test is the open test. For this test the suspected substance (fish, apple, carrot) is applied and gently rubbed on either normal-looking or slightly affected skin, usually the hand. The test site is observed for 60 min (Hannuksela, 1986). A positive result is seen as an edema and erythema reaction or as tiny intraepidermal spongiotic vesicles typical of acute eczema.

The use test requires the patient to handle the suspected agent precisely as handled when symptoms appeared. Wearing surgical gloves on wet hands to provoke contact urticaria to latex is a typical use test.

In the open test, 0. 1 ml of the test substance is spread on a 3×3 cm area of the skin of the upper back or on the extensor side of the upper arm. The test should first be performed on nondiseased skin and then, if negative, on previously or currently affected skin (Lahti and Maibach, 1986). Even in immunologic contact urticaria there may be a marked difference between skin sites in their capacity to elicit contact urticaria (Maibach, 1986). This is typical of nonimmunologic contact urticaria. The face has been considered the most sensitive skin area (Gollhausen and Kligman, 1985). Often it is desirable to apply contact urticants to skin sites suggested by the patient's history. The immunologic contact reactions usually appear within 15–20 min and nonimmunologic ones within 45–60 min after application. A positive reaction comprises a wheal-and-flare reaction and sometimes a vesicular eruption indistinguishable from that seen in eczema (Hjorth and Roed-Petersen, 1976).

42.4.2 Tests for immunologic contact urticaria (ICU)

Open application as already described is all that is required for most ICU agents. Prick testing is often the method of choice for testing patients with suspected allergic contact reactions when the open application method is negative.

The scratch test is a less standardized method than the prick test, but it is useful when nonstandardized allergens must be used (Paul, 1987). The allergen solutions in scratch testing are the same as those used in prick testing. Also,

CHAPTER 42

freeze-dried and other powdered allergens moistened with 0.1 N aqueous sodium hydroxide solution and fresh foods (e.g., potato, apple, carrot) can be used. When testing with poorly standardized or nonstandardized substances, control tests should be made on at least 20 people to avoid false interpretation of the test results.

The chamber scratch test was introduced for testing foods when commercial allergens with proven efficacy are not available (Hannuksela and Lahti, 1977). Potato, apple, and carrot lose their allergenicity when cooked, deep-frozen, or made into juice, and it is therefore best to use them fresh for skin testing.

In the chamber scratch test, the procedure is that of the ordinary scratch test but the scratch and the foodstuff are covered with a small aluminum chamber (Finn Chamber, Epitest Ltd Oy, Hyryla, Finland) for 15 min. The result is read 5 min after the removal of the chamber according to the criteria of the scratch test. Reactions at least the size of a similarly produced histamine reaction are usually clinically significant. Histamine hydrochloride (10 mg/ml) is the positive reference and aqueous 0.1 N sodium hydroxide the negative reference.

The Prausnitz-Kustner test or passive transfer test has been used in occupational dermatology for detecting immunologic contact urticaria to potato (Tuft and Blumstein, 1942) and to rubber (Kopman and Hannuksela, 1983). Today this would be generally limited to animal studies.

RAST is seldom needed for contact urticaria diagnosis, but RAST inhibition tests are used in investigating cross-allergenicity (Halmepuro and Løvenstein, 1985). For this purpose crossed radioimmunoelectrophoresis and its inhibition are also used.

Nonsteroidal anti-inflammatory drugs and antihistamines should not be taken by patients during tests for immediate contact reactions because these drugs may inhibit the reactions. Using the same test site repeatedly may result in the tachyphylaxis phenomenon and cause false negative results.

A positive open test (erythema alone or wheal and flare) is almost always of clinical significance in ICU, assuming that the same agent is not reactive in controls. With skin prick and scratch testing, great caution must be utilized to rule out non-specific reactions.

Caution: In testing for ICU when other organs are also involved, very small doses and dilute solutions are indicated to avoid reproducing systemic reactions (von Krogh and Maibach, 1982). Facilities for resuscitation should also be available.

When examining patients with a suspected allergic contact reaction, the prick, scratch, or scratch chamber tests may be done first because the test procedures are fast. The diagnosis should be based on the result of the open application test and interpreted by reviewing the clinical history and the background controls.

42.5 SUMMARY

In clinical practice, patients report immediate contact reactions after applying cosmetics or therapeutic agents and after handling food products. Not only have dermatologists and allergists been uncertain about the nature of these reactions, but manufacturers, their toxicologists, and other involved personnel have had difficulty in understanding this type of reaction and in developing less irritating products. Studies on the mechanisms of immediate contact reactions from different substances and the standardization of human and animal tests for these reactions are a challenge for future research. Dermatologists, allergists, toxicologists, and medical authorities need to combine their efforts to investigate the capacity of various environmental agents to produce immediate contact reactions, as was done in the past for delayed-type skin effects.

REFERENCES

AARONSON, C.M. (1969) Generalized urticaria from sensitivity to nifuroxime. *J. Am. Med. Assoc.* **210**, 557.

ADINOFF, A.D., TELLEZ, P. and CLARK, R.A. (1988) Atopic dermatitis and aeroallergen contact sensitivity. *J. Allergy Clin. Immunol.* **81**, 736–742.

AGRUP, G. and SJOSTEDT, L. (1985) Contact urticaria in laboratory technicians working with animals. *Acta Dermaro-Venereol. (Stockh.)* **65**, 111–115.

ANDERSEN, K.E. and MAIBACH. H.I. (1984) Multiple application delayed onset contact urticaria: Possible relation to certain unusual formalin and textile reactions. *Contact Dermatitis* **10**, 227–234.

ANDERSEN, C. (1988) Irritant contact reactions versus non-immunologic contact urticaria. *Acta DermatoVenereol. Suppl. (Stockh.)* **68**, 45–48.

APTED, J. (1988a) Acute contact urticaria from *Grevillea juniperina*. *Contact Dermatitis* **18**, 126.

APTED, J. (1988b) Acute contact urticaria from *Hakea suaveolens*. *Contact Dermatitis* **18**, 126.

ARCHER C.B. and CRONIN, E. (1986) Contact urticaria induced by pyridine carboxaldehyde. *Contact Dermatitis* **15**, 308–309.

ASSALVE, D., CICIONI, P., PERNO, P. and LISI, P. (1988) Contact urticaria and anaphylactoid reaction from cornstarch surgical glove powder. *Contact Dermatitis* **19**, 61.

AXELSSON, J.G.K., JOHANSSON, S.G.O. and WRANGSJO, K. (1987) IgE-mediated anaphylactoid reactions to rubber. *Allergy* **42**, 46–50.

BAES H. (1974) Allergic contact dermatitis to virginiamycin. *Dermarologica (Basel)* **149**, 231.

BARKER J.N.W.N., ALEGRE, V.A. and MacDONALD, D.M. (1988) Surface-bound immunoglobulin E on antigenpresenting cells in cutaneous tissue of atopic dermatitis. *J. Invest. Dermatol.* **90**, 117–121.

BERGQVIST-KARLSSON, A. (1988) Delayed and immediate-type hypersensitivity to chlorhexidine. *Contact Dermatitis* **18**, 84–88.

BERNSTEIN, D.I., GALLAGHER, J.S. and BERNSTEIN, I.L. (1983) Mealworm asthma: Clinical and immunological studies. *J. Allergy Clin. Immunol.* **72**, 475–480.

BERNSTEIN, J.E., SWIFT, R.M., KEYOUMARS, S. and LORINCZ, A.L. (1981) Inhibition of axon reflex vasodilatation by topically applied capsaicin. *J. Invest. Dermatol.* **76**, 394–395.

BLAIR, H. and PARISH, W.E. (1985) Asthma and urticaria induced by seminal plasma in a woman with IgE antibody and T-lymphocyte responsiveness to a seminal plasma antigen. *Clin. Allergy* **15**, 117–130.

BOSO, E.G. and BRESTEL, E.P. (1987) Contact urticaria to cow milk. *Allergy* **42**, 151–153.

BÖTTGER, E.M., MUCKE, C. and TRONNIER, H. (1981) Kontaktdermatitis auf neuere Ancikykotika und Kontakturtikaria. *Acta Dermato-Venereol. Suppl. (Stockh.)* **7**, 70.

BRUYNZEEL-KOOMEN, C. (1986) IgE on Langerhans cells: New insights into the pathogenesis of atopic dermatitis. *Dermatologica* **172**, 181–183.

BRUYNZEEL-KOOMEN, C., VAN WICHEN, D.F., TOONSTRA, J., BERRENS, J. and BRUYNZEEL, P.L.B. (1986) The presence of IgE molecules on epidermal Langerhans cells in patients with atopic dermatitis. *Arch. Dermatol. Res.* **278**, 199–205.

BURNS, D.A. (1987) Papular urticaria produced by the mite *Listrophorus gibbus*. *Clin. Exp. Dermatol.* **12**, 200–201.

BURRALL, B.A., HALPERN, G.M. and HUNTLEY, A.C. (1990) Chronic urticaria. *West. J. Med.* **152**(3), 268–276.

CAMARASA, J.G. (1986) Contact urticaria to naphthylacetic acid. *Contact Dermatitis* **14**, 113.

CAPRON, M., CAPRON, A., DESSAINT, J., JOHANSSON, S. and PRIN, L. (1981) Fc-receptors for IgE on human and rat eosinophils. *J. Immunol.* **126**, 2087–2092.

CARRILLO, T., CUEVAS, M., MUNOZ, T., HINOJOSA, M. and MONEO, I. (1986) Contact urticaria and rhinitis from latex surgical gloves. *Contact Dermatitis* **15**, 69–72.

DANNAKER, C.J., MAIBACH, H.I. and O'MALLEY, M. (1993) Contact urticaria and anaphylaxis to the fungicide chlorothalonil. *Cutis* **52**, 312–315.

DAROCZY, J. and TEMESVARI. E. (1988) Light microscopic and electron microscopic (EM) examination of contact urticaria. *Contact Dermatitis* **19**, 156–158.

DE GROOT, A.C. and GERKENS, F. (1989) Contact urticaria from a chemical textile finish. *Contact Dermatitis* **20**, 63–64.

DE HAAN, P., VON BLOMBERG-VAN DER FLIER, B.M., DE GROOT, J., NIEBOER, C. and BRUYNZEEL, D. P. (1994) The risk of sensibilization and contact urticaria upon topical application of fumaric acid derivatives. *Dermatology* **188**, 126–130.

DÍAZ SÁNCHEZ, C., LAGUNA MARTINEZ, J., IGLESIAS CADARSO, A. and VIDAL PAN, C. (1994) Protein contact dermatitis associated with food allergy to fish. *Contact Dermatitis* **31**, 55–57.

DOOMS-GOOSSENS, A., DEVEYLDER. H., DURON, C., DOOMS, M. and DEGREEF, H. (1986a) Airborne contact urticaria due to cinchona. *Contact Dermatitis* **15**, 258.

DOOMS-GOOSSENS, A., DURON, C., LONEKE, J. and DEGREEF, H. (1986b) Contact urticaria due to nylon. *Contact Dermatitis* **14**, 63.

DUCOMBS, G., LAMY, M., MICHEL, M., PRADINAUD, R., JAMET, P., VINCENDEAU, P., MALEVILLE, J. and TEXIER, L. (1983) La papillonite de Guyane Francaise. Etude clinique et épidémiologique. *Ann. Dermatol. Venereol.* **110**, 309–816.

EDWARDS, E.K. and EDWARDS, E.K. (1984a) Contact urticaria provoked by pickels. *Cutis* **33**, 230.

EDWARDS, E.K. and EDWARDS, E.K. (1984b) Contact unicaria and allergic contact dermatitis caused by paraphenylenediamine. *Cutis* **34**, 87–88.

EDWARDS, E.K., EDWARDS, E.K. and KOWALEZYK, A.P. (1986) Contact urticaria and allergic contact dermatitis to saddleback caterpillar with histologic correlation. *Int. J. Dermatol.* **25**, 467.

■ CHAPTER 42 ■

ELPERN, D.J. (1985a) The syndrome of immediate reactivities (contact urticaria syndrome). An historical study from a dermatology practice. I. Age, sex, race and putative substances. *Hawaii Med. J.* **44**, 426–439.

ELPERN, D.J. (1985b) The syndrome of immediate reactivities (contact urticaria syndrome). An historical study from a dermatology practice. II. The atopic diathesis and drug reactions. *Hawaii Med. J.* **44**, 466–468.

ELPERN, D.J. (1986) The syndrome of immediate reactivities (contact urticaria syndrome). An historical study from a dermatology practice. III. General discussion and conclusions. *Hawaii Med. J.* **45**, 10–12.

EMMONS, W.W. and MARKS, J.G. (1985) Immediate and delayed reactions to cosmetic ingredients. *Contact Dermatitis* **13**, 258–265.

ENGLISH, J.S.C., WINKELMANN, R.K., LOUBACK, J.B., GREAVES, M.W. and MACDONALD, D.M. (1987) The cellular inflammatory response in nicotinate skin reactions. *Br. J. Dermatol.* **116**, 341–349.

ESTLANDER, T., JOLANKI, R. and KANERVA, L. (1987) Contact urticaria from rubber gloves: a detailed description of four cases. *Acta Dermato-Venereol. Suppl. (Stockh.)* **134**, 98–102.

FISHER, A.A. (1987) Contact urticaria and anaphylactoid reaction due to corn starch surgical glove powder. *Contact Dermatitis* **16**, 224–225.

FISHER, A.A. (1989) Contact urticaria from chlorhexidine. *Cutis* **43**, 17–18.

FRANCOIS, A., HENIN, P., CARLI BASSET, C. and GINIES, G. (1970) Anaphylactic shock following applications of Milian's solution. *Bull. Soc. Fr. Dermatol. Syphiligr.* **77**, 834.

FREITAS, J.P. and BRANDÃO, F.M. (1986) Contact urticaria to chlorocresol. *Contact Dermatitis* **15**, 252.

FROSCH, P.J., WAHL, R., BAHMER, F.A. and MAASCH H.J. (1986) Contact urticaria to rubber gloves is IgE-mediated. *Contact Dermatitis* **14**, 241–245.

FUNK, J.O. and MAIBACH, H.I. (1994) Propylene glycol dermatitis: Re-evaluation of an old problem. *Contact Dermatitis* **31**, 236–241

GOLLHAUSEN, R. and KLIGMAN, A.M. (1985) Human assay for identifying substances which induce non-allergic contact urticaria: The NICU-test. *Contact Dermatitis* **13**, 98–106.

GONCALO, M., GONGALO, S. and MORENO, A. (1987) Immediate and delayed sensitivity to chlorocresol. *Contact Dermatitis* **17**, 46–47.

GOODFIELD, M.J.D. and SAIHAN E.M. (1988) Contact urticaria to naphtha present in a solvent. *Contact Dermatitis* **18**, 187.

GOTTMANN-LÜCKERATH, I. (1982) Kontakturticaria nach DermoxinR. *Soc. Proc. Dermatosen* **30**, 124.

GRATTAN, C.E.H. and HARMAN, R.R.M. (1985) Contact urticaria to strawberry. *Contact Dermatitis* **13**, 191–192.

GROB, J.J., POMMIER, G., ROBAGLIA, A., COLLET-VILLETTE, A.M. and BONERANDI, J.J. (1987) Contact urticaria from rifamycin. *Contact Dermatitis* **16**, 284–285.

GUILL, A., GOETTE, K., KNIGHT, C.G., PECK, C.C. and LUPTON, G.P. (1979) Erythema multiforme and urticaria. *Arch. Dermatol.* **115**, 742.

GUIN, J.D., MEYER, B.N., DRAKE, R.D. and HAFFLEY, P. (1984) The effect of quenching agents on contact urticaria caused by cinnamic aldehyde. *J. Am. Acad. Dermatol.* **10**, 45–51.

HALMEPURO, L. and LØVENSTEIN, H. (1985) Immunological investigation of possible structural similarities between pollen antigens and antigens in apple, carrot and celery tuber. *Allergy* **40**, 264–272.

HALMEPURO, L., VUONTELA, K., KALIMO, K. and BJORKSTEN, F. (1984) Cross-reactivity of IgE antibodies with allergens in birch pollen, fruits and vegetables. *Int. Arch. Allergy Appl. Immunol.* **74**, 235–240.

HANNUKSELA, M. (1980) Atopic contact dermatitis. *Contact Dermatitis* **6**, 30.

HANNUKSELA, M. (1986) Contact urticaria from foods. In ROE, D. (ed.) *Nutrition and the Skin.* New York: Alan R. Liss, 153–162.

HANNUKSELA, M. and LAHTI, A. (1977) Immediate reactions to fruits and vegetables. *Contact Dermatitis* **3**, 79–84.

HANNUKSELA, A., LAHTI, A. and HANNUKSELA, M. (1989) Nonimmunologic immediate contact reactions to three isomers of pyridine carboxaldehyde. In FROSCH, P.J., DOOMS-GOOSSENS, A., LACHAPELLE, J.M., RYCROFT, R.J.G. and SCHEPER, R.J. (eds) *Current Topics in Contact Dermatitis,* Berlin: Springer-Verlag, 448–452.

HATCH, K.L. and MAIBACH, H.I. (1985) Textile fiber dermatitis. *Contact Dermatitis* **12**, 1–11.

HELTON, J. and STORRS, F. (1994) The burning mouth syndrome: Lack of a role for contact urticaria and contact dermatitis. *J. Am. Acad. Dermatol.* **31**(2 Pt. 1), 201–205.

HENRY, J.C., TSCHEN, E.H. and BECKER, L.E. (1979) Contact urticaria to parabens. *Arch. Dermatol.* **115**, 1231.

HJORTH, N. and ROED-PETERSEN, J. (1976) Occupational protein contact dermatitis in foodhandlers. *Contact Dermatitis* **2**, 28–42.

CHAPTER 42

JOHANSSON, G. (1988) Contact urticaria from levomepromazine. *Contact Dermatitis* **19**, 304.

JOHANSSON, G. and LAHTI, A. (1988) Topical non-steroidal anti-inflammatory drugs inhibit non-immunologic immediate contact reactions. *Contact Dermatitis* **19**, 161–165.

JOLANKI, R., ESTLANDER. T. and KANERVA, L. (1987) Occupational contact dermatitis and contact urticaria caused by epoxy resins. *Acta Dermato-Venereol. Suppl. (Stockh.)* **134**, 90–94.

JOSEPH, M., TONNEL, A., CAPRON A. and VOISIN, C. (1980) Enzyme release and super oxide anion production by human alveolar macrophages stimulated with immunoglobulin E. *Clin. Exp. Immunol.* **40**, 416–422.

JOSEPH, M., AURIAULT, C., CAPRON, A., VORNG, H. and VIENS, P. (1983) A new function for platelets: IgE-dependent killing of schistosomes. *Nature (Lond.)* **303**, 810–812.

KALVERAM, K.-J., KASTNER, H. and FROCK, G. (1986) Detection of specific IgE antibodies in veterinarians suffering from contact urticaria. *Z. Hautkr.* **61**, 75–81.

KASSEN, B. and MITCHELL, J.C. (1974) Contact urticaria from a vitamin E preparation in two siblings. *Contact Derm. Newslett.* **16**, 482.

KAVLI, G. and MOSENG, D. (1987) Contact urticaria from mustard in fish stick production. *Contact Dermatitis* **17**, 153–155.

KELLER, K. and SCHWANITZ, H.I. (1993) Combined immediate and delayed type hypersensitivity to Mezlocillin. *H + G* **68**(3), 178–180.

KLEINHANS, D. (1985) Kontakt-Urtikaria. *Dermatosen* **33**, 198–203.

KLEINHANS, D. and ZWISSLER, H. (1980) Anaphylaktischer Schock nach Anwendung einer Benzocainhaltigen Salbe. *Z. Hautkr.* **55**, 945.

KOPMAN, A. and HANNUKSELA, M. (1983) Contact urticaria to rubber. *Duodecim* **99**, 221–224.

KREMSER, M. and LINDEMAYR, W. (1983) Celery allergy (celery contact urticaria syndrome) and relation to allergies to other plant antigens. *Wien. Klin. Wochenschr.* **95**, 838–843.

KUJALA, T. and LAHRI, A. (1989) Duration of inhibition of non-immunologic immediate contact reactions by acetylsalicylic acid. *Contact Dermatitis* **21**, 60–61.

KULZE, A. and GREAVES, M. (1988) Contact urticaria caused by stinging nettles. *Br. J. Dermatol.* **119**, 269–270.

LAHTI, A. (1980) Non-immunologic contact urticaria. *Acta Dermato-Venereol. (Stockh.)* 60(Suppl. 91), 1–49.

LAHTI, A. (1986a) Contact urticaria and respiratory symptoms from tulips and lilies. *Contact Dermatitis* 14, 317–319.

LAHTI, A. (1986b) Contact urticaria to plants. *Dermatol. Clin.* 4, 127–136.

LAHTI, A. (1987) Terfenadine (Hi-antagonist) does not inhibit non-immunologic contact urticaria. *Contact Dermatitis* 16, 220–223.

LAHTI, A. (1988) Non-immunologic contact urticaria. Animal tests and their relevance. *Acta DermatoVenereol. Suppl. (Stockh.)* 68, 43–44.

LAHTI, A. and MAIBACH, H.I. (1984) An animal model for nonimmunologic contact urticaria. *Toxicol. Appl. Pharmacol.* 76, 219–224.

LAHTI, A. and MAIBACH, H.I. (1985a) Contact urticaria from diethyl fumarate. *Contact Dermatitis* 12, 139–140.

LAHTI, A. and MAIBACH, H.I. (1985b) Species specificity of nonimmunologic contact urticaria: Guinea pig, rat and mouse. *J. Am. Acad. Dermatol.* 13, 66–69.

LAHTI, A. and MAIBACH, H.I. (1985c) Long refractory period after one application of nonimmunologic contact urticaria agents to guinea pig ear. *J. Am Acad. Dermatol.* 13, 585–589.

LAHTI, A. and MAIBACH, H.I. (1986) Immediate contact reactions (contact urticaria syndrome). In MAIBACH, H. (ed.) *Occupational and Industrial Dermatology*, 2nd ed., Chicago: Year Book Medical, 32–44

LAHTI, A. and MAIBACH, H.I. (1987) Immediate contact reactions: Contact urticaria syndrome. *Semin. Dermatol* 6, 313–320.

LAHTI, A., OIKARINEN, A., YLIKORKALA, O. and VIINIKKA, L. (1983) Prostaglandins in contact urticaria induced by benzoic acid. *Acta. Dermato-Venereol. (Stockh.)* 63, 425–427.

LAHTI, A., McDONALD, D.M., TAMMI, R. and MAIBACH, H.I. (1986) Pharmacological studies on nonimmunologic contact urticaria in guinea pig. *Arch. Dermatol Res.* 279, 44–49.

LAHTI, A., VAANANEN, A., KOKKONEN, E.-L. and HANNUKSELA, M. (1987) Acetylsalicylic acid inhibits non-immunologic contact urticaria. *Contact Dermatitis* 16, 133–135.

LARKÖ, O., LINDSTEDT, G., LUNDBERG, P. A. and MOBACKEN, H. (1983) Biochemical and clinical studies in a case of contact urticafla to potato. *Contact Dermatitis* 9, 108–114.

CHAPTER 42

LARMI. E. (1989) Systemic effect of ultraviolet irradiation on non-immunologic immediate contact reactions to benzoic acid and methyl nicotinate. *Acta Dermato-Venereol. (Stockh.)* **69**, 296–301.

LARMI, E., LAHTI, A. and HANNUKSELA, M. (1988) Ultraviolet light inhibits nonimmunologic immediate contact reactions to benzoic acid. *Arch. Dermatol. Res.* **280**, 420–423.

LARMI, E., LAHTI, A. and HANNUKSELA, M. (1989) Effects of capsaicin and topical anesthesia on nonimmunologic immediate contact reactions to benzoic acid and methyl nicotinate. In FROSCH, P.J., DOOMS-GOOSSENS, A., LACHAPELLE, J.-M., RYCROFT, R.J.G. and SCHEPER, R.J. (eds) *Current Topics in Contact Dermatitis*, Berlin: Springer-Verlag, 441–477.

LA ROSA, M., CREA, C.F., DI FRANCESCO, S., DI PAOLA, M. and CASTIGLIONE, N. (1986) Fennel allergy: Case report. Abstr. *3rd Int. Symp. Immunological and Clinical Problems of Food Allergy*, Taormina, Giardini Naxos. Italy. October 1–4.

LARSEN W.G. (1985) Perfume dermatitis. *J. Am. Acad. Dermatol.* **12**, 1–9.

LEUNG, D.Y., SCHNEEBERGER, E.E., SIRAGANIAN, R.P., GEHA, R.S. and BHAN, A.K. (1987) The presence of IgE on macrophages and dendritic cells infiltrating into the skin lesion of atopic dermatitis. *Clin. Immunol. Immunopathol.* **42**, 328–337.

LEWIS-JONES, M.S. (1985) Papular urticaria caused by *Dermestes maculatus* Degeer. *Clin. Exp. Dermatol.* **10**, 181.

LEZAUN, A., IGEA, J.M., QUIRCE, S., CUEVAS, M., PARRA, F., ALONSO, M.D., MARTIN, I.A. and CANO, M.S. (1994) Asthma and contact urticaria caused by rice in a housewife. *Allergy* **49**, 92–95.

LINDSKOV, R. (1982) Contact urticaria to formaldehyde. *Contact Dermatitis* **8**, 333.

LOMBARDI, P., GIORGINI, S. and ACHILLE. A. (1983) Contact urticaria from aminophenazone. *Contact Dermatitis* **9**, 428–429.

LOVELL, C.R. and RYCROFT, R.J.C. (1984) Contact urticaria from winged bean (*Psophocarpus tetragonolobus*). *Contact Dermatitis* **10**, 310–318.

LOVELL C.R., CRONIN, E. and RHODES, E.L. (1986) Photocontact urticaria from chlorpromazine. *Contact Dermatitis* **14**, 290–291.

LÖWENFELD, W. (1928) Uberempfindlichkeit gegen lodthion mit gleichzeitiger urtikarieller reaction. *Derm. Wochenschr.* **78**, 502.

MAIBACH, H.I. (1976) Immediate hypersensitivity in hand dermatitis: Role of food contact dermatitis. *Arch. Dermatol.* **112**, 1289–1291.

MAIBACH, H.I. (1986) Regional variation in elicitation of contact unicaria syndrome (immediate hypersensitivity syndrome): Shrimp. *Contact Dermatitis* **15**, 100.

MAIBACH, H.I. and JOHNSON, H.L. (1975) Contact urticaria syndrome to diethyl-taluamide (immediate type hypersensitivity). *Arch. Derm.* **111**, 726–730.

MELEWICZ, F. and SPIEGELBERG. H. (1980) Fc-receptors for IgE on a subpopulation of human peripheral blood monocytes. *J. Immunol.* **125**, 1026–1031.

MELINO, M., TONI, F. and RIGUZZI, G. (1987) Immunologic contact urticaria to fish. *Contact Dermatitis* **17**, 182.

MENNÉ, T. and MAIBACH, H.I., eds. (1994) *Hand Eczema.* Boca Raton. FL: CRC Press.

MITCHELL, E.B., CROW, J., WILLIAMS, G. and PLATTS-MILLS, T.A.E. (1986) Increase in skin mast cells following chronic house dust mite exposure. *Br. J. Dermatol.* **114**, 65–73.

MITTELBACH, F. (1983) Urticaria and Quincke's edema caused by *Chironomidae (Chirononius thummi thummi)* as fishfood. *Z. Hautkr.* **58**, 1548–1555.

MIZUTANI, H., OHYANAGI, S. and SHIMIZU, M. (1994) Anaphylactic shock related to occupational handling of Cefotiam dihydrochloride [letter]. *Clin. Exp. Dermatol.* **19**(5), 449.

MONK, B.E. (1988) Contact urticaria to locusts. *Br. J. Dermatol.* **118**, 707–708.

MORALES, C., BASOMBA A., CARREIRA, J. and SASTRE, A. (1989) Anaphylaxis produced by rubber glove contact. Case reports and immunological identi-fication of the antigens involved. *Clin. Exp. Allergy* **19**, 425–430.

MORREN, M.-A., JANSSENS, V., DOOMS-GOOSENS, A., VAN HOEYVELD, E., CORNELIS, A., DE WOLF-PEETERS, C. and HEREMANS, A. (1993) Alpha-amylase. a flour additive: An important cause of protein contact dermatitis in bakers. *J. Am. Acad. Dermatol.* **29**, 723–728.

Muñoz, D., LEANIZBARRUTIA, I., LOBERA, T. and DE CORRES, F. (1985) Anaphylaxis from contact with carrot. *Contact Dermatitis* **13**, 345–346.

NAGANO, T., KANAO, K. and SUGAI, T. (1984) Allergic contact urticaria caused by raw prawns and shrimps: Three cases. *J. Allergy Clin. Immunol.* **74**, 489–493.

NAJEM, N. and HULL, D. (1989) Langerhans cells in delayed skin reactions to inhalant allergens in atopic dermatitis—An electron microscopic studv. *Clin. Exp. Dermatol.* **4**, 218–222

CHAPTER 42

NETHERCOTT, J.R., LAWRENCE, M.J., ROY, A.-M. and GIBSON, B.L. (1984) Airborne contact urticaria due to sodium benzoate in a pharmaceutical manufacturing plant. *J. Occup. Med.* **26**, 734–736.

NIINIMAKI, A. (1987) Scratch-chamber tests in food handler dermatitis. *Contact Dermatitis* **16**, 11–20.

NILSSON, E. (1985) Contact sensitivity and urticaria in "wet" work. *Contact Dermatitis* **13**, 321–328.

NISHIOKA, K., DOI, T. and KATAYAMA, I. (1984) Histamine release in contact urticaria. *Contact Dermatitis* **11**, 191.

OLIVER, F., AMON, E.U., BREATHNACH, A., FRANCIS, D.M., SARATHCHANDRA, P., KOBZA BLACK, A. and GREAVES, M.W. (1991) Contact urticaria due to the common stinging nettle (*Urtica dioica*)—histological, ultrastructural and pharmacological studies. *Clin. Exp. Dermatol.* **16**, 1–7.

ORANJE, A.P., AARSEN, R.S., MULDER, P.G., VAN TOORENENBERGEN, A.W., LIEFAARD, G. and DIEGES, P.H. (1992) Food immediate-contact hypersensitivity (FICH) and elimination diet in young children with atopic dermatitis. Preliminary results in 107 children. *Acta Dermato-Venereol Suppl.* **176**, 41–44.

ORANJE, A.P., DE WAARD-VAN DER SPEK, F.B., VAN OOSTENDE, L., AARSEN, R.S.R., VAN TOORENENBERGEN, A.W. and DIEGES, P.H. (1994) Food-induced contact urticaria syndrome (CUS) in young children with atopic dermatitis: Practical consequences. *J. Eur. Acad. Dermatol. Venereol.* **3**, 295–301.

PAUL, E. (1987) Skin reactions to food and food constituents—Allergic and pseudoallergic reactions. *Z Hautkr. Suppl.* **62**, 79–87.

PAYERO, M.L.P., CORRECHER, B.L. and GARCIA-PEREZ, A. (1985) Contact urticaria and dermatitis from phosphorous sesquisulphide. *Contact Dermatitis* **13**, 126–127.

PECQUET, C. and LEYNADIER, F. (1993) IgE mediated allergy to natural rubber latex in 100 patients. *Clin. Rev. Allergy* **11**, 381–384.

PICARDO, M., ROVINA, R., CRISTAUDO, A., CANNISTRACI, C. and SANTUCCI, B. (1988) Contact urticaria from Tilia (lime). *Contact Dermatitis* **19**, 72—73.

PIGATTO, P.D., RIVA, F., ALTOMARE, G.F. and PAROTELLI, R. (1983) Short-term anaphylactic antibodies in contact urticaria and generalized anaphylaxis to apple. *Contact Dermatitis* **9**, 511.

PINOL, J. and CARAPETO, F.J. (1984) Contact urticaria to etofenamate. *Contact Dermatitis* **11**, 132–133.

QUIRCE, S., GARCIA-FIGUEROA, B., OLAGUIBEL, J.M., MURO, M.D. and TABAR, A.I. (1993) Occupational asthma and contact urticaria from dried flowers of *Limonium tataricum*. *Allergy* **48**, 285–290.

REITAMO, S., VISA, K., KAHONEN, K., KAYHKO, K., STUBB, S. and SALO, O.P. (1986) Eczematous reactions in atopic patients caused by epicucaneous testing with inhalant allergens. *Br. I. Dermatol.* **114**, 303–309.

REUNALA, T., BJORKSTEN, F., FORSTROM, L. and KANERVA, L. (1983) IgE-mediated occupational allergy to a spider mite. *Clin. Allery* **13**, 383–388.

RILLIET, A., HUNZIKER, N. and BRUN, R. (1980) Alcohol contact urticaria syndrome (immediate type hypersensitivity). *Dermatologica (Basel)* **161**, 361.

RIVERS, J.K. and RYCROFT, R.J.G. (1987) Occupational allergic contact urticaria from colophony. *Contact Dermatitis* **17**, 181.

RUDZKI, B. and REBANDEL, P. (1985) Occupational contact urticaria from penicillin. *Contact Dermatitis* **13**, 192.

RUDZKI, B., REBANDEL, P. and GRZYWA, Z. (1985) Incidence of contact urticaria. *Contact Dermatitis* **13**, 279.

SALO, O.P., MAKINEN-KILJUNEN, S. and JUNTUNEN, K. (1986) Milk causes a rapid urticarial reaction on the skin of children with atopic dermatitis and milk allergy. *Acta Dermato-Venereol. (Stockh.)* **66**, 438–442.

SANIUCCI, B., CRISTAUDO, A. and PICARDO, M. (1985) Contact urticaria from papain in a soft lens solution. *Contact Dermatitis* **12**, 233.

SCHEWACH-MILLET, M. and SHPIRO, D. (1985) Urticaria and angioedema due to topically applied chloramphenicol ointment. *Arch. Dermatol.* **121**, 587.

SEIFERT, H.U., WAHL, R., VOCKS, E., BORELLI, S. and MAASCH, H.J. (1987) Immunoglobulin E-mediated contact urticaria and bronchial asthma caused by household rubber gloves containing latex. 3 case reports [German]. *Dermatosen* **35**, 137–139.

SHELLEY, W.B., SHELLEY, E.D. and HO. A.K.S. (1983) Cholinergic urticaria: Acetylcholine-receptor dependent immediate-type hypersensitivity reaction to copper. *Lancet* **i**, 843–846.

SOSCHIN, D. and LEYDEN, J.J. (1986) Sorbic acid-induced erythema and edema. *J. Am. Acad. Dermatol.* **14**, 234–241.

SPANER, D., DOLOVICH J., TARLO, S., SUSSMAN, G. and BUTTOO, K. (1989) Hypersensitivity to natural latex. *J. Allergy Clin. Immunol* **83**, 1135–1137.

STEINMAN, H.K., LOVELL, C.R. and CRONIN, E. (1984) Immediate-type hypersensitivity to *Crataegus monogyna* (hawthorn). *Contact Dermatitis* **11**, 321.

CHAPTER 42

STERRY, W. and SCHMOLL. M. (1985) Contact urticaria and dermatitis from self-adhesive pads. *Contact Dermatitis* **13**, 284–285.

TACHIBANA, S., HORIO, T. and HAYAKAWA, M. (1977) Contact urticaria and dermatitis due to fiuocinonide cream. *Acta Dermatol. (Kyoto)* **72**, 141.

TANAKA, I., MORIWAKI, S. and HORIA, T. (1987) Occupational dermatitis with simultaneous immediate and delayed allergy to *Chrysanthemum*. *Contact Dermatitis* **16**, 152– 154.

TARVAINEN, K., KANERVA, I., TUPASELA, O., GRENQUIST-NORDEN, B., JOLANKI, R., ESTLANDER, T. and KESKINEN, H. (1991) Allergy from cellulase and xylanase enzymes. *Clin. Exp. Dermatol.* **21**, 609–615.

TEE, R.D., GORDON, D.J., HAWKINS, E.R., NUNN, A.J., LACEY, J., VENABLES, K.M., COOTER, R.J., McCAFFERY, A.R. and NEWMAN TAYLOR, A.J. (1988) Occupational allergy to locusts: An investigation of the sources of the allergen. *J. Allergy Clin. Immunol.* **81**, 517–525.

TEMESVARI, B. (1984) Contact urticaria from paraphenylenediamine. *Contact Dermatitis* **11**, 125.

TIGALONOWA, M., BRAATHEN, L.R. and LEA, T. (1988) IgE on Langerhans cells in the skin of patients with atopic dermatitis and birch allergy. *Allergy* **43**, 464–468.

TOSTI, A., BETTOLI, V., IANNINI, G. and FORLANI, L. (1986) Contact urticaria from polypropylene. *Contact Dermatitis* **15**, 51.

TOSTI, A., MELINO, M. and VERONESI, S. (1987) Contact urticaria to tobacco. *Contact Dermatitis* **16**, 225–226.

TRUNELL, T.N., WAISMAN, M. and TRUNELL, T.L. (1985) Contact dermatitis caused by *Brucella*. *Cutis* **35**, 379–381.

TUER, W.F., JAMES, W.D. and SUMMERS, R.J. (1986) Contact urticaria to Ophenylphenate. *Ann. Allergy* **56**, 19–21.

TUFT, L. and BLUMSTEIN, G.I. (1942) Studies in food allergy II. Sensitization to fresh fruits: Clinical and experimental observations. *J. Allergy* **13**, 574–581.

TURJANMAA, K. (1987) Incidence of immediate allergy to latex gloves in hospital personnel. *Contact Dermatitis* **17**, 270–275.

TURJANMAA, K. (1994) Hand eczema from rubber gloves. In MENNÉ, T. and MAIBACH, H.I. (eds) *Hand Eczema*, Boca Raton. FL: CRC Press, 255–260.

TURJANMAA. K. and REUNALA, T. (1988) Contact urticaria from rubber gloves. *Dermatol. Clin.* **6**, 47–51.

TURJANMAA, K. and REUNALA, T. (1989) Condoms as a source of latex allergen and cause of contact urticaria. *Contact Dermatitis* **20**, 360–364.

TURJANMAA, K., REUNALA, T., TUIMALA, R. and KARKKAINEN, T. (1988a) Allergy to latex gloves: Unusual complication during delivery. *Br. J. Dermatol.* **297**, 1029.

TURJANMAA, K., REUNALA, T. and RASANEN, L. (1988b) Comparison of diagnostic methods in latex surgical glove contact urticaria. *Contact Dermatitis* **19**, 241–247.

TURJANMAA, K., LAURILA, K., MAKINEN-KILJUNEN, S. and REUNALA, T. (1988c) Rubber contact urticaria. Allergenic properties of 19 brands of latex gloves. *Contact Dermatitis* **19**, 362–367.

TURJANMAA, K., RASANEN, L., LEHTO, M., MAKINEN-KILIUNEN, S. and REUNALA, T. (1989) Basophil histamine release and lymphocyte proliferation tests in latex contact urticaria. *Allergy* **44**, 181–186.

VALDIVIESO, R., MONEO, I., POLA, J., MUNOZ, T., ZAPATA, C., HINOJOSA, M. and LOSADA, B. (1989) Occupational asthma and contact urticaria caused by buckwheat flour. *Ann. Allergy* **63**, 149–152.

VALSECCHI, R. and CAINELLI, T. (1987) Contact urticaria from nickel. *Contact Dermatitis* **17**, 187.

VALSECCHI, R. and CAINELLI, T. (1989) Contact urticaria from dog saliva. *Contact Dermatitis* **20**, 62.

VALSECCHI, R., FOIADELLI, L., RESEGHETTI, A. and CAINELLI, T. (1986) Generalized urticaria from DNCB. *Contact Dermatitis* **14**, 254–255.

VAN DER MEEREN, H.L.M. and VAN ERP, P.E.J. (1986) Life-threatening contact urticaria from glove powder. *Contact Dermatitis* **14**, 190–191.

VAN HECKE, B. and SANTOSA, S. (1985) Contact urticaria to DNCB. *Contact Dermatitis* **12**, 282.

VARIGOS, G.A. and NURSE, D.S. (1986) Contact urticaria from methyl ethyl ketone. *Contact Dermatitis* **15**, 259–260.

VEIEN, N.K., HATTEL, T., JUSTESEN, O. and NORHOLM, A. (1987) Dietary restrictions in the treatment of adult patients with eczema. *Contact Dermatitis* **17**, 223–228.

VON KROGH, G. and MAIBACH, H.I. (1982) The contact urticaria syndrome— 1982. *Semin. Dermatol.* **1**, 59–66.

WAHL, R. and KLEINHANS, D. (1989) IgE-mediated allergic reactions to fruit gums and investigation of cross-reactivity between gelatine and modified gelatine-containing products. *Clin. Exp. Allergy* **19**, 77–80.

CHAPTER 42

WALLENEREN, J. and MOLLER, H. (1986) Effect of capsaicin on some experimental inflammations in human skin. *Acta Dermato-Venereol. (Stockh.)* **66**, 375–380.

WEISSENBACH, T., WUTRICH, B. and WEIHE, W.H. (1988) Allergies to laboratory animals. An epidemiological allergological study in persons exposed to laboratory animals. *Schweiz. Med. Wochenschr.* **118**, 930–938.

WHITE, I.R. and CRONIN, E. (1984) Irritant contact urticaria to diethyl fumarate. *Contact Dermatitis* **10**, 315.

WILKIN, J. K. and FORTNER, O. (1985) Ethnic contact urticaria to alcohol. *Contact Dermatitis* **12**, 118–120.

WRANGSJO, K., MELLSTROM, O. and AXELSSON, G. (1986) Discomfort from rubber gloves indicating contact urticaria. *Contact Dermatitis* **15**, 79–84.

WRANGSJO, K., WAHLBERG, J.E. and AXELSSON, I.G. (1988) IgB-mediated allergy to natural rubber in 30 patients with contact urticaria. *Contact Dermatitis* **19**, 264–271.

WUTHRICH, B. and DIETSCHI R. (1985) The celery-carrot-mugwort-condiment syndrome: Skin test and RAST results. *Schweiz. Med. Wochenschr.* **115**, 258–264.

YODOI, J. and ISKIZAKA, K. (1979) Lymphocytes bearing Fc-receptors for IgE. Presence of human and rat lymphocytes and Fc-receptors. *J. Immunol.* **122**, 2577–2583.

YOSHIKAWA, M. (1985) Skin lesions of papular urticaria induced experimentally by *Chyletus malaccensis* and *Chelacaropsis* sp. (*Acari. Cheyletidae*). *J. Med Entomol.* **22**, 115–117.

An Optimized In Vitro Approach to Assess Skin Irritation and Phototoxicity of Topical Vehicles

**BART DE WEVER, MARTIN ROSDY
AND ALAN M GOLDBERG**

Contents

43.1 Introduction

43.2 Human epidermis reconstituted in chemically defined medium: characteristics and advantages

43.3 *In vitro* analysis of epidermal toxicity based on Multiple Endpoint Analysis MEA

43.4 Conclusion

43.1 INTRODUCTION

Today's litigious social climate requires an extensive testing regimen for any new product that is placed on the market by industry. The acceptance of new products, cosmetics, household goods, industrial chemicals and pharmaceuticals is based in part on the use of non-animal testing methods to evaluate safety. Over the last 20 years, there has been many attempts to utilize *in vitro* approaches to replace whole animal methods. One problem has been the multiple approaches with each test to examining a single endpoint. In this chapter we propose an integrated strategy for *in vitro* skin irritation and photo-toxicity risk assessment based on the use of human epidermis, reconstituted *in vitro* in chemically defined medium, coupled to an optimized analytical evaluation of multiple *in vitro* toxicity parameters (MEA: Multiple Endpoint Analysis), including histology, epidermal tissue viability and the release of pro-inflammatory mediators by the epidermal keratinocytes. This approach increases the effectiveness and predictability of pre-clinical testing.

43.2 HUMAN EPIDERMIS RECONSTITUTED IN CHEMICALLY DEFINED MEDIUM: CHARACTERISTICS AND ADVANTAGES

In the 1980s it was generally accepted by the scientific community that epidermal tissue regeneration could not be accomplished without the presence of bovine serum (undefined mixtures of growth factors and lipids), supplemented to culture medium, and dermal components or fibroblasts-collagen matrices (Asselineau *et al.*, 1986; O'Keefe *et al.*, 1987; Prunièras *et al.*, 1983; Régnier *et al.*, 1988; Schürer *et al.*, 1989; Boyce *et al.*, 1990; Bell *et al.*, 1991; Tinois *et al.*, 1991; Gay *et al.*, 1992; Fleischmeyer *et al.*, 1993; De Wever *et al.*, 1994; Gibbs *et al.*, 1997). Three dimensional skin models produced in the presence of serum are however of limited success: they demonstrate major disadvantages because of their undefined manufacturing conditions resulting in uneven reproducibility, and the relevancy of the test results obtained with these epidermal models for skin toxicity, percutaneous absorption or skin efficacy, have been questioned (Lenoir *et al.*, 1990). As a result, many companies have been reluctant to adopt such "incomplete" models in their testing programs.

Improvement of the cell culture conditions and the use of chemically defined medium has led to the optimization of epidermal tissue models (Rosdy and Clauss, 1990): by cultivating second passage normal human keratinocytes in chemically defined modified MCDB-153 medium on inert filter substrates at the air-liquid interface for 17 days, a fully differentiated epithelium having features of normal epidermis has been obtained *in vitro*. In this model, the basal cells synthesize and secrete all major markers of hemidesmosomes, the lamina lucida, and a basement membrane-like structure is identifiable (Rosdy *et al.*, 1993). This suggests that the presence of added serum and dermal components are not required for epidermal reconstruction. In fact, a structurally and biochemically normal permeability barrier is obtained when no serum or sphingolipids are included in the defined medium (Rosdy *et al.*, 1996; Rosdy *et al.*, 1997; Doucet *et al.*, 1997).

Fartasch and Ponec described the maturation of the barrier function in these epidermal cultures as comparable to the ontogeny of epidermal barrier formation in mammalian skin *in vivo* (Fartasch *et al.*, 1996a, b). In the early stages of epidermal differentiation of this tissue model (day 2–4), hyperprolif- erative markers such as keratin-13 and 16 are clearly expressed and increasing thickening of the epidermal layers is observed; however at day 13–16 of culture, i.e. as soon as the formation of the barrier function is completed, epidermal thickness decreases, K13 and K16 are no longer expressed, and a normalization of the expression of differentiation and proliferation markers is seen. Additionally, biochemical analysis of epidermal lipids of the mature epidermal tissues shows a profile similar to *in vivo* human epidermis, with physiological amounts of free fatty acids and ceramides (Maria Ponec: personal communi- cations). The addition of Vitamin C analogs (Ponec *et al.*, 1997) assists in the equilibration of the relative amounts of ceramides (Ramdin *et al.*, 2001), the lipid structures which are responsible for the permeability barrier of the epidermis, which is a primary function of human skin *in vivo* and which is determining for any consequent skin reaction (Garcia *et al.*, 2002).

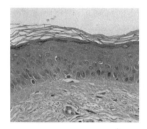 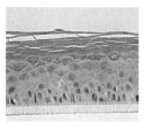 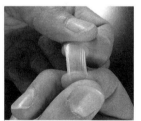

Figure 43.1: Human epidermis reconstituted *in vitro* in chemically defined medium Transversal section of human skin *in vivo* (a); human epidermis reconstituted *in vitro* in chemically defined medium on a polycarbonate substrate (b), and removed from the polycarbonate substrate after dispase treatment (c).

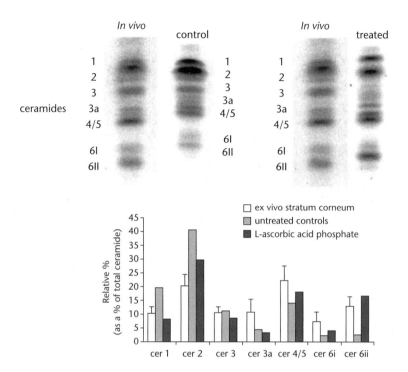

Figure 43.2: Epidermal lipid analysis of the *in vitro* tissue construct (control and ascorbic acid treated) and human epidermis *in vivo* (Ramdin *et al.*, 2001). Addition of ascorbic acid 2-phospate to the culture medium during epidermal tissue reconstruction normalizes the ceramide subspecies to a profile reminiscent of that shown in *ex-vivo* samples. The relative percentages of fatty acid:cholesterol:ceramides were unaffected by the treatment.

Recently, using a customized cDNA array system containing 475 skin-related genes, the gene expression pattern of reconstructed epidermis in chemically defined medium was compared with biopsies of normal human epidermis and with epidermal keratinocyte monolayers (Bernard *et al.*, 2002). The epidermal model was found to closely reproduce the gene expression profile of normal human epidermis, as opposed to keratinocyte monolayers. Additionally, topically applied retinoids induced gene expression modifications that confirmed previously reported retinoid effects, but also provided new insights into their pharmacological activity on human skin.

Another very important advantage of using human epidermis reconstituted in serum-free chemically defined medium is the minimal presence of growth factors and protein in the culture medium, which makes these living epidermal models the most suitable for detecting, with very high precision, even minor toxicological and/or pharmacological effects of any product intended to be in contact with the epidermis: For example, after topical application of test chemicals or finished products to the *in vitro* epidermal model at concentrations that would be used *in vivo*, a slightly irritating effect, typically occurring after prolonged 2 to 3 weeks repeat *in vivo* human clinical patch test application, can be measured objectively by quantifying pro-inflammatory mediators, released by the epidermal keratinocytes in the chemically defined culture medium underneath the epidermal tissue. Moreover, the quantification of these pro-inflammatory mediators, coupled to the analytical evaluation of other *in vitro* toxicity parameters including histology and tissue viability (we suggest the term MEA or Multiple Endpoint Analysis), provide an accurate prediction of skin irritation potential of the test product. Additionally, all parameters in the MEA can be quantified objectively and reproducibly, as opposed to the subjective measurements such as erythema and edema, often used in clinical evaluation.

In this manuscript all studies cited were performed on commercially available SkinEthic® reconstituted human epidermal tissue constructs.

43.3 *IN VITRO* ANALYSIS OF EPIDERMAL TOXICITY BASED ON MULTIPLE ENDPOINT ANALYSIS MEA

The bio-analytical analysis most frequently performed in toxicology and pharmacology screening tests using reconstituted human epidermal tissue models are based on biochemical parameters including tissue viability, either by mitochondrial enzymatic MTT conversion (Triglia *et al.*, 1991; Roguet *et al.*, 1994; Edwards *et al.*, 1994; Brozin *et al.*, 1997; Spielmann *et al.*, 2001), or cell membrane damage as measured by leakage of enzymes such as lactate dehydrogenase (Ponec *et al.*, 1995), tissue damage (histological evaluation using hematoxylin-eosin staining (HandE)), and the release of pro-inflammatory mediators by epidermal keratinocytes including interleukin-1alpha (Slivka and Zeigler, 1993; Doucet *et al.*, 1996; Corsini and Galli, 1997), interleukin-6 (Boxman *et al.*, 1993), interleukin-8 (Ponec *et al.*, 1995), prostaglandins (Roguet *et al.*, 1992; Roguet *et al.*, 1994; Rheins *et al.*, 1994; Lawrence *et al.*, 1997), hydroxy-eicosatreonates and leukotrienes (LTB4) (Dykes *et al.*, 1991). Each of these parameters (biological endpoints) provide very specific information on the toxicological or pharmacological effect of the test product in contact with the epidermal model.

The MTT test is widely used for cell viability assessment of single-cell monolayer cell cultures in comparison to negative and positive controls (Mosmann *et al.*, 1983). In three dimensional epidermal tissue cultures however, too often MTT is being used as a single parameter to assess the biocompatibility of test products and can induce false negative results. This incorrect outcome is the result of MTT being mainly converted by the basal cells of the epidermal tissue constructs and necrosis of the upper superficial layers of the tissue model is not detected (Figure 43.3). To date, this can only be observed by histological analysis.

Furthermore, a very common need in the safety assessment of finished products, is the ability to discriminate between mild and very slightly irritating products, which cannot be detected by MTT assay or histology since slightly irritating products often induce the release of pro-inflammatory mediators (interleukin-1alpha and interleukin-8) without affecting tissue integrity as measured by MTT and histology. Therefore, critical evaluation of each endpoint in the Multiple Endpoint Analysis (MEA) strategy (i.e.; tissue morphology, tissue viability and pro-inflammatory mediator release) is equally important for accurate *in vitro* cutaneous biocompatibility predictions (Figure 43.4). Different examples of the MEA approach are described below for assessing cutaneous irritation and phototoxicity.

43.3.1   *In vitro* skin irritation and phototoxicity prediction based on the MEA approach

The identification of test compounds that could potentially induce clinical skin irritation or phototoxicity are important steps in the product development phase of skin care products, and are very often performed in animal models such as the rabbit skin irritation test (Draize *et al.*, 1944), the maximization test

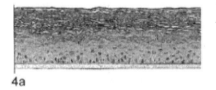 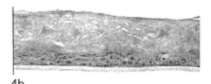

4a   4b

Figure 43.3: Histological analysis of *in vitro* reconstituted human epidermis: 4a untreated control and 4b treated with 2% SDS for 24 hours. Note the almost similar optical density readings (at 540 nm) after MTT assay: 0.944 ± 0.066 for the untreated control culture 4a, and 0.875 ± 0.040 or 92.2 percent of the untreated control tissue, whereas a clear necrosis of the upper epidermal cell layers can be observed in the 2% SDS treated tissue.

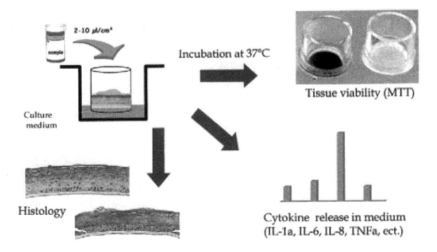

Figure 43.4: *In vitro* skin biocompatibility determination using the MEA approach: epidermal tissues are being dosed with 2–10 µg/cm² of test formulation for 24 and 72 hours and consequently analyzed for tissue viability, tissue morphology and the release of pro-inflammatory mediators interleukin-1alpha, interleukin-8 among others.

using guinea pigs (Magnusson and Kligman, 1969), the mouse local lymph node assay (Kimber and Weisenberger, 1989) and the mouse ear swelling test (Gad *et al.*, 1986). Because of structural and physiological differences between animal and human skin, the relevance of these methods to the human situation is limited and can lead to misclassification (Nixon *et al.*, 1975; Basketter *et al.*, 1996; York *et al.*, 1996). In recent decades, different *in vitro* skin models using de-epidermized dermis (Prunerias *et al.*, 1983; Regnier *et al.*,1990; Gibbs *et al.*, 1997), and collagen matrixes (Bell *et al.*, 1991; Ernesti *et al.*, 1992; Slivka and Zeigler, 1993; Ponec *et al.*, 1995; Augustin *et al.*, 1997) have been reported to be useful to predict skin irritation (Osborne and Perkins, 1994; Boelsma *et al.*, 1996, Roguet *et al.*, 1998, Fentem *et al.*, 2001).

Using human epidermis, reconstituted in chemically defined medium, a test method was validated against *in vivo* data from skin tolerability studies (De Fraissinette *et al.*, 1997; 1999). Based on Multiple Endpoint Analysis (MEA), i.e. *in vitro* epidermal tissue viability modulation, morphological changes (Figure 43.5(a)) and the release of pro-inflammatory mediators interleukin-1alpha and interleukin-8 during 3 days (Figure 43.5(b)), clinical skin reactions observed *in vivo* by visual scoring and biophysical measurement after repeat applications over 3 weeks could be predicted: all topical products that were non-irritating in the human clinical trial were non-cytotoxic *in vitro* and did not induce pro-inflammatory mediator release after 24 hours of exposure. All strong irritating controls demonstrated specific *in vitro* tissue viability changes and cytokine release patterns. Based on the lack of cytotoxicity but the presence of specific pro-inflammatory mediator release patterns after 72 hours of exposure, ranking of mild to moderate skin irritation potential, clinically observed after 3 weeks, could be established (De Wever *et al.*, 2000).

Using a similar testing approach and confirming previously reported data (De Wever *et al.*, 1999; Bernard *et al.*, 2000b), a model system was designed to predict *in vitro* the phototoxicity potential of test chemicals and finished products (Medina *et al.*, 2001). A set of well-known phototoxic and non-phototoxic compounds were tested using reconstituted human epidermis grown in

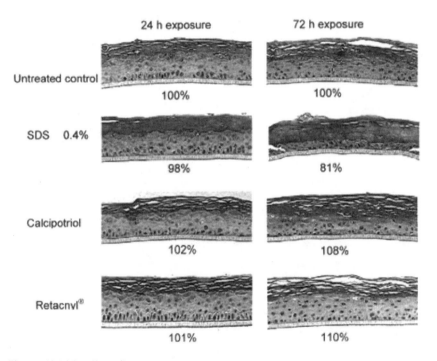

Figure 43.5(a): Effect of SDS, vitamin D3 analogue Calcipotriol and a retinoid based formulation Retacnyl®. *In vitro* epidermal tissues were dosed topically for 24 and 72 hours with 10 mg/cm² of the test chemicals and consequently analyzed using the MEA approach. Histology and tissue viability analysis. Note the SDS induced tissue necrosis at 72 hours. Calcipotriol induces increased epidermal differentiation, whereas Retacnyl® treated tissue showed disappearance of the stratum granulosum layers.

Interleukin-1alpha release

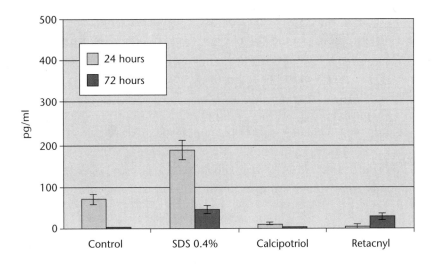

Interleukin-8 release

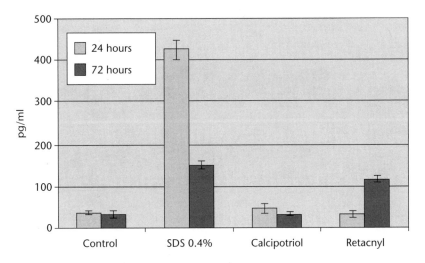

Figure 43.5(b): Pro-inflammatory release of interleukin-1alpha and interleukin-8 after topical treatment with SDS, Calcipotriol and Retacnyl®. The amount of mediator release correlates with the clinical trial data scored after 22 days: SDS 0.4 percent was irritating, Calcipotriol was innocuous and Retacnyl® moderately irritating (De Fraissinette *et al.*, 1999).

chemically defined medium. Test chemicals were topically applied for 24 hours, in the presence or absence of UVA light, and consequently analyzed for tissue viability (LDH release), tissue histology and the release and mRNA expression of the pro-inflammatory mediator interleukin-8. Using this MEA strategy, the phototoxic potential of all chemicals tested were classified correctly: strong phototoxicants were detected by LDH release and morphological changes, whereas the weak phototoxic products (such as 6-methyl coumarin) did not induce changes in tissue viability or morphology, but increased interleukin-8 release and mRNA expression.

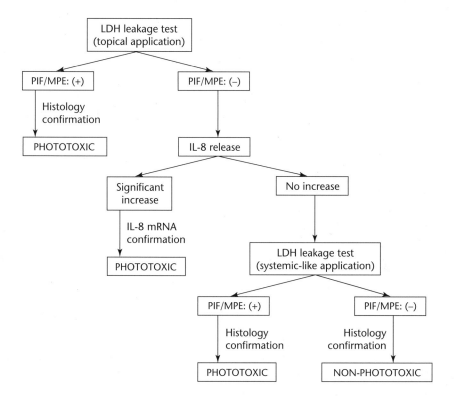

Figure 43.6: Tiered strategy for testing the phototoxic potential of test articles based on MEA (release of LDH, tissue morphology and release of interleukin-8 (Medina *et al.*, 2001).

■ CHAPTER 43 ■

43.3.2 Differentiating skin irritants from skin sensitizers based on the MEA approach

Both irritant and sensitizing compounds trigger clinical cutaneous responses that are very similar in terms of erythema, edema and epidermal scaling and thickening (acanthosis). The difference between a sensitizing and irritating compound lies in the ability of the sensitizer to induce a specific cutaneous response with immunological 'memory' (Coquette *et al.*, 1999a). In either cases, epidermal keratinocytes releasing pro-inflammatory cytokines play a key role in the cascade of cellular and biochemical events that will eventually activate dermal microvascular endothelial cells and initiate accumulation of specific mononuclear cells (Ansel *et al.*, 1990; Enk and Katz 1992a, b; Barker *et al.*, 1991; Barker, 1992; Ponec *et al.*, 1995; Knopp and Enk, 1995). In other words, the critical signals that will to lead to skin irritation and/or sensitization originate at the epidermal keratinocyte level and therefore the expression or release of such cytokines by reconstituted human epidermal models has been proposed as reliable signs to predict *in vivo* adverse reactions (McKenzie and Snauders, 1990; Roguet *et al.*, 1992; Dickson *et al.*, 1993, De Wever *et al.*, 1994; Wilmer *et al.*, 1994). However considering the complexity of the biochemical pathways underlying cutaneous cytokine production, the prediction of chemically induced contact dermatitis remains an area in which considerable effort is being directed toward the development of an *in vitro* test method that can replace the traditional *in vivo* assays.

Recent *in vitro* experimental data obtained using reconstituted human epidermis grown in chemically defined medium show that pro-inflammatory mediator interleukin-1alpha and interleukin-8 expression induced by topical exposure to irritants is different from the expression pattern following exposure to sensitizing chemicals (Berna *et al.*, 1998; Coquette *et al.*, 1999b; Coquette *et al.*, 2000). At the tested concentrations, the irritants (Triton x-100, Benzalkonium chloride and Tween-80) induced an elevated release of interleukin-1alpha, but not interleukin-8, but whereas DNCB, a well known sensitizer, did not induce an increase in interleukin-1alpha but it provoked interleukin-8 release. Based on these preliminary results, additional experiments with five sensitizers (nickel sulfate, DNCB, DNFB, oxazolone, and TNSB) and three irritants (SLS, Benzalkonium chloride and benzoic acid) tested at five different concentrations were performed. MEA analysis (tissue viability, histology and interleukin-1alpha and interleukin-8) demonstrated that indeed the sensitizers induced a dose dependent cytotoxicity, but with concomitant low interleukin-

1alpha release but a high interleukin –8 release, and the irritants exhibited a high interleukin-1alpha release but low interleukin-8 release when tested at doses that induced a cytotoxic response. Additional experiments are currently ongoing to provide further evidence to support these observations.

43.4 CONCLUSION

The improvement of tissue culture techniques that allow the reconstitution of human epidermis *in vitro* in chemically defined medium results in highly reproducible epidermal constructs that demonstrate much closer physiological features of normal human skin in terms of structural, biochemical and barrier function properties as compared to 'conventional' epidermal models reconstructed in the presence of serum or dermal components. Consequently their use as alternative test models to predict cutaneous toxicological and pharmacological reactions of topically applied agents has proven to be highly reliable and reproducible (Doucet *et al.*, 1996; 1998; Gysler *et al.*, 1999a; Gysler *et al.*, 1999b; Doucet *et al.*, 1999; Laugier *et al.*, 2000; Dagues *et al.*, 2001, Mavon and Raufast, 2001) as opposed to animal test methods.

Using these tissue constructs in an optimized *in vitro* analytical evaluation of morphological epidermal assessment, cell viability measurement and consequent pro-inflammatory mediator release by the epidermal keratinocytes (MEA or Multiple Endpoint Analysis), a very precise and reliable pre-clinical test method is provided to accurately predict cutaneous irritation and phototoxicity. It should be noted however that all *in vitro* parameters analyzed in MEA strategy are equally important for accurate data interpretation. To avoid misinterpretation leading to false negatives and false positives, one should not perform tissue viability testing based on MTT without performing histological analysis: MTT is mainly converted by basal cells of the epidermal construct and tissue necrosis occurring only in the upper epidermal cell layers will not be detected. Conversely, one should not assess interleukin-1alpha and/or interleukin-8 release without performing tissue viability testing or histology, as some pro-inflammatory mediators (for instance interleukin-8) will not be synthesized and consequently released when the epidermal tissue is necrotic. Additionally, assessing tissue histology and tissue viability without quantifying the release of pro-inflammatory mediators can lead to false negative results as slightly irritating or weekly phototoxic agents will induce interleukin-1alpha and/or interleukin-8 release without affecting tissue morphology and viability since their release are early signs of irritation or phototoxicity, undetected by either MTT or tissue morphology. Taken into account the MEA approach, human epidermis reconstituted *in vitro* in chemically defined medium represents a very useful model for assessing skin irritation and phototoxicity.

REFERENCES

ANSEL J., PERRY, P., BROWN, J., DAMM, D., PHAN, T., HART, C., LUGER, T. and HEFENEIDER, S. (1990) Cytokine modulation of keratinocyte cytokines. *J. of Investi. Dermatol.* **94**, 101s–107s.

ASSELINEAU, D., BERNARD, B., BAILLY, C., DARMON, M. and PRUNIÈRAS M. (1986) Human epidermis reconstructed by culture: Is it normal? *J. Invest. Dermatol.* **86**, 181–186.

AUGUSTIN, C., COLLOMBEL, C. and DAMOUR, O. (1997) Measurements of the protective effect of topically applied sunscreens using *in vitro* three-dimensional dermal and skin equivalents. *Photochem. Photobiol.* **66**(6), 853–859.

BARKER, J., MITRA, R., GRIFFITHS, C., DIXIT, V. and NICKOLOFF, B.J. (1991) Keratinocytes as initiators of inflammation. *The Lancet* **337**, 211–214.

BARKER J. (1992) Role of keratinocytes in allergic contact dermatitis. *Contact Dermatitis* **26**, 145–148.

BASKETTER, D., BLAIKIE, L and REYNOLDS, F. (1996) The impact of atopic status on a predictive human test of skin irritation potential. *Contact Dermatitis* **35**(1), 33–39.

BELL E., PARENTEAU, N., GAY, R., NOLTE, C., KEMP, P., BILBO, P., EKSTEIN, B. and JOHNSON, E. (1991) The living skin equivalent: its manufacture, its organotypic properties and its responses to irritants. *Toxicology In Vitro* **5**, 591–596.

BERNA, N., COQUETTE, A., VANDENBOSCH, A. and POUMAY, Y. (1998) Use of reconstructed epidermis to assess keratinocyte activation by skin irritant and sensitizing compounds. *J. Invest. Dermatol.* **110**(4, abstract), 1108.

BERNARD, F.-X., BARRAULT, C., DEGUERCY, A., DE WEVER, B. and ROSDY, M. (2000a) Expression of type 1 5a-reductase and metabolism of testosterone in reconstructed human epidermis (SkinEthic): a new model for screening skin-targeted androgen modulators. *International Journal of Cosmetic Science* **22**, 397–407.

BERNARD, F.-X., BARRAULT, C. DEGUERCY, A., DE WEVER, B. and ROSDY, M. (2000b) Development of a highly sensitive *in vitro* phototoxicity assay using the SkinEthic reconstructed human epidermis. *Cell Biology and Toxicology* **16**(6), 391–400.

BERNARD, F.-X., PREDETTI, N., ROSDY, M. and DEGUERCY, A. (2002) Comparison of gene expression profiles in human keratinocyte monolayer cultures, reconstituted human epidermis and normal human skin; transcriptional effects of retinoid treatments in reconstructed human epidermis. *Experimental Dermatology* **11**(1): 59–75.

BOELSMA E., TANOJO, H., BODDE, E. and PONEC, M. (1997) An *in vitro* study of the use of a human skin equivalent for irritancy screening of fatty acids. *Toxic. In Vitro* **11**, 365–376.

BOXMAN, I., LÖWIK, C., AARDEN, L., and PONEC, M., (1993) Modulation of IL-6 and IL-1 activity by keratinocyte-fibroblast interaction. *J. Invest. Dermatol.* **101**(3), 316–324.

BOYCE, S, MICHEL, S., REICHERT, U., SCHROOT, B. and SCHMIDT, R. (1990) Reconstructed skin from cultured human keratinocytes and fibroblasts on a collagen-glycosaminoglycan biopolymer substrate. *Skin Pharmacol.* **3**(2), 136–143.

BROSIN, A., WOLF, W., MATTHEUS, A. and HEISE, H. (1997) Use of XTT-assay to assess the cytotoxicity of different surfactants and metal salts in human keratinocytes (HACAT): A feasible method for *in vitro* testing of skin irritants. *Acta Dermatologica-Venereologica* **77**(1), 26–28.

COQUETTE, A., BERNA, N., VANDENBOSCH, A. and ROSDY, M., POUMAY, Y. (1999a) Differential expression and release of cytokines by an *in vitro* reconstituted human epidermis model following skin irritant and sensitizing compounds. *Toxicology In Vitro* **13**(6), 867–877.

COQUETTE, A., BERNA, N., POUMAY, Y. and PITTELKOW, M.R. (1999b) The keratinocyte in cutaneous irritation and sensitization. In: KYDONIEUS, A.F. and WILLE, J.J. (eds) *Biomedical Modulations of Skin Reactions in Dermal and Transdermal Drug Delivery*, CRC Press, 125.

COQUETTE, A., BERNA, N., VANDENBOSCH, A. and POUMAY, Y. (2000) Specific enhanced release of interleukin-8 and interleukin-1α in reconstructed human epidermis *in vitro* after simulation with different classes of skin irritants and contact sensitisers. In BALLS, M., VAN ZELLER, A.M. and HALDER, M. *Developments in Animal and Veterinary Sciences, 31B, Progress in the Reduction, Refinement and Replacement of Animal Experimentation*, Oxford: Elsevier. 653–664.

CHAPTER 43

CORSINI, E. and GALLI, C.L. (1997) Use of the *in vitro* reconstituted human epidermis, EPISKIN, to assess the molecular mechanisms of skin irritation and sensitization. In VAN ZUTPHEN, L.F.M. and BALLS, M. *Animal Alternatives, Welfare and Ethics*. Amsterdam: Elsevier Science. 575–582.

DAGUES, N., MONTBROUSSOU, E., DOMINGO, I., LE NET, J.L., BLANCK, O. and ALÉPÉE, N. (2001) Correlation of *in vivo* studies and *in vitro* human epidermis model for dermal xenobiotic-induced toxicity. *Toxicology Letters* **123**(suppl. 1) 21.

DE BRUGEROLLE DE FRAISINETTE, A., PICARLES, V., KOLOPP, M., MEINGASSNER, JG., POPP, X., GRASS, P., EBELIN, M.E., BURTIN, P., TRONNIER, H., RICHTER, F. and CORDIER, A. (1997) *In vitro* human skin models as predictive tools for the skin irritant potential of dermal formulations. Presented at the 19th World Congress of Dermatology, Sydney, Australia.

DE BRUGEROLLE DE FRAISINETTE, A., PICARLES, V., CHIBOUT, S., KOLOPP, M., MEDINA, J., BURTIN, P., EBELIN, M-E., OSBORNE, S., MAYER, F.K., SPAKE, A., ROSDY, M., DE WEVER, B., ETTLIN, R.A., and CORDIER, A. (1999) Predictivity of an *in vitro* model for acute and chronic skin irritation (SkinEthic) applied to the testing of topical vehicles. *Cell Biology and Toxicology* **15**(2), P. 121–135.

DE WEVER, B. and RHEINS, L.A. (1994) Skin 2TM: An *in vitro* skin analog. *Alternative Methods in Toxicology* **10**: 121–131.

DE WEVER, B., CAPPADORO, M., and ROSDY, M. (2000) Prediction of Acute and Chronic Skin Irritation using Human Epidermis Reconstituted *In Vitro* in Chemically Defined Medium. Alternative Toxicological Methods for the New Millenium: Science and Application. Maryland, USA: National Library of Medicine, Bethesda.

DICKSON, F.M., LAWRENCE, J.N. and BENFORD, D.J. (1993) Release of inflammatory mediators in human keratinocyte cultures following exposure to a skin irritant. *Toxicology In Vitro* **7**(4), 385–388.

DOUCET, O., ROBERT, C. and ZASTROW, L. (1996) Use of a serum-free reconstituted epidermis as a skin pharmacological model. *Toxicology In Vitro* **10**, 305–313.

DOUCET, O., GARCIA, N., ROSDY, M., FARTASH, M., ZASTROW (1997) Critical events in the barrier formation of reconstituted epidermis. *Perspectives in Percutaneous Penetration* **5B**, 141–144.

DOUCET, O., GARCIA, N. and ZASTROW, L. (1998) Skin culture model: a possible alternative to the use of excised human skin for assessing *in vitro* percutaneous absorption. *Toxicology In Vitro* **12**, 423–430.

DOUCET, O., GARCIA, N., ZASTROW, L. (1999) Potential of skin culture models for assessing *in vitro* percutaneous absorption. In: CLARCK, D.G., LISANSKY, S.G. and MACMILLAN, R. (Eds.), *Alternatives to Animal Testing II*, Cardiff, UK: CPL Press.

DRAIZE, J.H., WOODARD, G. and CALVERY, H.O. (1944) Methods for the study of irritation and toxicity of substances applied topically to the skin and mucous membranes. *Journal of Pharmacology and Experimental Therapeutics* **82**, 377–390.

DYKES, P., EDWARDS, M., DONOVANI, M., MERRET, V., MORGAN, H. and MARKS, R. (1991) *In vitro* reconstruction of human skin: the use of skin equivalents as potential indicators of cutaneous toxicity. *Toxicology In Vitro* **5**(1).

EDWARDS, S., DONNELLY, T., SAYRE, R. and RHEINS L. (1994) *European Medicine Research*, Fracchia, G. (Ed.) Amsterdam: IOS Press, 106–115. (1994)

ENK, A.H. and KATZ, S.I. (1992a) Early molecular events in the induction of contact sensitivity. *Proceedings of the National Academy of Sciences of the USA* **89**, 1398–1402.

ENK, A.H. and KATZ, S.I. (1992b) Identification and induction of keratinocyte-derived IL-10. *Journal of Immunology* **149**, 92–95.

ERNESTI, A.M., SWIDEREK, M. and GAY, R. (1992) Absorption and metabolism of topically applied testosterone in an organotype skin culture. *Skin Pharmacology* **5**(3), 146–153.

FARTASCH, M., PONEC, M. and ROSDY, M. (1996a) Development of a structurally competent epidermal barrier in air-exposed keratinocyte cultures: A time course study. *J. Invest. Dermatol.* **107**(4), 656.

FARTASCH, M. and ROSDY, M. (1996b) Maturation of the epidermal barrier in air-exposed keratinocyte cultures: A time course study. *J. Invest. Dermatol.* **107**(3), 518.

FENTEM, J., BRIGGS, D., CHESNE, C., ELLIOT, G., HARBELL, J., HEYLINGS, J., PORTES, P., ROGUET, R., VAN DE SANDT, J. and BOTHAM, P. (2001) A prevalidation study on *in vitro* tests for acute skin irritation. Results and evaluation by the Management Team. *Toxicol. In Vitro* **15**(1), 57–93.

FLEISCHMAJER, R., MACDONALD II, E., CONTARD, P. and PERLISH, J. (1993) Immunochemistry of a keratinocyte-fibroblast co-culture model for reconstruction of human skin. *J. of Histochemistry and Cytochemistry* **41**(9), 1359–1366.

GAD, S.C., DUNN, B.J., DOBBS, D.W., REILLY, C. and WALSH, R.D. (1986) Development and validation of an alternative dermal sensitization test: The mouse ear swelling test (MEST). *Toxicology and Applied Pharmacology* **84**, 93–114.

■ CHAPTER 43 ■

GARCIA, N., DOUCET, O., BAYER, M., ZASTROW, L., and MARTY, J.P. (2000) Use of reconstituted human epidermis cultures to assess the disrupting effect of organic solvents on the barrier function of excised human skin. *In Vitro and Molecular Toxicology* **13**(3), 159–171.

GARCIA, N., DOUCET, O., BAYER, M., FOUCHARD, D., ZASTROW, L. and MARTY, J.P. (2002) Characterization of the barrier function in a reconstituted human epidermis cultivated in chemically defined medium. *Intl. J. of Cosmetic Sciences* **24**, 25–34.

GAY, R., SWIDEREK, M., NELSON, D. and ERNESTI, A. (1992) The living skin equivalent as a model *in vitro* for ranking the toxic potential of dermal irritants. *Toxicology In Vitro* **6**(4), 303–315.

GIBBS, S., VICANOVA, J., BOUWSTRA, J., VALSTAR, D., KEMPENAAR, J. and PONEC, M. (1997) Culture of reconstructed epidermis in a defined medium at 33 degrees C shows a delayed epidermal maturation, prolonged lifespan and improved stratum corneum. *Arch. Dermatol. Res. Sep.* **289**(10), 585–595.

GYSLER, A., KOENIGSMANN, U., SCHAFER-KORTING, M. (1999a) Tridimensional skin models recording percutaneous absorption. *ALTEX 16*, 2, 67–72.

GYSLER, A., KLEUSER, B., SIPPL, W., LANGE, K., KORTING, H. C., HÖLTJE, H.-D. and SCHÄFER-KORTING, M. (1996b) Skin penetration and metabolism of topical glucocorticoids in reconstructed epidermis and excised human skin. *Pharmaceutical Research.* **16**, 9, 1386–1391.

KIMBER, I. and WEISENBERGER, C. (1989) A murine local lymph node assay for the identification of contact allergens. Assay development and results of an initial validation study. *Archives of Toxicology* **63**, 274–282.

KNOP, J. and ENK, A. (1995) Cellular and molecular mechanisms in the induction phase of contact sensitivity. *International Archives of Allergy and Immunology* **107**(1–3), 231–232.

LAUGIER, J-P., SHUSTER, S, ROSDY, M., CSÓKA, A.B., STERN, R. and MAIBACH, H. I. (2000) Topical hyaluronidase decreases hyaluronic acid and CD44 in human skin and in reconstituted human epidermis: evidence that hyaluronidase can permeate the stratum corneum. *British Journal of Dermatology* **142**, 226–233.

LAWRENCE, J., DICKSON, F., BENFORD, D. (1997) Skin irritant-induced cytotoxicity and prostaglandin E-2 release in human skin keratinocyte cultures. *Toxicology In Vitro* **11**(5), 627–631.

LENOIR, M. and BERNARD, B. (1990) Architecture of reconstructed epidermis on collagen lattices varies according to the method used: a comparative study. *Skin Pharmacol.* 3(2), 97–106.

MCKENZIE, R. and SNAUDERS, D. (1990) The role of keratinocytes cytokines in inflammation and immunity. *Journal of Investigative Dermatology* 95, 105S–107S.

MAGNUSSON, B. and KLIGMAN, A. (1969) The identification of contact allergens by animal assay. The guinea pig maximization test. *Journal of Investigative Dermatology* 52(3), 268–276.

MAVON, A. and RAUFAST, V. (2001) Assessment of the skin metabolism of two stable antioxidant precursors to a free tocopherol, tocopheryl-glucoside versus tocopherol acetate, in an epidermal equivalent and in human skin. European Society of Dermatological Research, Stockholm, September.

MEDINA, J., ELSAESSER, C., PICARLES, V., GRENET, O., KOLOPP, M., CHIBOUT, S. and DE BRUGEROLLE DE FRAISSINETTE, A. (2001) Assessment of the phototoxic potential of compounds and finished topical products using a human reconstructed epidermis. *In Vitro and Molecular Toxicology* 14(3), 157–168.

MOSMANN, T. (1983) Rapid colorimetric assay for cellular growth and survival: application to proliferation and cytotoxicity assays. *J. Immunol. Meth.* 65, 55–63.

NIXON, G.A., TYSON, C.A. and WERTZ, W.C. (1975) Interspecies comparison of skin irritancy. *Toxicology and Applied Pharmacology* 31, 481–490.

O'KEEFE, E., WOODLEY, D., FALK, R., GAMMON, W. and BRIGGAMAN, R. (1987) Production of fibronectin by epithelium in a skin equivalent. *J. Invest. Dermatol.* 88, 634–639.

OSBORNE, R. and PERKINS, M. (1994) An approach for development of alternative test methods based on mechanisms of skin irritation. *Food Chem. Toxicol.* 32(2), 133–142.

PONEC, M., WEERHEIM, A., KEMPENAAR, J., MOMMAAS, A.M. and NUGTEREN, D.H. (1988) Lipid composition of cultured keratinocytes in relation to their differentiation. *Journal of Lipid Research* 29, 949–962.

PONEC, M. (1991) Reconstruction of human epidermis on de-epidermized dermis: expression of differentiation specific protein markers and lipid composition. *Toxicology In Vitro* 5, 597–606.

PONEC, M. and KEMPENAAR, J. (1995) Use of human skin recombinants as an *in vitro* model for testing the irritation potential of cutaneous irritants. *Skin Pharmacology* 8, 49–59.

CHAPTER 43

PONEC, M., WEERHEIM, A., KEMPENAAR, J., MULDER, A., GOORIS, G.S., BOUWSTRA, J. and MOMMAAS, A.M. (1997) The formation of competent barrier lipids in reconstructed human epidermis requires the presence of vitamin C. *J. Invest. Dermatol. Sep.* **109**(3), 348–355.

PRUNIERAS, M., REGNIER, M. and WOODLEY, D. (1983) Methods for cultivation of keratinocytes with an air-liquid interface. *Journal of Investigative Dermatology* **81**, 28S-33S.

RAMDIN, L.S.P., RICHARDSON, J., HARDING, C.R. and ROSDY, M. (2001) The effect of ascorbic acid (Vitamin C) on the ceramide subspecies profile in the SkinEthic epidermal model. Poster presented at the Stratum Corneum Meeting, Basel, Switzerland, September.

REGNIER, M., DESBAS, C., BAILLY, C. and DARMON, M. (1988) Differentiation of normal and tumoral human keratinocytes cultured on dermis: reconstruction of either normal or tumoral architecture. *In Vitro Cell Dev. Biol.* **24**, 625–632.

REGNIER, M. and DARMON, M. (1989) Human epidermis reconstructed *in vitro*: a model to study keratinocyte differentiation and its modulation by retinoic acid. *In Vitro Cell Dev. Biol.* **25**(11), 1000–1008.

REGNIER, M., ASSELINEAU, D. and LENOIR, M.C. (1990) Human epidermis reconstructed on dermal substrates *in vitro*: an alternative to animals in skin pharmacology. *Skin Pharmacol.* **3**(2), 70–85.

RHEINS, L.A., EDWARDS, S.M., MIA, O. and DONELLY, T.A. (1994) Skin 2TM: an *in vitro* model to assess cutaneous immunotoxicity. *Toxicology In Vitro* **8**(5), 1007–1014.

ROGUET, R., DOSSOU, K.G. and ROUGIER, A. (1992) Use of *in vitro* skin recombinants to evaluate cutaneous toxicity: a preliminary study. *Journal of Toxicology-cutaneous and Ocular Toxicology* **11**, 305–315.

ROGUET, R., DOSSOU, K.G. and ROUGIER, A. (1994) A reconstructed human epidermis to assess cutaneous irritation, photoirritation and photoprotection *in vitro*. In ROUGIER, A., GOLDBERG, A.M. and MAIBACH, H.I. (eds) *In Vitro Skin Toxicology: Irritation, Phototoxicity, Sensitization*. New York: Mary Ann Liebert, 141–149.

ROSDY, M. and CLAUSS, L.C. (1990) Terminal epidermal differentiation of human keratinocytes grown in chemically defined medium on inert filter substrates at the air-liquid interface. *Journal of Investigative Dermatology* **95**(4), 409–414.

ROSDY, M., PISANI, A. and ORTONNE, J.P. (1993) Production of basement membrane components by a reconstructed epidermis cultured in the absence of serum and dermal factors. *British Journal of Dermatology* **129**, 227–234.

ROSDY, M., FARTASCH, M. and PONEC, M. (1996) Structurally and biochemically normal permeability barrier of human epidermis reconstituted in chemically defined medium. *J. Invest. Dermatol.* **107**(4), 664.

ROSDY, M., FARTASCH, M. and DARMON, M. (1997) Normal permeability barrier to tritiated water in reconstituted human epidermis. Abstract. Prediction of percutaneous penetration meeting. April 2–5, La Grande Motte, France.

ROSDY, M., BERTINO, B., BUTET, V., GIBBS, S., PONEC, M. and DARMON, M. (1997) Retinoic acid inhibits epidermal differentiation when applied topically on the stratum corneum of epidermis formed *in vitro* by human keratinocytes grown on defined medium. *In Vitro Toxicology* **10**, 39–47.

SCHÜRER, N., MONGER, D., HINCENBERGS, M. and WILLIAMS, M. (1989) Fatty acid metabolism in human keratinocytes cultivated at an air-medium interface. *J. Invest. Dermatol.* **92**, 196–202.

SLIVKA, S.R. (1992) Testosterone metabolism in an *in vitro* skin model. *Cell. Biol. and Toxicol.* **8**(4), 267–275.

SLIVKA, S.R. and ZEIGLER, F. (1993) Use of an *in vitro* skin model for determining epidermal and dermal contributions to irritant response. *Journal of Toxicology—Cutaneous and Ocular Toxicology* **12**(1), 49–57.

SPIELMANN, H. and LIEBSCH, M. (2001) Lessons learned from validation of *in vitro* toxicity tests: from failure to acceptance into regulatory practice. *Toxicol. In Vitro* **15**(4–5), 585–590.

TINOIS, E., TIOLLIER, J., GAUCHERAND, M., DUMAS, H., TARDY, M. and THIVOLET, J. (1991) *In vitro* and post-transplantation differentiation of human keratinocyte growth on human type IV collagen film of a bilayered dermal substitute. *Exp. Cell. Res.* **58**, 310–319.

TRIGLIA, D., BRAA, S., YONAN, C. and NAUGHTON, G.K. (1991) Cytotoxicity testing using neutral red and MTT assays on a three-dimensional human skin substrate. *Toxicology In Vitro.* **5**, 573–578.

WILMER, J., BURLESON, F., KAYAMA, F., KANNO, J. and LUSTER, M.I. (1994) Cytokine induction in human epidermal keratinocytes exposed to contact irritants and its relation to chemical-induced inflammation in mouse skin. *Journal of Investigative Dermatology* **102**(6), 915–922.

YORK, M., GRIFFITHS, H., WHITTLE, E., BASKETTER, D. (1996) Evaluation of a human patch test for the identification and classification of skin irritation potential. *Contact Dermatitis* **34**(3) 204–212.

Photoirritation (Phototoxicity) Testing in Humans

FRANCIS N MARZULLI AND HOWARD I MAIBACH

Contents

44.1   Definition

44.2   Screening

44.3   Spectral measurements

44.4   Precautions

44.5   Exploratory studies

44.6   Additional fundamentals

44.7   Lamp sources

44.8   Conclusions

44.1 DEFINITION

Photoirritation (phototoxicity) has been defined as a nonimmunologic sunlight-induced skin response (dermatitis) to a photoactive chemical, with the response being likened to an exaggerated sunburn (Marzulli and Maibach, 1970). The photoactive chemical may reach the target tissues either after direct application or indirectly via the blood stream, following ingestion or parenteral administration. The skin response is characterized by erythema and sometimes edema, vesiculation, and pigmentation.

44.2 SCREENING

Chemicals that are phototoxic are usually activated by the ultraviolet (UVR) portion of the sun's radiation, which involves wavelengths in the range 280–400 nm. Screening tests for evaluating phototoxic potential should therefore begin with an examination of the test chemical under UVR. Fluorescence under UVR examination suggests that the chemical may be photoirritating and may require further investigation. Additional screening can be performed with *in vitro* tests (Nilsson *et al.*, 1993). Finally, human tests should not be undertaken prior to familiarization with and performance of animal tests.

44.3 SPECTRAL MEASUREMENTS

The basic unit of radiant work energy emitted by a source is the joule (J). One joule delivered over 1 s is 1 watt (W) of radiant power. Radiant power, or irradiance, is reported in watts per square meter (often mW/m^2) and radiant exposure is reported in joules per square meter (often J/cm^2) skin. Optical radiation is measured with a radiometer. Other details about spectral measurements are given in the chapter on spectral equipment for photobiology.

44.4 PRECAUTIONS

The American Conference of Government Industrial Hygienists (1988) has established that total irradiance upon unprotected skin or eye should not exceed $1.0 \ mW/cm^2$ for exposure times greater than 16 mm and should not exceed $1.0 \ J/cm^2$ for exposure times less than 16 mm. Recommendations for other exposure periods are also given.

A report by the Commission Internationale de l'Eclairage (CIE) states that a review of a considerable amount of data suggests that the damage risk for UVR at 290 nm appears to be about 100 times higher than that at 320 nm (McKinlay and Diffey, 1987). The damage risk at 320 nm is about 10 times that at 340 nm and about 100 times that at 400 nm. These findings have resulted in a modification of one of the traditional terms (UVA) employed by the photobiologist to describe portions of the solar spectrum that are accorded special biologic attention. Besides UVA (320–400 nm), UVB (280–320 nm), and UVC (<280 nm), we now have UVA1 (340–400 nm), and UVA2 (320–340 nm). Other values for UVA, UVB, and UVC are given by the Commission de l'Eclairage (1970).

The upper atmosphere screens out some UVB radiation; however, in 1982, the National Bureau of Standards reported that radiation down to 286 nm was measured at Gainesville, FL.

Urbach (1989) emphasized the importance of spectral distribution as compared with intensity of the UVR source. He found that a 4 per cent reduction in total UVR produced by doubling the filter thickness (Schott WG 320) from 1 to 2 mm produced a 50 per cent decrease in erythema effectiveness because of change in spectral distribution of UVB.

44.5 EXPLORATORY STUDIES

Tests that rely on simple equipment can provide a satisfactory starting point. Marzulli and Maibach (1970) used this approach in identifying bergapten (5-methoxypsoralen) as the principal phototoxic component of oil of bergamot. The mouse, rabbit, guinea pig, and other mammalian species can be used for exploratory work, with humans as the ultimate test subjects. The rabbit has a large area of the back, which can be divided into four test sections, enabling a reduction in the number of test animals required.

A source of UVR with over 90 per cent of the UV radiation (300–400 nm) output at 365 nm was provided by a Hanovia Inspectolite (no longer available). When used with no. 16125, type EH-4 bulb, red purple Corning 7-39 (5874) filter, and frosted glass cutoff at 290 nm, total output at 10 cm from the source is about 3000 μW/cm^2 and about 1900 μW/cm^2 at 15 cm.

The test chemical (0.05 ml) is applied to skin, and after 5 mm it is irradiated for 25–40 mm (animals–humans) at a distance of 8–10 cm. The skin is examined for erythema and edema at 24 and 48 h and again at 7 d. Positive controls (using 0.01 percent 5-methoxypsoralen or 8-methoxypsoralen in 70 percent ethanol) and negative (vehicle) controls are similarly exposed for comparison.

Appropriate modification of the aformentioned basic scheme is needed for investigating orally administered chemicals, such as nonsteroidal anti-inflammatory drugs.

44.6 ADDITIONAL FUNDAMENTALS

Duplicating the sun's spectrum in the laboratory has been one of the challenges posed to scientists and engineers during the past 20 years.

Experimentalists currently engaged in photobiologic work need to report the source and output of radiation used in their experiments. They should employ sources with output of UVA and UVB and should specify exposure time and distance of source to the skin. The UVA should be about 10 J/cm^2 and the UVB about 0.1 J/cm^2.

Irradiance from the UVR source can be measured with a UV radiometer at an appropriate distance. For correct readings, the radiometer is calibrated by the supplier, with the intended source. Irradiance is measured in mW/cm^2; dose in J/cm^2; and exposure time *(t)* in minutes.

Urbach (1989) reported that:

> The sun emits a polychromatic continuum of different wavelengths; low pressure fluorescent sun lamps emit a continuum mainly in the UVB, or mainly in the UVA; high-pressure mercury arcs provide discontinuous line spectra; and high intensity solar simulators, based on xenon, xenon-mercury or doped tungsten may mimic solar UVR, but require special filtration to shape the UVB spectrum and remove intense visible and infrared radiation. The age of the lamp, temperature of the bulb or arc, and age of filters will influence both the spectral power distribution and irradiance (p. 178).

44.7 LAMP SOURCES

In the United States, General Electric Co. (Baltimore), Sylvania Corporation (Danvers, MA), Solar Light Co., Inc. (Philadelphia), and Elder Pharmaceuticals (Bryan, OH) market lamps with UVA and UVB outputs. Xenon Corp. (Wilmington, MA) manufactures solar simulators. Optronics (Orlando, FL), Eppley (Newport, RI) and G. Gamma Scientific (San Diego, CA) market radiometers. United Detector Tech. (California) calibrates radiometers. Schoeffel Co. (New Jersey) is a source for detectors and simulators (Anderson, 1986).

44.8 CONCLUSIONS

The literature on phototoxicity contains a large assortment of data involving a wide variety of compounds, test methods, equipment, and results. Maurer (1987) reviewed and studied the published findings on humans and animals and voiced concern about the complexities of phototoxicity testing and the limitations of the predictability of test results. Nilson *et al.* (1993) submitted to the Organization for Economic Cooperation and Development (OECD) a proposed standard protocol for topical and systemic phototoxicity testing in guinea pigs, which was evaluated and found satisfactory in a collaborative study involving six different laboratories. The method provides test details such as experimental design, irradiation sources, and scoring. The proposed method is similar to one employed by Lovell and Sanders (1992). It is suggested that these animal test methods be employed as part of the familiarization experience that is needed prior to exposing humans to UVR in laboratory tests.

REFERENCES

AMERICAN CONFERENCE of GOVERNMENT INDUSTRIAL HYGIENISTS. (1988) *Threshold limit values and biological exposure indices for 1988–1989*. Cincinnati. OH: ACGIH.

ANDERSON, T. F. (1986) Artificial light sources. In DE LEO, V. A. (eds) *Dermatologic Clinics*, Vol. 4, Philadelphia: W. B. Saunders, 203–215.

COMMISION DE L'ECLAIRAGE. (1970) Publication No. 17 defining UVA (315–380 nm), UVB (280–315 nm), and UVC (100–280 nm).

LOVELL, W. and SANDERS, (1992) Phototoxicity testing in guinea pigs. *Food Chem. Toxico.* **30**, 155–160.

MARZULLI, F. and MAIBACH, H. (1970) Perfume phototoxicity. *J. Soc Cosmet. Chem.* **21**, 695–715.

MAURER, T. (1987) Phototoxicity testing—*In vivo* and *in vitro. Food Chem. Toxicol.* **25**, 407–414.

MCKINLAY, A. and DIFFEY, B. (1987) A reference action spectrum for ultraviolet induced erythema in human skin. *CIE j.* **6**, 17–22.

NATIONAL BUREAU of STANDARDS (1982) Technical Note 910–15. Manual on Radiation Measurements, December.

NILSSON, R., MAURER, T. and REDMOND, N. (1993) Standard protocol for phototoxicity testing. *Contact Dermatitis* **28**, 285–290.

URBACH, F. (1989) Testing the efficacy of sunscreens: Effect of choice of source and spectral power distribution of ultraviolet radiation, and choice of endpoint. *Photodermatology* 6, 177–181.

ADDITIONAL READING

ARLETT, C., EARL, L., FERGUSON, J., GIBBS, N., HAWK, J., HENDERSON, L., JOHNSON, B., LOVELL, W., MENAGE, H., NAVARATNAM, S., PROBY, C., STEER, S. and YOUNG, A. (1995) British Photodermatology Group Workshop. Predictive *in vitro* methods for identifying photosensitizing drugs: A report. *Br. J. Dermatol.* 132, 271–274.

MAIBACH, H. and MARZULLI, F. (1986), Photoirritation (phototoxicity) from topical agents. In DeLeo, V. A. (ed.) *Dermatologic Clinics*, Vol. 4, Philadelphia: W. B. Saunders, 217–222.

MONTEIRO-RIVIERE, N. A., INMAN, A. O. and RIVIERE, J. (1994) Development and characterization of a novel skin model for cutaneous phototoxicology. *Photoderm. Photoimmunol. Photomed.* 10, 235–244.

SPIELMANN, H., LOVELL, W. W., HÖLZLE, B. E., MAURER, T., MIRANDA, M. A., PAPE, W. J. W., SAPORA, O. and SLADOWSKI, D. (1994) *In Vitro* Phototoxicity Testing (ECVAM Workshop Report 2). European Centre for the Validation of Alternative Methods, JRC Environment Institute, Ispra, Italy.

■ CHAPTER 44 ■

Measuring and Quantifying Ultraviolet Radiation Exposures

DAVID H SLINEY

Contents

45.1   Introduction

45.2   Optical radiation sources

45.3   UV measurement

45.4   General biophysical and photobiological factors

45.5   Determining action spectra

45.6   Conclusion

45.1 INTRODUCTION

Quantitative phototoxicology requires appropriate dosimetry. The important concepts, terminology and units of optical dosimetry required in photobiology are all too frequently not fully appreciated in experimental studies, leading to needless misinterpretation and error. The objective of this chapter is to familiarize scientists working in photodermatology with the basic concepts related to light measurement and light source characterization that are necessary for reproducible scientific tests. Hopefully this chapter will encourage the reader to look differently at the optical source being used and how correctly to express the exposure dose. Phototoxicological studies require knowledge of the optical and radiometric parameters of ultraviolet optical sources and geometrical exposure factors. This knowledge is required to accurately determine the irradiances (dose rates). In performing any phototoxicity study, it is imperative that the spectral characteristics of the optical source must be known. For a specific photobiological action spectrum, different light sources delivering the same optical power can produce completely different dermatological effects if the sources have differing spectra (Figure 45.1). Indeed, a photodermatologist will choose a specific ultraviolet (UV) source to match best a given biological action spectrum (if known) in order to achieve the greatest efficiency in delivering a photobiologically significant dose. Different applications require different light sources and a variety of measurement techniques may be in order when attempting to conduct different types of studies. Photochemical interaction mechanisms are normally most pronounced at short wavelengths (UV) where photon energies are greatest, and also will be most readily observed for lengthy exposure durations (Sliney and Wolbarsht, 1980; WHO, 1994).

The concepts of a photobiological dose evolved from applying standard physical measures of exposure (radiant exposure) and exposure rate (irradiance) used by physicists (CIE, 1987). The basic physical measures (termed *radiometric quantities*) were modified by applying the laws of photochemistry to employ action spectra, and by applying rules as the Bunsen-Roscoe Law—the rule of reciprocity. Because of the reciprocal relationship of irradiance (dose-rate in $W \cdot cm^{-2}$) and exposure duration (in seconds, s) to achieve a threshold photochemical radiant exposure (dose in $J \cdot cm^{-2}$), the cumulative exposures from either a single lengthy exposure or repeated exposures within a given time (usually a few hours) will be additive. Prior to any discussion of light sources and measurements, it is important to consider those physical quantities and units useful in photobiology. These quantities are termed radiometric (and spectro-radiometric),

■ CHAPTER 45 ■

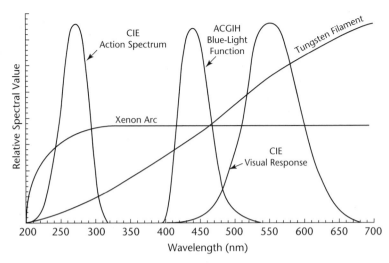

Figure 45.1: The effect of different light source spectra for delivering an effective dose relative to the same action spectrum. Two sources with the same total radiant power output are not equally effective in delivering a photobiologically effective dose.

and they should not be confused with the photometric system of measurements (lumens and candelas) used by lighting engineers. Radiometry is the science of measurement of optical radiation. Photometry is the science of measuring visible radiation, i.e., *light*. Radiometric quantities such as radiant power—used to describe the output power (not electrical input power) of a source in watts [W]—must be used to describe and quantify ultraviolet radiation (UVR). Photometric quantities such as luminous power—used to describe the luminous output of a lamp in lumens [lm]—are based upon the relative visibility of different spectral sources as seen by a human "standard observer." In illuminating engineering, light levels are spectrally weighted by the standard photometric visibility curve, which peaks at 550 nm for the human eye.

To quantify a photochemical effect it is not sufficient to specify the number of photons-per-square-centimeter (photon flux) or the irradiance (W·cm^{-2}) since the efficiency of the effect is highly dependent on wavelength. Generally, shorter-wavelength, higher-energy photons are more efficient. Photometric quantities are hybrid quantities that are defined by the action spectrum for vision—a photochemically initiated process. Photometric quantities have no value in photobiology except in describing visual processes and retinal photochemistry.

Unfortunately, since the spectral distributions of different light sources vary widely, there is no simple conversion factor between photometric (either photopic or scotopic) and radiometric quantities. This conversion may vary from 15 to 50 lumens·watt^{-1} (1m·W^{-1}) for an incandescent source to about 100 1m·W^{-1} for a xenon arc, to perhaps 300 to 400 lm·W^{-1} for a fluorescent source (Sliney and Wolbarsht, 1980). The fraction of radiant energy in the UV is much less still. Although the action spectra for erythema in normal human skin have been published by many investigators (Hausser 1928; Luckiesh *et al.*, 1930; Coblentz *et al.*, 1931; Everett *et al.*, 1965; Freeman *et al.*, 1966; Berger *et al.*, 1968; Urbach 1969; Sliney 1972, 1987; Willis *et al.*, 1972; Sliney and Wolbarsht 1980; Parrish *et al.*, 1982; Cole *et al.*, 1986; McKinlay and Diffey 1987; ACGIH 1994), the action spectra of photosensitized responses appear to be quite imprecise or even unknown (Fitzpatrick *et al.*, 1974; Parrish *et al.*, 1978; Diffey, 1982; Urbach and Gange, 1986; WHO, 1994). This suggests the need to specify the spectrum of the light source used as well as the irradiance levels if one is to compare experimental results from different studies.

45.1.1 Radiometric quantities

The following radiometric quantities may be used in photodermatology, and are briefly summarized here:

1 *Irradiance* (surface dose rate) and *radiant exposure* (surface dose) are units specifying power or energy incident upon a plane. As shown in Figure 45.1, these quantities are the dose rate (irradiance) and exposure dose (radiant exposure) that are the most fundamental dose quantities used in all of photobiology. The units most commonly used are W·cm^{-2} and J·cm^{-2}, respectively, 1 W = 1 J·s^{-1}.

2 *Fluence rate* and *fluence* are used in some very sophisticated studies, where the internal surface dose with backscatter is included. These quantities are used correctly most often in theoretical studies, but these terms are frequently misused to mean irradiance and radiant exposure because the units of W·cm^{-2} and J·cm^{-2} are the same.

3 *Radiance* (irradiance per solid angle) is an important quantity used by physicists in specifying a source. This quantity limits the ability of lenses and reflective optics in concentrating a light source. For, example, a xenon-arc lamp has a very high radiance and its energy can be focused to produce a very high irradiance on a target tissue. By contrast, a fluorescent lamp tube has a much lower radiance, and its energy cannot be focused to a high concentration. The units are W· cm^{-2}·sr^{-1}.

4   *Radiant intensity* (power per solid angle) is used to indicate how collimated a light source really is. Although useful for specifying searchlights, it normally has very limited use in photobiology. The units are $W \cdot sr^{-1}$.

5   *Spectral quantities* (units per wavelength) are used for specifying the energy, power or irradiance per wavelength interval. When calculating a *photo-biologically effective dose* the spectral quantity must be multiplied by the action spectrum. Examples: spectral radiant power, spectral irradiance, spectral radiant exposure, etc. The units for each quantity are modified by adding "per nanometer," e.g., $W \cdot cm^{-2}$ becomes $W \cdot cm^{-2} \cdot nm^{-1}$.

6   *Photon (Quantum) quantities* (units of photons) are used primarily in theoretical studies, and in photochemistry. In this case the radiant exposure is specified in $photons \cdot cm^{-2}$ and irradiance is specified in $photons \cdot cm^{-2} \cdot s^{-1}$.

45.1.2   Spectral band notations

When considering UVR bioeffects, it is useful to employ the convention of the International Commission on Illumination (CIE) for spectral bands. The CIE has designated 315–320 to 400 nm as UV-A, 280 to 315–320 nm as UV-B, and

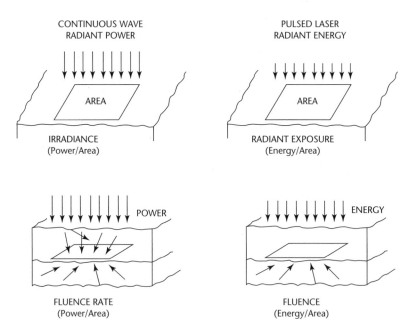

Figure 45.2: Radiometric quantities and units used in photodermatology.

100–280 nm as UV-C (CIE 1987). Wavelengths below 180 nm (vacuum UV) are of little practical significance since they are readily absorbed in air. The 308-nm UV wavelength is therefore in the UV-B spectral region. UV-C wavelengths are more photochemically active, because these wavelengths correspond to the most energetic photons, they are strongly absorbed in certain amino acids and therefore by most proteins (Harding and Dilley, 1976; Hillenkamp 1980; Grossweiner 1984; Smith 1989); whereas, UV-B wavelengths are less photo-chemically active, but are more penetrating in most tissues. UV-A wavelengths are far less photobiologically active, but are still more penetrating than UV-B wavelengths. UV-A wavelengths play an interactive (sometimes synergistic) role when exposure occurs following UV-B exposure (Willis *et al.*, 1972). UV-B radiation has been shown to alter enzyme activity in the lens (Tung *et al.*, 1988).

It is very important to keep in mind that these photobiological spectral bands are merely a useful "short-hand" notation, and they can be used to make general (but not absolute) statements about the relative spectral effectiveness of different parts of the UV spectrum in producing effects. The dividing lines, while not arbitrary, are certainly not fine dividing lines between wavelengths that may or may not elicit a given biological effect. One should always provide a wavelength band or spectral emission curve for the UV source being used and not rely totally on these spectral terms. There are also many authors who use 320 nm rather than the CIE-defined dividing line of 315 nm to divide UV-A from UV-B. Some authors also may divide the UV-A band into two regions: UV-A1 and UV-A2, with a division made at about 340 nm.

45.1.3 Radiometric principles

There are a number of general principles when help to avoid errors in dosimetry. Probably the most important first principle is the:

1 *Bunsen-Roscoe Law*, which specifies the reciprocity of photochemical reactions. Within the recovery time of the system (generally a few hours for erythema and photokeratitis), the product of the dose rate (irradiance) and the exposure duration results in a constant dose (radiant exposure) required to elicit a given effect. Therefore, a very high dose rate from a very intense source can result in the same effect within a very short time as a less intense source can produce in a much longer time.

2 *Critical Photon Energy*. To produce a photochemical effect in tissue, normally only one photon will alter one molecule, when we examine the process at

■ CHAPTER 45 ■

the molecular level. For this reason the individual photon energy must be sufficient to alter the molecule, or else the interaction results in imparting energy to the molecule that will probably result in vibrational motion (and in a temperature rise at the macroscopic level). For this reason, the long-wavelength cut-off for the action spectrum is normally fairly sharply pronounced. This also makes the measurement of a rapidly changing action spectrum quite difficult unless very narrow wavelength bands are used.

3   *Inverse Square Law and the "Rule of Ten."* For most sources that are not highly collimated (such as a laser), the well-known "Inverse Square Law" aids in extrapolating the irradiance to different distances from a small optical source. While the Inverse Square Law is strictly true only for a geometrical point source, the "Rule of Ten" allows us to apply it to practical lamp sources. One will have a very small error (less than 10 percent) if one begins the extrapolation at a distance of at least ten times the diameter of the source. For example, if one has a small mercury arc lamp with an arc size of 3 mm, then at ten times the 3 mm, i.e., at 30 mm, one would expect the measured irradiance to decrease inversely as the square of the distance beyond that point. For example, if that lamp source was specified to produce an irradiance of 10 mW·cm^{-2} at 20 cm, then at twice that distance the irradiance would drop to $(1/2^2)$ 1/4 its value, or to 2.5 mW·cm^{-2}. At four times that distance the irradiance would drop to $(1/4^2)$ 1/16 the value of 10 mW·cm^{-2}, or only 625 µW·cm^{-2}. Thus, without making detailed measurements at each distance, a wide range of dose rates can be established by merely moving to different distances from the source.

4   *Law of Conservation of Radiance (Brightness).* This principal derives from the physical law of conservation of energy. Basically, it states that no matter what optical focusing lenses one employs, the focal irradiance cannot exceed a value limited by the brightness of a source. Arc lamps and the sun are of nearly equivalent radiance, whereas a tungsten source has a much lower radiance. Lasers have by far the greatest radiance of any source, and their rays can be concentrated in a very high focal irradiance. The use of larger collecting optics can increase the size of the irradiation zone, but not the irradiance.

45.2   OPTICAL RADIATION SOURCES

There are many different types of optical sources that can be used in photo-dermatology. Even the sun has been employed in some studies, but the sun's changing spectrum from hour to hour makes it difficult to use for reproducible exposures. Artificial sources are therefore almost always used in laboratory studies, and these are generally high-intensity lamps.

Broad-band, polychromatic sources deliver much more irradiance than narrow band sources. With a monochromator or narrow-band filters, one can achieve nearly monochromatic (one-wavelength) sources of light or UVR by sacrificing the total power available. By the Bunsen-Roscoe Law, the same exposure dose would require a much longer time to deliver. Nevertheless, to determine an action spectrum for a given photobiological effect, one is forced to take this approach. If the action spectrum is known, or if one wishes simply to simulate sunlight with a *solar simulator*, one can achieve a threshold exposure dose in a far shorter time with broad-band sources. The continuous light sources used most frequently are:

1   tungsten lamps and tungsten-halogen lamps;
2   high pressure gas discharge lamps, e.g., deuterium lamps;
3   arc lamps, e.g., xenon, or mercury-xenon high pressure lamps; and
4   low-pressure discharge lamps, generally used for "line" sources.

Other continuous sources, such as LEDs, lasers and synchrotrons have generally not been of much value; although lasers have been used for rapid determination of action spectra. Pulsed sources, such as flashlamps, could be employed to achieve stepped doses, but this is rare.

The greatest pitfalls with regard to the optical exposure in phototoxicity studies relate to poor *source characterization*. Unfortunately, to properly characterize a light source is quite difficult. Some of the factors that should be considered are:

1   *Lamp envelope and filtration.* The spectral filtration of the glass or quartz envelope determines how much short-wavelength UV-C and UV-B are emitted by the lamp. A quartz envelope transmits down to approximately 180–200 nm and gives the broadest spectrum of UVR. Most glass envelopes filter out wavelengths below 310—320 nm. In addition, through the use of short-wavelength cutoff filters, the relative contribution of UV-B and UV-A can be controlled. Since the terrestrial solar spectrum has a cutoff between 295 and 305 nm (depending upon time of day), filters with cutoffs in this region are used in solar simulators.
2   *Source size and distance.* Through the use of the Inverse-Square Law, it is possible to produce a range of irradiances for a given experiment. However,

CHAPTER 45

if the source size is rather large (e.g., a UV-A "black-light" reflectorized spotlight), the irradiance will not decrease rapidly with increasing distance from the lamp. If a high-pressure arc lamp is used, the arc size may be only a couple of millimeters in diameter, and the inverse-square law would apply within a few centimeters from the source.

3   *Source uniformity.* The uniformity of the source can affect the uniformity of the irradiance patten, particularly if the source is focused. If the UV source is not readily visible, a fluorescent card may be used to visually examine the irradiance pattern at the point of the subject's exposure. An aperture can be positioned over the site of greatest uniformity in order to achieve reproducible exposure doses.

4   *Source stability.* Tungsten-halogen (and tungsten) lamps generally provide the most stable optical sources with little fluctuation with time. However, because relatively little UVR is emitted from these types of lamps (tungsten-halogen lamps emit more UVR because of higher operating temperature), a slight change in supply voltage can result in much greater changes in UV output. A stabilized power supply may therefore be necessary. Arc lamps typically produce some degree of flicker, which can be averaged over most practical exposure durations. The temporal stability of lasers varies greatly with the type used.

5   *Aging characteristics.* The aging characteristics of different sources vary considerably, but all sources will change with extensive use. It is therefore best to have at least an inexpensive monitor to measure the relative output of the source from day to day.

6   *Temperature and environmental sensitivities.* The sensitivities of different light sources to environmental changes, e.g., with temperature, are generally not great, but if the laboratory environment does change, the UVR monitor should be used to check for possible changes. The greatest change of output with temperature occurs during lamp warm-up. Mercury discharge lamps are particularly noted for this, and a five-minute warm-up period is generally advisable; one can check for this with the UVR monitor.

7   *Radiant efficiency.* The radiant efficiency of different light sources varies greatly with regard to the UV radiant power emitted for a given electrical input in watts. Arc lamps are probably the most UV efficient sources, but require special power supplies. Radio-frequency power supplies for arc lamps can also create substantial electromagnetic interference and disable electronic instruments and nearby computers. Gas discharge lamps such as sun-lamps require less expensive power supplies, or they can be operated

at main voltages. Lasers are notoriously inefficient, e.g., an argon laser emits less than 0.1 percent of the electrical input power; however, the mono-chromatic purity of the laser cannot be equalled.

45.3 UV MEASUREMENT

45.3.1 Types of UVR measurement instruments

There are a variety of different instruments that can be used to measure UV radiant power or irradiance. They vary greatly in cost and complexity (and accuracy). Depending upon the application a relatively inexpensive UV monitor may suffice, but the user must be aware of the limitations of the instrument.

Instruments are often grouped by the detector type used (e.g., a photo-multiplier tube (PMT), a photodiode, a photofluorescence detector, or a thermal detector). The PMT is by far the most sensitive; hence, it is used in instruments where very low irradiances must be measured, as with monochromators to measure the spectral distribution of a lamp.

Most simple instruments have a "broad-band" spectral response which may cover just a band in the UV or may include the visible. These meters use a photodiode. A special type of UV-B detector employs a fluorescent screen that is sensitive only to the short-wavelength UVR, and a photodiode measures the visible fluorescence, which is proportional to the actinic UVR. This seemingly complicated method is used to greatly reduce out-of-band response—a severe problem in UVR radiometry. Thermal detectors are seldom used, because these respond to all wavelengths from UV to infrared, although for certain calibrations they may be useful for an absolute measurement. Aside from arc lamps, most optical radiation sources such as the sun or general service fluorescent and incandescent lamps used for illumination emit only trace quantities of UVR. Indeed, the UV-B or UV-C emission is normally less than 0.1–1 percent of the total radiant power output. For this reason, attempting to measure UV-B in the presence of so much longer-wavelength radiant energy presents an incredible challenge. If a special UV lamp is in use, this may not be a problem, and a simple, less expensive instrument may suffice.

In addition to the broad-band instruments just described, it will be necessary to use a *spectroradiometer* to measure the spectrum of the incident UVR. These are rarely inexpensive or simple instruments, but are essential to obtain the spectrum of the lamp source being used, unless the spectrum can be obtained from the manufacturer. All spectroradiometers have three fundamental elements:

input optics, a monochromator (prism or diffraction grating to disperse the spectrum) and a detector. Spectroradiometers are too complex to describe in any detail here, and the reader is referred to any number of references (Kostowski, 1997; Sliney and Wolbarsht, 1980). It is important, nevertheless, to be familiar with the importance of using appropriate input optics for an experiment. The input optics are the lenses, optical fibers, diffusers, and apertures used between the point of measurement and the entrance slit of the monochromator. Frequently, substantial errors are introduced by a failure to understand the limits of the input optics in achieving a good "cosine response," and uniform spatial response. Some of the response factors that should be taken into account are: the linearity of response with increasing light input, the nature of the entrance aperture and whether it is smaller than the irradiation area being measured, the cosine response, the temperature response and the wavelength range. The most challenging problem of monochromators is the rejection of out-of-band radiation, or "stray light." A double grating or double prism monochromator is far better in stray light rejection than a single element monochromator. Again, this problem may not be significant if one is using a UVR source with little or no visible or infrared output.

45.3.2   Performing the measurement

Prior to using any UV meter or spectroradiometer, one should attempt to perform a general characterization of the instrument. It is most helpful to measure several types of sources where there exist published output and spectral data with which to compare. Since many radiometric errors originate from a failure to adequately appreciate the geometry of exposure, be sure that the input optics are appropriate for the measurement.

Calibration of the instrument should be traceable to a national laboratory and the type of secondary standard should be noted to see if it is at all similar to the light source you are using. If not, you may wish to inquire of the instrument manufacturer as to any special limitations of your instrument and whether it is appropriate for the task in mind. Some laboratories maintain some limited calibration capability, such as a reference lamp or a reference detector or standard meter. In general, calibration may be "reference source based" or "reference detector based." Examples of reference optical sources are the FEL tungsten-halogen lamp, a standard deuterium lamp (for UV-C), or even a laser. Reference detectors generally have a flat response, e.g., a pyroelectric detector or a disk calorimeter, although some reference silicon detectors are used in the ultraviolet spectral region. In any calibration procedure, the source specifications must be understood, and the uncertainty in the final calibration should be determined. The determination of the contribution of all errors in the process frequently is termed the "error budget."

Before purchasing an instrument, one should hopefully know what level of measurement accuracy the project requires. As noted before, a simple UVR monitor may suffice if one is using a well characterized lamp and there is little visible light to produce a stray-light problem. Also important is to estimate the level of measurement uncertainty that you can live with. For example, in a pass-fail situation, where one desires to determine if the measured level exceeds a limit of X and the measurements are typically at 50 percent of X, one can use an instrument with a 20–30 percent uncertainty, without being too concerned of passing a source that emits too much UVR. However, if the level is typically 95 percent of the limit, a very accurate measurement with an uncertainty less than 5 percent is required. For phototoxicity studies, one should be pleased if one can achieve a 20 percent accuracy in irradiance measurements.

For the instrument manufacturer to adequately assess the accuracy and stability of the instrument, a thorough study of the system and the sources and components of the system is required—a challenging task. In the end, the individual investigator must rely on the reputation of the manufacturer and the experience of colleagues with different instruments. Do not expect a simple instrument to perform the task required of a much more sophisticated instrument.

Special exposure equipment exists for phototoxicity testing, and the manufacturer provides the radiometric output characteristics and spectrum. Figure 45.3 shows one such instrument that features a multiple-port fiber delivery system to allow multiple simultaneous exposures of the skin at different irradiance levels.

45.4 GENERAL BIOPHYSICAL AND PHOTOBIOLOGICAL FACTORS

The purpose of this section is not to add another review of photobiology, but to consider the dosimetry required for adequate comparison of UVR effects being determined in various studies. While the great majority of investigators in phototoxicology have made UVR measurements designed to characterize the exposure conditions, the calculated levels of exposure that have been published in different studies often vary by more than a factor of ten amongst studies

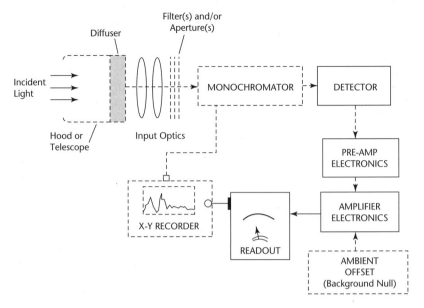

Figure 45.3: General diagram of a radiometer or spectroradiometer. The solid lines indicate the essential elements for any radiometer. The dashed lines indicate the two added elements required for a spectroradiometer: the monochromator and a spectral output in the form of a printer/X-Y recorder or CRT display to show the spectrum. Also, one normally wants to have a background null adjustment (lower left). Adapted from Sliney and Wolbarsht (1980), p. 352.

employing the same light sources. This chapter will hopefully reduce that problem.

For photobiologically induced injury of tissue occurring after prolonged exposure (i.e., greater than 10 s in the visible and UV-A; greater than at most 1 ms in the UV-B and C), it is generally agreed that the mechanism of injury is initiated by a photochemical event, rather than a thermal event. Two key factors distinguish a photochemical process from a thermal process. Thermal injury is a *rate process* and is dependent upon the volumic absorption of energy across the spectrum. By contrast, any photochemical process will have a long wavelength cutoff where photon energies are insufficient to cause the molecular change of interest. A photochemical reaction will also exhibit reciprocity between irradiance (exposure dose rate) and exposure duration. Repair mechanisms, recombination over long periods and photon saturation for extremely short periods will lead to reciprocity failure. For the lengthy exposures characteristic of phototoxicity studies, it is difficult to know what effective exposure time to use for an exposure calculation. Irradiance E in $W \cdot cm^{-2}$ times exposure duration t is equal to the radiant exposure H in $J \cdot cm^{-2}$, i.e., the exposure dose.

$$H = E \cdot t \tag{45.1}$$

Since most photobiological effects are photochemically initiated, it is necessary for the UV or visible photons to penetrate to the target molecules, the *chromophores*, to trigger the photochemical event. Therefore, the action spectrum for a given effect in the skin is actually not only the *in vitro* action spectrum for the target molecules, but is altered by the spectral transmission of the overlying tissue, such as the stratum corneum. UV-C wavelengths are strongly absorbed in proteins, are very photochemically interactive, and have the least penetration into biological tissue. In this regard, the ArF excimer laser wavelength of 193 nm provides the extreme case of a wavelength shown very clearly to produce damage to the cell wall without effectively penetrating to the nuclei of many cell types.

The *biologically effective irradiance* E_{eff} from an optical source is obtained by a mathematical weighting of the spectral irradiance $E\lambda$ and the normalized action spectrum $S(\lambda)$ which is unitless:

$$E_{eff} = \Sigma \ E\lambda \cdot S(\lambda)\Delta\lambda \tag{45.2}$$

where $\Delta\lambda$ is the spectral interval. The spectral region of summation would be from approximately 200 nm (or where the lamp envelope permitted emission) to at least 400 nm over the full range of the action spectrum. This effective irradiance is very useful, and some instruments have a spectral response function designed to mimic a common action spectrum such as erythema.

With regard to photocarcinogenesis, it is generally agreed that only a very narrow UV-B wavelength band is generally considered very effective in producing skin carcinogenesis (Cole *et al.*, 1986; Sterenborg and van der Luen, 1987)— and for that matter, severe sunburn (Hausser, 1928), and cataractogenesis in humans (Sliney and Wolbarsht, 1980). Even though we are concerned with immediate effects in the skin, a study of the delayed effects upon both dermal and ocular tissues from UVR, can provide a deeper insight into the potential for biological effects upon the skin as well as the eye in this wavelength region.

In *phototoxicity studies,* the exposure site can be limited for topical photo-sensitivity tests. Relative thresholds and altered action spectra can be tested on

■ CHAPTER 45 ■

the same subject at different skin sites for comparison. In this case, the multiple-port exposure system (shown in Figure 45.3) can be useful for more rapid testing. In such tests, it is presumed that the spectrum eliciting the phototoxity is sunlight, and this is one reasonable approach where an in-depth study of action spectra is not possible. However, it should be remembered that although the action spectrum of a photosensitizer might be the same as its absorption spectrum *in vitro*, as with some drugs, the photosensitizer may interact with proteins or DNA and produce an altered erythema spectrum. Obviously, the nature of the interaction in tissue and the resultant action spectrum can influence the results of a photosensitivity test depending upon the light source used.

45.5 DETERMINING ACTION SPECTRA

In phototoxicology, it is frequently necessary to determine an action spectrum for the photosensitization. Initially, a very crude action spectrum may suffice. This can be accomplished by use of several band-pass filters or short-wavelength filters to determine the band that appears to be most photosensitizing. However, for the purposes of basic photobiology or if the action spectrum is later to be used by engineers to determine the efficacy of different lamps in eliciting a response, a much more refined action spectrum will generally be necessary. In comparing action spectra obtained in different laboratories, scientists are frequently puzzled at apparent differences. The sources of these differences generally arise from the use of different means to obtain the monochromatic light. A tunable continuous-wave laser will provide the most precise and accurate result (Anders, 1995), but this is generally unavailable, and one must employ a number of narrow-band spectral filters to sample the spectrum or a tunable diffraction-grating monochromator to provide the selected narrow-bands to sample the region of interest (Diffey, 1975; Sliney and Wolbarsht, 1980; Young and Diffey, 1985). The choice of monochromator and selection of a sampling spectral bandwidth can greatly impact the resulting action spectrum (Sliney, 1998), and photobiologists frequently overlook this effect.

45.5.1 Choice of monochromator bandwidth

When determining action spectra using monochromators and a broadband UV source, a very narrow bandwidth is essential to obtain an accurate spectrum for further applications. This, however, is a very difficult challenge to the experimentalist. Typical UV sources that have been used in photobiological

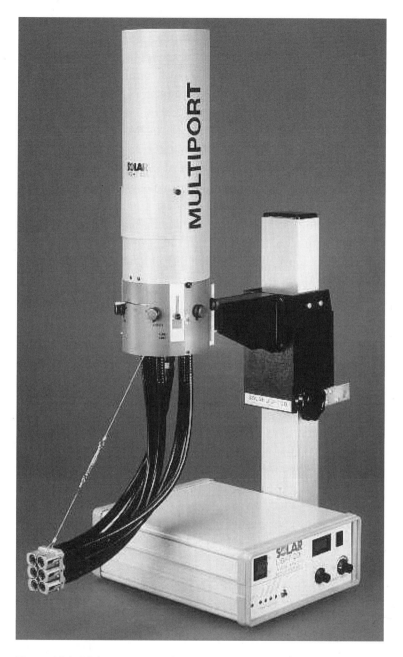

Figure 45.4: Multi-port UV irradiator. In this unit, an arc lamp source is filtered to simulate sunlight and multiple liquid light guides are used to provide more than one irradiation site with stepped irradiance (dose rate) values. Photo, courtesy of Solar Light Company, Philadelphia, PA.

threshold studies are low-pressure mercury lamps with filters or xenon-arc (or mercury-xenon-arc) high-pressure lamps with a grating monochromator. The spectral filters or the monochromator isolates the desired wavelengths. The disadvantage of the low-pressure lamp is that only a limited number of wavelengths are available. While the xenon arc monochromator is continuously tunable, it suffers from poor resolution, as the slit widths must be great enough to pass enough power. When analyzing any published action spectrum, it is necessary to consider the spectral bandwidth for all data and to consider also "stray radiation" and the sources of "stray radiation" in the instrument; e.g. stray light scattered from the gratings in monochromators, leaks in radiometric housing, etc.

The slit function is the spectral power distribution of radiant energy emitted at the given wavelength set on the monochromator (Kostkowski, 1997). For a perfect grating monochromator, the shape of the slit function is triangular, as shown in Figure 45.5. Although it would always be desirable to employ a high-resolution monochromator slit-width, such as 0.5 or 1.0 nm, the throughput is so low that a threshold exposure could require hours. In practice, much larger bandpass values of 5–10 nm are therefore used. Threshold data are frequently

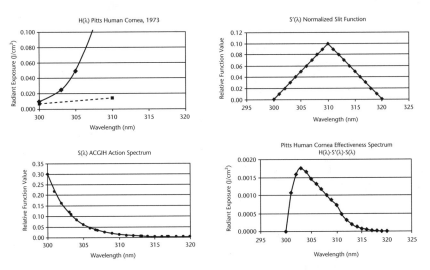

Figure 45.5: The upper left panel shows the ACGIH threshold limit value for the 300–320 nm region (solid line). The dashed line is the radiant exposure threshold at 310 nm as determined by Pitts' 1973 experimental data. The upper right panel is the normalized slit function; the lower left panel is the S(λ) action spectrum. When the slit function is weighted by the experimental data and the action spectrum, the effective wavelength shifts as shown in the lower right panel.

plotted against the center-wavelength of each spectral bandpass; however, significant plotting errors can be introduced into the true action spectrum when the slit width of the monochromator is not accounted for (Diffey, 1975; Sliney, 1998; Sliney and Wolbarsht, 1980; Young and Diffey, 1985). To derive a true action spectrum from the low-resolution threshold data obtained from monochromator studies, a mathematical convolution is required.

If the target molecule, or chromophore, is a protein or DNA, the most effective dose will normally come from the shorter wavelengths (i.e., those before the center wavelength of the slit function), since these will contribute much more to the effective dose than the longer wavelengths in the rapidly changing 300–320 nm region.

Published photobiological threshold data are frequently plotted as an action spectrum with relative response versus wavelength. The accuracy and resolution of the action spectrum are significantly influenced by the choice of the monochromatic source and the number of data points obtained. Measurements of UV action spectra for erythema or photokeratitis can be especially challenging in the 300–320-nm spectral region, as the UV hazard action spectrum, $S(\lambda)$, changes quite rapidly in this region, i.e., the limits increase by an order of magnitude between 303–310 nm, and another order of magnitude between 310–320 nm.

When the slit function covers a region where the true action spectrum varies greatly with wavelength, it is difficult to arrive at the "true" effective wavelength for proper plotting of the data points of the action spectrum. No mono-chromator really achieves a perfect, triangular slit function, but instead there is a "skirt" at the base of the triangle. For example, if the slit function in Figure 45.5 applies to taking a data point for photokeratitis (corneal UV damage) at a monochromator setting of 310 nm, the "310-nm threshold" would have an enormous error. At 300 nm the slit function had at least a 1 percent value, the effective wavelength shifts noticeably to the shorter wavelengths, because the true action spectrum, simulated by $S(\lambda)$ at 300 nm has a value 20 times more effective than at 310 nm.

In an effort to show the impact of monochromator bandwidth on threshold data, Chaney and Sliney studied the impact of bandwidth on effectiveness spectra of photokeratitis studies. They recalculated the effectiveness spectra using the bandwidths specified in the literature, and the revised action spectrum was remarkably steeper than that published by the authors of the original study (Chaney and Sliney, 2002).

■ CHAPTER 45 ■

45.6 CONCLUSION

While all reports of photosensitization contain some quantitative exposure information, important spectral information is often lacking. The careful development of an action spectrum for each type of interaction is an important research goal when dealing with a new target molecule. Radiometric and spectroradiometric measurements of lamps permit one to calculate the effective exposures.

When one considers the very small, but biologically significant, fraction of UVR in natural sunlight, one is struck by the fact that even fluorescent lamps and other lamps used in general indoor illumination also have a fraction of UVR that may be biologically significant. The enormous importance of considering both spectral and geometrical factors in phototoxicity experiments cannot be overstated.

REFERENCES

AMERICAN CONFERENCE OF GOVERNMENTAL INDUSTRIAL HYGIENISTS (ACGIH) (2002) *TLV's, Threshold Limit Values and Biological Exposure Indices for 2002*, Cincinnati: ACGIH.

ANDERS, A., ALTHEIDE, H., KNALMANN, M. and TRONNIER, H. (1995) Action spectrum for erythema in humans investigated with dye lasers. *Photochem. Photobiol.* **61**(2), 200–205.

BERGER, D., URBACH, F. and DAVIES, R.E. (1968) The action spectrum of erythema induced by ultraviolet radiation, in JADASSOHN, W. and SCHIRREN, C.G. (eds) *Preliminary Report XIII. Congressus Internationalis Dermatologiae, Munchen 1967*, New York: Springer-Verlag, 1112–1117.

CHANEY, E.K. and SLINEY, D.H. (2002) Spectral bandwidth used to determine UV action spectra, in HASTINGS, J.W. (ed.) *Abstracts of the 30th Annual Meeting of the American Society for Photobiology*, 86.

COBLENTZ, W.R., STAIR, R. and HOGUE, J.M. (1931) The spectral erythemic reaction of the human skin to ultraviolet radiation. *Proc. Nat. Acad. Sci. US* **17**, 401–403.

COLE, C.A., FORBES, D.F. and DAVIES, P.D. (1986) An action spectrum for UV photocarcinogenesis, *Photochem. Photobiol.* **43**(3), 275–284.

COMMISSION INTERNATIONALE DE L'ECLAIRAGE (INTERNATIONAL COMMISSION ON ILLUMINATION). (1987) *International Lighting Vocabulary*, 4th ed. Pub. CIE No. 17.4 (E-1.1). Paris: CIE.

CROKE, D.T., BLAU, W., OhUIGIN, C., KELLY, J.M. and MCCONNELL, D.J. (1988) Photolysis of phosphodiester bonds in plasmid DNA by high intensity UV laser irradiation, *Photochem. Photobiol.* **47**(4), 527–536.

DIFFEY, B. (1975) Variation of erythema with monochromator bandwidth, *Arch. Dermatol.* **111**, 1070–1071.

DIFFEY, B.L. (1982) *Ultraviolet Radiation in Medicine*, Bristol: Adam Hilger Ltd.

EVERETT, M.A., OLSEN, R.L. and SAYER, R.M. (1965) Ultraviolet erythema, *Arch. Dermatol.* **92**, 713–719.

FITZPATRICK, T.B., PATHAK, M.A., HARBER, L.C., SEIJI, M. and KUKITA, A. (eds) (1974) *Sunlight and Man, Normal and Abnormal Photobiologic Responses*, Tokyo, Japan: University of Tokyo Press.

FREEMAN, R.S., OWENS, D.W., KNOX, J.M. and HUDSON, H.T. (1966) Relative energy requirements for an erythemal response of skin to monochromatic wavelengths of ultraviolet present in the solar spectrum, *J. Invest. Dermatol.* **47**, 586–592.

GROSSWEINER, L.I. (1984) Photochemistry of proteins: a review, *Curr. Eye Res.* **3**(1), 137–144.

HAUSSER, K.W. (1928) Influence of wavelength in radiation biology, *Strahlentherapie* **28**, 25–44.

HARDING, J.J., DILLEY, K.J. (1976) Structural proteins of the mammalian lens: A review with emphasis on changes in development, aging and cataract, *Exp. Eye Res.*, **22**, 1–73.

HILLENKAMP, F. (1980) Interaction between laser radiation and biological systems, in HILLENKAMP, F., PRATESI, R. and SACCHI, C.A. (eds) *Lasers in Biology and Medicine*, New York: Plenum Press, 37–68.

KOSTKOWSKI, H.J. (1997) *Reliable Spectroradiometry*, La Plata, MD: Spectroradiometry Consulting, 89–120.

LUCKIESH, M.L., HOLLADAY, L., TAYLOR, A.H. (1930) Reaction of untanned human skin to ultraviolet radiation, *J. Opt. Soc. Am.* **20**, 423–432.

MCKINLAY, A.F. and DIFFEY, B.L. (1987) A reference action spectrum for ultraviolet induced erythema in human skin, in PASSCHIER, W.F. and BOSNJAKOVIC, B.F.M. (eds), *Human Exposure to Ultraviolet Radiation: Risks and Regulations*, New York: Excerpta Medica Division, Elsevier Science Publishers, 83–87.

PARRISH, J.A., ANDERSON, R.R., URBACH, F. and PITTS, D. (1978) *UV-A, Biological Effects of Ultraviolet Radiation with Emphasis on Human Responses to Longwave Radiation*, New York: Plenum Press.

PARRISH, J.A., JAENICKE, K.F. and ANDERSON, R.R. (1982) Erythema and melanogenesis action spectra of normal human skin, *Photochem. Photobiol.* **36**(2), 187–191.

PITTS, D.G. (1973) The ocular ultraviolet action spectrum and protection criteria, *Health Phys.* **25**(6), 559–566.

SLINEY, D.H. (1972) The merits of an envelope action spectrum for ultraviolet radiation exposure criteria, *Am. Ind. Hyg. Assoc. J.* **33**, 644–653.

SLINEY, D.H. (1987) Estimating the solar ultraviolet radiation exposure to an intraocular lens implant, *J. Cataract Refract. Surg.* **13**(5), 296–301.

Sliney, D.H. (1998) Photobiological action spectra-limits on resolution, in MATTHES, R. and SLINEY, D.H. (eds) *Measurements of Optical Radiation Hazards*, Geneva: CIE and ICNIRP, 41–47.

SLINEY, D.H. and WOLBARSHT, M.L. (1980) *Safety with Lasers and Other Optical Sources*, New York: Plenum Publishing Corp.

SMITH, K.C. (1989) *The Science of Photobiology*, New York: Plenum Press.

STERENBORG, H.J.C.M. and VAN DER LEUN, J.C. (1987) Action spectra for tumorigenesis by ultraviolet radiation, in PASSCHIER, W.F. and BOSNJAKOVIC, B.F.M. (eds) *Human Exposure to Ultraviolet Radiation: Risks and Regulations*, New York: Excerpta Medica Division, Elsevier Science Publishers, 173–191.

TUNG, W.H., CHYLACK, JR., L.T. and ANDLEY, U.P. (1988) Lens hexokinase deactivation by near-uv irradiation, *Curr. Eye Res.* **7**(3), 257–263.

URBACH, F. (ed.) (1969) *The Biologic Effects of Ultraviolet Radiation*, New York: Pergamon Press.

URBACH, F. and GANGE, R.W. (eds) (1986) *The Biological Effects of UV-A Radiation.* Westport, CT: Praeger Publishers.

WILLIS, I., KLIGMAN, A. and EPSTEIN, J. (1972) Effects of long ultraviolet rays on human skin: photoprotective or photoaugmentative, *J. Invest. Dermatol.* **59**, 416–420.

WORLD HEALTH ORGANIZATION (WHO) (1994) Environmental Health Criteria No. 160, Ultraviolet Radiation, joint publication of the United Nations Environmental Program, the International Radiation Protection Association and the World Health Organization, Geneva: WHO.

YOUNG, S. and DIFFEY, B. (1985) Influence of monochromator bandwidth on the erythema action spectrum in the UV-B region, *Photodermatology* **2**, 383–387.

CHAPTER

46

Use of Pig Skin Preparations in Novel Diffusion Cell Arrays to Measure Skin Absorption and to Evaluate Potential Chemical Toxicity

WILLIAM G REIFENRATH, VICTORIA L GARZOUZI
AND HAROLD O KAMMEN

Contents

46.1   Introduction

46.2   Test system

46.3   Formulation and skin permeation studies

46.4   Chemical toxicity studies

46.5   Summary

46.1 INTRODUCTION

The development of topical products generally requires the screening of large numbers of formulations in order to optimize drug disposition. Changes in vehicle can also result in local or systemic toxicity, and an early indication of potential toxicity will facilitate formulation development. To this end, a new *in vitro* test system was developed to efficiently determine skin absorption and potential chemical toxicity. Sheets of viable excised pig skin were sandwiched between two standard 24 well plates. The lower wells contained receptor fluid and a magnetic stirrer. The visceral side of the skin sample was bathed by tissue culture medium that maintained skin viability. The medium also served as a sink for skin penetrants, their metabolites, and excretion products from the skin. The upper wells were opened to the atmosphere for topical application.

Using ^{14}C-salicylic acid as a model compound, the effect of vehicle on skin absorption was determined. Using a number of known toxicants, alterations in skin metabolism were measured as potential markers of adverse effects.

46.2 TEST SYSTEM

Arrays of diffusion cells were created from polystyrene, 24-well tissue culture plates (Falcon Multiwell Primaria, Becton Dickinson and Co., Franklin Lakes, NJ). One plate, which served as a reservoir for receptor fluid, was modified by drilling a small off-center hole through the bottom of each well and fitting the hole with a plastic tapered luer plug. This hole allowed the addition or removal of receptor fluid following assembly. A second plate, which served as an array of donor chambers, was modified by removing the bottom of the wells. The lower plate contained a magnetic stirrer and approximately 3-ml of RPMI tissue culture medium prewarmed to 37°C.

Following euthanasia, skin was harvested from the upper back of young Yorkshire pigs. Pig skin was selected because it has been found to be a good model for the permeability properties of human skin (Reifenrath and Hawkins, 1986). Skin strips were processed with a dermatome to yield a thickness of 0.8-1.1 mm and were sandwiched between the donor and receptor wells (Figure 46.1). The upper plate, situated on the stratum corneum side of the skin strip, exposed the outer surface of the skin to the atmosphere and allowed topical applications. The width of the skin strip covered three of the four rows on a plate (18 wells per plate). Delrin rods, placed in the ends of the empty row, served to align the wells. The assemblies were placed in Plexiglas holders machined with

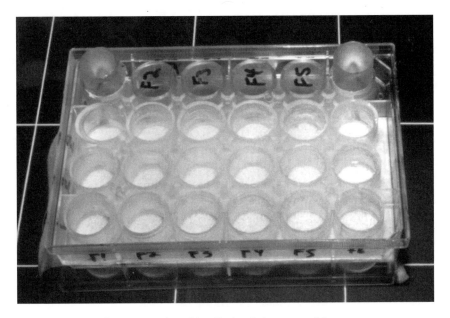

Figure 46.1: Pig skin mounted on 24 well plate/stirrer assembly.

a recess of the outer dimensions of the plates. Two thin bars, one between the second and third column of the plate and the other between the fourth and fifth column of the plate, were fastened to the Plexiglas holder with set screws to compress the skin strip between the plates. Three to four such assemblies are typically prepared to give 54–72 cells. The assemblies were positioned on top of a 15 position electronic stirrer (Variomag, Daytona Beach, FL), which allowed all the wells to be agitated.

46.3 FORMULATION AND SKIN PERMEATION STUDIES

Vehicle formulation is known to have a tremendous effect on topical-drug delivery. However, because every drug has unique physical chemistry and pharmacology, theoretical prediction of the optimal vehicle for a given drug is nearly impossible. The purpose of this study was to create topical-drug formulations from which correlations between vehicle and drug-delivery kinetics could be derived and to demonstrate the range of topical-delivery kinetics achievable for a model drug using a rapid, efficient *in vitro* method.

Formulation began with an evaluation of the chemistry and solubility of salicylic acid. Experiments were done to identify suitable solvents and solubilizers for the drug at the concentration being studied. These experiments also revealed materials in which salicylic acid was insoluble. Results of these experiments were then used to define and create a range of vehicle types that either dissolved, solubilized or suspended salicylic acid in the vehicle.

Seven experimental formulations of 0.5 percent salicylic acid were developed, consisting of three hydrophilic solutions (F1, F3, F4), one lipophilic solution (F2), an oil-in-water emulsion (F7), a water-in-oil emulsion (F8), and a lipophilic suspension (F6). These were compared with a commercial solution of 0.5 percent salicylic acid (F5, OXY Balance). The composition of each formula is given in Table 46.1.

46.3.1 Experimental procedures

Eight different formulations containing the radiolabeled salicylic acid were topically applied in order to obtain six replicates for each of the formulations. Twenty microliters or approximately 20 mg of formulation was applied to each cell. Since the formulations contained 0.5 percent (w/w) of salicylic acid, the chemical dose was approximately 100 µg of salicylic acid applied to 2 cm^2 of exposed skin in each cell (50 µg/cm^2). The plates were placed in an incubator oven maintained at skin surface temperature (32°C).

46.3.2 Radiometric analysis

Twenty-four hours after application, the skin surface was decontaminated with two dry wipes. The wipes were analyzed for radioactivity. Tissue culture medium was removed from the wells and subjected to radiometric analysis. The skin strips were positioned and pinned on a cutting board. The stratum corneum was harvested by tape stripping. Each skin strip was stripped 22 times using tape approximately 2.75 inches (7 cm) in width and approximately 6 inches (15 cm) long. Sets of three tape strips were affixed to mylar film mounted in a frame. Frames were mounted in a Packard Instruments Imager for determination of net CPM. CPMs were divided by the instrument's counting efficiency through the mylar film (2 percent) to obtain "Imager" DPMs. In separate experiments comparing DPMs determined by LSC and imaging, we have determined that radioactivity was further quenched by the presence of the stratum corneum tape strip. Imager DPMs were linearly related ($r = 0.998$) to LSC DPMs (Figure 46.2) by the following equation:

LSC (true) DPM = (Imager DPM)/0.60

CHAPTER 46

Table 46.1:

Salicylic acid formulations

No.	Formula type	Ingredients	% (w/w)
F1	Ethanol soln., non-aqueous, hydrophilic, volatile	Salicylic Acid SD Alcohol 40-B, 200 Proof	0.50 99.50
F2	Safflower oil soln., lipophilic, non-volatile	Salicylic Acid High Oleic Safflower	0.50 99.50
F3	Surfactant solution, aqueous, hydrophilic, volatile	Salicylic Acid Dimethyl Isosorbide Purified Water	0.50 20.00 79.50
F4	Glycerol Solution, Non-aqueous, hydrophilic, non-volatile	Salicylic Acid Glycerol, 99.5% USP	0.50 99.50
F5	OXY Balance, Hydroglycolic ethanol-surfactant soln.	Salicylic Acid Disodium Lauryl Sulfosuccinate Fragrance Glycerin Menthol Polyethylene Glycol Sodium Lauroyl Sarcosinate Sodium PCA Trisodium EDTA Water Alcohol	0.50(w/v) proprietary proprietary proprietary proprietary proprietary proprietary proprietary proprietary proprietary 22.00(w/v)
F6	Cyclomethicone suspension, lipophilic, volatile	Salicylic Acid Cyclomethicone (and) Polysilicone-ll	0.50 99.50
F7	Oil in water emulsion, drug dissolved in the internal phase	Salicylic Acid Purified Water High Oleic Safflower Oil Polyacrylamide (and) C13–14 Isoparaffin (and) Laureth-7	0.50 81.50 15.00 3.00
F8	Water in oil emulsion, drug dissolved in the external phase	Salicylic Acid Purified Water High Oleic Safflower Oil Polyglyceryl-4 Isostearate (and)Cetyl Dimethicone Copolyol (and) Hexyl Laurate Sodium Chloride	0.50 78.80 15.00 5.00 0.70

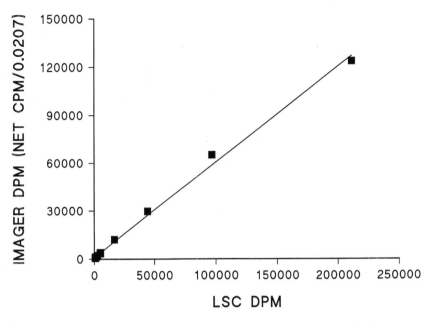

Figure 46.2: Relationship between DPOM determined by imaging and LSC

DPMs thus calculated were combined for tape strips 1 and 2, 3–7, 8–12, 13–17, and 18–22. The imager analyzed three 3×6 arrays of circular areas corresponding to the application areas (Figure 46.3). The remaining epidermis was heat separated from the dermis. The epidermis was peeled from the dermis and the two skin layers were placed in LSC vials containing tissue solubilizer for radiometric analyses.

46.3.3 Statistical analysis

Analyses were performed using BMDP statistical software. One way analysis of variance was conducted to determine the effect of formulation on the distribution of radioactivity on the skin surface, stratum corneum, epidermis, dermis and receptor fluid. When a significant F was observed, the Student-Newman-Keuls multiple range test was applied to determine which formulations were different. All analyses were conducted at the 0.05 level of significance.

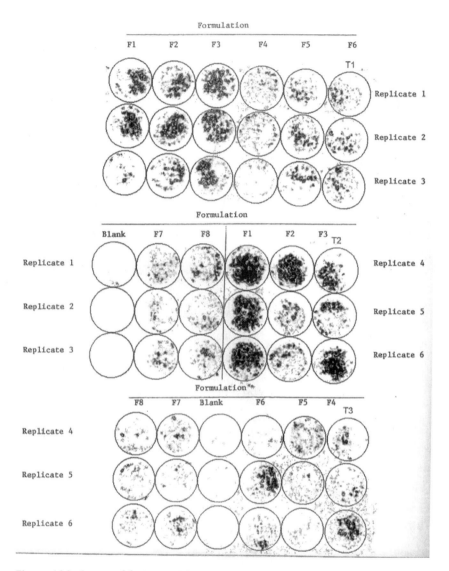

Figure 46.3: Image of first tape strip.

46.3.4 Results

The distribution of radiolabel (percent of applied radioactive dose) for the different formulations is given in Figures 46.4–46.8. Each bar represents the mean and standard deviation of 6 replicates. Columns designated with the same letter are not significantly different.

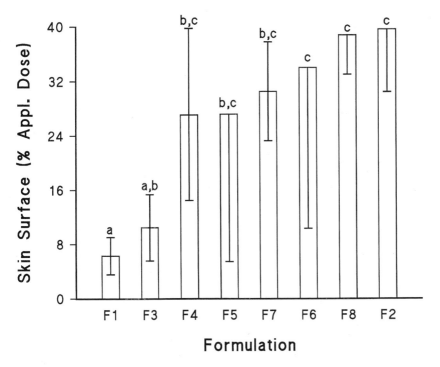

Figure 46.4: Effect of formulation on radiolabel at skin surface. Columns with the same letter are not significantly different. $N = 6$.

46.3.5   Discussion

Average overall recovery of label was 96 ± 16 percent of the applied radioactive dose. Formulation had a significant effect on the disposition of radioactivity in the upper layers of the skin (skin surface, stratum corneum tape strips), epidermis, dermis and receptor fluid at the $P = 0.05$ level of significance (ANOVA, Student Newman-Kuels multiple range test).

Formulation F1 had the lowest percentage of radioactivity recovered from the skin surface, as compared to the other formulations (Figure 46.4). The control salicylic acid formulation (OXY-Balance, F5) had approximately four times the percentage of radioactivity recovered from the skin surface (Figure 46.4). Formulation F1 had the highest percentage of radioactivity recovered from the tape strips (stratum corneum); the control formulation F5 was 50 percent lower (Figure 46.5). Formulation F4 had the lowest percentage of radioactivity (13 percent, Figure 46.6) recovered in the epidermis; the remaining formulations

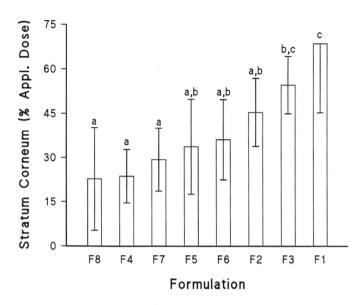

Figure 46.5: Effect of formulation on radiolabel in stratum corneum. Columns with the same letter are not significantly different. $N = 6$.

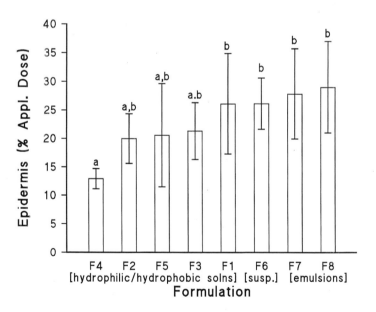

Figure 46.6: Effect of formulation on radiolabel in the epidermis. Columns with the same letter are not significantly different. $N = 6$.

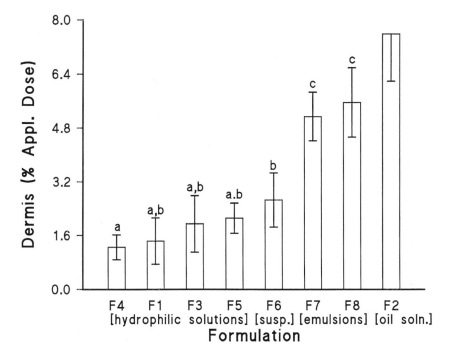

Figure 46.7: Effect of formulation on radiolabel in the dermis. Columns with the same letter are not significantly different. $N = 6$.

had values ranging from 20–29 percent and were not significantly different from each other. Radiolabel in the hydrophilic solutions (F1, F3, F4, F5) penetrated the least into the dermis and receptor fluid (Figures 46.7 and 46.8) with aqueous surfactant (F3), ethanol solution (F1) and glycerol solution (F4) being equivalent to the control formulation (F5). Radiolabel in the lipophilic solution (F2) had the greatest penetration into the dermis and receptor fluid. Radiolabel penetration into the dermis and receptor fluid from the oil-in-water (o/w, F7) and water-in-oil (w/o, F8) emulsions were equivalent.

Percutaneous absorption of compounds has typically been measured using individual diffusion cells (e.g. the Franz cell (Franz, 1978) or flow cells (Reifenrath *et al.*, 1994)). However, when replicate measurements are required for a large number of formulations, assembly time becomes lengthy. Additionally, proto- cols involving tape stripping would require a large number of samples to be processed separately. For example, 22 tape strips of 50 individual cells would result in 1100 samples. Using the methods described herein, 18 cells can be covered at once with a single piece of skin and 18 cells can be tape stripped

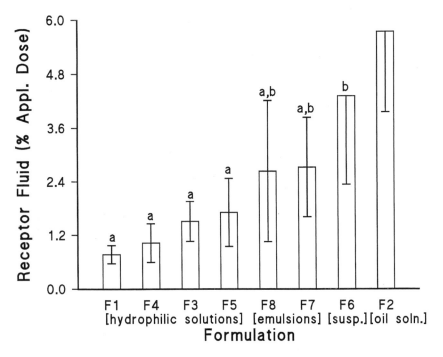

Figure 46.8: Effect of formulation on radiolabel in receptor fluid. Columns with the same letter are not significantly different. $N = 6$.

with a single piece of tape. Radiometric analysis of a tape strip from 50 cells can be done in the same time taken for LSC counting of one tape strip from a single cell. The reduced processing of individual cells greatly reduces labor and may improve reproducibility.

46.3.6 Conclusions

The results demonstrate the importance of vehicle in directing drug delivery using a test system designed to simultaneously evaluate large numbers of formulations. The lipophilic solution, the emulsions and (suprisingly) the lipophilic suspension resulted in a significantly greater percentage of radiolabel penetration into the epidermis, dermis and receptor fluid, as compared to the hydrophilic solutions (Table 46.2). Formulation F1 and F3 resulted in significantly less radiolabel on the skin surface and significantly more radiolabel in the stratum corneum, as compared for formulation F5 (OXY Balance, Table 46.2).

Table 46.2:

Summary of the influence of formulation on the skin disposition of radiolabeled salicylic acid.

Compartment	Formulation with highest amount of radiolabel (percent of appl. dose)		Formulation with lowest amount of radiolabel (percent of appl. dose)	
Skin surface	Lipophilic Soln.	(F2)	Hydrophilic Soln.	(F1)
Stratum Corneum	Hydrophilic Soln.	(F1)	W/O Emulsion	(F8)
Epidermis	W/O Emulsion	(F8)	Hydrophilic Soln.	(F4)
Dermis	Lipophilic Soln.	(F2)	Hydrophilic Soln.	(F4)
Receptor Fluid	Lipophilic Soln.	(F2)	Hydrophilic Soln.	(F1)

Thus, the clearest correlation demonstrated between vehicle and salicylic acid delivery was that lipophilicity of the vehicle encouraged deeper penetration of salicylic acid, while vehicle hydrophilicity discouraged drug penetration past the stratum corneum. The value of this process of formulation research and development, pharmacokinetic evaluation and correlation of the results is that it offers a quick, *in vitro* prediction of delivery kinetics in man, and can direct the development of an optimally-targeted topical drug formulation in the earliest stages of product development.

46.4 CHEMICAL TOXICITY STUDIES

Skin is a metabolically diverse, dynamically active tissue that undergoes constant turnover and replenishment of many of its cellular constituents. Because skin is exposed, either intentionally or unintentionally, to a wide variety of chemicals, we are developing general procedures to assess possible adverse effects. The use of pigskin preparations maintained on tissue culture media is appropriate for such efforts because of the many biochemical and physiological similarities to human skin (Meyer, 1978). We report a useful panel of methods suitable for systematic evaluation of hazards from various chemical exposures by addressing several different toxicological endpoints.

In considering the response of skin to a chemical challenge, we consider several major questions:

CHAPTER 46

1   How readily does the material permeate the skin and pass into the circulation or lymphatics? How are the chemical or its metabolites distributed in the various layers of the skin?

2   Does the chemical cause any local structural or metabolic damage to the skin itself? This can be addressed in two ways: by determining whether significant disruption of cell integrity occurs after exposure, releasing cellular contents into the medium; and from disruption or interference with major metabolic activities of skin, such as glycolytic or oxidative functions.

3   Has there been significant damage to the major informational macro-molecules in the tissue, particularly to the nucleic acids? Such damage could arise from specific targeting of nucleic acid components by the toxicant, but could also result from general structural cell damage that leads to macromolecular degradation.

4   Does the skin metabolize the chemical agent to products with toxic potential? Skin is an important site of extrahepatic metabolism of xenobiotic chemicals, and is known to play a key role in bioactivation of aromatic hydrocarbons, which ultimately can result in carcinogenicity. Therefore, a pertinent question is whether the skin can form mutagenic or carcinogenic metabolites or products after a chemical exposure.

46.4.1   Experimental procedures

We have employed a panel of methods to detect cellular damage by a variety of toxicological end-points as follows:

Release of lactic dehydrogenase (LDH)

Lactic dehydrogenase activity was evaluated as an indicator of cell lysis, by measuring the release of this normally cytoplasmic enzyme into the culture medium (Al Casey and Acosta, 1995). Injury to cell membranes releases the enzyme into the receptor fluid, and would be similar to its appearance in the serum of patients with clinical cardiac, liver or muscle damage.

The assays measured the pyruvate-dependent rate of oxidation of NADH from the change in absorbance at 340 nm for 1.0 ml reaction mixtures containing 6 mM Na pyruvate, 0.1 mM NADH (neutralized to pH 7.0) and 100 mM Tris-HCl buffer, pH 7.0. Control mixtures, lacking pyruvate, were run for all samples. The mixtures were incubated at 30°C and reactions were initiated by addition of up to 20 µl samples of receptor fluid. The absorbance at 340 nm was monitored every 30 seconds for up to 10 minutes; initial reaction rates were determined for the 5-minute interval from 2 to 7 minutes after enzyme addition. A Perkin-Elmer Lambda 3A spectrophotometer was used for absorbance measurements and enzyme assays.

Lactate production

Glycolytic activity is the main energy-producing pathway of the skin, and the rate of lactate produced from glucose in the culture medium was used to evaluate the functional integrity of the pathway as a whole (Frienkel, 1960). The procedure used an end-point assay to measure the amount of lactate, from the formation of hydrogen peroxide produced by a bacterial lactate oxidase. Up to 10 µl of receptor fluids were tested, using the methodology and reagents in the lactate assay kit from the Sigma Chemical Company.

Mitochondrial oxidative function

The status of mitochondrial oxidation is a good indicator of cell viability: a loss of metabolic reduction by viable cells would indicate interference with or loss of cellular respiration. For these tests, we employed the redox indicator, Alamar Blue (Accumed International, Westlake, OH), which changed color in the appropriate oxidation-reduction range relating to cellular metabolic reduction (Fields and Lancaster, 1993). The extent of color change which reflected the extent of cellular proliferation was determined from the absorbance of the dye at 570 nm (wave length maximum for absorbance by the reduced dye) and the absorbance at 600 nm (wavelength maximum for absorption by the oxidized dye). Since this dye does not interfere with electron transport at earlier steps, cellular toxicity from dye exposure was minimized.

Procedurally, a sterile solution of Alamar Blue was diluted 10-fold with RPMI medium, and the resulting blue solution was used to fill the receptor compartment of the skin penetration cells. Freshly obtained pigskins were attached to the cells, with a 3.9 cm^2 area of skin in contact with the medium. Absorbance readings of the medium were made at 2 h and 14 h after skin exposures to test chemicals or controls. After 14 h, the media were replaced. Final spectrophotometric readings were made at 18 h after the start of the experiment.

Application of commercial mutagenicity tests for analysis of receptor fluids

These tests were performed using the Xenometrix Ames II Assay kit (Xenometrix, Inc., Boulder, CO) following the manufacturer's recommended procedure, with modifications adapted for skin permeation studies. The kit contained a mixture of *Salmonella typhimurium* strains capable of screening for each of the six possible base transitions or transversions in a defined genetic background, and also included a tester strain (T-98) to detect frame shift mutations. The procedure was conducted with and without supplementation with a mammalian liver activation preparation (S9, Moltox, Boone, NC) and included 2-nitrofluorene, methyl methane sulfonate and 2-amino anthracene in dimethyl sulfoxide as positive controls, and RPMI Medium as a negative control. The assays measured the number of histidine-independent revertants obtained by exposing the tester strains to receptor fluid samples, both with and without the metabolic supplement (rat liver microsomes induced with Arochlor 1254). The results were expressed as the number of observed reversions obtained for a tested sample compared with the maximum possible number of reversions.

Analysis and excretion of RNA terminal metabolites in receptor fluids

Enormous advances in the past 30 years have elucidated the detailed structures and roles of many nucleic acid macromolecules. Two major facts pertinent to our efforts are the recognition that all cells contain many different types of RNA molecules and that, in addition to the prototypic nucleosides (uridine, cytidine, adenosine, guanosine), many RNA species also normally contain various modified derivatives of the nucleosides or their bases. More than 80 different modifications have been characterized in various RNAs and range from simple base or sugar methylations to complex multlifunctional groups (Bjork and Kohli, 1990). The modified derivatives are most abundant in transfer RNAs, but are common in various ribosomal RNAs, in the cap structures of messenger RNAs, and in many small ribonucleoprotein constituents. This panoramic distribution obviously requires a vast array of enzymes and regulatory controls to assure their proper assembly and functions.

In recent years, a wealth of new information has enlarged our perspectives about RNA structure and functions. We now know that plants, prokaryotes and eukaryotes contain many types of non-coding RNA species that are not part of the conventional repertoire of structural and messenger RNAs (Storz, 2002). They vary in size from very small (21–25 nucleotides) to many thousand nucleotides and participate in a remarkable variety of biological functions, including transcriptional regulation, translational control, RNA modification and processing, and genomic immune-like protective mechanisms (Plasterk, 2002; Storz, 2002; Zamore, 2002).

Several considerations underlie the efforts to evaluate cell damage by analysis of terminal nucleic acid metabolites. (a) Chemical agents that react with nucleic acid bases might affect the bases common to both DNA and RNA, although reaction rates might vary because of differences in secondary structure or in macromolecules associated with the nucleic acids. (b) In contrast with DNA damage, for which extensive repair and regulatory control systems exist, cells contain far fewer enzymatic and regulatory means to repair RNA damage: direct structural damage to RNA molecules will lead more readily to degradation of the RNA. Cellular damage that produces cell death would trigger autolytic reactions to degrade the RNAs and increase the production of terminal RNA metabolites. (c) Finally, the terminal metabolites of RNA breakdown include not only the major ribonucleosides and bases, but also include the modified nucleosides and bases derived from normal RNA components. But, in contrast with the metabolic end-products of the major ribonucleosides, the terminal metabolites of modified nucleosides and bases are not readily reutilized for macromolecular biosynthesis. Instead, they are typically excreted from cells, or converted to secondary metabolites. In the *in vitro* skin system employed here, most metabolites of the modified components are excreted into the receptor fluids.

With this rationale, our expectation was that the modified nucleosides and their derivatives would serve as unique markers to evaluate the metabolic turnover of RNA molecules as a tissue response to chemical, physical or biological damage. The main practical outgrowths of this analytical approach have been for clinical diagnosis and prognosis of cancer patients (Kuo *et al.*, 1990), but few systematic applications exist for toxicological monitoring.

In working with receptor fluids from pigskin preparations, our analytical procedures were based on existing methodology for separation of nucleic acid constituents (Buck, 1983, Schoch *et al.*, 1990). The approach involved affinity purification of ribonucleosides followed by resolution of the complex mixture of products using HPLC. The detailed procedure is outlined in Table 46.3 and involved initial sterile filtration of the receptor fluids. A known quantity of 3-methyl uridine was then added as an internal standard for evaluating sample

■ CHAPTER 46 ■

Table 46.3:

Analysis of terminal RNA metabolites

1. Preincubate split-thickness pigskin preparations with RPMI medium for 2 h before treatment.

2. Change medium. Expose skin epidermally or dermally to chemical challenge for 24 h or more; collect receptor media at timed intervals. Weigh receptor media; reserve and freeze aliquots at –20°C for later analyses. Add fresh medium and continue chemical exposures.

3. Analysis of RNA metabolites in receptor fluids:

    (a) Thaw and sterile filter receptor fluids (0.45 µ Acrodisc membranes).

    (b) Add known quantity (3–5 nmoles) of 3-Methyl uridine as Internal Standard to evaluate final recoveries after processing steps.

    (c) Deproteinize receptor fluids by centrifugal filtration at $6000 \times g$ through Centricon 10 membranes (10,000 Dalton cutoff).

    (d) Adjust pH of filtrates to 9.0, pass samples through Affigel 601 (boronate) affinity columns (2.0 cm × 1.0 cm) and wash columns with ammonium acetate, pH 8.8. Vicinal cis-diols, (e.g., ribonucleosides) are bound; free bases, 2'-O-methyl ribonucleosides and deoxyribonucleosides are not, and are collected in the breakthrough and washes. Pool breakthrough and washes and freeze at –20°C for later analysis.

    (e) Elution: Columns are washed with 2 column volumes of distilled water. Adsorbed products are eluted with 5–6 volumes of 0.02 N acetic acid and pH of eluates is adjusted to ~ 6 to minimize depurination. The eluates are lyophilized to dryness and residues are dissolved in 1.0 ml of water or initial chromatography buffer.

    (f) HPLC resolution of nucleosides required a C18 reversed phase column (Supelcosil LC-18S, 5 u, 250 × 4.6 mm), using a linear gradient (0.05 M sodium acetate, pH 6.0/1% methanol to 0.05 M sodium acetate, pH 5.1/20% methanol). Flow rate is 1.0 ml/min. Elution is monitored at 254 or 260 nm. Peaks are identified by elution position and by spiking with authentic standards.

4. Recovery of each metabolite is quantitated from the integrated peak area and the molar absorbancies at 254 or 260 nm, and is corrected for the recovery as determined from that of the internal standard.

losses in the ensuing analytical steps. After residual proteins were removed by centrifugal filtration, the terminal ribonucleosides were recovered after absorption to, and elution from Affigel 601 boronate gel. This gel retains ribonucleosides and compounds with vicinal diols; nucleic acid bases, most saccharides, deoxyribonucleosides and sugar-methylated nucleosides are not retained by the resin. After desorption from the affinity column, the nucleoside fractions were concentrated and quantitatively analyzed by reversed phase chromatography.

46.4.2 Materials

Nucleosides, modified nucleosides and bases, RPMI medium, acetonitrile, methanol and potassium phosphate were obtained from Sigma-Aldrich; thiodiglycol was from Fluka. Chemical and nucleoside test mixtures, RDX and 1,3,5-trinitrobenzene (TNB) were purchased from Supelco. N^6-carbamoyl threonyl adenosine (t^6A) was a generous gift from the late Barbara Vold, SRI International, Menlo Park, CA. Other chromatographic solvents and inorganic salts were obtained from Mallinckrodt Chemicals and Fisher Scientific Co.

46.4.3 HPLC analysis of nucleosides

For nucleoside analysis, 100–250 µl samples were injected into the analytical column (Supelcosil LC-18S, 5 u, 250×4.6 mm) using a Spectraphysics 8780XR autosampler with a 500 µl Alltech sample loop; pumping was regulated by a Spectra-physics 8800 ternary pump. The ribonucleosides were resolved using a linear methanol gradient (1 percent to 20 percent in 20 mM sodium acetate buffer, pH 6.0 to pH 5.1), at a flow rate of 1.0 ml/ml. Eluates were continuously monitored by a Milton Roy Spectromonitor III UV monitor set at 254 or 260 nm and data were collected, stored and processed using Perkin-Elmer TurboChrom analytical software.

The elution pattern for separation of ribonucleosides is shown in Figure 46.9, and the identity of the individual peaks is summarized in Table 46.4 with comments on their metabolic origins. Note that the peak areas in Figure 46.9 do not necessarily reflect the relative concentrations of each component, since the molar extinctions of individual nucleosides vary over a broad range. The most prominent products in the receptor fluids are the common unmodified nucleosides, uridine, cytidine, guanosine and inosine; relatively low levels of adenosine are found, probably due to its ready deamination in this tissue. Most striking is the presence of dozens of minor components, many of whose identities have been validated by co-migration with authentic samples of known modified nucleosides.

46.4.4 Statistical analysis

For replicate samples, the tabulated results refer to the molar quantities or mean total peak areas with their calculated standard deviations. Analysis of the variance (BMPD statistical software) was conducted to determine the effects of test

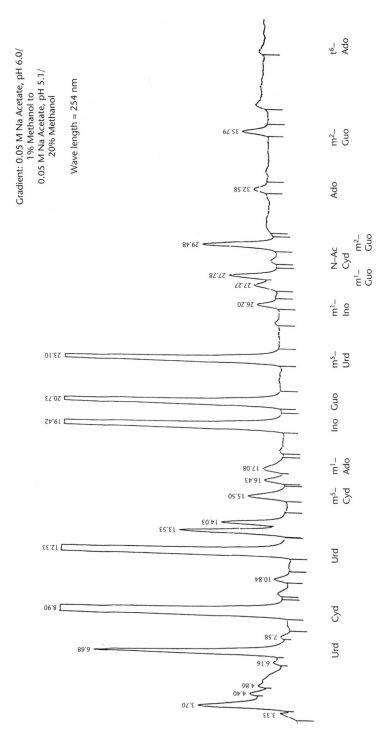

Figure 46.9: HPLC separation of ribonucleosides in receptor fluid from untreated pig skin.

Table 46.4:

Notes on the origins of nucleoside metabolites

Pseudouridine (Ψrd)—5-ribosyl uracil. Found in many RNA species (transfer, ribosomal, small nuclear RNAs). Best regarded as a "global indicator" of RNA breakdown. Prominent excretion product in mammalian urine.

Cytidine (Cyd)—derived from both RNA breakdown and nucleotide pools.

Uridine (Urd)—derived from both RNA breakdown and nucleotide pools.

5-methyl Cytidine (m^5C)—found in both transfer and ribosomal RNAs.

1-methyl Adenosine (m^1A)—found only in transfer RNAs.

Inosine (Ino)—formed by deamination of adenosine; thus, derived from both RNA breakdown and nucleotide pools.

Guanosine (Guo)—derived from both RNA breakdown and nucleotide pools.

3-Methyl Uridine (m^3U)—used as internal standard.

1-methyl Inosine (m^1I)—formed by deamination of 1-methyl adenosine.

1-methyl Guanosine (m^1G)—found in transfer RNA molecules only.

N4-acetyl Cytidine (ac^4C)—found in transfer RNAs at several locations.

2-methyl Guanosine (m^2G)—found only in transfer RNAs.

Adenosine (Ado)—from both RNA breakdown and nucleotide pools. Readily deaminated.

7-Methyl Guanosine (m^7G)—originates from messenger, transfer and ribosmal RNA turnover.

N2,N2-dimethyl Guanosine (m^2_2G)—found in many species of transfer RNA.

N6-carbamoyl threonyl Adenosine (t^6A)—found in a number of specific transfer RNA species

N6,N6-dimethyl Adenosine (m_2^6A)—present only in all ribosomal RNAs.

5-methyl Deoxycytidine (m^5Cdo)—the modified nucleoside in DNA from higher animals.

The corresponding modified bases are designated as follows:
    Thymine (Thy)—Base from Thymidine or Ribothymidine derivatives.
    Hypoxanthine (Hx)—Base for Inosine derivatives.
    Adenine (Ade)—Base for Adenine derivatives.
    Cytosine (Cyt)—Base for Cytosine derivatives.
    Uracil (Ura)—Base for Uracil derivatives.
    Xanthine (Xan)—metabolite from oxidation of Hypoxanthine.

compounds and skin sources on the level of nucleosides and base metabolites in the receptor fluids, and to compare *in vitro* results with published *in vivo* data (Demetrulias *et al.*, 1998). Where a significant F value was observed, the Student-Newman-Keuls multiple range test was applied to determine which entities were different. All analyses were conducted for the 0.05 level of significance.

46.4.5 Results of RNA metabolite feasibility study

To assess the feasibility of analyzing receptor fluids for the RNA metabolites, it was first necessary to determine which products of RNA breakdown were present in these fractions. Replicate samples of untreated pigskin were maintained on RPMI medium for a period of 24 hours, with changes of medium at 2 and 14 hours. Two or three pairs of duplicate samples of receptor fluid were combined for analysis and were subjected to the processing procedure for purification and concentration of the ribonucleosides (Table 46.3). The amounts of uridine, cytidine and pseudouridine were analyzed as representative products of the normal and modified nucleosides, respectively. These compounds eluted early in the resolving system as prominent, easily quantifiable peaks. The results (Table 46.5) indicated that each of these products was readily detected in receptor fluids from untreated pigskins, and that the sensitivity of the procedure was compatible with the selected sample size and the purification procedure. Each of these pyrimidine metabolites continued to accumulate throughout the 24-hour period, indicating their continuous production over this time. Subsequent work (see control samples, Tables 46.6 and 46.7), made it evident that accumulation of these products was not a result of ongoing cell lysis or loss of metabolic functions related to energy production. Instead, both the normal and modified nucleosides originated from the turnover of RNA species in the skin, and the quantitative pattern in control samples provided an endogenous baseline for skin. Exposure to toxicological agents that cause nucleic

Table 46.5:

Preliminary analysis of nucleosides in receptor fluids

		Total quantity (nmoles) of nucleosides in receptor fluids[a]						
Time	Pooled media	Pseudouridine		Cytidine		Uridine		
		Mean S.D.	N	Mean S.D.	N	Mean S.D.	N	
0–2 h	Sample 1	3.4 ± 0.6	3	29.3 ± 0.2	3	26.5 ± 0.7	3	
	Sample 2	3.5 ± 0.3	2	23.5 ± 0.3	3	23.8 ± 1.1	3	
2–14 h	Sample 1	6.3 ± 0.4	3	47.0 ± 1.8	3	31.0 ± 1.3	3	
	Sample 2	8.1 ± 0.4	3	47.3 ± 1.8	3	33.4 ± 0.9	3	
14–24 h	Sample 1	6.3 ± 0.4	10	48.1 ± 3.5	10	25.1 ± 3.2	10	
	Sample 2	7.5 ± 0.5	7	48.9 ± 3.1	7	27.8 ± 1.7	5	
	Sample 3	7.2 ± 0.2	4	49.5 ± 3.6	4	25.0 ± 1.7	4	

[a]Calculated from the combined volumes of receptor fluid for each set of samples.

acid breakdown or turnover should alter the relative levels of terminal RNA metabolites in the receptor fluids.

Table 46.6:

Release of Lactate dehydrogenase (LDH) into receptor fluids after chemical exposures

Exposure period (epidermal)	LDH released, milliunits/cm² per hour				
	Control (untreated)	Lead acetate	NaF	BAP	Infected skin
–2 hr—0 hr	18.9	14.54	21.31	19.94	17.96
0 hr—2 hr	2.31	1.94	2.11	1.83	3.01
2 hr –14 hr	0.53	<0.21	0.47	<0.21	3.98
14 hr –24 hr	<0.60	<0.25	0.57	0.26	3.46
Exposure period (dermal)					
–2 hr—0 hr	5.38	9.23	5.25	6.55	
0 hr—2 hr	3.48	5.25	1.60	7.85	
2 hr –14 hr	0.56	1.10	0.28	9.38	
14 hr –24 hr	<0.25	<0.25	0.29	2.74	

Table 46.7:

Production of lactate after chemical exposures

Exposure period (epidermal)	Lactate produced, milligrams/cm² per hour				
	Control (untreated)	Lead acetate	NaF	BAP	Infected skin
–2 hr—0 hr	11.77	10.11	10.53	12.03	11.77
0 hr—2 hr	8.1	6.8	9.95	8.46	6.74
2 hr –14 hr	10.5	9.28	10.81	9.91	7.9
14 hr –24 hr	11.43	9.62	11.57	10.96	9.5
Exposure period (dermal)					
–2 hr—0 hr	14.89	14.8	14.49	18.30	
0 hr—2 hr	15.77	13.83	10.93	17.6	
2 hr –14 hr	12.52	11.09	11.51	6.46	
14 hr –24 hr	12.39	11.42	11.46	2.71	

■ CHAPTER 46 ■

46.4.6   Results of known toxicants on biochemical measurements and RNA terminal metabolites

In these experiments, we determined whether skin exposures to different types of toxic chemicals would produce unique or informative patterns of nucleoside excretion. The chemical challenges tested included lead acetate, sodium fluoride, benzo(α)pyrene in hexane solution, and trinitrobenzene. The receptor fluids were also analyzed for lactic acid and LDH and, in some instances, mutagenicity of the receptor fluids. The results are shown in Figures 46.10—46.13 and Tables 46.6 and 46.7.

(a)   Skin exposures to lead acetate (5 mg/cm^2)and sodium fluoride (1 mg/cm^2) drastically curtailed excretion of uridine and cytidine (Figure 46.10), without comparable effects on cell integrity or glycolytic function (Tables 46.6 and 46.7). The formation of these nucleosides involved the action of specific pyrimidine-5-nucleotidases, many of which are membrane bound. The specificity of this effect for pyrimidine nucleosides was considered to be indicative of specific interference with the function of these nucleotidases, which are also inhibited by lead salts and fluoride. Only modest changes were found in the lactate production, and minor releases of LDH were evident in the first few hours of exposure, as was typical of controls.

(b)   Epidermal exposure of skin to benzo(α)pyrene led to increased excretion of uridine and cytidine (Figure 46.11) without significant changes in lactate production or release of LDH (Tables 46.6 and 46.7). Dermal exposures to benzo(α)pyrene (0.625 mg/ml, Figures 46.12A-C) caused major changes in nucleoside excretion, starting early after exposure (Figure 46.12A). Between 2–14 hours, the excretion of the common and modified nucleosides was greatly increased (Figure 46.12B) and was concurrent with evidence of cell lysis (Tables 46.6 and 46.7). This pattern clearly reflected extensive structural and functional damage to the skin, with increased cell lysis and loss of glycolytic capacity.

(c)   Microbial growth was found in the skin and culture medium for one control sample. Compared to controls, receptor fluid from this sample was found to have diminished lactic acid levels and increased cell lysis (Tables 46.6 and 46.7) and a large change in nucleoside excretion, especially for cytidine and uridine (Figure 46.13). The changes in the RNA metabolites were more pronounced than the other measured end-points.

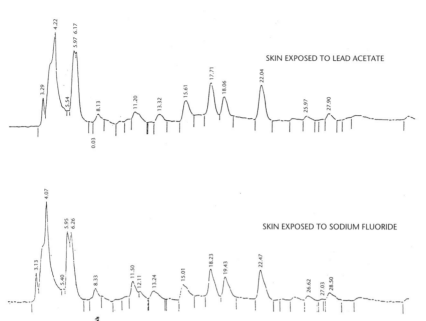

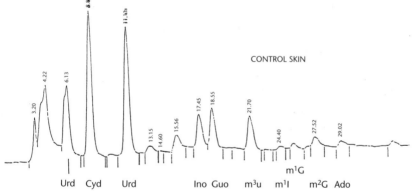

Figure 46.10: Nucleoside excretion patterns from receptor fluids 14-24 hours after topical exposure to lead acetate (5 mg/cm²) or sodium fluoride (1 mg/cm²). The control was untreated skin.

(d) Exposures to other potentially toxic chemicals. Skin exposures to thiodiglycol or the explosive, RDX, had no significant effect on cell integrity, glycolytic metabolism, or nucleoside excretion levels (data not shown). Treatment with 1,3,5-trinitrobenzene caused a general increase in excretion of both unmodified and modified nucleosides (Figure 46.14), especially after longer exposure periods (14–24 h). We attributed this to a general increase in RNA turnover, affecting many RNA species.

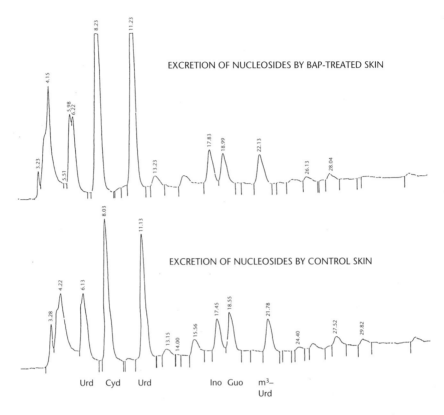

Figure 46.11: Nucleoside patterns in receptor fluids 14–24 hours after topical exposure to benzo(a)pyrene (BAP) in xylene (0.625 mg/ml). The control pattern was from untreated skin.

Mutagenicity assays after topical exposures to trinitrobenzene (TNB) revealed that TNB itself produced a strong mutagenic response with tester strain TA-98, but only in the presence of the S-9 rat liver activation system (data not shown). However, no significant mutagenicity was found with the tested samples of the receptor fluids, supporting the belief that only limited penetration of mutagenic metabolites of TNB had occurred into the receptor fluid, or that the mutagenic potencies of the metabolites in the receptor fluids were below the sensitivity limits of the assay.

(e) Skin exposure to surfactants may produce alterations in the formation and excretion of terminal RNA metabolites. To investigate this, we treated excised pig skin samples with five surfactants of known clinical irritancy: di-octyl sulfosuccinate, sodium salt, cocamide diethanolamine, polyoxyethylene sorbitan monolaurate (Tween 20), benzalkonium chloride, and

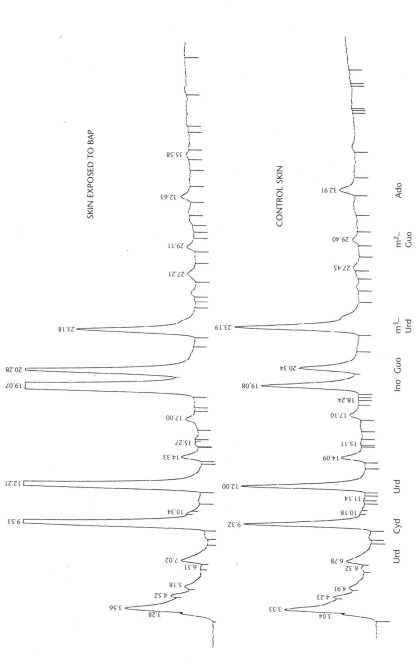

Figure 46.12A: Nucleosides in receptor fluid 0–2 hours after dermal exposure to benzo(a)pyrene (BAP). The control was from untreated skin.

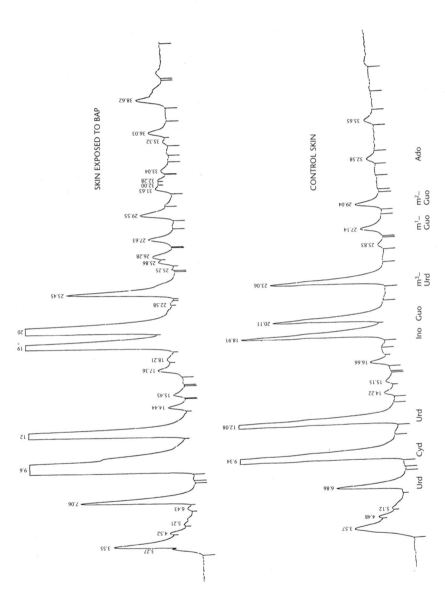

Figure 46.12B: Nucleosides in receptor fluid 2–14 hours after dermal exposure to benzo(α)pyrene (BAP). The control was from untreated

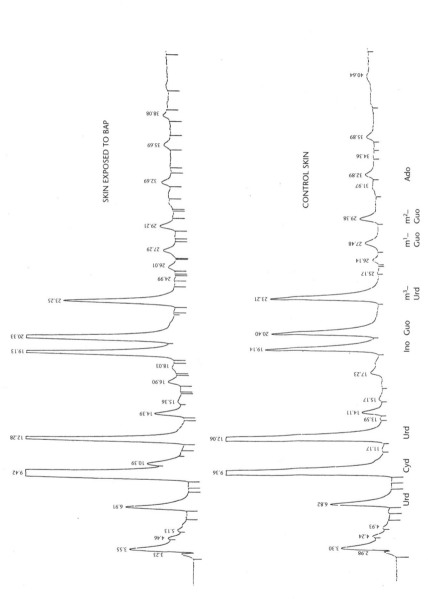

Figure 46.12C: Nucleosides in receptor fluid 14–24 hours after dermal exposure to benzo(α)pyrene (BAP). The control was from untreated skin.

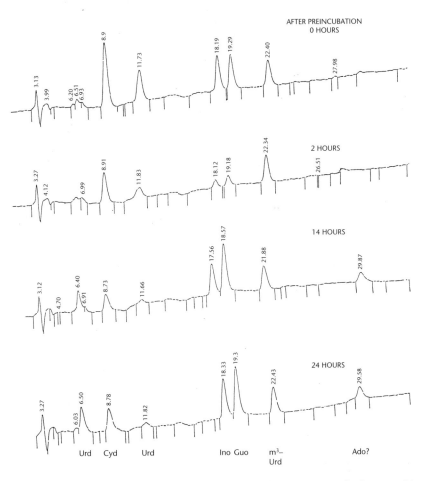

Figure 46.13: Effect of microbial growth on nucleosides in receptor fluid over a 24-hour period. Microbial growth took place on otherwise untreated pig skin.

sodium lauryl sulfate. Chemicals were applied and skin samples were maintained for 24 h at 32°C. Receptor fluids withdrawn and replenished after 2, 14 and 24 h after start of exposure to the irritants and were frozen at –20°C until processed for nucleoside analysis. We also determined whether other RNA terminal metabolites e.g., bases, modified bases, secondary metabolites or other products were excreted by the skin, and whether any of them were accumulated or depleted after exposure to the test compounds. The procedure for separating these products was was as follows. A known quantity of 3-methyl uridine was added as an internal marker to portions

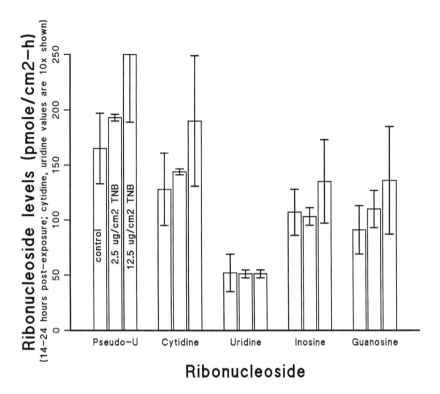

Figure 46.14: Effect of trinitrobenzene (TNB) exposure to excised pig skin on ribonucleoside levels.

of the flow-through fraction from the boronate affinity resin. An aliquot of this mixture was then injected into the Phenomenex resolving column (C18 Luna column, 5u, 150 × 4.6 mm). The components were resolved using a ternary solvent system of (a) 0.02 M potassium phosphate buffer, pH 6.0; (b) 40 percent methanol in distilled water; (c) 64 percent methanol in distilled water. More than 30 different peaks were separable in this way. Many peaks were heterogeneous (data not shown) and some of the contaminating or unresolved components were probably derived from minor contaminants in the solvents or column resins. Despite these difficulties, it was possible to define peaks for cytosine, uric acid, uracil, guanine /hypoxanthine, and several modified guanine bases, including 7-methyl guanine. However, there were no statistically significant changes in the accumulation of any nuceloside or nucleobase that correlated with the clinical irritancy scores of the surfactants.

46.4.7 Discussion

Measurements of various toxic endpoints appear to be a useful procedure for evaluating chemical toxicity with the use of the *in vitro* pigskin test system. The release of LDH during pigskin exposures clearly indicated that a small but consistent release of this enzyme occurs at early time points. We attribute this to the mechanical damage and tissue injury from the handling and dermatoming of the skin after its removal from the animals. The release of LDH soon reaches a very low baseline within about 2 hours after the exposure of the tissue to the culture media (Tables 46.6 and 46.7) indicating that little additional trauma or cell lysis normally occurs after this time. Releases of LDH above the baseline level would be substantive evidence for lytic effects on the tissue.

RNA turnover is an ongoing process in skin, even in the absence of chemical exposures. Pseudouridine and many methylated ribonucleosides in receptor fluids originated only from the breakdown of various RNAs. They are excreted into receptor fluids in the absence of significant cell lysis (release of LDH). Thus, their production is not merely the result of lytic cell damage leading to RNA breakdown.

Altered levels of the common major nucleosides (cytidine, uridine, guanosine, adenosine and inosine), can arise from several sources: (a) changes in synthesis or turnover of nucleotide pools; (b) membrane changes affecting their transport or permeability, and (c) changes in the rate of RNA turnover. The changes in production and excretion of these RNA metabolites can be more sensitive and may occur sooner than the traditional end-points used to measure skin toxicity (lactate production and release of LDH).

Because most of the modified nucleosides and bases are handled metabolically as one-way end products and are excreted (mostly unchanged) from cells, their accumulation should reflect the composition and overall turnover rates of the RNA species from which they originate. Many modified bases or nucleosides originate from only one class of RNA molecules (e.g., transfer RNA), and their production should reflect the turnover rate for that class of RNA. Other modified nucleosides or bases originate from two or more classes of RNA and their production would represent a weighed composite of the composition and turnover of these classes of RNA. Pseudouridine is a notable metabolite because it is normally present in many kinds of RNA, which accounts for the fact that it is the most abundant modified nucleoside metabolite in human urine. Based on this specificity, procedures have been developed (Schoch *et al.*, 1990) for evaluating *in vivo* turnover rates for various classes of RNA using excretion measurements for a small panel of terminal urinary metabolites. Such an approach may be feasible for estimations of RNA turnover in skin.

The main limitations in the use of *in vitro* skin preparations for toxicological evaluations arise from several sources. One source is the intrinsic variability of skin itself. Skin is a complex tissue with glandular-secretory, proliferative, barrier, supportive and regenerative cellular functions. Not all regions of the skin are identical or homogeneous: considerable variation exists in the thickness, cell types and population densities of cells in the stratum corneum, epidermis, dermis and glands. This structural variability emphasizes the need for appropriate experimental design.

A second major limitation is the lack of a circulatory system for *in vitro* experiments with skin. Receptor fluid serves as a quasi-surrogate for a physiological circulation, but this is predominantly for the removal of metabolites and cellular wastes. The receptor fluids generally do not usually deliver humoral or other factors at controllable time intervals or in response to physiological signals. This limitation narrows the utility of *in vitro* systems for investigating processes such as immune reactivity, inflammation, chemokine responses, etc.

While this work indicates the potential value of RNA metabolite response to toxic chemical exposures, much more information is needed for expanding our knowledge of the patterns of response to broader groups of toxic chemicals that affect various cell functions.

46.5 SUMMARY

A new skin permeation test system has been developed to permit rapid screening of formulations for their effect on the skin disposition of radiolabeled drug. The system is now routinely used in our laboratory to evaluate a wide variety of topical drug formulations.

Biochemical analysis of receptor fluid derived from the test system can potentially be used to detect toxic effects of compounds or formulations that come in contact with the skin. The system allowed detection of deleterious effects involving energy production, cell integrity, mutagenicity and several types of damage to nucleic acids or membrane transport mechanisms involved in nucleoside/nucleotide metabolic pathways. The results warrant further efforts to calibrate and quantitate this test system with chemicals of known toxicity, in order to establish more clearly the significance and predictive range of these responses.

CHAPTER 46

REFERENCES

AL CASEY, S. and ACOSTA, D. (1995) Dermal irritancy induced by SDS and TWEEN-20, anionic and non-ionic surfactants, in rat keratinocyte cultures. *Toxicologist* **15**, 123.

BJORK, G.R. and KOHLI, J. (1990) Synthesis and function of modified nucleosides in t-RNA. In GEHRKE, G.W. and KUO, K.C. (eds) *Chromatography and Modification of Nucleosides, Part B: Biological Roles and function of modifications.* Amsterdam: Elsevier, B13–B67.

BUCK, M., CONNICK, M. and AMES, B.N. (1983) Complete analysis of tRNA modified nucleosides of *Salmonella typhimurium* and *Escherichia coli* tRNA. *Analyt. Biochem.* **129**, 1–13.

DEMETRULIAS, J., DONELLY, T., MORHENN, V. JESSEE, B., HAINSWORTH, S., CASTERTON, P., BERNHOFER, L. MARTIN, K. and DECKER, D. (1998) Skin²—an *in vitro* human skin model: the correlation between *in vivo* and *in vitro* testing of surfactants. *Exp. Dermatol.* **7**, 18–26.

FRANZ, T.J. (1978) The finite dose technique as a valid *in vitro* model for the study of percutaneous absorption in man. In SIMON, G.A., PASTER, Z., KLINGBERG, M.A. and KAYE, M. *Current Problems in Dermatology, Vol. 7: Skin: drug application and evaluation of environmental hazards.* Basel: Karger, 58–68.

FRIENKEL, R.K. (1960) Metabolism of glucose by human skin *in vitro*. *J. Invest. Dermatol.* **34**, 37–42.

KUO, K.C., PHAN, D.T., WILLIAMS, N., GEHRKE, G.W. (1990) Ribonucleosides in biological fluids by a high-resolution quantitative RPLC-UV method. In: GEHRKE, G.W. and KUO, K.C. (eds) *Chromatography and Modification of Nucleosides, Part C: Modified nucleosides in cancer and normal metabolism methods and applications,* Amsterdam: Elsevier, C41–C113.

FIELDS, R.D. and LANCASTER, M.V. (1993) Dual-attribute continuous monitoring of cell proliferation/cytotoxicity. *American Biotech. Lab.* **11**(4), 48–50.

MEYER, W., SCHWARZ, R. and NEURAND, K. (1978) The skin of domestic mammals as a model for the human skin, with special reference to the domestic pig. In SIMON, G.A., PASTER, Z., KLINGBERG, M.A. and KAYE, M. (eds) *Current Problems in Dermatology, Vol 7, Skin: drug application and evaluation of environmental hazards.* Basel: Karger, 39–52.

PLASTERK, R.H. (2002) RNA silencing: the genome's immune system. *Science.* **296**, 1263–1265.

REIFENRATH, W.G. and HAWKINS, G.S. (1986) The weanling Yorkshire pig as an animal model for measuring percutaneous penetration. In: TUMBLESON, M.E. (ed.) *Swine in Biomedical Research*. New York: Plenum, 673–680.

REIFENRATH, W.G., LEE, B., WILSON, D.R. and SPENCER, T.S. (1994) A comparison of *in vitro* skin-penetration cells. J. *Pharm. Sci.* **83**, 1229–1233.

SCHOCH, G., SANDER, G., TOPP, H., and HELLER-SCHOCH, G. (1990) Modified nucleosides and nucleobases in urine and serum as selective markers for whole-body turnover of tRNA, rRNA and mRNA-Cap—Future prospects and impact. In: GEHRKE, G.W. and KUO, K.C. (eds) *Chromatography and Modification of Nucleosides, Part C: Modified nucleosides in cancer and normal metabolism methods and applications*. Amsterdam: Elsevier, C389–C442.

STORZ, G. (2002) An expanding universe of non-coding RNAs. *Science*. **296**, 1260–1263.

ZAMORE, P.D. (2002) Ancient pathways programmed by small RNAs. *Science*. **296**, 1265–1269.

CHAPTER 46

Determination of Subclinical Changes of Barrier Function

VÉRANNE CHARBONNIER, MARC PAYE AND
HOWARD I MAIBACH

Contents

47.1   Introduction

47.2   Measurement of sub-clinical barrier changes by
       evaporimetry (TEWL)

47.3   Assessment of sub-clinical barrier alterations by
       squamometry

47.4   Conclusions

47.1 INTRODUCTION

The epidermis serves as a barrier to the outside world. Through its external layer, the stratum corneum (SC), the epidermis plays a mechanical protective role and minimizes the exchange of materials between our body and the environment. One of the major functions of the SC layer is to prevent excessive evaporation of water from the viable cell layers. Removal of the SC results in a significant increase in the rate of water loss from the skin (Eriksson and Lamke, 1971). The SC mainly consists of protein-enriched corneocytes embedded in a highly organized lamellar bilayer of lipids (Schurer and Elias, 1991). It is generally assumed that this cutaneous barrier is disrupted through intercellular lipid reorganizations, through lipid removal, or through protein alterations (Grubauer et al., 1989). The "barrier" maintains SC functionality by preventing fluid loss and by minimizing the penetration of exogenous substances.

However, the epidermis is not an inert membrane since it undergoes a continuous proliferation-desquamation process. Basal cells at the junction with the dermis continuously divide and move toward the surface. During this migration, the cell morphology changes and lipids and proteins are both synthesized and modified by enzymatic reactions. During the final stages of the proliferation process, lipids are excreted into the intercellular space to provide a unique structure that defines the skin's permeability properties (Elias, 1983). These lipids as well as proteinic bridges called desmosomes play a role in insuring inter-cellular cohesion. Desmosomes are found between the keratinocytes and corneosomes and corneo-desmosomes are found between corneocytes (Chapman and Walsh, 1990). In the non-palmo-plantar SC, the density of these "bridges" significantly decreases and they only remain at the periphery of corneocytes to weaken the cohesion between cells (Chapman and Walsh, 1990). In the most external layers of the SC, sometimes defined as the stratum disjunctum, proteolytic enzymes degrade the corneosomes, and isolated corneocytes detach and are released from the surface of the skin (Suzuki et al., 1993). Cell turnover, from division to desquamation, lasts about four weeks in normal conditions. If any of these maturation or renewal steps is impaired, for instance by contact with skin irritants, the desquamation rate and pattern, and the water impermeability barrier properties are affected (Rawlings et al., 1994). Corneocyte release does not occur anymore in the form of isolated cells, but rather as clusters of corneocytes forming scales or flakes. Moreover, water is not retained by the SC anymore, but evaporates at a much increased rate.

Human skin irritation is classically evaluated by clinical (visual and/or tactile) scoring. Bioengineering methods measuring skin surface capacitance, color, transepidermal water loss, and blood flow have been introduced over the last 25 years to get more objective measurements and have been widely used (Berardesca, 1988; Tupker *et al.*, 1989; Wilhelm *et al.*, 1989; Agner and Serup, 1990; Tupker, 1994; De Boer *et al.*, 1995; Wilhelm and Maibach, 1995). But the identification of the effect of substances of low or sub-clinical irritation potential still remains problematic in some instances. In order to detect and quantify the "invisible" irritation effects, these bioengineering techniques have also been of great help (Paye and Morrison, 1996). Changes of the electrical properties of the SC are very early predictors of skin surface alterations (Paye and Morrison, 1996; Rizvi *et al.*, 1996a, b), and evaporimetry measurements allow early discrimination between surfactant-based products in irritation tests. These measurements detect differences earlier than those observed visually by trained evaluators (Simion *et al.*, 1991).

An increasing interest has been observed for techniques focusing on the stratum corneum. Cellophane, and related tape forms used to remove and analyze the stratum corneum, have been developed with numerous applications: quantifying stratum corneum desquamation (Marttin *et al.*, 1996; Dreher *et al.*, 1998), barrier function pertubation (Schatz *et al.*, 1993; Welzel *et al.*,1996) or percutaneous penetration (Coderch *et al.*, 1996), observing histological changes (Gerritsen *et al.*, 1994; van der Molen *et al.*, 1997), and testing cosmetics and drugs effects (Pershing *et al.*, 1992; Letawe *et al.*, 1996). To evaluate non-erythematous irritant dermatitis, squamometry has recently appeared to be a sensitive complementary method to conventionnal skin color, transepidermal water loss (TEWL), and hydration measurements (Charbonnier *et al.*, 1998; Charbonnier and Maibach, 1999; Charbonnier *et al.*, 2000; 2001a, b; in preparation).

This chapter mainly focuses on two types of methods to evaluate sub-clinical barrier changes: transepidermal water loss (TEWL) which is the most conventional technique, and squamometry (SQM), a more recent technique that has shown a lot of promise. TEWL mainly measures the effect of the alteration of the barrier, while SQM investigates the origin and prior interactions with the SC that have caused the barrier to be altered.

47.2 MEASUREMENT OF SUB-CLINICAL BARRIER CHANGES EVAPORIMETRY (TEWL)

The barrier's integrity seems to be a key factor in determining the responsivity of the skin to external aggressions. Patients with atopic dermatitis have been

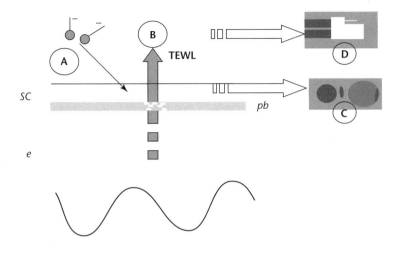

Figure 47.1: Skin barrier sub-clinical alterations.
Anionic surfactants interact with the stratum corneum (A) which can be assessed by squamometry (C). This interaction causes an alteration of the permeability barrier (*pb*) of the stratum corneum (*sc*) and as a result, transepidermal water loss (TEWL) increases, as measured by evaporimetry (D). *e* is the epidermis.

reported to have elevated TEWL values (Werner and Lindberg, 1985) and are more readily irritated by detergents than non-atopic subjects (Van der Valk *et al.*, 1985). Similarly, in a normal population, subjects with the highest TEWL values were reported to be the most susceptible to surfactant irritation (Pinnagoda *et al.*, 1989; Tupker *et al.*, 1989). In experimental test models, skin is sometimes compromised by sub-irritant treatment with SLS in order to pre-damage the cutaneous barrier (Allenby *et al.*, 1993). In such cases, TEWL is enhanced and skin responsiveness to mild irritants increased (Paye, personal data). In all these situations, evaporimetry measurements proved to be very sensitive in detecting damages to the skin barrier associated with reduced skin protection caused by external irritants.

Measurement of water loss from the skin has also been widely used to investigate and compare the irritation potential of products (mostly surfactant-containing) entering into contact with the surface of the skin (Van der Valk *et al.*, 1984; 1985; Simion *et al.*, 1991). This is the case for hygiene products like soaps, shower gels, foam baths, etc. as well as for a multitude of detergent products such as hand dishwashing liquids, household cleaners or even fabrics cleaners. In occlusive patch tests with surfactant-based products, the stratum corneum barrier function is impaired before any erythema is induced (Simion *et al.*, 1991). This is expected as occlusion is known to affect the barrier properties of the skin by itself (Ramsing and Agner, 1996). Furthermore, the test product first encounters the stratum corneum and alter the barrier function before reaching deeper skin layers to induce erythema. When very mild products are tested under such conditions, it is typical to observe impairment of the barrier function in the absence of an erythematous reaction. In contrast, for very irritating products or substances, the skin barrier can be very quickly damaged. The resulting inflammation occurs immediately and predominates over the TEWL readings. Evaporimetry measurements of SC alterations are thus mostly appropriate for comparing very mild products to each other when no or minimal erythema is induced. Clinical evaluation of the erythematous reaction is often preferable when one wants to compare harsh products. TEWL can be used to monitor barrier damage as well as to follow the recovery of the barrier integrity during the repair phase following a skin challenge (Wilhelm *et al.*, 1994). There is thus a great deal of evidence supporting the use of evaporimetry measurements to study cutaneous alterations at a sub-clinical level. However, due to the high sensitivity of the measurements and to the numerous factors that can affect the water evaporation rate of subjects, a lot of caution must be considered to obtain accurate measurements.

47.2.1   Principle of TEWL measurements

Water diffusion from the skin may involve several components: the sweat-gland activity, the evaporation of water from the surface of the skin, and the evaporation of body water through the SC. This latter component is usually referred to as the transepidermal water loss and, providing that the two other components are controlled and minimized, can be used to monitor changes in the water permeability barrier function of the SC. Several instrumental methods have been investigated to measure TEWL from local skin sites; however the major progresses were made since the description by Nilsson (1977) of a method based on the estimation of the vapor-pressure gradient immediately adjacent to the surface of the skin in an open, ventilated, chamber. Using this kind of chamber, the skin is exposed to normal ambient air and the development of a warm and humid microclimate at the measurement site is avoided.

In the probe of the measuring device, two vapor-pressure sensitive sensors are placed at a specific distance from each other. When the probe is placed horizontally to the surface of the skin, these sensors are able to determine the vapor-pressure gradient above the skin surface. This gradient is then translated into the amount of water crossing the SC per hour and square meter of skin (g of water/h.m^2). This value, measured below the sweating temperature and in non-stressful conditions, is relatively low (usually between 4 and 10 g/h.m^2 depending on the body site) when the skin barrier is intact, while it can grow up by 10 to 30 times when the barrier is severely damaged.

Two instruments are quite popular for measuring TEWL, the ServoMed Evaporimeter® and the Courage & Khazaka Tewameter®. Both are based on the same principle and have been described and compared elsewhere (Barel and Clarys, 1995). More recently, a third instrument has been described, the Derma-Lab® system (Cortex Technology, Hadsund, Denmark), which has a TEWL probe. The DermaLab® system has been compared to the Evaporimeter® and very good agreement has been observed (Grove *et al.*, 1999a). It is based on the same principle as an open chamber and measures a water vapor gradient. Temperature and humidity at the level of each of the two sensors are constantly displayed during measurements, and the system can be linked to a computerized program (Grove *et al.*, 1999b). Due to the low number of publications currently available on this system, its performance should however be confirmed in more evaluation conditions.

The ServoMed Evaporimeter® is probably the one that has been the most widely used to measure TEWL, being the first one on the market place. It is easy to handle and to carry, and provides instant measurements of the TEWL from the skin. Its main advantage, on top of the quality of the instrument, is its large usage around the world rendering comparison of data between laboratories quite easy. One of the main disadvantages is the time required before the displayed value stabilizes (usually between 30 seconds and one minute depending on the extent of barrier alteration); an internal integration system of the values for 10, 20 or 30 seconds exists to minimize those fluctuations and recently it has been made possible to link the Evaporimeter® to a computerized program (cyberDERM®, Media, PA, USA or ServoMed®, Kinna, Sweden) to register the evolution of the measured values and integrate them on a certain period of time after TEWL has reached stability. This makes the use of this instrument much easier and the precision of the measurements much greater. More details can be found in a specialized book (Elsner *et al.*, 1994).

The Tewameter® has also been designed so that it is easy to use and to carry, and directly provides integration values and graphic representations of the evolution of the measurements on the computer screen. Information about temperature and humidity values of the probe is also recorded during the measurement and could be of some importance for the accuracy of TEWL measurement (Rodrigues and Pereira, 1998). The sensitivity of the Tewameter(r) and of the Evaporimeter® has been compared with some advantages for both of them depending on the extent of the barrier alteration.

47.2.2 Cautions for TEWL measurements

Due to the sensitivity of the TEWL measurements and the numerous factors that can affect water evaporation, a lot of parameters must be carefully controlled for evaporimetry measurements. Those parameters reviewed in previous publications (Pinnagoda *et al.*, 1990; Paye, 1999; Rogiers and the EEMCO Group, 2001) may be related to the individuals (e.g. extreme age, anatomical site, menstrual cycle periods, circadian rhythm, sweating characteristics, . . .), to environmental factors (e.g. ambient temperature or humidity, air convection, . . .), to measurement or instrument variables (e.g. calibration, temperature of the probe, positioning of the probe, . . .), or to test variables (e.g. occlusion, moisture in the vehicle for leave-on products, delay between product application and measurement, . . .). For all these reasons, several guidelines for a proper assessment of TEWL and a proper interpretation of results have been published by several expert groups (Pinnagoda *et al.*, 1990; Rogiers and the EEMCO Group, 2001). When those guidelines are strictly followed, TEWL measurement is unequivocally an excellent method to measure the effect of sub-clinical changes in the integrity of the skin barrier.

47.3 ASSESSMENT OF SUB-CLINICAL BARRIER ALTERATIONS BY SQUAMOMETRY

Few human *in vivo* studies have been described relating to assessing sub-clinical surfactant-induced irritation (Paye and Morrison, 1996; Charbonier *et al.* 1998; 2000; 2001a). In those studies that have, open models were used in order to better approximate consumer surfactant use. Our goal was to determine whether we could differentiate between various surfactant solutions in terms of their skin surface effect. Squamometry provided some insight into changes of irritation (sub-erythematous irritation) not readily discerned with clinical readings and bioengineering instruments.

47.3.1 Squamometry-methodology

The use of the adhesive D-SQUAME® disk as a harvesting method for the superficial desquamating layer of the stratum corneum has been discussed in detail (Miller, 1995) and guidelines for their analysis have been published by the EEMCO (European group for the Efficacy Measurement of Cosmetics and Other topical products) (Pierard, 1996). Stratum corneum (SC) tape strippings may be rated by visual examination after placing the sample on a black bottom, by weighting, by optical measurement with or without specific staining, by image analysis, and by morphometry (Pierard, 1996; Pierard and Pierard-Franchimont, 1996).

In this section, we focus our attention on an optical measurement method and on morphometric changes of stained SC tape strippings. Squamometry is a non-invasive, protein-dependent, colorimetric evaluation of the level of alteration in the corneocyte layer collected by clear adhesive-coated disks. Xerotic and irritant changes in the stratum corneum can also be quantified (Pierard *et al.*, 1992; Pierard and Pierard-Franchimont, 1996). The disks are applied onto the skin under controlled pressure. A short application time (15 seconds) enables the harvesting of the superficial corneocytes (superficial squamometry) and a long application time (1 hour) enables the collection of a thicker layer of corneocytes (deep squamometry) (Pierard, 1996; Pierard and Pierard-Franchimont, 1996). The disks are stained for 30 seconds with a solution of toluidine blue and basic fushsin in 30 percent alcohol (Polychrome Multiple Stain, PMS; Delasco, IA, USA), applied to the surface, and gently rinsed in water. Tape strippings are placed on a transparent microscope slide which is itself placed on the calibration white plate of the Chromameter® (Chromameter®, Minolta, Japan). Measurements of the color of the samples in the L*a*b* mode are made using a reflectance colorimeter according to Pierard *et al.* (1992). Calculation of the Chroma C* values is done after $(a^{*2}+b^{*2})^{1/2}$. This parameter combines the values of the red and blue chromacities, predominant colors of the PMS. The Chroma C* value has been shown to be related to the amount of stratum corneum harvested in xerotic situation (Pierard *et al.*, 1992). The calculation of the Colorimetric Index of Mildness (CIM), with CIM=L*-C*, was performed (Pierard and Pierard-Franchimont, 1996) where L* is a measure of the luminance (Pierard *et al.*, 1992). A trained person scores the disks with a microscope at (X20) magnification according to the following scoring scales (Paye *et al.*, 1995; Paye and Morrison, 1996):

■ CHAPTER 47 ■

Intercorneocyte cohesion:

0 = large sheet;
1 = large clusters + few isolated cells;
2 = small clusters + many isolated cells;
3 = clusters in disruption, most cells isolated;
4 = all cells isolated, many cases of lysis.

Amount and distribution of dye found in cells:

0 = no staining;
1 = staining between cells or slight staining in cells;
2 = moderate staining in cells;
3 = large amount of dye in cells, but uniform;
4 = important staining in all cells, often with grains.

An illustration of a stained disk is presented in Figure 47.2. This methodology has been used into the studies mentioned below.

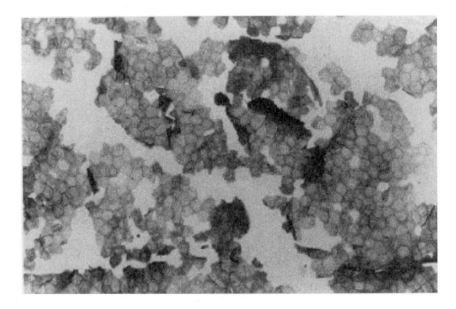

Figure 47.2: Illustration of a stained disk with PMS

47.3.2 Sub-clinical alterations of the stratum corneum with surfactant

After a single occlusive application (24 h patch-test), low concentrations of sodium lauryl sulfate (SLS, 0.5 percent in water) can cause irritation, dryness, tightness and barrier alterations (Wilhelm *et al.*, 1994; Treffel and Gabard, 1996; Tupker et al., 1997). These occlusive tests are, however, too severe to observe sub-clinical damage, since erythema and skin barrier alterations predominate. Furthermore, occlusion plays a significant role in the barrier alterations that can hide the effect of the test product at that level. In typical use, the consumer contact with surfactant is brief, via hand washing or personal cleansing and repetitive. The open application model becomes relevant when phenomena, such as dryness and sub-clinical (i.e. non-visible) irritation, especially cumulative faint alterations of the skin surface barrier, are induced. SLS can induce sub-clinical skin damage in a repetitive open application test method (exaggerated model hand wash) as well as in a short exposure patch tests. Analysis of the skin surface via squamometry offers a unique way of measuring skin changes when traditional methods do not. It also permits exploration of sub-clinical surfactant irritation and stratum corneum alterations (Charbonnier *et al.*, 1998; Morrison *et al.*, 1998).

In two of the studies (Charbonnier *et al.*, 1998), we performed four successive stratum corneum tape disk strippings on the dorsal hand in order to estimate the penetration pattern of the surfactant solution in terms of the skin barrier damage effect measured via squamometry. Data on dye fixation per cell revealed differences between SLS solutions at 0.75 percent an 2.25 %w/w in water as early as the first day (out of four treatment days) on the upper two tape strips. Thereafter, differences appeared on all days for each of the four tape strippings successively collected on a same site. In such an application mode, dryness manifested itself first in the uppermost stratum corneum (two most superficial tape strippings) before appearing in the lower layers (third and fourth tape strippings) after more washings. Overall, there was an increased dying of the tape strips from the first up to the fourth day. Thus, the 24 h patch test and the open test are disparate: skin response to an SLS challenge indicates inflammation and dryness in the occlusive patch while only faint, non-visible alteration due to surface interactions occurs in the open assay.

A single skin challenge with an irritant is a momentary reflection of skin susceptibility with little bearing on the cumulative effect of irritation or the associated repair mechanisms. An occlusive application of surfactant enhances

■ CHAPTER 47 ■

the penetration of the irritant into or through the stratum corneum and permits to investigate the interaction of the surfactant with deeper skin layers than in an open test. More importantly, the occlusive application test is not appropriate to study and conclude on the effect of an irritant on the skin barrier function. In real life, consumers are exposed to surfactants mainly through skin washing. The contact time of the surfactant with the skin is thus short, non-occlusive, and followed by a rinsing phase. The surfactant can thus in most cases only interact with the stratum corneum without reaching deeper layers.

In test models, squamometry allows one to assess irritation effects under more realistic test conditions without causing any overt irritation (Paye and Cartiaux, 1999). To refine the exaggerated hand washing model (Charbonnier et al., 1998), we tried to move from exaggerated hand washing to more consumer realistic conditions. The exaggerated hand washing procedure was replaced by three daily controlled washes at the laboratory for five days, one wash on day 7 after the week-end, and volunteer use at home for one week (instructions and gloves were provided for other products use at home over the test period) (Charbonnier et al., 2000). The two surfactants compared were SLS and SLES. Based on the results of this study, squamometry was able to document sub-clinical non-erythematous effects. The data also suggested that differences existed between SLS and SLES at 5 %w/w both by chroma C*, CIM and microscopic examination of cell cohesion and dye fixation per cell. Even if most differences were observed one hour after the day 7 wash in the laboratory, the CIM (the higher, the milder) and the chroma C* (the lower, the milder) statistical analysis also revealed a significant difference between SLS and SLES before the controlled-laboratory wash on day 7, which was after volunteers were self-dosed over the week-end. Encouraged by these results, an open assay, using only volunteer washing (whole body wash) at home as usual, was tested. Bioengineering measurements, squamometry and clinical assessments were performed after three washes and after a week's usage at home (Charbonnier et al., 2001a). The conventional techniques of erythema and dryness, capacitance and evaporimetry were not capable of distinguishing between the effects on skin of the two surfactants after the first three washings while squamometry clearly and significantly showed that SLS was more damaging to the stratum corneum than SLES by chroma C* measurements and microscope assessment of corneocytes cohesion loss and dye fixation per cell. Even if it was expected that protected sites (i.e., forearm) could be more discriminating in a home use assay, squamometry proved also to be sensitive enough to differentiate between the effect of surfactant solution on any skin site after as few as the three first home washes. Details have been reported elsewhere (Charbonnier and Maibach, 2001).

47.3.3   Conclusion

An open application method seems essential, particularly in the detection of sub-clinical skin surface alterations occurring during test methodologies relevant with the normal consumer practice. Within this respect, it is crucial for the clinician to have, at his/her disposal, very sensitive techniques used to evaluate the stratum corneum. Squamometry appears to be a robust and facile complementary method to conventional skin color, TEWL, and hydration measurements, particularly in the detection of subclinical alterations. This section only briefly described a few applications of squamometry in open test models; however, several other usages have so far been published where squamometry has been used to investigate xerotic conditions (Pierard *et al.*, 1992; Pierard, 1996), the interaction of body cleansing products (Pierard *et al.*, 1994; Pierard and Pierard-Franchimont, 1996), shampoos (Goffin *et al.*, 1996) or dishwashing liquids (Paye *et al.*, 1999a) with the skin, differences of corneocytes cohesion between sensitive and non-sensitive hands subjects (Paye *et al.*, 1999b), and the effect of skin barrier protectants (Shimizu and Maibach, 1999) or of topical drugs (Pierard *et al.*, 1993). With so many potential applications and its extension of use in many different groups, squamometry seems to represent a choice method for investigating the effect of irritants on stratum corneum integrity.

47.4   CONCLUSIONS

This chapter briefly reviews two different methods used to study at a sub-clinical level the alteration of the skin protective barrier. With the current trend to develop test models on volunteers which are more respectful of volunteers' skin condition and closer to consumer use habits of the products, it has been mandatory to design assessment methods able to detect "invisible irritation." Evaporimetry measurements, even if not a new bioengineering method, obviously fulfills those requirements to quantify the consequences of the barrier disruption in terms of transepidermal water loss. Easy to use, the method, however, requires a lot of precautions to provide meaningful information. More recently described is squamometry. Unlike evaporimetry, the technique does not measure the effects of barrier integrity modifications. Instead, it documents

■ CHAPTER 47 ■

the alterations caused to the stratum corneum, and hence to the cutaneous barrier, by surfactants or other irritants. Although still a new technique, squamometry has shown numerous applications through several testing procedures, for several types of products and is already being used in several laboratories.

Targeting two different phases of the skin barrier alteration process, evaporimetry and squamometry may be regarded as two complementary tools to follow and understand sub-clinical skin changes.

REFERENCES

AGNER, T. and SERUP, J. (1990) Sodium lauryl sulfate for irritant patch testing: a dose response study using bioengineering methods for determination of skin irritation. *J. Invest. Dermatol.* **95**, 543–547.

ALLENBY, C.F., BASKETTER, D.A., DICKENS, A. BARNES, E.G. and BROUGH, H.C. (1993) An arm immersion model of compromised skin. (I) Influence on irritation reactions. *Contact Dermatitis* **28**, 84–88.

BAREL, A.O. and CLARYS, P. (1995) Study of the stratum corneum barrier function by transepidermal water loss measurements: comparison between two commercial instruments: Evaporimeter and TEWAmeter. *Skin Pharmacol.* **8**, 186–195.

BERARDESCA, E. and MAIBACH, H.I. (1988) Bioengineering and the patch test. *Contact Dermatitis* **18**, 3–9.

CHAPMAN, S.J. and WALSH, A. (1990) Desmosomes, corneosomes and desquamation. An ultrastructural study of adult pig epidermis. *Arch. Dermatol.* **282**, 304–310.

CHARBONNIER, V. and MAIBACH, H.I. (1999) Non-erythematous irritation. *Allured's Cosmetics and Toiletries* **114** (June) 39–40.

CHARBONNIER, V. and MAIBACH, H.I. (2001) Site sensitivity of non-erythematous irritation. *Allured's Cosmetics and Toiletries* **116**, 6, 20–23.

CHARBONNIER, V., MORRISON, JR, B.M., PAYE, M. and MAIBACH, H.I. (1998) Open application assay in investigation of sub-clinical irritant dermatitis induced by SLS in man: Advantage of squamometry, *Skin Research and Technology* **4**, 244–250.

CHARBONNIER, V., MORRISON, JR, B.M., PAYE, M. and MAIBACH, H.I. (2000) An open assay model to induce subclinical non-erythematous irritation. *Contact Dermatitis* **42**, 207–211.

CHARBONNIER, V., MORRISON, JR, B.M., PAYE, M. and MAIBACH, H.I. (2001a) Subclinical, non-erythematous irritation with an open model (washing): sodium lauryl sulfate versus sodium laureth sulfate. *Food and Chemical Toxicology* **39**, 3, 279–286.

CHARBONNIER, V., MORRISON, JR, B.M., PAYE, M. and MAIBACH, H.I. (2001b) Quantification of non-erythematous irritant dermatitis. In: MAIBACH, H.I. (ed.) *Toxicology of Skin.* Taylor & Francis Publ, New York, 31–37.

CHARBONNIER, V., MORRISON, JR, B.M., PAYE, M. and MAIBACH, H.I. (in preparation) Hand dryness by an exaggerated wash procedure *in vivo* with sodium lauryl sulfate, sodium laureth sulfate and sodium alpha olefin sulfonate.

CODERCH, L., OLIVA, M., PONS, A., DE LA MAZA, A., MANICH, A.M. and PARRA, J.L. (1996) Percutaneous penetration of liposome using the tape stripping technique. *Intl J. Pharmac.* **139**, 197–203.

DE BOER, E.M. and BRUYNZEEL, D.P. (1995) Irritancy. In: BERARDESCA, E., ELSNER, P. and MAIBACH, H.I. (eds) *Bioengineering of the Skin: Cutaneous Blood Flow and Erythema.* CRC Press, Boca Raton 199–215.

DREHER, F., ARENS, A., HOSTYNEK, J.J., MUDUMBA, S., ADEMOLA, J. and MAIBACH, H. (1998) Colorimetric method for quantifying human stratum corneum removed by adhesive-tape-stripping. *Acta Derm. Venereol. Stockholm* **78**, 1–4.

ELIAS, P.M. (1983) Epidermal lipids, barrier function and desquamation, *J. Invest. Dermato.* **80**, 44–49.

ELSNER, P., BERARDESCA, E. and MAIBACH, H.I. (eds). (1994) *Bioengineering and the Skin: Water and the Stratum Corneum.* CRC Press, Boca Raton.

ERIKSSON, G. and LAMKE, L. (1971) Regeneration of human epidermal surface and water barrier function after stripping. *Acta. Derm. Venereol.* Stockholm, **51**, 169–178.

GERRITSEN, J.P., VAN ERP, P.E.J., VAN VLIJMEN-WILLEMS, I.M.J.J., LENDERS, L.T.M. and VAN DE KERKHOF, C.M. (1994) Repeated tape stripping of normal skin: histological assessment and comparison with events in psoriasis. *Arch. Dermatol. Res.* **286**, 455–461.

GOFFIN, V., PIÉRARD-FRANCHIMONT, C. and PIÉRARD, G.E. (1996) Anti-dandruff shampoos and the stratum corneum. *J. Dermatological Treatment* **7**, 215–218.

GROVE, G., GROVE, M.J., ZERWECK, C. and PIERCE, E. (1999a) Comparative metrology of the Evaporimeter and the DermaLab TEWL Probe. *Skin Res. Technol.* **5**, 1–8.

CHAPTER 47

GROVE, G., GROVE, M.J., ZERWECK, C. and PIERCE, E. (1999b) Computerized evaporimetry using the DermaLab TEWL Probe. *Skin Res. Technol.* **5**, 9–13.

GRUBAUER, G., FEINGOLD, K.R., HARRIS, R.M., ELIAS, P.M. (1989) Lipid content and lipid type as determinants of the epidermal permeability barrier. *J. Lipid Res.* **30**, 89–96.

LETAWE, C., PIERARD-FRANCHIMONT, C. and PIERARD, G.E. (1996) Squamometry in rating the efficacy of topical corticosteroids in atopic dermatitis. *Eur. J. Clin. Pharmacol.* **51**, 253–257.

MARTTIN, E., NEELISSEN-SUBNEL, M.T.A., DE HAAN, F.H.N. and BODDE, H.E. (1996) A critical comparison of methods to quantify stratum corneum removed by tape stripping. *Skin Pharmacol.* **9**, 69–77.

MILLER, D.L. (1995) Sticky slides and tape techniques to harvest stratum corneum material. In: SERUP, J. and JEMEC, G.B.E. (eds) *Handbook of Non-invasive Methods and the Skin.* CRC Press, Boca Raton, Chapter 7.2.

MORRISON, B.M. JR, CARTIAUX, Y., PAYE, M., CHARBONNIER, V. and MAIBACH, H.I. (1998) Demonstrating Invisible (Sub-clinical) Sodium Lauryl Sulfate Irritation with Squamometry. American Academy of Dermatolology, 56th annual meeting, Feb 27–Mar 4. Poster session, Orlando, FL, USA.

NILSSON, G.E. (1977) Measurement of water exchange through skin. *Med. Biol. Eng. Comput.* **15**, 209–218.

PAYE, M. (1999) Models for studying surfactant interactions with the skin. In: BROZE G. (ed.) *Handbook of Detergent,* New York: Marcel Dekker Inc. Publ. 469–509.

PAYE, M. and MORRISON JR, B.M. (1996) Non visible skin irritation, Proc. the Fourth World Surfactant Congress, Barcelona, **3**, 3–7 June: 42–51.

PAYE, M. and CARTIAUX, Y. (1999) Squamometry: A tool to move from exaggerated to more and more realistic application conditions for comparing human skin compatibility of surfactant based products. *International Journal of Cosmetic Science* **21**, 59–68.

PAYE, M., GOFFIN, V., CARTIAUX, Y., MORRISON, B.M. JR and PIÉRARD, G.E. (1995) D-squame strippings in the assessment of intercorneocyte cohesion. *Allergologie* **18**, S 462 (abstract).

PAYE, M., GOMES, G., ZERWECK, C.R., PIÉRARD, G.E. and GROVE, G.L. (1999a) A hand immersion test under laboratory-controlled usage conditions: the need for sensitive and controlled assessment methods. *Contact Dermatitis* **40**, 133–138.

PAYE, M., DALIMIER, C., CARTIAUX, Y. and CHABASSOL, C. (1999b) Consumer perception of sensitive hands: what is behind? *Skin Res. Technol.* **5**, 28–32.

PERSHING, L.K., LAMBERT, L.D., SHAH, V.P. and LAM, S.Y. (1992) Variability and correlation of chromameter and tape-stripping methods with visual skin blanching assay in the quantitative assessment of topical 0.05% betamethasone dipropionate bioavailability in humans. *Intl. J. Pharm.* **86**, 201–210.

PIERARD, G.E. (1996) EEMCO guidance to the assessment of dry skin (xerosis) and ichtyosis: evaluation by stratum corneum strippings. *Skin Res. Technol.* **2**, 3–11.

PIERARD, G.E. and PIERARD-FRANCHIMONT, C. (1996) In: MAIBACH, H.I. (ed.) *Dermatology Research Technique: Drug and cosmetic evaluations with skin strippings.* CRC Press, Boca Raton, 132–149.

PIERARD, G.E., PIERARD-FRANCHIMONT, C., SAINT-LEGER, D. and KLIGMAN, A.M. (1992) Squamometry: The assessment of xerotic by colorimetry of D-squame adhesive discs. *J. Soc. Cosmet. Chem.* **47**, 297–305.

PIÉRARD, G.E., PIÉRARD-FRANCHIMONT, C. and ARRESE, E.J. (1993) Comparative study of the activity and lingering effect of topical antifungals. *Skin Pharmacol.* **6**, 208–214.

PIÉRARD, G.E., GOFFIN, V. and PIÉRARD-FRANCHIMONT, C. (1994) Squamometry and corneosurfametry for rating interactions of cleansing products with stratum corneum. *J. Soc. Cosmet. Chem.* **45**, 269–277.

PINNAGODA, J., TUPKER, R.A., COENRAADS, P.J. and NATER, J.P. (1989) Prediction of susceptibility to an irritant response by transepidermal water loss. *Contact Dermatitis* **20**, 341–346.

PINNAGODA, J., TUPKER, R.A., AGNER, T. and SERUP, J. (1990) Guidelines for transepidermal water loss (TEWL) measurement. *Contact Dermatitis* **22**, 164–178.

RAMSING, D.W. and AGNER, T. (1996) Effect of glove occlusion on human skin (II) Long-term experimental exposure. *Contact Dermatitis* **34**, 258–262.

RAWLINGS, A-V., WATKINSON, A., ROGERS, J., MAYO, A.-M., HOPE, J. and SCOTT, I.R. (1994) Abnormalities in stratum corneum structure, lipid composition and desmosome desquamation in soap-induced winter xerosis. *J. Soc. Cosmet. Chem.* **45**, 203–220.

RIZVI, P.Y., MORRISON, B.M. JR, GROVE, M.J. and GROVE, G.L. (1996a) Instrumental evaluation of skin irritation. *Cosmet. Toilet.* **111** (9), 39–42.

■ CHAPTER 47 ■

RIZVI, P.Y., MORRISON, B.M. JR, GROVE, M.J. and GROVE, G.L. (1996b) Determination of the Irritation Potential of Mild and Ultra Mild Products by Surface Characterization through Impedance Monitoring (SCIM). *Skin Res. Technol.* **2**, 226 (abstract).

RODRIGUES, L. and PEREIRA, L.M. (1998) Basal transepidermal water loss: right/left forearm difference and motoric dominance. *Skin Res. Technol.* **4**, 135–137.

ROGIERS, V. and the EEMCO GROUP (2001) EEMCO guidance for the assessment of the transepidermal water loss (TEWL) in cosmetic sciences. *Skin Pharm. and Appl. Skin Physiol.* **14**, 117–128.

SCHATZ, H., KLIGMAN, A.M., MANNING, S. and STOUDEMAYER, T. (1993) Quantification of dry (xerotic) skin by image analysis of scales removed by adhesive discs (D-Squames). *J. Soc. Chem.* **44**, Jan/Feb 53–63.

SCHURER, N.Y. and ELIAS, P.M. (1991) Biochemistry and function of stratum corneum lipids. *Adv. Lipid Res.* **24**, 27–56.

SHIMIZU, T. and MAIBACH, H.I. (1999) Squamometry: an evaluation method for a barrier protectant (tannic acid). *Contact Dermatitis* **40**, 189–191.

SIMION, F.A., RHEIN, L.D., GROVE, G.L., WOJTKOWSKI, J.M., CAGAN, R.H. and SCALA, D.D. (1996) Sequential order of skin responses to surfactants during a soap chamber test. *Contact Dermatitis* **25**, 242–249.

SUZUKI, Y., NOMURA, J., HORI, J., KOYAMA, J., TAKAHASHI, M. and HORII, I. (1993) Detection and characterization of endogenous protease associated with desquamation of stratum corneum. *Arch. Dermatol. Res.* **285**, 372–377.

TREFFEL, P. and GABARD, B. (1996) Measurements of Sodium Lauryl Sulfate-induced skin irritation, *Acta Derm. Venereol.* **76**, 341–343.

TUPKER, R.A. (1994) Prediction of irritancy. In: ELSNER, P., BERARDESCA, E. and MAIBACH, H.I. (eds) *Bioengineering of the Skin: Water and the Stratum Corneum.* CRC Press, Boca Raton 73–85.

TUPKER, R.A., COENRAADS, P.J., PINNAGODA, J. and NATER, J.P. (1989) Baseline transepidermal water loss (TEWL) as a prediction of susceptibility to sodium lauryl sulfate. *Contact Dermatitis* **20**, 265–269.

TUPKER, R.A., PINNAGODA, J., COENRAADS, P.J. and NATER, J.P. (1989) The influence of repeated exposure to surfactants on the human skin as determined by transepidermal water loss and visual scoring. *Contact Dermatitis* **20**, 108–113.

TUPKER, R.A., VERMEULEN, K., FIDLER, V. and COENRAADS P.J. (1997) Irritancy testing of Sodium Lauryl Sulfate and other anionic detergents using an open exposure model. *Skin Research and Technology* **3**, 133–136.

VAN DER MOLEN, R.G., SPIES, F., VAN'T NOORDENDE, J.M., BOELSMA, E., MOMMAAS, A.M. and FOERTEN, H.K. (1997) Tape stripping of human stratum corneum yield cell layers that originate from various depths because of furrows in the skin. *Arch. Dermatol. Res.* **289**, 541–518.

VAN DER VALK, P.G.M., NATER, J.P. and BLEUMINK, K. (1984) Skin irritancy of surfactants as assessed by water vapor loss measurements. *J. Invest. Dermatol.* **82**, 291–294.

VAN DER VALK, P.G.M., NATER, J.P. and BLEUMINK, E. (1985) Vulnerability of the skin to surfactants in different groups of eczema patients and controls as measured by water vapor loss. *Clin. Exp. Dermatol.* **10**, 98–103.

WELZEL, J., WILHELM, K.P. and WOLFF, H.H. (1996) Skin permeability barrier and occlusion: no delay of repair in irritated human skin. *Contact Dermatitis* **35**, 163–168.

WERNER, Y. and LINDBERG, M. (1985) Transepidermal water loss in dry and clinically normal skin in patients with atopic dermatitis. *Acta Dermato.-Venereol.* **65**, 102–105.

WILHELM, K.P., SURBER, C. and MAIBACH, H.I. (1989) Quantification of sodium lauryl sulfate irritant dermatitis in man: comparison of four techniques— skin color reflectance, transepidermal water loss, laser doppler flow measurement and visual scores. *Arch. Dermatol. Res.* **281**, 293–295.

WILHELM, K.-P., FREITAG, G. and WOLFF, H.H. (1994) Surfactant-induced skin irritation and skin repair. Evaluation of the acute human irritation model by noninvasive techniques. *J. Am. Acad. Dermatol.* **30**, 944–949.

WILHELM, K.P. and MAIBACH, H.I. (1995) Evaluation of irritation tests by chromametric measurements. In: BERARDESCA, E., ELSNER, P. and MAIBACH, H.I. (eds) *Bioengineering of the Skin: Cutaneous Blood Flow and Erythema.* CRC Press, Boca Raton 269–280.

General readings

ELSNER, P. and MAIBACH, H.I. (eds) (1995) *Irritant Dermatitis: New Clinical and Experimental Aspects*, Karger, vol. **23**.

VAN DER VALK, P.G.M. and MAIBACH, H.I. (eds) (1996) *The Irritant Contact Dermatitis Syndrome*, CRC Press, Boca Raton.

CHAPTER 47

Assessing the Validity of Alternative Methods for Toxicity Testing

**LH BRUNER, GJ CARR, M CHAMBERLAIN
AND RD CURREN**

Contents

48.1   Introduction

48.2   The definition of validation

48.3   Confirming alternative method reliability in a
       validation study

48.4   Assessing alternative method relevance

48.5   Discussion

48.1 INTRODUCTION

Toxicologists have developed an array of animal-based tests that are used to assess the toxicity of chemicals and mixtures of chemicals during the last half century. These methods have been adopted by regulatory agencies throughout the world to provide data that are ultimately used to protect public health and to warn chemical users of potential health dangers. For the most part, these methods have provided adequate information for the protection of plant workers and the general public.

The use of animals for routine toxicity testing is now questioned by a growing segment of society. The expression of this concern is seen with particular clarity in the 6th Amendment to the European Union (EU) Cosmetics Directive 93/35/EEC (Anonymous, 1994). This Directive contains a provision stating that it will become illegal to market cosmetic products in EU countries if they contain ingredients or mixtures of ingredients that have been tested in animals (to meet the purposes of the Directive) unless there are no valid alternatives to replace the animal tests.

If currently used animal tests are to be successfully replaced, it is important to demonstrate that the alternative methods provide chemical hazard data equivalent to that now available from animal-based tests. Additionally, in order for toxicologists to take the best advantage of new technologies that are constantly evolving it is important that the validation process be conducted in a manner that efficiently and definitely characterizes the performance of new test methods.

The performance of numerous alternative methods have been assessed in recent validation programs (Booman *et al.*, 1989; Gettings *et al.*, 1991; Bagley *et al.*, 1992; Spielmann *et al.*, 1993; 1994; 1995; 1996; 1998; 2000; Balls *et al.*, 1995b; Balls and Fentem, 1997; Brantom *et al.*, 1997; Fentem *et al.*, 1998). These programs have provided a great deal of information about the validation process and the utility of the alternative methods. Additionally, there has been significant discussion on the theoretical and practical aspects of the validation process (Balls *et al.*, 1990; 1995a; Frazier, 1990; Curren *et al.*, 1995; Bruner *et al.*, 1996b; 1997; 2000; 2002a, b, c; Balls and Fentem, 1997). The purpose of this review is to summarize some of the important lessons that have been acquired during this work, and to provide recommendations of design factors that should be considered in future validation programs. The role of validation studies in obtaining objective measures of alternative method performance is reviewed. Additionally, we present a multistep process that may guide the design,

CHAPTER 48

execution, and evaluation of validation studies. Finally, we review factors that must be considered when the relevance of an alternative method is assessed. The validation of alternative methods for eye irritation testing is used as a specific example to illustrate important points associated with the validation process.

48.2 THE DEFINITION OF VALIDATION

Validation has been defined as "the process by which the reliability and relevance of an alternative method is established for a particular purpose" (Balls *et al.*, 1990). We therefore begin with a discussion of what is meant by reliability and relevance from a test user's point of view, and provide a perspective on how these elements may be assessed in the validation process.

48.2.1 Reliability

Toxicologists must rely on results obtained from an alternative method if it is to serve as a replacement for an *in vivo* toxicity test. Two measures of alternative method performance must be known in order to define reliability from a test user's point of view. First, a toxicologist must know it is possible to consistently reproduce the data obtained from the alternative method over long periods of time. A test that does not provide the same results on the same test substance repeatedly would not be useful in the safety assessment process. Second, it must be possible to consistently predict *in vivo* toxicity endpoints at a known level of accuracy and precision. These measures of reliability are objective endpoints that can be measured experimentally. The part of the validation process that provides the data needed to confirm the reliability of an alternative method as proposed by its developers is the validation study.

48.2.2 Relevance

In practical terms, the assessment of relevance addresses the following question: Given the information known about the alternative method, are the data provided by the assay good enough to allow its acceptance as a replacement for a given *in vivo* test? In order to answer this question, all of the available information related to performance, operation, and mechanistic basis of an alternative method and the *in vivo* toxicity test it is intended to replace must be thoroughly reviewed. The benefits and risks associated with the adoption of the new method must also be defined. Once this information is available, it must be synthesized in a manner that allows those involved in a validation process to render a judgment that the performance of the alternative method is acceptable or not as a replacement for the *in vivo* toxicity test.

Based on the preceding discussion, it is clear that the processes used to establish the reliability and relevance of an alternative method are distinct. The confirmation of alternative method reliability is an objective process, since it provides data measured in the laboratory during a validation study. The assessment of relevance is a subjective process, since it is based on the evaluation and integration of information and requires judgment. Since these processes are distinct, we review them separately. The discussion begins with a review of the validation study process and how it is used to obtain measures of a test's reliability. Following this discussion, we review the information that must be considered in order to establish relevance.

48.3 CONFIRMING ALTERNATIVE METHOD RELIABILITY IN A VALIDATION STUDY

As noted already, the tool used to obtain the data that provides objective measures of an alternative method's reliability is the validation study. Experience shows that conducting validation studies is complex. In order to provide a clear review of the steps that need to be considered, we have organized our discussion around the flow chart depicted in Figure 48.1. We begin with a consideration of the information that must be available about the performance of an alternative method before it is included in a validation study.

48.3.1 Step 1. Define the performance measures to be confirmed in the validation study (Figure 48.1)

In order to more easily design and ultimately interpret the results of a validation study, it is important to define two factors that define the reliability of an alternative method before the study starts. These factors are reproducibility and predictive capability of the alternative method. It is of critical importance these performance factors are clearly stated before a validation study starts. When these performance characteristics are defined beforehand, they provide critical information needed to design the study so that it includes the appropriate number of laboratories, an acceptable set of test substances, and the appropriate range of toxicity. They also provide benchmarks that can be used to set the criteria an alternative method must meet in order to be considered reliable. If

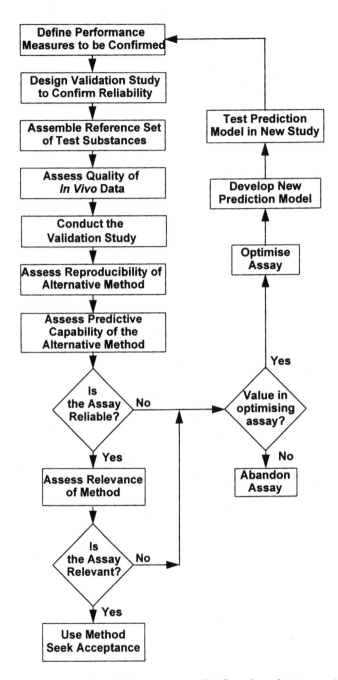

Figure 48.1: The validation process: The flow chart depicts a series of steps that may be used as a guide to design and conduct a validation program. The steps proceeding down the left side of the chart represent the actual validation process. The steps

the data obtained from the study meet or exceed these predefined performance criteria, then it confirms that the alternative method performs as described by its developers. If the method fails to perform at a level equivalent to the criteria set at the start of the study, then its performance cannot be confirmed.

Preliminary evidence of an alternative method's reproducibility is usually generated during its initial development. This information may be further supported by data obtained from formal method development programs that involve the collaboration of several laboratories. A discussion on how such programs may be conducted has been elaborated in detail elsewhere (Curren *et al.*, 1995).

Evidence demonstrating the predictive capability of an alternative method is usually also generated early in its development. This evidence is obtained by evaluating a subset of test substances of known toxicity in the alternative method. The results from the alternative method are directly compared with the *in vivo* toxicity data from each test substance. If this comparison reveals the existence of a definable relationship between the two data sets, it indicates that the alternative method may be useful for predicting *in vivo* toxicity.

An example of a definable relationship between alternative method and *in vivo* test data is illustrated in Figure 48.2. This plot shows that the results from a hypothetical alternative method are directly related to the level of toxicity measured *in vivo*. In this case, the relationship may be described in terms of the standard equation for a line, $y = mx + b$, where m is the slope of the regression line, and b represents the value of the y intercept of the regression line. If this algorithm is true for all test materials, then any result x, from this alternative method could be incorporated into the algorithm, $y = mx + b$, to obtain an output, y, that represents the prediction of toxicity *in vivo*. Other, non-mathematical approaches, like binary classification schemes, can be used to define the relationship between two tests (Bruner *et al.*, 1996a, b).

Since such algorithms constitute models that convert the results from an alternative method into a prediction of toxicity observed *in vivo*, they have been called *prediction models* (Bruner *et al.*, 1996b). A prediction model is essential because it defines exactly how an alternative method is used to predict *in vivo* toxicity. Therefore, if an assay does not have an adequate prediction model,

proceeding up the right side of the chart depict the steps associated with improving the performance of the alternative method and defining another prediction model prior to inclusion of the method in a new validation study.

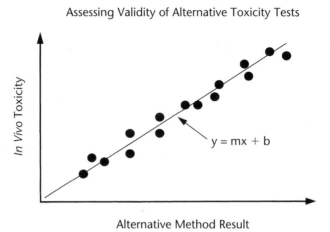

Figure 48.2: Plot showing a hypothetical relationship between a specific toxic endpoint measured *in vivo* and corresponding results from an alternative method. In order for an alternative method to be useful, there must be a consistent and definable relationship between toxicity measured *in vivo* and corresponding results in the alternative method. In this ca se, the relationship may be described in terms of a mathematical algorithm, $y = mx + b$. If this algorithm is true for all test materials, then any result, x, from this alternative method could be put in the algorithm $y = mx + b$, to obtain an output, y, which represents the prediction of toxicity *in vivo*. Such algorithms can be incorporated into Prediction Models that translate the results from an alternative method into a prediction of toxicity *in vivo*.

there is no way to confirm the assay's reliability (Bruner *et al.*, 1996a, b; Worth and Balls, 2001a). We now describe in detail the key elements that make up an adequate prediction model.

A prediction model is adequate when it defines three elements (Figure 48.3). These elements include a definition of all the possible results that may be obtained from an alternative method (inputs), an algorithm that allows a conversion of each result into a prediction of the *in vivo* toxicity endpoints (outputs), and a description of the types of test materials for which the prediction model may be used (Bruner *et al.*, 1997).

A prediction model must define all of the possible results that may be obtained from the alternative method. This is important since there are many different types of data available from typical alternative methods. Examples of data types include quantitative data, censored data, qualitative data, descriptive data, default values, and nonqualified data. *Quantitative data* are specific numerical values obtained as endpoints from the assays. These data are most

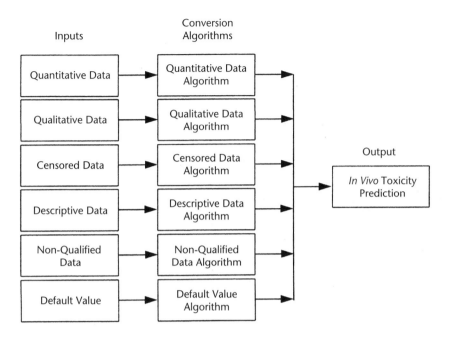

Figure 48.3: Elements of the prediction model: In order for an alternative method to predict toxicity *in vivo*, there must be a way to convert the results of the alternative method into a correct prediction of toxicity *in vivo*. The description of how to perform this conversion is called the prediction model. The conversion process followed must be input into the conversion algorithm that will lead to a prediction of toxicity as an output. A prediction model must define each of the data types available from the alternative method, an algorithm useful for converting the results of the alternative method into a prediction of toxicity, and the chemical classes, product categories, and physical forms for which the prediction model is valid.

commonly ED50s, but may be any other numerical values specifically measured in the assay. *Censored data* occur in assays that have maximum or minimum obtainable quantitative data. The result ">10,000 μg/ml" is a specific example of a censored datum. Censored data usually occur due to technical restraints that limit the dynamic range of a particular procedure. *Qualitative data* represent a classification of the effects caused by the test substance on the target of the assay. A result described as "irritant," "moderate irritant," or "nonirritant" is an example of qualitative data. *Descriptive data* are written phrases that characterize an observed effect of the test substance in the test system. The result "test substance causes coagulation of the chorioallantoic membrane" is an example of descriptive data. *Default values* result when two or more outputs obtained from an alternative method at the same time are combined to make a prediction. For example, two results from an alternative method at the same time are combined to make a prediction. For example, two results from an alternative method such as "the ED50 is greater than 10,000 µg/ml" and "no denaturation of proteins" may be combined to give the default value of "not irritating." *Nonqualified data* represent values obtained from an assay that cannot be used due to some kind of technical incompatibility of the test substance with the assay. For example, the buffering capacity of the tissue culture medium might neutralize an acid test substance. If the toxic effect of the test substance depends on its acidity, the result obtained from testing the material should not be considered an accurate indicator of the test substance toxicity. Other types of data in addition to these examples may be available. If so, each type must be defined in the prediction model.

Second, a prediction model must adequately define the conversion algorithms that translate each alternative method result into a prediction of the toxicity *in vivo* (Figure 48.3). The example illustrated in Figure 48.2 depicts an alternative method where the quantitative data algorithm, $y = mx + b$, is used to predict an *in vivo* toxicity, y, given any alternative method result, x. The conversion algorithms do not necessarily need to be mathematical equations. For example, algorithms may describe how to convert the alternative method data into classifications that fit a particular *in vivo* toxicity test classification scheme. No matter what approach is used, each algorithm must provide an unambiguous description of how to arrive at a prediction of *in vivo* toxicity given any possible result obtained from an alternative method. Any reasonably trained individual should be able to perform this translation. In addition to providing a prediction, it is important that the prediction model provide an indication of the variability associated with any prediction.

Third, the prediction model should define the chemical classes, product categories, and physical forms of test substance for which it is valid. For example, a particular alternative method may be useful (or validated) only for predicting the toxicity of surfactant-containing liquids. If so, these limitations must be defined.

48.3.2 Step 2. Design a validation study to test the validity of the prediction model (Figure 48.1)

Once the performance measures of an alternative method have been defined in terms of reproducibility and predictive capability, the next step in the process is to design a validation study that will test whether or not the alternative method actually performs as described. The design of a validation study is crucial to its success, not only in terms of testing reliability but also in retaining credibility and gaining acceptance by regulatory agencies. The factors that need to be considered include how the validation study will be managed, the nature and competence of the participating laboratories, the protocols and standard operating procedures (SOPs) to be used, how test substances will be coded and distributed, how data will be collected and analyzed, how well laboratories comply with the principles of good laboratory practice (GLP), and what data will be needed in order to confirm the reliability of the alternative method.

Management structure

In order to be successful, large and complex validation studies must have a well-defined management structure. This structure is required in order to assure the study principles and overall design are followed as agreed by the sponsors of the study. Responsibilities of managers and participating laboratories should be defined to assure the program accomplishes the mandates outlined in the goals of the study.

Participating laboratories

Ideally, all participating laboratories should be independent in order to ensure the integrity of separate data sets. If more than one laboratory is in the same large organization, the laboratories should be able to demonstrate local management structure and operational as well as financial independence. In the case of commercial enterprises, the design of the study should ensure that their participation is as unbiased as any other. If it is necessary for technical staff to undergo a period of training to ensure use of common methods, such training should be undertaken and documented.

Establishment of common protocols and standard operating procedures

It is essential that all factors relevant to the conduct of the alternative method that may affect the results, the collection of data, and interpretation of the alternative method results be clearly defined before the study begins. These are best documented in the study protocol and standard operating procedures

(SOPs) that define the alternative methods. In order to assess the adequacy of the SOPs, they should be examined to determine if they contain three key elements. First, each SOP must have a detailed step-by-step description of how to conduct the assay. Enough details need to be provided such that any appropriately trained and competent laboratory technician need use only this document as the guide to run the assay. Second, the SOP must indicate the steps used to calculate the endpoint of the assay and the number of replicates necessary. Any data transformation or algorithms applied to the data should be clearly documented and consistently applied across all laboratories conducting a particular assay. Third, the protocol must specifically describe the prediction model being tested in the validation study.

Test material selection, coding and distribution

The reference set of test substances (RSTS) included in the study should be commensurate with the prediction model being tested in the validation study (discussed more fully in step 3). The substances should be obtained with a specification stating source, purity, and whether there are any contaminants. These specifications should be identical to those of the material actually used to generate the *in vivo* data. If identical substances are not available, the potential effect that such discrepancies may have on a test substance toxicity must be assessed. In the case of formulated products, the ingredients and their levels in the product should be identified so that the formulation can be made again if necessary. Commercial sources of all single substances should be stated so that substances of the same or similar specification may be purchased in the future. Since testing usually occurs under conditions where participants do not know the identity of the reference substances, procedures need to be established to distribute substances under a randomly generated code. The system established to code and distribute the test samples should be evaluated to assure the coding is done correctly and that participants do not have access to the codes. Each laboratory should receive substances under different codes in order to assure that results generated in each laboratory are independent.

Data collection and analysis

The methods for the submission of results from the participants should be established to assure that all the necessary information has been provided to the study statistician. The mechanisms used to assure there are no errors in transcription should also be established in order to ensure that all data are accurately entered into the analysis.

Good laboratory practice

Acceptance of results and conclusions from a validation study may be compromised if the principles of GLP are not applied during the study. While this is unlikely to be an issue for industrial laboratories, it may be a more important concern in academic laboratories where adherence to GLP traditionally has been less of a concern. All efforts should be made to ensure that the principles of GLP were adhered to in all participating laboratories. This in large part can be achieved by determining whether common protocols, SOPs, and data reporting procedures were followed by the participants.

48.3.3 Step 3. Assemble an RSTS appropriate for confirming the reliability of the alternative method (Figure 48.1)

The next step in the process is to assemble an RSTS appropriate for assessing the reliability of the alternative method. The factors that need to be considered are the chemical classes, physical form, distribution of toxicity, and the number of materials that need to be included.

Chemical classes included in the RSTS

The chemical and physical forms of the substances included must be consistent with the stated prediction model. For example, if the prediction model indicates the alternative method is valid for assessing the eye irritation potential of mild, moderate, and severely irritating liquid, surfactant-based formulations, then the RSTS should contain liquid surfactant-based substances of the relevant class that cover a range of toxicity from mild to severe. Quantitative structure-activity relationships may be useful in helping selection of relevant test chemicals (Barratt, 1995; Chamberlain and Barratt, 1995).

Distribution of toxicity in the RSTS

The toxicity of the substances in the RSTS should be distributed as uniformly as possible across the range of interest. This is important because a nonuniform distribution of test substance toxicity in an RSTS may not allow an effective assessment of alternative method performance. Potential effects of non-uniform test substance distribution are illustrated in Figure 48.4. The ideal situation is shown in Figure 48.4B. In this example, the test substances are uniformly distributed across the range of possible toxicity. If such results were obtained from an alternative method, it would strongly suggest that it could be used to predict toxicity across the full range of possible responses. In Figure 48.4A, the substances in the RSTS are not uniformly distributed, but rather are either mildly or strongly toxic. The problem with such an RSTS is that it is impossible to determine whether the method is useful for predicting the toxicity of the moderately toxic materials. In fact, recent work has shown that the distribution of toxicity included in an RSTS can have profound effects on the performance statistics obtained from a validation study (Bruner *et al.*, 2002b). If the distribution of toxicity used in a validation study were indeed similar to that shown in Figure 48.4A, it is good test performance. However, when materials of mild and moderate toxicity are tested, the measures of performance may be considerably poorer. It may be found that the performance is more similar to those shown in Figures 48.4C or 48.4D. Alternative methods performing similar to the former two examples are less useful than one similar to Figure 48.4B. The best way to distinguish between the possible outcomes illustrated in Figures 48.4B, C, and D is to evaluate an RSTS having a uniform distribution of toxicity across the entire range of interest.

Number of test substances in the RSTS

The number of test substances included in the RSTS must also be evaluated. Although it has been suggested that a RSTS should contain up to 250 substances (Balls *et al.*, 1990), requiring such a large number is impractical for several reasons. First, it has proven extremely difficult to identify such a large set of test substances that have been evaluated in a common toxicity test procedure. Hence, it is unlikely that a set containing 250 substances can be assembled without conducting additional *in vivo* testing. Second, experience has shown that the cost of conducting a validation study using such a large RSTS is prohibitive. Third, there is a diminishing returns phenomenon after the RSTS reaches a certain size.

In order to gain a better understanding of how many test substances would be acceptable, we used a computer simulation based on the Draize eye irritation test to investigate the effects of changing sample size on the precision of future predictions of an *in vivo* test result from an alternative method test score. For

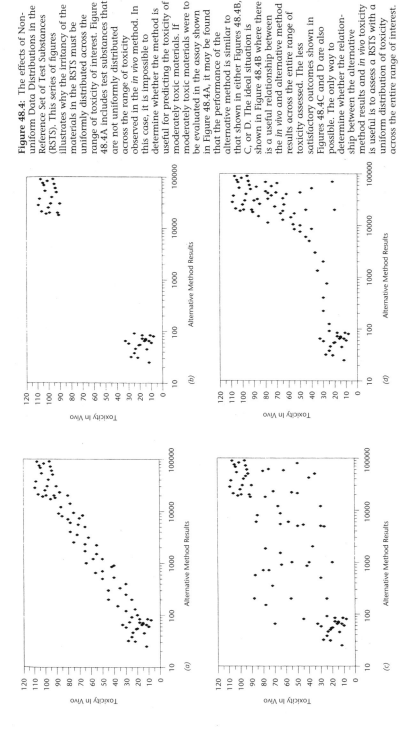

Figure 48.4: The effects of Non-uniform Data Distributions in the Reference Set of Test Substances (RSTS). This series of figures illustrates why the irritancy of the materials in the RSTS must be uniformly distributed across the range of toxicity of interest. Figure 48.4A includes test substances that are not uniformly distributed across the range of toxicity observed in the *in vivo* method. In this case, it is impossible to determine whether the method is useful for predicting the toxicity of moderately toxic materials. If moderately toxic materials were to be evaluated in the assay shown in Figure 48.4A, it may be found that the performance of the alternative method is similar to that shown in either Figures 48.4B, C, or D. The ideal situation is shown in Figure 48.4B where there is a useful relationship between the *in vivo* and alternative method results across the entire range of toxicity assessed. The less satisfactory outcomes shown in Figures 48.4C and D are also possible. The only way to determine whether the relationship between the alternative method results and *in vivo* toxicity is useful is to assess a RSTS with a uniform distribution of toxicity across the entire range of interest.

this simulation, it was assumed that the relationship between a hypothetical alternative method response, X, and a corresponding eye irritation response, Y, has the linear form:

$$Y = (1.1)X \tag{48.1}$$

where we restricted the alternative response X to be on the range [0–100], so that the *in vivo* response Y is on the usual maximum average scores (MAS) scale [0–110].

Values for X were chosen with a uniform distribution across the range of interest. Corresponding Y values were then calculated using Eq. (48.1). Since there is inherent variability in both alternative method and *in vivo* data, random error was added to the X and Y values, respectively. This was achieved through the use of independent beta distributions (Vose, 1996) scaled to give a specified coefficient of variation. The coefficient of variation applied to the alternative method response, X, was maintained constant on the full range 0 to 100. The coefficient of variation applied to the *in vivo* response, Y, was based on the distance of a particular Y value from the closest end of the 110 point Draize scale. This was done because the variability in eye irritation scores decreases as the score approaches either extreme of the Draize irritation scale (DeSousa *et al.*, 1984; Talsma *et al.*, 1988). Data from Weil and Scala (1971) provided a basis for assigning a level of variability to the Y values. Maximum average scores (MAS) defined by Draize*et al.* (1944) were computed using data given in the original Weil and Scala (1971) publication. The coefficient of variation for the MAS was also calculated for each test substance. The degree of variation among the laboratories conducting the Draize eye irritation test on the same substances was strikingly large, ranging between 40 and 60 percent for a 6-animal rabbit eye irritation test. The variability in alternative method data is typically less than the *in vivo* test, with coefficients of variation (CV) ranging between 10 and 25 percent (Table 48.1).

Data sets were generated containing hypothetical RSTS sample sizes of 10, 20, 50, 100, or 250, each having defined levels of error added to the X and Y terms. The 95 percent confidence interval (Forthofer and Lee, 1995; Snedecor and Cochran, 1980) for the prediction of a single future observation of a maximum average score of 55 (95% CI_{pred}) and the standard deviation of the 95% CI_{pred} values were then calculated for each data set.

The effects of the RSTS size on the precision of a prediction derived from an alternative method are summarized in Table 48.2. Each of the tabled 95% CI_{pred}

TABLE 48.1:

Intralaboratory reproducibility

Eye irritation test alternative method	Positive control	n	Endpoint units	Mean	SD	CV (%)
Bovine corneal opacity[a]	Acetone	119	units	156.50	18.800	12.0
Bovine corneal opacity	Ethanol	44	units	54.30	9.000	16.0
Bovine corneal opacity	Imidazol	20	units	113.60	17.400	15.3
MICROTOX[b]	Phenol	123	µg/ml	20.10	3.900	19.4
Silicon microphysiometer[b]	SLS	163	µg/ml	78.60	12.200	15.5
Neural red uptake[b]	SLS	191	µg/ml	4.24	0.920	21.7
SIRC plaque forming assay[c]	SLS	205	µg/ml	24.50	4.170	17.0
Neural red release[d]	Triton X-100	26	mg/ml	0.20	0.038	19.0
CORROSITEX[e]	NaOH	44	minutes	11.74	1.120	9.5
ZK1200 topical application[f]	SLS	44	% viability	45.40	11.800	26.0

Note. The coefficient of variation following multiple runs using the indicated positive control test substances in one laboratory is shown. The overall average of the intralaboratory CVs listed is approximately 17 percent. n is the number of times the assay has been conducted with the indicated control material; units indicates the measurement units obtained from the alternative method; mean indicates the average value obtained for all the indicated runs; SD is the standard deviations calculated associated with the mean of the alternative method sources; CV is the coefficient of variation (mean/SD); SLS is sodium lauryl sulfate.

[a] As described by Gautheron *et al.* (1992).
[b] As described by Bruner *et al.* (1991).
[c] As described by North-Root *et al.* (1982, 1985).
[d] As described by Reader *et al.* (1989).
[e] As described by Gordon *et al.* (1993).
[f] As described by Osborn *et al.* (1995).

values and standard deviations are based on 1000 simulations conducted for each sample size. In the first case (ideal conditions, Table 48.2) the imposed variation is relatively low. As expected, the 95% CI_{pred} values are relatively narrow, ranging from ±7 to ±16. As the number of test substances included in the RSTS increases from 10 to 250, the 95% CI_{pred} decreases slightly and the standard deviations of the 95% CI_{pred} decrease by about fourfold.

In the second case (typical conditions, Table 48.2), the CVs applied to the data are more consistent with those observed in the Draize test and currently available alternative methods. Under these circumstances, the 95% CI_{pred} is significantly wider, ranging from approximately 54 to 28 depending on the sample size and imposed variation. Again, the prediction intervals tend to be narrower as the sample size increases, but this improvement is not substantial when $n > 20$. Also, the standard deviation of the 95% CI_{pred} decreases approximately four- to eightfold.

These simulations therefore indicate that the width of the 95% CI_{pred} does not improve with larger RSTS sizes. Rather, the real benefit of increasing sample

TABLE 48.2:

95% Confidence intervals for the prediction of an *in vivo* eye irritation score of 55 from an alternative method (95% CI_{pred})

Coefficient of variation Alternative method	In vivo	Sample size n=10 95% CI_{pred}	SD* of 95% CI_{pred}	Sample size n=20 95% CI_{pred}	SD* of 95% CI_{pred}	Sample size n=50 95% CI_{pred}	SD* of 95% CI_{pred}	Sample size n=100 95% CI_{pred}	SD* of 95% CI_{pred}	Sample size n=250 95% CI_{pred}	SD* of 95% CI_{pred}
Ideal conditions											
0.05	0.05	8.4	2.4	7.5	1.4	7.1	0.8	7.0	0.5	7.0	0.3
0.10	0.10	16.3	4.5	14.9	2.9	14.2	1.5	13.9	1.1	13.8	0.7
Typical conditions											
0.10	0.40	34.0	9.2	30.5	5.0	28.9	2.9	28.3	2.1	27.9	1.3
0.10	0.50	41.8	11.6	37.1	6.4	34.7	3.9	34.0	2.6	33.6	1.6
0.10	0.60	48.5	12.9	43.3	7.7	40.7	4.5	39.9	3.0	39.6	2.0
0.20	0.40	41.8	10.6	37.5	6.1	34.9	3.4	34.5	2.4	34.3	1.5
0.20	0.50	46.8	12.4	43.0	7.3	40.0	4.1	39.4	2.9	39.1	1.8
0.20	0.60	53.1	14.2	47.9	8.1	45.6	4.6	44.7	3.2	44.3	2.0
0.40	0.40	56.4	14.2	50.5	8.0	48.0	4.5	46.9	3.2	46.5	2.0
0.40	0.50	60.4	15.4	54.7	8.9	51.7	5.0	50.6	3.3	50.1	2.1
0.40	0.60	66.0	16.0	59.3	9.2	56.0	5.2	54.8	3.6	54.3	2.3

Note. The mean 95% CI_{pred} is shown for different numbers of materials in the Reference Set of Test Substances (RSTS). The 95% CI_{pred} for a predicted *in vivo* score of 55 were obtained from computer simulations designed to assess the effect of changing the size of the RSTS on the uncertainty in predictions obtained from an alternative method. The variability in the 95% CI_{pred} is indicated as the standard deviation of the 95% CI_{pred}. Each of the values shown are based on 1000 runs of the simulation. This simulation shows that the 95% CI_{pred} is relatively wide given the variability associated with the *in vivo* eye irritation test and current alternative methods. For example, if an alternative method having a CV = 0.2 predicts a Maximum Average Score of 55, the 95% CI_{pred} is ±40 if the CV = 0.5 for the *in vivo* data and the RSTS n = 50.

* SD – Standard Deviation

size is that the 95% CI_{pred} estimation is more precisely defined. This is because increasing the sample size improves estimation of the confidence interval endpoints. This is because statistical theory assures that in arbitrarily large samples the estimated endpoints converge to the true endpoint values.

The simulations also indicate that the overall width of the 95% CI_{pred} is limited by the variability in the *in vivo* response. Low levels of variability in the populations are needed in order to predict individual responses both accurately and precisely. High levels of variability in individual predictions cannot be overcome by simply increasing the size of the RSTS. The quality of the *in vivo* data, therefore, is more important than the quantity of substances included in a validation study.

48.3.4   Step 4. Evaluate the quality of the *in vivo* toxicity data (Figure 48.1)

The quality of the *in vivo* data available for the substances in the RSTS must be reviewed. This is important. If the quality of the *in vivo* data is poor, then the results of comparison between the *in vivo* data and the alternative method results will be difficult to assess definitely.

It is difficult to obtain a set of test substances that has consistent, high-quality toxicity data (Balls *et al.*, 1995a). The difficulty arises because many different schemes are used for measuring and classifying toxicity endpoints. The situation is made worse by the fact that there is no consistent source for the information that currently exists. This has meant that toxicity data used in validation studies have often come from many laboratories that have used different protocols and produced different kinds of data.

Some of these problems have been addressed through the efforts of organizations such as the European Chemical Ecology and Toxicology Centre (ECETOC). This organization established a committee that developed a reference data bank containing 55 chemicals with *in vivo* eye irritation data that were generated using tests conforming to OECD (Organization for Economic Cooperation and Development) Guideline 405 (ECETOC, 1992; 1998). The ECETOC criteria provide a useful example of an approach that can be taken to assemble sets of test substances for which there is a uniform quality of *in vivo* data. The criteria the test substances had to meet in order to be included in the eye irritation data bank are shown in Table 48.3. If it is not possible to identify a set of test substances where the data meet such a set of standards, then it may be necessary to generate new *in vivo* data. If that is not possible, then all the

TABLE 48.3:

Acceptance criteria for *in vivo* data

All test materials should be defined entities available at a known high level of purity of specification.

Each material should be chemically stable.

In vivo data generated recently (since 1981 when GLP were introduced).

Good Laboratory Practices followed in generation of *in vivo* data.

Studies carried out according to OECD Guideline 405:

    At least 3 rabbits evaluated per test material.

    A volume of 0.1 ml or the equivalent weight of test substance was instilled into the conjunctival sac.

    Topical anaesthesia was *not* used (Durham *et al.*, (1992) 535–541).

    Observations made at least at 24, 48, and 72 hours.

    Enable reversibility/irreversibility to be assessed.

    Scoring done using the scheme of (Draize *et al.* (1944) 377–390) so that corneal opacity and area affected, iris inflammation, and conjunctival redness, swelling, and discharge data are available for each test substance at each time point evaluated.

Chemicals tested undiluted, except where testing materials undiluted would likely lead to severe effects.

Note. The *in vivo* data available for materials in the reference set of test substances should meet a minimum quality standard before they are used in a validation program. An example of a set of criteria established for the selection of test substances is provided in the ECETOC Eye Irritation Chemicals Data Bank (ECETOC, 1992). The factors considered important by the Technical Committee who prepared the ECETOC Technical Report are listed here. Reprinted with permission.

shortcomings associated with the *in vivo* data in the RSTS must be documented and factored into the overall assessment of the performance of the alternative method at the end of the study. ECETOC have also prepared reference chemicals data banks for skin and respiratory sensitizes (ECETOC, 1999) and for skin irritation and corrosion (ECETOC, 1995).

48.3.5 Step 5. Conduct the validation study (Figure 48.1)

Once an adequate RSTS has been assembled and characterized, the next step is to test each of the materials in the alternative method. Many logistical issues need to be carefully monitored during this phase of typical large validation studies. Although these issues have been thoroughly reviewed elsewhere (Balls *et al.*, 1995a; Worth and Balls, 2001b), a few are particularly important. First, careful communication between the participants is essential. Those involved in validation studies must never underestimate the possibility for misunderstanding. Second, preliminary runs of the alternative methods using a small subset of test substances are particularly useful in helping to identify and solve start-up problems that invariably occur. Third, managers of validation studies must carefully monitor the progress being made throughout the study to assure the program proceeds as planned.

48.3.6   Step 6. Assess the reproducibility of the alternative method (Figure 48.1)

Once the testing of the RSTS materials in the alternative method is completed, the next step in the validation process is to assess the reproducibility of the data generated by the participating laboratories. This analysis is important because it provides the half of the data needed to confirm the reliability of the alternative method.

Many validation studies use a nested or hierarchical design (Figure 48.5). These studies usually involve several laboratories that independently conduct the same alternative method on all the substances in a RSTS. There are four sources of variability in such studies. These include variation in the test substances, variation within experiments within a laboratory (intraexperiment variability), variation between experiments within a laboratory (intralaboratory variability), and variation between laboratories (interlaboratory variability). We now review the nature and importance of each. The differences between chemicals are ignored in this discussion since they can generally be minimized with well-controlled test article distribution and storage. Attention is concentrated on the variability in results obtained by testing a single chemical in a number of different laboratories.

Definitions (Figure 48.5)

During a validation study, each participating laboratory generally carries out a number of separate executions of an alternative method on each material in the RSTS. Each of these independent executions is a *repeat experiment*. Often, within each repeat experiment, duplicate, triplicate, or quadruplicate measures are obtained. These are *replicate measurements*. The mean of results from several repeat experiments gives the *laboratory mean*, and the mean of several laboratory means gives the *overall laboratories mean*. The importance of variation in the replicate measures, repeat experiments, and overall laboratories mean and how these measurements should be assessed is described in the following sections.

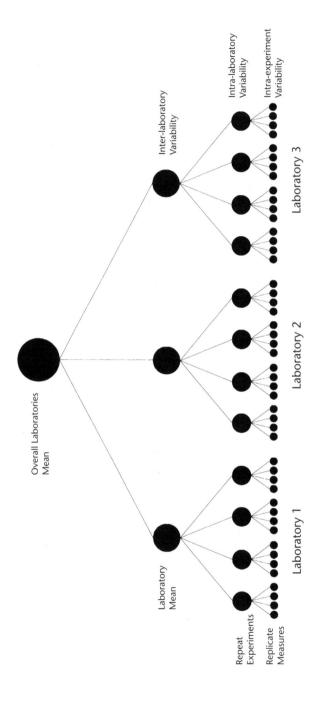

Figure 48.5: Hierarchical design of a validation study. The different levels of repeated measures obtainable from assays treated in a validation study are shown. The descriptions on the left side indicate the names of the endpoints at each level, and the descriptions of the right side indicate the variability term associated with each level.

Intraexperiment variability (Figure 48.5)

The intraexperiment variability is evaluated by examining the variation in the replicate measures obtained within a given repeat experiment. This value is most useful for workers within a laboratory, since it is an indicator of the performance of a particular assay on a specific day. While useful for internal monitoring, this value does not provide a particularly good indication of how an assay performs over time. This is because replicate measures are obtained under conditions where sources of variability such as different technical staff, preparation of the test substances, preparation of cell cultures, and preparation of media are tightly controlled. Because of this control, results obtained from a group of replicate measures best represent a *precise* estimate of test variability at the particular time under the particular conditions when the test was run. It is not necessarily an *accurate* reflection of a test's performance over multiple runs. Thus, the performance of an assay over time within one laboratory is best measured at the level of the repeat experiment.

Intralaboratory variability (Figure 48.5)

Intralaboratory variability is assessed by evaluating the results obtained from repeat experiments conducted on the same substance in the same laboratory over a reasonable period of time. This assessment will be most representative if it is performed using data from several repeat experiments conducted completely independent of each other in terms of substances, batches of chemicals, and possibly even the technical staff who performed the work.

What are the limits of interlaboratory variation that should be considered acceptable for a given alternative method? The consideration of this question must be done on a case-by-case basis. The example illustrated in Figure 48.6 shows the results obtained from a test substance that has a laboratory mean score of 100 (bold horizontal line) in an alternative method that produces scores ranging between 0 and 200. Two diagonal lines indicate the upper and lower 95 percent confidence limits for the laboratory mean when the alternative method CV ranges from 0 to 50 percent. As the CV increases, the width of the 95 percent confidence interval for the laboratory mean score increases. Eventually this interval becomes so wide that the results obtained from the test become meaningless relative to the entire response range of the alternative method. As the CV reaches 20 percent in this example, the width of the 95 percent confidence interval is ±40 (dotted horizontal lines, Figure 48.6). Because

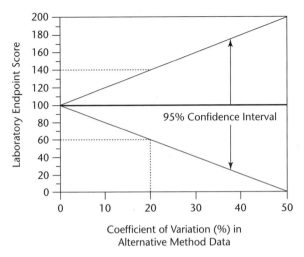

Figure 48.6: The effect of varying the coefficient of variation in the width of the 95 percent confidence interval is shown. The alternative method illustrated in this example has a laboratory mean score of 100. As the CV increases from 0–50 percent, the width of the confidence interval decreases. In this specific example, when the CV = 20 percent, the 95 percent confidence interval is ±40. An acceptable level of variability for an alternative method depends on the range of responses obtained from the alternative method and the effect of this variability on the precision of *in vivo* predictions.

the ±40 covers 40 percent of the total range of possible responses from the alternative method, if the CV is consistently greater than 20 percent, a good case could be made that this alternative method is not acceptably reproducible. On the other hand, if the range of responses from the alternative method covers several orders of magnitude, a CV of 20 percent might not cause concern. This is because an alternative method response in the range of 100 ± 40 may correspond to only a small percentage of the total possible range of responses *in vivo*. Ultimately, the toxicologist who uses the alternative method for making decisions in a safety assessment must define the level of uncertainty in a prediction that is acceptable for the purpose at hand.

Interlaboratory variability (Figure 48.5)

Interlaboratory variability gives an assessment of how well results can be reproduced across several independent laboratories. This level of reproducibility measurement is of greatest importance when assessing the reliability of a toxicity test to be used for regulatory purposes since regulators will receive results generated from any number of laboratories across the world. This value can be determined by evaluating results derived from the same alternative method protocol on the same test substances across several laboratories. An approach often used to assess interlaboratory reproducibility is to calculate the correlation coefficient that relates the results from different laboratories (Bagley *et al.*, 1992). Although this statistic provides useful information, it has some limitations. For example, the results of an alternative method in one laboratory may differ across the entire range of results by an order of magnitude compared to a second laboratory. Thus, even though the laboratories did not duplicate each other's results (i.e., poor interlaboratory reproducibility), the data will be highly correlated. Correlation, therefore, should be used with caution when comparisons between laboratories is required (Bland and Altman 1986; 1995a; 1995b; 1999). Satisfactory evidence of interlaboratory variability could also be obtained by considering the CV obtained from the results of all the participating laboratories (i.e., the CV associated with the overall laboratories mean). As noted in the discussion of intralaboratory variation, the acceptability of a particular CV must be assessed on a case-by-case basis. The effect of the variability on the uncertainty in predictions must also be considered. This issue is discussed later relative to the assessment of alternative method relevance.

Number of participating laboratories

The number of laboratories that need to be included in a validation study in order to obtain a precise assessment of reproducibility is dependent on the level of variability associated with the alternative method being evaluated. This is illustrated in Figure 48.7. The figure shows the relationship between the width of the 95 percent confidence interval for the overall laboratories mean and the number of laboratories included in a determination of the overall laboratories mean. Each curve shows the results obtained when the CV of the laboratory means range from 5 to 60 percent. These curves were calculated using a model that assumed the true laboratory mean score is 100 and that, on average, each laboratory is able to obtain this value. These calculations demonstrate that as the variability in the laboratory means decreases, and as the number of laboratories included in the study increases, the 95 percent confidence interval for the overall laboratories mean becomes narrower. The 95 percent confidence interval is especially wide when tests are highly variable (i.e., laboratory means CVs > 20 percent). This is particularly true when the number of participating laboratories is low (note the ordinate in Figure 48.7 is a log scale). For example,

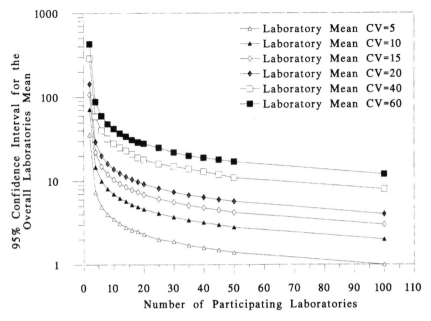

Figure 48.7: Number of laboratories in an interlaboratory variability assessment. This figure shows the relationship between the width of the 95 percent confidence interval for the overall laboratories mean and the number of laboratories participating in a validation study. Each curve shows the results obtained when the CV of the laboratory means range from 5 to 60 percent. The curves where calculated using a model that assumes the true laboratory mean score is 100. As the laboratory mean CV decreases, and as the number of laboratories included in the evaluation increases, the width of the 95 percent confidence interval of the overall laboratories mean becomes narrower.

the width of the 95 percent confidence interval for the overall laboratories mean of 100 is ±59 if the four laboratories have a laboratory mean CV = 40 percent. If only two laboratories participate, the 95 percent confidence interval is so wide (±287) that such results would have to be viewed with considerable caution. The choice of how many laboratories to include in a validation study ultimately becomes a trade-off between reducing the variability in the estimate of interlaboratory variation versus the cost of including more laboratories. Certainly there is a diminishing returns aspect to number of laboratories used. The largest benefits occur with smaller sizes: There is a large benefit to using three instead of two, and five instead of three.

48.3.7   Step 7. Assess the predictive capability of the alternative method (Figure 48.1)

The next step in the process is to assess the predictive capability of the alternative method. This many be done by confirming that alternative method data input into the predefined prediction models provide outputs that predict *in vivo* toxicity at the level of both accuracy and precision defined at the beginning of the study. Once the data are available from the validation study, each result from the alternative method should be converted by the algorithm(s) in the prediction model into a prediction of *in vivo* toxicity. Then the predicted toxicity should be directly compared with the actual toxicity of each test substance. If the method predicts toxicity within the limits defined by the prediction model, then it would provide strong evidence supporting the predictive capability of the assay. If the results from the alternative method poorly predict *in vivo* toxicity, then there would be little evidence supporting the utility of the method.

If the conclusion reached is that the method is reliable in terms of reproducibility (see step 6) and predictive capability, then the results of the validation study may be used in the next part of the validation process which is the determination of relevance (discussed next). If the methods are shown not to be reliable, then two courses of action may be followed (Figure 48.1). If it appears there is merit in further developmental work (test method optimization), then additional research should be undertaken. When the assay is adequately modified and/or a new prediction model is developed, it may be evaluated in a subsequent validation study. Alternatively, the method may be abandoned if it is apparent that additional effort is unlikely to be fruitful.

48.4   ASSESSING ALTERNATIVE METHOD RELEVANCE

Once the reliability of an alternative method has been confirmed in a validation study, its relevance as a replacement for an *in vivo* toxicity test must be assessed. As noted earlier, the assessment of relevance addresses the question: Is the performance of the method good enough to allow its acceptance as a replacement for a given *in vivo* test? Answering this question requires assembly and review of as much information as possible about the performance of the alternative method and the *in vivo* test it is intended to replace. This review process must ultimately allow the formulation of a judgment that the alternative method is acceptable or not for its intended use. We now review the information that must be considered in order to judge the relevance of an alternative method, and provide recommendations on how to establish objective benchmarks that can be used to help make this judgment.

The factors that must be considered in defining the relevance of an alternative method include an assessment of (1) the best performance that can be expected from an alternative method given the performance characteristics of both the alternative method and the *in vivo* test it is intended to replace, (2) the performance of the *in vivo* test being replaced, and (3) the supplemental data available for use in conjunction with the alternative method during a safety assessment. Each of these factors is next reviewed.

48.4.1 Assessing the best performance that can be expected from an alternative method

Ideally, alternative method results should provide nearly perfect predictions of the toxic endpoints measured in the *in vivo* method. However, there are important technical factors that prevent this ideal from being reached. One of the most important is the variability in the *in vivo* and alternative method data. If perfect prediction is unrealistic, then what is the best performance that can be expected from an alternative method? One approach that can be taken to answer this question is to use computer simulations based on the known performance characteristics of the *in vivo* test and the alternative method to create a picture that describes how the results from the validation study will appear if the prediction model is true. The results of these simulations can be used as benchmarks for objectively judging the acceptability of the alternative method that was measured in the validation study. In order to provide a practical example of this process, we again return to the assessment of eye irritation alternatives. In order to assess the performance that may be expected from an alternative method evaluated in a validation program, we used a computer simulation based on the simple linear relationship of Eq. (48.2):

$$Y = (1.1)X \tag{48.2}$$

The effect of variability on the overall performance of the method was assessed by adding an error term to X and Y in each run of the simulation as described earlier (see Step 3). After a large number of data points were simulated for each set of alternative method and *in vivo* test CVs, the Pearson's correlation coefficient was calculated in order to determine the correlation between the X and Y values. A second set of X values ranging from 0 to 40 were also run to simulate results for eye irritation scores that might be observed with a more restricted set of test substances such as cosmetics products.

Results from the simulations are summarized in Table 48.4 and Figure 48.8. Each of the correlations shown in Table 48.4 is based on 10,000 simulated

TABLE 48.4:

Expected Pearson correlation coefficients when the error *in vivo* and alternative method data are considered

Imposed coefficient of variation		Expected Pearson's correlation coefficient	
Alternative method	*In vivo*	Full range (x=1–100)	Restricted range (x=1–40)
Ideal conditions			
0.05	0.05	0.994	0.990
0.10	0.10	0.975	0.960
Typical conditions			
0.20	0.40	0.860	0.719
0.20	0.50	0.828	0.652
0.20	0.60	0.803	0.608
0.40	0.40	0.719	0.604
0.40	0.50	0.690	0.542
0.40	0.60	0.672	0.504
Theoretical best conditions			
0.00	0.40	0.930	0.787
0.00	0.50	0.891	0.706
0.00	0.60	0.862	0.647
Alternative method equivalent to *in vivo* method			
0.40	0.40	0.719	0.604
0.50	0.50	0.635	0.490
0.60	0.60	0.543	0.403

Note. Computer simulations were used to assess the effects of variablity in eye irritation test and alternative method data on the correlation coefficients expected between the data sets. The model used in the simulation assumed that the algorithm, $y = (1.1)x$, describes the relationship between the *in vivo* and alternative method data. Values for $x = 0$–100 were used to simulate responses across the entire Draize eye irritation scale. The simulations were conducted with test substances having the full range of response ($x = 1$–100) and for a restricted range representing the least irritating part of the eye irritation scale ($x = 1$–40). Each result is based on 10,000 runs of the simulation. Results are shown for the simulations where the variability is set relatively low (ideal conditions), and where the variability was set at a level consistent with performance of currently available alternative methods and the *in vivo* test (practical conditions). Additionally, simulations were conducted where the variability was set at zero for the alternative method (theoretical best conditions) and where the variablity of the alternative method was set equivalent to the eye irritation test (alternative method equivalent to *in vivo*). The results of these simulations demonstrate that variability in the data sets can have a significant effect on the performance of the alternative method in predicting the *in vivo* response. Thus, the effect of variability must be taken into account when the performance of an alternative method is assessed.

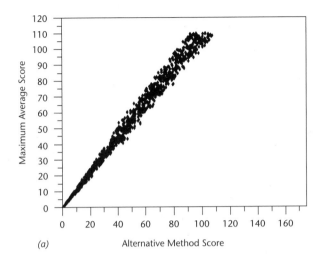

(a)

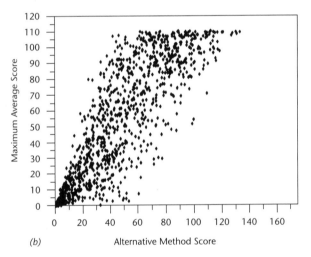

(b)

Figure 48.8: Effects of variability in the Draize test and alternative methods on correlation. Computer simulations were used to assess the effects of variability in the eye irritation test and alternative method data on the relationship between the two data sets. Figure 48.8A: The CVs applied to both the *in vivo* and alternative method data were 5 percent. Figure 48.8B: The CVs applied to the *in vivo* and alternative method data were 50 percent and 20 percent respectively. Figure 48.8C: The CVs applied to the *in vivo* and alternative method data were 50 percent and 0 percent respectively. Figure 48.8D: The CVs applied to the *in vivo* and alternative method data were 50 percent and 40 percent, respectively.

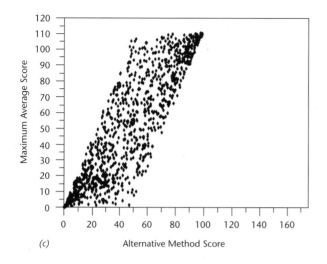

(c)

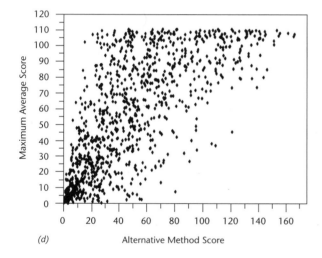

(d)

Figure 48.8: C and D.

responses. The effects on the size of the Pearson correlation coefficient due to error imposed on the *in vivo* alternative method responses are shown under several conditions. In general, we know that a tight linear relationship with nearly perfect correlation will exist when there are negligible levels of error in either X or Y. As error is introduced into either X or Y the expected level of correlation will be reduced. In the first case (ideal conditions, Table 48.4, Figure 48.8A), the imposed variation is set relatively low. As expected, Pearson correlation coefficients are large, ranging between 0.97 and 0.99. Furthermore, restricting the alternative method results to the least irritating portion of the Draize scoring scheme ($X = 0$–40) has little effect on the correlation coefficients. In the second case (typical conditions, Table 48.4, Figure 48.8B), the CVs applied to the data (*in vivo* CV = 50 percent, alternative method CV = 20 percent) are consistent with those observed in the Draize test. Under these circumstances, the correlation is still high (>0.8). Importantly, restricting the range of alternative method responses to the least irritating materials ($X = 0$–40) results in a decrease in the correlation coefficient to an approximate range of 0.6–0.7. Setting the imposed CV for the alternative method at 0.4 further decreases the correlation coefficients (Table 48.4). If an alternative method could be perfected technically, its CV would approach 0. Third case shows the effect of setting the CV = 0 (theoretical best conditions, Table 48.4, Figure 48.8C). Under these conditions, the expected Pearson correlation coefficients range between 0.85 and 0.95 when $X = 0$–100. When the alternative method results are restricted to the least irritating substances ($X = 0$–40) the correlation coefficients are lower, ranging from approximately 0.65 to 0.80. Finally, in the fourth simulation, the alternative method CV was set to a level equivalent to that observed in the Draize eye irritation test. Under these conditions, the simulations estimate that the correlation coefficients will range from approximately 0.5 to 0.7 when all levels of alternative method response ($X = 0$–100) are included (alternative method equivalent to the *in vivo* method, Table 48.4, Figure 48.8D). When the alternative method results are restricted to the least irritating range ($X = 0$–40), the coefficients are lower, ranging from 0.4 to 0.6.

It is important to note that these simulation studies were conducted under idealized conditions. The underlying assumption is that the relationship between the *in vivo* and alternative method data is linear. Also, the number of substances included in the simulations was large (10,000). Hence, the results of the simulations shown in Table 48.4 and Figure 48.8 represent a long-run average of the most optimistic correlations. In practical terms, even if all of the assumptions were true, the observed correlation might be higher or lower than the long-run average. Other deviations from the conditions assumed in these simulations, such as nonlinearity or nonuniform distribution of responses, can also be expected to reduce the level of correlation. Since it is unlikely the results from an alternative method are so simply related to a particular *in vivo* toxicity, it can be expected that validation studies will result in lower correlation coefficients, even for those alternative methods that may actually be reasonably predictive of the *in vivo* response.

Once completed, the results of the simulations may be used as benchmarks to objectively compare against the actual results obtained in the validation study. If the data from the validation study meet or exceed the simulated benchmarks, a strong case could be made that the method performs at an acceptable level. For example, if an eye irritation alternative method has a prediction model algorithm of $Y = (1.1)X$ and a CV = 20 percent, and if the *in vivo* test has a CV = 50 percent, then the best performance that may be expected would appear as follows: The relationship between the *in vivo* and alternative method data would look similar to that shown in Figure 48.8B, the correlation coefficients would be within the range of approximately 0.6–0.8 (Table 48.4), and 95% CI_{pred} for a MAS prediction of 55 would be in the range of ±40 ($n = 50$, Table 48.2). A method performing at these levels should be considered a reasonable performer. If the alternative method performance is less than such a simulated benchmark, then there would be little evidence supporting its relevance.

48.4.2 Assess the performance of the *in vivo* test that will be replaced

Once estimates of the best possible performance of the methods are defined, another useful benchmark that can be used to assess the relevance of an alternative method is to compare its performance against that of the *in vivo* toxicity test it will replace. If the capability of the alternative method to predict an *in vivo* toxicity endpoint is at least equivalent to the capability of the *in vivo* test to predict its own result, then it would provide strong evidence supporting the relevance of the alternative method.

The capability of an *in vivo* method to predict results across multiple laboratories can be determined if its performance characteristics are known. If these data do not exist, then the interlaboratory variability terms needed to define the performance characteristics can be obtained by testing a common set of substances in several independent laboratories as was done for the irritation tests by Weil and Scala (1971). If an alternative method is capable of predicting toxicity at a level equivalent to or better than the test it is intended to replace, then it would provide strong evidence supporting the contention that the alternative method can substitute for the *in vivo* toxicity test. Returning to our specific example of assessing the validity of eye irritation alternatives, the results of simulations we have conducted to assess the capability of the Draize test to predict results across laboratories are similar to those obtained from the simulations presented in Tables 48.2 and 48.4 and Figure 48.8B. Thus, if the capability of the Draize test to predict eye irritation responses is used as the criterion for judging the relevance of eye irritation alternatives, then methods that perform similar to or better than those illustrated under typical conditions in Tables 48.2 and 48.4 and Figure 48.8B should be considered adequate performers.

48.4.3 Assessing supplemental data available for use in conjunction with the alternative method during a safety assessment

Once the performance of the alternative method is compared against the appropriate benchmarks (such as the computer simulations described earlier), there are other factors that need to be considered when assessing the relevance of an alternative method. One factor considered particularly important is the mechanistic basis supporting the alternative method (Flint, 1992; Frazier, 1994). Having an understanding of the mechanistic basis is important because it increases the probability that predictions of *in vivo* toxicity by the alternative methods are correct. Unfortunately, the science of toxicology has not progressed to the point that all toxic mechanisms are well understood. Thus, if alternative methods are to be accepted in the foreseeable future, they will be used under conditions where a full understanding of mechanisms is not available. Therefore, it is important to consider the approaches the developers of an alternative method recommend following in order to compensate for this lack of knowledge.

Toxicologists who use alternative methods in the safety assessment process generally utilize three approaches to help decrease the uncertainty of the predictions when mechanistic understanding is weak. The first is to restrict the use of an alternative method to the same chemical classes that were used to develop the prediction model. This is important because similar materials are more likely to act by the same mechanisms of action. If the materials tested diverge significantly from those used to develop the prediction model, then the reliability of the predictions will decrease (see, e.g., Chamberlain and Barratt, 1995). This will occur because the divergent materials may exert effects through different toxic mechanisms that should perhaps be tested in different alternative methods that are sensitive to different chemical parameters and that use different prediction models.

The second approach commonly used to decrease the uncertainty of predictions is to compare the results obtained from an unknown test substance with one or two similar benchmark substances tested in the alternative method at the same time. If a material is intermediate in toxicity between two well-known benchmark standards in the alternative method, then it provides evidence that the material will be intermediate in toxicity *in vivo*. This approach provides greater confidence in a prediction than can be derived from testing isolated test substances on an absolute scale without any reference to other materials (O'Brian *et al.*, 1994).

The third approach used to decrease the uncertainty associated with the predictions is to define specific limitations on the use of the assay. For example, developers may recommend restricting the use of a particular method to specific physical forms of test materials (liquids only or solids only) or for predicting limited ranges of irritancy (mild irritancy or severe irritancy only). These limitations may depend on many factors, especially specific technical incompatibilities associated with testing certain kinds of substances.

Next, it is important to consider whether the width of the 95% CI_{pred} from the alternative method is small enough to provide an acceptably precise prediction of *in vivo* toxicity. The analysis presented earlier demonstrated that the 95% CI_{pred} from an alternative method may be large. A benchmark that can be used to assess the acceptability of a large 95% CI_{pred} could be derived from an examination of the precision of toxicity measurements obtained from the *in vivo* toxicity test. If an alternative method provides predictions as precise as those obtained from the *in vivo* method it is intended to replace, then it would provide evidence that the 95% CI_{pred} alternative method is acceptable (for more information on the utility of the 95% CI_{pred}, see (Bruner *et al.*, 2002a).

The margin of safety provided by a prediction from an alternative method compared to that obtained from the *in vivo* method must be considered. *In vivo* tests, such as the Draize eye irritation test, significantly overpredict the human response (Griffith *et al.*, 1980). This has been considered important because use of an overpredictive method decreases the probability of false negative results that may be associated with a highly variable test. Establishing an acceptable margin of safety for an alternative method will depend on finding an appropriate balance between the risks to humans associated with possible underprediction due to variability versus the losses associated with a higher incidence of false positive results that invariably results from setting more stringent cut-offs.

Finally, it is important to consider the experience that has been gained in use of the alternative method outside formal validation programs. Although the

■ CHAPTER 48 ■

quality of data from other sources may be variable and not collected under blind conditions, it may provide additional useful insights into an alternative method's performance. If these additional data are consistent with the results obtained from a validation study, it would provide further evidence supporting the relevance of the alternative method.

Once all of this information is assembled and assessed, the participants in the validation study must render a final judgment on whether or not the method is relevant for the stated purpose. If the measurement of method reliability from a validation study, the actions take to compensate for lack of mechanistic understanding, the performance of the method relative to calculated benchmarks, the width of the 95% CI_{pred}, the margin of safety, and the breadth of experience toxicologists have with the method are judged to be adequate, this would provide strong evidence supporting the relevance of the alternative method.

If the alternative method is judged both reliable and relevant at the end of this process, then the new assay should be considered validated. Once validated, the alternative method may be used routinely in the safety assessment process and should be considered for acceptance by regulatory authorities (Figure 48.1). If the alternative method is judged not relevant, then it should not be used or considered for acceptance by regulatory authorities. The reasons for the rejection should be clearly stated so that the deficiencies can be identified and resolved in followup research if such work is likely to be fruitful.

48.5 DISCUSSION

The development of an alternative method begins with the creation of a test followed by generation of a database that supports its utility. This work provides the preliminary evidence that a method is reproducible and has predictive capability. Once available, this information can be used to construct a prediction model that describes how to convert the results from an alternative method into predictions of toxicity *in vivo*. When a method has been technically advanced to this point, it may be assessed in the validation process.

Relative to the development of valid toxicity tests, the assessment of a toxicity test's validity is a relatively simple matter. Validation is relatively simple when the studies are designed to test the performance of an alternative method relative to performance criteria established prior to the start of the study. Defining a prediction model prior to the commencement of the study allows those evaluating an alternative method to construct a clear picture of what the results from a valid assay will look like before the study begins. When the results from the validation study become available, objective comparisons can be made between the predetermined picture and the actual study results. If the results are consistent with this picture, it provides strong evidence that the alternative method is reliable. If the results do not fit the picture, it provides evidence that either further developmental work on the alternative method is needed or that the method should be abandoned. Such an approach has the advantage that it allows an objective evaluation of the data, while avoiding post hoc data fitting that does not provide definitive answers on alternative method validity.

Once the reliability of an alternative method has been confirmed in a validation study, the next step in the process is to review the relevance of the alternative method. This requires thorough consideration of all the performance data related to both the alternative method and the *in vivo* test it will replace. Ultimately, those conducting a validation program must take this information and render a judgment on whether the performance is good enough to allow replacement of the alternative method.

REFERENCES

ANONYMOUS (1994) Council Directive 93/35/EEC of 14 June, 1993 amending for the 6th time Directive 76/768/EEC on the approximation of the laws of the Member States relating to cosmetic products, *Official Journal of the European Communites* **L151**, 32–36.

BAGLEY, D.M., BRUNER, L.H., DE SILVA, O., COTTIN, M., O'BRIEN, K.A., UTTLEY, M. and WALKER, A.P. (1992) An evaluation of five potential alternatives *in vitro* to the rabbit eye irritation test *in vivo*, *Toxicol. in Vitro* 6(4) 275–284.

BALLS, M., BLAAUBOER, B., FENTEM, J.H., BRUNER, L.H., COMBES, R., EKWALL, B., FIELDER, R.J., GUILLOUZO, A., LEWIS, R.W., LOVELL, D.P., REINHARDT, C.A., REPETTO, G., SLADOWSKI, D., SPIELMANN, H. and ZUCCO, F. (1995a) Practical aspects of the validation of toxicity test procedures, *Alternatives to Laboratory Animals* **23**, 129–147.

BALLS, M., BLAAUBOER, B., FRAZIER, J.M., LAMB, D., PEMBERTON, M., REINHARDT, C., ROBERFROID, M., ROSENKRANZ, H., SCHMID, B., SPIELMANN, H., STAMMATI, A.-L. and WALUM, E. (1990) Report and Recommendations of the CAAT/ERGATT Workshop on the Validation of Toxicity Test Procedures, *Alternatives to Laboratory Animals* **18**, 313–336.

BALLS, M., BOTHAM, P.A., BRUNER, L.H. and SPIELMANN, H. (1995b) The EC/HO international validation study on alternatives to the Draize eye irritation test, *Toxicology In Vitro* 9(6) 871–929.

BALLS, M. and FENTEM, J.H. (1997) Progress toward the validation of alternative methods, *Alternatives to Laboratory Animals* 25, 33–43.

BARRATT, M.D. (1995) Quantitative structure activity relationships for skin corrosively of organic acids, bases, and phenols, *Toxicol. Lett.* 75, 169–176.

BLAND, J.M. and ALTMAN, D.G. (1986) Statistical methods for assessing agreement between two methods of clinical measurement, *Lancet* 1(8476), 307–310.

BLAND, J.M. and ALTMAN, D.G. (1995a) Calculating correlation coefficients with repeated observations: Part 1—Correlation within subjects, *BMJ* 310(6977), 446.

BLAND, J.M. and ALTMAN, D.G. (1995b) Comparing two methods of clinical measurement: a personal history, *Int. J. Epidemiol.* 24(Suppl 1), S7–14.

BLAND, J.M. and ALTMAN, D.G. (1999) Measuring agreement in method comparison studies, *Stat. Methods Med. Res* 8(2) 135–160.

BOOMAN, K.A., DEPROSPO, J., DEMETRULIAS, J., DRIEDGER, A., GRIFFITH, J.F., GROCHOSKI, G., KONG, B., McCORMICK, W.C., NORTH-ROOT, H., ROZEN, M.G. and SEDLAK, R.I. (1989) The SDA alternatives programme: Comparison of *in vitro* data with Draize test data., *J. Toxicol. Cutaneous Ocular Toxicol.* 8, 35–39.

BRANTOM, P.G., BRUNER, L.H., CHAMBERLAIN, M., DE SILVA, O., DUPUIS, J., EARL, L.K., LOVELL, D.P., PAPE, W.J., UTTLEY, M., BAGLEY, D.M., BAKER, F.W., BRACHER, M., COURTELLEMONT, P., DECLERCQ, L., FREEMAN, S., STEILING, W., WALKER, A.P., CARR, G.J., DAMI, N., THOMAS, G., HARBELL, J.W., JONES, P.A., PFANNENBECKER, U., SOUTHEE, J.A., TCHENG, M., ARGEMBEAUX, H., CASTELLI, D., CLOTHIER, R., ESDAILE, D.J., ITAGAKI, I., JUNG, K., KASI, Y., KOJIMA, H., KRISTEN, U., LARNICOL, M., LEWIS, R.W., MARENUS, K.D., MORENO, O., PETERSON, A., RASMUSSEN, E.S., ROBLES, C. and STERN, M. (1997) A summary report of the COLIPA International validation study on alternatives to the Draize rabbit eye irritation test, *Toxicol. in Vitro* 11, 141–179.

BRUNER, L.H., CARR, G.J., CHAMBERLAIN, M. and CURREN, R.D. (1996a) No prediction model, no validation study, *Alternatives to Laboratory Animals* 24, 139–142.

BRUNER, L.H., CARR, G.J., CHAMBERLAIN, M. and CURREN, R.D. (1996b) Validation of alternative methods for toxicity testing, *Toxicology In Vitro* 10(4), 479–501.

BRUNER, L.H., CARR, G.J., CHAMBERLAIN, M. and CURREN, R.D. (1997) A practical approach to the validation of alternative methods for toxicity testing, in

MARZULLI, F.N. and MAIBACH, H.I. (eds) *Dermatotoxicology Methods: The laboratory worker's vade mecum*, Washington, DC: Taylor and Francis, 353–377.

BRUNER, L.H., CARR, G.J. and CURREN, R.D. (2000) Is it good enough? Objective assessment of toxicity test method performance in validation studies, in BALLS, M., ZELLER, A.-M. and HALDER, M. (eds) *Progress in the Reduction, Refinement and Replacement of Animal Experimentation*, Amsterdam: Elsevier Science, 375–384.

BRUNER, L.H., CARR, G.J., HARBELL, J.W. and CURREN, R.D. (2002a) An investigation of new toxicity test method performance in validation studies: 1. Toxicity test methids which have predictive capacity no greater than chance, *Hum. Exp. Toxicol.* **21**, 312.

BRUNER, L.H., CARR, G.J., HARBELL, J.W. and CURREN, R.D. (2002b) An investigation of new toxicity test method performance in validation studies: 2. Comparative assessment of three measures of toxicity test performance, *Hum. Exp. Toxicol.* **21**, 313–323.

BRUNER, L.H., CARR, G.J., HARBELL, J.W. and CURREN, R.D. (2002c) An investigation of new toxicity test method performance in validation studies: 3. Sensitivity and specificity are not independent of prevalence or distiribution of toxicity, *Hum. Exp. Toxicol.* **21**, 325–334.

BRUNER, L.H., KAIN, D.J., ROBERTS, D.A. and PARKER, R.D. (1991) Evaluation of seven *in vitro* alternatives for ocular safety testing, *Fundam. Appl. Toxicol.* **17**(1), 136–149.

CHAMBERLAIN, M. and BARRATT, M.D. (1995) Practical application of QSAR to *in vitro* toxicology illustrated by consideration of eye irritation, *Toxicol. in Vitro*, **9**, 543–547.

CURREN, R.D., SOUTHEE, J.A., SPIELMANN, H., LIEBSCH, M., FENTEM, J.H. and BALLS, M. (1995) The role of prevalidation in the development, validation and acceptance of alternative methods, *Alternatives to Laboratory Animals* **23**, 211–217.

DESOUSA, D.J., ROUSE, A.A. and SMOLON, W.J. (1984) Statistical consequences of reducing the number of rabbits utilized in eye irritation testing: data on 67 petrochemicals, *Toxicol. Appl. Pharmacol.* **76**(2), 234–242.

DRAIZE, J.H., WOODARD, G. and CALVERY, J.O. (1944) Methods for the study of irritation and toxicity of substances applied topically to the skin and mucous membranes, *Journal of Pharmacology and Experimental Pharmacology* **82**, 377–390.

DURHAM, K.A., SAWYER, V.L., KELLER, W.F. and WHEELER, C.A. (1992) Topical ocular anesthetics in ocular irritancy testing: a review *Lab. Anim. Sci.* **42**, 535–541.

ECETOC (1992) *Eye Irritation, Technical Report No. 48*. Reference Chemicals Data Bank, Brussels

ECETOC (1995) *Technical Report No. 66. Skin Irritation and Corrosion*. Reference Chemicals Data Bank, Brussels.

ECETOC (1998) *Technical Report No.48 (2). Eye Irritation*. Reference Chemicals Data Bank (Second Edition), Brussels

ECETOC (1999) *Technical Report No. 77. Skin and Respiratory Sensitisers*. Reference Chemicals Data Bank, European Centre for Ecotoxicology and Toxicology of Chemicals, Brussels,

FENTEM, J.H., ARCHER, G., BALLS, M., BOTHAM, P.A., CURREN, R.D., EARL, L.K., ESDAILE, D.J., HOLZHUTTER, H.-G. and LIEBSCH, M. (1998) The ECVAM International Validation Study on *in vitro* tests for skin corrosivity. 2. Results and evaluation by the management team, *Toxicology In Vitro* **12**(4), 483–524.

FLINT, O. (1992) *In vitro* test validation: A house built on sand, *ATLA* **20**, 196–198.

FORTHOFER, R.N. and LEE, J. (1995) *Introduction to Biostatistics. A Guide to Design, Analysis, and Discovery* San Diego: Academic Press, Inc.

FRAZIER, J.M. (1990) *Scientific Criteria for Validation of In Vitro Toxicity Tests*, 36th edn, Paris: Organisation for Economic Co-operation and Development (OECD).

FRAZIER, J.M. (1994) The role of mechanistic toxicology in test method validation, *Toxicol. in Vitro* **8**, 787–791.

GAUTHERON, P., DUKIC, M., ALIX, D. and SINA, J.F. (1992) Bovine corneal opacity and permeability test: an *in vitro* assay of ocular irritancy, *Fundam. Appl. Toxicol.* **18**(3), 442–449.

GETTINGS, S.D., BAGLEY, D.M., DEMETRULIAS, J.L., DIPASQUALE, L.C., HINTZE, K.L., ROZEN, M.G., TEAL, J.J., WEISE, S.L., CHUDKOWSKI, M., MARENUS, K.D., PAPE, W.J.W., RODDY, M.T., SCHNETZINGER, R., SILBER, P.M., GLAZA, S.M. and KURTZ, P.J. (1991) The CTFA Evaluation Alternatives Program: An evaluation of *in vitro* alternatives to the Draize primary eye irritation test. (Phase I) Hydro-alcoholic formulations; (part 2) Data analysis and biological significance, *In Vitro Toxicol.* **4**, 247–288.

GORDON, V.C. (1992) Utilization of biomacromolecular *in vitro* assay systems in the prediction of *in vivo* toxic responses, *Lens Eye Toxic. Res.* **9**(3–4), 211–227.

GORDON, V.C. and BERGMAN, H.C. (1987) Eytex: an *in vitro* method for evaluation of ocular irritantcy, *Alternative Methods in Toxicology* 5, 87–90.

GRIFFITH, J.F., NIXON, G.A., BRUCE, R.D., REER, P.J. and BANNAN, E.A. (1980) Dose-response studies with chemical irritants in the albino rabbit eye as a basis for selecting optimum testing conditions for predicting hazard to the human eye, *Toxicol. Appl. Pharmacol.* 55(3), 501–513.

NORTH-ROOT, H., YACKOVICH, F., DEMETRULIAS, J., GACULA, M., JR. and HEINZE, J.E. (1982) Evaluation of an *in vitro* cell toxicity test using rabbit corneal cells to predict the eye irritation potential of surfactants, *Toxicol. Lett.* 14(3–4), 207–212.

NORTH-ROOT, H., YACKOVICH, F., DEMETRULIAS, J., GACULA, M., JR. and HEINZE, J.E. (1985) Prediction of the eye irritation potential of shampoos using the *in vitro* SIRC cell toxicity test, *Food Chem. Toxicol.* 23(2), 271–273.

O'BRIAN, K.A.F., BASKETTER, D.A., JONES, P.A. and DIXIT, M.B. (1994) An *in vitro* study of the eye irritation potential of new shampoo formulations, *Toxicol. in Vitro* 8, 257–261.

OSBORNE, R., PERKINS, M.A. and ROBERTS, D.A. (1995) Development and intralaboratory evaluation of an *in vitro* human cell-based test to aid ocular irritancy assessments, *Fundam. Appl. Toxicol.* 28(1), 139–153.

READER, S., BLACKWELL, V., O'HARA, R., CLOTHIER, R.H., GRIFFIN, G. and BALLS, M. (1989) A vital dye release method for assessing the short term cytotoxic effects of chemicals and formulations, *Alternatives to Laboratory Animals* 17, 28–37.

SNEDECOR, G.W. and COCHRAN, W.G. (1980) *Statistical Methods*, 7th edn, Ames, IA, USA: Iowa State University Press

SPIELMANN, H., BALLS, M., BRAND, M., DOERING, B., HOLZHUETTER, H.G., KALWEIT, S., KLECAK, G., EPLATTENIER, H.L., LIEBSCH, M., LOVELL, W.W., MAURER, T., MOLDENHAUER, F., MOORE, L., PAPE, W.J., PFANENBECKER, U., POTTHAST, J., DE SILVA, O., STEILING, W. and WILLSHAW, A. (1994) EEC/COLIPA project on *in vitro* phototoxicity testing: First results obtained with a BALB/C 3T3 cell phototoxicity assay, *Toxicology In Vitro* 8(4), 793–796.

SPIELMANN, H., BALLS, M., DUPUIS, J., PAPE, W.J., PECHOVITCH, G., DE SILVA, O., HOLZHUETTER, H.-G., CLOTHIER, R., DESOLLE, P., GERBERICK, F., LIEBSCH, M., LOVELL, W.W., MAURER, T., PFANENBECKER, U., POTTHAST, J.M., CSATO, M., SLADOWSKI, D., STEILING, W. and BRANTOM, P. (1998) The International EU/COLIPA *in vitro* Phototoxicity Validation Study: Results of phase II (Blind Trial): Part 1: The 3T3 NRU phototoxicity test, *Toxicology In Vitro* 12(3), 305–327.

■ CHAPTER 48 ■

SPIELMANN, H., KALWEIT, S., LIEBSCH, M., WIRNSBERGER, T., GERNER, I., BERTRAM-NEIS, E., KRAUSER, K., KREILING, R., MILTENBURGER, H.G. and ET, A.L. (1993) Validation study of alternatives to the draize eye irritation test in Germany: Cytotoxicity testing and HET-CAM test with 136 industrial chemicals, *Toxicology In Vitro* **7**(4), 505–510.

SPIELMANN, H., LIEBSCH, M., DOERING, B. and MOLDENHAUER, F. (1996a) First results of the EU/COLIPA validation trial *in vitro* phototoxicity testing, *In Vitro Toxicology* **9**(3), 325–338.

SPIELMANN, H., LIEBSCH, M., KALWEIT, S. MOLDENHAUER, F., WIMSBERGER, T., HOLZHÜTTER, H.G., SCHNEIDER, B., GLASER, S., GERNER, I., PAPE, W.J.W., KREILING, R., KRAUSER, K., MILTENBURGER, H.G., STEILING, W., LUEPKE, N.P., MÜLLER, N., KREUZER, W., MÜRMANN, P., SPENGLER, J., BERTRAM-NELS, E., SEIGEHUND, B. and WIEBEL, F.J. (1996b) Results of a validation study in Germany on two *in vitro* alternatives to the Draize eye irritation test, the HET-CAM test and the 3T3-NRU cytotoxicity test, *Alternatives to Laboratory Animals* **24**, 741–858.

SPIELMANN, H., LIEBSCH, M., PAPE, W.J., BALLS, M., DUPUIS, J., KLECAK, G., LOVELL, W.W., MAURER, T., DE SILVA, O. and STEILING, W. (1995) EEC/COLIPA *in vitro* photoirritancy program: results of the first stage of validation, *Curr. Probl. Dermatol.* **23**, 256–264.

TALSMA, D.M., LEACH, C.L., HATOUM, N.S., GIBBONS, R.D., ROGER, J.C. and GARVIN, P.J. (1988) Reducing the number of rabbits in the Draize eye irritancy test: a statistical analysis of 155 studies conducted over 6 years, *Fundam. Appl. Toxicol.* **10**(1), 146–153.

VOSE, D. (1996) *Monte Carlo Simulations: A Guide to Monte Carlo Simulation Modelling.* New York: John Wiley and Son.

WEIL, C.S. and SCALA, R.A. (1971) Study of intra- and interlaboratory variability in the results of rabbit eye and skin irritation tests, *Toxicol. Appl. Pharmacol.* **19**(2), 276–360.

WORTH, A.P. and BALLS, M. (2001a) The importance of the prediction model in the validation of alternative tests, *Altern. Lab. Anim.* **29**(2), 135–144.

WORTH, A.P. and BALLS, M. (2001b) The role of ECVAM in promoting the regulatory acceptance of alternative methods in the European Union. European Centre for the Validation of Alternative Methods, *Altern. Lab. Anim.* **29**(5), 525–535.

Animal Models for Immunologic and Nonimmunologic Contact Urticaria

ANTTI LAUERMA AND HOWARD I MAIBACH

Contents

49.1 Introduction

49.2 Immunologic contact urticaria: mechanisms

49.3 Respiratory chemical allergy as an animal model for immunologic contact urticaria

49.4 Contact chemical allergy as an animal model for immunologic contact urticaria

49.5 Protein allergy as an animal model for immunologic contact urticaria

49.6 Nonimmunologic contact urticaria: mechanisms

49.7 Animal models for nonimmunologic contact urticaria

49.8 Conclusions

49.1 INTRODUCTION

Contact urticaria is a skin disease with an increasing importance. The usefulness of products made from natural rubber latex has caused an increase in allergic (immunologic) contact urticaria, often causing occupational disability. Other forms of contact urticaria continue to be rather common. The symptoms experienced in contact urticaria range from local tingling to systemic anaphylaxis. The common factor in urticaria is the release of inflammatory mediators from cutaneous mast cells, which causes pruritus and swelling of the skin tissue.

Contact urticaria is seen as two different entities: immunologic contact urticaria (ICU) and nonimmunologic contact urticaria (NICU). These two forms are separate in their mechanisms and etiology, while some differences in their clinical pictures may be seen. The most important distinguishing factor is the role of immunologic memory in these diseases. ICU occurs only in patients sensitized previously to the causative agent, whereas NICU does not require immunologic memory and may occur in any person. Due to these differences, the diagnostic procedures in patients are also different.

As an increasing number of new substances, especially chemicals, enter the fields of skin medication and care, contact urticarias to the new substances are a constant threat. To avoid such problems, predictive tests to exclude the possibility that the new substance causes contact urticaria, are needed. Additionally, as ICU and NICU are common skin problems, medications are also needed. To develop new medications for contact urticarias, models of NICU and ICU would be highly desirable. As of today, *in vitro* models for ICU and NICU are not available. Therefore, this chapter will concentrate on *in vivo* models, i.e. animal models.

49.2 IMMUNOLOGIC CONTACT URTICARIA: MECHANISMS

Immunologic contact urticaria is mediated through IgE antibodies that identify molecules entering the body through skin and perceived as foreign. The molecule has to penetrate epidermal layers including the stratum corneum, as well as basement membrane, before it is able to attach to IgE bound on mast cell surfaces in the dermis. The responsible molecules have to have sufficient size and contain amino acid sequences to be able to bind to IgE. Therefore the most usual molecules causing ICU are proteins or large-molecule-size polypeptides. Smaller peptides or chemicals have to bind to a carrier protein to

CHAPTER 49

be able to trigger immune response. After the responsible molecule binds to the IgE on mast cell, the cell releases inflammatory mediators, which cause itch, inflammation and swelling in the skin. The swelling is seen as edema, the principal feature of urticaria (Lauerma and Maibach, 1997).

49.3 RESPIRATORY CHEMICAL ALLERGY AS AN ANIMAL MODEL FOR IMMUNOLOGIC CONTACT URTICARIA

Anhydrides cause asthmatic-like symptoms in persons that have been exposed to them, trimellitic anhydride (TMA) being well-studied (Zeiss *et al.*, 1977). The immunologic reactions in lungs of experimental animals and patients feature anaphylactic (Type I), complement-mediated (Type II), antibody-complex-mediated (Type III) and cell-mediated (Type IV) reactions. Nonimmunologic (irritant) reactions may also participate (Hayes *et al.*, 1992), possibly due to degradation of trimellitic anhydride to trimellitic acid.

TMA causes skin reactions if sensitization is done through skin contact (Dearman *et al.*, 1992b). The skin reactions appear in two phases, i.e. immediate and delayed, implying that both Type I and IV reactions are involved (Dearman *et al.*, 1992b; Lauerma *et al.*, 1997).

Sensitization of experimental animals can be done through airways (Obata *et al.*, 1992) or skin. Cutaneous sensitization can be done intradermally (guinea pigs) (Hayes *et al.*, 1992) or topically (mice) (Dearman *et al.*, 1992b). Cutaneous sensitization seems to induce both immediate and delayed skin reactions when an animal sensitized to TMA encounters the chemical next time.

Intradermal sensitization of guinea pigs can be done with TMA 30 percent in corn oil at 0.1 ml dose. The guinea pigs can be used for challenges 3–4 weeks after the injection.

Topical sensitization with TMA has been done in mice. BALB/C mice have been sensitized topically on shaven skin on the trunk that has been tape-stripped prior to application. The first dose has been 100 µl TMA at 500 mg/mL. To enhance development of anti-TMA-IgE-antibodies, a second sensitization has been performed with 50 µl TMA at 250 mg/ml at the same site. The animals have been used for elicitation 1 week after the second dosing.

In mice sensitized to TMA a first immediate-type reaction due to reapplication is seen at 1 hour after dosing and a second delayed-type swelling reaction is seen at 24 hours. A dose-dependent swelling is also seen in nonsensitized animals (Lauerma *et al.*, 1997), which can be caused by trimellitic acid, a hydrolization product of TMA (Patterson *et al.*, 1982). Such reactions could possibly be a form of NICU.

Mice sensitized to topical TMA can be used for study of topical immuno-modulating drugs. In one study an antihistamine suppressed early, a glucocorticosteroid suppressed both early and delayed and a nonsteroidal anti-inflammatory drug enhanced early skin reaction, in line with the clinical findings seen in patients in practice when these medications have been given in atopic IgE-mediated diseases (Lauerma *et al.*, 1997).

Other haptens capable of inducing respiratory allergy, such as diphenyl-methane-4,4-diisocyanate (MDI) and phtalic anhydride are respiratory hapten allergens that possibly could also be used to establish an animal model for ICU.

49.4 CONTACT CHEMICAL ALLERGY AS AN ANIMAL MODEL FOR IMMUNOLOGIC CONTACT URTICARIA

When BALB/C mice are repeatedly sensitized for up to 48 days with strong contact allergen 2,4,6-trinitro-1-chlorobenzene (TNCB), an immediate-type reaction kinetic emerges at the expense of the more typical delayed-type response to this contact allergen. Such reaction kinetic shift coincided with an increase of the number of mast cells in the skin area used for sensitization and elicitation. Antigen-specific IgE was also seen, and the reactions were dependent on the increased number of mast cells on the site of application used (Kitagati *et al.*, 1995).

49.5 PROTEIN ALLERGY AS AN ANIMAL MODEL FOR IMMUNOLOGIC CONTACT URTICARIA

Rabbits sensitized through airways or through skin with natural rubber latex show wheal-and-flare responses when prick tested (Reijula *et al.*, 1994). Therefore it could be that such animals can be used as an animal model for ICU to study its pathogenesis and possible medications to it. However, it has not been studied whether open application could be sufficient for ICU in this model as the rate of cutaneous penetration of natural rubber latex proteins has not been established. Also mice exposed to NRL have elevated IgE levels and eosinophilia (Kurup *et al.*, 1994). Other proteins, such as ovalbumin, that is able to cause Type I IgE-mediated reactions (Spergel *et al.*, 1998), should be studied to see if they could be used in a similar manner.

49.6   NONIMMUNOLOGIC CONTACT URTICARIA: MECHANISMS

Nonimmunologic immediate contact reactions range from erythema to urticaria and occur in individuals that have not necessarily been previously exposed to them and who are also not sensitized to them. It is likely that nonimmunologic contact urticaria reactions are more common than immunologic contact urticaria reactions. The reactions arise most likely from the causative agent's ability to induce release of histamine and/or leukotrienes from skin tissue, being therefore pharmacological in its nature. The agents causing NICU are numerous and include, among others, benzoic acid, sorbic acid, cinnamic aldehyde and nicotinic acid esters. Provocative skin tests for NICU include the rub test and open test. The kinetics of NICU reactions are somewhat slower than those of ICU, i.e. the peak being at 45–60 minutes instead of 15–20 minutes (Gollhausen and Kligman, 1984).

49.7   ANIMAL MODELS FOR NONIMMUNOLOGIC CONTACT URTICARIA

Animal models have been searched in the hope to find a suitable screening method for compounds causing NICU (Lahti and Maibach, 1984). The different agents causing NICU have often different mechanisms (the NICU reactions are pharmacological rather than immunological in aetiology) and therefore an *in vivo* end-point, i.e. thickness of ear pinnae, has been utilized.

Guinea pigs are more sensitive to NICU than mice and rats, and therefore guinea pigs have been used in most studies (Lahti and Maibach, 1985). Substances studied are applied openly on guinea pig ear lobe, and edema is quantified with micrometer. The reactions are seen at their maximum after approximately 50 minutes after the application, the largest swellings being two-fold. NICU model can be also used to study pharmacological agents to treat it (Lahti *et al.*, 1986).

49.8   CONCLUSIONS

It seems that mice sensitized to TMA and possibly also other respiratory chemical allergens may be used as animal models for ICU. For NICU the guinea pig ear lobe method may be most useful. These models need more refinement and standardization. Alternative methods may include *in vitro* mast cell cultures with specific IgE obtained from patients for ICU; for NICU several tissue culture systems should be tried. If *in vitro* methods are used also percutaneous absorption of the responsible agents should be studied, as it is the prerequisite for both ICU and NICU.

REFERENCES

DEARMAN, R.J., BASKETTER, D.A. and KIMBER, I. (1992a) Variable effects of chemical allergens on serum IgE concentration in mice. Preliminary evaluation of a novel approach to the identification of respiratory sensitizers. *J. Appl. Toxicol.* **12**(5), 317–323.

DEARMAN, R.J., MITCHELL, J.A., BASKETTER, D.A. and KIMBER, I. (1992b) Differential ability of occupational chemical contact and respiratory allergens to cause immediate and delayed dermal hypersensitivity reactions in mice. *Int. Arch. Allergy Immunol.* **97**(4), 315–321.

GOLLHAUSEN, R. and KLIGMAN, A.M. (1985) Human assay for identifying substances which induce non-allergic contact urticaria: the NICU-test. *Contact Dermatitis* **13**(2), 98–106.

HAYES, J.P., DANIEL, R., TEE, R.D., BARNES, P.J., TAYLOR, A.J. and CHUNG, K.F. (1992) Bronchial hyperreactivity after inhalation of trimellitic anhydride dust in guinea pigs after intradermal sensitization to the free hapten. *Am. Rev. Respir. Dis.* **146**(5 Pt 1), 1311–1314.

KARUP, V.P., KUMAR, A., CHOI, H., MURALI, P.S., RESNICK, A., KELLY, K.J. and FINK, J.N. (1994) Latex antigens induce IgE and eosinophils in mice. *Int. Arch. Allergy Immunol.* **103**, 370–377.

KITAGATI, H., FUJISAWA, S., WATANABE, K., HAYAKAWA, K. and SHIOHARA, T. (1995) Immediate-type hypersensitivity response followed by a later reaction is induced by repeated epicutaneous application of contact sensitizing agents in mice. *J. Invest. Dermatol.* **105**, 749–755.

LAHTI, A. and MAIBACH H.I. (1984) An animal model for nonimmunologic contact urticaria. *Toxicol. Appl. Pharmacol.* **76**(2), 219–224

LAHTI, A. and MAIBACH, H.I. (1985) Species specificity of nonimmunologic contact urticaria: guinea pig, rat, and mouse. *J. Am. Acad. Dermatol.* **13**(1), 66–69.

LAHTI, A., McDONALD, D.M., TAMMI, R. and MAIBACH, H.I. (1986) Pharmacological studies on nonimmunologic contact urticaria in guinea pigs. *Arch. Dermatol. Res.* **279**(1), 44–49.

■ CHAPTER 49 ■

LAUERMA, A.I., FENN, B. and MAIBACH, H.I. (1997) Trimellitic anhydride-sensitive mouse as an animal model for contact urticaria. *J. Appl. Toxicol.* **17**(6), 357–360.

LAUERMA, A.I. and MAIBACH, H.I. (1997) Model for immunologic contact urticaria. In: AMIN, S., LAHTI, A. and MAIBACH H.I. (eds) *Contact Urticaria Syndrome*, Boca Raton: CRC Press, 27–32.

OBATA, H., TAO, Y., KIDO, M., NAGATA, N., TANAKA, I. and KUROIWA, A. (1992) Guinea pig model of immunologic asthma induced by inhalation of trimellitic anhydride. *Am. Rev. Respir. Dis.* **146**(6), 1553–1558.

PATTERSON, R., ZEISS, C.R. and PRUZANSKY, J.J. (1982) Immunology and immunopathology of trimellitic anhydride pulmonary reactions. *J. Allergy Clin. Immunol.* **70**(1), 19–23.

REIJULA, K.E., KELLY, K.J., KURUP, V.P., CHOI, H., BONGARD, R.D., DAWSON, C.A. and FINK, J.N. (1994) Latex-induced dermal and pulmonary hypersensitivity in rabbits. *J. Allergy Clin. Immunol.* **94**(5), 891–902.

SPERGEL, J.M., MIZOGUCHI, E., BREWER, J.P., MARTIN, T.R., BHAN, A.K. and GEHA, R.S. (1998) Epicutaneous sensitization with protein antigen induces localized allergic dermatitis and hyperresponsiveness to methacholine after single exposure to aerosolized antigen in mice. *J. Clin. Invest.* **101**(8), 1614–1622.

ZEISS, C.R., PATTERSON, R., PRUZANSKY, J.J., MILLER, M.M., ROSENBERG, M. and LEVITZ, D. (1977) Trimellitic anhydride-induced airway syndromes: clinical and immunologic studies. *J. Allergy Clin. Immunol.* **60**(2), 96–103.

Diagnostic Tests in Dermatology: Patch and Photopatch Testing and Contact Urticaria

50

SMITA AMIN, ANTTI LAUERMA
AND HOWARD I MAIBACH

Contents

50.1   Introduction

50.2   Drug eruptions

50.3   Contact dermatitis

50.4   Contact urticaria syndrome: immediate contact reactions

50.5   Subjective irritation

50.1 INTRODUCTION

Diagnostic *in vivo* skin tests are used in dermatology to detect and define the possible exogenous chemical agent that causes a skin disorder, and hence are critical in their scientific documentation. Such chemical agents often cause skin disorders by hypersensitivity mechanisms, which can thus be diagnosed by a provocative test (Lauerma and Maibach, 1995). The anatomical advantage of studying skin disorders is that the skin is the foremost frontier of the human body and therefore easily accessible for testing. Although it has been shown that differences in the reactivity of different skin sites exist, many causative agents may be tested locally on one skin site, thus exposing only limited areas of skin to the diagnostic procedures. Such procedures include patch, intradermal, prick, scratch, scratch-chamber, open, photo, photopatch, and provocative use tests. In cases of some generalized skin reactions, however, systemic exposure to the external agent may be necessary for diagnosis.

The value of diagnostic tests is identification of the causative agent, which enables restarting of those chemicals and/or medications not responsible for the eruption. This chapter briefly describes the *in vivo* test methods used for making diagnoses of skin disorders. The skin disorders in which such tests are useful include drug eruptions, contact dermatitis and immediate contact reactions (contact urticaria), and possibly sensory (subjective) irritation (Table 50.1).

50.2 DRUG ERUPTIONS

Drug eruptions are a heterogeneous class of adverse skin reactions due to ingestion or injection of therapeutic drugs. The drug eruptions should ideally be diagnosed through systemic rechallenge, because many factors (e.g., systemic drug metabolism) may contribute to the process, and skin tests therefore are not as reliable. Because systemic challenge is not always easy to perform, skin tests may, however, precede such challenges, according to reaction type. If skin tests do not provide information about the causative agent and a medication needs to be restarted, the next step is a controlled drug rechallenge, preferably in a hospital environment (Kauppinen and Alanko, 1989).

The choice of provocation protocols depends on the type of reaction involved. Although much work has been directed toward classifying drug eruptions and elucidating their mechanisms, they are still not well understood. Many of them are presumably mediated by immunological mechanisms, but there are also *nonimmunological drug eruptions*, idiosyncrasies, in genetically

■ CHAPTER 50 ■

TABLE 50.1:

Chemically related skin disorders diagnosable through diagnostic testing

Disorder	Mechanism	Test method
Drug eruption	Type I	Prick test or open test Scratch rest Intradermal test Systemic challenge
	Type II	Patch test Systemic challenge
	Type III	Intradermal test Systemic challenge
	Type IV	Patch test Systemic challenge
	Nonimmunological	Systemic challenge
Allergic contact dermatitis	Type IV	Patch test Intradermal test Open test or provocative use test (repeated open application test)
Contact urticaria syndrome (immediate contact reaction)	Type I	Open test (single application) Prick test Scratch test Scratch-chamber test
	Nonimmunological	Open test (single application)
Subjective irritation	Unknown	Lactic acid test Open test (single application)

^aTypes I–IV: Coombs–Gell classification of immunological mechanisms.

predisposed persons. In cases of nonimmunological drug eruptions, skin tests are usually negative, and systemic provocations are also often negative (Tables 50.2 and 50.3). Immunological drug eruptions may be classified into the four reaction types according to Coombs and Gell (Bruynzeel and Ketal, 1989).

Anaphylactic (Coombs–Gell type I) reactions include anaphylaxis. urticaria, and angioneurotic edema. They are usually mediated by immunoglobulin E (IgE) antibodies. Penicillin is one well-known causative agent for type I reactions. Prick (Table 50.4) and scratch (Table 50.5) tests are used in diagnosis of type I reactions and are a relatively safe way of detecting the causative agent. Intradermal tests (Table 50.6) may also be used in such cases, although a much larger amount of the antigen is introduced into the body, which makes systemic reactions more likely. Also, *in vitro* tests such as the radioallergosorbent test (RAST) are used in diagnosis (Bruynzeel and Ketel, 1989). Because type I reactions are potentially life-threatening, systemic challenges (Tables 50.2 and 50.3) (Kauppinen and Alanko, 1989), if done, should be performed

TABLE 50.2:

Systemic challenge: Protocol

The patient should be monitored under hospital conditions and emergency resuscitation equipment should be available throughout the study. Especially if the initial drug eruption was strong, challenge should be started at a low dose, that is, no more than one-tenth of the initial dose.

A dose of the suspected drug is given orally in the morning. The patient's skin, temperature, pulse, and other signs are followed at 1-h intervals for 10 h and recorded.

If no reactions appear during 24 h, the challenge is repeated at a higher dose (e.g., one-third of the initial dose) the next morning.

If no reactions appear on d 1 and 2, then on the third morning a full therapeutic dose is given as a third challenge. If necessary, different drug challenges may be repeated every 24 h.

Note: See Kauppinen and Alanko (1989) for detailed instructions. The publication provides an unequaled clinical experience, and offers many valuable short-cuts in making scientifically based diagnoses.

TABLE 50.3:

Systemic challenge: Precautions

Challenge is not advisable if the patient has had:
    Anaphylaxis
    Toxic epidermal necrolysis (TEN)
    Stevens–Johnson syndrome and/or erythema multiforme
    Systemic lupus erythematosus-like reaction

Extreme care should be exercised if the patient has had:
    Urticaria
    Asthma
    Any other immediate-type reaction
    Fixed drug eruption or its most severe form: generalized bullous fixed drug eruption (special variant of TEN)

Usually performed 1–2 mo after the original eruption, except in severe reactions, when a longer interval (6 mo-1 yr) is advisable.

Minimum provocative dose is generally less than one single therapeutic dose, except that in cases of severe bullous fixed drug eruption the initial test dose must be smaller (i.e., one-tenth to one-fourth of a single therapeutic dose).

Note: See Kauppinen and Alanko (1989) for detailed instructions.

with extreme care, starting with very low doses, under hospital conditions. A physician should always be readily available, and the patient should be monitored frequently.

Cytotoxic (type II) reactions are mediated by cytotoxic mechanisms: quinine and quinidine are examples of causative agents. Patch tests (Table 50.7) may be attempted before systemic challenges (Tables 50.2 and 50.3) (Kauppinen and

TABLE 50.4:

Prick test

Materials:	(1) Allergens in vehicles. (2) Vehicle (negative control). (3) Histamine in 0.9% NaCl (positive control). (4) Prick lancets.
Method:	One drop of each test allergen, vehicle, and histamine control is applied to the volar aspects of forearms. The test site is pierced with a lancet to introduce the allergen into the skin.
Reading time:	15–30 min
Interpretation:	An edematous reaction (wheal) of at least 3 mm in diameter and at least half the size of the histamine control is considered positive, in the absence of such reaction in the vehicle control.
Precautions:	General anaphylaxis not very likely, because of the small amount of allergen introduced, but a physician should always be available for such occurrences. The patient should not leave the premises during the first 30 min after the test.
Controls:	Required.

TABLE 50.5:

Scratch test

Materials:	(1) Allergens in vehicles. (2) Vehicle (negative control). (3) Histamine in 0.9% NaCl (positive control). (4) Needles.
Method:	One drop of each test allergen, vehicle, and histamine control is applied to the volar aspects of forearms or back, and needles are used to scratch the skin slightly at these sites.
Reading time:	Up to 30 min
Interpretation:	Difficult because of unstandardized procedure. Edematous reaction at least as wide as the histamine control is considered positive in the absence of such reaction in the vehicle control.
Precautions:	As with prick test.
Controls:	Required.

Alanko, 1989), for example. in the case of thrombocytopenic purpura caused by carbromal or bromisovalum (Bruynzeel and Ketel, 1989).

Immune complex-mediated (type II) reactions include Arthus and vasculitic reactions. Type III reactions are mediated by immunoglobulins, complement, and the antigen itself, which form complexes. For example, sulfa preparations, pyrazolones, and hydantoin derivatives have caused vascular purpura via type

TABLE 50.6:

Intradermal test

Materials:	(1) Allergens in isotonic solution vehicles. (2) Solution vehicle (negative control). (3) Tuberculin (1 cc) syringes and needles.
Method:	0.05–0.1 ml of allergen solution and vehicle solution is applied intradermally to the skin of the volar aspects of forearms.
Reading time:	30 min, 24 h, and 48 h
Interpretation:	Erythematous and edematous reaction at 30 min is suggestive of immediate type (type I) allergy in the absence of such a reaction in the vehicle control.
	Arthus reaction with polymorphonuclear leukocyte infiltration appearing in 2–4 h, which may progress into necrosis in hours or days, suggests cytotoxic (type III) reaction.
	Erythema and edema of at least 5 mm in diameter at 48 h indicates delayed-type hypersensitivity (type IV), for example, contact allergy.
Precautions:	The risk of general anaphylaxis is higher than in prick or scratch tests because of larger amount of allergen introduced; therefore, a physician should always be available for such occurrences. The risk is greater in asthmatic patients. The patient should not leave the premises during the first 30 min after the test.
Controls:	Required.

TABLE 50.7:

Patch test

Materials:	(1) Allergens in vehicle (e.g., petrolatum, ethanol, water). (2) Vehicles. (3) Aluminum chambers (Finn chamber), Scanpor tape, and filter papers (for solutions). OR: (1) Ready-made patch test series (TRUE test).
Method:	Patches on tape or ready-made patch test series are applied on intact skin of the back. Filter papers are used for solutions: 17 µl of allergen in vehicle is used for each patch. Ready-made patch series is applied as is on similar skin sites. The patches are removed after 48 h.
Reading time:	48 h and 96 h
interpretation:	Erythema and edema or more is positive. Distinguishing between allergic and irritant reaction is important. If the reaction spreads across the boundaries of the patch site, the reaction is more likely to be allergic, if the reaction peaks at 48 h and starts to fade rapidly after that, it may be irritant.
Precautions:	Intense skin reactions possible: these can be treated with topical glucocorticosteroids. Active sensitization possible.
Controls:	Required.

III mechanisms. Intradermal tests (Table 50.6) may be tried for diagnosis before systemic challenges (Tables 50.2 and 50.3) (Bruynzeel and Ketel. 1989).

Delayed hypersensitivity (type IV) reactions are cell-mediated immune reactions involving the antigen, antigen-presenting cells, and T lymphocytes. Drug reactions of this type are often maculopapular or eczematous, although photoallergic reactions and fixed drug eruptions are also presumably mediated by type IV mechanisms. Other type IV reactions include some cases of erythroderma, exfoliative dermatitis, lichenoid and vesicobullous eruptions, erythema exudativum multiforme, and toxic epidermal necrolysis. Type IV reactions may be detected by patch tests with the causative agent (Table 50.7) (Calkin and Maibach, 1993). In the case of a fixed drug eruption, in which the reaction reoccurs in the same skin site every time the drug is ingested, the patch test should be done in that particular skin site for a positive result (Alanko *et al.*, 1987). For photosensitivity reactions, photo (Table 50.8) or photopatch tests (Table 50.9) should be done (Rosen, 1989). A negative patch test does not rule

TABLE 50.8:

Photo test

Materials:	Ultraviolet (UV) radiation source.
Method:	Minimal erythema dose (MED) of UVA or UVB is measured (1) while the subject is taking the suspected medication and (2) after discontinuing the same medication.
Interpretation:	If MED (UVA or UVB) is much lower while the subject is taking the medication, this suggests a photosensitive (phototoxic or photoallergic) reaction to the drug.

TABLE 50.9:

Photopatch test

Materials:	(1) Ultraviolet (UV) radiation source. (2) Patch test materials (see Table 50.8).
Method:	Two sets of patch test are applied for 48 h. After removal, one set is irradiated with UVA at a dose below minimal erythema dose (MED) (5–10 J/cm² or 50% of MED, whichever is smaller), and the other set is protected from UV Dose.
Reading time:	48 and 96 h
Interpretation:	Reaction only at irradiated site suggests photoallergy. Reaction at both sites suggests contact allergy. Reaction at both sites and a much stronger reaction at the irradiated site suggests both contact allergy and photoallergy.
Controls:	Required.

out the possibility that the tested drug may be causative. This is because patch testing involves potential limitations, such as insufficient penetration. In this case a systemic provocation (Tables 50.2 and 50.3) should be considered (Kauppinen and Alanko, 1989).

50.3   CONTACT DERMATITIS

Contact dermatitis is commonly divided into irritant contact dermatitis and allergic contact dermatitis. *Irritant contact dermatitis*, the more common of the two, is initiated by nonimmunological toxic mechanisms and is not diagnosed by patch testing, while allergic contact dermatitis is. In *allergic contact dermatitis* the patient becomes topically sensitized to a low-molecular-weight hapten and in subsequent topical contact develops an eczematous skin reaction, which is mediated by delayed hypersensitivity (type IV) mechanisms. Allergic contact dermatitis is diagnosed with patch tests (Table 50.7), intradermal tests (Table 50.6), or open tests (repeated application) (Table 50.10).

Of these three methods, patch testing is the most common and standardized. The problems involved in patch testing are insufficient penetration of the allergenic compound, which may result in false-negative results, and irritation from the test compound, which may cause a false-positive result. Also, patch testing may cause a worsening of eczema in other skin sites (excited skin syndrome) or active sensitization to patch compounds (Fischer and Maibach, 1990).

Two widely used methods for patch testing exist, the Finn chamber and TRUE test methods. Both have been shown to be reliable, especially when stronger

■ CHAPTER 50 ■

TABLE 50.10:
Provocative use test (open test or repeated open application test)

Materials:	(1) Allergen in vehicle (petrolatum, ethanol, water). (2) Vehicle. (3) Cotton-tipped applicators or other devices to spread the preparations.
Method:	Patient applies allergen and vehicle on antecubital fossa (outpatient) or shoulder regions of upper back, 2 times a day, for 14 d or until a positive reaction appears.
Reading time:	Patient reports whether positive reaction appears. At 7 and 14 d the patient returns for reading of the test site.
Interpretation:	Erythema and edema or more is positive.
Precautions:	Active sensitization possible, but not yet documented.
Controls:	May be required.

reactions (contact allergies) are investigated (Ruhneck-Forsbeck *et al.*, 1988). The TRUE Test is somewhat easier to handle. as it is ready to use. However, the Finn chamber method provides more flexibility for the dermatologist and the allergist to test substances not in routine patch test use. Regardless of the test method, the most important factor in successful patch testing is the experience and skill of the interpreter.

A standard patch test series is shown in Table 50.11. It is the standard series of the International Contact Dermatitis Research Group and the European Environmental and Contact Dermatitis Research Group (Andersen *et al.*, 1991). A standard patch test series has been compiled to represent the most commonly encountered contact allergens, and it is meant to act as a screening tray. Its content is subject to change due to research findings about contact allergy (Andersen *et al.*, 1991). A multitude of other patch test series are available when the causative agents of the individual patient's contact dermatitis are known better; these include, for example, patch test series for preservatives, rubber

TABLE 50.11:

Standard patch test series

Potassium dichromate	0.50% pet.
Neomycin sulfate	20.0% pet.
Thiuram mix	1.0% pet.
p-Phenylenediamine free base	1.0% pet.
Cobalt chloride	1.0% pet.
Benzocaine	5.0% pet.
Formaldehyde	1.0% aq.
Colophony	20.0% pet.
Quinoline mix	6.0% pet.
Balsam of Peru	25.0% pet.
PPD-black rubber mix	0.6% pet.
Wool alcohols (lanolin)	30.0% pet.
Mercapto mix	2.0% pet.
Epoxy resin	1.0% pet.
Paraben mix	15.0% pet.
p-*tert*-Butylphenol-formaldehyde resin	1.0% pet.
Fragrance mix	8.0% pet.
Ethylenediamine dihydrochloride	1.0% pet.
Quaternium 15	1.0% pet.
Nickel sulfate	5.0% pet.
Kathon CG	0.01% aq.
Mercaptobenzothiazole	2.0% pet.
Primin	0.01% pet.

Note: pet. = petrolatum vehicle; aq. = aqueous vehicle. Series is standard for the International Contact Dermatitis Research Group and the European Environmental and Contact Dermatitis Research Group.

chemicals, topical drugs, and clothing chemicals. There are also special series to investigate occupational contact allergies in, for example, dental personnel or hairdressers.

Patch tests should be applied on the back for 48 h and be read after removal. A second reading 24–48 h after patch removal is necessary, as irritant reactions, which are often easily misinterpreted as allergic, often tend to fade during the third and fourth days, while allergic reactions tend to persist. Additionally, with some allergens, such as corticosteroids and neomycin, late reactions often occur, possibly because of low percutaneous penetration. Therefore, a third reading approximately 1 wk after patch application may be advisable, although this may be difficult to do routinely in practice.

Intradermal testing (Table 50.6) has recently been shown to be of value in diagnosing hydrocortisone contact allergy (Wilkinson *et al.*, 1991); see Herbst *et al.* (1993) for a review of intradermal testing for allergic contact dermatitis. Open tests or repeated open application tests (Table 50.10) are not as sensitive as patch or intradermal tests, possibly because of insufficient penetration of the compound under unoccluded conditions (Hannuksela and Salo, 1986; Hannuksela, 1991).

50.4   CONTACT URTICARIA SYNDROME: IMMEDIATE CONTACT REACTIONS

Contact urticaria syndrome includes a group of skin reactions, that is, immediate contact reactions, that usually appear within 1 h of skin contact with the causative agent. Immediate skin reactions are divided into immunological [immunoglobulin E (IgE) mediated] and nonimmunological immediate contact reactions. The symptoms range from mere itching and tingling to local wheal and flare. In cases of intense sensitivity, a generalized urticaria, systemic symptoms, and even anaphylaxis (contact urticaria syndrome) may occur (Lahti and Maibach, 1992).

Immunological immediate contact reactions are usually urticarial, although they may range from mere tingling in the skin to a generalized anaphylactic reaction in the whole body. Immunological immediate reactions are Coombs–Gell type I reactions mediated mainly via allergen-specific IgE bound to skin mast cells. Coupling of membrane-bound IgE by allergen causes mast cells to liberate histamine, which with other inflammatory mediators makes skin vessels permeable, and edema (urticaria) results. The sensitization in IgE-mediated contact urticaria may occur through skin or possibly the respiratory or gastrointestinal tract. Exposure through skin is the most likely route in occupational latex allergy in health personnel. The provocative *in vivo* methods usually performed first are a prick test (Table 50.4), scratch test (Table 50.5), and scratch-chamber test (Table 50.12). However, the test method simulating the clinical contact situation more realistically is the open application test (single application) (Table 50.13). A previously affected skin site is more sensitive to immunological skin reactions than a nonaffected site. In addition to *in vivo* methods, the diagnosis of immunological immediate contact reactions can be done with RAST, which detects antigen-specific IgE molecules from the patient's serum (Lahti and Maibach, 1992).

Nonimmunological immediate contact reactions range from erythema to urticaria and occur in persons not sensitized to the compounds (Lahti and Maibach,

TABLE 50.12:

Scratch-chamber test

Materials:	(1) Scratch test materials (see Table 50.5). (2) Chambers.
Method:	As with scratch test, but scratch sites are covered with aluminum chambers for 15 min.
Reading time:	30 min
Interpretation:	See Table 50.5.
Precautions:	As with prick and scratch tests.
Controls:	Required.

TABLE 50.13:

Open test (single application) for contact urticaria syndrome immediate contact reactions

Materials:	(1) Allergen in vehicle (petrolatum, ethanol, water). (2) Vehicle. (3) Cotton-tipped applicators or other devices to spread the preparations.
Method:	Allergen and vehicle are applied to skin.
Reading time:	Up to 1 h
Interpretation:	Urticarial reaction is positive.
Precautions:	See Table 4.
Controls:	Required to aid in disciminating immunological (ICU) from nonimmunological contact urticaria (NICU); in NICTJ, the reaction will be noted in most controls.

1992). Nonimmunological contact reactions are probably more common than immunological contact reactions. They are possibly due to the causative agent's ability to release inflammatory mediators, such as histamine, prostaglandins, and leukotrienes, from skin cells, without the participation of IgE molecules. Agents capable of causing nonimmunological contact reactions are numerous: the most potent and best-studied agents are benzoic acid, sorbic acid, cinnamic aldehyde, and nicotinic acid esters. The test for diagnosis of nonimmunological contact urticaria is the open application test (single application) (Table 50.13).

50.5 SUBJECTIVE IRRITATION

Although sensory (subjective) irritation is not fully characterized, there is evidence for a group of such persons, known as "stingers" (Maibach *et al.*, 1989). The lactic acid test (Table 50.14) has been used experimentally to distinguish between "stingers," who more often have subjective irritation, and "non-stingers" (Lammintausta *et al.*, 1988).

TABLE 50.14:

Lactic acid test: Model for sensory irritation

Materials:	(1) Facial sauna.
	(2) 5% Lactic acid in water.
	(3) Vehicle (water).
	(4) Soap, paper towels, cotton-tipped applicators.
Method:	Facial area below eyes is cleansed with soap, paper towels, and water, rinsed with water, and patted dry. Face is exposed to sauna heat for 15 min. Moisture of face is blotted away. Lactic acid in water is rubbed on one side of face (cheek) and water on other. Face is exposed to sauna again.
Reading time:	2 and 5 min after second sauna exposure.
Interpretation:	Any subjective sensation is graded by patient: 0 = none; 1 = slight; 2 = moderate; 3 severe. If cumulative score of two time points is 3 or more, patient is a "stinger."
Precautions:	Irritation may occur.

CHAPTER 50 ■

REFERENCES

ALANKO, K., STUBB, S. and REITAMO, S. (1987) Topical provocation of fixed drug eruption. *Br. J. Dermatol.* **116**, 561–567.

ANDERSEN, K., BURROWS, D. and WHITE, I.R. (1991) Allergens from the standard series. In RYCROFT, R.J.G., HENNE, T., FROSCH, P.J. and BENEZRA, C. (eds) *Textbook of Contact Dermatitis*. Berlin: Springer-Verlag, 416–456.

BRUYNZEEL, D.P. and KETEL, W.G.V. (1989) Patch testing in drug eruptions. *Semin. Dermatol.* **8**, 196–203.

CALKIN, J.M. and MAIBACH, H.I. (1993) Delayed hypersensitivity drug reactions diagnosed by patch testing. *Contact Dermatitis* **29**, 223–233.

FISCHER, T. and MAIBACH, H. (1990) Improved, but not perfect. patch testing. *Am. J. Contact Dermatitis* **1**, 73–90.

HANNUKSELA, M. (1991) Sensitivity of various skin sites in the repeated open application test. *Am. J. Contact Dermatitis* **2**, 102–104.

HANNUKSELA, M. and SALO, H. (1986) The repeated open application test (ROAT). *Contact Dermatitis* **14**, 221–227.

HERBST, R.A., LAUERMA, A.I. and MAIBACH. H.I. (1993) Intradermal testing in the diagnosis of allergic contact dermatitis—A reappraisal. *Contact Dermatitis* **29**, 1–5.

KAUPPINEN, K. and ALANKO, K. (1989) Oral provocation: Uses. *Semin. Dermatol.* **8**, 187–191.

LAHTI, A. and MAIBACH, H.I. (1992) Contact urticaria syndrome. In MOSCHELLA, S.L. and HURLEY, H.J. *Dermatology*. Philadelphia: W. B. Saunders, 433–440.

LAMMINTAUSTA, K., MAIBACH, H.I. and WILSON, D. (1988) Mechanisms of subjective (sensory) irritation. Propensity to non-immunologic contact urticaria and objective irritation in stingers. *Dermatosen* **36**, 45–49.

LAUERMA, A.I. and MAIBACH, H.I. (1995) Provocative tests in dermatology. In SPECTOR, S.L. (ed.) *Provocation in Clinical Practice*, New York: Marcel Dekker, 749–760.

MAIBACH, H.I., LAMMINTAUSTA, K., BERARDESCA, E., and FREEMAN, S. (1989) Tendency to irritation: Sensitive skin. *J. Am. Acad. Dermatol.* **21**, 833–835.

ROSEN, C. (1989) Photo-induced drug eruptions. *Semin. Dermatol.* **8**, 149–157.

RUHNEK-FORSBECK, M., FISCHER, T., MEDING, B., PETTERSON, L., STENBERG, B., STRAND, A., SUNDBERG, K., SVENSSON, L., WAHLBERG, I.E., WIDSTRÖM, L., WRANGSJÖ, K. and BILLBERG, K. (1988) Comparative multi-center study with TRUE test and Finn chamber patch test methods in eight Swedish hospitals. *Acta Dermat.-Venereol. (Stockh.)* **68**, 123–128.

WILKINSON S.M., CARTWRIGHT, P.H. and ENGLISH, J.S.C. (1991) Hydrocortisone: An important cutaneous allergen. *Lancet* **337**, 761–762.

Cosmetic Reactions

51

SARA P MODJTAHEDI, JORGE R TORO,
PATRICIA ENGASSER, AND HOWARD I MAIBACH

Contents

51.1   Introduction

51.2   Cutaneous reactions

51.3   Ingredient patch testing

51.4   Cosmetic products

51.5   Cosmetic intolerance syndrome

51.6   Occupational dermatitis: hairdressers

51.1 INTRODUCTION

The term "cosmetic" is familiar, and its meaning has been expanded by an increase in the variety and complexity of substances used for cosmetic purposes. There are numerous ways to define and describe cosmetics. The Food, Drug and Cosmetic Act, which the Food and Drug Administration (FDA) administers, defines cosmetics in the following manner:

> The term "cosmetic" means articles intended to be rubbed, poured, sprinkled, or sprayed on, introduced into, or otherwise applied to the human body or any part thereof for cleansing, beautifying, promoting attractiveness, or altering the appearance, and (Jackson, 1991) articles intended for use as a component of any such articles: except the term shall not include soap.
>
> (Code of Federal Regulations, 1986: 20201(I), paragraph 40)

Definitions pertaining to Europe and Japan are found in Barel *et al.* (2001), Elsner and Maibach (2000), Elsner *et al.* (1999), Baran and Maibach (1998). Note two important aspects of this legal definition of cosmetics. First, in the United States, cosmetics in theory do not contain "active drug" entities of any type nor can they be promoted as altering any physiological state either in disease or health. Many countries do not recognize this legal distinction. The US FDA classifies products into cosmetics, OTC (over-the-counter) drugs, and prescription drugs. By the US definition, antiperspirants are OTC drugs regulated by the FDA through the OTC drug monograph system, while deodorants are cosmetics. The second aspect of the US definition of cosmetics is the so-called soap exemption. Soap in the classic sense, as made of natural ingredients, is the type of soap that is excepted by the definition above. However, if the soap product is made of detergent chemicals (synthetic surfactants) the product is regulated by the Consumer Product Safety Commission under the Federal Hazardous Substances Act, as a household product. If the soap contains a therapeutic ingredient for a medical condition it is regulated as a prescription drug (Jackson, 1991). Likewise the classification of cosmetics is equally complex. The cosmetic industry itself divides the products into more general categories oriented as to their purpose as described in the definition.

Reactions to cosmetics constitute a small but significant portion of the cases of contact dermatitis seen by dermatologist in the United States. In a five-year study, the North American Contact Dermatitis Group found that 5.4 percent of 13,216 patients tested were identified as having reactions caused by cosmetics (Adams and Maibach, 1985. This is an under-representation of the true incidence because most patients who experience reactions to newly purchase cosmetics seldom consult a physician and just stop using the suspected cosmetic. In addition, they reported that 59 percent of the reactions caused by cosmetics occurred on the face including the periorbital area and 79 percent were females. Half of the cases later proven to evoke reactions to cosmetics were initially unsuspected. Reactions to cosmetics can have a variety of presentations. including subjective and objective irritation, allergic contact dermatitis, contact uriticaria, photosensitive reactions, pigmentation and, hair and nail changes.

51.2 CUTANEOUS REACTIONS

51.2.1 Irritant dermatitis

Objective irritation

Skin irritation has been described by exclusion as localized inflammation not mediated by either sensitized lymphocytes or by antibodies, e.g., that which develops by a process not involving the immune system. Skin irritation depends on endogenous and exogenous factors (Lammintausta and Maibach, 1988). Predictive testing in human beings and rabbits can reliably detect strong or moderate irritants as ingredients in cosmetics or the products themselves. This allows manufacturers to test thoroughly to eliminate these potential hazards before marketing. There is recent evidence that no significant difference across skin types exists (McFadden et al., 1998). Because the stratum corneum of the facial skin is penetrated easily, more irritant reactions occur but always recognized clinically because of the complex biology of the human face. Many supposedly non irritating moisturizers or emollient creams contain surfactants and emulsifiers that are mild irritants. These cosmetics are applied frequently to facial or inflamed skin resulting in irritant reactions. In product use testing, reproducing an irritant reaction may be difficult because penetrability of the stratum corneum varies with environmental conditions; and small panel testing may not account for the complexity and variance of the human genome. Provocative use testing may be performed at the original site of the reactions.

Application of some chemicals may directly destroy tissue, producing skin necrosis at the application site. Chemicals producing necrosis that results in formation of scar tissue are described as corrosive. Chemicals may disrupt cell functions and/or trigger the release, formation, or activation of autocoids that produce local increases in blood flow, increase vascular permeability, attract white blood cells in the area, or directly damage cells. The additive effects of the mediators result in local skin inflammation. A number of as yet poorly defined pathways involving different processes of mediator generation appear to exist. Although no agent has yet met all the criteria to establish it as a mediator of skin irritation, histamine, 5-hydrotryptamine, prostaglandins, leukotrienes, kinins (Effendy and Maibach, 2001), complement, reactive oxygen species, and products of white blood cells have been implicated as mediators of some irritant reactions (Protty, 1978). Chemicals that produce inflammation as a result of a single exposure are termed acute or primary irritants.

Some chemicals do not produce acute irritation from a single exposure but may produce inflammation following repeated application, i.e., cumulative irritation, to the same area of skin. Because of the possibility of skin contact during transport and use of many chemicals, regulatory agencies have mandated screening chemicals for the ability to produce skin corrosion and acute irritation. These studies are conducted in animals, using standardized protocols. However, the protocols specified by some agencies vary somewhat. It is not routinely appropriate to conduct screening studies for corrosion in humans, but acute irritation is sometimes evaluated in humans after animal studies have been completed. Tests for predicting irritation in both animals and humans have been widely utilized. Predictive irritation assay in animals includes modified Draize test repeated application patch tests, the guinea pig immersion test and mouse ear test. Predictive human irritation assay includes many forms of the single application patch test, cumulative irritation assays, chamber scrarification test and exaggerated exposure test. These predictive assays have been reviewed (Marzulli and Maibach, 1991). Currently *in vitro* skin corrosion test methods are being developed that avoid using animal models (Robinson and Perkins, 2002). Sensitive bioengineering equipment used to evaluate pathophysiology of skin irritation includes transepidermal water loss (Effendy *et al.*, 1995), dielectric characteristics, skin impedance, conductance, resistance, blood flow velocity skin pH, O_2 resistance and CO_2 effusion rate (Fluhr *et al.*, 2001). Several textbooks describe these methods in detail (Berardesca *et al.*, 1994; 1995a, b; 2002; Wilhelm *et al.*, 1997). Also, irritant contact dermatitis can be avoided by prevention methods (Loffler and Effendy, 2002).

CHAPTER 51

Sensory or subjective irritation

Application of a cosmetic causing burning, stinging, or itching without detectable visible or microscopic changes, is designated as subjective irritation. This reaction is common in certain susceptible individuals occurring most frequently on the face. Some of the ingredients that cause this reaction are not generally considered irritants and will not cause abnormal responses in non-susceptible individuals. Materials that produce subjective irritation include dimethyl sulfoxide, some benzoyl peroxide preparations, and the chemicals salicylic acid, propylene glycol, amyl-dimethyl-amino benzoic acid, and 2-ethoxy ethyl-methoxy cinnamate, which are ingredients of cosmetics and over-the-counter (OTC) drugs. Pyrethroids, a group of broad-spectrum insecticides, produce a similar condition that may lead to paraesthesia (Cagen *et al.*, 1984) at the nasolabial folds, cheeks, periorbital areas, and ears.

Only a portion of the human population seems to develop nonpyrethroid subjective irritation, and ethnic variations in self-perceived sensitive skin has been noted (Jourdain *et al.*, 2002). Frosch and Kligman (1977a) found that they needed to prescreen subjects to identify "stingers" for conducting predictive assays. Only 20 percent of subjects exposed to 5 percent aqueous lactic acid in a hot, humid environment developed stinging response. All stingers in their series reported a history of adverse reactions to facial cosmetics, soaps, etc. A similar screening procedure by Lammintausta *et al.* (1988) identified 18 percent of their subjects as stingers. Prior skin damage, e.g., sunburn, pretreatment with surfactants, and tape stripping, increase the intensity of responses in stingers, and persons not normally experiencing a response report pain on exposure to lactic acid or other agents that produce subjective irritation (Fosch and Kligman, 1977b). Attempts to identify reactive subjects by association with other skin descriptors, e.g., atopy, skin type, or skin dryness, have not yet been fruitful. However, Lammintausta *et al.* (1988) showed that stingers develop stronger reactions to materials causing nonimmunologic contact urticaria and some increase in transepidermal water loss and blood flow following application of irritants via patches than those of non-stingers.

The mechanisms by which materials produce subjective irritation have not been extensively investigated. Pyrethroids directly act on the axon by interfering with the channel gating mechanism and impulse firing (Vivjeberg and VandenBercken, 1979). It has been suggested that agents causing subjective irritation act via a similar mechanism because no visible inflammation is present. An animal model was developed to rate paraesthesia to pyrethroids and may be useful for other agents (Cagen *et al.*, 1984). Using this technique, it was possible to rank pyrethroids for their ability to produce paraesthesia. Lammintausta *et al.* (1988) and Berardesca *et al.* (1991) suggested that patients with subjective irritation have more responsive blood vessels. Assays and tests have been developed to quantify subjective irritation (Herbst, 2001; Pelosi *et al.*, 2001).

As originally published, in human subjective irritation assay volunteers were seated in the chamber (110°F (65°C) and 80 percent relative humidity) until a profuse facial sweating was observed (Frosch and Kligman, 1977a). Sweat was removed from the nasolabial fold and cheek; then a 5 percent aqueous solution of lactic acid was briskly rubbed over the area. Those who reported stinging for 3 to 5 minutes within the first 15 minutes were designated as stingers and were used for subsequent tests. Lammintausta *et al.* (1988) used a 15-min treatment with a commercial facial sauna to produce facial sweating. The facial sauna technique is less stressful to both subjects and investigators and produces similar results.

51.2.2   Allergic contact dermatitis

Although allergic contact dermatitis is the most frequently diagnosed reaction to cosmetics and its incidence is rising (Kohl *et al.*, 2002), it is clinically suspected initially in less than half the proven cases. Most cosmetics are a complex mixture containing perfumes, preservatives, stabilizers, lipids, alcohols, pigments, etc. Frequently, these components are responsible for cosmetic allergy (Ale and Maibach, 2001). The clinical relevance of allergic contact dermatitis has been described (Ale and Maibach, 1995).

Allergic contact dermatitis is cell-mediated. This type of skin response is often referred to as delayed type contact hypersensitivity because of the relatively long period (–24 h) required for the development of the inflammation following exposure. Lymphocytes are responsible for producing delayed-type hypersensitivity (DTH) and for regulation of the immune system. Lymphocytes leaving the lymphoid organs are "programmed" to recognize a specific chemical structure via a receptor molecule(s). If, during circulation through body tissues, a cell encounters the structure it is programmed to recognize, an immune response may be induced. To stimulate an immune response, a chemical must be presented to lymphocytes in an appropriate form (Landsteiner and Jacobs, 1935). Chemicals are usually haptens, which must conjugate with proteins in the skin or in other tissues in order to be recognized by the immune system. Haptens conjugate with proteins to form a number of different antigens that may stimulate an allergic response (Polak *et al.*, 1974). Hapten protein conjugates are processed by macrophages or other cells expressing proteins on their surface. Although the exact nature of this process is not completely understood, it is known that physical contact between macrophage and T cells is required (Unanue, 1984). In the skin, keratinocytes produce interleukin (Cunningham-Rundles, 1981), an important regulatory protein for induction of DTH. Langerhans cells express Ia antigen and may act as antigen presenting cells (Lever and Schaumberg-Lever, 1983). Histologically, the DTH response has been described as a hyperproliferative epidermis with intracellular edema, spongiosis, intraepidermal vesiculation, and mononuclear cell infiltrate by 24 h. The dermis shows perivenous accumulation of lymphocytes, monocytes, and edema. No reaction occurs if the local vascular supply is interrupted and the appearance of epidermal changes follows the invasion of monocytes. The histology of the response varies somewhat by species.

Many factors modulate development of DTH in experimental animals and humans. The method of skin exposure and rate of penetration influence the rate of sensitization, The effects of vehicle and occlusion are well documented (Magnussun and Kligman, 1970; Franklin, 2001). Vehicle choice determines in part the absorption of the test material and can influence sensitization rate, ability to elicit response at challenge, and the irritation threshold. Application of haptens to irritated or tape stripped skin, the dose per unit area, repeated applications to the same site (Magnussun and Kligman, 1969), increased numbers of exposures (this applies through 10–15 exposures only), an interval of 2–6 days between exposures (Magnussun and Kligman, 1969) and treatment with adjutant increase sensitization rates (Maguire, 1974). The development of DTH is under genetic control; all individuals do not have the capability to respond to a given hapten. In addition, the status of the immune system determines if an immune response can be induced. For example, young animals may become tolerant to a hapten, and pregnancy may suppress expression of allergy (Magnussun and Kligman, 1969). The intrinsic biological variables controlling sensitization can be influenced only by selection of animals likely to be capable of mounting an immune response to the hapten. Thresholds in contact sensitization using immunological models and experimental evidence have been described (Boukhman and Maibach, 2001). The extrinsic variables of dose, vehicle, route of exposure, adjuvant, etc., can be manipulated to develop sensitive predictive assays.

Appropriate execution of predictive sensitization assays is critical. All too often techniques are discredited when, in fact, the performance of the tests was inferior or study design, e.g., choice of dose, was inappropriate. A common error in choosing an animal assay is using Freund's complete adjuvant (FCA) when setting dose response relationships. The adjuvant provides such sensitivity that dose effect relationships are muted. Although the dose must be high enough to ensure penetration, it must be below the irritation threshold at challenge to avoid misinterpretation of irritant inflammation as allergic. For instance, the quaternary ammonium compounds, e.g., benzalkonium chloride, rarely sensitize but have been identified as allergens in some guinea pig assays. Knowing the irritation potential of compounds and choosing an appropriate experimental design will allow the investigator to design and execute these studies appropriately. John Draize developed the first practical animal assay to predict the proclivity of a chemical or a final product to produce allergic contact dermatitis. This test is widely used and forms the basis for current testing. Modifications to this test include the Buhler method, Freud's adjuvant, the Freud's complete adjuvant test and the open epicutaneous test. An extensive review of this assay is found in Maibach and Marzulli (1991). If done properly, these tests will identify most of the contact allergens. Human testing supplements animal testing but most sensitization studies have been done in animals

The Draize repeated insult patch test is the standard human assay to identify the propensity of a chemical to induce ACD Modifications to this test have been developed. A complete review of assays is found in Maibach and Marzulli (1991). Patch testing of patients with suspected cosmetic contact dermatitis is discussed later in this chapter, and the scientific basis of patch testing can be found in Ale and Maibach (2002). Recent Prevention and treatment of allergic contact dermatitis has been discussed (Wille and Kyclonieus, 2001).

51.2.3 Contact urticaria syndrome

Contact urticaria has been defined as a wheel-and-flare response that develops within 30 to 60 min after exposure of the skin to certain agents (von Krogh and Maibach, 1982). Symptoms of immediate contact reactions can be classified according to their morphology and severity. Itching, tingling, and burning with erythema is the weakest type of immediate contact reaction. Local wheel-and-flare with tingling and itching represents the prototype reaction of contact urticaria. Generalized urticaria after local contact is rare but can occur. Signs and symptoms in other organs can appear with the skin symptoms in cases of immunologic contact urticaria syndrome. This includes asthma, angioedema and anaphylaxis.

The strength of the reactions may greatly vary, and often the whole range of local symptoms—from slight erythema to strong edema and erythema—can be seen from the same substance if different concentrations are used in skin tests (Lahti and Maibach, 1980). Not only the concentration but also the site of the skin contact affects the reaction. A certain concentration of contact urticant may produce strong edema and erythema reactions on the skin of the back and face but only erythema on the volar surfaces of the lower arms or legs. In some cases, contact urticaria can be demonstrated only on damaged or previously eczematous skin. Some agents, such as formaldehyde, produce urticaria on healthy skin following repeated but not single applications to the skin. Differentiation between nonspecific irritant reactions and contact urticaria may be difficult. Strong irritants, e.g., hydrochloric acid, lactic acid, cobalt chloride, formaldehyde, and phenol, can cause clear-cut immediate whealing if the concentration is high enough, but the reactions do not usually fade away within a few hours. Instead, they are followed by signs of irritation; erythema, scaling, or crusting are seen 24 h later. Some substances have only urticant properties (e.g., benzoic acid, nicotinic acid esters). Diagnosis of immediate contact urticaria is based on a thorough history and skin testing with suspected substances. Skin tests for human diagnostic testing are summarized by Von Krogh and Maibach (1982), and patch testing and photopatch testing for contact urticaria has been described (Amin and Maibach, 2001). Because of the risk of systemic reactions, e.g., anaphylaxis, human diagnostic tests should only be performed by experienced personnel with facilities for resuscitation on hand. Contact urticaria has been divided into two main types on the basis of proposed pathophysiological mechanisms, nonimmunologic and immunologic (Maibach and Johnson, 1975). Recent reviews list agents suspected to cause each type of urticarial response (Lahti and Maibach, 1985; Harvel *et al.*, 1994). Some common urticants are listed in Table 51.1. A flow sheet designed by von Krogh and Maibach (1982) (46) can be used to approach testing in suspected cases (Table 51.2).

Nonimmunologic contact urticaria

Nonimmunologic contact urticaria is the most common form and occurs without previous exposure in most individuals. The reaction remains localized and does not cause systemic symptoms or spread to become generalized urticaria. Typically, the strength of this type of contact urticaria reaction varies from sensory complaints of sting, itch or burn to an urticarial response,

Table 51.1:

Some agents reported to cause urticaria in humans

Immunologic mechanisms
- Bacitracin
- Ethyl and methyl parabens
- Seafood (high molecular weight protein extracts)

Nonimmunologic mechanisms
- Cinnamic aldehyde
- Balsam of Peru
- Benzoic acid
- Ethyl aminobenzoate
- Dimethyl sulfoxide

Unknown mechanisms
- Epoxy resin
- Lettuce/endive
- Cassia oil
- Formaldehyde
- Ammonium persulfate
- Neomycin

Table 51.2:

Test procedures for evaluation of immediate-type reactions in recommended order

1. *Open application*
   - Nonaffected normal skin:
     Negative

   - Slightly affected (or previously affected) skin:
     Negative Positive → positive diagnosis

2. *Occlusive application (infrequently needed)*
   - Nonaffected normal skin:
     Negative

   - Slightly affected (or previously affected) skin:
     Negative

3. *Invasive (inhalant, prick, scratch, or intradermal injection)**

* When invasive methods are employed (especially scratch and inhalant testing) adequate controls are required.

depending on the concentration, skin site and substance. The mechanism of nonimmunologic contact urticaria has not been delineated, but a direct influence on dermal vessel walls or a non-antibody-mediated release of histamine prostaglandins, leukotrienes, substance P, or other inflammatory mediators represents possible mechanisms. Lahti and Maibach (1985) suggested that nonimmunologic urticaria produced by different agents may involve different combinations of mediators. Common non-immunological urticans can be inhibited by oral acetylsalicylic acid and indomethacin (Lahti *et al.*, 1983; 1986) and by topical dicloferac and naproxene gel, but not hydroxyzine or terfenadine (Lahti, 1987) and capsaicin. This suggests that prostaglandins and leukotrienes may play a role in the inflammatory response.

The most potent and best studied substances producing nonimmunologic contact urticaria are benzoic acid, cinnamic acid, cinnamic aldehyde, and nicotinic esters. Under optimal conditions, more than half of a random sample of individuals show local edema and erythema reactions within 45 min of application of these substances if the concentration is high enough. Benzoic acid and sodium benzoate are used as preservatives for cosmetics and other topical preparations at concentrations from 0.1 percent to 0.2 percent and are capable of producing immediate contact reactions at the same concentrations (Marzulli and Maibach, 1974). Cinnamic aldehyde at a concentration of 0.01 percent may elicit an erythematous response associated with a burning or stinging feeling in the skin. Mouthwashes and chewing gums contain cinnamic aldehyde at concentrations high enough to produce a pleasant tingling sensation in the mouth and enhance the sale of the product. Higher concentrations produce lip swelling or typical contact urticaria in normal skin. Eugenol in the mixture may inhibits contact sensitization to cinnamic aldehyde and inhibits nonimmunologic contact urticaria from this same substance, The mechanism of the putative quenching effect is not certain, but a competitive inhibition at the receptor level may be an explanation (Guin *et al.*, 1984). Provocative testing patients suspected of non-immunologic urticaria with individual ingredients such as benzoic acid, sorbic acid and sodium benzoate, commmon preservatives found in cosmetics, frequently will reproduce patients symptoms.

Immunologic contact urticaria

Immunologic contact unicaria is an immediate Type I allergic reaction in people previously sensitized to the causative agent (von Krogh and Maibach, 1982).

It is more prevalent in atopic patients than in non-atopic patients (Fisher, 1990). The molecules of a contact urticant react with specific IgE molecules attached to mast cell membranes. The cutaneous symptoms are elicited by vasoactive substances, i.e, histamine and others, released from mast cells. The role of histamine is conspicuous, but other mediators of inflammation, e.g., prostaglandins, leukotrienes, and kinins, may influence the degree of response. Immunologic contact urticaria reaction can extend beyond the contact site, and generalized urticaria may be accompanied by other symptoms, e.g., rhinitis, conjunctivitis, asthma, and even anaphylactic shock. The term "contact urticaria syndrome" was therefore suggested by Maibach and Johnson (1975). The name generally has been accepted for a symptom complex in which local urticaria occurs at the contact site with symptoms in other parts of the skin or in target organs such as the nose and throat, lung, and gastrointestinal and cardiovascular systems. Anaphylactic reactions may result from substances that induce a strong hypersensitivity response or easily absorbed from the skin (Lahti and Maibach, 1987). Fortunately, the appearance of systemic symptoms is less common than the localized form, but it may be seen in cases of strong hypersensitivity or in a widespread exposure and abundant percutaneous absorption of an allergen. Foods are common causes of immunologic contact urticaria (Table 51.1). The orolaryngeal area is a site where immediate contact reactions are frequently provoked by food allergens, most often among atopic individuals. The actual antigens are proteins or protein complexes. As a proof of immediate hypersensitivity, specific IgE antibodies against the causative agent can typically be found in the patient's serum using the RAST technique and skin test for immediate allergy. In addition, the prick test can demonstrate immediate allergy. The passive transfer test (Prausnitz-Kustner test) also often gives a positive result. This is now performed in the monkey rather than man.

51.2.4 Acne and comedones

Acnegenesis and comedogenesis are distinct but often related types of adverse skin reactions to facial, hair and other products. Acnegenesis refers to the chemical irritation and inflammation of the follicular epithelium with resultant loose hyperkeratotic material within the follicle and inflammatory pustules and papules. Comedogenesis refers to the noninflammatory follicular response that leads to dense compact hyperkeratosis of the follicle. Mills and Berger (1991) indicated that the time courses for the development of facial acne and comedones are different. While facial acne will appear in a matter of days, comedone formation in the human back and rabbit model takes longer to occur.

Classes of ingredients such as the lubricants isopropyl myristate and some analogs, lanolin and its derivatives, detergents, and D&C red dyes have been incriminated by the rabbit ear test (Fulton *et al.*, 1984). Fulton (1989) published a report about the comedogenicity and irritancy of commonly used cosmetics. Lists of comedogenic agents are not necessarily meaningful. Although they are important for pharmaceutical research and for the formulation of nonacnegenic products, they cannot alone predict the defects of the final product. The concentrations used in testing are often much greater than those in the final product. Thus it is possible to use concentrations that are lower that the minimal acnegenic level. In addition, the vehicles in finished products can increase or decrease the acnegenic potential of individual compounds. In the final analysis, what is important is the testing of the finished product for its acnegenic and irritancy potential. When only inadequate data are available, elimination regimen remains the only constructive approach to treat patients with suspected acne or comedones secondary to cosmetic use.

The rabbit ear assay is the mayor predictive animal model available. Kligman and Mills (1972) developed the value of testing cosmetics and its ingredients by the rabbit ear assay. However, several improvements in the model have been proposed (Tucker *et al.*, 1986). The test is not standardized. The AAD Invitational Symposium on Comedogeninity Panel (1989) suggested some guidelines for maximizing the usefulness of the rabbit ear model.

In 1972, Kligman and Mills showed production of microcomedones in the backs of black men after testing cosmetics with occlusion. One test for evaluating comedogenicity in humans is the occlusive-patch application to the back followed by a cyanoacrylate follicular biopsy as described by Mills and Kligman (1982). The test material previously positive in the rabbit ear assay is applied for 4 weeks under occlusion to the upper portion of the back of people with large follicles. This test needs refinement. However, if this occlusive patch test is negative, it provides additional assurance that the test material may be nonacnegenic.

Bronaugh and Maibach (1982) reported that results of the rabbit ear test correlate well with pustule formation noted in use tests of cosmetics performed on women's faces. They noted that some cosmetics may produce papulopustules after 3 to 7 days of use. The products were strongly positive in the rabbit ear model. This may represent a manifestation of primary irritancy. Correlative studies with rabbit pustulogenicity assay should be performed. The acute onset papulopustules are often described by the patient as a "breakout." The cause and effect relationship to cosmetics is strong but is often missed by the dermatologist. Jackson and Robillard (1982) proposed the ordinary clinical-usage test. This test, conducted for 4–6 weeks, may not provide reliable information on comedogenesis. However, follicular inflammation may be noted within 1 to 2 weeks of applications done twice a day to the face of people with acne-prone oily skin.

It is not known how long the applications need to be continue to observe true comedogenesis. Clinical observations should be done at least weekly for the first 2 weeks of using the product to detect folliculitis. The acute papulo-pustular form will be identified in short term testing (days, in contradistinction to months). However, to conclusively incriminate cosmetics as a cause of comedonal acne, long-term testing using a single cosmetic on the faces of women will have to be conducted and the disease produced. Lines of cosmetics will ideally be manufactured which are screened with an appropriate rabbit ear test and then tested definitively in panels of acne-prone women for long term.

Wahlberg and Maibach (1981) attempted to brige the gap between comedo identified in the rabbit ear assay and the more common acute papulo-pustule by developing an animal model. The rabbit's back is pierced with a needle and dosed topically. The resulting lesion closely resembles that seen in man. Unfortunately, for several reasons including reluctance to performed animal testing, identification of acnegenicity premarketing remains a weak link in the of dermatotoxicology. The lesion occurs not only from cosmetics ingredients but also from topical and systemic drugs.

51.2.5 Pigmentation

Hyperpigmentation of the face caused by contact dermatitis to ingredients in cosmetics occurs more frequently in dark complexioned individuals (Rorsman, 1982). An epidemic of facial pigmentation reported in Japanese women was attributed to "coal tar" dyes principally Sudan I, a contaminant of D&C Red No. 31 (Kozuka et al., 1980). The following fragrance ingredients have also been implicated-benzyl salicylate, ylang-ylang oil, cananga oil, jasmin abso-lute, hydroxycitronellal, methoxycitronellal, sandalwood oil, benzyl alcohol, cinnanuc alcohol, lavender oil, geraniol, and geranium oil (Nakayama et al., 1976). Histologic examination shows hydropic degeneration of the basal layer, pigment incontinence and little evidence of inflammation (Lahti and Maibach, 1987). Mathias (1982) reported pigmented cosmetic contact dermatitis due to contact allergy to chromium hydroxide used as a dye in toilet soap, and Maibach (1978) reported hyperpigmentation in a black man sensitive to petrolatum. Dermatologists should search scrupulously for a causative agent in patients with hyperpigmentation. Eliminating the product results frequently in gradual fading of the pigment. Unfortunatly, until a predictive assay is 14 identified, most patients will be incorrectly indentified as idiopathic.

Cosmetic chemicals have infrequently been associated with leukoderma. Nater and de Groot (1985) and de Groot (1988) listed chemicals associated with leukoderma. Recently, Taylor and colleagues (1993) added seven more chemicals. Although Riley (1971) reported that low concentrations of butylated hydroxyanisole were toxic in culture guinea pig melanocytes, Gellin *et al.* (1979) could not induce depigmentation in guinea pigs or black mice by appying butylated hydroxyanisole. In addition, Maibach and colleagues (1975) were unable to produce depigmentation after a 60-day occlusive application of hydroxytoluene to darkly pigmented men. The Cosmetic Ingredient Review panel (1984) concluded that is safe to use BHA in the present practices of use.

Hydroquinone has produced depigmentation in humans. Although it is a weak depigmenter at 2 percent concentration, it is a stronger depigmenter at higher concentrations and with different vehicles. Hydroquinone, used as a bleaching agent, has caused postinflammatory hyperpigmentation in South African Blacks. Findlay *et al.* (1975) from South Africa reported a long-term complication of the use of hydroquinone-deposits of ochronotic pigment in the skin along with colloid milia. The melanocyte, despite intense hydro-quinone use, escaped destruction and the site of the injury shifted to the dermis and the fibroblast. Polymeric pigment adhered to thickened, abnormal collagen bundles. In 1983, Cullison *et al.* reported that an American black woman developed this complication after intense use of a 2 percent hydroquinone cream. Prolonged use of hydroquinone followed by sun exposure may lead to exogenous ochronosis with colloid milium production. In addition, a few cases of persistent hypopigmentation have incriminated topical hydroquinone (Fisher, 1983). Pyrocatechol has similar structure and effects to hydroquinone. The most frequent use of hydroquinone and pyrocatechols is in rinse-off type hair dyes and colors in which the use concentration is 1 percent concen-tration or less. The Cosmetic Ingredient Review panel declared hydroquinone and pyrocatechol safe for cosmetic use at 1 percent concentration or less. Monobenzyl ether of hydroquinone is a potent depigmenting agent and is not approved for cosmetic use in the United States. The only approved use for monobenzyl ether of hydroquinone is as a therapeutic agent for patients with vitiligo. P-hydroxyanisole is a potent depigmenting agent in black guinea pigs at concentrations near ones used in cosmetics. It may cause depigmentation at distant sites from application in humans.

Angenilli and co-worker (1993) reported depigmentation of the lip margins from p-tertiary butyl phenol in a lip liner. The p-tertiary butyl phenol patch test site also depigmented and the presence of p-tertiary butyl phenol was confirmed by gas chromatography with mass spectroscopy. Most recently, Taylor and co-workers (1993) reported four cases of chemical leukoderma associated with the application of semipermanent and permanent hair colors and rinses. They identified benzyl alcohol and paraphenylenediamine in three of the four cases. Depigmentation occurred at the hair color patch test sites in three of the four cases.

Mathias *et al.* (1980) reported perioral leukoderma in a patient who used a cinnamic aldehyde-containing toothpaste. Wilkenson and Wilkin (1990) reported that azelaic acid is a weak depigmenter and its esters do not depigment pigmented guinea pig skin.

51.2.6 Photosensitivity

Contact photosensitivity results from UV-induced excitation of a chemical applied to the skin. Contact photosensitivity is divided into phototoxic and photoallergic reactions. Phototoxic reactions may be experienced by any individual, provided that ultraviolet light contains the appropriate wave lengths to activate the compound and that the UV dose and the concentration of the photoreactive chemical are high enough. Clinically, it consists of erythema followed by hyperpigmentation and desquamation. Sunburn is the most common phototoxic reaction. However, photoallergic reactions require a period of sensitization. The reactions are usually delayed, manifesting days to weeks or years after the UV exposure. The major problem with photoallergic reactions is that the patient may develop persistent light reaction for many years after the chemical has been removed. These patients tend to be exquisitely sensitive to the sun and usually have very low UV-B and UVA minimal erythema doses. With the exception of the epidemic caused by halogenated salicylanides in soap in the 1960s, photosensitivity accounts for a small number of cosmetic adverse reactions. Maibach and colleagues (1988) reported only nine of 713 patients with photoallergic and photosensitive reactions. Musk ambrette, a fragrance in some aftershaves, has been reported as a major cause of cosmetic photosensitivity reactions.

Predictive testing in human skin is not always definitive. In the 1960s, identification of TCSA and related phenolic compounds was accomplished by photopatch testing clinically involved patients. Subsequently, Willis and Kligman (1968) induced contact photoallergy to certain agents in normal human subjects using a modification of the maximization test which was developed for evaluating the potential of chemicals to produce contact dermatitis (Kligman, 1966).

Kaidbey and Kligman (1980) and Kaidbey (1983) modified the photo-maximization procedure. They were able to sensitize normal human volunteers readily to certain methylated coumarins derivatives, e.g., TCSA, 3,5-DBS, chlorpromazine and sodium omadine. A smaller number of positive induction responses was noted with TBS contaminated with 47 percent DBS, 4,5-DBS, Jadit and bithionol. Negative results were obtained with para-aminobenzoic (PABA) and musk ambrette, which have produced photoallergic contact dermatitis clinically. To date there is no proven effective predictive testing model for photoallergic contact dermatitis in that most of the known photo-allergens have been identified clinically and not in toxicologic assays. Furthermore, the refinement of risk assessment (not hazard identification) may be difficult, e.g., sodium omadine is positive in the assay but not yet clinically in spite of extensive use.

Photopatch testing

The criteria for separating allergic contact and allergic photocontact dermatitis utilizing patch-testing techniques are imprecise. General criteria and their interpretation are listed in Table 51.3. Often, the results are not all-or-none, as implied in the table. Frequently, there is a difference in response intensity, with either the contact or photocontact response being greater. All too infrequently serial dilutions are performed with either the putative antigen or the amount of ultraviolet light employed. Until a significant number of patients are so studied, it will be unclear how many of them represent contact versus photocontact sensitization.

Wennersten et al. (1986) recommended that patients with suspected photocontact allergy be phototested prior to implementation of patch testing. The aim of this preliminary light testing is to detect any abnormal sensitivity to UVA and UVB wavebands. It is generally agreed that UVA sources are adequate and sufficient to elicit responses, an important convenience as UVA does not produce erythema in normal fair-skinned subjects until a dose of

Table 51.3:

Patch and photopatch testing

Contact test site response	Photocontact test site response	Interpretation
Positive	Positive	Allergic contact dermatitis
Negative	Positive	Photoallergic dermatitis
Negative	Negative	Non sensitized

20–30 J/cm^2 is delivered. High doses of UVA such as 10–15J/cm^2 for photopatch testing are unnecessary. Such doses increase the possibility of adverse reactions and increase the incidence of phototoxic reactions. Despite widespread use, there is little standardization in the UVA dosage used in photopatch testing. Doses may range from 1J/cm^2–15J/cm^2 at various centers (Holzle *et al.*, 1988). The Scandinavian Photodermatitis Group was the first to formulate a protocol using 5 J/cm^2 of UVA in photosensitive patients, half their UVA MED for the prodedure. Most photoallergies will be defined with a far smaller dose (e.g. 1 J/cm^2). Duguid *et al.* (1993) showed that positive responses occur at 1.0, 1.0 and 0.7 J/cm^2 for Eusolex 8020, benzophenone-10 and benzophenone-3 respectively. In addition Duguid and coworkers (1993) confirmed the adequacy of 5 J/cm^2 or less as a photoelicitation dose. Although some data on the dose of light required to elicit a response exists, this remains incomplete and must be studied in context with the dose of antigen and the vehicle. Until the light and antigenic intensities are more fully defined, most physicians utilize a PUVA unit, a bank of UVA bulbs in a diagnostic unit or a hot quartz (Kromayer) unit, with an appropriate filter to remove any light with wavelengths below 320 nm (UVB). The effect of UV irradiation on photopatch test substances *in vitro* has been reported by Bruze *et al.* (1985). It appears that 5 J of UVA is almost always adequate. All thirteen photoactive compounds formed photoproducts after UVA irradiation; eight substances were decomposed by both UVA and UVB radiation; five by UVA alone. It is also possible that some patients may require UVB to elicit photoallergic dermatitis. However, since UVB testing is not done routinely, it may be some time before this is clarified. Epstein (1963) observed that many patients are so sensitive to light that the dose delivered under an ordinary patch will elicit reactions. He provided details of testing the nonexposed site, utilizing a large light-impermeable black patch applied in a dimly lit room.

■ CHAPTER 51 ■

Commercial sources of appropriately diluted sunscreen antigens are not presently available in the United States. On request, many thoughtful manufacturers provide patch-test kits of individual ingredients for their products. A "standard" series of sunscreen antigens has been proposed by the International Contact Dermatitis Research Group (ICDRG). In Europe, these test kits are commercially available. These sunscreen antigens are available in 2 percent concentrations, although the maximum nonirritating doses of putative antigens in a given vehicle have not been defined. Maibach *et al.* (1980) and de Groot (1994) reported the test concentrations and vehicles for the dermatological testing of many cosmetic ingredients that may be in sunscreen formulations. We currently lack adequate virgin controls for the high concentrations used in contemporary formulations. When high concentrations are required to elicit allergic contact dermatitis, an impurity or a photoproduct may be the actual allergen.

The specific vehicle in which the allergens are dissolved or suspended is important (Fisher and Maibach, 1986; Tanglersampan and Maibach, 1993). The ICDRG list employs petrolatum as diluent. This vehicle appears to be adequate to elicit reactions in many patients. It is clear, however, that the bioavailability of the antigen may be too limited in some cases. Thus Mathias *et al.* (1978) required ethanol to demonstrate PABA sensitivity, and Schauder and Ippen (1988) noted more pronounced test reactions to avobenzone in isopropylmyristate than petrolatum. This topic remains an area of investigation. Presumably each ingredient may require an optimal vehicle and concentration for eliciting a reaction.

Some patients develop dermatitis that appears allergic or photoallergic in a morphologic and historic sense, yet fails to demonstrate a positive patch or photopatch test, in spite of seemingly appropriate testing. Such false-negative reactions are more difficult to identify than false positive reactions (Rycroft, 1986). Table 51.4 provides the basic strategy employed in attempting to help these patients. Unfortunately, in some patients, even these extensive work-ups fail to elicit the etiology of their reactions.

Many of the reported positives test to date, and especially the cross-reaction studies, may well represent false-positives due to the Excited Skin Syndrome. This state of skin hyperirritability often induced by a concomitant dermatitis is responsible for many nonreproducible patch tests. Bruynzeel and Maibach (1986) detail strategies for minimizing such false-positives.

Table 51.4:

Strategy for identifying the cause when routine patch testing is negative

Intervention	Comment
Increase UVA dose	Avoid UVA erythema Use UVA control
Increase concentration of sunscreen	Upper limit of nonirritating dose not completely defined
Alter vehicle	Ethanol has been found to be effective
Test other components	Sunscreen manufactures often helpful in providing test kits
Add suberythemogenic doses of UVB	
Perform provocative-use test on final formulation	
Consider "compound" allergy	

51.2.7 Nail changes

Paronychia, onycholysis (Draelos, 2001), nail destruction and discoloration are some of the most common cosmetic adverse reactions found in the nails. The physician should obtain a detailed description of the nail grooming habits in patients who have paronychia, onycholysis, nail destruction, or nail discoloration because any of these problems may be caused by nail cosmetic usage. Nail discoloration has been reported with the use of hydroquinone bleaching creams and hair dyes containing henna (Fitzpatrick *et al.*, 1966; Samman, 1977).

51.2.8 Hair changes

Permanents and hair straighteners are intended to break the disulfide bonds that give hair keratin its strength. Improper usage or incomplete neutralization of these cosmetics causes hair breakage. Hair that has been damaged by previous applications of permanent waves, straighteners, oxidation type dyes, bleaches, or excessive exposure to sunlight and chlorine is more susceptible to this damage. The dermatologist should always take a complete history in these cases, including a detailed account of the use of drugs, to detect any causes of telogen or anagen effluvium. Careful examination of the hair shafts is essential to detect any pre-existing abnormalities. Saving a sample of these hairs in the patient

CHAPTER 51

record may be invaluable should litigation against the beautician or supplier occur (Whitmore and Maibach, 1984).

51.3 INGREDIENT PATCH TESTING

The diagnosis and treatment of reactions to cosmetics has been facilitated by the Food and Drug Administration's (FDA) regulation (1975) requiring the ingredient labeling of all retailed cosmetics.

The European Community has also endorsed such labeling. The ingredients are listed in order of descending concentration. Because of the complexity of the composition of fragrances, their compositions are not given but are listed simply as "fragrance." The regulation was designed to aid the consumer in identifying ingredients at the time of purchase; therefore, the list is often placed on the outer package, which may be discarded, rather than the container. Correspondence with the manufacturer or a trip to the cosmetic counter, however, can bring the needed information. This regulation, besides identifying ingredients, is helpful to dermatologists because it mandated a uniform nomenclature for cosmetic ingredients. The CTFA *Ingredient Dictionary* published by the Cosmetic Toiletries and Fragrance Association (1993) is the source for the official names This dictionary provides a brief description of the chemical, alternative names, and names of suppliers: Without this key reference book the dermatologist is at a distinct disadvantage in advising patients in this area.

The standard screening patch test tray includes some ingredients that are allergens found in cosmetics (De Groot, 2000). Imidazolidinyl urea, diazalidinyl urea, thimerosal, formaldehyde, and quaternium 15 are preservatives. Patch testing balsam of Peru screens for approximately 50 percent of the known allergic reactions to fragrance in the United States. Colophony and its constituents are used in the manufacture of eye cosmetics, transparent soap, and dentifrice (Rapaport, 1980). If a patient has a positive patch-test reaction to one of these chemicals, clinicians should consider allergic contact dermatitis to cosmetics a possible diagnosis. We emphasize that cosmetic contact dermatitis can often be unsuspected. Any positive patch tests should be interpreted cautiously because many cosmetics are mild irritants and Excited Skin State may cause false positive results. Ideally, a positive patch test should should be confirmed with a repeat test several weeks later or with a provocative-use test. Reassessment of the patient's history and presenting findings and patch testing with the patient's cosmetics may establish the diagnosis.

Once a product or products has been implicated with patch testing, pin pointing the offending ingredient is an important part of the work-up so that the patient may spare recurring reactions. Cosmetic ingredient patch testing is complicated because the proper concentration for closed patch testing is known only for a small percentage of these ingredients. Patch test concentrations and vehicles has been proposed for less than 450 of the nearly 2000 cosmetic ingredients listed (Bruze *et al.*, 1985). The texts by Nater and de Groot (1993) and by Cronin (1980) are important sources for clinicians seeking information on cosmetic ingredient patch testing.

Screening fragrance trays provides the most common fragrance allergens in the United States. Further information for patch testing fragrance ingredients is reviewed in several articles (Larsen, 2000; Launder and Kansky, 2000). When the clinical history, appearance of the reaction, or patch test results lead the clinician to conclude that a cosmetic has caused an adverse reaction, it is important to obtain the ingredients for patch testing. The Cosmetic, Toiletry, and Fragrance Association publishes a pamphlet called "Cosmetic Industry On Call." This pamphlet lists the names of members of the industry who are willing to answer questions about their products. Physicians can contact these persons requesting specific ingredients for patch testing and information about patch-test concentrations. If the patient does or does not prove to have a reaction due to the cosmetics, the manufacturer should be notified of your results. Manufacturers will not always send materials for patch testing, and the patient cannot be treated successfully and counseled on how to avoid recurrences. On occasion "fractionated" samples will be sent for patch testing. Because irritant concentrations of ingredients may be present in these samples, they are often not suitable to use for closed patch testing. Some manufacturers will supply individual ingredients in the concentration that they appear in the product. These are often unsatisfactory for patch testing because the nonstandardized concentrations may be too low to provoke an allergic response or may be high enough to elicit irritation under occlusion.

51.4 COSMETIC PRODUCTS

51.4.1 Preservatives

After fragrances, preservatives are the next most common cause of cosmetic reactions (Adams and Maibach, 1985). The ten most frequently used preservatives are listed in Table 51.5 (FDA, 1993). A large number of specific studies

Table 51.5:

Preservative frequency of use (FDA data)*

Chemical Name	No. of products using chemical
Methylparaben	6738
Propylparaben	5400
Propylene glycol	3922
Citric acid	2317
Imidazolidinyl urea	2312
Butylparaben	1669
Butylated hydroxyanisole (BHA)	1669
Butylated hydroxytoluene (BHT)	1610
Ethylparaben	1213
5-Choro-2-methyl-4-isothiazolin-3-one (methylchloroisothiazoline)	1042

* Adapted from preservative frequency of use. Cosmetic and Toiletries (1993) 108: 97–98

have focused on individual preservatives as being identified as potential sensitizers and directly responsible for a number of adverse reactions.

Paraben Esters (Methyl, Propyl, Butyl, and Ethyl) are nontoxic and nonirritating, preservatives that protect well against gram-positive bacteria and fungi, but poorly against several gram-negative bacteria including pseudomonads (White *et al.*, 1982). Parabens, the most widely used preservatives in topical products, have long been known to be contact allergens, when at relatively high concentrations and at a low frequency (Schubert *et al.*, 1990). However, their potential for being the causative agents in cosmetic adverse reactions has not diminished their use, and in fact, it is on the increase. Fortunately, parabens compared to total use (tons × years) have a remarkable safety record. Although parabens may be sensitizers occasionally when applied to eczematous skin, cosmetics containing parabens infrequently cause clinical difficulties when they are applied to normal skin. Fisher (1980a) called this phenomenon the "paraben paradox." It is not known how often this phenomenon represents the Excited Skin State (due to high concentration of paraben in the patch-test mixture) rather than the paraben paradox.

Imidazolidinyl Urea (Germall 115) has low toxicity and is nonirritating. It has a broad antimicrobial activity especially when used in combination with parabens. Although formaldehyde is released on hydrolysis, the levels are too low to cause reactions in many formaldehyde-sensitive patients clinically or during patch testing. Diazolidinyl urea is a related preservative, whose use is increasing.

Quaternium-15 is active against bacteria but less active against yeast and molds. It is a formaldehyde releaser. A patient who has simultaneous positive patch test readings to quaternium-15 and formaldehyde should be studied carefully, as this may require special instructions. The patient may be allergic to both ingredients or sensitive only to formaldehyde reacting to its release by this preservative in the occlusive patch test. In the latter situation, quaternium-15 may or may not be tolerated by the patient when present in cosmetics at a 0.02 to 0.3 percent concentration. A product use test should clarify the situation. A negative test relates to the product tested and not to all products due to differences in bioavailability.

Formaldehyde as a preservative is used almost exclusively in wash-off products such as shampoos. Used in this manner, formaldehyde is seldom a cause of sensitization in the consumer and is only infrequently problematic for the beautician (Lynde and Mitchell, 1982; Bruynzeel *et al.*, 1984).

Bronopol (2-Bromo-2-nitropropane-1,3-diol) has a broad spectrum of activity, most effective against bacteria. It is a formaldehyde releaser and may pose a problem for the formaldehyde-sensitive patient. In addition, this preservative may interact with amines or amides to produce nitrosamines or nitroamides: suspected carcinogens. Patch testing with standard concentrations may produce marginal irritations responses. Positives are best retested and if positive followed by a provocative use test.

Benzoisothiazides have developed great popularity as preservatives. Kathon CG (5-chloro-2-methyl-4-isothiazolin-3-one and 2-methyl-4-isothiazolin-3-one) has been a preservative of choice by many formulators because of its broad application and ease of formulation it is incorporated in many popular rinse off products, and some leave on cosmetics under concentration restrictions. In spite of inducing sensitivity in guinea pigs at levels down to 25 ppm and elicitation levels down to 100 ppm and less, this preservative has infrequently produced sensitization from shampoo usage (Chan *et al.*, 1983). Methylchoroisothiazolinone and methylisothiazolinone has been the subject of several adverse reaction investigations. It has shown significant rates of sensitization at concentrations from 2 to 5 percent (Shuster and Shapiro, 1976; Hjorth and Roed-Peterson, 1986; Patcher and Hunziker, 1989). Diagnostic testing should be performed at 100 ppm in water bacause 300 ppm in water induces active sensitization (Bjorker and Fregert, personal communication). Possibly 150–200 ppm might be more appropiate, but this requires additional study.

■ CHAPTER 51 ■

51.4.2 Preservation of the future

The cosmetic industry experiences two major challenges: the elimination of all animal testing and the development of preservative-free cosmetics. In recent years, a strong socio-economic pressure has focused interest and research on developing preservative free products and preservation based upon natural extracts. Both of these approaches while seemingly sound scientifically and from a marketing position, are fraught with problems. Natural preservatives are often complex mixtures with many unknown chemicals. It is likely that some of these active materials may present with sensitization rates equal or greater than synthetic materials. The Sixth Amendment of the EC Cosmetic Directive has called for the elimination of all animal testing of personal care products and ingredients by 2002, unless alternative methods cannot be developed by then. While most new raw materials will be able to use new, alternative safety testing methods, preservatives will experience difficulty complying with existing requirements for chronic safety studies such as mutagenicity and teratogenicity, without relying on animals. Almost all regulatory agencies currently require the use of *in vivo* methods to confirm the safely of biocidal ingredients. *In vitro* tests will most likely be used first as prescreening test. At the present time, this may reduce the need for some animal testing. However, it is unlikely that all *in vivo* methods of biocide safety will be replaced in the short term. Before *in vitro* assays can replace animal testing they should be validated against the known *in vivo* testing. This is an unfortunate drawback of increasing the safety testing cost since the cost of acute *in vitro* testing is as high as acute *in vivo*.

51.4.3 Emulsifiers

Creams and lotions require the presence of an emulsifier to allow the combination of water and oil. Emulsifiers may act as mild irritants especially if applied to slightly damaged skin. Pugliese (1983) suggested that increased epidermal cell renewal or "plumping" of the skin may be due to mild irritant effects of nonionic surfactants. Hannuksela *et al.* (1976) patch tested over 1200 eczematous patients with common emulsifiers.

Another emulsifier, stearamidoethyl diethylamine phosphate, has been implicated in four cases of cosmetic contact dermatitis (Taylor *et al.*, 1984). Irritant reactions are seen at the same concentration as allergic responses. When 5 percent triethanolamine stearate in petrolatum was tested, 9.5 percent of the patch tests showed irritant reactions. Even positive reactions to 1 percent triethanolamine in petrolatum should be confirmed by retesting and the provocative-use testing.

51.4.4 Lanolin

Lanolin is a mixture of esters and polyesters of high molecular weight alcohols and fatty acids. This naturally occurring wax varies in its composition depending on its source. Adams and Maibach (1985) reported in the NACDG study that lanolin and its derivatives remains among the ingredients that most commonly cause allergic contact dermatitis in cosmetics. Because of its superior emollient properties, lanolin is a popular ingredient for cosmetics.

Sulzberger *et al.* (1953) patch tested over 1000 patients suspected of having contact dermatitis, 1 percent reacted to anhydrous lanolin. The allergen or allergens which have not been identified are found in the alcoholic fraction of lanolin. Patch testing is done most accurately using 30 percent wool alcohols in petrolatum. Kligman (1983) tested 943 healthy young women with hydrous lanolin and 30 percent wool wax alcohol. The results were interpreted as follows: no positive allergic patch tests were read, but irritant reactions to wool alcohols were common. Clark *et al.* (1981) estimated that the incidence of lanolin allergy in the general population is 5.5 per million. Lanolin is an important sensitizer when it is applied to eczematous skin eruptions, especially stasis dermatitis. However, cosmetics containing lanolin applied to normal skin are generally harmless. Cronin (1980) reported only 26 cases of lanolin-cosmetic dermatitis seen between 1966 to 1976 in women.

In all of these cases, the lanolin-cosmetic dermatitis affected the face at some time during its course; almost half showed eyelid involvement. The history was of intermittent eruptions often with swelling and edema.

51.4.5 Eye makeup preparations

Mascara, eyeliner, eye shadow, and eyebrow pencil or powders are the most commonly used eye-area makeups. The upper eyelid dermatitis syndrome is complex and often frustrating to the patient and dermatologist, because of chronicity and failure to respond to our well-intentioned assistance. Causes that we have documented included in Table 51.6.

Although patients often consider this a reaction to eye makeup, the association is seldom proven. In the North American Contact Dermatitis Group study 12 percent of the cosmetic reactions occurred on the eyelid but only 4

Table 51.6:

Some causes of upper-eyelid dermatitis syndrome

- Irritant dermatitis
- Allergic contact dermatitis
- Photoallergic contact dermatitis
- Phototoxic dermatitis
- Contact urticaria
- Seborrheic dermatitis
- Rosacea diathesis
- Psoriasis
- Collagen vascular diseases
- Conjunctivitis
- Blepharitis
- Dysmorphobia

percent of the reactions were attributed to eye makeup (Adams and Maibach, 1985). A workup of patients with eyelid dermatitis includes a careful history of all cosmetic usage, because facial, hair, and nail cosmetic reactions appear frequently on the eyelids (Sher, 1979). Reactions to cosmetics on the eyelid are often the irritant type; and to further complicate their diagnosis, they may be due to cumulative irritancy—the summation of several, mild irritants (climatic, mechanical, or chemical).

When the history does not clearly incriminate certain cosmetics, test with the screening patch-test trays as well as all cosmetics that may reach the eye area directly or indirectly. Occlusive patch tests with eyeliner or mascara may give an irritant reaction, thus weakly positive results are interpreted cautiously. Waterproof mascaras must be dried thoroughly for 20 minutes to volatilize hydrocarbon solvents before occluding, and even with this precaution. Epstein (1965) noted some irritant reactions. Positive patch tests are repeated for confirmation, and individual ingredient patch testing should be carried out whenever possible. Patch testing cosmetics used in the eye area may occasionally give false-negative results when testing is done on the back or extremities (Sher, 1979). A provocative use test performed in the antecubital fossa or the eyelid itself may ultimately prove the diagnosis.

In the United States, the pigments used in eye area cosmetics are restricted. No coal-tar derivatives may be incorporated; only purified natural colors or inorganic pigment or lakes of low allergic potential are used. Nickel contamination of iron oxide pigments has been implicated as a cause of allergic reaction to these cosmetics in the nickel-sensitive user (Van Ketel and Liem, 1981). Eye cosmetics are seldom fragranced, but other known allergens are used in these cosmetics. Almost all eye area cosmetics are preserved with parabens combined with a second preservative such as phenyl mercuric acetate, imidazolidinyl urea, quaternium-15, or potassium sorbate. The following antioxidants are sensitizers found in eye cosmetics: butylated hydroxytoluene, butylated hydroxyanisole (Turner, 1977), propyl gallate (Cronin, 1980), ditert-butyl hydroquinone (Calnan, 1973), resins: colophony (Cronin, 1980) and dihydroabietyl alcohol (Doons-Gossens *et al.*, 1979), bismuth oxychloride (Eierman *et al.*, 1982), and lanolin (Schorr, 1973). Propylene glycol may act as an irritant or sensitizer. Soap emulsifiers, surfactants, and solvents are all potential irritants used in these cosmetics. Allergic contact dermatitis from shellac (Le Coz *et al.*, 2002), prime yellow carnauba wax and coathylene (Chowdhury, 2002), and black iron oxide (Saxena *et al.*, 2001) found in mascara has been reported.

Infected corneal ulcers due to abrasions from mascara resulted when the mascaras were not properly preserved (Wilson *et al.*, 1979). These preservation problems appear to be solved and reports of infected corneal ulcers have decreased. Patients should be urged to use their eye cosmetics hygienically and advised not to use eye cosmetics inside the lash line.

51.4.6 Hair preparations (non-coloring)

Permanents

Permanent waves are cosmetics that alter the disulfide bonds of hair keratin so that hair fiber configuration can be changed. The disulfide bonds of cystine are broken in the first step when the waving solution is applied to the hair wound around mandrels. In the second step, with neutralization, new disulfide bonds are formed by locking in the curl configuration of the hair.

The waving solutions contain reducing agents that can cause irritant reactions when allowed to run incautiously on the skin surrounding the scalp. Irritant reactions range from erythema to bullous dermatitis. Hair breakage and loss may result when permanent waves are used improperly—in too concentrated a form, for too long a time, or on hair previously damaged by dyes, straighteners, or permanent waves. Old-fashioned hot waves occasionally caused chemical burns, which scarred the scalp producing permanent alopecia, but modern permanents can cause breakage, which results in temporary loss.

In 1973, "acid permanents" were introduced for beauty salon use (Brauer, 1984). Acid permanents are the most widely used perm preparation today. These waving lotions, which contain anhydrous glyceryl monothioglycolate in acid form, are mixed at the time of application with a water-based ammonium hydroxide solution to produce a neutral solution. The hair is covered with a plastic cap and placed under a hair dryer. Since the introduction of "acid perms," irritant and allergic reactions have been noted to occur on the hands of hairdressers and the face, neck, scalp, and hair line of their customers from use of these permanents (Storrs, 1984). Patch testing can be carried out with 1.0 percent glyceryl thioglycolate (glyceryl monothioglycolate) in petrolatum or water (freshly prepared).

When clients are suspected of contact sensitization, glyceryl mono-thioglycolate (GMT) is one of the most likely sensitizers. Frosch *et al.* (1993) stated that sensitization seems to be much less frequent in clients than in hairdressers due to less exposure.; this was evident with ammonium persulfate (APS) (0 percent in clients versus 8 percent in hairdressers) Guerra *et al.* (1992) studied 261 hairdresser's clients and reported similar results. They reported the mean frequencies of sensitization as follows: p-phenylenediamine (PPD) 7 percent, O-nitro-p-phenylenediamine (ONPPD) 5 percent, GMT 3 percent ammonium thioglycolate (AMT) 1 percent and APS 3 percent. Morrison and Storrs (1988) indicated that the identification of GMT sensitization in a patient is of particular importance, as the clinical symptoms may continue for months even if the use of acid permanents waves is stopped. The allergen clings to the hair and during shampooing, it is liberated in sufficient amounts to maintain the dermatitis. This may elicit dermatitis on the face and neck, which may be confused with allergy or irritancy to shampoo. The operational definition for allergic contact dermatitis has not been fulfilled. It is likely that most if not all patch test reactions are irritant rather than allergic.

The "cold waves" contain thioglycolic acid combined with ammonia or another alkali to raise the pH. The concentration of the thioglycolic acid and alkali can be varied to change the products' speed of action or to suit the type of hair to be waved, i.e., hard to wave, normal, or easy to wave. The neutralizer contains hydrogen peroxide or sodium bromate. These permanents have been alleged to rarely cause allergic reactions. Ammonium thioglycolate can be patch tested as 1 or 2.5 percent in petrolatum (FDA, 1975). Positives should be confirmed with serial dilution patch testing and provocative use testing. Another type of permanent used primarily at home is the sulfite wave. Although the sulfite wave produces less strong curls and is slower, the odor is more pleasant. Neutralization is done usually with bromates. Occasional allergic reactions have been alleged with these permanents. It is recommended to use 1 percent sodium bisulfite in water for patch testing (Schorr, 1983).

Straighteners

Straightening hair involves using a heated comb with petrolatum or a mixture of petrolatum, oils, and waxes. The petrolatum or "pressing oils" act as a heat modifying conductor, which reduces friction when the comb travels down the hair fibers. Mechanical and heat damage can cause hair breakage. Over the years, the heated oils can injure the hair follicles leading to scarring alopecia.

Chemical straighteners containing sodium hydroxide, "lye," cleave the disulfide bonds of keratin thoroughly and straighten hair permanently. Experience and caution in applying these straighteners are important to avoid hair breakage and chemical burns. Similar products that contain guanidine carbonate mixed with calcium hydroxide are reputed to be milder. It is necessary to straighten new growth every several months. Care is taken not to "double process" the distal hair, which is already straightened. Some manufacturers advise against using permanent hair colors that require peroxide on chemically straightened hair to avoid damage. Sulfite straighteners, chemically similar to sulfite permanents, are best suited to relaxing curly Caucasian hair. "Soft Curls" have become a fashionable way of styling black hair. Ammonium thioglycolate and a bromate or peroxide neutralizer are used to achieve restructuring of the hair.

Shampoos

When shampoos are used, they have generally a short contact time with the scalp and are diluted and rinsed off quickly. These factors reduce their sensitizing potential. Consumers' complaints are commonly directed at their eye stinging and irritating qualities (Nater and de Groot, 1993). The importance of eye safety testing for these products became apparent 35 years ago when shampoos based on blends of cationic and nonionic detergents caused blindness in some users.

Modern shampoos are detergent-based with a few containing small amounts of soap for conditioning. Anionic detergents and amphoteric detergents are occasional sensitizers (Sylvest *et al.*, 1975; Van-Hoote and Dooms-Goosens, 1983). Fatty acid amides used in shampoos as thickeners and foam stabilizers have caused allergic contact dermatitis in other products (Hindson and Lawler, 1983). Formaldehyde or formaldehyde releasers may be used as a preservative in shampoos but formaldehyde rarely causes contact dermatitis in hairdressers or consumers related to use of shampoos (Lynde and Mitchell, 1982; Bruynzeel *et al.*, 1984). Other new preservatives used in shampoos include 5-cloro-2-methyl-4-isothozoline-3-one and 2-methyl-4-isothiazoline-3-one. Individual ingredient patch testing is necessary to incriminate allergens in shampoos. They produce false negative results because they are diluted in the final product.

51.4.7 Hair coloring preparations

Over 30 million Americans color their hair using five different types of dye: Permanent hair dyes (Type I) are mixtures of colorless aromatic compounds that act as primary intermediates and couplers. The primary intermediates, phenylenediamine (PPD), toluene-2,5 diamine (p-toluenediamine), and p-ami-nophenol are oxidized by couplers to form a variety of colors that blend to give the desired shade. These reactions take place inside the hair shaft accounting for the fastness of these dyes. Permanent dyes are the most popular in the United States because of the variety of natural colors they can achieve. Semipermanent hair dyes (Type II) contain low molecular weight nitro-phenylenediamine and anthroquinone dyes which penetrate the hair cortex to some extent. Their color lasts-through approximately five shampoos. Temporary rinses (Type III) are mixtures of mild, organic acids and certified dyes that coat the hair shaft. These rub and shampoo off easily Vegetable dyes (Type IV) in the United States contain henna, which only colors hair red. Metallic dyes (Type V) contain lead acetate and sulfur. When they are combed through the hair daily they deposit insoluble lead oxides and sulfides that impart colors that range from yellow-brown to dark gray.

Types I and II contain "coal tar" hair dyes, and in the United States they must bear a label warning about adverse reactions. Instructions for open patch testing are given. The law requires patch testing be performed before each application of dye; in practice, this is seldom carried out in homes or salons. "Coal tar" dyes are added occasionally to temporary rinses; these rinses must also bear a warning label and patch-test instructions.

A persistent and significant number of reactions to hair dyes are seen by dermatologists each year. Seven percent of the reactions to cosmetics diagnosed by the North American Contact Dermatitis Group were caused by hair dyes (Adams and Maibach, 1985). Their severity ranges from mild erythema at the hair line, ears to swelling of the eyelids and face, to an acute vesicular eruption in the scalp that requires prompt medical attention.

Most reactions to "coal tar" dyes are reactions to PPD. Independent sensitization to toluene-2,5diamine or 2-nitro-p-phenylenediamine dyes or resorcinol occurs rarely, but positive patch tests to toluene-2,5-diamine or 2-nitro-p-phenylenediamine dyes result generally from cross-sensitization to PPD.

One percent PPD in petrolatum is used in the standard closed patch test Occasionally patients 32 who have a +1 reaction to PPD do not have a significant reaction when they dye their hair, but stronger patch-test results should warn patients not to use these hair dyes. P-phenylenediamine is a colorless compound. Patch-test material gradually darkens as PPD oxidizes, and it should be stored in dark containers and should be made fresh at least yearly.

The products of PPD's oxidation are not allergenic. Reiss and Fisher (1974) studied the allergenicity of dyed hair. Twenty patients sensitive to PPD were tested to freshly dyed hair in closed patch tests and all were negative. The findings of this study are important particularly to hairdressers, sensitive to PPD, who may work with dyed hair all day. Occasional case reports have appeared that suggested contact reactions occurred to another person's dyed hair (Cronin, 1973; Hindson, 1975; Warin, 1976; Foussereau et al., 1980). We assume that the dyeing process must not have been carried out properly and that the unoxidized products remained on the hair.

Patients sensitive to PPD should be warned about possible cross-reactions with local anesthetics (procaine and benzocaine), sulfonamides, and para-aminobenzoic acid sunscreens. It is estimated that 25 percent of patients who are PPD-sensitive will react to semipermanent hair dyes. Patients who wish to try these as a substitute, should do an open patch test with the dye first.

Several patients have been reported who experienced immediate hyper-sensitivity reactions to PPD, and this spectrum of reactions to hair dyes should now be considered as a diagnostic possibility in appropriate patients (Engrasser and Maibach, 1985). Some patients complain of scalp irritation after dyeing their hair, but we are unaware of published data that study the potential of these dyes for irritation. Some hair-dye reactions occur most prominently in light-exposed areas, but the phototoxic and photoallergic potential of "coal tar" dyes has not been investigated. Severe reactions to hair dyes are uncommon, but not impossible, as even fatal anaphylactic reactions to hair dyes have been reported (Belton and Chira, 1997).

Henna has not been reported to cause allergic contact dermatitis when used as a hair dye, but a case has been reported from coloring the skin with henna (Pasricha et al., 1980). Cronin (1979) described a hairdresser who noted wheezing and coryza when she handled henna; this patient had a positive prick test to henna. Edwards (1982) reported a case of contact dermatitis due to lead acetate in the metallic dyes.

When hair is bleached ammonium persulfate is added to hydrogen peroxide to obtain the lightest shades. Ammonium persulfate has several industrial uses and it is known commonly to cause irritant reactions and allergic contact dermatitis occasionally. Methods of testing for immediate hypersensitivity include rubbing a saturated solution of ammonium persulfate on intact skin; scratch tests or intracutaneous tests using 1 percent aqueous solution of ammonium persulfate; and inhalation of 0.1 µg of ammonium persulfate powder. All of these methods can cause immediate hypersensitivity reactions including urticaria, facial edema, asthma, and syncope so they should be performed only when emergency treatment for anaphylaxis is available. These reactions are histamine mediated, but it is not clear whether or not immunologic mechanisms are involved (Fisher and Dooms-Goosens, 1976). Hairdressers should be instructed that clients who develop hives, generalized itching, facial swelling, or asthma when the hair is bleached should not have the process repeated using persulfate. Clients experiencing such reactions should receive immediate medical attention.

51.4.8   Facial makeup preparations

Eleven percent of the reactions to cosmetics in the NACDG Study were attributed facial make-up products, which includes lipstick, rouge, makeup bases, and facial powder (Adams and Maibach, 1985). Prior to 1960, allergic reactions to lipsticks were common: most were caused by D&C Red 21 (eosin), an indelible dye used in longlasting deeply colored lipsticks. The sensitizer in eosin proved to be a contaminant; improved methods of purification have reduced its sensitizing potential. Because eosin is strongly bound to keratin, patch tests are performed with 50 percent eosin in petrolatum.

Other dyes have occasionally been reported as sensitizers. Cronin (1980) reported reactions to D&C Red 36, D&C Red 31, D&C Red 19, D&C Red 17, and D&C Yellow 11. The latter is a potent sensitizer seldom used in lipsticks, but reported also as a sensitizing agent in eye Cream (Calnan *et al.*, 1976) and rouge as well as lipstick (Calnan, 1976a). D&C Red 17 not permitted in lipstick in US D&C Yellow 10, produced by the sulfonation of D&C Yellow 11, is not a potent sensitizer (Sato *et al.*, 1984). Other sensitizers reported in lipsticks include castor oil acting as a pigment solvent (Sai, 1983) antioxidants propyl gallate and monotertiarybutylhydroquinone (van Joost *et al.*, 1984), sunscreens phenyl salicylate and amyldimethyl aminobenzoic acid (Calnan, 1981; Calnan *et al.*, 1981), lanolin (Schorr, 1973), and fragrance.

Although reactions to lipstick are uncommon, dermatologists should consider this diagnosis even when the eruption has spread beyond the lips, because the sensitizing chemical may be present in cosmetics other than the lipstick. Do not neglect to test each lipstick that the patient uses closed as well as performing photopatch tests, because some of the dyes used may be photoallergens.

Rouge or "blush" is manufactured in various forms—powder, cream, liquid, stick, or gel. It is designed to highlight the cheeks with color. The composition is not unique: powders are similar to face powder, and creams and liquids are similar to foundation. To achieve bright shades, organic colors are added to rouges as they are to lipsticks. D&C Yellow 11 caused allergic reactions to rouges as well as lipsticks (Chowdhury, 2002). Some women may use lipstick to color their cheeks in place of rouge, or rouge may be used all over the face to achieve a healthy glow. These practices need to be taken into account when evaluating patterns of contact dermatitis on the face.

Facial makeups or foundations are applied to the skin to give an appearance of uniform color and texture and to disguise blemishes or imperfections. They are produced in a variety of forms—emulsions of water and oil, oil-free lotions, anhydrous sticks, poured powders, and pancake makeups and the amount of coverage given is determined by the titanium dioxide (TiO2) content. Because TiO2 reflects light, some ordinary makeups achieve sun protection factor (SPF) values of 2 or even 4 (Laznet, 1982). In recent years, sunscreening agents have been added to some foundations to increase these SPF values. When sunscreening claims are made for these cosmetics, the US government will consider these products as OTC drugs also. PABA derivatives, fragrances, emulsifiers, preservatives, propylene glycol, and lanolin are chemicals with significant sensitizing potential used in these makeups. Synthetic esters, such as isopropyl myristate and lanolin derivatives added to these makeups, have been implicated as causes of acne by the rabbit's ear test (Kligman and Mills, 1972). However, most cosmetic reactions, such as contact allergy, are due to fragrance mixtures and formaldehyde (Held *et al.*, 1999).

Calnan (1975) described a woman who had a positive patch test to her foundation on two occasions, and her facial eruption flared when she used this foundation. However, patch testing the individual ingredients of this foundation was negative. Calnan raised the possibility of compound allergy— the allergen is produced by a combination of more than one ingredient. Despite some noted advers reactions to cosmetics, facial cosmetics are considered safe consumer products (Scheman, 2000).

■ CHAPTER 51 ■

51.4.9 Sunscreen

Sunscreens can be classified into two major types: chemical and physical (Food and Drug Administration, 1978). Physical sunscreens such as titanium dioxide and zinc oxide reduce the amount of light penetrating the skin by creating a physical barrier that reflects, scatters, or physically blocks the ultraviolet light reaching the skin surface. Chemical sunscreens, on the other hand, reduce the amount of light reaching the stratum corneum by absorbing the radiation. Examples of chemical sunscreens include para-amino benzoic acid (PABA) and PABA derivatives such as Padimate 0, cinnamates, benzophenones, salicylate derivatives, and dibenzoylmethane derivatives.

Because chemical sunscreens are applied topically to the skin in relatively high concentrations (up to 26 percent), contact sensitization can occur (Cook and Freeman, 2001; Nixon *et al.*, n.d.). Similarly, because these chemicals absorb radiation, they have the potential to cause photosensitization. Both types of sensitization can occur with not only the various sunscreening agents but also with excipients such as emulsifiers, antioxidants, and preservatives that are included in the various hydroalcoholic lotions, ointments, oil-in-water or water-in-oil emulsions. Despite extensive sunscreen use, there have been infrequent published reports of sunscreen-induced side effects, including allergic/ photoallergic reactions, but we have inadequate data to accurately predict the degree of hypersensitivity to sunscreening agents due to the lack of a well-developed adverse reaction reporting system.

Numerous sunscreening preparations are currently sold in the United States. Table 51.7 lists examples of the sunscreen formulations sold in the United States together with the active ingredients and their sun protection factors (SPF), a measure of sunscreen protection against sunburn. Most of the formulations that are combination sunscreens contain one or more UVB absorbers and a UVA absorber to provide much needed protection against the damaging effects of UVA. Several sunscreens also include physical blockers such as titanium dioxide.

In general, as the SPF of the sunscreen formulation increases, the number of active ingredients increases to three or four, and in some cases the total amount of active sunscreens increases up to 26 percent. Not all formulations list the specific concentrations of the active ingredients, and it is possible that some may contain higher concentrations. As with many chemicals, increasing the concentrations of the active ingredients may increase the likelihood of sensitization (Thompson, 1977). The majority of sunscreens contain octyl dimethyl PABA

Table 51.7:

Selected sunscreen formulations available the United States

Trade name	SPF	Active ingredients
Four sunscreening ingredients		
Coppertone (Plough)	30	Padimate 0, Parsol MCX, octyl salicylate, oxybenzone
Sundown (Johnson & Johnson)	30	Parsol MCX, octyl salicylate, oxybenzone, titanium dioxide
	20	Padimate 0, Parsol MCX, octyl salicylate, oxybenzone
Cancer Garde (Eclipse Labs)	30	Padimate 0, Parsol MCX, oxybenzone, titanium dioxide
T/I Screen (T/I Pharmaceuticals)	30+	Parsol MCX, octocrylene, octyl salicylate, oxybenzone
Block Out (Carter Products)	30	Parsol MCX, padimate 0, octyl salicylate, oxybenzone
Supershade (Plough)	44	Parsol MCX, padimate 0, homosalate, oxybenzone
Three sunscreening ingredients		
Solbar (Person and Covey)	50	Parsol MCX, octocrylene, oxybenzone
PreSun for Kids (Westwood)	39	Parsol MCX, octyl salicylate, oxybenzone
PreSun 29	29	Parsol MCX, octyl salicylate, oxybenzone
Bain de Soleil (Bain de Soleil)	30	Padimate 0, Parsol MCX, oxybenzone
Ultrashade (Plough)	23	Padimate 0, Parsol MCX, oxybenzone
Total Eclipse (Eclipse Labs)	15	Padimate 0, octyl salicylate, oxybenzone
Sundown (Johnson & Johnson)	15	Padimate 0, Parsol MCX, oxybenzone
Two sunscreening ingredients		
Supershade (Plough)	8, 15	Parsol MCX, oxybenzone
Coppertone (Plough)	4, 6, 8, 15	Padimate 0, oxybenzone
Shade (Plough)	4, 6	Padimate 0, oxybenzone
PreSun (Westwood)	8, 15	Padimate 0, oxybenzone
Water Babies (Plough)	15	Parsol MCX, oxybenzone
Sundown (Johnson & Johnson)	4, 6, 8	Padimate 0, oxybenzone
Block Out (Carter Products)	15	Padimate 0, oxybenzone
Photoplex (Herbert Labs)	15	Padimate 0, avobenzone
One sunscreening ingredient		
Coppertone (Plough)	2	Octyl salicylate
Bain de Soleil (Bain de Soleil)	2, 4	Padimate 0
Eclipse (Eclipse Labs)	5	Padimate 0
	10	Glyceryl PABA

■ CHAPTER 51 ■

(Padimate 0) as the main UVB absorber. The cinnamate derivative, octyl methoxycinnamate (Parsol MCX), is also used as a UVB absorber.

Most sunscreens with more than one ingredient contain oxybenzone as the additional ingredient. The absorption peak of this compound lies in the UVB region and extends partially into the UVA. Other agents that absorb in the

UVA region include sulisobenzone, dioxybenzone, menthyl anthranilate and avobenzone. The latter chemical, which has an absorption maximum in the middle of the UVA region (358 nm), has been approved in the United States in two sunscreen formulations (Photoplex, Herbert Laboratories, Santa Ana, CA and Coppertone, Sun and Shade) (Table 51.7).

Published reports of contact and photocontact sensitization and contact urticaria induced by sunscreening agents are listed in Table 51.1. Representatives of all major sunscreen categories including PABA derivatives, anthranilates, salicylates, cinnamates, and benzophenones have caused allergic reactions are described as follows:

Para Amino Benzoic Acid (PABA) In 1975, Willis (1975) suggested that the sensitization potential of p-amino benzoic acid was minimal. Wennersten (1984) reported that a total of 73/1883 (3.9 percent) subjects tested with 5 percent PABA in alcohol in the Scandinavian Standard Photopatch Tray had either allergic or photoallergic responses to PABA. These subjects represent 73 percent of the total number of subjects with contact and photocontact sensitization to PABA (Table 51.1). The use of PABA as a sunscreening agent in Europe and the United States has decreased significantly in recent years. PABA has been replaced by ester derivatives such as Padimate 0 that, unlike PABA, are not water soluble and tend to remain on the surface layer with less than 10 percent penetrating the corneum even after 24 hours (Weller and Eireman, 1984). These PABA esters appear to be less sensitizing than PABA; however, there is no data to substantiate this impression.

PABA derivatives

Sensitization to glyceryl PABA have been reported for the last 30 years (Marmalzat and Rapaport, 1976; Caro, 1978). Many of the cases of glyceryl PABA sensitization showed uniform strong reactions to benzocaine, suggesting that the sensitization may be due to the presence of impurities in the glyceryl PABA. This suggestion was first made by Fisher (1976) and has since been confirmed (Hjorth *et al.*, 1978). Benzocaine impurities (1–18 percent) occurred in many commercial sources of glyceryl PABA. Thus many of the early reports of contact allergy to glyceryl PABA may have falsely implicated glyceryl PABA as the sensitizer. Thune (1984) reported two cases of allergic/photoallergic reactions to glyceryl PABA in which there was no reaction to benzocaine, suggesting true allergy to the PABA derivative. However, no allergic responses were observed when these subjects were patched with glyceryl PABA which had been purified via high-pressure liquid chromatography (Bruze *et al.*, 1988). This suggests the presence of an, as yet, unknown impurity (or impurities) other than benzocaine as the sensitization source. This shows the importance of utilizing purified raw materials in the manufacture of consumer products and the need for careful interpretation of patch test results.

Other PABA derivatives that have caused sensitization/photocontact sensitization include octyl dimethyl PABA (Padimate 0), amyl dimethyl PABA (Padimate A), and ethyl dihydroxy PABA. The number of case reports of sensitization/photocontact sensitization with Padimate 0 is less than that reported with PABA and glyceryl PABA suggesting a lower sensitization potential with this derivative. This may be because Padimate 0 is not a true PABA ester since it does not contain the NH2 grouping present in glyceryl PABA, PABA, and benzocaine (Fisher, 1977a).

Although Padimate A was included (FDA, 1978) as a safe and effective sunscreening agent, this derivative can cause phototoxicity and may have accounted for the erythemal response observed by Katz (1970) 30 minutes after sun exposure. This compound is no longer used in sunscreens in the United States. In addition to benzocaine impurities in the glyceryl PABA raw materials, some PABA esters contain 0.2 to 4.5 percent PABA (Bruze *et al.*, 1984). It possible that PABA impurities may account for some of the reports of sensitization to the PABA derivatives.

Salicylates

There are two cases of contact allergy and two reports of photocontact allergy to homomenthyl salicylate in the literature (Rietschel and Lewis, 1978) and no reports of sensitization to octyl salicylate, the major salicylate derivative in many sunscreens.

Cinnamates

Cinnamates are chemically related to or are found in balsam of Peru, balsam of Tolu, coca leaves, cinnamic acid, cinnamic aldehyde and cinnamon oil, ingredients used in perfumes, topical medications, cosmetics, and flavoring. Thune (1984) reported eight cases of sensitivity to cinnamates, two cases of photoallergy to 2-ethoxyethyl-p-cinnamate, and six subjects with contact allergy to other cinnamates such as amyl cinnamaldehyde, amyl cinnamic acid, and cinnamon oil. Calnan (1976b) reported cross-sensitization among cinnamon derivatives.

■ CHAPTER 51 ■

Benzophenones

There have been reported cases of photocontact allergy (Thune, 1984) and contact allergy (Camarasa and Serra-Baldrich, 1986) to oxybenzone; and reports of contact allergy (Adams and Maibach, 1985) and photocontact allergy to sulisobenzone. Benzophenone-10 (Mexenone), a benzophenone derivative not used in sunscreens in the United States, can also cause contact and photocontact dermatitis (Bury, 1980; De Groot and Wegland, 1987).

Dibenzoylmethanes

Dibenzoylmethane derivatives such as isopropyldibenzoylmethane (Eusolex 8020) and butyl dibenzoylmethane (avobenzone) have been incorporated in European sunscreens as UVA absorbers since 1980. Instances of contact allergy/ photoallergy to sunscreens and lipsticks containing dibenzoylmethanes or these derivatives have been reported, although the majority of reports have been associated with the isopropyl derivative (English and White, 1986; Schander and Ippen, 1986; De Groot et al., 1987). As a result, manufacturers stopped incorporating Eusolex 8020 into their products (Roberts, 1988; Alomar and Cerda, 1989). Recently, the manufacturers of Eusolex 8020 withdrawn from the market.

There have been fewer reports of contact allergy/photoallergy to the butyl dibenzoylmethane derivative, avobenzone. It is possible that some of these reactions to avobenzone may have been cross-reactions resulting from prior exposure to the isopropyl derivative (Held et al., 1999). Greater utilization of these compounds with appropriate testing should help clarify their relative sensitization potential.

Camphor derivatives

3-(4-Methyl-benzylidene) camphor (Eusolex 6300) is a sunscreening agent used extensively in Europe, often in combination with Eusolex 8020, but it is not approved for use in the United States. There have been several reports of allergic and photoallergic reactions to sunscreens containing this agent (FDA, 1978).

Miscellaneous

Other chemical sunscreens that have caused allergic reactions include diagalloyl trioleate (Sams, 1956), the glycerol ester of o-aminometa (2,3 dihydroxyproxy) benzoic acid (van Ketel, 1977), a dioxane derivative (Fagerlund *et al.*, 1983); and 2-phenyl-methyl-benzoazol (witisol) (Mork and Austad, 1984). None of these ingredients are approved for use in sunscreens in the United States.

Titanium dioxide

Physical blockers such as titanium dioxide and zinc oxide have the advantage of not being sensitizers, but may be so occlusive that they can cause miliaria (Fisher, 1973). Kaminester (1981) reported that the inclusion of titanium dioxide in a PABA sunscreen blocked the appearance of photoallergy. It is possible that the reflection and scattering of light by titanium dioxide reduced the amount of UV light that penetrated the skin and elicited photoallergy.

Excipients

Contact allergy can also be caused by excipients included in sunscreens. These chemicals include mineral oil, petrolatum, isopropyl esters, lanolin derivatives, aliphatic alcohols, triglycerides, fatty acids, waxes, propylene glycol, emulsifiers, thickeners, preservatives, and fragrances. An extensive list of vehicle constituents in cosmetics that can cause allergic responses has been published (Nater and De Groot, 1993). De Groot *et al.* (1988) indicated that preservatives, fragrances, and emulsifiers are the main classes of ingredients responsible for cosmetic allergy, with Kathon CG producing contact allergic reactions in 27.7 percent of subjects tested. Sunscreens available in the United States provide a complete list of ingredients including the excipients. The listing of all ingredients in sunscreens should be encouraged so that consumers, especially those with known sensitivities to chemicals, are fully informed about the composition of the formulation prior to the purchase and application of the product to the skin.

51.4.10 Manicuring preparations

In the past, adverse reactions have been reported to numerous nail cosmetics that have been removed subsequently from the market because of reported hazards. Nail hardeners containing formaldehyde are in this category. In the United States, this type of hardener is permitted for use only on the free edge of the nail when the skin is protected from contact with the hardener. Some manufacturers sell products called hardeners but they have merely increased the resin content of ordinary nail enamel. Nail enamels including base coats and top coats have a similar composition. The concentration of each of these chemicals depends on the quality to be achieved in the final product. The base coat will have increased amounts of resin to improve adhesion to the nail plate, but the top coat has increased nitrocellulose and plasticizers to enhance gloss and abrasion resistance.

Toluene sulfonamide/formaldehyde resin (TSFR) is responsible for contact dermatitis around the nails but also at sites distant from the fingers, commonly eyelids, around the mouth and chin, sides of the neck, on the genitalia, and rarely a generalized eruption. In contrast free formaldehyde in nail hardeners causes mostly local reactions. Cronin (1980) recommends 10 percent toluene sulfonamide/formaldehyde in petrolatum to perform a closed patch test. Norton (1991) reported that free formaldehyde (FF) hardeners are the most common cause of nail cosmetric reaction followed by methacrylate and cyanoacrylate resins, TSFR, acetone removers and sodium and potassium hydroxide removers. Norton also reported onychomycosis, chromonychia, anonychia and pterigum inversum unguis, secondary to FF nail hardeners. A small amount (0.1 to 0.5 percent) of free formaldehyde is in the resin (Calnan, 1975). Fisher (1977) proposed that patients who are allergic to this resin may wear nail polish without problems if they allow it to dry thoroughly with their hands quietly at rest. Those who find this inconvenient can be advised to purchase certain "hypoallergenic" brands of nail polish, which substitute alkyd or other resins. Ask the patient to check the ingredient list for toluene sulfonamide/formaldehyde resin as a precaution. The durability and abrasion resistance of these other resins is said to be inferior to toluene sulfonamide/formaldehyde resin. Although onycholysis has been attributed to reactions to toluene sulfonamide/formaldehyde resin, no published data firmly support this (Braur, 1980; Paltzik and Enscoe, 1980). A new nail enamel compound has been introduced by Almay and Revlon. The toluenesulfonamide/folmaldehyde resin, the principal allergic sensitizer in nail enamels have been replaced by glyceryl tribenzoate. In addition, these new enamels are toluene-free. The new enamel also replaces dibutyl phthalate for glyceryl triacetate. This new plasticizer, polymer that prevents brittleness, provides longer wearability. Another very recent innovation is quick-drying suspensions. Two recent patents employing acetone and halogenated hydrocarbons provide for a reduction time from 50–70 percent over conventional nail enamel compositions without adversely affecting the other desirable properties of the coating. Environmental safe nail enamels are a real challenge for the cosmetic industry. Water-based nail polish with adhesion, gloss and drying qualities will be developed (Mitchell *et al.*, 1992). A water-dilutable nail polish was developed containing a mixture of poly-urethanes, vinyl and/or acrylic ester (Yamazaki and Tanaka, 1990).

Yellow pigmentation of the nail plate, darkest at the distal end, occurs commonly in women who wear colored nail polish. Samman (1977) reproduced this staining with the following colors: D&C Red No. 7, D&C Red No. 34, D&C Red No. 6, and FD&C Yellow No. 5 lake. Nail enamel removers are mixtures of solvents such as acetone, amyl, butyl, or ethyl acetate to which fatty materials may be added (Wilkinson and Moore, 1982). These can be irritating to the skin and can strip the nail plate. Cuticle removers contain alkaline chemicals, frequently sodium or potassium hydroxide to break the disulfide bonds of keratin. They should not be left on for prolonged periods or be used by people who are susceptible to paronychia. Cuticle removers are irritants.

"Sculptured nails" have become popular in recent years because they build an attractive artificial nail on the nail plate. Sculpture nails are prosthetic nails with a fresh acrylic mixture of methyl methacrylate monomer liquid and polymer powder. They are molded within a metabolized paperboard template on the natural nail surface to produce nails of desired thickness and length. When hardened, the template is removed, the prosthesis filed and the surface is polished. Acrylate sculptured nails are of two varieties: methacrylate monomers and polymers that polymerized in the presence of hydroquinone in ordinary light, Photo-bonded acrylate sculptured nails based on acrylates that are photobonded. Allergic reactions consist of paronychia, onychia, and severe and prolonged paresthesia. Fisher (1980b) reported a patient developed a severe reaction to methyl methacrylate monomers resulting in permanent loss of all her fingernails. Fisher and Baran (1991) reported that cyanoacrylates do not cross-react with other acrylates.

Unfortunately irritant and allergic reactions to the liquid monomers as well as secondary infections may be painful and long-lasting. Paronychia, onycholysis, onychia, and dermatitis of the finger and distant sites may occur. Fisher *et al.* (1977) reported allergic sensitization to the methyl methacrylate monomers in sculptured nails. In 1974, the FDA banned the use of methyl methacrylate in these cosmetics. However, analysis of 31 products sold between 1975 and 1981 revealed this monomer was present in nine of them (Fuller, 1982). Sensitization has also been reported to other monomers, and cross-reactions between acrylate monomers does occur (Marks *et al.*, 1979). Patch testing to 1.0 to 5.0 percent monomer in petrolatum or olive oil can help confirm the diagnosis of an allergic sensitization. Controls may be required if the patient responds to 5 percent and not to 1 percent of the monomer.

Performed plastic nails may be designed to cover the nail plate or extended tips. Their prolonged use causes mechanical damage to the nail, and those covering the entire nail plate may cause injury by occlusion (Baran, 1982). Sensitization to p-tertiary butylphenol formaldehyde resin in the nail adhesive and tricresyl ethyl phthalate of the artificial nail has been reported (Burrows and Rycroft, 1981). Nail mending and wrapping kits often help women grow the longer nails they desire with few adverse reactions. A split nail can be repaired with cyanoacrylate glue with a negligible risk of sensitization. The repair is splinted with papers affixed by a nitrocellulose containing glue. These papers, or in some cases linen or silk, are wrapped over the free edge of the nail to protect it from trauma. Use of more sensitizing glues, of course, increases the risk of adverse reactions. The paper or cloth should not cover a large portion of the attached nail plate to avoid complications of occlusion.

51.4.11   Oral hygiene product

Dentifrices and mouthwashes are incriminated infrequently as causing allergic contact reactions. This may be due to the short exposure time these products have with the skin and mucous membrane under ordinary use situations. If sensitization occurs inside the mouth, patch testing on the skin usually shows a positive reaction. Many of the products contain detergents and are unsuitable for closed patch testing. To avoid irritant reactions, test open in the antecubital fossa and confirm positive results with tests in controls. To help patients avoid further reactions, ingredient patch testing should be done. Fisher (1970) reviewed concentrations for patch testing ingredients found in toothpastes and mouthwashes. If the physician suspects allergic contact dermatitis and negative patch tests on the skin do not reflect mucosal sensitivity, ingredients may be incorporated in Orabase (Squibb). This material can be held against the inside of the lip for 24 hours, and then examined for erythema. Reports of allergic sensitization to toothpastes in the last decade have primarily involved flavoring agents (Andersen, 1978). Cinnamic aldehyde has been the most frequent offender, because it was introduced in a relatively high concentration in toothpaste sold in several countries (Drake and Maibach, 1976). A case of contact dermatitis to cinnamic aldehyde resulted in depigmentation about the vermilion border (Ale and Maibach, 2001).

51.4.12 Personal cleanliness products

The action of bacteria upon sterile apocrine secretions produces a characteristic odor. Labows *et al.* (1982) reported lipophilic diptheroids as the organisms that produce unique axillary odors. Although deodorants are considered cosmetics, antiperspirants are regulated as over-the-counter (OTC) drugs as well as cosmetics. Many of these products have been reformulated in the last decade because of government regulations (Jass, 1982). Hexachlorophene was banned because of its neurotoxicity and halogenated salicylanilides because of their photoallergic nature. Chlorofluorocarbon propellants were removed from aerosols because of their role in depleting the stratosphere of ozone. The chlorofluorocarbons have been replaced by hydrocarbon propellants—isobutane, butane, and propane—which are flammable. The FDA OTC Antiperspirant Review Panel recommended the removal of zirconium-containing chemicals from aerosol antiperspirants because of the potential for formation of granuloma in the lung. Sodium zirconium acetate salts had caused granulomatous lesions in the skin of the axilla, have been removed from antiperspirants.

Simple deodorants reduce the number of bacteria in the axilla. Most deodorants contain triclosan as an active ingredient. Triclosan is an antimicrobial agent used in soaps and shampoos. Draize testing showed a low-sensitizing potential for this chemical (Marzulli and Maibach, 1973). Allergic contact dermatitis to this chemical have been reported, but this requires confirmation (FDA, 1975). We recommend patch testing with 1 to 2 percent triclosan in petrolatum in suspected cases. The OTC Review Panel published a list of aluminum and aluminum-zirconium chemicals permitted in antiperspirants. These chemicals are not regarded us sensitizers. Irritant reactions to aluminum salts in antiperspirants are common because of the environmental heat, moisture, and friction and the inflammation caused by shaving in the axilla. Dermal penetration of calcium salts and calcinosis cutis has been studied (Soileau, 2001). Allergic reactions are due to the other chemicals in the antiperspirants; most frequently the fragrance ingredients. Similarly, feminine hygiene sprays are primarily fragrance products that cause irritant reactions when sprayed at too close a range.

51.4.13 Baby products

These products are marketed primarily to use on the skin and scalps of infants. Some experimental data suggest that infants are less easily sensitized than adults are. However, Epstein (1961) reported that 44 percent of infants under 1 year of age could be sensitized to pentadecyl catechol, but that 87 percent of children over 3 years of age were sensitized in the same experiment. In clinical practice, allergic contact dermatitis is diagnosed infrequently in young children (Hjorth, 1981). Patch testing with ingredients in standard concentrations may result in a higher incidence of irritant reactions in young children (Marcussen, 1963). Because the diaper area is a frequent site of irritant contact dermatitis, careful attention should be paid to the products used in this area.

Generally, baby products are fragranced. Baby oil, talc, and corn starch have simple compositions with little sensitizing potential beside the fragrances. Baby lotions or creams may contain fragrance, preservatives, lanolin, or propylene glycol which are common sensitizers (Eierman *et al.*, 1982). Propylene glycol, present in these lotions and the moistened towelettes marketed for cleansing the diaper area, is a common irritant. In the treatment of infants with diaper rash, it is important to examine the ingredients of the cosmetics used on the diaper area.

51.4.14   Bath preparations

Adverse reactions to bubble bath reported to the FDA include skin eruptions, irritation of the genitourinary tract, eye irritation, and respiratory disorders (Simmons, 1955). The genitourinary tract reactions in children have been the most serious; many children have been subjected to extensive urologic workups before the cause was established. The skin eruptions are assumed usually to be irritant reactions due to the detergent content of this cosmetic.

51.4.15   Other skin care preparations

Depilatories

Most depilatories today contain mercaptans such as calcium thioglycolate 2.5 to 4.0 percent in conjunction with an alkali to bring the pH to between 10 and 12.5 (Wilkinson and Moore, 1982). The keratin of the cortex is more vulnerable before it emerges from the follicle, and depilatories attack it there leaving a soft rather than sharp end For this reason, the use of depilatories in place of shaving can prevent pseudofolliculitis barbae in some black men. Powdered facial depilatories, produced for beard removal, contain barium or strontium sulfide because these chemicals are quicker acting. Unfortunately, these chemicals cause more irritation and produce an unpleasant odor. In order to use the less malodorous thioglycolate depilatories for coarser beard removal, hair accelerators such as thiourea, melamine, or sodium metasilicate are added. Depilatories cannot be patch tested directly and these thioglycolates are seldom sensitizers.

Epilating waxes

Epilating waxes are usually warmed to soften, and they harden and enmesh the hair after application. When the wax is pulled off, the hair is removed by the root. Some modified waxes do not have to be warmed and can be applied with a backing material. These cosmetics may contain beeswax, rosin (colophony), fragrance, or rarely benzocaine as potential sensitizers (Wilkinson and Moore, 1982). The problems usually seen with these epilating cosmetics are due to mechanical irritation.

51.5   COSMETIC INTOLERANCE SYNDROME

Fisher (1980c) coined the term "status cosmeticus" for the condition in which a patient is no longer able to tolerate the use of many or any cosmetic on the face. Patients complain of itching or stinging, facial burning and discomfort. This group seriously challenges our diagnostic skills as well as our ability to be empathetic because the severity of patients' symptoms does not match objective signs of disease. Most of these patients have only subjective symptoms, but some may have mild inflammation. The Cosmetic Intolerance Syndrome is not a single entity, but rather a symptom complex due to multiple factors, exogenous and endogenous (Polak *et al.*, 1974). Therefore, these patients need a thorough history, physical examination and workup. Some patients have occult allergic contact dermatitis, allergic photocontact dermatitis, or contact urticarial reactions, and the causal agents are documented by careful clinical review and patch testing.

Others who have a seborrheic or rosacea diathesis with or without inflammation seem to have flared this condition by by overusing cleansing creams and emollients. Both of these conditions may be accompanied by facial erythema or scaling. Some patients require anti-inflammatory therapy, as do a atopic patients who develop this state. Fisher found that itching or stinging or both can be produced in patients with "status cosmeticus." He recommended that whenever possible these chemical should be avoided by these patients.

Table 51.8:

Management of patients who are intolerant to cosmetic usage

1. Examine every cosmetic and skin care agent
2. Patch and photopatch test to rule out occult allergic and photoallergic contact dermatitis, or contact urticaria
3. Limit skin care to
   - Water washing without soap or detergent
   - Lip cosmetics
   - Eye cosmetics (if the eyelids are not symptomatic)
   - Face powder
   - Glycerol and rose water as moisturizer (only if needed)
   - 6–12 months of avoidance of other skin care agents and cosmetics
4. Watch for and test, if necessary, depression and other neuropsychiatric aspects

When the offending agent cannot be found prolonged elimination of cosmetics seems to help some women who after 6 to 12 months or more are able to gradually return to the use of other cosmetics (Table 51.8). Additions of skin care products should be made one at a time and no more frequently than every 2 weeks. The final program should be simple and limited in the number and frequency of cosmetics used. Golbenberg and Safrin (1977) suggested that stinging effects of cosmetics irritants may be neutralized by anti-irritants. They proposed three possible mechanisms of action of anti-irritants: to complex the anti-irritant, to block the reactive sites in the skin and to prevent physical contact with the skin.

51.6 OCCUPATIONAL DERMATITIS: HAIRDRESSERS

Cosmeticians may perform a variety of personal care tasks including hair grooming, manicuring, and applying makeup. It is primarily the hair care tasks that account for the high rate of occupational hand dermatitis. Cronin (1982) noted that beauticians frequently develop a dry, scaling dermatitis over the metacarpophalangeal joints, however individuals vary in their ability to react to irritants (Smith et al., 2002). Novice beauticians and those in training are required to shampoo many customers each day, and the resulting irritation is frequently the initial cause of hand dermatitis. These hairdressers have a good chance of improving as they learn to protect and lubricate their hands. However, patients with atopic eczema may have a particularly difficult time with hand dermatitis as hairdressers, although we do believe they should not be barred from this career. Young atopic patients who are contemplating career choices should be appraised of the occupational hazards of hairdressing.

When beauticians with hand dermatitis are patch tested at different centers the percentage of reactions varies. PPD is usually the leading offender when allergy is present (Wahlberg, 1975). Frosch and co-workers (1993) reported that the major contact sensitizer of hairdressers in Europe was GMT. Sensitization is at least as frequent to PPD; in some countries (Germany, UK, Spain) sensitization frequencies, were high. This has to be emphasized in comparison to the relatively low frequencies to AMT. The recently introduced acid permanents waves pose a higher risk of sensitization to hairdressers than the alkaline permanent waves that have been used since the early 1940s. The low figures for GMT sensitization in some centers may be explained by lower usage in salons or by more careful handling. In Denmark, most hairdressers wear gloves when dyeing and permanent waving. In Germany, most hairdressers protect their hands only against hair dyes. There is still a strong prejudice against the use of gloves in this occupation. Guerra *et al.* (1992) confirmed this attitude in Italy: only 12.5 percent of 240 hairdressers wore gloves for permanent waving, whereas 51 percent wore them for hair dying. This group found a relatively low sensitization to GMT, attributing this to its infrequent usage in Italy. They demonstrated that vinyl gloves may not always suppress the reaction to GMT in sensitized individuals. They found 3 of 8 patients patch tested with GMT through vinyl gloves were positive after 3 days. Better plastic materials must be looked for, if GMT continues to be used in European salons. Furthermore, it must be kept in mind that wearing gloves over a prolonged time poses its own risks. The primary goal in the prevention of occupational dermatitis must be reduction of exposure to highly sensitized agents. They reported GMT was the number one sensitizer. After the series described by Storrs (1984), the German CDRG reported sensitization to GMT in 38 percent of 87 patients in 1989, and in 31 percent of a second series of 178 patients (Frosch, 1989). Holness and Nethercott (1990) found 23.5 percent of 34 patients positive to GMT. GMT sensitization may become increasingly frequent if no further action is taken.

Hairdressers need to be instructed to handle this type of permanent wave with caution. Direct skin contact should be avoided, Gloves and improved handling technique may lead to a decrease in the frequency of sensitization, which may, in comparison to hair dyes, be acceptable to this occupational group.

Rietschel *et al.* (1984) and other investigators have shown that allergens can penetrate gloves. Fisher reported that polyethylene laminate glove (4-H glove;

Safety 4 Company, Denmark) protect allergic patients from epoxy resin and acrylic monomers. McCain and Storrs (1992) in a placebo-controlled double-blind patch test study reported that 4-H glove was effective in preventing allergic contact dermatitis in GMT sensitized volunteers, protecting four of four patients after an 8 h exposure and two of three after 48 h. Melstran *et al.* (1994) provides extensive documentaion aboout protectives gloves. Frosch and co-workers (1993) found PPD the 2nd sensitizer very closed to GMT. However, PPD derivatives were considerably lower and ranged from 375. In the Italian study, the figures were similar for PPD but higher for the derivatives. Frosch and colleagues (were unable to conclude that ONPPD had the lowest sensitization risk. They stated that pyrogallol and resorcinol are the least frequent sensitizers in the hairdressers' series.

Nickel, preservatives such as (cloro) methylisothiazolinone and formaldehyde, surface active agents such as cocamidopropylbetaine and hydrolyzed animal proteins as well as perfume ingredients, may also be responsible for dermatitis in hairdressers. To work-up hairdressers with hand eczema, we use the standard hairdressers screening series. This series includes resorcinol, p-toluenediamine sulfate, glyceryl monothioglycolate, ammonium thioglycolate, ammonium persulfate, p-aminodiphenylamine hydrochloride pyrogallol and 0-nitro-p-phenylenediamine. At the same session, we apply 1.0 percent glyceryl thioglycolate in petrolatum, and pieces of the hairdresser's protective glove applied on both sides.

Hairdressers who are nickel-sensitive also have a serious challenge. There is evidence that permanent solutions may leach nickel out of metal objects (Dahlquist *et al.*, 1979). Fastidious care in the selection of stainless steel tools and use of dimethyl glyoxide for testing pins, clips, and other paraphernalia allows some patients to continue in this career. Hairdressers with allergic contact dermatitis need to be told that protective gloves may not provide an absolute barrier to allergens (Frosch *et al.*, 1993).

Tomb and co-workers (1993) reported a young hairdresser who developed acute periorbital eczema and marked edema of eyelids, lip erosions and eczema of her fingertips to two instant glues used to attach false hair. Patch test was strongly positive to ethyl cyanoacrylate adhesive. Ingredient labeling of retailed cosmetics in the United States has greatly aided dermatologists in caring for patients with contact dermatitis. There is no regulation requiring similar labeling for cosmetics used in beauty salons. However preventive strategies for occupational skin diseases in hairdressers are known and can be rarely successful (Dickel *et al.*, 2002).

REFERENCES

ADAMS, R.M. and MAIBACH, H.I. (1985) A five year study of cosmetic reactions. *J. Am. Acad. Dermatol.* **13**, 1062–1069.

ALE, S.I. and MAIBACH, H.I. (1995) Clinical relevance in allergic contact dermatitis: an algorithmic approach. *Dermatosen* **43**, 119–121.

ALE, S.I. and MAIBACH, H.I. (2001) Operational definition of allergic contact dermatitis. In: HAYES, A.W., THOMAS, J.A., GARDNER, D.E. and MAIBACH, H.I. (eds) *Toxicology of the Skin*. London: Taylor and Francis.

ALE, S.I. and MAIBACH, H.I. (2002) Scientific basis of patch testing. *Dermatologie in Beruf and Umwelt Occupational Environmental Dermatology* **50** (2), 43–50.

ALOMAR, A. CERDA, M.T. (1989) Contact allergy to Eusolex 8021. *Contact Dermatitis* **20**, 74–75.

AMIN, S. and MAIBACH, H.I. (2001) Diagnostic tests in dermatology: patch and photopatch testing and contact uriticaria. In: HAYES, A.W., THOMAS, J.A., GARDNER, D.E. and MAIBACH, H.I. (eds) *Toxicology of the Skin*. London: Taylor and Francis.

ANDERSEN, K.E. (1978) Contact allergy to toothpaste flavors. *Contact Dermatitis* **4**, 195–198.

ANGELINI, E., MARINARO, C., CARROZZO, A.M. *et al.* (1993) Allergic contact dermatitis of the lip margins from para-tertiary butylphenol in a lip liner. *Contact Dermatitis* **28**, 146–148.

BARAN, R. (1982) Pathology induced by the application of cosmetics to the nail. In: FROST, P. and HORWITZ, S.N. (eds) *Principles of Cosmetics for the Dermatologist*. St Louis, MO: CV Mosby.

BARAN, R. and MAIBACH, H.I. (eds) (1998) *Textbook of Cosmetic Dermatology*. (2nd edition). London: Martin Dunitz.

BAREL, A.O., PAYE, M. and MAIBACH, H.I. (2001) *Handbook of Cosmetic Science and Technology*. New York: Marcel Deckker, Inc.

BELTON, A.L. and CHIRA, T. (1997) Fatal anaphylactic reaction to hair dye. *Am. J. Forensic Med. Pathol.* **18**(3), 290–292.

BERARDESCA, E., CESPA, M., FARINELLI, N., *et al.* (1991) *In vivo* transcutaneous penetration of nicotinates and sensitive skin. *Contact Dermatitis* **25**, 35–38.

BERARDESCA, E., ELSNER, P. and MAIBACH, H.I. (1994) *Bioengineering of the Skin: Water and the Stratum Corneum*. Boca Raton: CRC Press Inc.

BERARDESCA, E., ELSNER, P. and MAIBACH, H.I. (1995a) *Bioengineering of the Skin: Cutaneous Blood Flow and Erythema*. Boca Raton: CRC Press Inc.

BERARDESCA, E., ELSNER, P., WILHELM, K-P. and MAIBACH, H.I. (1995b) *Bioengineering of the Skin: Methods and Instrumentation*. Boca Raton: CRC Press Inc.

BOUKHMAN, M.P. and MAIBACH, H.I. (2001) Thresholds in contact sensitization: Immunologic mechanisms and experimental evidence in humans—an overview. *Food and Chemical Toxicology* **39**, 1125–1134.

BRAUER, E.W. (1980) Onycholysis secondary to toluene sulfonamide formaldehyde resin used in a nail hardener mimicking onychomycosis. *Cutis* **26**, 58.

BRAUER, E.W. (1984) Cosmetics for the dermatologist. In: DENNIS, D.J. and McGUIRE J. (eds) *Clinical Dermatology*, Vol 4. Philadelphia: Harper and Row.

BRONAUGH, R.L. and MAIBACH, H.I. (1982) Primary irritant, allergic contact, phototoxic, and photoallergic reactions to cosmetics and tests to identify problem products. In: FROST, P. and HORWITZ, S.N. (eds) *Principles of Cosmetics for the Dermatologist*. St Louis, MO: CV Mosby.

BRUYNZEEL, D.P. and MAIBACH, H.I. (1986) Excited skin syndrome (angry back). *Arch. Dermatol.* **122**, 323–328.

BRUYNZEEL, D.P., VAN KETEL, W.G. and DE HAAN, P. (1984) Formaldehyde contact sensitivity and the use of shampoos. *Contact Dermatitis* **10**, 179–180.

BRUZE, M., FREGRET, S. and LUGGREN, B. (1985) Effects of ultraviolet irradiation of photopatch test substances *in vitro*. *Photodermatology* **2**, 32–37.

BRUZE, M., FREGERT, S. and GRUVBERGER, B. (1984) Occurrence of *para*-aminobenzoic acid and benzocaine as contaminants in sunscreen agents of *para*-aminobenzoic acid type. *Photodermatology* **1**, 277–285.

BRUZE, M., GRUVBERGER, B. and THUNE, P. (1988) Contact and photocontact allergy to glyceryl *para*-aminobenzoate. *Photodermatology* **5**, 162–165.

BURROWS, D. and RYCROFT, R.J.G. (1981) Contact dermatitis from PTBP resin and tricresyl ethyl phthalate in plastic nail adhesive. *Contact Dermatitis* **7**, 336–367.

BURY, J.N. (1980) Photoallergies from benzophenones and β-carotene in sunscreens. *Contact Dermatitis* **6**, 211–239.

CAGEN, S.Z., MALLOY, L.A., PARKER, C.M. *et al.* (1984) Pyrrethroid mediated skin sensory stimulation characterized by a new behavioral paradigm. *Toxicol. Appl. Pharmacol.* **76**, 270–279.

CALNAN, C.D. (1973) Ditertibarybutylhydroquinone in eyeshadow. *Contact Dermatitis Newsl.* **13**, 368.

CALNAN, C.D. (1975) Compound allergy to a cosmetic. *Contact Dermatitis* **1**, 123.

CALNAN, C.D. (1976a) Quinazoline yellow SS in cosmetics. *Contact Dermatitis* **2**, 160–166.

CALNAN, C.D. (1976b) Cinnamon dermatitis from an ointment. *Contact Dermatitis* **2**, 167–170.

CALNAN, C.D. (1981) Amyldimethylamino benzoic acid causing lipstick dermatitis. *Contact Dermatitis* **6**, 233.

CALNAN, C.D., CRONIN, E. and RYCROFT, R.J.G. (1981) Allergy to phenyl salicylate. *Contact Dermatitis* **7**, 208–211.

CALNAN, C.D., FISHER, A.A. And DOOMS-GOOSENS, A. (1976) Persulfate hair bleach reactions. Cutaneous and respiratory manifestations. *Arch. Dermatol.* **112**, 1407–1409.

CAMARASA, J.G. and SERRA-BALDRICH, E. (1986) Allergic contact dermatitis to sunscreens. *Contact Dermatitis* **15**, 253–254.

CARO, I. (1978) Contact allergy/photoallergy to glyceryl PABA and benzocaine. *Contact Dermatitis* **4**, 381–382.

CHAN, P.K., BALDWIN, R.C., PARSONS, R.D. *et al.* (1983) Kathon biocide: manifestation of delayed contact in guinea pigs is dependent on the concentration of induction and challenge. *J. Invest. Dermatol.* **81**, 409–411.

CHOWDHURY, M.M. (2002) Allergic contact dermatitis from prime yellow carnauba wax and coathylene in mascara. *Contact Dermatitis* **46**(4), 244.

CLARK, E.W., BLONDEEL, A., CRONIN, E. *et al.* (1981) Lanolin of reduced sensitizing potential. *Contact Dermatitis* **7**, 80–83.

COOK, N. and FREEMAN, S. (2001) Report of 19 cases of photoallergic contact dermatitis to sunscreens seen at the skin and cancer foundation. *Australas. J. Dermatol.* **42**(4), 257–259.

CRONIN, D. (1973) Dermatitis from wife's dyed hair. *Contact Dermatitis Newl.* **13**, 363.

CRONIN, D. (1979) Immediate-type hypersensitivity to henna. *Contact Dermatitis* **5**, 198–199.

CRONIN, E. (1980) *Cosmetic Dermatitis.* New York: Churchill Livingstone.

CRONIN, E. (1982) Dermatitis of the hands of beauticians. In: MAIBACH, H.I. and GELLIN, G.A. (eds) *Occupational and Industrial Dermatology.* New York: Year Book Medical Publishers, 215.

■ CHAPTER 51 ■

CRONIN, E. (1980) Lipstick dermatitis due to propyl galate. *Contact Dermatitis* 6, 231–214.

CULLISON, D., ABELE, D.C. and O'QUINN, J.L. (1983) Localized exogenous ochronosis. *J. Am. Acad. Dermatol.* 8, 882–889.

CUNNINGHAM-RUNDLES, S. (1981) Cell-mediated immunity. In: SAFAI, B. and GOOD, R.A. (eds) *Immunodermatology.* New York: Plenum, 233.

DAHLQUIST, I. and FREGERT, S. GRUYBERGER, B. (1979) Release of nickel from plated utensils on permanent wave liquids. *Contact Dermatitis* 5, 52–53.

DE GROOT, A.C. (1988) *Adverse Reactions to Cosmetics.* Thesis, State University of Groningen.

DE GROOT, A.C. (1994) *Patch Testing: Test Concentrations and Vehicles for 3700 Chemicals.* 20th edition. Amsterdam: Elsevier Science BV.

DE GROOT, A.C. and WEYLAND, J.W. (1987) Contact allergy to butyl methoxydibenzoylmethane. *Contact Dermatitis* 16, 278.

DE GROOT, A.C. (2000) Allergic contact dermatitis: cosmetics. In: PAMHAM, M.J. (ed.) *Progress in Inflammation Research.* Basel Switzerland: Birkhauser Verlag.

DE GROOT, A.C. VAN DER WALLE, H.B. JAGTMAN, B.A. and WEYLAND, J.W. (1987) Contact allergy to 4-isopropyldibenzoylmethane and 3-(4-methylbenzylidene) camphor in sunscreen Eusolex 8021. *Contact Dermatitis* 16, 249–254.

DICKEL, H., KUSS, O., SCHMIDT, A., and DREPGEN, T.L. (2002) Impact of preventative strategies on trend of occupational skin disease in hair dressers: population based register study. *MBJ* 324(7351), 1422–1423.

DOOMS-GOOSENS, A., DEGREEF, H. and LUYTENS, E. (1979) Dihydroabieyl alcohol (Abitol), a sensitizer in mascara. *Contact Dermatitis* 5, 350–353.

DRAELOS, Z.D. (2001) Nail cosmetics. *Emedicine Journal* 2(11), 1–10.

DRAKE, T.E. And MAIBACH, H.I. (1976) Allergic contact dermatitis and stomatitis caused by cinnamic aldehyped-flavored toothpaste. *Arch. Dermatol.* 112, 202–203.

DUGUID, C., O'SULLIVAN, D. and MURPHY, G.M. (1993) Determination of threshold UV-A elicitation dose on photopatch testing. *Contact Dermatitis* 29, 192–194.

EDWARDS, E.K. JR. and EDWARDS, E.K. (1982) Allergic contact dermatitis to lead acetate in hair dye. *Cutis* 30, 629–630.

EFFENDY, I. and MAIBACH, H.I. (2001) Cytokines and irritant dermatitis syndrome. In: HAYES, A.W., THOMAS, J.A., GARDNER, D.E. and MAIBACH, H.I. (eds) *Toxicology of the Skin*. London: Taylor and Francis.

EFFENDY, I., LOFFLER, H. and MAIBACH, H.I. (1995) Baseline Transepidermal water loss in patients with acute and healed irritant contact dermatitis. *Contact Dermatitis* **333**, 371–374.

EIERMAN, H.J., LARSEN, W., MAIBACH, H.I. and TAYLOR, J.S. (1982) Prospective study of cosmetic reactions: 1977–1980. *J. Am. Acad. Dermatol.* **6**, 909–917.

ELSNER, P. and MAIBACH, H.I. (eds) (2000) *Cosmeceuticals: drugs vs. Cosmetics.* New York: Marcel Deckker, Inc.

ELSNER, P., BERARDESCA, E., WILHELM, K-P. and MAIBACH, H.I. (2002) *Bioengineering of the Skin: Skin Biomechanics*. Boca Raton: CRC Press LLC.

ELSNER, P., MERK, H.F. and MAIBACH, H.I. (eds) (1999) *Cosmetics: Controlled Efficacy Studies and Regulation*. Berlin Heidelberg: Springer-Verlag.

ENGLISH, J.S.C. and WHITE, I.R. (1986) Allergic contact dermatitis from isopropyl dibenzoylmethane. *Contact Dermatitis* **15**, 94.

ENGRASSER, P.G. and MAIBACH, H.I. (1985) Cosmetics and dermatology: hair dye toxicology. In: ROOK, A.J. and MAIBACH, H.I. (eds) *Recent Advances in Dermatology*, Vol. 6, New York: Churchill Livingstone, 127.

EPSTEIN, W.L. (1961) Contact-type delayed hypersensitivity in infants and children: Induction of rhus sensitivity. *Pediatrics* **27**, 51–53.

EPSTEIN, S. (1963) Masked photopatch tests. *Contact Dermatitis* **41**, 369.

EPSTEIN, E. (1965) Misleading mascara patch test. *Arch Dermatol* **91**, 615–616.

FAGERLUND, V-L., KALIMO, K. and JANSEN, C. (1983) Valonsuojaaineet fotokontaktiallergian aiheuttajina. *Duodecin* **99**, 146–153.

FINDLAY, G.H., MORISON, J.G.L. and SIMSON, I.W. (1975) Exogenous ochronosis and pigmented colloid millium from hydroquinone bleaching creams. *Br. J. Dermatol.* **93**, 613–622.

FISHER, A.A. (1970) Patch tests of allergic reactions to dentifrices and mouthwashes. *Cutis* **6**, 554–561.

FISHER, A.A. (1973) *Contact Dermatitis,* 2nd edn. Philadelphia: Lea & Febiger.

FISHER, A.A. (1976) Sunscreen dermatitis due to glyceryl PABA: significance of cross-reactions to this PABA ester. *Cutis* **18**, 495–496, 500.

FISHER, A.A. (1977a) Dermatitis due to benzocaine present in sunscreens containing glyceryl PABA (Escalol 106). *Contact Dermatitis* **3**, 170–171.

■ CHAPTER 51 ■

FISHER, A.A. (1977b) Suppression of reactions to certain cosmetics. *Cutis* **20**, 170, **176**, 182–187.

FISHER, A.A. (1980a) Cosmetic dermatitis, II. Reaction to some commonly used perservatives. *Cutis* **26**, 136–137, 141–142, 147–148.

FISHER, A.A. (1980b) Cross reaction between methyl methacrylate monomer and acrylic monomers presently used in acrylic nail preparations. *Contact Dermatitis* **6**, 345–347.

FISHER, A.A. (1980c) Current contact news (cosmetic action and reactions: therapeutic irritant, and allergic). *Cutis* **26**, 22–24, 29–30, 32.

FISHER, A.A. (1983) Current contact news. Hydroquinone uses and abnormal reactions. *Cutis* **31**, 240–244, 250.

FISHER, A.A. (1990) Management of facial irritation due to cosmetics in patients with "status cosmeticus" (cosmetic intolerance). *Cutis* **46**, 291–293.

FISHER, A.A. and BARAN, R. (1991) Adverse reactions to acrylate sculpture nails with particular reference to prolonged paresthesia. *Am. J. Contact Dermatitis* **2**, 38–42.

FISHER, T. and MAIBACH, H.I. (1986) Patch testing in allergic contact dermatitis: an update. *Semin. Dermatol.* **5**, 214–224.

FISHER, A.A. and DOOMS-GOOSENS, A. (1976) Persulfate hair bleach reactions. Cutaneous and respiratory manifestations. *Arch. Dermatol.* **112**, 1407–1409.

FISHER, A.A. FRANKS, A. and GLICK, H. (1977) Allergic to sensitization skin and nails to acrylic plastic nails. *.J. Allergy* **28**, 84–88.

FITZPATRICK, T.B., ARNDT, K.A., EL MOFTY, A.M. and PATHAK, M.A. (1966) Hydroquinone and psoralens in the therapy of hypermelanosis and vitiligo. *Arch. Dermatol.* **93**, 589–600.

FLUHR, J.W., KUSS, O., DIEPGEN, T., LAZZERINI, S., PELOSI, A., GLOOR, M. and BERARDESCA, E. (2001) Testing for irritation with a multifactorial approach: comparison of 8 non-invasive measuring techniques on 5 different irritation types. *Br. J. Dermatol.* **145**(5), 696–703.

FOOD and DRUG ADMINISTRATION (1975) Food, Drug, and Cosmetic Products Warning Statements. *Federal Register* **40**, 8912.

FOOD and DRUG ADMINISTRATION (1978) Sunscreen drug products for the over-the-counter human drugs: proposed safety, effective and labeling conditions. *Federal Register* **43**, 38-206.

FOUSSEREAU, J., REUTER, G. and PETITJEAN, J. (1980) Is hair dyed with PPD-like dyes allergenic? *Contact Dermatitis* **6**, 143.

FRANKLIN, S. (2001) Dose-response studies in the guniea pig allergy test. In: HAYES, A.W., THOMAS, J.A., GARDNER, D.E. and MAIBACH, H.I. (eds) *Toxicology of the Skin*. London: Taylor and Francis.

FROSCH, P.J. (1989) Aktuelle Kontaktallergerne. *Hautarzt* 41(Suppl 10) 129–133.

FROSCH, P.J. and KLIGMAN, A.M. (1977a) A method for appraising the stinging capacity of topically applied substances. *J. Soc. Cosmet. Chem.* **28**, 197–207.

FROSCH, P.J., and KLIGMAN, A. (1977b) The chamber scarification test for assessing irritancy of topically applied substances. In: DRUKK, V.A. and LAZAR, P. (eds). *Cutaneous Toxicology* New York: Academic Press 127–144.

FROSCH, D.B., CAMARASA, J.G., DOOMS-GOOSENS, A. *et al.* (1993) Allergic reactions to a hair dressers' series: results from 9 European centers. *Contact Dermatitis* **28**, 180–183.

FULLER, M. (1982) Analysis of paint-on artificial nails. *J. Soc. Somset. Chem.* **33**, 51–53.

FULTON, J.E. (1989) Cosmedogenicity and irritancy of commonly used ingredients in skin care products. *J. Soc. Cosmet. Chem.* **40**, 321–333.

FULTON, J.E., PAY, S.R. and FULTON, J.E. (1984) Cosmedogenicity of current therapeutic products, cosmetics, and ingredients in the rabbit ear. *J. Am. Acad. Dermatol.* **10**, 96–105.

GELLIN, G.A., MAIBACH, H.I., MISISAZXEK, M.H. *et al.* (1979) Detection of environmental depigmenting substances. *Contact Dermatitis* **5**, 201–213.

GOLDENBERG, R.L. and SAFRIN, L. (1977) Reduction to topical irritiation. *J. Soc. Cosmet.* **28**, 667–701.

GUERRA, L., BARDAZZI, F. and TOSTI, A. (1992) Contact dermatitis in hairdressers' clients. *Contact Dermatitis* **26**, 108–111.

GUERRA, L., TOSTI, A., BARDAZZI, F. *et al.* (1992) Contact dermatitis in hairdressers: the Italian experience. *Contact Dermatitis* **26**, 101–107.

GUIN, J.D., MEYER, B.N., DRAKE, R.D. and HAFFLEY, P. (1984) The effects of quenching agents on contact urticaria caused by cinnamic aldehyde. *J. Am. Acad. Dermatol.* **10**, 45–51.

HANNUKESELA, M., KOUSA, M. and PIRILA, V. (1984) *Contact Dermatitis* **10**, 74–76.

HARVEL, J., BASON, M. and MAIBACH, H.I. (1994) Contact urticaria and its mechanisms. *Food and Chem. Toxicol.* **32**, 103–112.

HELD, E., JOHANSEN, J.D., AGNER, T. and MENNE, T. (1999) Contact allergy to cosmetics: testing with patients' own products. *Contact Dermatitis* **40**(6), 310–315.

HERBST, R.A. (2001) Assay to quantify subjective irritation caused by pyrethroid irritation caused by the pyrethroid insecticide alpha-cypermethrin. In: HAYES, A.W., THOMAS, J.A., GARDNER, D.E. and MAIBACH, H.I. (eds) *Toxicology of the Skin.* London: Taylor and Francis.

HINDSON, C. and LAWLOR, F. (1983) Coconut diethanolamide in hydraulic mining oil. *Contact Dermatitis* 9, 168.

HINDSON, C. (1975) o-Nitro-*para*phenylenediamine in hair dye—an unusual dental hazard. *Contact Dermatitis* 1, 333.

HJORTH, N. (1981) Contact dermatitis in children. *Acta Derm. Venerol. (Stockh.)* 95, 36–39.

HJORTH, N. and ROED-PETERSON, J. (1986) Patch testing to Kathon CG. *Contact Dermatitis* 14, 155–157.

HJORTH, N. WILKINSON, D. MAGNUSSON, B. *et al.* (1978) Glyceryl *p*-aminobenzoate patch testing in benzocaine-sensitive subjects. *Contact Dermatitis* 4, 46–48.

HOLNESS, D.L. and NETHERCOTT, J.R. (1990) Dermatitis in hair-dressers. In: ADAMS, R.M. and NETHERCOTT, J.R. (eds) *Dermatology Clinics*, Vol 8. Philadelphia: Saunders, 119–126.

HOLZLE, E., NEUMANN, N., HANSEN, B. *et al.* (1988) Photopatch testing: the 5-year experience of the German, Australian, and Swiss Photopatch Test Group. *J. Am. Acad. Dermatol.* 18, 1044–1047.

JACKSON, E.M. (1991) Cosmetics: substantiating safety. In: MARZULLI, N. and MAIBACH, H.I. (eds) *Dermatoxicology*, 4th edn New York: Hemisphere.

JACKSON, E.M. and ROBILLARD, N.F. (1982) The controlled use test in a cosmetic product safety substantiation program. *J. Toxicol.-Cutan. Ocular Toxicol.* 1, 117–132.

JASS, H.E. (1982) Rationale of formulations of deodorants and antiperspirants. In: FROST, P. and HORWITZ, S.N. (eds) *Principles of Cosmetics for the Dermatologist.* St Louis, MO: CV Mosby, 98.

JOURDAIN, R., DE LACHARRIERE, O., BASTEIN, P. and MAIBACH, H.I. (2002) Ethnic variations in self-perceived sensitive skin: epidemiological survey. *Contact Dermatitis* 46(3), 162–169.

KAIDBEY, K.H. (1983) The evaluation of photoallergic contact sensitizers in humans. In: MARZULLI, F.N. and MAIBACH, H.I. (eds) *Dermatoxicology*, 2nd edition. Washington DC: Hemisphere, 405–414.

KAIDBEY, K.H. and KLIGMAN, A.M. (1980) Photomaximization test for identifying photoallergic contact sensitizers. *Contact Dermatitis* 6, 161–169.

KAMINESTER, L.H. (1981) Allergic reaction to sunscreen products. *Arch. Dermatol.* **117**, 66.

KATZ, S.I. (1970) Relative effectiveness of selected sunscreens. *Arch. Dermatol.* **101**, 466–468.

KLIGMAN, A.M. (1966) The identificaion of contact allergens by human assay. II. Factors influencing the induction and measurement of allergetic contact dermatitis. *J. Invest. Dermatol.* **47**, 375–392.

KLIGMAN, A.M. (1983) Lanolin allergy crisis or comedy. *Contact Dermatitis* **9**, 99.

KLIGMAN, A.M. and MILLS, O.H. (1972) Acne cosmetica. *Arch. Dermatol.* **106**, 843–850.

KOHL, L., BLONDEEL, A. and SONG, M. (2002) Allergic contact dermatitis cosmetics. Retrospective analysis of 819 patch-tested patients. *Dermatology* **204**(4), 334–337.

KOZUKA, T., TASHIRO, M. and SANO, S. *et al.* (1980) Pigmented cosmetic dermatitis from azo dyes. I. Cross-sensitivity in humans. *Cosmetic Dermatitis* **6**, 330–336.

LABOWS, J.N., MCGINLEY, K.Z.J. and KLIGMAN, A.M. (1982) Axillary odor: current status. In: FROST, P. and HORWITZ, S.N. (eds) *Principles of Cosmetics for the Dermatologist.* St Louis, MO: CV Mosby, 98.

LAHTI, A. (1987) Terfenadine does not inhibit non-immunologic contact urticaria. *Contact Dermatitis* **16**, 220–223.

LAHTI, A. and MAIBACH, H.I. (1980) Nonimmunologic contact urticaria. *Acta Derm. Venereol. (Stockh.) Suppl.* **60**(91), 1–49.

LAHTI, A. and MIABACH, H.I. (1985) Species specificity of non-immunologic contact urticaria: guinea pig, rat, and mouse. *J. Am. Acad. Dermatol.* **13**, 66.

LAHTI, A. and MAIBACH, H.I. (1987) Immediate contact reaction: contact urticaria syndrome. *Semin. Dermatol.* **6**, 313–320.

LAHTI, A., MCDONALD, D.M., TAMMI, R. and MAIBACH, H.I. (1986) Pharmacological studies on non-immunologic contact urticaria in guinea pigs. *Arch. Dermatol. Res.* **279**, 44–49.

LAHTI, A., OIKARINEN, A., VIINIKKA, L. *et al.* (1983) Prostaglandins in contact urticaria induced by benzoic acid. *Acta Derm. Venereol. (Stockh.)* **63**, 425–427.

LAMMINTAUSTA, K. and MAIBACH, H.I. (1988) Exogenous and endogenous factors in skin irritation. *International Journal of Dermatology* **27**, 213–222.

LAMMINTAUSTA, K., MAIBACH, H.I, and WILSON, D. (1988) Mechanisms of subjective irritation: propensity of nonimmunologic contact urticaria and objective irritation in stingers. *Derm. Beruf. Unwelt.* **36**, 45–49.

LANDSTEINER, K. and JACOBS, J. (1935) Studies on the sensitization of animals with simple chemical compounds. II. *J. Exp. Med.* **64**, 626–629.

LARSEN, W.G. (2000) How to test for fragrance allergy. *Cutis* **65**(1) 39–41.

LAUNDER, T. and KANSKY, A. (2000) Increase in contact allergy to fragrances: patch testing results 1989–1998. *Contact Dermatitis* **43**(2) 107–109.

LAZNET, M. (1982) Modern formulations of coloring agents: facial and eye. In: FROST, P. and HORWITZ, S.N. (eds) *Principles of Cosmetics for the Dermatologist.* St. Louis, MO: CV Mosby, 133.

LE COZ, C.J., LECLERE, J.M., ARNOULT, E., RAISON-PEYRON, N., PONS-GUIRAUD, A. and VIGAN, M. (2002) Allergic contact dermatitis from shellac in mascara. *Contact Dermatitis* **46**(3), 149–152.

LEVER, W.F. and SCHAUMBURG-LEVER, G. (1983) *Histopathology of the Skin,* 6th edition. Philadelphia: Lippincott.

LOFFLER, H. and EFFENDY, I. (2002) Prevention of irritant contact dermatitis. *Eur. J. Dermatol.* **12**(1), 4–9.

LYNDE, C.W. and MITCHELL, J.C. (1982) Patch test results in 66 hairdressers 1973–81. *Contact Dermatitis* **8**, 302–307.

MAGNUSSUN, B. and KLIGMAN, A.M. (1969) The identification of contact allergens by animals assay. The guinea pig maximization test. *J. Invest. Dermatol.* **52**, 268–276.

MAGNUSSUN, B. and KLIGMAN, A.M. (1970) *Allergic Contact Dermatitis in the Guinea Pig.* Springfield, Il: Charles C Thomas.

MAGUIRE, H.C. (1974) Alteration in the acquisition of delayed hypersensitivity with adjuvant in the guinea pig. *Monogr. Allergy* **8**, 13–26.

MAIBACH, H.I. and ENGASSER, P. (1988) Management of cosmetic syndrome. *Clinics Dermatol.* **6**, 102–107.

MAIBACH, H.I. and JOHNSON, H.L. (1975) Contact hypersensitive urticaria syndrome. Contact urticaria to diethyltoluamide (immediate-tivity). *Arch. Dermatol.* **111**, 726–730.

MAIBACH, H.I., ALKERSON, J.M., MARZULLI, F.N. *et al.* (1980) Test concentrations and vehicles for dermatological testing of cosmetic ingredients. *Contact Dermatitis* **6**, 369–404.

MAIBACH, H.I., GELLEN, G. and RING, M. (1975) Is the antioxidant butylated hydroxytoluene depigmenting agent in man? *Contact Dermatitis* **1**, 295–296.

MAIBACH, H.I. (1978) Chronic dermatitis and hyperpigmentation from pertrolatum. *Contact Dermatitis* **4**, 62.

MARCUSSEN, P.V. (1963) Primary irritant patch-test reactions in chlidren. *Arch. Dermatol.* **87**, 378–382.

MARKS, J.F. BISHOP, M.E. and WILLIS, W.F. (1979) Allergic contact dermatitis to sculptured nails. *Arch. Dermatol.* **115**, 100.

MARMELZAT, J. and RAPAPORT, J.M.J. (1980) Photodermatitis with PABA. *Contact Dermatitis* **6**, 230–231.

MARZULLI, F.N. and MAIBACH, H.I. (1974) The use of graded concentration in studying skin sensitizers: experimental contact sensitization in man. *Food Cosmet. Toxicol.* **12**, 219–227.

MARZULLI, F.N. and MAIBACH, H.I. (eds) (1991) *Dermatoxicology*, 4th edition. New York: Hemisphere.

MARZULLI, F.N. and MAIBACH, H.I. (1973) Antimicrobials: experimental contact sensitization in man. *J. Soc. Cosmet. Chem.* **24**, 399–421.

MATHIAS, C.G. (1982) Pigmented cosmetic dermatitis from contact allergy to a toilet soap containing chromium. *Contact Dermatitis* **8**, 29–31.

MATHIAS, C.G. and MAIBACH, H.I. (1978) Dermatoxicology monographs I. Cutaneous irritation: factors influencing the response to irritants. *Clin. Toxicol.* **13**, 333–346.

MATHIAS, C.G., MAIBACH, H.I. and CONANT, M.A. (1980) Perioral leukoderma simulation vitiligo from use of a toothpaste containing cinnamic aldehyde. *Arch. Dermatol.* **116**, 1172–1173.

MCCAIN, D.C. and STORRS, F.J. (1994) *Am. J. Contact Dermatitis* **3**, 201–205.

MCFADDEN, J.P., WAKELIN, S.H. and BASKETTER, D.A. (1998) Acute irritation thresholds in subjects with Type I-Type V1 skin. *Contact Dermatitis* **38**, 147–149.

MELSTRAN, G.A., WAHLBERG, J.E. and MAIBACH, H.I. (eds). (1994) *Protective Gloves for Occupational Use.* Boca Raton, FL: CRC Press.

MILLS, O.H. and BERGER, R.S. (1991) Defining the susceptibility of acne prone and sensitive skin populations to extrinsic factors. *Dermatol. Clin.* **9**, 93–98.

MILLS, O.H. JR and KLIGMAN, A.M. (1982) A human model for assessing comedogenic substances. *Arch. Dermatol.* **118**, 903–905.

■ CHAPTER 51 ■

MITCHELL, L., SCHOLOSSMAN, M.L. and WIMMER, E. (1992) Advances in nail enamel technology. *J. Sco. Cosmet. Chem.* **43**, 331–337.

MORK, N-J. AUSTAD, J. (1984) Contact dermatitis from witisol, sunscreen agent. *Contact Dermatitis* **10**, 122–123.

MORRISON, L.H., STORRS, F.J. (1988) Persistance of an allergen in hair after glyceryl monothioglycolate-containing permanent wave solutions. *J. Am. Acad. Dermatol.* **19**, 52–59.

NAKAYAMA, H., HARADA, R. and TODA, M. (1976) Pigmented cosmetic dermatitis. *Int. J. Dermatol.* **15**, 673–675.

NATER, J.P. and DE GROOT, A.C. (1993) *Unwanted Effects of Cosmetics and Drugs Used in Dermatology*, (3rd edition). New York: Elsevier.

NIXON, R.L., FROWEN, K.E. and LEWIS, A.E. (n.d.) Skin reactions to sunscreens. *Australas. J. Dermatol.* **38**(Suppl 1), 583–585.

NORTON, L.A. (1991) Common and uncommon reactions to formaldehyde-containing nail hardeners. *Semin. Dermatol.* **10**, 29–33.

PALTZIK, R.L. and ENSCOE, I. (1980) Onycholysis secondary to toluene sulfon-amide formaldehyde resin used in a nail hardener mimicking onychomycosis. *Cutis* **25**, 647–648.

PASRICHA, I.S., GUPTA, R. and PANJWANI, S. (1980) Contact dermatitis to henna (*Lawsonia*). *Contact Dermatitis* **6**, 288–289.

PATCHER, F. and HUNZIKER, N. (1989) Sensitization to Kathon CG in Switzerland. *Contact Dermatitis* **20**, 115–119.

PELOSI, A., LAZZERINI, S., BERARDESCA, E. and MAIBACH, H.I. (2001) Test for sensitive skin. In: BAREL, A.O., PAYE, M. and MAIBACH, H.I. (eds) *Handbook of Cosmetic Science and Technology* . Marcel Dekker, Inc., New York, NY. Part 9: Cosmetic Claims, Chapter 68, 823–828.

POLAK, L., POLAK, A. and FREY, J.R. (1974) The development of contact sensitivity to DNFB in guinea pigs genetically differing in their response to DNP-skin protein conjugate. *Int. Arch. Appl. Immunol.* **46**, 417–426.

PROTTEY, C. (1978) The molecular basis of skin irritation. In: BREUER, M.M. (ed.) *Cosmetic Science*, Vol I. London: Academic Press.

PUGLIESE, P.T. (1983) Cell renewal—an overview. *Cosmet. Toiletries* **98**, 61–65.

RAPAPORT, M.J. (1980) Sensitization to abitol. *Contact Dermatitis* **6**, 137.

REISS F and FISHER, A.A. (1972) Is hair dyed with paraphenylenediamine allergenic. Arch. 73. Mitchell JC. Allergic contact dermatitis from paraphenylenediamine presenting as nummular eczema. *Contact Dermatitis Newsl.* **11**, 270.

RIETSCHEL, H.L., HUGGINS, L. LEVY, ?. *et al.* (1984) *In vivo* and *in vitro* testing of gloves for protection against UV-curable acrylate resin systems. *Contact Dermatitis* **11**, 279–282.

RIETSCHEL, R.L. and LEWIS, C.W. (1978) Contact dermatitis to homomenthyl salicylate. *Arch Dermatol* **114**, 442–443.

RILEY, P.A. (1971) Acquired hypomelanosis. *Br. J. Dermatol.* **84**, 290–293.

ROBERTS, D.L. (1988) Contact allergy to Eusolex 8021. *Contact Dermatitis* **8**, 302.

ROBINSON, M.K. and PERKINS, M.A. (2002) A strategy for skin irritation testing. *Am. J. Contact Dermat.* **13**(1), 21–29.

RORSMAN, H. (1982) Riehl's melanosis. *Int. J. Dermatol.* **21**, 75–78.

RYCROFT, R.J.G. (1986) False reactions to non-standard patch test. *Semin. Dermatol.* **5**, 225–230.

SAI, S. (1983) Lipstick dermatitis caused by ricinoleic acid. *Contact Dermatitis* **9**, 524.

SAMMAN, P.D. (1977) Nail disorders caused by external influences. *J. Soc. Cosmet. Chem.* **28**, 351–356.

SAMS, W.M. (1956) Contact photodermatitis. *Arch. Dermatol.* **73**, 142–148.

SATO, Y., KUTSUNA, H., KOBAYASHI, T. and MITSUI, T. (1984) D&C nos. 10 and 11: chemical compositions analysis and delayed contact hypersensitivity testing in guinea pig. *Contact Dermatitis* **10**, 30–38.

SAXENA, M., WARSHAW, E. and AHMAD, D.D. (2001) Eyelid allergic contact dermatitis to black iron oxide. *Am. J. of Contact Dermatitis* **12**(1), 38–39.

SCHAUDER, S. and IPPEN, H. (1986) Photoallergic and allergic contact dermatitis from dibenzoylmethanes. *Photodermatology* **3**, 140–147.

SCHAUDER, S. and IPPEN, H. (1988) Photoallergic and allergic contact eczema caused by dibenzoylmethane compounds and other sunscreening agents. *Der Hautarzt* **39**, 435–440.

SCHEMAN, A. (2000) Adverse reactions to cosmetic ingredients. *Dermatol. Clin.* **18**(4), 685–698.

SCHORR, W.F. (1973) Lip gloss and gloss-type cosmetics. *Contact Dermatitis Newsl.* **14**, 408.

SCHORR, W.F. (1983) Multiple injuries from permanents. Presented at Cosmetic Symposium, American Academy of Dermatology. December 3, Chicago, IL.

CHAPTER 51

SCHUBERT, H., BAUMBACH, N., PRATER, E., *et al.* (1990) Patch testing with parabens. *Contact Dermatitis* 23, 245–246.

SHER, M.A. (1979) Contact dermatitis of the eyelids. *S. Afr. Med. J.* 55, 511–513.

SHUSTER, S. and SHAPIRO, J. (1976) Measurement of risk of sensitization and its application to Kathon. *Contact Dermatitis* 17, 299–302.

SIMMONS, R.J. (1955) Acute vulvovaginitis caused by soap products. *Obstet. Gynecol.* 6, 447–448.

SMITH, H.R., ARMSTRONG, D.K., HOLLOWAY, D., WHITTAM, L., BASKETTER, D.A. and McFADDEN, .JP. (2002) Skin irritation thresholds in hairdressers: implications for the development of dermatitis. *Br. J. Dermatol.* 146(5), 849–852.

SOILEAU, S.D. (2001) Dermal penetration of calcium salts and calcionis cutis. In: HAYES, A.W., THOMAS, J.A., GARDNER, D.E. and MAIBACH, H.I. (eds) *Toxicology of the Skin.* London: Taylor and Francis.

STORRS, F.J. (1984) Permanent wave contact dermatitis: contact allergy to glyceryl monothioglycolate. *J. Am. Acad. Dermatol.* 11, 74–85.

SULZBERGER, M.B., WARSHAW, T. and HERMANN, F. (1953) Studies of hyper-sensitivity to lanolin. *J. Invest. Dermatol.* 29, 33–43.

SYLVEST, B., HJORTH. N. and MAGNUSSON, B. (1975) Lauryl ether sulfate dermatitis in Denmark. *Contact Dermatitis* 1, 359–362.

TANGLERSAMPAN, C. and MAIBACH, H.I. (1993) The role of vehicles in diagnostic patch testing: A reappraisal. *Contact Dermatitis* 29(4), 169–174.

TAYLOR, J.S., JORDAN, W.P. and MAIBACH, H.I. (1984) Allergic contact dermatitis from stearamidoethyl diethylamine phosphate: a cosmetic emulsifier. *Contact Dermatitis* 10, 74–76.

TAYLOR, J.S., MAIBACH, H.I., FISHER, A.A. and BERGELD, W.F. (1933) Contact leukoderma associated with the use of hair colors. *Cutis* 52, 273–280.

THOMPSON, G., MIABACH, H. and EPSTEIN, J. (1977) Allergic contact dermatitis from sunscreen preparations complicating photodermatitis. *Arch. Dermatol.* 113, 1252–1253.

THUNE, P. (1984) Contact and photocontact allergy to sunscreens. *Photo-dermatology* 1, 5–9.

TOMB, R.R., LEPOITTEVIN, J., DUREPAIRE, F. *et al.* (1993) Ectopic contact dermatitis from ethyl cyanoacrylate instant adhesives. *Contact Dermatitis* 23, 206–208.

TUCKER, S.B., FLANNIGAN, S.A., DUNBAR, M. JR and DROTMAN, R.B. (1986) Development of an objective cosmedogenicity assay. *Arch. Dermatol.* 122, 660–702.

TURNER, T.W. (1977) Dermatitis from butylated hydroxyanisol. *Contact Dermatitis* **3**, 282.

UNANUE, E.R. (1984) Antigen-presenting function of the macrophage. *Annu. Rev. Immunol.* **2**, 395–428.

VAN HOOTE, N., DOOMS-GOOSENS, A. (1983) A shampoo dermatitis due to cocobetaine and sodium lauryl ether sulphate. *Contact Dermatitis* **9**, 169.

VAN JOOST, T., LIEM, D.H. and STOLZ, E. (1984) Allergic contact dermatitis to monotertiary-butylhydroquinone in lip gloss. *Contact Dermatitis* **10**, 189–190.

VAN KETEL, W.G. and LIEM, D.H. (1981) Eyelid dermatitis from nickel contaminated cosmetics. *Cosmetic Dermatitis* **7**, 217.

VAN KETEL, W.G. (1977) Allergic contact dermatitis from an aminobenzoic acid compound used in sunscreens. *Contact Dermatitis* **3**, 283.

VIVJEBERG, H.P. and VANDEN BERCKEN, J. (1979) Frequency dependent effects of the pyrethroid insecticide decamethrin in frog myelinated nerve fibers. *Eur. J. Pharmacol.* **58**, 501–515.

VON KROGH, G. and MAIBACH, H.I. (1982) The contact urticaria syndrome. *Semin. Dermatol.* **1**, 59–66.

WAHLBERG, J.E. (1975) Nickel allergy and atopy in hair-dressers. *Contact Dermatitis* **1**,161–165.

WAHLBERG, J.E. and MAIBACH, H.I. (1981) Sterile cutaneous pustules: a manifestation of primary irritancy? Identification of contact pustulogens. *J. Invest. Dermatol.* **76**, 381–383.

WARIN, A. (1976) Contact dermatitis to partner's hair dye. *Clin. Exp. Dermatol.* **1**, 283.

WELLER, P. and EIREMAN, S. (1984) Photocontact allergy to octyldimethyl PABA. *Aust. J. Dermatol.* **25**, 73–76.

WENNERSTEN, G., THUNE, P., JANSEN, C.T. and BRODHAGEN, H. (1986) Photocontact dermatitis: Current status with emphasis on allergic contact photosensitivity (CPS) occurrence, allergens, and practical phototesting. *Semin. Dermatol.* **5**, 277–289.

WENNERSTEN, G., THUNE, P.. BROADTHAGEN, H. *et al.* (1984) The Scandinavian multicenter photopatch study: preliminary results. *Contact Dermatitis* **10**, 305–309.

WHITE, I.R., CATCHPOLE, H.E. and RYCROFT, R.J.G. (1982) Rashes among persulfate workers. *Contact Dermatitis* **8**, 168–172.

WHITMORE, C.W. and MAIBACH, H.I. (1984) *Courtroom Medicine: The Skin*. New York: Mathew Bender.

WILHELM, K-P., ELSNER, P., BERARDESCA, E. and MAIBACH, H.I. (1997) *Bioengineering of the Skin: Skin Surface Imaging and Analysis*. Boca Raton: CRC Press Inc.

WILKENSON, M.G. and WILKIN, J.K. (1990) Azelic acid esters do not depigment pigmented guinea pigs. *Arch. Dermatol.* **126**, 252–253.

WILKINSON, J.B. MOORE, R.J. (1982) *Harry's Cosmetology*. New York: Chemical Publishing.

WILLE, J.J. and KYDONIEUS, A.F. (2001) Novel topical agents for prevention and treatment of allergic and irritant contact dermatitis. In: HAYES, A.W., THOMAS, J.A., GARDNER, D.E. and MAIBACH, H.I. (eds) *Toxicology of the Skin*. London: Taylor and Francis.

WILLIS, I. (1975) Photosensitivity. *Int. J. Dermatol.* **14**, 326–337.

WILLIS, I. and KLIGMAN, A.M. (1968) The mechanism of photoallergic contact dermatitis. *J. Invest. Dermatol.* **51**, 378–384.

WILSON, L.A., REID, F.R. and WOOD, T.O. (1979) *Pseudomonas* corneal ulcer. The causative role of contaminated eye cosmetics. *Arch. Ophthalmol.* **97**, 1640–1641.

YAMAZAKI, K. and TANAKA, M. (1990) Development of a new w/o emulsion-type nail enamel. In: *Preprints 16th IFSCC Congress, 1990*, Vol 1: 464–495.

Evaluating Efficacy of Barrier Creams: In Vitro and In Vivo Models

HONGBO ZHAI AND HOWARD I MAIBACH

Contents

52.1   Introduction

52.2   Testing methodology

52.3   Conclusions

52.1 INTRODUCTION

Contact dermatitis (CD) including irritant contact dermatitis (ICD) and allergic contact dermatitis (ACD) is a major occupational disease, with a significant medical, economical, and social impact. To avoid these annoying substances (irritants and allergens) may not be practicable for some occupational requirements. Therefore, barrier creams (BC) are utilized in the prevention of CD. Their efficacy in reducing the developing ICD and ACD have been documented *in vitro* and *in vivo* experimental studies (Frosch *et al.*, 1993a; Lachapelle, 1996; Zhai and Maibach, 1996a; Wigger-Alberti and Elsner, 1998; Zhai and Maibach, 1999; Wigger-Alberti and Elsner, 2000a, 2000b; Maibach and Zhai, 2000; Zhai and Maibach, 2002). However, some reports indicate that the inappropriate BC application may induce a deleterious rather than a beneficial effect (Goh, 1991a, b; Frosch *et al.*, 1993a, b, c, d; Treffel *et al.*, 1994; Zhai and Maibach, 1996b; Lachapelle, 1996). Two major reasons might generate these divergent results: one is the design defect of the BC; another possibility relates to the testing models. Thus, the methodology is important and hence the accuracy of results depends on the choice of proper models.

Several *in vitro* and *in vivo* methods have been developed to evaluate efficacy, and this subject has been reviewed (Frosch *et al.*, 1993a; Lachapelle, 1996; Zhai and Maibach, 1996a; Wigger-Alberti and Elsner, 1998; Zhai and Maibach, 1999; Wigger-Alberti and Elsner, 2000a; Maibach and Zhai, 2000; Zhai and Maibach, 2000; Wigger-Alberti and Elsner, 2000b; Zhai and Maibach, 2001; Zhai and Maibach, 2002). This chapter briefly introduces recent updated data.

52.2 TESTING METHODOLOGY

52.2.1 *In Vitro* Methods

Treffel *et al.* (1994) measured the effectiveness of BC on human skin against dyes (eosin, methylviolet and oil red O) with varying n-octanol/water partition coefficients (0.19, 29.8 and 165, respectively). BC effects were assayed by measurements of the dyes in the epidermis of protected skin samples after 30 minutes. Some BC showed efficacy but several revealed data contrary to manufacturers' claims. No correlation existed between the galenic (pharmaceutic) parameters of the assayed products and protection level, indicating that neither the water content nor the consistency of the formulations influenced effectiveness.

Fullerton and Menne (1995) tested the protective effect of ethylene-diaminetetraacetate barrier gels against nickel contact allergy. Thirty milligrams of barrier gel was applied on the epidermal side of the skin *in vitro* and a nickel disk applied above the gel. After 24 h, the nickel disk was removed and the epidermis separated from the dermis. Nickel content in epidermis and dermis was quantified by adsorption differential pulse voltammetry. The amount of nickel in the epidermal skin layer on barrier gels treated skin was significantly reduced compared to the untreated control.

Shah and Kirchner (1997) evaluated moisture penetration through a thin film of skin protectants *in vivo* and *in vitro* utilizing Fourier transform infrared spectroscopy. Petrolatum offered some protection against water penetration; a hydroactive polymer system (protectant) prevented moisture penetration.

Goffin *et al.* (1998) assessed the efficacy of BC to surfactants and organic solvents with shielded variants of corneosurfametry and corneoxenometry method. Petrolatum exhibited the best protection being a blocker for sodium lauryl sulfate (SLS) and also provided protection against hexane-methanol.

Zhai *et al.* (1999a) utilized an *in vitro* diffusion system to measure the protective effective of 3 quaternium-18 bentonite (Q18B) gels to prevent 1 percent 35S-SLS penetration by human cadaver skin. The accumulated amount of 35S-SLS in receptor cell fluid were counted to evaluate the efficacy of the model Q-18B gels over 24 h. These test gels significantly decreased SLS absorption when compared to the unprotected skin control samples. Protection effect (percent) of 3 Q18B was 88 percent, 81 percent and 65 percent, respectively.

van Der Bijl *et al.* (2000) conducted an *in vitro* study of the permeability of tritiated water through fresh and frozen human skin in the presence and absence of two different BC in a flow-through diffusion system. Buffer/tritiated water was collected from the acceptor chambers at 2-h intervals for a total of 20 h and counted in a liquid scintillation counter. Both BC lowered the average flux rates of tritiated water through fresh and frozen skin, but no significant differences could be detected between the two.

52.2.2 *In Vivo* Methods

Mahmound and Lachapelle (1985) and Lachapelle *et al.* (1990) developed a guinea pig model to evaluate the protective value of BC and/or gels by laser Doppler flowmetry (blood flow) and histological assessment. The histopathological damage after 10 min of toluene contact was mainly confirmed to the epidermis. Dermal blood flow changes were relatively high on the control site compared to the gel pretreated sites.

Fullerton and Menne (1995) performed an *in vivo* patch testing with nickel-sensitive patients by using nickel disks with and without barrier gels. Test preparations and nickel disks were removed 1-day post application, and the test sites evaluated. Barrier gel treated sites significantly reduced the positive test reactions.

Frosch *et al.* (1993b, 1993c, 1993d, 1994) established the repetitive irritation test (RIT) in the guinea pig and in humans to evaluate the efficacy of BC using series bioengineering techniques. The cream pretreated and untreated test skin (guinea pig or humans) were exposed daily to the irritants for 2 weeks. The resulting irritation was scored on a visual scale and assessed by biophysical (bioengineering) techniques' parameters. Some test creams suppressed irritation with all test parameters; some even increased irritation.

Grunewald *et al.* (1995) utilized a SLS repetitive washing model to evaluate the protective effects of BC by measuring with bioengineering techniques on 15 human volunteers. All BC reduced the deterioration of skin functions following one week repetitive washing. Subsequently, they also found urea- and glycerol oil-in-water emulsions provided a greater protection against a lipophilic irritant (toluene) after 7 days' repetitive irritation (Grunewald *et al.*, 1996).

Marks *et al.* (1995) investigated a topical lotion containing 5 percent Q18B in the prevention of experimentally induced poison ivy and poison oak ACD in susceptible volunteers. One hour before both forearms were patch tested with urushiol, 5 percent Q18B lotion was applied on one forearm. The test patches were removed after 4 h and the sites interpreted for reaction 2, 5, and 8 days later. The test sites pretreated with Q18B lotion had absent or significantly reduced reactions to the urushiol compared with untreated control sites (p<0.0001) on all test days.

Zhai and Maibach (1996b) measured the effectiveness of BC in an *in vivo* human model to against dye indicator solutions: methylene blue in water and oil red O in ethanol, representative of model hydrophilic and lipophilic compounds. Solutions of 5 percent methylene blue and 5 percent oil red O were applied to untreated and BC pretreated skin with the aid of aluminum occlusive chambers, for 0 h and 4 h. Post application time, materials were removed, and consecutive skin surface biopsies obtained. The amount of dye penetrating into each strip was determined by colorimetry. Two model creams exhibited effectiveness, but one enhanced the cumulated amount of dye.

Schlüter-Wigger and Elsner (1996) assessed four commercially-available BC against four standard irritants: 10 percent SLS, 1 percent sodium hydroxide (NaOH), 30 percent lactic acid (LA), and undiluted toluene (TOL) in the RIT in humans for 12 days. Irritation was assessed by visual scoring, transepidermal water loss (TEWL), and colorimetry. All products were very effective against SLS irritation. No BC provided significant protection against TOL. Three products showed a partially protective effect against all ionic irritants, while the fourth showed less protection against SLS and NaOH, and even amplification of inflammation by TOL. Wigger-Alberti and Elsner (1997) evaluated petrolatum utilizing the above model; petrolatum was effective against SLS, NaOH, and LA irritation, and provided a moderate protection against TOL. Wigger-Alberti *et al.* (1998) also examined three other BC and petrolatum against 10 percent SLS, 0.5 percent NaOH, 15 percent LA, and undiluted TOL in the RIT in humans for 9 days. All BC exhibited a significant protective effect against irritation by SLS, NaOH, and LA. Less efficacy was observed against TOL. In another 12-days RIT study (Wigger-Alberti *et al.*, 1999), white petrolatum provided a significant protective effect against SLS, NaOH, and TOL but with less protective effect against LA irritation.

de Fine Olivarius *et al.* (1996) determined BC efficacy in protecting against water, based on evaluation of color intensities when an aqueous solution of crystal violet is applied to the skin, after pretreatment with different creams. The BC with particles gave the best immediate protection (dorsal 76 percent, volar 69 percent). The moisturizer was intermediately protective (dorsal 57 percent, volar 34 percent), while little protection was found for the silicone-containing cream (dorsal 16 percent, volar 10 percent).

Fartasch *et al.* (1998) investigated protective capacity of a lipophilic BC on acute ICD by TEWL measurement. Application of the BC before and during irritation showed a decrease of TEWL by 58 percent (back) and 49 percent (arm).

Elsner *et al.* (1998) evaluated perfluoropolyethers containing BC against a set of four irritants: 10 percent SLS, 0.5 percent NaOH, 15 percent LA, and undiluted TOL in the RIT on the humans back. Irritation was assessed by visual scoring, TEWL, and colorimetry. All PFPE preparations significantly suppressed irritation by SLS and NaOH. However, only the 4 percent PFPE preparation was significant against LA and TOL.

Zhai *et al.* (1998) introduced a facile approach to screening protectants *in vivo* in human subjects. Two acute irritants and one allergen were selected: SLS, the combination of ammonium hydroxide (NH4OH) and urea, and Rhus. The model irritants and allergen were applied with an occlusive patch for 24 h.

Inflammation was scored with an expanded 10 point scale at 72 h post-application. Most test protectants statistically suppressed SLS irritation and Rhus allergic reaction but not NH4OH and urea induced irritation. They further utilized this model to evaluate the putative skin-protective formulations (Zhai *et al.*, 1999b). All formulations failed to inhibit NH4OH and urea irritation. Only paraffin wax in cetyl alcohol statistically ($p<0.01$) reduced Rhus-ACD. Three commercial formulations markedly ($p<0.001$) suppressed SLS-ICD.

Shimizu and Maibach (1999) used squamometry method to evaluate a barrier protectant (tannic acid). Five percent tannic acid and distilled water (as a control) were applied to forearms for 30 min; these pretreated sites were dosed with different concentrations of SLS for 24 h. Squamometric evaluation indicated the skin damage increased with SLS concentration in a dose-dependent manner, and tannic acid significantly reduced the damage ($p<0.01$).

Vidmar and Iwane (1999) assessed the ability of the topical skin protectant (TSP) to protect against to urushiol (Rhus)-ACD. Open urushiol patch testing was conducted on 50 rhus-sensitive subjects. After 96 h, dermatitis severity scores were compared between TSP protected and TSP unprotected sites by using a nine-point dermatitis scale. Results showed that TSP protected sites had mean dermatitis scores about two points lower than TSP unprotected sites ($p<0.001$).

Patterson *et al.* (1999) determined the preventive effect of a skin protectant containing dimethicone and glycerin with various inactive ingredients in an aerosol foam against SLS-ICD and poison ivy and poison oak (urushiol)-ACD. Skin reaction was assessed periodically for 10 days by using a 0 to 7 point dermatitis scale. The formulation was significantly effective in reducing SLS irritation but did not prevent urushiol-ACD.

Zhai *et al.* (2000) evaluated the efficacy of a dimethicone skin protectant lotion against SLS-ICD by clinical visual grading and bioengineering techniques in humans. Both forearms were pretreated either with the testing protectant lotion or with its vehicle control prior to contact with SLS. Thirty minutes later, 0.5 percent SLS was applied to each pretreated site for 24 h. One additional site received SLS only. The efficacy of protective effect was determined by visual scoring (VS), TEWL, skin color (a* value), and cutaneous blood flow volume (BFV). VS and TEWL data showed a significant decrease on the protectant lotion pretreated site in comparison to SLS only treated site as well as to vehicle control site. But, BFV and a* values did not show a statistically difference between either treated sites.

Berndt *et al.* (2000) investigated the efficacy of a BC and its vehicle in a field setting: two panels of 25 hospital nurses with mild signs of skin irritation were asked to use one of the test products (BC or its vehicle) and especially to use before contact with skin irritants over 4 weeks. Effects of both preparations were studied weekly by clinical examination and bioengineering measurements. Results showed no significant differences between BC and its vehicle. In both groups, clinical skin status improved and stratum corneum hydration increased significantly. They concluded that the vehicle alone is capable of positively influencing skin status.

Schnetz *et al.* (2000) introduced a standardized test procedure for the evaluation of skin protective products. A repeated short-time occlusive irritation test (ROIT) with a standardized protocol has been evaluated in two phases (12 days and 5 days protocol) in several clinical centers. Skin was treated by two irritants (0.5 percent SLS and toluene, twice a day for 30 min). Inflammation was measured by bioengineering methods (TEWL and colorimetry) and clinical scoring. The 5-day protocol was sufficient to achieve significant results. Furthermore, in spite of the expected inter-center variations due to heterogeneity of the individual threshold of irritation, interpretation of clinical score, and inter-instrumental variability, the ranking of the vehicles regarding reduction of the irritant reaction was consistent in all centers.

McCormick *et al.* (2000) measured the efficacy of a BC and an oil-containing lotion for protecting the hands of health care workers with severe hand irritation. Objective and subjective parameters for scaling, cracking, weeping, bleeding, and pain were scored by two blinded investigators weekly for 4 weeks. Subjects in both groups experienced marked improvement in overall hand condition (each, $p<0.02$), particularly in scaling, cracking, and pain. Volunteers randomized to use the oil-containing lotion showed the greatest improvement.

Sun *et al.* (2000) utilized laser-induced breakdown spectroscopy (LIBS) to evaluate the effect of BC on human skin; three representatives of commercial BC advertised as being effective against lipophilic and hydrophilic substances were evaluated by measuring zinc absorbed through the stratum corneum. Four consecutive SSBs were taken from biceps of the forearms of six volunteers at time periods of 0.5 h and 3 h after BC application. The BC provided appreciable protection against the penetration of both $ZnCl_2$ and ZnO into the skin when compared with control skin (without BC treated).

Allmers (2001) tested two types of latex gloves with and without the use of a BC on subjects who had Type I hypersensitivity reactions to natural rubber latex gloves. One hand received BC for 10 min, before both hands utilized gloves for 30 min. BC decreased latex gloves-induced contact urticaria syndrome.

Zhai *et al.* (2002) evaluated prevention of a model lipid emulsion against wearing occlusive glove-induced ICD. Test emulsion was applied to one hand, while the opposite hand remained untreated. Thirty minutes later, both hands were gloved for 3 h. Skin conditions were evaluated by visual scoring, water sorption-desorption test, TEWL, and skin capacitance. This procedure was repeated for 5 days. Emulsion treated hands showed significantly greater water holding capacity and lower TEWL values when compared to untreated hands. They concluded the test emulsion minimized glove induced-ICD.

Table 52.1 summarizes the recent experimental models and BC efficacy.

52.3 CONCLUSIONS

BC have shown the efficacy to diminish the development of CD from *in vitro* and *in vivo* methods described above. However, their actual benefits should be evaluated in the workplace as a supplement to model experiments. Additionally, many factors may influence the actual effectiveness of the BC (Packham *et al.*, 1994; Wigger-Alberti *et al.*, 1997a, 1997b).

These *in vitro* and *in vivo* models have been well developed; they provide insight into mechanisms as well as greater discriminatory potential. *In vitro* models are widely used to test the effects of BC because they are simple, rapid, and safe. In particular, they are recommended as a screening procedure for BC candidates. Radiolabeled methods may determine the accurate protective and penetration results even with lower levels of chemicals due to the sensitive of radiolabeled counting. Animal experiment may be used to generate kinetic data because of a closer similarity between humans and some animals (pigs and monkeys) in percutaneous absorption and penetration for some compounds. But no one animal, with its complex anatomy and biology, will simulate penetration in humans for all compounds. Therefore, the best estimate of human percutaneous absorption is determined by *in vivo* studies in humans. Histological assessments may define what layers of skin are damaged or protected, and may provide insight in BC mechanisms. Noninvasive bioengineering techniques provide accurate, highly reproducible, and objective observations in quantifying the inflammation response to various irritants and allergens; they can assess subtle differences to supplement traditional clinical studies.

Though BC may act against many irritants or allergens, their benefits are individual, i.e., to specific kinds of chemical. Regarding testing method, there is no standardized procedure so far. The testing quality or the reproducibility of results remains incompletely developed. We believe that a sensible,

CHAPTER 52

Table 52.1:

BC efficacy and testing models from recent experiments

Models		Irritants or allergens	BC	Efficacy	Authors and References
In Vitro	*In Vivo*				
Human skin		Dyes (eosin, methyl-violet, oil red O)	16 BC	Protection varied	Treffel *et al.* (1994)
Human skin	Nickel-sensitive patients	Nickel disk	(EDTA) gels	Significantly reduced the amount of nickel in the epidermis *in vitro*, and significantly reduced positive reactions *in vivo*	Fullerton and Menne (1995)
Thin protective product film	Humans	Moisture penetration	Petrolatum and a protectant	Petrolatum offered some protection against water penetration and a hydroactive polymer system (protectant) prevented moisture penetration	Shah and Kirchner (1997)
Human skin		SLS and a mixture of hexane and methanol	6 products	Petrolatum exhibited the best protective effect against SLS and also provided good protection to organic solvents	Goffin *et al.* (1998)
Human skin		[35S]-SLS	3 Q18B gels	Protection effect (percent) was 88 percent, 81 percent and 65 percent, respectively	Zhai *et al.* (1999a)
Fresh and frozen human skin		Tritiated water	2 BC	Both BC lowered the average flux rates of tritiated water through fresh and frozen skin	van Der Bijl *et al.* (2000)
	Guinea pig	TOL, n-hexane, and trichlorethylene	Antisolvent gel and other 3 BC	Dermal blood flow changes were relatively high on the control site compared to the gel pretreated sites. They found that BC can against TOL, n-hexane but not trichlorethylene	Mahmound and Lachapelle (1985); Lachapelle *et al.* (1990)
	Guinea pigs and humans	SLS, sodium hydroxide, TOL, and LA	Several BC	Some suppressed irritation, some failed, and some exacerbated	Frosch *et al.* (1993b, 1993c, 1993d, 1994)

Humans	TOL	Several BC	All tested BC markedly reduced the irritating effect of repetitive toluene contact	Grunewald et al. (1995)
Humans with a history of allergic to poison ivy/oak	Urushiol	Q18B lotion	Q-18B lotion significantly reduced reactions to the urushiol	Marks et al. (1995)
Humans	Dyes (methylene blue and oil red O)	3 BC	Two exhibited effectiveness; one enhanced cumulative amount of dye	Zhai and Maibach (1996b)
Humans	10 percent SLS, 1 percent NaOH, 30 percent LA, and TOL	4 BC and white petrolatum	Different protective effects were detectable. All products were effective against SLS irritation	Schlüter-Wigger and Elsner (1996)
Humans	Water	2 BC and a moisturizer	BC with particles provided the greatest immediate protection (dorsal 76 percent, volar 69 percent)	de Fine Olivarius et al. (1996)
Humans	SLS	A lipophilic BC	A decrease of TEWL by 58 percent (back) and 49 percent (arm)	Fartasch et al. (1998)
Humans	SLS, NaOH, LA, and TOL	BC containing PFPE	All BC significantly suppressed irritation by SLS and NaOH. Only the 4 percent PFPE-containing preparation was significant against LA and TOL	Elsner et al. (1998)
Humans	SLS, NH⁴OH and urea, Rhus	Several protectants	Most suppressed SLS irritation and Rhus ACD, but failed to NH⁴OH and urea irritation	Zhai et al. (1998)
Humans	SLS	A barrier protectant (tannic acid)	Tannic acid significantly reduced SLS induced damage	Shimizu and Maibach (1999)
Rhus-sensitive subjects	Urushiol	TSP	TSP protected sites had lower dermatitis scores than TSP unprotected sites	Vidmar and Iwane (1999)

Table 52.1:
(Continued)

Models	Irritants or Allergens	BC	Efficacy	Authors and References
In Vitro				
In Vivo				
Humans and Rhus-sensitive subjects	SLS-ICD and poison ivy and poison oak (urushiol)-	A formulation containing dimethicone and glycerine	Test formulation significantly effective in reducing the irritation from SLS but did not prevent urushiol-ACD	Patterson *et al.* (1999)
Humans	SLS	A dimethicone containing skin protectant lotion	VS and TEWL data showed a significant decrease on the protectant lotion pretreated site in comparison to SLS only treated site as well as to vehicle control site	Zhai *et al.* (2000)
Nurses with mild signs of skin irritation	Occupational risk exposures	A test BC or its vehicle	No significant differences between BC and its vehicle. In both groups, clinical skin status improved and stratum corneum hydration increased significantly during the study	Berndt *et al.* (2000)
Humans	SLS and TOL	3 BC	Various protective effects were detectable with 5-day study protocol to achieve significant results	Schnetz *et al.* (2000)
Health care workers with severe hand irritation	Working environments	1BC and an oil-containing lotion	Subjects in both groups experienced marked improvement in overall hand condition, but use of the oil-containing lotion showed greater improvement	McCormick *et al.* (2000)
Humans	Zinc	Three representatives commercial BC	BC provided appreciable protection against the penetration of both ZnCl$_2$ and ZnO into skin	Sun *et al.* (2000)
Humans	2 types of latex gloves	A test BC	BC decreased latex gloves-induced contact urticaria syndrome	Allmers (2001)
Human	Latex glove	A model lipid emulsion	The test emulsion minimized glove induced-ICD.	Zhai *et al.* (2002)

standardized and hopefully widely accepted method will accelerate product development.

REFERENCES

ALLMERS, H. (2001) Wearing test with 2 different types of latex gloves with and without the use of a skin protection cream. *Contact Dermatitis* **44**, 30–33.

BERNDT, U., WIGGER-ALBERTI, W., GABARD, B. and ELSNER, P. (2000) Efficacy of a barrier cream and its vehicle as protective measures against occupational irritant contact dermatitis. *Contact Dermatitis* **42**, 77–80.

DE FINE OLIVARIUS, F., HANSEN, A.B., KARLSMARK, T. and WULF, H.C. (1996) Water protective effect of barrier creams and moisturizing creams: a new *in vivo* test method. *Contact Dermatitis* **35**, 219–225.

ELSNER, P., WIGGER-ALBERTI, W. and PANTINI, G. (1998) Perfluoropolyethers in the prevention of irritant contact dermatitis. *Dermatology* **197**, 141–145.

FARTASCH, M., SCHNETZ, E. and DIEPGEN, T.L. (1998) Characterization of detergent-induced barrier alterations—effect of barrier cream on irritation. *Journal of Investigative Dermatology* **3**, 121–127.

FROSCH, P.J. and KURTE, A. (1994) Efficacy of skin barrier creams. (IV). The repetitive irritation test (RIT) with a set of 4 standard irritants. *Contact Dermatitis* **31**, 161–168.

FROSCH, P.J., KURTE, A. and PILZ, B. (1993a) Biophysical techniques for the evaluation of skin protective creams. In: FROSCH, P.J. and KLIGMAN, A.M. (eds) *Noninvasive Methods for the Quantification of Skin Functions,* Berlin: Springer-Verlag, 214–222.

FROSCH, P.J., KURTE, A. and PILZ, B. (1993b) Efficacy of skin barrier creams. (III). The repetitive irritation test (RIT) in humans. *Contact Dermatitis* **29**, 113–118.

FROSCH, P.J., SCHULZE-DIRKS, A., HOFFMANN, M. and AXTHELM, I. (1993c) Efficacy of skin barrier creams. (II). Ineffectiveness of a popular "skin protector" against various irritants in the repetitive irritation test in the guinea pig. *Contact Dermatitis* **29**, 74–77.

FROSCH, P.J., SCHULZE-DIRKS, A., HOFFMANN, M., AXTHELM, I. and KURTE, A. (1993d) Efficacy of skin barrier creams. (I). The repetitive irritation test (RIT) in the guinea pig. *Contact Dermatitis* **28**, 94–100.

FULLERTON, A. and MENNE, T. (1995) *In vitro* and *in vivo* evaluation of the effect of barrier gels in nickel contact allergy. *Contact Dermatitis* **32**, 100–106.

■ CHAPTER 52 ■

GOFFIN, V., PIÉRARD-FRANCHIMONT, C. and PIÉRARD, G.E. (1998) Shielded corneosurfametry and corneoxenometry: novel bioassays for the assessment of skin barrier products. *Dermatology* **196**, 434–437.

GOH, C.L. (1991a) Cutting oil dermatitis on guinea pig skin. (I). Cutting oil dermatitis and barrier cream. *Contact Dermatitis* **24**, 16–21.

GOH, C.L. (1991b) Cutting oil dermatitis on guinea pig skin. (II). Emollient creams and cutting oil dermatitis. *Contact Dermatitis* **24**, 81–85.

GRUNEWALD, A.M., GLOOR, M., GEHRING, W. and KLEESZ, P. (1995) Barrier creams. Commercially available barrier creams versus urea—and glycerol—containing oil-in-water emulsions. *Dermatosen* **43**, 69–74.

GRUNEWALD, A.M., LORENZ, J., GLOOR, M., GEHRING, W. and KLEESZ, P. (1996) Lipophilic irritants: protective value of urea—and of glycerol—containing oil-in-water emulsions. *Dermatosen* **44**, 81–86.

LACHAPELLE, J.M. (1996) Efficacy of protective creams and/or gels. In: ELSNER, P., LACHAPELLE, J.M., WAHLBERG, J.E. and MAIBACH, H.I. (eds) *Prevention of Contact Dermatitis. Current Problem in Dermatology*, Basel: Karger, 182–192.

LACHAPELLE, J.M., NOUAIGUI, H. and MAROT, L. (1990) Experimental study of the effects of a new protective cream against skin irritation provoked by the organic solvents n-hexane, trichlorethylene and toluene. *Dermatosen* **38**, 19–23.

MAHMOUD, G. and LACHAPELLE, J.M. (1985) Evaluation of the protective value of an antisolvent gel by laser Doppler flowmetry and histology. *Contact Dermatitis* **13**, 14–19.

MAIBACH, H.I. and ZHAI, H. (2000) Evaluations of barrier creams. In: WARTELL, M.A. KLEINMAN, M.T. HUEY, B.M. and DUFFY, L.M. (eds) *Strategies to Protect the Health of Deployed US Forces. Force Protection and Decontamination*, Washington DC: National Academy Press, 217–220.

MARKS, J.G. JR., FOWLER, J.F. JR., SHERETZ, E.F., RIETSCHEL, R.L. (1995) Prevention of poison ivy and poison oak allergic contact dermatitis by quaternium-18 bentonite. *Journal of the American Academy of Dermatology* **33**, 212–216.

MCCORMICK, R.D., BUCHMAN, T.L. and MAKI, D.G. (2000) Double-blind, randomized trial of scheduled use of a novel barrier cream and an oil-containing lotion for protecting the hands of health care workers. *American Journal of Infection Control* **28**, 302–310.

PACKHAM, C.L., PACKHAM, H.L. and RUSSELL-FELL, R. (1994) Evaluation of barrier creams: an *in vitro* technique on human skin (letter). *Acta Dermato-Venereologica* **74**, 405–406.

PATTERSON, S.E., WILLIAMS, J.V. and MARKS, J.G. JR. (1999) Prevention of sodium lauryl sulfate irritant contact dermatitis by Pro-Q aerosol foam skin protectant. *Journal of the American Academy of Dermatology* **40**, 783–785.

SCHLÜTER-WIGGER, W. and ELSNER, P. (1996) Efficacy of 4 commercially available protective creams in the repetitive irritation test (RIT). *Contact Dermatitis* **34**, 278–283.

SCHNETZ, E., DIEPGEN, T.L., ELSNER, P., FROSCH, P.J., KLOTZ, A.J., KRESKEN, J., KUSS, O., MERK, H., SCHWANITZ, H.J., WIGGER-ALBERTI, W. and FARTASCH, M. (2000) Multicentre study for the development of an *in vivo* model to evaluate the influence of topical formulations on irritation. *Contact Dermatitis* **42**, 336–343.

SHAH, S. and KIRCHNER, F. (1997) *In vitro* and *in vivo* evaluation of water penetration through skin protectant barriers. *Skin Research and Technology* **3**, 114–120.

SHIMIZU, T. and MAIBACH, H.I. (1999) Squamometry: an evaluation method for a barrier protectant (tannic acid). *Contact Dermatitis* **40**, 189–191.

SUN, Q., TRAN, M., SMITH, B. and WINEFORDNER, J.D. (2000) In-situ evaluation of barrier-cream performance on human skin using laser-induced breakdown spectroscopy. *Contact Dermatitis* **43**, 259–263.

TREFFEL, P., GABARD, B. and JUCH, R. (1994) Evaluation of barrier creams: An *in vitro* technique on human skin. *Acta Dermato-Venereologica* **74**, 7–11.

VAN DER BIJL, P., VAN EYK, A.D., CILLIERS, J. and STANDER, I.A. (2000) Diffusion of water across human skin in the presence of two barrier creams. *Skin Pharmacology and Applied Skin Physiology* **13**, 104–110.

VIDMAR, D.A. and IWANE, M.K. (1999) Assessment of the ability of the topical skin protectant (TSP) to protect against contact dermatitis to urushiol (Rhus) antigen. *American Journal of Contact Dermatitis* **10**, 190–197.

WIGGER-ALBERTI, W. and ELSNER, P. (1997) Petrolatum prevents irritation in a human cumulative exposure model *in vivo*. *Dermatology* **194**, 247–250.

WIGGER-ALBERTI, W. and ELSNER, P. (1998) Do barrier creams and gloves prevent or provoke contact dermatitis? *American Journal of Contact Dermatitis* **9**, 100–106.

WIGGER-ALBERTI, W. and ELSNER, P. (2000a) Barrier creams and emollients. In: KANERVA, L., ELSNER, P., WAHLBERG, J.E. and MAIBACH, H.I. (eds) *Handbook of Occupational Dermatology*, Berlin: Springer, 490–496.

CHAPTER 52

WIGGER-ALBERTI, W. and ELSNER, P. (2000b) Protective creams. In: ELSNER, P. and MAIBACH, H.I. (eds) *Cosmeceuticals. Drugs vs. Cosmetics,* New York: Marcel Dekker, 189–195.

WIGGER-ALBERTI, W., CADUFF, L., BURG, G. and ELSNER, P. (1999) Experimentally induced chronic irritant contact dermatitis to evaluate the efficacy of protective creams *in vivo. Journal of the American Academy of Dermatology* **40**, 590–596.

WIGGER-ALBERTI, W., MARAFFIO, B., WERNLI, M. and ELSNER, P. (1997a) Self-application of a protective cream. Pitfalls of occupational skin protection. *Archives of Dermatology* **133**, 861–864.

WIGGER-ALBERTI, W., MARAFFIO, B., WERNLI, M. and ELSNER, P. (1997b) Training workers at risk for occupational contact dermatitis in the application of protective creams: Efficacy of a fluorescence technique. *Dermatology* **195**, 129–133.

WIGGER-ALBERTI, W., ROUGIER, A., RICHARD, A. and ELSNER, P. (1998) Efficacy of protective creams in a modified repeated irritation test. Methodological aspects. *Acta Dermato-Venereologica* **78**, 270–273.

ZHAI, H. and MAIBACH, H.I. (1996a) Percutaneous penetration (Dermatopharma-cokinetics) in evaluating barrier creams. In: ELSNER, P., LACHAPELLE, J.M., WAHLBERG, J.E. and MAIBACH, H.I. (eds) *Prevention of Contact Dermatitis. Current Problem in Dermatology,* Basel: Karger, 193–205.

ZHAI, H. and MAIBACH, H.I. (1996b) Effect of barrier creams: human skin *in vivo. Contact Dermatitis* **35**, 92–96.

ZHAI, H. and MAIBACH, H. I. (1999) Efficacy of barrier creams (skin protective creams). In: ELSNER, P., MERK, H.F. and MAIBACH, H.I. (eds) *Cosmetics. Controlled Efficacy Studies and Regulation,* Berlin: Springer, 156–166.

ZHAI, H. and MAIBACH, H.I. (2000) Models assay for evaluation of barrier formulations. In: MENNÉ, T. and MAIBACH, H.I. (eds) *Hand Eczema,* 2nd edition, Boca Raton: CRC Press, 333–337.

ZHAI, H. and MAIBACH, H.I. (2001) Tests for skin protection: barrier effect. In: BAREL, A.O., MAIBACH, H.I. and PAYE, M. (eds) *Handbook of Cosmetic Science and Technology,* New York: Marcel Dekker, Inc., 823–828.

ZHAI, H. and MAIBACH, H.I. (2002) Barrier creams—skin protectants: can you protect skin? *Journal of Cosmetic Dermatology* **1**, 20–23.

ZHAI, H., WILLARD, P. and MAIBACH, H.I. (1998) Evaluating skin-protective materials against contact irritants and allergens. An *in vivo* screening human model. *Contact Dermatitis* **38**, 155–158.

ZHAI, H., BUDDRUS, D.J., SCHULZ, A.A., WESTER, R.C., HARTWAY, T., SERRANZANA, S. and MAIBACH, H.I. (1999a) *In vitro* percutaneous absorption of sodium lauryl sulfate (SLS) in human skin decreased by Quaternium-18 bentonite gels. *In Vitro and Molecular Toxicology* **12**, 11–15.

ZHAI, H., WILLARD, P. and MAIBACH, H.I. (1999b) Putative skin-protective formulations in preventing and/or inhibiting experimentally-produced irritant and allergic contact dermatitis. *Contact Dermatitis* **41**, 190–192.

ZHAI, H., BRACHMAN, F., PELOSI, A., ANIGBOGU, A., RAMOS, M.B., TORRALBA, M.C. and MAIBACH, H.I. (2000) A bioengineering study on the efficacy of a skin protectant lotion in preventing SLS-induced dermatitis. *Skin Research and Technology* **6**, 77–80.

ZHAI, H., SCHMIDT, R., LEVIN, C., KLOTZ, A. and MAIBACH, H.I. (2002) Prevention and therapeutic effects of a model emulsion on glove induced irritation and dry skin in man. *Occupational and Environmental Dermatology* **4**, 134–138.

53

Light-Induced Dermal Toxicity: Effects on the Cellular and Molecular Levels

ANDRIJA KORNHAUSER, WAYNE G WAMER
AND LARK A LAMBERT

Contents

53.1   Introduction

53.2   Light characteristics

53.3   Fundamental concepts in photochemistry

53.4   Cellular targets and mechanisms of
       phototoxicity

53.5   Specific molecular alterations in cells

53.6   Cellular mediators induced by light

53.7   Photoimmunology

53.8   Alterations in gene expression induced by light

53.9   Epilogue

53.1 INTRODUCTION

Die Sonne ist auch da wenn die Wolken schwarz und undurchdringlich scheinen.

Ernst Jucker (1957)*

Toxicology has evolved as a multidisciplinary field of study and is still in rapid evolutionary development. As such, toxicology overlaps many other basic biomedical disciplines, including biochemistry, pharmacology, and physiology. A recent event in this development has been the intersection of toxicology with photobiology, opening the field of phototoxicology.

Sunlight is the most potent environmental agent influencing life on the earth. Historically, exposure to the sun has been believed to be healthful and beneficial. It has only recently become apparent that many of the effects of solar radiation are detrimental. In a broad sense, therefore, the evolution of life can be regarded a continuous adaptation to light by simultaneously utilizing solar energy and protecting against its detrimental effects.

Modern civilization presents a challenge for basic phototoxicologic research. This challenge arises from alterations in the life-styles of a large portion of the population, including holiday trips, clothing styles, and particularly the fashion of suntanning among Caucasians. It is also possible that environmental factors may change the spectral characteristics of light reaching the earth's surface. Many of these factors lead to an essentially increased exposure to light for a large segment of the population (Fitzpatrick et al., 1974; Urbach, 1989). Furthermore, in the past decade, phototoxic reactions to drugs, cosmetics and many industrial and environmental chemicals have become an important health problem.

Definitions of phototoxicity are numerous and frequently inconsistent. In the broadest sense, any toxicity induced by photons can be termed photosensitivity. Photosensitivity may involve either photoallergies or nonimmunologic photoinduced skin reactions. Phototoxicity is used to describe all nonimmunologic light-induced toxic skin reactions. Sunburn is the most frequently occurring phototoxic reaction, requiring only the interaction of ultraviolet (UV) light with skin. In most cases of phototoxicity, however, we deal with an endogenous or exogenous chemical (chromophore) that absorbs light and

* "The sun is still present even when the clouds seem dark and impenetrable." From *Ein gutes Wort zur rechten Zeit*, Bern: Verlag Paul Haupt.

transfers the energy to, or reacts in the excited state with, cellular components. Such toxic reactions would most properly be termed chemical phototoxicity.

Chronic phototoxic exposure can lead to neoplastic changes. It is established that the consequence of lifelong enhanced exposure to light is a significant increase in skin tumors (Urbach *et al.*, 1974), including basal and squamous cell carcinomas and, to a certain extent, malignant melanomas. This is confirmed by the pronounced increase in frequency of skin cancers in that part of the population, particularly those Celts and Teutons, that in the course of history settled in regions with higher solar irradiation (Africa, Australia, and North America).

Phototoxicity studies, particularly those related to human disorders, have so far been based predominantly on gross anatomic or histological procedures. Although our knowledge of the molecular events that occur during these processes is rapidly growing, much basic research remains to be done. In this chapter we discuss some molecular and cellular events that take place on exposure to light.

53.2 LIGHT CHARACTERISTICS

Aside from artificial light sources, solar radiation is the primary source of light that elicits biological effects. A portion of the solar spectrum containing the biologically most active region (290–700 nm) is shown in Figure 53.1.

The UV part of the spectrum includes wavelengths from 200 to 400 nm. Portions of the UV spectrum have distinctive features from both the physical and medical points of view. The accepted designations for the biologically important parts of the UV spectrum are UVA, 320–400 nm; UVB, 290–320 nm; and UVC, 220–290 nm (Figure 53.2).

Wavelengths less than 290 nm (UVC) do not occur at the earth's surface, since they are absorbed, predominantly by ozone, in the stratosphere. The most thoroughly studied photobiological reactions that occur in skin are induced by UVB. Although UVB wavelengths represent only approximately 1.5 percent of the solar energy received at the earth's surface (World Health Organization, 1979), they elicit most of the known biological effects. Light distributed over these wavelengths inhibits cell mitosis, makes vitamin D, and induces sunburn, skin aging and skin cancer. The UVA region elicits most of the known chemical phototoxic and photoallergic reactions. It has been proposed that the longer wavelengths of the UVA spectrum (UVA I: 340–400 nm) are less detrimental than the shorter UVA wavelengths (UVA II: 320–340 nm) (National Institutes

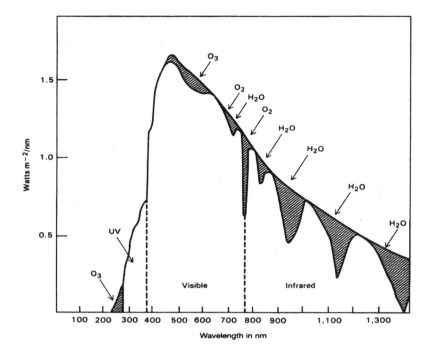

Figure 53.1: Spectrum of solar energy received at the earth's surface. The absorption bands of atmospheric O_2, O_3, and H_2O are shown. Modified from Hynek (1951), p. 272, with permission.

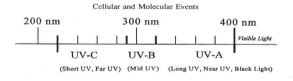

Figure 53.2: The UV regions of the solar spectrum.

of Health Consensus Development Conference Statement, 1989). Recent studies conducted on the influence of UVA on biological systems show that a great variety of effects are induced by these wavelengths. The findings of these studies have become increasingly important because of the popularity of indoor tanning which can involve high UVA doses from powerful UVA sources. Research has shown that within the UVA spectrum lies the peak response for immediate pigment darkening (Irwin *et al.*, 1993). Skin cancer, once thought to be induced solely by UVB also results from UVA exposure (Sterenborg and Van Der Leun, 1990). In addition, protein kinase C, which has been linked to chemical tumor promotion, and may play a role in UV-induced tumor promotion, was shown to be induced by UVA in cultured mouse fibroblasts (Matsui and DeLeo, 1990). Similarities have been found between UVA and ionizing radiation with respect to DNA damage induction. Unlike single-strand breaks, which are efficiently repaired by normal cells, DNA double-strand breaks are thought to be a critical lethal lesion. UVA, as well as UVB, UVC, and ionizing radiation have been shown to induce double-strand breaks in DNA of cultured human epithelioid cells (Peak and Peak, 1990). UVA, not UVB, caused mouse skin to become highly resistant to solubilization by pepsin digestion, possibly as a result of increased cross-linking of dermal collagen (Kligman and Gebre 1991). UVA effects not shared with UVB or UVC have been reported for nonnuclear damage and cell lysis in three strains of murine lymphoma cell lines (Beer *et al.*, 1993) and for the oxidation of cytoplasmic components causing adverse cytoskeleton effects resulting in hemolysis of sheep red blood cells (Godar *et al.*, 1993).

The visible portion of the spectrum, representing about 50 percent of the sun's energy received at sea level, includes wavelengths from 400 to 700 nm. Visible light is necessary for such biological events as photosynthesis, circadian cycles, and vision. Furthermore, visible light in conjunction with certain chromophores (e.g., dyes, drugs, and endogenous compounds) and molecular oxygen induces photodynamic effects.

Understanding the toxic effects of light impinging on the skin requires knowledge of the skin's optical properties. Skin may be viewed as an optically nonhomogeneous medium, composed of three layers that have characteristic refractive indices, chromophore distributions, and light-scattering properties. Light of wavelengths between 250 and 3000 nm entering the outermost layer of the skin, the stratum corneum, is in part reflected approximately 4–7 percent due to the difference in refractive index between air and stratum corneum (Fresnel reflection) (Anderson and Parrish, 1981).

Absorption by urocanic acid (a deamination product of histidine), melanin, and proteins containing the aromatic amino acids tryptophan and tyrosine in the stratum corneum produces further attenuation of light, particularly at shorter UV wavelengths. Approximately 40 percent of the UVB is transmitted through the stratum corneum to the viable epidermis (Everett *et al.*, 1966). The light entering the epidermis is attenuated by scattering and, predominantly, absorption. Epidermal chromophores consist of proteins, urocanic acid, nucleic acids, and melanin. Passage through the epidermis results in appreciable attenuation of UVA and particularly UVB radiation. The transmission properties of the dermis are largely due to scattering, with significant absorption of visible light by melanin, carotenoids, and blood-borne pigments such as bilirubin, hemoglobin, and oxyhemoglobin. Light traversing these layers of the skin is extensively attenuated, most drastically for wavelengths less than 400 nm. Longer wavelengths are more penetrating. It has been noted that there is an "optical window," that is, greater transmission for light at wavelengths of 600–1300 nm, which may have important biological consequences (Anderson and Parrish, 1981). These features are presented in Figure 53.3.

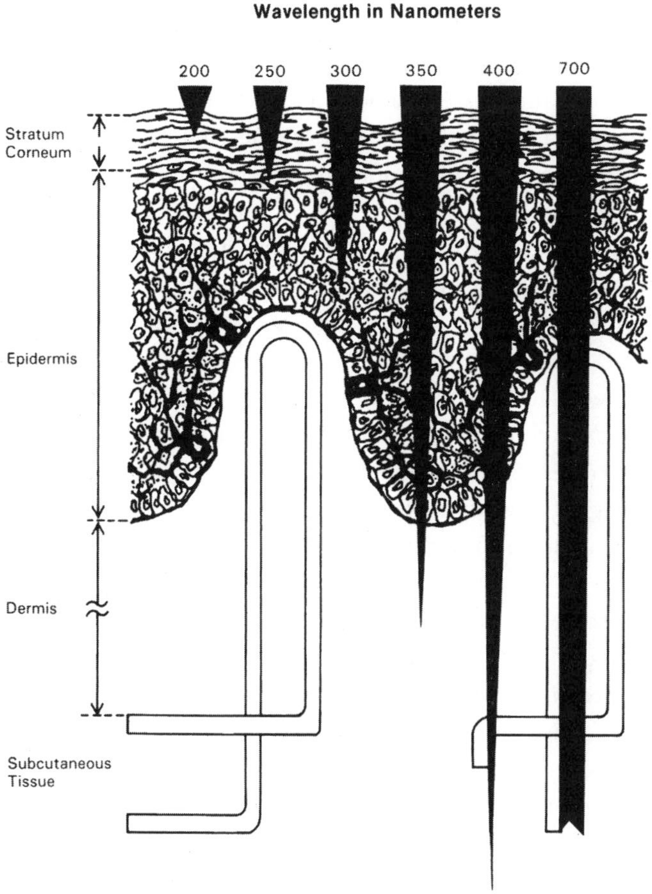

Figure 53.3: Schematic representation of light penetration into skin.

Normal variations in the skin's melanin content may result in changes in the attenuation of light, particularly in those wavelengths between 300 and 400 nm, by as much as 1.5 times more in Negroes than in Caucasians (Pathak, 1967). Alterations in the amount or distribution of other natural chromophores account for further variations in the skin's optical properties.

Urocanic acid deposited on the skin's surface during perspiration (Anderson and Parrish, 1981) and UV-absorbing lipids excreted in sebum (Beadle and Burton, 1981) may significantly reduce UV transmission through the skin. Epidermal thickness, which varies over regions of the body and increases after exposure to UVB radiation, may significantly modify UV transmission (Soffen and Blum, 1961; Parrish and Jaenicke, 1981).

Certain disease states also produce alterations in the skin's optical properties. Alteration of the skin's surface, such as by psoriatic plaques, decreases transmitted light. This effect may be lessened by application of oils whose refractive index is similar to that of skin (Anderson and Parrish, 1981). Disorders such as hyperbilirubinemia, porphyrias, and blue skin nevi result in increased absorption of visible light due to accumulation or altered distribution of chromophoric endogenous compounds.

The penetration of light into and through dermal tissues has important consequences. Skin, as the primary organ responsible for thermal regulation, is overperfused with blood relative to its metabolic requirements (Anderson and Parrish, 1981). It is estimated that the average cutaneous blood flow is 20–30 times that necessary to support the skin's metabolic needs. The papillary boundaries between epidermis and dermis allow capillary vessels to lie close to the skin's surface, permitting the blood and important components of the immune system to be exposed to light. The equivalent of the entire blood volume of an adult may pass through the skin, and potentially be irradiated, in 20 minutes. This corresponds to the time required to receive 1–2 minimal erythema doses (MEDs).* The accessibility of incident radiation to blood has been exploited in such regimens as phototherapy of hyperbilirubinemia in neonates, where light is used as a therapeutic agent. However, in general there is a potential for light-induced toxicity due to irradiation of blood-borne drugs and metabolites.

Of course light-induced damage is not confined to the skin. Ocular injury and aging of the eye can result from oxidative stress in tissues caused by radiant

---

* The minimal erythema dose (MED) is defined as the minimal dose of UV radiation that produces definite, but minimally perceptible, redness 24 h after exposure.

energy. Due to various molecular species in the eye, different parts of the eye absorb different wavelengths; the cornea absorbs UVB, the lens absorbs the majority of UVA and some UVB, and the retina and pigment epithelium absorb all the blue light (Zigman, 1993).

53.3 FUNDAMENTAL CONCEPTS IN PHOTOCHEMISTRY

Damage to cells through a photoreaction is initiated at the site where the chromophore absorbs specific wavelengths of light. Absorption of UV or visible photons results in electronically excited molecules; dissipation of this energy may result in an adverse phototoxic effect on the cell. The sequence of events initiated by light absorption is shown in Figure 53.4.

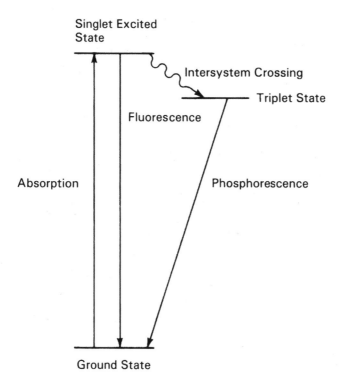

Figure 53.4: Electronic energy diagram of physical events accompanying the absorption of a photon.

The transition of a ground-state molecule to an excited singlet electronic state accompanies absorption of a visible or UV photon. Molecules in their singlet excited states exist for only about 10^{-8}–10^{-9} s before either returning to the ground state or converting (intersystem crossing) to a long-lived (10^{-4}–10^{1} s) metastable triplet state. Both excited singlet and triplet states relax to the ground state through (1) transfer of energy to another molecule and (2) emission of light (fluorescence or phosphorescence) or release of heat.

Alternatively, the excited molecule may undergo photochemistry such as cis-trans isomerization, fragmentation, ionization, rearrangement, and intermolecular reactions. The probability that an excited molecule will choose any given path to the ground state depends on both its molecular structure and its environment and may be determined experimentally (Turro, 1965).

All these factors, such as light absorption, the nature of the excited states, the extent of intersystem crossing, and photochemical reactions, will finally determine the phototoxic potential of an endogenous or exogenous compound. However, we are not yet able to predict the phototoxic potential of a compound from its molecular structure alone. Reliable predictive tests are still required to evaluate suspected compounds. Several lists of compounds that are phototoxic in humans have appeared (e.g., Parrish *et al.*, 1979). Classes of compounds known to be phototoxic in humans are:

Psoralens	Sulfonamides
Sulfonylureas	Phenothiazine
Tetracyclines	Coal tar
Anthracene	Acridine
Phenanthrene	Fluoroquinolones

The mechanisms through which absorption of light causes a chemical alteration in the chromophore, eventually resulting in a phototoxic response, are shown in Figure 53.5.

Compounds such as psoralens may react directly in their excited states with a biological target. Because of the short lifetimes of most excited states, direct reactions require close association, or complex formation, between the chromophore and the target before light absorption. Alternatively, a stable toxic photoproduct may be formed after absorption of light. Chlorpromazine and protriptyline are examples of this mechanism (Kochevar, 1981). The phototoxicity of these compounds is in large part the result of the toxicity of their photoproducts.

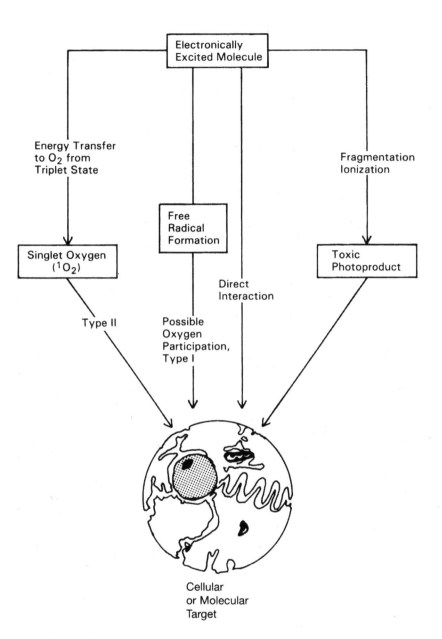

Figure 53.5: Diagram of basic phototoxicity mechanisms. The electronically excited molecule, located within or near a cell, may elicit a phototoxic response through several mechanisms.

The other mechanisms shown in Figure 53.5 are frequently categorized as photodynamic mechanisms. Photodynamic reactions usually involve compounds that absorb UVA or visible light. In type I photodynamic reactions the chromophore, in an excited triplet state, is reduced either by an electron or by hydrogen transfer from a compound in the environment. This reduction results in the generation of highly reactive free radicals, whose subsequent attack on biological substrates may result in toxicity. In type II photodynamic reactions the chromophore transfers its energy to O_2, generating singlet oxygen ($^1O_2$), an active oxidizing agent. A large body of evidence now supports the involvement of $^1O_2$ in photodynamic reactions. Recently, investigators have demonstrated photosensitized formation of $^1O_2$ in *in vitro* as well as *in vivo* studies (Baker and Kanofsky, 1991; Baker and Kanofsky, 1993; Oelckers *et al.*, 1999; Niedre *et al.*, 2002).

53.4 CELLULAR TARGETS AND MECHANISMS OF PHOTOTOXICITY

A vigorous effort is under way to discover the biological targets in phototoxicity. Cellular injury by photons may be studied on either the histological or the molecular level. The characteristic histological change induced by photons is the appearance of the so-called sunburn cell (SBC) (Daniels *et al.*, 1961), a dyskeratotic cell with bright eosinophilic cytoplasm and a pyknotic nucleus. SBCs appear 24–48 h after UVB irradiation (Woodcock and Magnus, 1976) and may persist 1 week or longer (Parrish *et al.*, 1979). The mechanisms of SBC formation are still obscure, although its morphological and biochemical characteristics have been investigated (Danno and Horio, 1980; Olson *et al.*, 1974). The primary chromophore for sunburn cell production is not known; however, Young and Magnus (1981) found evidence that DNA may be an important chromophore. They detected SBCs in mouse epidermis after administration of 8-methoxypsoralen (8-MOP) followed by UVA irradiation (psoralen + UVA is abbreviated PUVA). They speculated that since the primary molecular lesion in PUVA treatment is in DNA, the fact that PUVA can promote SBC formation supports the view that DNA may be a significant chromophore in SBC induction.

The mechanisms by which photosensitized cells are damaged are in most cases poorly understood. On the subcellular level, the primary targets in a phototoxic reaction include nucleic acids, proteins, and plasma and organelle membranes. Subcellular effects may differ depending on the photosensitizer's structure and intracellular localization. Sensitizers such as rose bengal, porphyrin, and anthracene accumulate selectively in cell plasma membranes (Ito, 1978). Acridine orange and psoralens accumulate in the cell nucleus (Van de Vorst and Lion, 1976; Pathak *et al.*, 1974; Bredberg *et al.*, 1977). Recently, it was reported that psoralens also accumulate in cell membranes. These membrane-bound psoralens may initiate important biological effects (Laskin *et al.*, 1985). Some photosensitizers may become concentrated in lysosomes and on irradiation may induce lysosomal rupture (Allison *et al.*, 1966). Table 53.1 shows results from some studies of the mechanisms of action for several important classes of phototoxic compounds.

It includes two endogenous photosensitizers, porphyrins and kynurenic acid. As reflected in Table 53.1, most compounds that evoke chemical phototoxicity are thought to act through a photodynamic mechanism. Further, it appears that a compound may elicit a phototoxic response through several modes. Studies are needed to correlate specific molecular alterations (such as DNA cross-linking and photooxidation of enzymes and of DNA) with cell toxicity and mutagenesis. To date, the mechanism of psoralen phototoxicity is relatively well understood. Much more remains to be learned about the mode of action for other groups of photosensitizers.

53.5 SPECIFIC MOLECULAR ALTERATIONS IN CELLS

On the molecular level, DNA is the most critical target in a cell exposed to UV light. As previously discussed, other cellular constituents may also be affected, generally with less severe consequences for the cell.

53.5.1 Thymine Photoproducts

Cyclobutane-type pyrimidine dimers in DNA are the best studied lesions induced in cells by UV. They are formed predominantly at wavelengths less than 300 nm (Rothman and Setlow, 1979; Rosenstein and Setlow, 1980; Kantor *et al.*, 1980, Yamada and Hieda, 1992), although they have also been found in human skin exposed *in situ* to UV wavelengths of 340–400 nm (Freeman *et al.*, 1987a). These dimers result from the formation of covalent bonds between adjacent pyrimidines of the same DNA strand and interfere with normal DNA function. Beukers and Berends (1960) first demonstrated the formation of these dimers *in vitro*, and Wacker *et al.* (1960) found them in DNA from UV-irradiated bacteria. These findings marked the beginning of a new era in molecular biology.

Table 53.1:
Mechanisms and targets of selected groups of phototoxic compounds

Compound	Structure	Mechanism of phototoxicity	Cellular target	Reference
Psoralen		Direct addition	DNA	Pathak et al. (1974)
		Photodynamic	DNA, membranes, proteins, ribosomes	de Mol et al. (1981), Poppe and Grossweiner (1975), Singh and Vadasz (1978), Pathak (1982)
Phenothiazines		Stable (toxic) photoproduct	DNA	Kochevar (1981)
		Photodynamic	DNA, membrane	Kochevar (1981), Copeland et al. (1976)
Porphyrins		Photodynamic	DNA, membranes proteins	Spikes (1975), Verweij et al. (1981), Jori and Spikes (1981)

Dyes	Photodynamic	DNA, membranes, proteins	Hass and Webb (1981), Ito (1978), Wacker et al. (1964), Wagner et al. (1980)
Kynurenic acid	Photodynamic	Membranes	Wennersten and Brunk (1977, 1978), Pileni and Santus (1978)
Anthracene	Photodynamic	DNA, membranes	Allison et al. (1966), Blackburn and Taussig (1975)
Fluoroquinolones	Photodynamic	DNA, membranes	Rosen et al. (1997), Ouedraogo et al. (1999)

Pyrimidine dimers were later shown to occur in a number of higher systems, including mammalian (Pathak *et al.*, 1972) and human skin (Freeman *et al.*, 1987b) after UV irradiation.

Studies initiated by Cleaver and Trosko (1970) demonstrated the involvement of thymine dimers (TT) (Figure 53.6a) in the disorder xeroderma pigmentosum (XP). This finding represents one of the rare cases in which a specific molecular lesion can be correlated with a malignant process. In another approach, Hart *et al.* (1977) used cell extracts from UV-irradiated Amazon mollies (small fish) and reported evidence that pyrimidine dimers in DNA gave rise to tumors.

Until recently, sensitive assays for pyrimidine dimers required use of radio-isotopes. However, additional techniques have now been developed for measuring pyrimidine dimers. These methods include radioimmunoassays (Mitchell and Clarkson, 1981) and endonuclease digestion followed by determination of DNA chain length (D'Ambrosio *et al.*, 1981; Freeman *et al.*, 1986), which have made quantitation of pyrimidine dimers in human biopsies feasible.

Several possible reaction mechanisms for the sensitized photodimerization of pyrimidines have been suggested, including population of the triplet state of a suitable sensitizer (Lamola, 1968). Our previous work showed that a Schenck type of mechanism (Schenck, 1960) involving a complex-forming reaction is highly favored in photosensitized thymine dimer formation (Kornhauser and Pathak, 1972; Kornhauser *et al.*, 1974). Also, we found that only a few of the

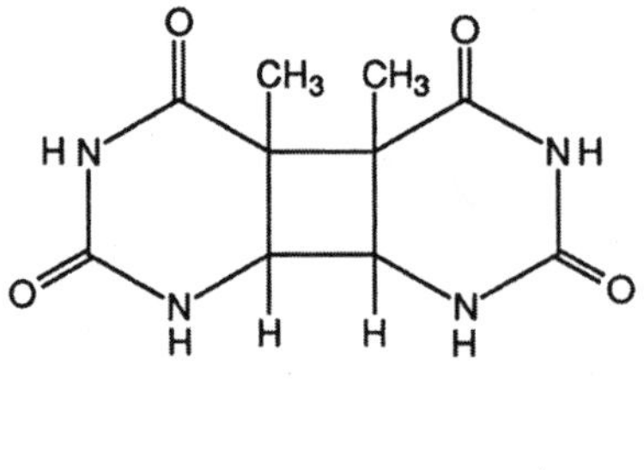

(a) 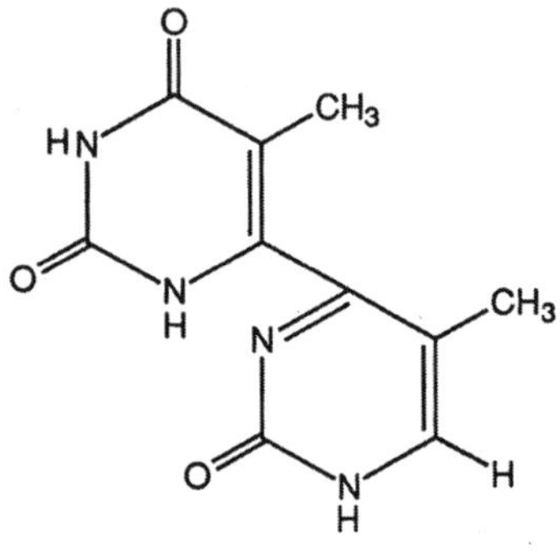   **(b)**

Figure 53.6: Structures of (a) the thymine dimer (*cis, syn*) and (b) the (6–4) photo-product.

potential sensitizers caused measurable thymine dimerization. A small amount (1–2 percent) of thymine dimer was detected after UV irradiation, even in the absence of a sensitizer. Acetone, ethyl acetoacetate, and dihydroxyacetone were more potent sensitizers than acetophenone and benzophenone (Table 53.2).

The following conclusions can be derived from our results:

1   The sensitized energy transfer taking place during thymine dimerization most likely does not occur through a simple physical mechanism. The ability of the sensitizer in its excited state to form a complex with the pyrimidine molecule appears to be a prerequisite for this type of photosensitization.

2   Ethyl acetoacetate and dihydroxyacetone, molecules that are commonly present in any viable cell and were not previously known to be photo-sensitizers, proved as effective as acetone or acetophenone. On the other hand, urocanic acid, a major UV-absorbing compound in mammalian skin, did not show sensitizing ability in inducing thymine dimerization. The UV energy absorbed by urocanic acid is believed to induce its cis-trans isomerization (Baden and Pathak, 1967).

3   Topical preparations containing acetone, dihydroxyacetone, or other acetone derivatives should be used cautiously, since they might damage

TABLE 53.2:

Formation of thymine dimers (TT) after irradiation of [2–^{14}C] thymine in the presence of different sensitizers

Number	Sensitizer	TT Formed (%)
1	None	1–2
2	Acetone	30–40
3	Dihydroxyacetone	25–30
4	Acetophenone	5–10
5	Benzophenone	5–8
6	4-Methoxyacetophenone	2–4
7	Ethyl acetoacetate	35–45
8	Phenyl cyanide	1–3
9	Carbazole	3–6
10	Fluorene	2–3
11	Naphthalene	1–3
12	Xanthene-9-one	1–3
13	Urocanic acid	1–3

Note. Solutions of [2–^{14}C]thymine (2×10^3 *M*) were irradiated with a total UV (≤ 300 nm) dose of 1.2 J/cm^2. Irradiations were carried out in water (sensitizers 1, 2, 3, and 13), water and ethanol (3:1) (sensitizers 4 and 6–12), and water and diozane (3:1) (sensitizers 5 and 12).

■ CHAPTER 53 ■

the epidermal DNA when skin is exposed to UV radiation. Interestingly, one of these compounds, dihydroxyacetone, has been used in cosmetics, notably as the active component in "sunless" tanning lotions (Maibach and Kligman, 1960).

The studies discussed above have practical application for correlating the structure of a potential phototoxic agent with its ability to induce pyrimidine dimerization or other molecular lesions in cells.

Other interesting photoproducts of DNA have been isolated and characterized. When a solution of DNA or a frozen thymine solution is irradiated, a new absorption peak at 320 nm appears. This is due to the photochemical formation of new products, the (6–4) adducts. In the case of thymine, 6,4'-(5'-methyl-pyrimidin-2'-one)-thymine is formed (Figure 53.6b) (Franklin *et al.*, 1982). These compounds cannot be split by reirradiation at short wavelengths as can cyclobutane-type pyrimidine dimers. An additional diagnostic property of these compounds is their instability in hot alkali (Franklin *et al.*, 1982). The (6–4) photoproducts are also generally produced less efficiently than are pyrimidine dimers (Franklin *et al.*, 1982). More recently, there has been an increased interest in the (6–4) adduct type lesions as they have been shown to play a major role in UV induced mutagenesis at specific sites in DNA (Franklin and Haseltine, 1986). They used the application of DNA sequencing procedures in *Escherichia coli* to demonstrate that the (6–4) adduct was the mutagenic lesion at certain "hot spots" in the *lacI* gene, a mutation that was previously ascribed to cyclobutane pyrimidine dimers. The relative importance of (6–4) adducts in the lethal and mutagenic effects of UV-light, as well as current methods for detection and quantitation, have been discussed in a review (Mitchell and Nairn, 1989).

53.5.2   DNA-Protein Cross-Links

The previous discussion focused on the reaction between bases, specifically thymine, within a strand of DNA to form an adduct. However, DNA in the cell has a complex and varied environment, making possible additional light-induced reactions.

Heteroadducts of DNA are those adducts formed by the covalent attachment of different types of compounds to DNA. These adducts may involve cellular constituents such as proteins, or exogenous compounds such as drugs, food additives, and cosmetics. Heteroadducts may have profound effects on cells. Artificially produced covalent linkages like DNA-protein cross-links, of the type not observed in normal viable cells, may result in a phototoxic response or be expressed as mutagenic or carcinogenic events.

The chemical nature of the DNA-protein cross-links is not yet known. An *in vitro* photochemical reaction between thymine and cysteine has been observed (Schott and Shetlar, 1974) and may be one of the mechanisms for covalent linking of DNA to protein *in vivo* (Smith, 1974). Similarly, it has been reported that irradiation of thymine-labeled DNA and lysine in aqueous solvent produces a photoproduct that behaves like a thymine-lysine adduct (Shetlar *et al.*, 1975). Furthermore, 11 of the common amino acids combine photochemically with uracil in different model systems (Smith, 1974). These pyrimidine-amino acid adducts are regarded as models for the coupling sites between proteins and DNA. In addition to reactions directly induced by UV, model systems provide evidence that acetone and acetophenone are effective photosensitizers for the covalent addition of amino acids to pyrimidine bases (Fisher *et al.*, 1974). It is reasonable to assume that suitable chromophores present in drugs, cosmetics, etc., will also be able to photosensitize the cross-linking of proteins and nucleic acids *in vitro* and *in vivo*.

The cross-linking of DNA and protein in bacteria was the first *in vivo* photochemical heteroadduct reaction reported (Smith, 1962). Several studies of UV-induced DNA and protein cross-links in mammalian cells *in vitro* have been based mainly on reduced DNA extractability after UV irradiation (Todd and Han, 1976). Evidence that this lesion plays a significant role in killing UV-irradiated cells has been obtained under several experimental conditions.

Mammalian (eukaryotic) cells, in general, represent a suitable model for the cross-linking reaction. Within the nuclei of eukaryotic cells, DNA is in intimate contact with proteins responsible for structurally organizing DNA and controlling macromolecular synthesis. Such a DNA-protein complex is commonly referred to as chromatin. The proximity of nuclear proteins to DNA should facilitate the formation of UV-induced DNA-protein covalent bonds. Todd and Han (1976) studied the general features of UV-induced (254 nm) DNA-protein cross-links in asynchronous and synchronous HeLa cells. Cross-linking was demonstrated by the detection of unextractable DNA in irradiated cells. Fornace and Kohn (1976), using a sensitive alkaline elution assay, measured UV-induced DNA-protein cross-links in both normal and xeroderma pigmentosum human fibroblasts. They noted that normal cells exhibit a repair phase lacking in XP cells. Similarly, Peak and Peak (1989) have reported DNA-protein cross-linking in cells exposed to UVA, UVB, or UVC radiation. These workers reported the relative importance of several DNA lesions (thymine dimers, single-strand breaks and DNA-protein cross-links) for each spectral region. DNA-protein cross-links were found to be the lesion most efficiently produced by UVA-irradiation of cells.

No *in vivo* data on DNA-protein cross-linking in mammalian skin, other than our preliminary work, have been reported. To study the possible role of the DNA-protein cross-links in epidermis, we focused on the isolation of chromatin from irradiated and nonirradiated guinea pig skin (Kornhauser, 1976; Kornhauser *et al.*, 1976a). The epilated backs of guinea pigs were irradiated with a moderate physiological dose (80 mJ/cm^2; 290–350 nm) that corresponds to approximately four times the minimal erythema dose in an average fair-skinned Caucasian. Epidermis was obtained from both the irradiated and the control (nonirradiated) sites on the same animal and was homogenized. Chromatin was isolated from the homogenates by using Sepharose B-4 and DEAE cellulose chromatography and density gradient centrifugation. Its biological activity was determined by chemical and biochemical methods (Kornhauser *et al.*, 1976a). We were able to obtain 4–5 mg of extractable DNA which was free of protein, from 1 g wet epidermal tissue. Immediately after UV irradiation, the yield of extractable DNA was reduced by 20–30 percent, presumably as a result of DNA-protein cross-linking and possibly of DNA strand breakage. The latter molecular lesion is consistent with previous findings (Zierenberg *et al.*, 1971). In this experiment we found (1) a significant breakdown of the high-molecular-weight DNA fraction and the presence of low-molecular-weight DNA fragments on top of the sucrose gradient after UV-irradiation, and (2) an increment in the high-molecular-weight DNA isolated 60 minutes after irradiation (the regeneration or repair phase).

The results discussed above can be summarized as follows:

1   UV irradiation, at physiological doses (4 MED) of 290–350 nm, decreased the actual amount of dissociable chromosomal DNA by 20–30 percent as a result of DNA strand breakage and cross-linking of DNA to protein.
2   A comparison of corresponding elution profiles from Sepharose columns of dissociable DNA isolated from UV-irradiated and nonirradiated epidermal specimens indicated cross-linking of protein to DNA.
3   UV irradiation caused significant breakdown of the high-molecular-weight DNA that was isolated after irradiation.
4   In the regeneration phase, an active repair of strand breaks and possibly DNA-protein heteroadducts was operating in the viable cells of the epidermis.

So far, no other evidence for the cellular repair of DNA-protein heteroadducts has been found *in vivo*. It is conceivable that cells exposed to light have evolved a repair system for eliminating this type of heteroadduct. It is likely that this system is different from photoreactivation, which is specific for pyrimidine dimers (Setlow and Setlow, 1963).

All these findings suggest that UV radiation, even in moderate doses, can induce measurable alterations of the chromosomal material chromatin in mammalian skin. At present, it is not known what biochemical changes accompany light-induced lesions in chromatin. It is possible that damage by photons may alter such important chromatin functions as regulation of gene expression. Thus further studies of lesions in chromatin are indispensable for a complete understanding of light-induced effects on cells.

53.5.3 Phototoxicity

In addition to DNA-protein cross-linking, cross-links between DNA strands are possible. Because of the distance between bases in the DNA double helix, light-induced cross-linking is not observed without a bridging molecule such as a drug or component of a cosmetic, etc. Psoralens, a class of furocoumarins, are important cross-linking agents. Psoralens are a group of naturally occurring and synthetic substances that, when added to biological systems and irradiated with UVA, produce various biological effects. These effects are not observed with either psoralens or light alone.

The photobiological reactions of psoralens with DNA have received widespread attention in recent years. On the molecular level, the following facts are known:

1   Psoralens intercalate into DNA, that is, slip in between adjacent base-pairs by forming molecular complexes involving weak chemical interactions ("dark reaction").

2   UVA irradiation of the DNA-psoralen complex, *in vivo* or *in vitro*, results in covalent bond formation between a pyrimidine base and the furocoumarin molecule (C_4 cycloaddition). Because of their structure, psoralens in this reaction can react either at their 3,4 double bond or at their corresponding 4′,5′ site, yielding monoadducts (in the former case the product is not fluorescent, and in the latter case it is).

3   The absorption of an additional photon may result in a further chemical reaction yielding a "cross-linked DNA." Thus psoralens can behave as

photoreactive bifunctional agents; one psoralen molecule reacting with two pyrimidines in opposite strands of DNA. The structures of psoralen mono- and di-adducts with thymine are shown in Figure 53.7. Figure 53.8 schematically shows DNA cross-linked by a psoralen molecule. The result is a cross-linked DNA in which the individual strands cannot be separated by standard denaturation conditions. Both types of lesions, the monofunctional adduct and the cross-linked product, can be repaired *in vivo* (Pathak and Kramer, 1969; Baden *et al.*, 1972) and *in vitro* (Friedburg, 1988).

Dall'Acqua (1977) showed that the photoaddition of furocoumarins to DNA is not a random process. Specific sites exist in DNA for the photochemical

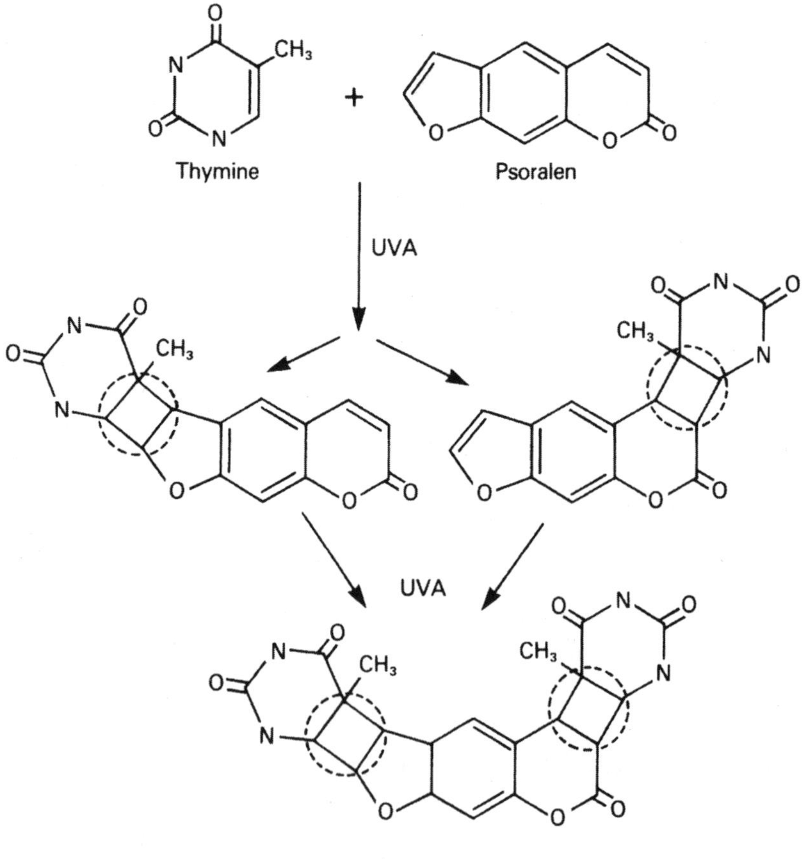

Figure 53.7: Photoaddition products of psoralen with thymine after UV irradiation.

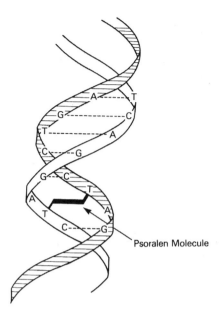

Figure 53.8: Schematic representation of DNA cross-linked by a psoralen molecule.

interaction with psoralens. The sites that can be considered specific receptors for the photobiological activity of psoralens are represented by alternating sequences of adenine and thymine in each complementary strand of the polynucleotide. Psoralen has a greater photoreactivity toward thymine than it has toward cytosine. The receptor sites have a high capacity for intercalation and subsequent photoreaction with psoralens (Dall'Acqua, 1977). It has been shown that flanking sequences, in addition to the adenine and thymine content of DNA, determine cross-linking (Boyer *et al.*, 1988).

The covalent addition of psoralens to DNA, particularly the cross-linking reaction, is usually believed to be responsible for the major effects of psoralen photosensitization. These include mutation and lethality in prokaryotic and eukaryotic systems, inhibition of DNA synthesis, sister chromatid exchange, and carcinogenesis. However, the relationship between psoralen photoaddition to DNA and the appearance of erythema remains to be elucidated. From early studies it appeared that erythema, the basic phototoxic effect induced by psoralens, correlated well with the *in vitro* capacity of psoralen derivatives to bind covalently to DNA (Vedaldi *et al.*, 1983). Neither the specific photoproduct(s) required for initiating psoralen-induced erythema nor the

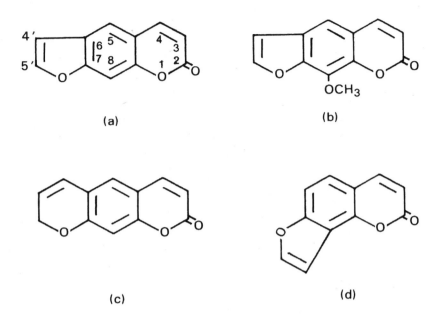

Figure 53.9: Structures of some furocoumarins and a pyranocoumarin: (a) psoralen; (b) 8-methoxypsoralen (8-MOP) ; (c) pyranocoumarin; (d) angelicin.

subsequent molecular events (e.g., mediators involved) have been definitely established.

Initially, the ability to sensitize cutaneous tissue appeared to be a unique characteristic of the psoralen ring system; for instance, pyranocoumarins, which have a similar linear tricyclic ring system, are found to lack photosensitizing activity (Pathak *et al.*, 1967). Furthermore, cutaneous phototoxicity is usually expressed only with linear derivatives; the angular furocoumarin, angelicin, does not photosensitize mammalian skin (Dall'Acqua *et al.*, 1981). Small changes in the structure of psoralen may produce dramatic changes in photosensitizing ability. Unsubstituted psoralen causes the most severe phototoxicity. This photobiological activity is reduced by adding methyl (on carbon 3) or halogen substituents (Pathak *et al.*, 1967). The structures of some furocoumarins and pyranocoumarin are shown in Figure 53.9.

The correlation of the structure of psoralen photoproducts to their photobiological effects has been the topic of several investigations. A large number of synthetic and natural furocoumarins have been subjected to systematic studies. From this work it has been concluded that the erythemogenic effect correlates with the capacity of a furocoumarin to form cross-links rather than monoadducts to DNA (Vedaldi *et al.*, 1983). This fact was confirmed by several investigators by preparing a relatively large number of monofunctional furocoumarin derivatives and testing their photobiologic properties (Rodighiero *et al.*, 1984).

In general, the monofunctional compounds do not induce erythema in human and guinea pig skin. Although this fact has been experimentally verified in many cases, exceptions to this rule seem to exist. A few 4-methyl angelicin derivatives are able to strongly photoreact with DNA without forming cross-links. When tested on guinea pig skin they were able, under certain experimental conditions, to induce a mild erythema (Baccichetti *et al.*, 1981, 1984). We must point out, however, that those experiments involved topical application of the compound in a relatively high concentration and with a high UVA dose. Also, great care must be taken in these experiments to ensure that the sample is free from bifunctional psoralen impurities, as they can easily yield false positives. In summary, a simple concept such as cross-links = erythema, monoadduct = no erythema, has yet to be established.

Various derivatives of psoralen, some with photosensitizing activity, have been synthesized. The synthesis of these derivatives is largely driven by the need to find new agents for improving current photochemotherapeutic treatment regimens. These derivatives include benzopsoralens and their tetrahydro-derivatives, pyrrolocoumararins, azapsoralens, thiopsoralens and khellin and related methylfurochromones (Dall'Acqua, 1989; Vedaldi *et al.*, 1997). The photobiological activity of many of these novel compounds has be investigated. Several derivatives (such as 1-thiopsoralen, 4-hydroxymethyl-4'-methylpsoralen, azapsoralens, and benzopsoralens) exhibit the ability to inhibit cellular growth, while eliciting no, or mild, erythemal responses (Conconi *et al.*, 1996; Bordin *et al.*, 1992; Chilin *et al.*, 1999; Dalla Via *et al.*, 1999). These compounds could potentially provide effective photochemotherapeutic treatment without adverse effects such as erythema. The driving force behind these investigations is to find new agents with the potential for improving current photochemotherapeutic treatment regimens.

Alternative mechanisms for the induction of erythema by psoralens and UV light that do not involve photoaddition to DNA have been suggested. One alternative mechanism is derived from the observation that there is a relationship between erythema production and the ability of a compound to form $^1O_2$ (Pathak, 1982). This correlation suggests that $^1O_2$ may be a mediator in psoralen-induced erythema. The involvement of $^1O_2$ in psoralen phototoxicity, however, has yet to be conclusively proven. Indeed, it has been pointed out that both the production of $^1O_2$ and the monoadduct and, particularly, the diadduct formation proceed by way of a common intermediate, the psoralen triplet state (de Mol *et al.*, 1981). Thus, psoralens that undergo efficient intersystem crossing should readily photosensitize the formation of $^1O_2$ as well as photoreact with DNA, unless low DNA binding or steric constraints predominate. It is, therefore, understandable that reports of correlation between both $^1O_2$ formation and erythema production (Pathak and Joshi, 1984) as well as DNA photobinding and erythema production (Vedaldi *et al.*, 1983) have appeared. However, the causal relationship between these two photoproducts ($^1O_2$ or DNA adducts) and erythema production is still under active investigation. Another alternative mechanism, not involving direct addition to DNA, has been proposed (Laskin *et al.*, 1986). It was demonstrated *in vitro* that 8-MOP binds to a specific cell surface receptor, thus inhibiting epidermal growth-factor binding. This work demonstrated for the first time that 8-MOP in combination with UVA irradiation can modify cell surface receptors in a variety of human and mouse cell lines. This alteration may play an important role in the mechanism of psoralen phototoxicity.

Two studies have been completed in our laboratory that have focused on psoralen + UVA (PUVA) induced phototoxicity. Both involved the micronutrient β-carotene, a naturally occurring pigment and vitamin A precursor found in many green and yellow-orange fruits and vegetables. Beta-carotene is a well-established quencher of $^1O_2$ and photooxidation (Krinsky and Deneke, 1982). In the first experiment, we studied the potential of β-carotene to influence PUVA-induced erythema in rats (Giles *et al.*, 1985). The rats were fed a β-carotene-fortified diet for approximately 14 weeks before treatment. Levels of β-carotene accumulated in the skin were measured by high performance liquid chromatography (HPLC). The rats were then orally dosed with 8-MOP (20 mg/kg body weight, in corn oil) and were irradiated 2 h later with a single dose of UVA (5 J/cm²). We found that the animals on the β-carotene fortified diet were significantly protected against PUVA-induced erythema. Furthermore, those rats having the highest β-carotene skin levels showed no perceptible erythema, indicating a correlation between β-carotene skin levels and a protective effect. No such protective effect was observed against UVB-induced erythema.

In the second experiment we investigated the potential of β-carotene for decreasing PUVA-induced melanogenesis (Kornhauser *et al.*, 1989). One of the side effects of PUVA therapy is tanning of the skin caused by an increase in the number of epidermal melanocytes (Blog and Szabo, 1979). Melanin is formed by an oxidative process. Previous *in vitro* studies indicated a role of activated-oxygen species in melanin synthesis (Kornhauser *et al.*, 1976b). Therefore, we reasoned that β-carotene might be able to influence melanogenesis *in vivo*. The animal of choice was the C57 BL/6 mouse, since the tail-skin had been found to be a good model for melanogenesis in human skin (Szabo *et al.*, 1982). Mice were fed standard rodent chow diets supplemented with either 1 percent β-carotene beadlets or 1 percent placebo beadlets for 10 weeks before treatment and throughout the treatment period. Mice were divided into UVA-treated and PUVA-treated groups. PUVA-treated mice received 20 mg/kg body weight of 8-MOP in corn oil orally by intubation, followed 2 h later with 3 J/cm^2 of UVA irradiation of the tail. The body of the animal was shielded from the light. UVA-treated mice received 3 J/cm^2 of UVA only. Mice received two, four, or five treatments within a 3-week period. Selected mice from each group were euthanized after these treatments and the tail-skin epidermis was removed for dihydroxyphenylalanine (DOPA) histochemical processing (Staricco and Pinkus, 1957). Melanogenesis was evaluated by counting the number of DOPA-positive melanocytes. As expected, the PUVA treatment resulted in an increase in the number of DOPA-positive melanocytes counted in each tail-skin epidermal section. An increase was also observed in the UVA-treated mice. However, mice fed β-carotene in both the UVA- and PUVA-treated groups had significantly fewer ($p < 0.05$, Student's *t*-test) DOPA-positive melanocytes than the corresponding placebo-fed animals at all three time points. The results are presented in Figure 53.10.

The most direct interpretation of the results described in both of these experiments would be that PUVA treatment involves photooxidation via $^1O_2$ or free radicals. It is well known that β-carotene is an effective quencher of these reactive intermediates (Krinsky and Deneke, 1982; Burton and Ingold, 1984). However, there is an alternative explanation for the observed protective effect, which involves the quenching of the psoralen triplet state by β-carotene (Giles *et al.*, 1985). In summary, the role of $^1O_2$ and related species in the induction of PUVA-induced erythema and other photobiological effects needs to be more extensively investigated before definitive conclusions can be drawn.

Some interesting studies on the mechanism of PUVA-induced melanogenesis involving photoreactions between furocoumarins and membrane unsaturated fatty acids (UFAs) have been performed (Dall'Acqua and Martelli, 1991). The C4-cycloaddition between one of the olefinic bonds of UFAs and the pyrone-side double bond of psoralen takes place after UV-irradiation at a wavelength

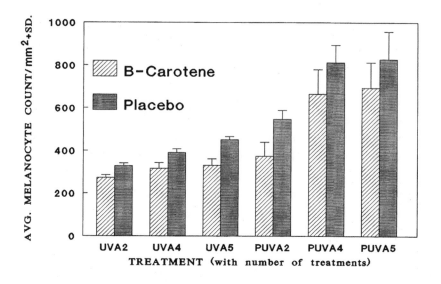

Figure 53.10: Average melanocyte counts as a measure of the effects of diet and treatment on DOPA-processed tail-skin epidermis of C57BL/6 mice. Averages are shown with the corresponding standard deviation. Mice were fed either ß-carotene- or placebo-fortified diets. Treatment groups: UVA-light treated (UVA), and oral 8-methoxypsoralen + UVA-light treated (PUVA). Mice received two, four, or five treatments. The numbers of DOPA-positive melanocytes were counted using a light microscope.

of 365 nm. This photoreaction also occurs between psoralen and the UFAs in lecithin *in vitro* and is indicated by indirect evidence *in vivo*. Caffieri *et al.* (1994) suggested that these lesions of cell membrane components may play a role as a second messenger, mimicking diacylglycerol (DAG). Recognizing the structural similarity between DAG and the psoralen-UFA cycloadducts, these investigators compared DAG's effective activation of protein kinase C (PKC) to that of the cycloadducts for activation of PKC in human platelets. Treatment of intact platelets with DAG resulted in the activation of PKC as measured by phosphorylation of a 47 kilodalton protein which is the major substrate for PKC. Results from the same platelet system showed that phosphorylation was induced to a similar extent by substituting DAG with the psoralen-linoleic acid cycloadduct. Gordon and Gilchrest (1989) reported previously that DAG stimulated melanogenesis in cultured melanocytes. In summary, these studies suggest that psoralen UFA-photoadducts may affect melanogenesis and that this mechanism may play an important role in PUVA-induced tanning.

Skin photosensitization is one of the most widely studied properties of furocoumarins. Several types of photodermatoses occur when skin comes into contact with plant or vegetable products containing psoralens and is later exposed to sunlight. Much less is known about potential adverse cutaneous effects resulting from chronic ingestion of foods that contain furocoumarins, such as figs, limes, parsnips, and cloves.

Although furocoumarins are potent phototoxic compounds, they are also used as therapeutic agents. Because of their ability to induce melanogenesis, psoralen derivatives have been applied clinically to treat vitiligo (leukoderma) and increase the tolerance of human skin to solar radiation. A new clinical discipline, photochemotherapy (PCT), is increasingly being introduced to treat psoriasis and other skin disorders (Parrish *et al.*, 1974; Wolff *et al.*, 1976; Gilchrest *et al.*, 1976).

Photochemotherapy involves the controlled interaction of light and orally administered drugs in order to produce beneficial effects. Psoralen PCT has entered the medical terminology as PUVA. The PUVA regimen is effective, clean, and acceptable to patients. However, some problems persist; these include possible induction of cataracts (Cloud *et al.*, 1960; Stern, 1994), hematologic effects (Friedmann and Rogers, 1980), alteration of the immune response (Strauss *et al.*, 1980; Aubin and Humbert, 1998) and skin aging (Bergfield, 1977). In addition, epidemiologic studies have demonstrated that extended treatment with PUVA can increase the patient's risk of basal cell carcinoma and malignant melanoma (Stern *et al.*, 1979, 1989; Stern, 2001; Hönigsmann *et al.*, 1980).

The use of psoralens in PCT has raised some additional questions concerning their phototoxicity. The structurally similar psoralens, 8-MOP, 5-methoxypsoralen (5-MOP), and 4, 5′, 8-trimethylpsoralen (TMP) have similar topical phototoxicity. However, when they are orally administered, the phototoxicity of TMP and 5-MOP is greatly diminished compared to that of 8-MOP (Mandula *et al.*, 1976; Hönigsmann *et al.*, 1979). This has been exploited by two European teams, who introduced 5-MOP as an alternative to 8-MOP, in the PCT of psoriasis (Hönigsmann *et al.*, 1979; Grupper and Berretti, 1981). Although the clearing of psoriatic lesions was comparable with 5-MOP and 8-MOP, acute side effects (including phototoxicity) were significantly reduced in the 5-MOP regimen. As more has been learned about the biotransformations of psoralens (Mandula *et al.*, 1976), it appears that metabolism may play a central role in determining the relative oral phototoxicity of substituted psoralens. However, it has not been established that reduced delivery of the phototoxic psoralen to the epidermis, due to metabolism or lack of absorption, is the basis for the observed differences in oral phototoxicity.

We have reported serum and epidermal levels of 5-MOP and 8-MOP in guinea pigs (Kornhauser *et al.*, 1982). Determinations of psoralen levels in the epidermis, the primary target organ for phototoxicity, had not previously been reported for either humans or an animal model. For this study we chose a guinea pig model system that we and others (Harber, 1969) have found to be reliable for predicting phototoxicity in humans. Our results indicated that, after equivalent oral dosing, metabolism and/or absorption constrains 5-MOP to lower epidermal levels than 8-MOP. Therefore, by orally administering 5-MOP it should be possible to maintain epidermal drug concentrations at lower levels than in an 8-MOP regimen.

Because psoralens, as used in PCT, react covalently with DNA, there is a potential risk of mutagenicity and oncogenicity. Indeed, in an *in vitro* study, 8-MOP and 5-MOP exhibited essentially the same activity in inducing chromosome damage in human cells (Natarajan *et al.*, 1981). Furthermore, it was reported that topical 5-MOP combined with UVA induced carcinogenesis in mice comparable to that observed with 8-MOP (Zajdela and Bisagni, 1981). These two studies suggest that 5-MOP and 8-MOP have a similar oncogenic potential when topically administered.

Extrapolating our findings with orally dosed guinea pigs to clinical applications, we suggest that a 5-MOP therapeutic regimen may minimize damage to epidermal DNA, reducing the risk of carcinogenesis that is suspected in 8-MOP PCT. For this reason, and because of the reduced acute side effects in a 5-MOP regimen, we feel that 5-MOP should be tested further, along with other psoralen derivatives, as alternatives to 8-MOP in PCT.

An additional application of psoralen phototoxicity, extracorporeal photophoresis, is increasingly being used for management of disorders such as cutaneous T-cell lymphoma (Edelson, 1988). Photophoresis involves oral administration of 8-MOP, then withdrawal of 1 unit of blood 2 h later. The blood is separated into its components by centrifugation. Plasma and leukocytes are combined with saline. This suspension is then passed as a thin film between twin banks of high-intensity UVA lamps. After irradiation, the erythrocytes are recombined with the remainder of the blood and retransfused into the patient. It has been reported that photophoresis is an effective treatment in many instances (Edelson *et al.*, 1987; Oliven and Shechter, 2001). The mechanism of this therapy appears to be complex, not merely involving cytotoxicity but also immunologic effects.

53.5.4   Photosensitized Oxidations

Many phototoxic compounds, such as porphyrins and dyes, affect biological substrates through photosensitized oxidations. These substances absorb light (both in long-wavelength UV and visible regions) and sensitize photooxidization from their triplet excited states. Following excitation, there are two distinct mechanisms (type I and type II) that result in photooxidation (Figure 53.11).

Although opinion is divided, type II is probably the more common mechanism producing $^1O_2$, a highly reactive oxidizing agent. A unique feature of $^1O_2$ involvement in photodynamic action is the fact that the generation and reaction sites may be different, the diffusion range of $^1O_2$ in cytoplasm being in the order of 0.1μm (Moan *et al.*, 1979). In contrast, in the type I (radical) mechanism the sensitizer and substrate must be closer at the time of photon absorption. The major processes involving $^1O_2$ are photooxidative loss of histidine, methionine, tryptophan, tyrosine, and cysteine in proteins; photooxidation of guanine bases in DNA; and formation of hydroperoxides with unsaturated lipids.

It has been recognized for decades that membrane damage plays a role in the photoinactivation of cells, especially in the presence of photodynamic sensitizers (Raab, 1900; Blum, 1941). The mechanism of cell membrane damage and disruption has been extensively studied for several photodynamic sensitizers. Photohemolysis of red blood cells sensitized by protoporphyrin (metal-free porphyrin) has been studied extensively because in several inheritable diseases of porphyrin metabolism (porphyrias), the red cells contain unusually high levels of photosensitizing porphyrins. Oxygen is required for protoporphyrin-photosensitized red cell lysis. On the molecular level, it is known that $^1O_2$, formed by energy transfer from triplet state protoporphyrin in red blood cell membranes, oxidizes unsaturated lipids (Lamola *et al.*, 1973; Golstein and Harber, 1972). Incorporation of cholesterol hydroperoxides, such as those formed in cholesterol photooxidation by protoporphyrin, leads to increased osmotic fragility and hemolysis of red blood cells (Lamola *et al.*, 1973). Protoporphyrin has also been shown to photosensitize protein cross-linking in membranes (Verweij *et al.*, 1981). It has been suggested that additional, more subtle, membrane functions, such as active transport of small molecules, are altered by membrane protein cross-linking (Kessel, 1977; Lamola and Doleiden,

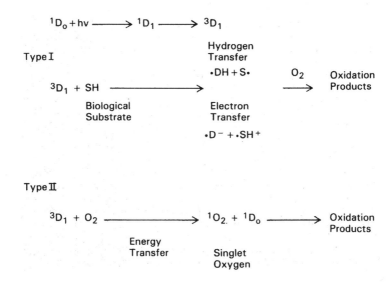

Figure 53.11: Mechanisms of photosensitized oxidation. The ground state sensitizer ($^1D_0$) is excited to the lowest excited singlet state ($^1D_1$) and undergoes intersystem crossing to the lowest excited triplet state ($^3D_1$).

1980). Indeed, later *in vitro* studies have shown that photodynamic sensitizers such can inactivate single ion channels and, also, transport of sugars and amino acids across cellular membranes (Kunz and Stark, 1997; Specht and Rodgers, 1991; Paardekooper *et al.*, 1993).

Photooxidation of cell membrane components and proteins is not the only mode of photodynamic damage. Various photodynamic sensitizers were found to be mutagenic in bacteria (Gutter *et al.*, 1977), yeast (Kobayashi and Ito, 1976), and mammalian cells (Gruener and Lockwood, 1979; Paardekooper *et al.*, 1997; Takeuchi *et al.*, 1997; Jeffrey *et al.*, 2000). Thus direct photodynamic damage to DNA is suspected, although alternative mechanisms for photodynamic mutagenesis have been proposed (Mukai and Goldstein, 1976).

There is now abundant evidence that bases in DNA may be oxidized by photodynamic sensitizers in the presence of light. Wacker *et al.*, 1964, presented the earliest direct evidence of photooxidative damage to guanine in DNA. Subsequent studies have demonstrated that, to differing degress, all nucleobases in DNA are susceptible to damage by photochemically generated radicals (i.e. type I photooxidation) (Cadet *et al.*, 1997). However, because guanine is the nucleobase with the lowest ionization potential, oxidative damage to guanine frequently predominates. Photosensitization through a type II mechanism, in which singlet oxygen is formed, has been shown to result in oxidative damage only to guanine bases in DNA (Cadet *et al.*, 1997). Because photosensitized oxidation through both type I and type II mechanisms results in damage to guanine bases, photoproducts of guanine have been widely used as markers for photooxidative damage in DNA. A number of products of the photooxidation of guanine have been isolated and characteized (Cadet and Teoule, 1978). The predominant decomposition product of guanine oxidation in DNA has been found to be 8-oxo-7,8-dihydro-2'-deoxyguanosine (8-oxodG) (Cadet *et al.*, 1997). With the development of sensitive and rapid methods for quantifying its formation (Floyd *et al.*, 1986), 8-oxodG has become the most widely used biomarker for oxidative damage to DNA. To date, this approach has been used to investigate a variety of photosensitizers including methylene blue (Floyd *et al.*, 1989), hematophorphyrin D (Floyd *et al.*, 1990), riboflavin (Yamamoto *et al.*, 1992), rose bengal (Schnieder *et al.*, 1993), fluoroquinolones (Rosen *et al.*, 1997), and titanium dioxide (Wamer *et al.*, 1997). These studies promise to better define the role of photooxidative damage to DNA in photo-toxicity and photomutagenesis.

The detailed mechanism of photooxidation of bases in DNA is not fully understood. When cells are in an environment containing a photodynamically active chromophore, such as a porphyrin or toluidine blue and exposed to visible light, damage to DNA from $^1O_2$ might be expected to result from an extracellular as well as an intracellular sensitizer. However, it has been found that toluidine blue, which is not taken up by cells, does not damage DNA (Ito and Kobayashi, 1977). Porphyrins, on the other hand, accumulate in cells and the efficiency of inducing DNA lesions follows the cellular uptake curve (Moan and Christensen, 1981). It is generally felt that accessibility of the sensitizing dye to DNA is a major factor in determining photomutagenic potential.

Both type I and type II mechanisms have been proposed for the photooxidation of DNA. The major pathway will be determined by the structure of the photosensitizing compound, the extent and type of binding to DNA, the oxygen concentration, and the polarity of the cellular environment (Kochevar, 1981; Ito, 1978).

Recent research has clearly shown that UV radiation can induce oxidative damage in skin without exposure to exogenous photodynamic sensitizers. It has been shown that:

1 UV induces the formation of free radicals in skin. Electron spin resonance spectrometry has been used to demonstrate that superoxide radical anion

CHAPTER 53

and/or hydroxyl radicals are generated in UV-irradiated whole skin (Pathak and Stratton, 1968) and skin homogenates (Ogura and Sugiyama, 1993).

2   The concentrations and oxidation state of antioxidants and antioxidant enzymes are altered after UV irradiation. Shindo *et al.* (1994) have reported that cutaneous antioxidants (glutathione, tocopherol, and ubiquinone) and antioxidant enzymes (particularly superoxide dismutase and catalase) are partially depleted in the skin of UV-irradiated mice. Depletion of these antioxidant defenses is measurable immediately after irradiation and is therefore not associated with the inflammatory response.

3   The level of oxidatively damaged molecules is elevated in UV-irradiated skin. Lipid peroxidation is significantly elevated after irradiation of mouse (Shindo *et al.*, 1994) or human (Punnonen *et al.*, 1991) skin *in vivo*. In addition, oxidative damage to DNA, measured as the formation of 8-hydoxy-2′-deoxyguanosine, is detected in the skin of UV-irradiated mice (Hattori-Nakakuki *et al.*, 1994).

These observations strongly indicate that UV radiation induces a state of oxidative stress in the skin. The identity of the endogenous photosensitizer(s) in the skin, whose excitation leads to photooxidation, is presently unknown. In addition, the relative importance of photooxidative damage caused by UV irradiation of skin and other molecular lesions (such as thymine dimers and DNA-protein cross-links) is at present unclear. Evidence is emerging that photooxidative stress in the skin may play a significant role in chronic disorders such as photocarcinogenesis (Black and Mathews-Roth, 1991) and photoaging (Bryce, 1993). However, the causal connection between photooxidation in the skin and significant adverse effects remains to be proven.

Selective photosensitized oxidative damage to cells has effectively been employed in photodynamic therapy (PDT) of solid tumors including eye, bladder, skin, and endobronchial tumors (Dougherty, 1987). PDT involves the use of hematoporphyrin (HP) derivatives as the photosensitizer. The HP derivatives, when injected, localize in tumors. Tissue is then irradiated with intense visible light, usually obtained by using a dye laser conjoined with fiber optics. The therapy described, which involves light activation of therapeutic agents, has the clear advantage of selectivity, that is, only the irradiated tissue is affected.

53.5.5   Mutations and Changes in Cellular Phenotype

The described classes of light-induced damage (thymine dimers, (6–4) adducts, DNA-protein cross-links, psoralen-DNA adducts, and oxidation of bases) represent potential premutational sites in DNA. High-fidelity repair of these DNA lesions would eliminate adverse cellular effects. As discussed, repair mechanisms have been found for many light-induced changes in DNA. Alternatively, unrepaired (or incorrectly repaired) DNA damage may lead to a range of cellular outcomes, including no effect (if the genetic alteration is unexpressed), cell death, or transformation to a neoplastic phenotype. The complex sequence of molecular events that determine these cellular outcomes is now becoming understood through the techniques of molecular biology.

Errors in DNA repair, or replication of a damaged DNA template result in the fixation of a DNA mutation. Several types of light-induced DNA mutations have been reported. Point mutations, involving single nucleotide base pair replacements, have been characterized in bacterial systems (Hutchinson and Wood, 1988; Cebula and Koch, 1990), well-defined plasmid sequences (Drobetsky *et al.*, 1989), and in mammalian genes (Bohr and Okumoto, 1988). Frameshift mutations, resulting from the addition or deletion of one or more base pairs, have also been studied (Cebula *et al.*, 1989). Techniques used to define mutational spectra (i.e., types of mutation and specific location within a DNA sequence) include hybridization with highly specific probes (Cebula and Koch, 1990; Pierceall *et al.*, 1991), direct DNA sequencing (Hutchinson and Wood, 1988; Cebula *et al.*, 1989), and analysis of altered restriction endonuclease sites (Drobetsky *et al.*, 1989). Use of polymerase chain reaction (PCR), to amplify DNA sequences within genes of interest, has allowed rapid and sensitive detection of UV-induced mutations in mammalian genes (Brash *et al.*, 1991; Tornaletti and Pfeifer, 1994).

The derived mutation spectra have proven useful for tracing the etiology of skin cancer and understanding mechanistic steps in UV-induced mutations. Brash *et al.* (1991) have described a point mutation in DNA isolated from human squamous cell carcinomas which may be characteristic of UV-induced carcinogenesis. Using PCR to amplify selected exons in the *p53* tumor suppressor gene, followed by direct sequencing of amplified exons, they demonstrated that the characteristic mutations were CC→TT double base substitutions. This observation of distinctive mutations produced by UV radiation has been subsequently confirmed by several investigators (Kress *et al.*, 1992; Dumaz *et al.*, 1994). This molecular epidemiological approach has significantly increased our

CHAPTER 53

understanding of the etiology of human skin cancers. The use of molecular biological techniques has also led to a clearer understanding of factors that predispose genes to mutation by UV radiation. As a corollary to the observation that CC→TT mutations occur after irradiation with UV, it has been observed that pyrimidine-rich DNA sequences have increased sensitivity to mutations induced by UV radiation (Brash *et al.*, 1991). In addition, it has been shown that UV-induced mutations in DNA derived from human skin carcinomas predominate on the nontranscribed strand of DNA (Dumaz *et al.*, 1993). Tornaletti and Pfeifer (1994) have definitively shown that rates of DNA repair are highly variable within a mammalian gene. Furthermore, they demonstrated that slowly repaired regions of DNA, such as nontranscribed DNA strands, are hot spots for UV-induced mutations. These insights into the factors predisposing UV-damaged DNA to mutation are essential for understanding the mechanism(s) of UV-induced mutations.

In the past decade, our understanding of the genetic basis of cancer has dramatically increased largely because of the discovery of specific genes, proto-oncogenes, whose normal function is vital for appropriate regulation of cellular growth and differentiation. Alteration of proto-oncogene structures or the regulation of their expression may lead to cancer (Bishop, 1983).

It is now well established that DNA damage, such as point mutations, can activate oncogenes. The role of oncogenes in UV-induced carcinogenesis is currently under active investigation. UV-induced mutations in Ha-ras proto-oncogene and *p53* tumor suppressor gene have been the most extensively studied. Attention has been focused on these genes since mutations in *Ha-ras* and *p53* are frequently observed in DNA derived from skin carcinomas (Daya *et al.*, 1994). The protein coded by *Ha-ras* proto-oncogene is associated with the cellular membrane and is critical for extracellular stimulation of cellular division (Khosravi-Far and Der, 1994). Several animal studies indicate that activation of *Ha-ras* oncogene is associated with photocarcinogenesis. Strickland *et al.* (1985) have reported activation of *Ha-ras* by a single treatment of Sencar mice with UVB or PUVA. In addition, Husain *et al.* (1990) have reported that UVB induces amplification and overexpression of *Ha-ras* proto-oncogene in mouse skin papillomas and carcinomas. In these animal studies, UV irradiation can definitively be associated with both the formation of morphological changes (i.e., papillomas and carcinomas) and activation of oncogenes(s). Mutations in *Ha-ras* are frequently detected in human skin tumors. Mutations have been reported in up to 45 percent of human skin squamous cell carcinomas biopsied from sun-exposed areas (Kanjilal *et al.*, 1993; Daya-Grosjean *et al.*, 1993). The incidence of mutations in *Ha-ras* is significantly lower in basal cell carcinomas and melanomas (Kanjilal *et al.*, 1993; Ananthaswamy *et al.*, 1988; Gerrit van der Schroeff *et al.*, 1990).

The *p53* tumor suppressor gene encodes a nuclear phosphoprotein which plays an important role in the control of cellular proliferation (Levine *et al.*, 1991). The normal or "wild type" *p53* protein acts as a powerful suppressor of cellular growth. Mutations of *p53* gene are frequently observed in animal and human skin tumors. Kress *et al.* (1992) have found mutations in *p53* gene in up to 50 percent of squamous cell carcinomas induced by UVB radiation of mice. In addition, all mutations occurred at dipyrimidine sequences and most frequently involved C→T single base and CC→TT double base mutations. As previously discussed, these base substitutions have been found to be characteristic of UVB-induced mutations. Mutations in *p53* gene are also frequently observed in DNA derived from human skin carcinomas. Shea *et al.* (1992) found overexpression of a mutant *p53* protein in 83 percent of basal cell carcinomas of the head and neck. In addition, Brash *et al.* (1991) found mutations of *p53* gene in 58 percent of human skin cancers. As previously discussed, a detailed analysis of these mutations suggested a distinctive UV-signature in the mutation type. Basset-Seguin *et al.* (1994) have reviewed evidence that mutation of *p53* may be involved in tumor progression from papilloma to carcinoma, providing further insight into the mechanistic role of *p53* mutations in photocarcinogenesis. Following a review of reports of mutations in *p53* gene, Harris and Hollstein (1993) have suggested that therapy, based on the renewal of *p53* function, may have future clinical importance. It is clear that application of these techniques of modern molecular biology has resulted in a major leap forward in our understanding of the etiology and possible treatment of photocarcinogenesis.

53.6 CELLULAR MEDIATORS INDUCED BY LIGHT

We have reviewed various sensitized and unsensitized light-induced reactions, such as pyrimidine dimer formation, DNA-protein cross-linking, and various photooxidations. It is still not fully known how these molecular events are involved in the complex physiological processes that give rise to erythema in sunburn or phototoxic reactions. Generally, a UV-induced effect in tissue may be a direct photon effect or may be mediated by diffusible substances induced by photons. Such substances include prostaglandins (PGs), cytokines, histamines, kinins, lysosomal enzymes, and activated oxygen species (e.g., $^1O_2$ and superoxide radical). Research in this field has focused primarily in two areas, prostaglandins and cytokines. Prostaglandins (PGs, eicosanoids) have been implicated in many physiological processes. The almost ubiquitous occurrence of the PG synthetase enzyme (cyclooxygenase) system and the presence of its substrate fatty acids in membrane phospholipids of mammalian cells suggest that PGs can be formed in most types of cells, where they can act as intracellular messengers (Silver and Smith, 1975).

The role of PGs in cutaneous pathology and inflammation is well established (Goldyne, 1975). PGs were found in whole rat skin homogenates; when the epidermis was separated from the dermis, most of the PG activity was located in the epidermis. The realization that PGs are important in cellular control mechanisms has motivated a great deal of research on their possible role in the etiology of cancer (Snyder and Eaglstein, 1974).

A tentative pathway for PG formation and its interrelation with the adenylate cyclase system in cutaneous tissue after UV irradiation is shown in Figure 53.12. Tissue (specifically membrane) damage, induced by light makes membrane phospholipids "accessible" to the enzyme, phospholipase. This is the first step in inducing the arachidonic acid cascade, which results in PG production (Cohen and DeLeo, 1993). In addition the signal transduction mechanism for

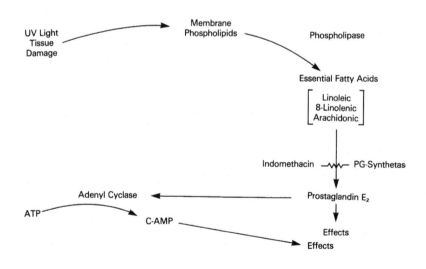

Figure 53.12: Tentative pathway of prostaglandin formation and its interrelation with the adenylate cyclase system in cutaneous tissue following UV irradiation.

UV-induced prostaglandin (PGE2) synthesis has been indicated to involve tyrosine kinases (Miller *et al.*, 1994).

The importance of PGs as mediators of delayed erythema is supported by the observation that inhibitors of PG synthetase such as indomethacin and aspirin can suppress UVB-induced erythema (Snyder and Eaglstein, 1974). On the other hand, erythema due to psoralen phototoxicity (PUVA) cannot be suppressed with indomethacin (Morison *et al.*, 1977) and no increase in PG activity is found in exudate from PUVA-inflamed skin (Greaves, 1978). For these reasons, mediators other than PGs are likely to be involved in the pathogenesis of PUVA-induced inflammation.

PGs are rapidly metabolized near the site of their synthesis, which increases the difficulty of studying their role in inflammation. A metabolite of PGE_2, 13,14-dihydro-15-keto-PGE_2 (PGE_2-M), is much more stable and accumulates in plasma, where it can be measured (Tashjian *et al.*, 1977). The introduction of a specific assay for the measurement of PGE_2-M provides an opportunity to examine, in a relatively noninvasive manner, the systemic levels of PGE_2 after a single acute UV injury.

After exposure to UVB, human suction blister aspirates showed metabolites of arachidonic acid, prostaglandin E_2 (PGE_2), PGD_2, $PGF_{2\forall}$, and 12-HETE. A contribution of mast cells to UVB-induced inflammation was indicated by the production of PGD_2 as was prostacyclin, a likely derivative of the vascular endothelium (Hruza and Pentland, 1993). UV-light has also been shown to induce increased synthesis of prostaglandins by increasing phospholipase activity in human keratinocyte cultures (Kang-Rotondo *et al.*, 1993), and through increasing the sensitivity of keratinocytes to various inflammatory mediators such as bradykinin (Pentland and Jacobs, 1991). The role of histamine in UV-induced erythema response has also been studied (Gilchrest *et al.*, 1981) and its suggested mechanism of action, by stimulation of prostaglandin release, was reported (Pentland *et al.*, 1990).

The second major area of interest involving cellular mediators is the study of cytokines and their role in cutaneous immune or inflammatory responses. These cytokines include interleukins (IL), hematopoietic colony stimulating factors (CSF), tumor necrosis factors (TNF), and interferons (INF). Although the role UV-light plays in inducing mutagenesis and carcinogenesis is still the focus of much research, the finding that UV-light induces the production of cytokines in cell culture or skin (Ansel *et al.*, 1983; Gahring *et al.*, 1984) has resulted in greater attention to the role of these mediators in acute and chronic effects in skin.

CHAPTER 53

Cytokines are small, soluble, polypeptides that are released by a variety of cells including monocytes, macrophages, lymphocytes, fibroblasts, neutrophils, brain cells, and keratinocytes as well as other cells of the skin. In the skin, cytokines bind to specific cell surface receptors and the signal is transduced by complex protein interactions, such as protein kinase C, to the nucleus where gene expression is altered, thus regulating the proliferation and functions of various target cells or the cytokine-producing cells themselves.

The cytokine environment in *in vitro* experiments may differ substantially from that found *in vivo*. It is important to remember that the biological and pathological responses induced by cytokines depend on the balance between cytokine induction, expression of specific receptors, modulation of cytokine effects by a cascade of cellular events including complex interactions of other cytokines, and by the presence of inhibitors (di Giovine and Duff, 1990).

A number of studies have suggested that UVB-induced inflammation involving epidermal keratinocytes and dermal fibroblasts results in the synthesis and release of "primary" cytokines, such as interleukin-1α (IL-1α) and tumor necrosis factor α (TNFα), which can stimulate their own production as well as that of a variety of secondary cytokines. Also, IL-1α and TNFα together have been shown to mediate UVB-induced prostaglandin release (Grewe *et al.*, 1993). IL-1, found as two distinct forms (IL-1α and IL-1β) is involved in many biological responses, including cellular proliferation, chemoattraction, and the induction of other cytokines involved in immune regulation, inflammatory responses, growth, and cellular differentiation (Cork *et al.*, 1993).

Epidermal keratinocytes are a major source of IL-1. It is suggested that this large reservoir of IL-1 may provide a protective mechanism against skin injury by its ability to activate a rapid inflammatory response to combat infection and promote wound healing (Gahring *et al.*,1985). Keratinocytes in normal epidermis also contain inhibitors that are necessary to control the action of IL-1 and other pro-inflammatory cytokines. If uncontrolled, these cytokines themselves can cause extensive tissue damage. The type I, IL-1 receptor antagonist (IL-1ra) competes with the cytokine for binding to the IL-1 receptor. Soluble type II inhibitor proteins, shed from cell surfaces, are also present and can bind to a cytokine and prevent it from binding to receptors on target cells. Keratinocytes express only a few high-affinity receptors for IL-1, but the number of these receptors is increased in response to UVB-radiation and trauma. Physical injury or UV-radiation damage to keratinocytes can activate keratinocytes to produce secondary cytokines such as granulocyte macrophage colony stimulating factor (GM-CSF), IL-6, IL-8, macrophage colony stimulating factor (M-CSF), granulocyte colony stimulating factor (G-CSF), and additional IL-1. These cytokines initiate the production of inflammatory infiltrates and activate fibroblasts to proliferate and produce collagen for wound healing. T-cell-derived interferon γ (IFNγ) induces expression of IL-1 receptors, thus increasing the biological effect of the IL-1 released from the keratinocytes (Cork *et al.*, 1993).

TNFα also plays an important role in both humoral and cell-mediated immune and inflammatory responses to infection and injury, including damage induced by UV-light. This cytokine has been found to alter surface properties of endothelial cells, stimulate fibroblasts and neutrophils, and increase production of collagenase and prostaglandin E_2. TNFα is a mediator of cachexia, the severe wasting of the body in certain malignant diseases. At high concentrations, TNFα has been shown to play a major role in potentially fatal endotoxic shock. TNFα can also activate polymorphonuclear leukocytes and macrophages, increase their chemotaxis, and stimulate the release of reactive oxygen intermediates including superoxide anion and hydrogen peroxide (Sherry and Cerami, 1988). Significant amounts of TNFα were detected in culture supernatants after normal human keratinocytes and human epidermoid carcinoma cell lines were irradiated by UV-light. After UVB exposure to humans, TNFα was detected in the serum of these volunteers (Köck *et al.*, 1990).

Other important events induced by cytokines that are stimulated or suppressed by UV-light include the expression of surface molecules such as the intercellular adhesion molecule-1 (ICAM-1), which regulates the migration, adhesion, and retention of leukocytes into traumatized sites (Krutmann *et al.*,1990; Norris *et al.*, 1990; Cornelius *et al.*, 1994).

Epidemiological evidence implicates the contribution of excessive exposure of UV-light on unprotected skin in Caucasians to the great increase in skin cancers that has been reported in recent years. In addition to its carcinogenic effect, UV-radiation has also been found to be immunosuppressive. UVB-induced immunosuppression is one of a variety of factors that may be a reasonable mechanism for skin cancer. Yoshikawa *et al.* (1990) reported that susceptibility to tolerance of a topically applied hapten after low-dose UVB exposure to the skin was found only in patients with a proved history of non-melanoma skin cancer. Shimizu and Streilein (1994) suggest that UVB-radiation converts *trans*- to *cis*-urocanic acid in the epidermis, which in turn causes the production of excessive amounts of TNFα. They reported that the mechanism of UVB-induced tolerance to the hapten dinitrofluorobenzene is separate and distinct from the mechanism that impairs contact sensitivity. Their data suggested that suppressor cells were generated in UV-irradiated mice even though the animals did not display *in vivo* tolerance.

Another significant cytokine, IL-10, has been found to be a suppressive cytokine produced by the TH2 subset of T-helper cells, and keratinocytes, B-cells, mast cells, and monocytes. IL-10 has been shown to have a wide range of activities among which is the ability to block the production of TNFα and IL-1β (Cassatella *et al.*, 1993). IL-10 also blocks natural killer cell stimulatory factor (IL-12), a cytokine of antigen presenting cells and Langerhans cells, and a powerful stimulator of TH1 cells, another subset of helper T-cells, to produce IFN((D'Andrea *et al.*, 1993). In addition, Langerhans cells exposed to IL-10 failed to cause TH1 cell proliferation and instead induced clonal anergy in these cells (Enk *et al.*, 1993). The synthesis of cytokines by TH1 cells is also regulated by the IL-10 cytokine (Mosmann, 1991).

Suppression of delayed type hypersensitivity was induced in mice after they were injected with supernatants containing IL-10 from UV-irradiated murine keratinocytes. Contrary to the findings of others, no TNFα was detected in the UV-irradiated keratinocyte culture fluid (Rivas and Ullrich, 1992). However, Kang *et al.* (1994) reported that although human keratinocytes accumulated intracellular IL-10 after *in vivo* exposure of volunteers to four minimal erythema doses (MEDs) of UVB, IL-10 was most potently produced and secreted by macrophages. The authors suggested that since macrophages produce IL-10, and immunosuppressive tolerance-inducing macrophages populate the skin after UV exposure, macrophages may play a role in down-regulating the UV-induced inflammatory response.

Yoshikawa *et al.* (1992) studied the effects of TNFα and low-dose UVB on dinitrochlorobenzene (DNCB)-induced contact hypersensitivity (CH). The authors used two strains of mice; those in which UVB-irradiation impaired the induction of CH to DNCB (UVB-susceptible) and those in which UVB-irradiation did not (UVB-resistant). Intradermal injection of TNFα at the ear challenge site before hapten application yielded an amplified CH reaction, even in the UVB-susceptible strain. Anti-TNFα antibodies given to UVB-susceptible mice neutralized the enhanced CH response to dinitrofluorobenzene (DNFB) but did not affect the CH response of UVB-resistant mice. The results indicated that TNFα, released from UVB-exposed epidermal cells, was a critical mediator of the effects of UVB radiation on both the induction and expression of CH. In addition these authors found that topically applied DNFB profoundly depleted the epidermis of Langerhans cells, whereas, DNFB applied to UVB-irradiated or TNFα-treated skin was less effective at eliminating these cells. This indicated that

TNFα immobilized Langerhans cells transiently within the epidermis. It was proposed that this immobilization had the paradoxical effects of (1) interfering with sensitization (low-dose UVB-irradiation has been found to impair the ability to *induce* CH) by preventing hapten-bearing Langerhans cells from migrating to the draining lymph nodes and, (2) amplifying CH (low-dose UVB-irradiation of previously immunized mice was found to exaggerate the *expression* of CH) by increasing the duration of retention and presentation of the hapten to the epidermis.

The pathological and physiological mechanisms involved in UV-induced immune and inflammatory responses remain poorly understood. Recent advances in this field, however, especially those involving the complex interactions of UV-induced cellular mediators such as prostaglandins and cytokines, have provided a framework of hypotheses to address the important issues concerning these UV-induced reactions.

53.7 PHOTOIMMUNOLOGY

In a broad sense, immunology is the study of how and why the body reacts against anything that is foreign and how an organism can recognize the difference between self and nonself. That UV-light can significantly influence the immune system is a relatively recent discovery. In recent years exceptional activity, development, and progress in this field has occurred resulting in a new understanding of the connection between light, skin, and the immune system. A complete discussion of these findings is beyond the scope of this section. The interested reader is advised to consult some of the many publications on this subject (Streilein, 1983; Kripke, 1986; Edelson and Fink, 1985; Morison, 1989).

The discipline of photoimmunology began with two important observations: (1) UVB induced suppression of contact hypersensitivity (CHS) in mice evoked by dinitrochlorobenzene or similar compounds, and (2) UV-light induced alterations in immune functions are involved in the pathogenesis of photo-carcinogenesis in mice (Kripke, 1980). UVB-induced tumors in mice are highly antigenic; they are immunologically rejected when transplanted into normal syngeneic recipients, but grow progressively in immunosuppressed animals. Subtumorigenic doses of UVB produce specific systemic alterations, which permit progressive growth of these highly antigenic tumors after transplantation.

The mechanism(s) of these phenomena are still incompletely understood. The evidence indicates that UV inhibition of CHS responses and of tumor rejection processes involve suppressor T lymphocytes that inhibit normal immunologic reactions. Recent investigations suggest that the suppressor lymphocytes may be regulatory T cells secreting IL-10 and TGFß (Schwarz, 2000) or NK T cells (Moodycliffe, 2000). UVB-mediated alteration of antigen presenting cells may be a critical event in the generation of suppressor T cells (Beissert *et al.*, 2001). The available evidence suggests that both CHS responses and tumor rejection processes involve suppressor T lymphocytes that inhibit normal immunologic reactions.

Evidence for the involvement of the immune system in the etiology of photocarcinogenesis in humans is now established. It is possible that chronic exposure to UV causes nonspecific immunosuppression and thus leads to the development of light-induced skin tumors. Long-term clinical treatment with PUVA also induces immunosuppression (Morison *et al.*, 1979), and this may be one of the mechanisms of PUVA-mediated carcinogenesis. The role of UV immunosuppression in melanoma skin cancer is still not established, and has until recently been inaccessible to experimentation. A recent transgeneic mouse model of junctional melanoma initiated by UV irradiation of neonatal mice, may rectify this deficit (Noonan, 2001).

The immune system involves complex molecular and cellular interactions, which are now being gradually revealed. A major breakthrough, as a result of studies in the fields of photobiology and immunology, has yielded new understanding of the skin as an active element of the immune system. The majority of the cells in the epidermis, Langerhans and Granstein cells, both dendritic populations of the epidermis, and even keratinocytes, have been shown to be active immunologically (Edelson and Fink, 1985). Furthermore, it was shown that certain types of T cells can undergo maturation in the epidermis. To emphasize the connection of these epidermal components to the total immune system, the term skin-associated lymphoid tissue (SALT), has been coined (Streilein, 1983). The concept of immune surveillance, which has undergone ups and downs in its history, has been reformulated: it is presently believed that immune surveillance does exist but is limited to the lymphoreticular and cutaneous systems (Streilein, 1983).

These diverse observations dramatically demonstrate the relevance of photobiology to dermatology and studies of carcinogenesis. An important insight from these findings is the demonstration that both direct (i.e., DNA damage) and indirect (modification of the immune system) effects influence the development of primary skin cancers. Aside from virus-associated cancers, this might be the only experimental carcinogenesis system in which the immune system has been shown to play a role in the carcinogenic process (Kripke, 1986).

Some interesting observations have been made about the mechanism(s) of the photoimmunologic response and the potential mediators involved, including genetic factors (Noonan and Hoffman, 1994). One of the experimental models that has attracted widespread attention is the UVB-suppression of the CHS response in rodents. The CHS method has also been used in human subjects and UV immunosuppression has been demonstrated (Selgrade, 2001). In addition this phenomenon has also been studied in various *in vitro* systems (CHS is commonly referred to as contact allergy in humans). Mediators produced by keratinocytes exposed to UV may be involved.

Another important approach to this problem was to identify the chromophore responsible for various photoimmunologic responses. However, the identity of the molecular target in the skin for the immunosuppressive effects of UV radiation continues to be controversial. Two schools of thought are currently predominant. The first, elaborated mainly by Kripke *et al.* (1992), states that DNA is the primary photoreceptor for UV-induced immunological changes. The experimental approach of these authors and of Yarosh *et al.* (1994), which led to this conclusion is extremely interesting and inventive. In one set of experiments, after C3H mice were exposed to UV-radiation, T4-endonuclease V, encapsulated in liposomes was used to deliver a dimer-specific excision repair enzyme into the epidermis *in situ*. The fate of the liposome membrane was followed by using a fluorescent, lipophilic dye, and the T4 enzyme was traced by immunogold labeling, followed by fluorescent or transmission electron microscopy. It was found that *in vivo*, liposomes penetrated the stratum corneum where they were localized in the epidermis inside basal keratinocytes (Yarosh *et al.*, 1994). Furthermore, ultrastructural studies demonstrated the presence of liposomes in the cytoplasm of cells in the epidermis. The T4 enzyme was present in both nucleus and cytoplasm of keratinocytes and Langerhans cells. These results confirmed that liposomes could deliver encapsulated enzymes into cells of the skin. In addition, the application of T4 liposomes to UV-irradiated mouse skin decreased the number of cyclobutane pyrimidine dimers in the epidermis and prevented suppression of both delayed and contact hypersensitivity responses. Control, heat-inactivated endonuclease encapsulated in liposomes had no effect. This treatment did not affect immunosuppression induced by 8-MOP plus UVA radiation.

Additional studies by Kripke and Yarosh (1994) involved the marsupial *Monodelphis domestica*, which has an active photorepair enzyme system. The authors demonstrated that both local and systemic types of photoimmunosuppression could be abrogated by exposing the animals to photoreactivating light immediately after UVB irradiation. The photorepair enzyme system is known to be specific for direct removal of cyclobutane pyrimidine dimers.

The studies mentioned above suggest that DNA is the photoreceptor in UV-induced immunosuppression and that the primary molecular event mediating this process is the formation of pyrimidine dimers. Furthermore, they illustrate that the delivery of lesion-specific DNA repair enzymes to *in vivo* skin is possible and is an effective tool for restoring immune function and possibly preventing other disorders caused by DNA damage.

The second school of thought concerning the photoreceptor for immuno-suppression evolved from the correlation of the action spectrum for UV-induced suppression of CHS with the absorption spectrum of components in the skin which suggested that urocanic acid (UCA), a molecule present in stratum corneum, may play this role (DeFabo *et al.*, 1981). DeFabo and Noonan (1983) presented additional evidence that the UVB-induced immunosuppression in mice is initiated by the photoisomerization of UCA. They predicted that the cis isomer is the natural immunosuppressant, and as such may play an important role as the "mediator" between the environment (UVB) and the immune system. Since that time, additional support for an immunoregulatory role for *cis*-UCA has been provided in a number of experimental systems. Administration of *cis*-UCA *in vivo* has been found to decrease the function of splenic antigen presenting cells (Noonan *et al.*, 1988). Furthermore, topical application of UCA during UV-induced carcinogenesis resulted in an increase in both the tumor number and the degree of malignancy (Reeve *et al.*, 1989). Applying *cis*-UCA to mice without UV irradiation, mimicked the photoimmune suppression effect (Noonan and DeFabo, 1992). In other experiments by Reilly and DeFabo (1991), increasing the UCA levels in mice by feeding its metabolic precursor, histidine, increased the susceptibility to UV suppression in these mice. These findings provide the first evidence that UV-induced immunosuppression can be enhanced by a dietary component (L-histidine).

Research efforts to identify the molecular target for UCA are continuing. It has been shown that cis-UCA inhibits induction of cAMP in fibroblasts (Bouscarel, 1998). Most recently evidence has been derived that UCA may in fact act via the neural system in the skin since cis-UCA stimulated the release of neuropeptides from sensory neurons (Khalil, 2001). This observation would link *cis*-UCA, sensory neurons, neuropeptides and mast cells in immuno-suppression. It has been shown that both histamine and *trans*-UCA up-regulate the cAMP formation in human skin fibroblasts in a dose-dependent fashion. *Cis*-UCA effectively downregulates this induction. These observations are consistent with the action of UCA via a histamine-like receptor, but the possibility of specific receptors for UCA isomers cannot be excluded. These studies link UCA to a major secondary cell signalling system (Palaszynski *et al.*, 1992). Complementing the role of UCA in these processes, an antibody to *cis*-UCA has been shown to prevent UV-induced immunosuppression (Moodycliffe, 1996). Administration of this antibody decreases UV carcinogenesis, consistent with a role for *cis*-UCA immunosuppression in skin cancer.

All these observations strongly suggest that at least two different mechanisms are involved in the UV-modification of the mammalian immune system. The results from the studies on UCA came from experiments performed in *in vitro* systems or in rodents. Although at this time there is no direct evidence that *cis*-UCA is immunosuppressive in humans, the fact that UCA is present in human skin and also isomerizes in response to UVB suggests that it may play the same immunoregulating role in humans. The importance of these findings is increased by the fact that the UV wavelengths (UVB) most affected by depletion of the stratospheric ozone layer are those known to be the most immunosuppressive in animals.

These studies also indicate that light-induced modification of the immune system will be important in the future, with broad applications for managing disorders such as graft rejection, allergies, and autoimmune diseases.

53.8 ALTERATIONS IN GENE EXPRESSION INDUCED BY LIGHT

Any discussion of the cellular and molecular effects of light on the skin is incomplete without reference to the induction of gene expression by light. Through the methods of modern molecular biology, we are now beginning to understand how light can alter the complex program of gene expression within the cell. The discussion to follow will deal with transient changes in gene expression following exposure of cells or skin to light rather than changes in gene expression resulting from mutations and altered cellular phenotype. It will, however, include only a portion of the large body of information on altered gene expression following irradiation that has appeared within the last decade. Recent reviews provide more comprehensive treatments of this subject (Ronai *et al.*, 1994; Holbrook and Fornace, 1991). To date, only alterations in gene expression following UV irradiation in the absence of photosensitizers have been widely studied.

Changes in cellular levels of messenger RNA (mRNA) and related proteins occur within minutes after exposure of cells or skin to UV. The immediate changes following UV exposure have been called the mammalian cell *UV response* (Devary *et al.*, 1992). This immediate UV response involves changes in cellular transcription factors, which are those proteins whose function it is to alter the transcription or expression of other cellular genes. The immediate UV response involves two distinct types of changes: (1) modification of pre-existing transcription factor proteins, resulting in their increased activities, and (2) resultant elevation of levels of cellular transcription factors through increased transcription of their mRNA. Modification of pre-existing transcription factors requires initial UV-induced activation of cytoplasmic proteins including *src* (Devary *et al.*, 1992), *raf-1* and *MAP-2* (Radler-Pohl *et al.*, 1993) by their phosphorylation. Activated *raf-1* leads to the phosphorylation and the resultant activation, of the pre-existing transcription factor, *c-jun* (Radler-Pohl *et al.*, 1993). Cytoplasmic activation of *c-jun* is an early and essential step in the UV response. Activation of *c-jun* initiates the second phase of the UV response in which levels of transcription factors dramatically increase. The events in this phase of the UV response occur within the nucleus and require formation of mRNA coding for transcription factors including *c-jun* and *c-fos*. Significant increases in the expression of *c-jun* and *c-fos* have been found in cells (Devary *et al.*, 1991), rat skin (Gillardon *et al.*, 1994) and human skin (Roddey *et al.*, 1994) following UV irradiation. The first phase of the UV response, occurring in the cytoplasm, allows a rapid and transient cellular response without mRNA or protein synthesis. The second phase results in a more sustained response to UV irradiation.

Many unanswered questions remain concerning the detailed mechanism connecting UV-induced cellular damage and altered gene expression of transcription factors. There is strong evidence that UV-induced damage to DNA initiates the UV response (Stein *et al.*, 1989; Yamaizumi and Sugano, 1994). However, as noted, the most immediate changes following exposure to UV are cytoplasmic. How UV-induced DNA damage triggers this cytoplasmic response remains to be elucidated and is currently the subject of vigorous research.

The transcription or expression of a wide array of genes is affected by increases in cellular levels of *c-jun* and *c-fos*, which combine to form the heterodimer, activator protein-1 (*AP-1*) (Angel and Karin, 1991). It is *AP-1* that orchestrates the expression of functionally diverse genes within the mammalian cell. AP-1 responsive genes induced by UV radiation include genes associated with protection from oxidative damage, such as metallothioneins I and II

(Fornace *et al.*, 1988b), and hemeoxygenase (Keyse and Tyrrell, 1989). AP-1 responsive genes which play a role in repair of the extracellular matrix in the dermis, such as collagenase (Petersen *et al.*, 1992), are also induced by UV radiation. Ornithine decarboxylase, a central enzyme in polyamine metabolism and stimulation of cell proliferation, is similarly an AP-1 responsive gene induced by UV radiation (Verma *et al.*, 1979).

Many of the important effects induced by UV irradiation of the skin result from alterations in the cell cycle of epidermal cells. These effects include UV-induced hyperplasia and sunburn cell formation (Danno and Horio, 1982). During passage through the cell cycle, the mammalian cell must pass through two critical check points: the G_1-S transition where DNA synthesis commences and the G_2-M transition where mitosis begins (Figure 53.13).

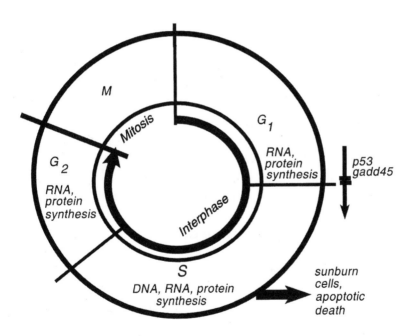

Figure 53.13: Diagram of stages in the mammalian cell cycle. Important regulatory stages, or check points, are at the $G_1 \rightarrow S$ and $G_2 \rightarrow M$ transitions. UV radiation induces *p53* and *gadd45* which are involved with inhibition at the $G_1 \rightarrow S$ transition.

Retardation of progression through these cell cycle checkpoints ostensibly permits repair of UV-damaged DNA before cell division, avoiding propagation of genetic damage. The checkpoint located at the G_1-S transition is critical in assuring that UV-damage is repaired before DNA synthesis and cell division. At least two genes, *p53* and *gadd45*, are involved with arresting the growth of cells containing UV-damaged DNA at this check point in the cell cycle (Kuerbitz *et al.*, 1992; Fornace *et al.*, 1988a). Increases in *p53* and *gadd45* cellular levels are closely linked to DNA damage in cells (Kastan *et al.*, 1991; Yamaizumi and Sugano, 1994; Fornace *et al.*, 1988a). It was also shown that increased levels of these two proteins results in arrest of growth at the G_1 phase of the cell cycle. Recently, it has been shown that the levels of *p53* are dramatically elevated in human skin following moderate levels of UV irradiation. Healy *et al.* (1994) have shown that sub-erythemal doses of UVB elicits a significant increase in epidermal *p53* levels. Similar results have been reported by Campbell *et al.* (1993) with UVA, UVB, or UVC. There is now evidence that *p53* and *gadd45* genes act in concert to arrest cell growth at the G_1 phase. Kastan *et al.* (1992) provided evidence that *p53* acts as a transcription factor whose activity leads to increased expression of *gadd45*.

53.9   EPILOGUE

Since its beginning around the turn of the century, the science of photobiology has had various stages of development. At a very early stage, through the classical experiments by Raab (1900) and others, it was shown that many dyes and pigments can sensitize various cells and organisms to visible light. The introduction of phototherapy by Niels R. Finsen dates from the same period. These developments extended the boundaries of photobiology to physicists, biologists, and clinicians.

The past three decades marked the beginning of molecular photobiology. An early milestone was the isolation of thymine dimers from living systems exposed to UV. Also, the molecular basis of a genetic disease, xeroderma pigmentosum, was established. The rapid expansion of molecular photobiology significantly contributed to the development of molecular biology and related disciplines and led to the advent of a new clinical discipline, photochemotherapy.

One of the objectives of photobiology will be to shed more light on the relation between phototoxicity and photocarcinogenesis, which is poorly established. It is still believed that chronic phototoxicity can lead to carcinogenesis. In at least a few cases, however, such as chronic phototoxicity evoked by anthracene or porphyrins, no carcinogenic developments were observed. A possible explanation for this phenomenon is that the primary targets of anthracene and other photodynamic sensitizers are molecules not directly involved in the transmission of genetic information.

One of the major conceptual advances in photobiology in the past few years is the perception that photon toxicity is not limited to skin; it can, and often does, induce significant systemic alterations. Therefore, the significance of photobiology exceeds that of dermatology. Basic photobiology should become common knowledge in all branches of basic and clinical medicine.

In all civilizations humans have worshiped the sun. They have recognized that the sun is the most important of the factors that sustain life on the earth, and that many of our daily rhythms are dependent on the cycles of sunlight. We know today that sunlight is also one of the most potent carcinogens present in the environment. To survive the insult of photons, humans have evolved a group of defense mechanisms. These include keratinization (thickening of the stratum corneum), production of melanin (the most important protective pigment in the skin), and synthesis of urocanic acid (an absorber of UV). The dietary carotenoid pigments also provide some protection by quenching singlet oxygen and various active radical species.

The protective mechanisms evolved against the detrimental effects of the sun are, in a growing number of cases, inadequate because of our modern life-styles. We must, therefore, increase our understanding of light-induced toxic reactions and judiciously use this knowledge to protect the public health.

CHAPTER 53

REFERENCES

ALLISON, A.C., MAGNUS, I.A. and YOUNG M.R. (1966) Role of lysosomes and of cell membranes in photosensitization. *Nature (Lond.)* **209**, 874–878.

ANANTHASWAMY, H.N., PRICE J.E., GOLDBERG, L.H. and BALES, E.S. (1988) Detection and identification of activated oncogenes in human skin cancers occuring on sun-exposed body sites. *Cancer Res.* **48**, 3341–3346.

ANDERSON, R.R. and PARRISH, J.A. (1981) The optics of skin. *J. Invest. Dermatol.* **77**, 13–19.

ANGEL, P. and KARIN, M. (1991) The role of jun, fos and the AP-1 complex in cell-proliferation and transformation. *Biochim. Biophys. Acta* **1072**, 129–157.

ANSEL, J.C., LUGER, T.A. and GREEN, I. (1983) The effect of *in vitro* UV irradiation on the production of ETAF activity by human and murine keratinocytes. *J. Invest. Dermatol.* **81**, 519–523.

AUBIN, F., and HUMBERT, P. (1998) Immunomodulation induced by psoralen plus ultraviolet A radiation. *Eur. J. Dermatol.* **8**, 212–213.

BACCICHETTI, F., BORDIN, F., CARLASSARE, F., RODIGHIERO, P., GUITTO, A., PERON, M., CAPOZZI, A. and DALL'ACQUA, F. (1981) 4'-Methylangelicin derivatives: A new group of highly photosensitizing monofunctional furocoumarins. *Il Farmaco, Ed. Sci.* **36**, 585–597.

BACCICHETTI, F., CARLASSARE, F., BORDIN, F., GUIOTTO, A., RODIGHIERO, P., TAMARO, M. and DALL'ACQUA, F. (1984) 4,4',6-Trimethylangelicin, a new very photoreactive and non skin-phototoxic monofunctional furocoumarin. *Photochem. Photobiol.* **39**, 525–529.

BADEN, H.P. and PATHAK, N.A. (1967) The metabolism and function of urocanic acid in skin. *J. Invest. Dermatol.* **48**, 11–17.

BADEN, H.P., PARRINGTON, J.M., DELHANTY, J.D.A. and PATHAK, M.A. (1972) DNA synthesis in normal and xeroderma pigmentosum fibroblasts following treatment with 8-methoxypsoralen and long wave ultraviolet light. *Biochim. Biophys. Acta* **262**, 247–255.

BAKER, A. and KANOFSKY, J. R. (1991) Direct observation of singlet oxygen phosporescence at 1270 nm from L1210 leukemia cells exposed to poly-porphyrin and light. *Arch. Biochem. Biophys.* **186**, 70–75.

BAKER, A. and KANOFSKY, J. R. (1993) Time-resolved studies of singlet-oxygen emission from L1210 leukemia cells labeled with 5-(N-hexadecanoyl) amino eosin: a comparison with a one-dimensional model of singlet-oxygen diffusion and quenching. *Photochem. Photobiol.* **57**, 720–727.

BASSET-SEGUIN, N., MOLES, J.P., MILS, V., DEREURE, O. and GUILHOU, J.J. (1994) *Tp53* tumor suppressor gene and skin carcinogenesis. *J. Invest. Dermatol.* **103**, 102S-106S

BEADLE, P.C. and BURTON, J.L. (1981) Absorption of ultraviolet radiation by skin surface lipid. *Br. J. Dermatol.* **104**, 549–551.

BEISSERT, S., RUHLEMANN, D., MOHAMMAD, T., GRABBE, S., EL-GHORR, A., NORVAL. M., MORRISON, H., GRANSTEIN, R.D., SCHWARZ, T. (2001) IL-12 prevents the inhibitory effects of *cis*-urocanic acid on tumor antigen presentation by Langerhans Cells: implications for photocarcinogenesis. *J. Immunol.*, **167**, 6232–6238.

BEER, J.Z., OLVEY, K.M., MILLER, S.A., THOMAS, D.P. and GODAR, D.E. (1993) Non-nuclear damage and cell lysis are induced by UVA, but not UVB or UVC, radiation in three strains of L5178Y cells. *Photochem. Photobiol.* **58**, 676–681.

BERGFELD, W.F. (1977) Histopathologic changes in skin after photo-chemotherapy. *Cutis* **20**, 504–507.

BEUKERS, R. and BERENDS, W. (1960) Isolation and identification of the irradiation product of thymine. *Biochim. Biophys. Acta* **41**, 550–551.

BISHOP, J.M. (1983) Cellular oncogenes and retroviruses. *Ann. Rev. Biochem.* **52**, 301–354.

BLACK, H.S. and MATHEWS-ROTH, M.M. (1991) Protective role of butyrated hydroxytoluene and certain carotenoides in photocarcinogenesis. *Photochem. Photobiol.* **53**, 707–716.

BLACKBURN, G.M. and TAUSSIG, P.E. (1975) The photocarcinogenicity of anthracene: Photochemical binding to deoxyribonucleic acid in tissue culture. *Biochem. J.* **149**, 289–291.

BLOG, F.B. and SZABO, G. (1979) The effects of psoralen and UVA (PUVA) on epidermal melanocytes of the tail in C57BL mice. *J. Invest. Dermatol.* **73**, 533–537.

BLUM, H.F. (1941) *Photodynamic Action and Diseases Caused by Light.* New York: Reinhold.

BOHR, V.A. and OKUMOTO, D.S. (1988) Analysis of pyrimidine dimers in defined genes. In FRIEDBURG, E.C. and HANAWALT, P.C. (eds) *DNA Repair,* Vol. 3, New York: Marcel Dekker, 347–366.

BORDIN, F., CARLASSARE, F., CONCONI, M.T., CAPOZZI, A., MAJONE, F., GUIOTTO, A., and BACCICHETTI, F. (1992) Biological properties of some benzopsoralen derivatives. *Photochem. Photobiol.* **55**, 221–229.

BOUSCAREL, B., NOONAN, F., CERYAK, S., GETTYS, T.W., PHILLIPS, T.M. and DEFABO, E.C. (1998) Regulation of stimulated cyclic AMP synthesis by urocanic acid. *Photochem. Photobiol.* **67**, 324–331.

BOYER, V., MOUSTACCHI, E. and SAGE, E. (1988) Sequence specificity in photoreactions of various psoralen derivatives with DNA: role in biological activity. *Biochemistry* **27**, 3011–3018.

BRASH, D.E., RUDOLPH, J.A., SIMON, J.A., LIN, A., MCKENNA, G.J., BADEN, H.P., HALPERIN, A.J. and PONTEN, J. (1991) A role for sunlight in skin cancer: UV-induced *p53* mutations in squamous cell carcinoma. *Proc. Natl. Acad. Sci. USA.* **88**, 10124–10128.

BREDBERG, A., LAMBERT, B., SWANBECK, G. and THYRESSON-HOK, M. (1977) The binding of 8-methoxypsoralen to nuclear DNA of UVA irradiated human fibroblasts *in vitro. Acta Derm. Venereol.* **57**, 389–391.

■ CHAPTER 53 ■

BRYCE, G.F. (1993) The effects of UV radiation on skin connective tissue. In FUCHS, J. and PACKER, L. (eds) *Oxidative Stress in Dermatology*, New York: Marcel Dekker, 105–125.

BURTON, G.W. and INGOLD, K.U. (1984) β-Carotene: An unusual type of lipid antioxidant. *Science* **224**, 569–573.

CADET, J. and TEOULE, R. (1978) Comparative study of oxidation of nucleic acid components by hydroxyl radicals, singlet oxygen and superoxide anion radicals. *Photochem. Photobiol.* **28**, 661–667.

CADET, J., BERGER, M., DOUKI, T., RAVANAT, J.-L. (1997) Oxidative damage to DNA: Formation, measurement and biological significance. *Rev. Physiol. Biochem. Pharmacol.* **131**, 1–26.

CAFFIERI, S., RUZZENE, M., GUERRA, B., FRANK, S., VEDALDI, D. and DALL'ACQUA, F. (1994) Psoralen-fatty acid cycloadducts activate protein kinase C (PKC) in human platelets. *J. Photochem. Photobiol.B* **22**, 253–256.

CAMPBELL, C., QUINN, A.G., ANGUS, B., FARR, P.M. and REES, J.L. (1993) Wavelength specific patterns of *p53* induction in human skin following exposure to UV radiation. *Cancer Res.* **53**, 2697–2699.

CASSATELLA, M.A., MEDA, L., BONORA, S., CESKA, M. and CONSTANTIN, G. (1993) Interleukin 10 (IL-10) inhibits the release of proinflammatory cytokines from human polymorphonuclear leukocytes. Evidence for an autocrine role of tumor necrosis factor and IL-1β in mediating the production of IL-8 triggered by lipopolysaccharide. *J. Exp. Med.* **178**, 2207–2211.

CEBULA, T.A., KOCH, W.H. and LAMPEL, K.A. (1989) Polymerase chain reaction (PCR) amplification of spontaneous and PUVA-induced mutations. *Photochem. Photobiol.* **49** (Suppl.):111s.

CEBULA, T.A. and KOCH, W.H. (1990) Analysis of spontaneous and psoralen-induced *Salmonella typhimurium hisG46* revertants by oligodeoxyribonu-cleotide colony hybridization: use of psoralens to cross-link probes to target sequences. *Mutat. Res.* **229**, 79–87.

CHILIN, A., MARZANO, C., GUIOTTO, A., MANZINI, P., BACCICHETTI, F., CARLASSARE, F., and BORDIN, F. (1999) Synthesis and biological activity of (hydroxymethyl)- and (diethylaminomethyl)benzopsoralens. *J. Med. Chem.* **42**, 2936–2945.

CLEAVER, J.E. and TROSKO, J.E. (1970) Absence of excision of ultraviolet-induced cyclobutane dimers in xeroderma pigmentosum. *Photochem. Photobiol.* **11**, 547–550.

CLOUD, T.M., HAKIM, R. and GRIFFIN, A.C. (1960) Photosensitization of the eye with methoxsalen. I. Chronic effects. *Arch. Ophthalmol.* **64**, 346–351.

COHEN, D. and DELEO, V.A. (1993) Ultraviolet radiation-induced phospholipase A$_2$ activation occurs in mammalian cell membrane preparations. *Photochem. Photobiol.* **57**, 383–390.

CONCONI, M.T., VALENTI, F., MONTESI, F., BASSANI, V., DE ANGELI, S., and PARNIGOTTO, P.P. (1996) Effects of benzopsoralen derivatives on HL60 and HeLa cells. *Pharmacol. Toxicol.* **79**, 340–346.

COPELAND, E.S., ALVING, C.R. and GRENAN, M.M. (1976) Light-induced leakage of spin label marker from liposomes in the presence of phototoxic phenothiazines. *Photochem. Photobiol.* **24**, 41–48.

CORK, M.J., MEE, J.B. and DUFF, G.W. (1993) Cytokines. In PRIESTLEY, G.C. (ed.) *Molecular Aspects of Dermatology*, New York: John Wiley & Sons, 129–146.

CORNELIUS, L.A., SEPP, N. LI, L-J., DEGITZ, K., SWERLICK, R.A., LAWLEY, T.J. and CAUGHMAN, S.W. (1994) Selective upregulation of intercellular adhesion molecule (ICAM-1) by ultraviolet B in human dermal microvascular endothelial cells. *J. Invest. Dermatol.* **103**, 23–28.

DALL'ACQUA, F. (1977) New chemical aspects of the photreaction between psoralen and DNA. In CASTELLANI, A. (ed.) *Research in Photobiology*, New York: Plenum Press, 245–255.

DALL'ACQUA, F. (1989) New psoralens and analogs. In FITZPATRICK, T.B., FORLOT, P., PATHAK, M.A. and URBACH, M.A. (eds) *PSORALENS Past, Present and Future of Photochemoprotection and other biological activities*, Paris: John Libbey Eurotex, 237–250.

DALL'ACQUA, F. and MARTELLI P. (1991) Photosensitizing action of furocoumarins on membrane components and consequent intracellular events. *J. Photochem. Photobiol.B.* **8**, 235–254.

DALL'ACQUA, F., VEDALDI, D., CAFFIERI, S., GUIOTTO, A., RODIGHIERO, P., BACCICHETTI, F., CARLASSARE, F. and BORDIN, F. (1981) New monofunctional reagents for DNA as possible agents for the photchemotherapy of psoriasis: Derivatives of 4,5'-dimethylangelicin. *J. Med. Chem.* **24**, 178–184.

DALLA VIA, L., GIA, O., MARCIANI MAGNO, S., SANTANA, L., TEIJEIRA, M., and URIARTE, E. (1999) New tetracyclic analogues of photochemotherapeutic drugs 5-MOP and 8-MOP; synthesis, DNA interaction, and antiproliferative activity. *J. Med. Chem.* **42**, 4405–4413.

D'AMBROSIO, S.M., WHETSTONE, J.W., SLAZINSKI, L. and LOWNEY, E. (1981) Photorepair of pyrimidine dimers in human skin *in vivo*. *Photochem. Photobiol.* **34**, 461–464.

D'ANDREA, A., ASTE-AMEZAGA, M., VALIANTE, N.M., MA, X., KUBIN, M. and TRINCHIERI, G. (1993) Interleukin 10 (IL-10) inhibits human lymphocyte interferon-α production by suppressing natural killer cell stimulatory factor/IL-12 synthesis in accessory cells. *J. Exp. Med.* **178**, 1041–1048.

DANIELS, F., JR., BROPHY, D. and LOBITZ, W.C., JR. (1961) Histochemical responses of human skin following ultraviolet irradiation. *J. Invest. Dermatol.* **37**, 351–357.

DANNO, K. and HORIO, T. (1980) Histochemical staining of cells for sulphhydryl and disulphide groups: A time course study. *Br. J. Dermatol.* **102**, 535–539.

DANNO, K. and HORIO, T. (1982) Formation of UV-induced apoptosis relates to the cell cycle. *Br. J. Dermatol.* **107**, 423–428.

DAYA, N., STARY, A., SOUSSI, T., DAYA-GROSJEAN, L. and SARASIN, A. (1994) Can we predict solar ultraviolet radiation as the causal event in human tumors by analyzing the mutation spectra of the *p53* gene? *Mutat. Res.* **307**, 375–386.

DAYA-GROSJEAN, L., ROBERT, C., DROUGARD, C., SUAREZ, H. and SARASIN, A. (1993) High mutation frequency in ras genes of skin tumors. *Cancer Res.* **53**, 1625–1629.

DEFABO, E.C. and NOONAN, F.P. (1983) Mechanism of immune suppression by ultraviolet radiation *in vivo*. I. Evidence for the existence of a unique photoreceptor in skin and its role in photoimmunology. *J. Exp. Med.* **158**, 84–98.

DEFABO, E.C., NOONAN, F.P. and KRIPKE, M.L. (1981) An *in vivo* action spectrum for ultraviolet radiation-induced suppression of contact sensitivity in BALB/c mice. *9th Annu. Meet. Am. Soc. Photobiol. Program Abstr.* 185.

DE MOL, N.J. and BEIJERSBERGEN VAN HENEGOUWEN, G.M.J. (1981) Relation between some photobiological properties of furocoumarins and their extent of singlet oxygen production. *Photochem. Photobiol.* **33**, 815–819.

DEVARY, Y., GOTTLIEB, R.A., LAU, L.F. and KARIN, M. (1991) Rapid and preferential activation of the c-jun gene during the mammalian UV response. *Mol. Cell. Biol.* **11**, 2804–2811.

DEVARY, Y., GOTTLIEB, R.A., SMEAL, T. and KARIN, M. (1992) The mammalian ultraviolet response is triggered by activation of src tyrosine kinases. *Cell* **71**, 1081–1091.

DI GIOVINE, F.S. and DUFF, G.W. (1990) Interleukin 1, the first interleukin. *Immunol. Today* **11**, 13–21.

DOUGHERTY, T.J. (1987) Photosensitizers: therapy and detection of malignant tumors. *Photochem. Photobiol.* **45**, 879–890.

DROBETSKY, E.A., GROSOVSKY, A.J., SKANDALIS, A. and GLICKMAN, B.W. (1989) Perspectives on UV light mutagenesis: investigation of the CHO aprt gene carried on a retroviral shuttle vector. *Somat. Cell Mol. Genet.* **16**, 401–408.

DUMAZ, N., DROUGARD, C., SARASIN, A. and DAYA-GROSIEAN, L. (1993) Specific UV-induced mutation spectrum in the *p53* gene of skin tumors from DNA-repair-deficient xeroderma pigmentosum patients. *Proc. Natl. Acad. Sci. USA.* **90**, 10529–10533.

DUMAZ. N., STARY, A., SOUSSI, T., DAYA-GROSIEAN, L. and SARASIN, A. (1994) Can we predict solar ultraviolet radiation as the causal event in human tumors by analyzing the mutation spectra of eh *p53* gene? *Mutation Res.* **307**, 375–386.

EDELSON, R.L. (1988) Light-activated drugs. *Sci. Am.* **Aug**, 68–75.

EDELSON, L.E. and FINK, J.M. (1985) The immunologic function of skin. *Sci. Am.* **June**, 46–53.

EDELSON, R.L. and 19 OTHER PARTICIPATING INVESTIGATORS. (1987) Treatment of cutaneous T-cell lymphoma by extracorporeal phototherapy. *N. Engl. J. Med.* **316**, 297–303.

ENK, A.H., ANGELONI, V.L., UDEY, M.C. and KATZ, S.I. (1993) Inhibition of Langerhans cell antigen-presenting function by IL-10. *J. Immunol.* **151**, 2390–2398.

EVERETT, M.A., YEARGERS, E., SAYRE, R.M. and OLSON, R.L. (1966) Penetration of epidermis by ultraviolet rays. *Photochem. Photobiol.* **5**, 533–542.

FISHER, G.J., VARGHESE, A.J. and JOHN, H.E. (1974) Ultraviolet induced reactions of thymine and uracil in the presence of cysteine. *Photochem. Photobiol.* **20**, 109–120.

FITZPATRICK, T.B., PATHAK, M.A., HARBER, L.C., SEIJI, M. and KUKITA, A. (1974) An introduction to the problem of normal and abnormal responses of man's skin to solar radiation. In PATHAK, M.A., HARBER, L.C., SEIJI, M. and KUKITA, A. (eds) *Sunlight and Man,* Tokyo: University of Tokyo Press, 3–14.

FLOYD, R.A., WATSON, J.J., WONG, P.K., ALTMILLER, D.H. and RICHARD, R. C. (1986) Hydroxyl free radical adduct of deoxyguanosine: sensitive detection and mechanism of formation. *Free Rad. Res. Commun.* **1**, 163–172.

FLOYD, R.A., WEST, M.S., ENEFF, K.L. and SCHNEIDER, J.E. (1989) Methylene blue plus light mediates 8-hydroxyguanine formation in DNA. *Arch. Biochem. Biophys.* **273**, 106–111.

FLOYD, R.A., WEST, M.S., SCHNEIDER, J.E., WATSON, J.J. and MAIDT, M. L. (1990) Hematoporphryin D plus light mediates 8-hydroxyguanosine formation in DNA and RNA. *Free Radic. Biol. Med.* **9**, **76** (Abstract).

FORNACE, A.J. and KOHN, K.W. (1976) DNA-protein cross-linking by ultraviolet radiation in normal human and xeroderma pigmentosum fibroblasts. *Biochim. Biophys. Acta* **435**, 95–103.

FORNACE, A.J., JR., ALAMO, I. and HOLLANDER, M.C. (1988a) DNA damage induction transcripts in mammalian cells. *Proc. Natl. Acad. Sci. USA* **85**, 8800–8804.

FORNACE, A.J.. JR., SCHALCH, H. and ALAMO, I., JR. (1988b) Coordinate induction of metallothioneins I and II in rodent cells by UV irradiation. *Mol. Cell. Biol.* **8**, 4716–4720.

FRANKLIN, W.A. and HASELTINE, W.A. (1986) The role of the (6–4) photoproduct in ultraviolet light-induced transition mutations in *E. coli*. *Mutat. Res.* **165**, 1–7.

FRANKLIN, W.A., MING LO, K. and HASELTINE, W.A. (1982) Alkaline lability of fluorescent photoproducts produced in ultraviolet light-irradiated DNA. *J. Biol. Chem.* **257**, 13535–13543.

FREEMAN, S.E., BLACKETT, A.D., MONTELEONE, D.C., SETLOW, R.B., SUTHERLAND, B.M. and SUTHERLAND J.C. (1986) Quantitation of radiation-, chemical-, or enzyme-induced single strand breaks in nonradioactive DNA by alkaline gel electrophoresis: application to pyrimidine dimers. *Anal. Biochem.* **158**, 119–129.

FREEMAN, S.E., GANGE, R.W., SUTHERLAND, J.C., MATZINGER, E.A. and SUTHERLAND, B.M. (1987a) Production of pyrimidine dimers in DNA of human skin exposed *in situ* to UVA radiation. *J. Invest. Dermatol.* **88**, 430–433.

FREEMAN, S.E., GANGE, R.W., SUTHERLAND J.C. and SUTHERLAND, B.M. (1987b) Pyrimidine dimer formation in human skin. *Photochem. Photobiol.* **46**, 207–212.

FRIEDBURG, E.C. (1988) Deoxyribonucleic acid repair in the yeast *Saccharomyces cerevisiae*. *Microbiol. Brief Rev.* **52**, 70–102.

FRIEDMAN, P.S. and ROGERS, S. (1980) Photochemotherapy of psoriasis: DNA damage in lymphocytes. *J. Invest. Dermatol.* **74**, 440–443.

GAHRING, L., MARILYN, B., PEPYS, M.B. and DAYNES, R. (1984) Effect of ultraviolet radiation on production of epidermal cell thymocyte-activating factor/ interleukin 1 *in vivo* and *in vitro*. *Proc. Natl. Acad. Sci.* **81**, 1198–1202.

GAHRING, L.C., BUCKLEY, A. and DAYNES, R.A. (1985) Presence of epidermal-derived thymocyte activating factor/interleukin 1 in normal human stratum corneum. *J. Clin. Invest.* **76**, 1585–1591.

GERRIT VAN DER SCHROEFF, J., EVERS, L.M., BOOT, J.M. and BOS, J.L. (1990) Ras oncogene mutations in basal cell carcinomas and squamous cell carcinomas of human skin. *J. Invest. Dermatol.* **94**, 423–425.

GILCHREST, B., PARRISH, J.A., TANNENBAUM, L., HAYNES, H. and FITZPATRICK, T.B. (1976) Oral methoxsalen photochemotherapy of mycosis fungoides. *Cancer (Philadelphia)* **38**, 683–689.

GILCHREST, B.A., SORTER, N.A., STOFF, J.S. and MIHM, M.A. (1981) The human sunburn reaction: Histologic and biochemical studies. *J. Am. Acad. Dermatol.* **5**, 411–422.

GILES, A., JR., WAMER, W. and KORNHAUSER, A. (1985) The *in vivo* protective effect of β-carotene against psoralen phototoxicity. *Photochem. Photobiol.* **41**, 661–666.

GILLARDON, F., ESCHENFELDER, C., UHLMANN, E., HARTSHUH, W. and ZIMMERMANN, M. (1994) Differential regulation of c-fos, fosB, c-jun, junB, bcl-2 and bax expression in rat skin following single or chronic ultraviolet irradiation and *in vivo* modulation by antisense oligodeoxynucleotide superfusion. *Oncongene* **9**, 3219–3226.

GODAR, D.E., THOMAS, D.P., MILLER, S.A. and LEE W. (1993) Long-wavelength UVA radiation induces oxidative stress, cytoskeletal damage and hemolysis. *Photochem. Photobiol.* **57**, 1018–1026.

GOLDSTEIN, B.D. and HARBER, L.C. (1972) Erythropoietic protoporphyria: Lipid oxidation and red cell membrane damage associated with photochemolysis. *J. Clin. Invest.* **51**, 892–902.

GOLDYNE, M.E. (1975) Prostaglandins and cutaneous inflammation. *J. Invest. Dermatol.* **64**, 377–385.

GORDON, P.R. and GILCHREST, B.A. (1989) Human melanogenesis is stimulated by diacylglycerol (DAG). *J. Invest. Dermatol.* **93**, 700–702.

GREAVES, M.W. (1978) Does ultraviolet-evoked prostaglandin formation protect skin from actinic cancer? *Lancet* **i**:189.

GREWE, M., TREFZER, U., BALLHORN, A., GYUFKO, K., HENNINGER, H. and KRUTMANN, J. (1993) Analysis of the mechanism of ultraviolet (UV) B radiation-induced prostaglandin E2 synthesis by human epidermoid carcinoma cells. *J. Invest. Dermatol.* **101**, 528–531.

GRUENER, N. and LOCKWOOD, M.P. (1979) Photodynamic mutagenicity in mammalian cells, *Biochem. Biophys. Res. Commun.* **90**, 460–465.

GRUPPER, C. and BERRETTI, B. (1981) 5-MOP in PUVA and RE-PUVA-a mono-centric study: 250 patients with a follow-up of three years. Presented at the 3rd International Symposium on Psorasis, Stanford, Calif.

GUTTER, B., SPECK, W.T. and ROSENKRANZ, H.S. (1977) A study of the photo-induced mutagenicity of methylene blue. *Mutat. Res.* **44**, 177–182.

HARBER, L.C. (1969) Use of guinea-pigs in photobiologic studies. In URBACH, F. (ed.) *The Biologic Effects of Ultraviolet Radiation,* New York: Pergamon Press, 291–295.

HARRIS, C.C. and HOLLSTEIN, M. (1993) Clinical implications of the *p53* tumor-suppressor gene. *N. Engl. J. Med.* **329**, 1318–1327.

HART, R.W., SETLOW, R.B. and WOODHEAD, A.D. (1977) Evidence that pyrimidine dimers in DNA can give rise to tumors. *Proc. Natl. Acad. Sci. USA* **74**, 5574–5578.

HASS, B.S. and WEBB, R.B. (1981) Photodynamic effects of dyes on bacteria. *Mutat. Res.* **81**, 277–285.

HATTORI-NAKAKUKI, Y., NISHIGORI, C., OKAMOTO, K., IMAMURA, S., HIAI, H. and TOYOKUNI, S. (1994) Formation of 8-hydroxy-2'-deoxyguanosine in epidermis of hairless mice exposed to near-UV. *Biochem. Biophys. Res. Commun.* **201**, 1132–1139.

HEALY, E., REYNOLDS, N.J., SMITH, M.D., CAMPBELL, C., FARR, P.M. and REES, J.L. (1994) Dissociation of erythema and *p53* protein expression in human skin following UVB irradiation, and induction of *p53* protein and mRNA following application of skin irritants. *J. Invest. Dermatol.* **103**, 493–499.

HOLBROOK, H.J. and FORNACE, A.J., JR. (1991) Response to adversity: Molecular control of gene activation following genotoxic stress. *New Biol.* **3**, 825–833.

HÖNIGSMANN, H., JASCHKE, E., GSCHNAIT, W.B., FRITSCH, P. and WOLFF, K. (1979) 5-Methoxypsoralen (Bergapten) in photochemotherapy of psorasis. *Br. J. Dermatol.* **101**, 369–378.

HÖNIGSMANN, H., WOLFF, K., GSCHNAIT, F., BRENNER, W. and JASCHKE, E. (1980) Keratoses and nonmelanoma skin tumors in long-term photochemotherapy (PUVA). *J. Am. Acad. Dermatol.* **3**, 406–414.

HRUZA, L.L. and PENTLAND, A.P. (1993) Mechanisms of UV-induced inflammation. *J. Invest. Dermatol.* **100**, 35s-41s.

HUSAIN, Z., YANG, Q. and BISWAS, D.K. (1990) cHa-ras proto-oncogene: amplification and overexpression in UV-B-induced mouse skin papillomas and carcinomas. *Arch. Dermatol.* **126**, 324–330.

HUTCHINSON, F. and WOOD, R.D. (1988) Determination of sequence changes induced by mutagenesis of the cI gene of lambda phage. In FRIEDBURG, E.C. and HANAWALT, P.C. (eds) *DNA Repair*, Vol. 3, New York: Marcel Dekker, 219–233.

HYNEK, J.A. (1951) *Astrophysics; a topical symposium commemorating the fiftieth anniversary of the Yerkes Observatory and a half century of progress in astrophysics.* 1st Ed. New York: McGraw-Hill.

IRWIN, C., BARNES, A., VERES, D. and KAIDBEY, K. (1993) An ultraviolet radiation action spectrum for immediate pigment darkening. *Photochem. Photobiol.* **57**, 504–507.

ITO, T. (1978) Cellular and subcellular mechanisms of photodynamic action: The $^1O_2$ hypothesis as a driving force in recent research. *Photochem. Photobiol.* **28**, 493–508.

ITO, T. and KOBAYASHI, K. (1977) A survey of *in vivo* photodynamic activity of xanthenes, thiazines, and acridine in yeast cells. *Photochem. Photobiol.* **26**, 581–587.

JORI, G. and SPIKES, J.D. (1981) Photosensitized oxidations in complex biological structures. In RODGERS, M.A.J. and POWERS, E.L. (eds) *Oxygen and Oxy-Radicals in Chemistry and Biology*, New York: Academic Press, 441–457.

JEFFREY, A.M., SHAO, L., BRENDLER-SCHWAAB, S.V., SCHLUTER, G., and WILLIAMS, G.M. (2000) Photochemical mutagenicity of phototoxic and photochemically carcinogenic fluoroquinolones in comparison with the photostable moxifloxacin. *Arch. Toxicol.* **74**, 555–559.

KANG, K., HAMMERBERG, C., MEUNIER, L. and COOPER K.D. (1994) CD11b⁺ macrophages that infiltrate human epidermis after *in vivo* ultraviolet exposure potently produce IL-10 and represent the major secretory source of epidermal IL-10 protein. *J. Immunol.* **153**, 5256–5264.

KANG-ROTONDO, C.H., MILLER, C.C., MORRISON, A.R. and PENTLAND, A.P. (1993) Enhanced keratinocyte prostaglandin synthesis after UV injury is due to increased phospholipase activity. *Am. J. Physiol.* **264**, C396-C401.

KANJILAL, S., PEIRCEALL, W. E. and ANANTHASWAMY, H. N. (1993) Ultraviolet radiation in the pathogenesis of skin cancers: Involvement of ras and *p53* genes. *Cancer Bull.* **45**, 205–211.

KANTOR, G.J., SUTHERLAND, J.C. and SETLOW, R.B. (1980) Action spectra for killing non-dividing normal human and xeroderma pigmentosum cells. *Photochem. Photobiol.* **31**, 459–464.

KASTAN, M.B., ONYEKWERE, O., SIDRANSKY, D., VOGELSTEIN, B. and CRAIG, R.W. (1991) Participation of *p53* protein in the cellular response to DNA damage. *Cancer Res.* **51**, 6304–6311.

KASTAN, M.B., ZHAN, Q., EL-DEIRY, W.S., CARRIER, F., JACKS, T., WALSH, W.V., PLUNKETT, B.S., VOGELSTEIN, B. and FORNACE. A.J., JR. (1992) A mammalian cell cycle checkpoint pathway utilizing *p53* and *GADD45* is defective in Ataxia-Telangiectasia. *Cell* **71**, 587–597.

KESSEL, D. (1977) Effects of photoactivated porphyrins at the cell surface of leukemia L1210 cells. *Biochemistry* 16, 3443–3449.

KEYSE, S.M. and TYRRELL, R.M. (1989) Heme oxygenase is the major 32-kDa stress protein induced in human skin fibroblasts by UVA radiation, hydrogen peroxide, and sodium arsenite. *Proc. Natl. Acad. Sci. USA* **86**, 99–103.

KHALIL, Z., TOWNLEY, S.L., GRIMBALDESTON, M.A., FINLAY-JONES, J.J. and HART, P.H. (2001) cis-Urocanic acid stimulates neuropeptide release from peripheral sensory nerves. *J. Invest. Dermatol.* **117**, 886–891.

KHOSRAVI-FAR, R. and DER, C.J. (1994) The ras signal transduction pathway. *Cancer and Metathesis. Rev.* **13**, 67–89.

KLIGMAN, L.H. and GEBRE, M. (1991) Biochemical changes in hairless mouse skin collagen after chronic exposure to ultraviolet-A radiation. *Photochem. Photobiol.* **54**, 233–237.

KOBAYASHI, K. and ITO, T. (1976) Further *in vivo* studies on the participation of singlet oxygen in the photodynamic inactivation and induction of genetic changes in *Saccharomyces cerevisiae*. *Photochem. Photobiol.* **23**, 21–28.

KOCHEVAR, I. (1981) Phototoxicity mechanisms: Chlorpromazine photo-sensitized damage to DNA and cell membranes. *J. Invest. Dermatol.* **77**, 59–64.

KÖCK, A., SCHWARZ, T., KIRNBAUER, R., URBANSKI, A., PERRY, P., ANSEL, J.C. and LUGER T.A. (1990) Human keratinocytes are a source for tumor necrosis factor α: Evidence for synthesis and release upon stimulation with endotoxin or ultraviolet light. *J. Exp. Med.* **172**, 1609–1614.

KORNHAUSER, A. (1976) UV-induced DNA-protein cross-links *in vivo* and *in vitro*. *Photochem. Photobiol.* **23**, 457–460.

KORNHAUSER, A. and PATHAK, M.A. (1972) Studies on the mechanism of the photosensitized dimerization of pyrimidines. *Z. Naturforsch. Teil B* **27**, 550–553.

KORNHAUSER, A. BURNETT, J.B. and SZABO, G. (1974) Isotope effects in the photosensitized dimerization of pyrimidines. *Croat. Chem. Acta* **46**, 193–197.

KORNHAUSER, A., PATHAK, M.A., ZIMMERMANN, E. and SZABO, G. (1976a) The *in vivo* effect of ultraviolet irradiation (290–350 nm) on epidermal chromatin. *Croat. Chem. Acta* **48**, 385–390.

KORNHAUSER, A., GARCIA, R.I., SZABO, G., STANFORD, D. and KRINSKY, N.I. (1976b) Possible role of singlet oxygen in melanin biosynthesis. *Fourth Annual Meeting Am. Soc. Photobiology.* Denver, CO.

KORNHAUSER, A., WAMER, W.G. and GILES, A.L., JR. (1982) Psoralen phototoxicity: correlation with serum and epidermal 8-methoxypsoralen and 5-methoxypsoralen in the guinea pig. *Science* **217**, 733–735.

KORNHAUSER, A., WAMER, W.G., LAMBERT, L.A. and KOCH, W.H. (1989) Are activated oxygen species involved in PUVA-induced biological effects *in vivo*? In FITZPATRICK, T.B., FORLOT, P., PATHAK, M.A. and URBACH, F. (eds) *Psoralens: Past, Present and Future of Photochemoprotection and Other Biological Activities*, Paris: John Libbey Eurotex, 251–260.

KRESS, S., SUTTER, C., STRICKLAND, P.T., MUKHTAR, H., SCHWEIZER, J. and SCHWARZ, M. (1992) Carcinogen-specific mutational pattern in the *p53* gene in ultraviolet B radiation-induced squamous cell carcinomas of mouse skin. *Cancer Res.* **52**, 6400–6403.

KRINSKY, N.I. and DENEKE, S.M. (1982) Interaction of oxygen and oxy-radicals with carotenoids. *J. Natl. Cancer Inst.* **69**, 205–210.

KRIPKE, M.L. (1980) Immunologic effects of UV radiation and their role in photocarcinogenesis. *Photochem. Photobiol. Rev.* **5**, 257–292.

KRIPKE, M.L. (1986) Photoimmunology: The first decade. *Curr. Prob. Dermatol.* **15**, 164–175.

KRIPKE, M.L. and YAROSH, D.B. (1994) DNA is a photoreceptor for UVR-induced immunologic changes. *Photochem. Photobiol.* **59**, 38s

KRIPKE, M.L., COCK, P.A., ALAS, L.G. and YAROSH, D.B. (1992) Pyrimidine dimers in DNA initiate systemic immunosuppression in UV-irradiated mice. *Proc. Natl. Acad. Sci. USA.* **89**, 7516–7520.

■ CHAPTER 53 ■

KRUTMANN, J., KÖCK, A., SCHAUER, E., PARLOW, F., MÖLLER, A., KAPP, A., FÖRSTER, E., SCHÖPF, E. and LUGER T.A. (1990) Tumor necrosis factor β and ultraviolet radiation are potent regulators of human keratinocyte ICAM-1 expression. *J. Invest. Dermatol.* **95**, 127–131.

KUERBITZ, S.J., PLUNKETT, B.S., WALSH, W.V. and KASTAN, M. B. (1992) Wild-type *p53* is a cell cycle checkpoint determinant following irradiation. *Proc. Natl. Acad. Sci. USA* **89**, 7491–7495.

KUNZ, L. and STARK, G. (1997) Photodynamic membrane damage at the level of single ion channels. *Biochim. Biophys. Acta* **1327**, 1–4.

LAMOLA, A.A. (1968) Excited state precursors of thymine photodimers. *Photochem. Photobiol.* **7**, 619–632.

LAMOLA, A.A. and DOLEIDEN, F.H. (1980) Cross linking of membrane proteins and protoporphyrin-sensitized photohemolysis. *Photochem. Photobiol.* **31**, 597–601.

LAMOLA, A.A., YAMANE, T. and TROZZALO, A.M. (1973) Cholesterol hydro-peroxide formation in red cell membranes and photochemolysis in erythropoietic protoporphyria. *Science* **179**, 1131–1133.

LASKIN, J.D., LEE, E., YURKOW, E.J., LASKIN, D.L. and GALLO, M. A. (1985) A possible mechanism of psoralen phototoxicity not involving direct interacton with DNA. *Proc. Natl. Acad. Sci. USA* **82**, 6158–6162.

LASKIN, J.D., LEE, E., LASKIN, D.L. and GALLO, M.A. (1986) Psoralens potentiate ultraviolet light-induced inhibition of epidermal growth factor binding. *Proc. Natl. Acad. Sci. USA* **83**, 8211–8215.

LEVINE, D.P., MOMAND, J. and FINLAY, C.A. (1991) The *p53* tumour suppressor gene. *Nature* **351**, 453–456.

MAIBACH, H.I. and KLIGMAN, A.M. (1960) Dihydroxyacetone: A suntan-stimulating agent. *Arch. Dermatol.* **82**, 505–507.

MANDULA, B.B., PATHAK, M.A. and DUDEK, G. (1976) Photochemotherapy: Identification of a metabolite of 4,5',8-trimethylpsoralen. *Science* **193**, 1131–1134.

MATSUI, M.S. and DeLEO, V.A. (1990) Induction of protein kinase C activity by ultraviolet radiation. *Carcinogenesis* **11**, 229–234.

MILLER, C.C., HALE, P. and PENTLAND, A.P. (1994) Ultraviolet B injury increases prostaglandin synthesis through a tyrosine kinase-dependent pathway. *J. Biol. Chem.* **269**, 3529–3533.

MITCHELL, D.L. and CLARKSON, J.M. (1981) The development of a radio-immunoassay for the detection of photoproducts in mammalian cell DNA. *Biochim. Biophys. Acta* **655**, 40–54.

MITCHELL, D.L. and NAIRN, R.S. (1989) The biology of the (6–4) photoproduct. *Photochem. Photobiol.* **49**, 805–820.

MOAN, J. and CHRISTENSEN, T. (1981) Photodynamic effects on human cells exposed to light in the presence of hematoporphyrin. Localization of the active dye. *Cancer Lett.* **11**, 209–214.

MOAN, J., PETTERSEN, E.O. and CHRISTENSEN, T. (1979) The mechanism of photodynamic inactivation of human cells *in vitro* in the presence of hematoporphyrin. *Br. J. Cancer* **39**, 398–407.

MOODYCLIFFE, A., NGHIEM, D., CLYDESDALE, G. and ULLRICH, S.E. (2000) Immune supression and skin cancer development: regulation by NKT cells. *Nat. Immunol.* **1**, 521–525.

MORISON, W.L. (1989) Effects of ultraviolet radiation on the immune system in humans. *Photochem. Photobiol.* **50**, 515–524.

MORISON, W.L., PAUL, B.S. and PARRISH, J.A. (1977) The effects of indomethacin on long-wave ultraviolet-induced delayed erythema. *J. Invest. Dermatol.* **68**, 120–133.

MORISON, W.L., PARRISH, J.A., BLOCK, K.J. and KRUGLER, J.I. (1979) Transient impairment of peripheral blood lymphocyte function during PUVA therapy. *Br. J. Dermatol.* **101**, 391–397.

MOSMANN, T.R. (1991) Regulation of immune responses by T cells with different cytokine secretion phenotypes: role of a new cytokine, cytokine synthesis inhibitory factor (IL10). *Int. Arch. Allergy Appl. Immunol.* **94**, 110–115.

MUKAI, F. and GOLDSTEIN, B. (1976) Mutagenicity of malonaldehyde, a decomposition product of peroxidized polyunsaturated fatty acids. *Science* **191**, 868–869.

NATARAJAN, A.T., VERDEGAAL-IMMERZEEL, E.A.M., ELLY, A.M., ASHWOOD-SMITH, M.J. and POULTON, G.A. (1981) Chromosomal damage induced by furocoumarins and UVA in hamster and human cells including cells from patients with ataxia telangiectasia and xeroderma pigmentosum. *Mutat. Res.* **84**, 113–124.

NATIONAL INSTITUTES OF HEALTH CONSENSUS DEVELOPMENT CONFERENCE STATEMENT (1989) *Sunlight, Ultraviolet Radiation, and the Skin.* Volume 7, Number 8, May 8–10.

■ CHAPTER 53 ■

NIEDRE, M., PATTERSON, M. S., and WILSON, B. C. (2002) Direct near-infrared luminescence detection of singlet oxygen generated by photodynamic therapy in cells *in vitro* and tissues *in vivo*. *Photochem. Photobiol.* **75**, 382–391.

NOONAN, F.P. and DEFABO, E.C. (1992) Immunosuppression by ultraviolet B radiation: Initiation by urocanic acid. *Immunol. Today* **13**, 250–254.

NOONAN, F.P. and HOFFMAN, H.A. (1994) Susceptibility to immunosuppression by ultraviolet B radiation in the mouse. *Immunogenetics* **39**, 29–39.

NOONAN, F.P., DEFABO, E.C. and MORRISON, H. (1988) *Cis* urocanic acid, a product formed by ultraviolet-B irradiation of the skin, initiates an antigen presentation defect in splenic dendritic cells *in vivo. J. Invest. Dermatol.* **90**, 92–99

NOONAN, F.P., RECIO, J.A., TAKAYAMA, H., DURAY, P., ANVER, M.R., RUSH, W.L., DEFABO, E.C. and MERLINO, G. (2001) Neonatal sunburn and melanoma in mice. *Nature* **413**, 271–272.

NORRIS, D.A., LYONS, B.M., MIDDLETON, M.H., YOHN, J.J. and KASHIHARA-SAWAMI, M. (1990) Ultraviolet radiation can either suppress or induce expression of intercellular adhesion molecule 1 (ICAM-1) on the surface of cultured human keratinocytes. *J. Invest. Dermatol.* **95**, 132–138.

OGURA, R. and SUGIYAMA, M. (1993) Reactive oxidants in skin: UV-induced lipid peroxidation. In FUCHS, J. and PACKER, L. (eds) *Oxidative Stress in Dermatology*, New York: Marcel Dekker, 49–68.

OLIVEN, A., and SHECHTER, Y. (2001) Extracorporeal photophoresis: a review. *Blood Rev.* **15**, 103–108.

OLSON, R.L., GAYLOR, J. and EVERETT, M.A. (1974) Ultraviolet-induced individual cell keratinization. *J. Cutan. Pathol.* **1**, 120, 125.

PAARDEKOOPER, M., DE BRUIJNE, A.W., VAN STEVENINCK, J., and VAN DEN BROEK, P.J. (1993) Inhibition of transport systems in yeast by photodynamic treatment with toluidine blue. *Biochim. Biophys. Acta* **1151**, 143–148.

PAARDEKOOPER, M., DE BRUIJNE, A. W., VAN GOMPEL, A. E., VERHAGE, R. A., AVERBECK, D., DUBBELMAN, T. M., and VAN DEN BROEK, P. J. (1997) Single strand breaks and mutagenesis in yeast induced by photodynamic treatment with chloroaluminum. *J. Photochem. Photobiol. B.* **40**, 132–140.

PALASZYNSKI, E.W., NOONAN, F.P. and DEFABO, E.C. (1992) *Cis* urocanic acid down-regulates the induction of adenosine 3', 5'-cyclicmonophosphate by either *trans*-urocanic acid or histamine in human dermal fibroblasts *in vitro*.

Photochem. Photobiol. **55**, 165–171.

PARRISH, J.A. and JAENICKE, K.F. (1981) Action spectrum for phototherapy of psoriasis. *J. Invest. Dermatol.* **76**, 359–362.

PARRISH, J.A., FITZPATRICK, T.B., TANNENBAUM, L. and PATHAK, M.A. (1974) Photochemotherapy of psoriasis with oral methoxsalen and long-wave ultraviolet light. *N. Engl. J. Med.* **291**, 1207–1222.

PARRISH, J.A., WHITE, H.A.D. and PATHAK, M.A. (1979) Photomedicine. In FITZPATRICK, T.B. EISEN, A.Z. WOLFF, K. FREEDBERG, I.M. and AUSTEN, K.F. (eds) *Dermatology in General Medicine,* New York: McGraw-Hill, 942–994.

PATHAK, M.A. (1967) Photobiology of melanogenesis: Biophysical aspects. In MONTAGNA, W. and HU, F. (eds) *Advances in Biology of Skin,* vol 8, *The Pigmentary System,* New York: Pergamon Press, 400–419.

PATHAK, M.A. (1982) Molecular aspects of drug photosensitivity with special emphasis on psoralen photosensitization reaction. *J. Natl. Cancer Inst.* **69**, 163–170.

PATHAK, M.A. and JOSHI, P.C. (1984) Production of active oxygen species ($^1O_2$ and O^-_2) by psoralens and ultraviolet radiation (320–400 nm). *Biochim. Biophys. Acta* **798**, 115–126.

PATHAK, M.A., WORDEN, L.R. and KAUFMAN, K.D. (1967) Effect of structural alterations on the potency of furocoumarins (psoralens) and related compounds. *J. Invest. Dermatol.* **48**, 103–118.

PATHAK, M.A. and STRATTON, K. (1968) Free radicals in the human skin before and after exposure to light. *Arch. Biochem. Biophys.* **123**, 468–476.

PATHAK, M.A. and KRAMER, D.M. (1969) Photosensitization of skin *in vivo* by furocoumarins (psoralens). *Biochim. Biophys. Acta* **195**, 197–206.

PATHAK, M.A., KRAMER, D.M. and GUNGERICH, U. (1972) Formation of thymine dimers in mammalian skin by ultraviolet radiation *in vivo*. *Photochem. Photobiol.* **15**, 177–185.

PATHAK, M.A., KRAMER, D.M. and FITZPATRICK, T.B. (1974) Photobiology and photochemistry of furocoumarins (psoralens). In PATHAK, M.A., HARBER, L.C., SEIJI, M. and KUKITA, A. (eds) *Sunlight and Man,* Tokyo: University of Tokyo Press, 335–368.

PEAK, M.J. and PEAK, J.G. (1989) Solar-ultraviolet-induced damage to DNA. *Photodermatology* **6**, 1–15.

PEAK, J.G. and PEAK, M.J. (1990) Ultraviolet light induces double-strand breaks

CHAPTER 53

in DNA of cultured human P3 cells as measured by neutral filter elution. *Photochem. Photobiol.* **52**, 387–393.

PENTLAND, A.P. and JACOBS, S.C. (1991) Bradykinin-induced prostaglandin synthesis is enhanced in keratinocytes and fibroblasts by UV injury. *Am. J. Physiol.* **261**, R543–R547.

PENTLAND, A.P., MAHONEY, M., JACOBS, S.C. and HOLTZMAN, M.J. (1990) Enhanced prostaglandin synthesis after ultraviolet injury is mediated by endogenous histamine stimulation. *J. Clin. Invest.* **86**, 566–574.

PETERSEN, M. J., HANSEN, C. and CRAIG, S. (1992) Ultraviolet A irradiation stimulates collagenase production in cultured human fibroblasts. *J. Invest. Dermatol.* **99**, 440–444.

PIERCEALL, W.E., GOLDBERG, L.H., TAINSKY, M.A., MUKHOPADHYAY, T. and ANANTHASWAMY, H. N. (1991) Ras gene mutation and amplification in human nonmelanoma skin cancers. *Mol. Carcinogen.* **4**, 196–202.

PILENI, M. and SANTUS, R. (1978) On the photosensitizing properties of N-formyl kynurenine and related compounds. *Photochem. Photobiol.* **28**, 525–529.

POPPE, W. and GROSSWEINER, L.I. (1975) Photodynamic sensitization by 8-methoxypsoralen via the singlet oxygen mechanism. *Photochem. Photobiol.* **22**, 217–219.

PUNNONEN, K., AUTIO, P., KIISTALA, U. and AHOTUPA, M. (1991) *In-vivo* effects of solar-simulated ultraviolet irradiation on antioxidant enzymes and lipid peroxidation in human epidermis. *Br. J. Dermatol.* **125**, 18–20.

RAAB, O. (1900) Uber die Wirkung Fluorescierender Stoffe auf Infusoriera. *Z. Biol.* **39**, 525–535.

RADLER-POHL, A., SACHSENMAIER, C., GEBEL, S., AUER, H., BRUDER, J.T., RAPP, U., ANGEL, P., RAHMSDORF, H.J. and HERRLICH, P. (1993) UV-induced activation of AP-1 involves obligatory extranuclear steps including Raf-1 kinase. *EMBO* **12**, 1005–1012.

REEVE, V.E., GREENOAK, G.E., CANFIELD, P.J., BOEHM-WILCOX, C. and GALLAGHER, C.H. (1989) Topical urocanic acid enhances UV-induced tumor yield and malignancy in the hairless mouse. *Photochem. Photobiol.* **49**, 459–464.

REILLY, S.K. and DeFABO, E.C. (1991) Dietary histidine increases mouse skin urocanic acid levels and enhances UVB-induced immune suppression of contact hypersensitivity. *Photochem. Photobiol.* **53**, 431–438.

RIVAS, J.M. and ULLRICH, S.E. (1992) Systemic suppression of delayed-type hypersensitivity by supernatants from uv-irradiated keratinocytes. *J. Immunol.* **149**, 3865–3871.

RODDEY, P.K., GARMYN, M., PARK, H., BHAWAN, J. and GILCHREST, B. A. (1994) Ultraviolet irradiation induces c-fos but not c-Ha-ras proto-oncogene expression in human epidermis. *J. Invest. Dermatol.* **102**, 296–299.

RODIGHIERO, G., DALL'ACQUA, F. and PATHAK, M.A. (1984) Photobiological properties of monofunctional furocoumarin derivatives. In SMITH, K.C. (ed.) *Topics in Photomedicine*, New York: Plenum Press, 319–397.

RONAI, Z., RUTBERG, S. and YANG, Y.M. (1994) UV-responsive element (TGACAACA) from rat fibroblasts to human melanomas. *Environ. Mol. Mut.* **23**, 157–163.

ROSEN, J.E., CHEN, D., PRAHALAD, A.K., SPRATT, T.E., SCHLUTER, G. and WILLIAMS, G.M. (1997) A fluoroquinolone antibiotic with a methoxy group at the 8 position yields reduced generation of 8-oxo-7, 8-dihydro-2'-deoxyguanosine after ultraviolet-A irradiation. *Toxicol. Appl. Pharmacol.* **145**, 381–387.

ROSENSTEIN, B.S. and SETLOW, R.B. (1980) Photoreactivation of ICR 2A frog cells after exposure to monochromatic ultraviolet radiation in the 252–313 nm range. *Photochem. Photobiol.* **32**, 361–366.

ROTHMAN, R.H. and SETLOW, R.B. (1979) An action spectrum for cell killing and pyrimidine dimer formation in hamster V-79 cells. *Photochem. Photobiol.* **29**, 57–61.

SCHENCK, G.O. (1960) Selektivitat und typische Reaktions-mechanismen in der Strahlenchemie. *Z. Electrochem.* **64**, 997–1011.

SCHNEIDER, J.E., PHILIPS, J.R., PYE, G., MAIDT, M.L., PRICE, S. and FLOYD, R.A. (1993) Methylene blue and rose bengal photoactivation of RNA bacterio-phages: Comparative studies of 8-oxoguanine formation in isolated RNA. *Arch. Biochem. Biophys.* **301**, 91–97.

SCHOTT, H.N. and SHETLAR, M.D. (1974) Photoaddition of amino acids to thymine. *Biochem. Biophys. Res. Commun.* **59**, 1112–1116.SETLOW, J.K. and SETLOW, R.B. (1963) Nature of the photoreactivable ultra-violet lesion in deoxyribonucleic acid. *Nature (Lond.)* **197**, 560–562.

SETLOW, J.K. AND SETLOW, R.B. (1963) Nature of the photoreactivable ultra-violet lesion in deoxyribonucleic acid. *Nature (Lond.)* **197**, 560–562.

SHEA, C.R., MCNUTT, N.S., VOLKENANDT, M., LUGO, J., PRIOLEAU, P.G. and

CHAPTER 53

ALBINO, A.P. (1992) Overexpression of *p53* protein in basal cell carcinomas of human skin. *Am. J. Pathol.* **141**, 25–29.

SHERRY, B. and CERAMI, A. (1988) Cachectin/tumor necrosis factor exerts endocrine, paracrine, and autocrine control of inflammatory responses. *J. Cell Biol.* **107**, 1269–1277.

SHETLAR, M.D., SCHOTT, H.N., MARTINSON, H.G. and LIN, E.T. (1975) Formation of thymine-lysine adducts in irradiated DNA-lysine systems. *Biochem. Biophys. Res. Commun.* **66**, 88–93.

SHIMIZU, T. and STREILEIN, J.W. (1994) Evidence that ultraviolet B radiation induces tolerance and impairs induction of contact hypersensitivity by different mechamisms. *Immunology* **82**, 140–148.

SHINDO, Y., WITT, E., HAN, D. and PACKER, L. (1994) Dose-response effects of acute ultraviolet irradiation on antioxidants and molecular markers of oxidation in murine epidermis and dermis. *J. Invest. Dermatol.* **102**, 470–475.

SILVER, M.J. and SMITH, J.B. (1975) Prostaglandins as intracellular messengers. *Life Sci.* **16**, 1635–1648.

SINGH, H. and VADASZ. J.A. (1978) Singlet oxygen: A major reactive species in the furocoumarin photosensitized inactivation of *E. coli* ribosomes. *Photochem. Photobiol.* **28**, 539–546.

SMITH, K.C. (1962) Dose-dependent decrease in extractability of DNA from bacteria following irradiation with ultraviolet light or with visible light plus dye. *Biochem. Biophys. Res. Commun.* **8**, 157–163.

SMITH, K.C. (1974) Molecular changes in nucleic acids produced by ultraviolet and visible radiation. In PATHAK, M.A., HARBER, L.C., SEIJI, M. and KUKITA, A. (eds) *Sunlight and Man,* Tokyo: University of Tokyo Press, 57–66.

SNYDER, D.S. and EAGLSTEIN, W.H. (1974) Intradermal antiprostaglandin agents and sunburn. *J. Invest. Dermatol.* **62**, 47–50.

SOFFEN, G.A. and BLUM, H.F. (1961) Quantitative measurements of cell changes following a single dose of ultraviolet light. *J. Cell. Comp. Physiol.* **58**, 81–96.

SPECHT, K.G. and RODGERS, M.A. (1991) Plasma membrane depolarization and calcium influx during cell injury by photodynamic action. *Biochim. Biophys. Acta* **1070**, 60–68.

SPIKES, J.D. (1975) Porphyrins and related compounds as photodynamic sensitizers. *Ann. N.Y. Acad. Sci.* **44**, 496–508.

STARICCO, R.J. and PINKUS, H. (1957) Quantitative and qualitative data on the pigment cells of adult human epidermis. *J. Invest. Dermatol.* **28**, 33–45.

STEIN, B., RAHMSDORF, H.J., STEFFAN, A., LITFIN, M. and HERRLICH, P. (1989) UV-induced DNA damage is an intermediate step in UV-induced expression of human immunodeficiency virus type 1, collagenase, c-fos, and metallothionein. *Mol. Cell. Biol.* **9**, 5169–5181.

STERENBORG, H.J.C.M. and VAN DER LEUN, J.C. (1990) Tumorigenesis by a long wavelength UV-A source. *Photochem. Photobiol.* **51**, 325–330.

STERN, R.S., THIBODEU, L.A., KLEINERMAN, R.A., PARRISH, J.A., FITZPATRICK, T.B. and 22 PARTICIPATING INVESTIGATORS (1979) Risk of cutaneous carcinoma in patients treated with oral methoxsalen photochemotherapy for psoriasis. *N. Engl. J. Med.* **300**, 809–813.

STERN, R.S. (1989) PUVA: its status in the United States. In FITZPATRICK, T.B., FORLOT, P., PATHAK, M.A. and URBACH, F. (eds) *PSORALENS Past, Present and Future of Photochemoprotection and other biological activities*, Paris: John Libbey Eurotex, 367–376.

STERN, R.S. (1994) Ocular lens findings in patients treated with PUVA. Photochemotherapy Follow-Up-Study. *J. Invest. Dermatol.* **103**, 534–538.

STERN, R.S. (2001) The risk of melanoma in association with long-term exposure to PUVA. *J. Am. Acad. Dermatol.* **44**, 755–761.

STRAUSS, G.H., GREAVES, M., PRICE, M., BRIDGES, B.A., HALL-SMITH, P. and VELLA-BRIFFA, D. (1980) Inhibition of delayed hypersensitivity reaction in skin (DNCB test) by 8-methoxypsoralen photochemotherapy. *Lancet* ii:556–559.

STREILEIN, J.W. (1983) Skin-associated lymphoid tissues (SALT): Origins and functions. *J. Invest. Dermatol.* **80**, 12–16s.

STRICKLAND, P.T., KELLEY, S.M. and SUKUMAR, S. (1985) Cellular transforming genes in mouse skin carcinomas induced by UVB or PUVA. *Photochem. Photobiol.* **41**, Suppl.:110S.

SZABO, G., BLOG, F.B. and KORNHAUSER, A. (1982) Toxic effect of ultraviolet light on melanocytes: Use of animal models in pigment research. *J. Natl. Cancer Inst.* **69**, 245–250.

TAKEUCHI, T., MATSUGO, S., and MORIMOTO, K. (1997) Mutagenicity of oxidative DNA damage in Chinese hamster V79 cells. *Carcinogenesis* **18**, 2051–2055.

TASHJIAN, A.H. JR., VOELKEL, E.F. and LEVINE, L. (1977) Plasma concentrations of 13,14-dihydro-15-keto-prostaglandin E_2 in rabbits bearing the VX_2 carcinoma:

Effects of hydrocortisone and indomethacin. *Prostaglandins* **14**, 309–317.

TODD, P. and HAN, A. (1976) UV-induced DNA to protein cross-linking in mammalian cells. In Smith, K.C. (ed.) *Aging, Carcinogenesis, and Radiation Biology,* New York: Plenum Press, 83–104.

TORNALETTI, S. and PFEIFER, G.P. (1994) Slow repair of pyrimidine dimers at *p53* mutation hotspots in skin cancer. *Science* **263**, 1436–1438.

TURRO, N.J. (1965) *Molecular Photochemistry.* Reading, Mass.: Benjamin.

URBACH, F. (1989) Potential effects of altered solar ultraviolet radiation on human skin cancer. *Photochem. Photobiol.* **50**, 507–513.

URBACH, F., EPSTEIN, J.H. and FORBES, P.D. (1974) Ultraviolet carcinogenesis: Experimental, global and genetic aspects. In PATHAK, M.A., HARBER, L.C., SEIJI, M. and KUKITA, A. (eds) *Sunlight and Man,* Tokyo: University of Tokyo Press, 259–283.

VAN DE VORST, A. and LION, Y. (1976) Indirect EPR evidence for the production of singlet oxygen in the photosensitization of nucleic acid constituents by proflavine. *Z. Naturforsch.* **31C**, 203–204.

VEDALDI, D., DALL'ACQUA, F., GENNARO, A. and RODIGHIERO, G. (1983) Photosensitized effects of furocoumarins: The possible role of singlet oxygen. *Z. Naturforsch.* **38c**, 866–869.

VEDALDI, D., PIAZZA, G., MORO, S., CAFFIERI, S., MIOLO, G., ALOISI, G.G., ELISEI, F., and DALL'ACQUA, F. (1997) 1-Thiopsoralen, a new photobiologically active heteropsoralen. Photophysical, photochemical and computer aided studies. *Farmaco* **52**, 645–652.

VERMA, A.K., LOWE, N.J. and BOUTWELL, R.K. (1979) Induction of mouse epidermal ornithine decarboxylase activity and DNA synthesis by ultraviolet light. *Cancer Res.* **39**, 1035–1040.

VERWEIJ, H., DUBBELMAN, T. and VAN STEVENINCK, J. (1981) Photodynamic protein cross-linking. *Biochim. Biophys. Acta* **647**, 87–94.

WACKER, A., DELLWEG, H. and WEINBLUM, D. (1960) Strahlenchemische Veranderung der bakterien-Deoxyribonucleinsaure *in vivo. Naturwissenschaften* **47**, 447.

WACKER, A., DELLWEG, H., TRAGER, L., KORNHAUSER, A., LODENMANN, E., TURK, G., SELZER, R., CHANDRA, P. and ISHIMOTO, M. (1964) Organic photochemistry of nucleic acids. *Photochem. Photobiol.* **3**, 369–395.

WAGNER, S., TAYLOR, W.D., KEITH, A. and SNIPES, W. (1980) Effects of acridine plus near ultraviolet light on *Escherichia coli* membranes and DNA *in vivo.*

Photochem. Photobiol. **32**, 771–780.

WAMER, W.G., TIMMER, W.C., WEI, R.R., MILLER, S.A. and KORNHAUSER, A. (1995) Furocoumarin-photosensitized hydroxylation of RNA and DNA. *Photochem. Photobiol.* **61**, 336–340.

WAMER, W. G., YIN, J-J., and WEI, R. R. (1997) Oxidative damage to nucleic acids photosensitized by titanium dioxide. *Free Radic. Biol. Med.* **23**, 851–858.

WENNERSTEN, G. and BRUNK, U. (1977) Cellular aspects of phototoxic reactions induced by kynurenic acid I. *Acta Derm. Venereol.* **57**, 201–209.

WENNERSTEN, G. and BRUNK, U. (1978) Cellular aspects of phototoxic reactions induced by kynurenic acid II. *Acta Derm. Venereol.* **58**, 297–305.

WOLFF, K., FITZPATRICK, T.B., PARRISH, J.A., GSCHNAIT, F., GILCHREST, B., HÖNIGSMANN, H., PATHAK, M.A. and TANNENBAUM, L. (1976) Photochemotherapy for psoriasis with orally adminstered methoxsalen. *Arch. Dermatol.* **112**, 943–950.

WOODCOCK, A. and MAGNUS, J.A. (1976) The sunburn cell in mouse skin: Preliminary quantitiative studies on its production. *Br. J. Dermatol.* **95**, 459–468.

WORLD HEALTH ORGANIZATION. (1979) *Ultraviolet Radiation, Environmental Health Criteria* **14**, 18. Geneva: World Health Organization.

YAMADA, H. and HIEDA, K. (1992) Wavelength dependence (150–290 nm) of the formation of the cyclobutane dimer and the (6–4) photoproduct of thymine. *Photochem. Photobiol.* **55**, 541–548.

YAMAIZUMI, M. and SUGANO, T. (1994) UV-induced nuclear accumulation of *p53* is evoked through DNA damage of actively transcribed genes independent of the cell cycle. *Oncogene* **9**, 2775–2784.

YAMAMOTO, F., NISHIMURA, S. and KASAI, H. (1992) Photosensitized formation of 8-hydroxydeoxyguanosine in cellular DNA by riboflavin. *Biochem. Biophys. Res. Commun.***187**, 809–813.

YAROSH, D., BUCANA, C., COX, P., ALAS, L., KIBITEL, J. and KRIPKE, M.L. (1994) Localization of liposomes containing a DNA repair enzyme in murine skin. *J. Invest. Dermatol.* **103**, 461–468.

YOSHIKAWA, T., RAE, V., BRUINS-SLOT, W., VAN DEN BERG., J-W. and TAYLOR, J.R. (1990) Susceptibility to effects of UVB radiation on induction of contact hypersensitiviey as a risk factor for skin cancer in humans. *J. Invest. Dermatol.* **95**, 530–536.

YOSHIKAWA, T., KURIMOTO, I. and STREILEIN, J.W. (1992) Tumor necrosis factor-alpha mediates ultraviolet light B-enhanced expression of contact hypersensitivity. *Immunol.* **76**, 264–271.

YOUNG, A.R. and MAGNUS, I.A. (1981) An action spectrum for 8-MOP induced sunburn cells in mammalian epidermis. *Br. J. Dermatol.* **104**, 541–547.

ZAJDELA, F. and BISAGNI, E. (1981) 5-Methoxypsoralen, the melanogenic additive in sun-tan preparations, is tumorigenic in mice exposed to 365 nm UV radiation. *Carcinogenesis* **2**, 121–127.

ZIERENBERG, B.E., KRAMER, D.M., GEISERT, M.G. and KIRSTE, R.G. (1971) Effects of sensitized and unsensitized longwave UV-irradiation on the solution properties of DNA. *Photochem. Photobiol.* **14**, 515–520.

ZIGMAN, S. (1993) Ocular light damage. *Photochem. Photobiol.* **57**, 1060–1068.

Index

A

Absorption (*See* Percutaneous absorption)
ACD (*See* Allergic contact dermatitis)
Acetone delipidization, 535
ACH (aluminium chlorohydrate), 331
Acnegenesis, cosmetics, 1033–1035
Acneiform irritant dermatitis, 187
Action spectra, ultraviolet, 894–897
Activator protein (AP-1), 1152
Active transdermal drug delivery systems, 641–642
Acute exposure, irritation testing, 679–681
Acute irritant contact dermatitis, 231, 240
Acute irritant dermatitis, 183–184
Acute reactions, 184–185, 485, 487
AD (*See* Atopic dermatitis)
Adhesive tapes (*See* Tape stripping)
Adhesives, transdermal drug delivery systems, 660
ADIS-4030, 158
ADME studies, 425–426, 621–630
Advance Depolarizing Pulse Iontophoretic System (ADIS-4030), 158
Africans, irritation, 199–200
Ageing skin
    barrier function, 57–59
    blood flow, 58
    irritation, 198–199
    permeability, 328
    sodium lauryl sulfate, 491
    water irritation, 475
Agrochemicals, permeability, 8–11
Airborne irritation, 193–194
Alcohol, 304
Alkylating agents, sulfur mustard, 389–408

All-trans-retinoic acid (ATRA), 422–423, 432–433
Allantoin, 512
Allergenic chemicals, 231, 253–255
Allergic contact dermatitis (ACD), 229–235
    animals, 725–727
    barrier creams, 509, 1087–1099
    bonding, 268–271
    clinical features, 240–243
    conformational analysis, 279–281
    cosmetics, 1027–1029
    cross-allergy, 278–281
    cytokines, 246–252
    diagnostic tests, 1015–1017
    excited skin syndrome, 772
    haptens, 267, 273–281
    histology, 243–246
    immunohistochemical studies, 243–246
    immunotoxicology testing, 253–255
    versus irritant contact dermatitis, 237–263
    metabolism, 275–277
    molecular basis, 265–284
    molecular modeling, 279
    patch tests, 184
    prohaptens, 275–277
    prospective testing, 775–792
    reactivity, 270–275
    sensitization mechanism, 795
    standard allergen tests, 770–771
    test methods in humans, 763–774
    transdermal drug delivery systems, 144–145, 633, 634, 636–640, 650
    water irritation, 476
    (*See also* Sensitization)
Allergic reactions, 125, 636

(*See also* Allergic contact dermatitis;
Immunologic contact urticaria)
Alprenolol, 305
Alternative toxicity testing
best performance, 984–989
data collection and analysis, 968–969
good laboratory practice, 969
in vivo toxicity data, 975–976
performance, 961–966, 989–990
prediction models, 963–969, 983
relevance, 960–961, 983–992
reliability, 960, 961–983
reproducibility, 963, 977–982
standard operating procedures,
967–968
supplemental data, 990–992
test substances, 968, 969–975, 977
validation, 957–998
(*See also In vitro* methods)
Aluminium chlorohydrate (ACH), 331
Aluminum hydroxide gel, 512
Amino acids
hapten selectivity, 273–275
ocular phototoxicity, 460
p-Amino compounds, 292–293
p-Aminobenzoic acid (PABA)
isolated perfused porcine skin flaps,
574
skin metabolism, 625
sunscreens, 1056–1059
Amiodarone, 345
Ammonium hydroxide, 1092–1093
Ammonium persulfate, 1053–1054
Amnion fluid, 828
Anaphylactic (Type I) reactions
diagnostic tests, 1010–1011
immediate contact agents, 820
transdermal drug delivery systems,
636
Anatomical differences
barrier function, 43–70
iontophoresis, 165–166
irritation, 195–196
permeability, 328–329
retinoids, 424–425
sodium lauryl sulfate, 492
Anchoring filament protein (GB-3),
397–400
Angelicin, 1127
Animal models
Buehler test, 739–741

contact allergen prospective testing,
777–787
contact dermatitis, 725–762
contact urticaria, 999–1006
cumulative contact enhancement
test, 744–745
ear/flank test, 752–753
epicutaneous maximization test,
745–746
footpad test, 749–750
Freund's complete adjuvant test, 656,
665–666, 736–737, 779–780,
1029
in vitro alternatives, 851, 855–856,
861
irritation testing
cumulative irritation assays,
681–683
Draize rabbit assay, 679–681
immersion assay, 683
mouse ear model, 683–684
transdermal drug delivery
systems, 660–661
local lymph node assays, 793–816
modified Draize test, 737–739
modified guinea pig maximization
test, 742–744
nonimmunologic contact urticaria,
831–832
open epicutaneous test, 741–742
optimization test, 734–736
sensitization factors, 729
sensitization testing, transdermal
drug delivery systems,
634–635, 656, 660–661,
664–668
single-injection adjuvant test,
746–748
split adjuvant technique, 732–734
tierexperimenteller nachweis test,
748–749
transdermal drug delivery systems,
634–635, 656, 664–668
(*See also* Guinea pig; Murine; Rabbit)
Animal use reduction, PB-PK models,
592
Animal welfare, local lymph node
assays, 800, 806
Animal-triggered contact dermatitis,
725–762
Antabuse, 294

Antibiotics, 291–292
Anticancer drugs, 781–782
Anticholinergic action, 634
Antihistamines, 292
Antiperspirants, 1065
Antisolvent gels (*See* Barrier creams)
AP-1 (activator protein), 1152
Apoptosis, sulfur mustard, 401
Appetite suppressants, 366–367
Aqueous (*See* Water)
Aroclor 1242, 555–556, 558
Aroclor 1254, 555–556, 558
Aromatic hydrocarbon solvents,
    358–359
Arsenic, 556–557, 558
Asians, irritation, 199–200
Atopic dermatitis (AD), 125, 126–128
    evaporimetry, 940–941
    irritation, 201–202
    sodium lauryl sulfate, 495
    transdermal drug delivery systems,
        633–634
ATRA (all-trans-retinoic acid), 422–423,
    432–433
Atrazine, 5–7
Autooxidative tissue damage, 211
Azone self-enhanced percutaneous
    absorption, 92–93

B

Baboon syndrome, 291
Baby products, 1065–1066
Bacitracin, 291
Bacterial DNA, 787
Balanced salt solutions, 624
Balsam of Peru, 233, 302–303
BAP (*See* Benzo(a)pyrene)
Barrier creams, 507–516, 1087–1103
    animal models, 681–682
    application method, 511
    definition, 509–510
    effective duration, 510–511
    efficacy, 511
    human models, 689–690
    ideal properties, 512–513
    in vitro models, 1089–1090
    in vivo models, 1090–1095
    mechanism of action, 510–511
    US FDA identified protectants,
        511–512

utilization reasons, 510
Barrier function, 13–28
    aging, 57–59
    anatomical factors, 43–70
    blood flow, 55–57
    dermis, 45, 49–50
    diseases, 59–60
    epidermis, 45–49, 697
    evaporimetry, 940–944
    hair follicles, 53–55
    lipid role, 73
    occlusion, 16–18
    powdered human stratum corneum,
        112–113
    quantification, 18–21
    regional differences, 50–53
    sebaceous glands, 53–55
    skin structure, 45–49
    species differences, 50–53
    squamometry, 944–949
    subclinical changes, 937–955
    sweat glands, 53–55
Bath preparations, 1066
Benzene, 605, 606
Benzo[a]pyrene (BAP)
    diffusion cell arrays, 927–929
    percutaneous absorption, 86–87,
        95–97, 553–555, 556, 558
    skin metabolism, 627
Benzocaine, 625–626
Benzoic acid, 625
Benzoisothiazides, 1045
Benzophenones, 1060
Benzyl alcohol, 626–627
Bergapten (5-MOP), 344, 874,
    1132–1133
Berlock dermatitis, 344
Best performance, validation testing,
    984–989
Bikini dermatitis, 343
Binding, PB-PK models, 600, 609
Bioavailability, multiple dosing, 89–90
Bioengineering, 488–490, 690
Biologic endpoints, 485–491
Biologically effective irradiance, 893
Biomarkers, 570–572
Biopsies, 573
Biotransformation, cutaneous, 578–579
Birch pollen allergies, 828
Bleaches, hair products, 1053–1054
Bleomycin, 363

Blister agents (*See* Vesicants)
Blood flow
    aging, 58
    barrier function, 55–57
    lag time, 88
Bone, retinoids, 433–434
Borates, skin permeability, 7–8
BPA (bullous pemphigoid antigen),
    397–400
Breast implants, 362
Bronopol, 1045
Buehler test, 739–741
Bullous pemphigoid antigen (BPA),
    397–400
Bunsen-Roscoe Law, 881, 885
Butylated hydroxyanisole, 304

C

C. parvum (Propionibacterium acnes),
    780
Cadaver stratum corneum, 704–712, 713
Cadmium, 86–87, 556–567, 558
Cadmium sulfide, 345
Calamine, 512
Camphors, 1060
Cancer chemotherapy drugs, 781–782
Capacitance, occlusion, 19
Carbon chain length, sodium lauryl
    sulfate, 482
Carcinogenesis
    dietary factors, 413–415
    genetic disposition, 413
    immunity, 413
    prevention, 414–415
    research trends, 409–418
    ultraviolet, 411–412, 893
    viruses, 412–413
β-Carotene, 1131
Cashew nuts, 302
Caucasians
    irritation, 199–200
    sensitive skin, 128, 129–131
CCET (cumulative contact enhancement
    test), 744–745
Cell culture
    human epidermis, 851–862
    ocular phototoxicity, 462
    transdermal drug delivery systems,
    661–663
Cellular mediators, 1141–1147

Censored data, 965
Central nervous system (CNS), 434
Ceramides, 75–77
CFA (*See* Complete Freund's adjuvant)
Chamber scarification tests, 688
Chamomile, 303
Chemical decontamination, 114–115
Chemical partitioning, 105–121
Chemical toxicity studies, 913–933
Chemical-specific parameters, 604–606
Chemically defined media, 851–854, 861
Chemically induced scleroderma,
    353–373
    environmental agents, 355–356
    iatrogenic agents, 362–365
    nonprescription drugs, 365–367
    occupational agents, 357–362
Chemicals in clothing, 97–98
Chemokines, 246–248
Chemoprevention, 414–415
Chemotherapy drugs, 781–782
China, cosmetics, 441–448
Chlordane, 553–555, 556, 558
Chlorpromazine, 343
Cholesterol, 76
Chromatin, 1123–1125
Chromium, 299–301, 329
Chromophores, 893
Chronic contact dermatitis, 240
Chronic phototoxic exposure, 1108
Cinnamates, 1059
Cinnamic aldehyde, 1031, 1032
Cisplatin, 363
Clonidine, 145, 634–636, 650–651
Clothing
    percutaneous absorption, 97–98
    problems wearing, 510
CMC (critical micelle concentration),
    711–712
CNS (central nervous system), 434
Coal-tar derivatives, 345, 1048–1049,
    1052–1054
Cobalt, 299–301
Cocaine, 367
Cocoa butter, 512
Colony stimulating factors (CSF),
    247–450, 1143
Color (*See* Pigmentation)
Colorimetry, 19, 489, 536
Coloring preparations (*See* Dyes)
Comedogenesis, cosmetics, 1033–1035

Commercial mutagenicity tests, 916
Compartments choice, PB-PK models,
    607–608
Competing ions, iontophoresis, 163–164
Complete Freund's adjuvant (CFA),
    736–737, 1029
    contact allergen prospective testing,
        779–780
    transdermal drug delivery systems,
        656, 665–666
Complex chemical mixtures
    interaction levels, 31–34
    interaction types, 34–38
    percutaneous absorption, 29–41
Compliance, transdermal drug delivery,
    144
Computer simulations, PB-PK models,
    606
Concentration effects, 163
Concentration profiles, 142
Condylomata acuminata, 475
Conformational analysis, 279–281
Contact allergens, 775–792
Contact chemical allergy, 1003
Contact dermatitis
    animal models, 725–726
    barrier creams, 1087–1099
    diagnostic tests, 1015–1017
    (See also Allergic contact dermatitis;
        Irritant contact dermatitis)
Contact sensitization (See Allergic
        contact dermatitis;
        Sensitization)
Contact urticaria
    animal models, 999–1006
    contact chemical allergy, 1003
    diagnostic tests, 1007–1020
    drug eruptions, 1009–1015
    mechanisms, 1001–1002, 1004
    patch testing, 1010, 1013, 1014–1015
    photopatch testing, 1014
    protein allergy, 1003
    respiratory chemical allergy,
        1002–1003
    subjective irritation, 1019
Contact urticaria syndrome (CUS),
    817–848
    agents causing, 820–826
    cosmetics, 1029–1033
    definition of terms, 819–820
    diagnostic tests, 833–835

immediate contact reactions,
    819–820, 1017–1019
immunologic contact urticaria,
    826–828
nonimmunologic contact urticaria,
    829–832
protein contact dermatitis, 828–829
    (See also Eczema)
Contaminated soil/water, 549–561
Coordinate bonds, 269
Core biopsies, 573
Corneal damage, 463
Corneocytes, 533, 939, 945, 949
Corrositex®, 685–686
Corrosive chemicals, 679
Corticosteroids, 279–281, 293–294
Cosmetic contact dermatitis, 443–444
Cosmetic intolerance syndrome,
    1067–1068
Cosmetic photosensitive dermatitis, 444
Cosmetics, 1021–1086
    acnegenesis, 445, 1033–1035
    allergic contact dermatitis,
        1027–1029
    baby products, 1065–1066
    bath preparations, 1066
    China, 441–448
    comedogenesis, 1033–1035
    contact urticaria syndrome,
        1029–1033
    cutaneous reactions, 1024–1042
    depilatories, 1066–1067
    emulsifiers, 1046–1047
    epilating waxes, 1067
    eye makeup, 1047–1049
    facial makeup, 1054–1055
    guinea pig allergy test, 750–752
    hair, 445–446, 1041–1042,
        1049–1054, 1068–1070
    immunologic contact urticaria,
        1032–1033
    ingredient testing, 750–752,
        1042–1043
    irritation, 1024–1027
    lanolin, 1047
    nails, 446, 1041, 1061–1064
    nonimmunologic contact urticaria,
        1030–1032
    objective irritation, 1024–1026
    occupational dermatitis, 1068–10670
    oral hygiene products, 1064

patch testing, 1042–1043
personal hygiene products, 1065
photosensitivity, 1037–1041
pigmentation, 444–445, 1035–1037,
     1063
preservatives, 1043–1046
sensitive skin, 128, 129–131
subjective irritation, 1026–1027
sunscreens, 1056–1061
Costus resinoid, 303
Counter ions, permeability, 325, 330
Covalent bonds, 268–269
Crenotherapy, 476
Critical micelle concentration (CMC),
     711–712
Critical photon energy, 885–886
Cross-allergy, 278–281
Crystal violet, 1092
CSF (colony stimulating factors),
     247–250, 1142–1143
Cumulative contact enhancement test
     (CCET), 744–745
Cumulative irritation, 186, 473
     animal models, 681–683
     human models, 687–688
     sodium lauryl sulfate, 481, 482, 485,
          487
Current density, iontophoresis, 164–165
Cutaneous biotransformation, 578–579
Cutaneous efflux profile prediction, 576
Cutaneous hyperthermia, 641
Cutaneous reactions, cosmetics,
     1024–1042
Cy (cyclophosphamide), 781
Cyclobutane-type pyrimidine dimers,
     1118–1121, 1123
Cyclophosphamide (Cy), 781
Cytochrome P450, 426
Cytokines
     allergic contact dermatitis, 232–233,
          246–252
     immunoadjuvants, 782–787
     irritant contact dermatitis, 239,
          246–252
     phototoxicity, 1142–6
     water irritation, 476
Cytotoxic (Type II) reactions, 1011–1012

D

D-Squame tape, 536, 537, 538–539

2,4-D, 553–555, 556, 558, 559
DAG (diacylglycerol), 1131
DDT, 85–87, 95–97, 553–555, 556, 558
Decontamination, chemical, 114–115
Delayed, acute irritant contact dermati-
     tis, 184
Delayed hypersensitivity (Type IV)
     reactions, 1014–1015
Delayed type contact sensitivity, 170
Delayed type hypersensitivity (DTH),
     1027–1028
     immunoadjuvants, 777–780, 782
     transdermal drug delivery systems,
          633
Delayed type reactions, 232
Delipidization, 534–535, 539, 540
Delirium, transdermal scopolamine, 634
Dendritic cells, 246
Dentifrices, 1064
Deodorants, 1065
Depigmentation, 375–387
     agents, 377–382
     hydroquinone, 379, 1036–1037
     mechanism, 382–384
Depilatories, 1066–1067
Depot formation, 327
Dermal risk assessment, 581–582
Dermatopharmacokinetics, 575–578,
     581–582
Dermatophytosis complex, 475
Dermis, 33, 45, 49–50
Descriptive data, 965
Desmosomal protein, 397–400
Desmosomes, 939
Detergents, 360
     (See also Sodium lauryl sulfate;
          Surfactants)
Diabetes, reverse iontophoresis, 171
Diacylglycerol (DAG), 1131
Diagnostic tests
     contact dermatitis, 1015–1017
     contact urticaria, 1007–1020
     contact urticaria syndrome,
          1017–1019
     drug eruptions, 1009–1015
     reverse iontophoresis, 171–172
     skin sensitization potential, 767, 772
     subjective irritation, 1019
Diaper rashes, 475
Diazinon, 98–99
Dibenzoylmethanes, 1060

Dietary factors, carcinogenesis, 413–415
Diethyl hexyl phthalic acid, 574
Diethylpropion, 366
Differentiation, lipids, 73, 74
Diffusion cells
    chemical toxicity studies, 913–933
    in vitro methods, 521–523
    lactate production, 915
    lactic dehydrogenase, 914–915
    mitochondrial oxidation, 915
    mutagenicity tests, 916–933
    nucleoside analysis, 919
    RNA terminal metabolites, 916–933
    skin viability maintenance, 624
    statistical analysis, 907–908, 919–921
    test system, 903–904
    vehicle formulation, 904–913
Dihydroxyacetone, 1120
Dihydroxyphenylalanine (DOPA), 382,
    1130
Dimethicone, 512
Dimethyl-*p*-aminobenzoic acid, 344
2,4-Dimethylamine, 574
Dinitrochlorobenzene (DNCB), 254,
    1145
Dinitrofluorobenzene (DNFB), 251, 1145
Dipolar bonds, 268
Diseases
    barrier function, 59–60
    irritation, 201–203
    powdered human stratum corneum,
        113
    sodium lauryl sulfate, 495–496
    vinyl chloride, 357
Disulfuram, 294
DNA
    gene expression, 1150–1153
    immunostimulatory, 787
    mutations in cellular phenotype,
        1137–1140
DNA-protein cross-links, 1121–114
DNCB (dinitrochlorobenzene), 254,
    1145
DNFB (dinitrofluorobenzene), 251, 1145
DOPA (dihydroxyphenylalanine), 382,
    1130
Doppler blood flow, 488–489
Dosimetry, ultraviolet, 881–883,
    891–894
5-Doxyl stearic acid (5-DSA), 701–703,
    704, 705

Draize tests
    human patch tests, 687
    modified, 737–739
    rabbit irritation assays, 679–681
    transdermal drug delivery systems,
        660–661, 663
Dressings, 16
Drug delivery (*See* Iontophoresis;
        Transdermal drug delivery
        systems)
Drug detection, tape stripping, 539–541
Drug eruptions, contact urticaria,
    1009–1015
Drug induced ocular phototoxicity,
    449–470
Drug–drug interactions, 29–41
5-DSA (5-Doxyl stearic acid), 701–703,
    704, 705
DTH (*See* Delayed type hypersensitivity)
Dyes, 1052–1054
Dyslipidemias, 430–432

E

Ear/flank test, 752–753
ECVAM (*See* European Centre for the
        Validation of Alternative
        Methods)
Eczema, 125
    clinical features, 240
    contact urticaria, 819–820, 833
    irritation, 202–203
    protein contact dermatitis, 828–829
    sodium lauryl sulfate, 495
Eczema rubrum, 287
Edema, 874
EEC toxicity testing, 664, 667
Electric shock, iontophoresis, 169
Electrically-assisted transdermal drug
        delivery systems, 641–642
Electrode materials, iontophoresis,
        159–160
Electron microscopy, 571
Electron paramagnetic resonance (EPR)
    membrane structure, 698
    ocular phototoxicity, 458–459
    principles, 698–700
    reading spectra, 703–704
    spectrometers, 700–701
    spin labeling method, 698, 701–705,
        717

stratum corneum measurement,
704–715
technique, 698–704
Electron spin resonance (ESR) (*See*
Electron paramagnetic
resonance)
Electroosmosis, 154, 156
Electrophiles, sulfur mustard, 389–408
Electroporation, 146
Emulsifiers, 1046–1047
(*See also* Sodium lauryl sulfate)
Enhanced topical formulation, 115–116
Environmental contaminants
chemically induced scleroderma,
355–356
complex chemical mixtures, 34–38
irritation, 192–193
percutaneous absorption, 51–52,
85–87, 95–98
powdered human stratum corneum,
113–114
skin permeability, 9–11
Eosinophilia-myalgia syndrome,
365–366
Epicutaneous maximization test,
745–746
EpiDerm™, 685–686
Epidermal barrier function, 45–49, 697
Epidermal cell cultures, 662–663,
849–877
Epilating waxes, 1067
EPISKIN™, 685–686
Epoxy resins, 359–360
EPR (*See* Electron paramagnetic resonance)
Ergot methysergide, 364–365
Erythema
iontophoresis, 170
phototoxicity, 874, 1127–1130
sulfur mustard, 401–403
systemic contact dermatitis, 290
transdermal drug delivery systems,
143, 635, 637, 640
ESCD guidelines, 485, 486
ESR (electron spin resonance) (*See*
Electron paramagnetic
resonance)
Essential fatty acids, 60
Estradiol, 638–639, 650–651
Estrogen/progesterone, 640, 651
Ethosuximide, 364

Ethyl aminobenzoate (benzocaine),
625–626
Ethylacetoacetate, 1121
Ethylenediaminetetraacetate, 1090
Eugenol, 1032
European Centre for the Validation of
Alternative Methods (ECVAM),
801
European Society of Contact Dermatitis
(ESCD), 485, 486
Evaluation periods, sodium lauryl sulfate
reaction, 484
Evaporimetry, 489, 940–944
Exanthema, 300
Excited skin syndrome, 494–495, 772
Excoriation, 635
Excretion, PB-PK models, 600
Explosions, nitroglycerin patches, 637
Exposure times, ultraviolet, 873–874
Exsiccation eczema, 125, 187–188
Extrapolation, PB-PK models, 592–593,
610–612
Eyes
cosmetics, 1047–1049
structure/function, 451–453
transdermal scopolamine delivery
systems, 634
(*See also* Ocular phototoxicity)

F

Facial makeup, 1054–1055
Fatty acids, 76
FCA (*See* Freund's complete adjuvant)
FDA (*See* US Food and Drug
Administration)
Fentanyl, 640–641, 650–651
FF (free formaldehyde) hardeners, 1062
Fibronectin, 397–400
Fick's first law of membrane diffusion,
332–333
Fingertip dermatitis, 473
Finn chambers, 483, 485
Flare-up reactions, 287–288, 289–290,
292–293
Flow-through diffusion cells, 521–523
Fluence (rate), 883
Flux equations, 599–600
Foam insulation, 356
Follicles (hair), 53–55, 160–162
Follicular spongiosis, 244

Foods
carcinogenesis, 413–415
immunologic contact urticaria,
821–822, 828
nonimmunologic contact urticaria,
825, 830
Footpad test, 749–750
Formaldehyde, 1045
Fragrances, patch testing, 1042–1043
Free formaldehyde (FF) hardeners, 1062
Freund's complete adjuvant (FCA),
736–737, 1029
contact allergen prospective testing,
779–780
transdermal drug delivery systems,
656, 665–666
Friction dermatitis, 188–189
Furocoumarins, 1124, 1127, 1131–1133

G

gadd45 gene, 1153–1154
Gamma-interferon (IFN-gamma),
782–784
Garlic, 304
GB-3 (anchoring filament protein),
397–400
Gel electrophoresis, 460
Gell and Coombs classification, 231
Gender
iontophoresis, 165–166
irritation, 201
sodium lauryl sulfate, 491–492
Gene expression
epidermal cell culture, 853
phototoxicity, 1150–1153
Genetic disposition, carcinogenesis, 413
German chamomile, 303
Gloves, problems wearing, 510
GLP (good laboratory practice), 969
Glucose utilization, 570, 624–625
Glucowatch® Biographer, 171–172
Glutathione reductase, 384
Glycerin, 512
Glyceryl monothioglycolate (GMT),
1050, 1069–1070
Glyphosphate, 97–98
GM-CSF (granulocyte-macrophage
colony-stimulating factor),
247–250, 1143
GMT (glyceryl monothioglycolate),

1050, 1069–1070
Gold, 301
Goldenrod, 303
Goldman constant field approximation,
156
Good laboratory practice (GLP), 969
GPMT (guinea pig maximization test),
731–732, 742–744
Granulocyte-macrophage colony-
stimulating factor (GM-CSF),
247–250, 1144
Grape skins, 413
Growth factors, 246–248
Guinea pig maximization test (GPMT),
731–732
modified, 742–744
Guinea pig models
contact allergy tests, 727–729,
750–752, 777–781
cosmetic ingredients, 750–752
cumulative irritation assays, 681–683
ear swelling test, 831–832
immersion assays, 683
immunoadjuvants, 778–780, 781
murine local lymph node assay, 796,
800
non-adjuvant methods, 777–778
nonimmunologic contact urticaria,
831–832
transdermal drug delivery systems,
634, 656, 660–661, 664–666

H

Ha-ras proto-oncogene, 1139
Hair, cosmetics, 445–446, 1041–1042,
1049–1054
Hair follicles
barrier function, 53–55
iontophoresis, 160–162
species differences, 54
Hairdressers, occupational dermatitis,
184–185, 1068–1070
Halothane, 605, 606
Hands
eczema, 495
fingertip dermatitis, 473
Hapten–protein bond, 275
Haptens, 267, 273–281
Hazard identification, 796–802
Hazardous substances, 85–87, 549–561

HDL (high density lipoproteins), 430–432
Healing phase, 490–491
Heavy metals, 86–87, 299–301
Hematogenic eczema, 125
Hematoporphyrin (HP), 1137
Henna, 1053
Hexachlorobenzene, 356
Hexachlorophene, 323
Hexane, 605, 606
High density lipoproteins (HDL), 430–432
High pressure liquid chromatography (HPLC), 461, 919
Hispanics, irritation, 199–200
Histamine, 830
Histological analysis, 854–857, 859, 861–862
Histopathologic changes, 485, 487–488
Homeostatic controls, 329
Host-related factors, 491–496
HP (hematoporphyrin), 1137
HPLC (high pressure liquid chromatography), 461, 919
Human papillomaviruses (HPV), 412–413
Humans
    allergic contact dermatitis, test methods, 763–774
    epidermal *in vitro* tests, 849–869
    extrapolation to, PB-PK models, 610–612
    irritation tests, 686–690, 849–869
    phototoxicity tests, 849–869
    surfactant effects on stratum corneum, 705, 712–715
Hydrating agents, 146, 210
Hydration, sodium lauryl sulfate, 493
Hydration dermatitis, 17–18, 19
Hydrocortisone
    cross-allergy, 280–281
    multiple dosing, 92–93
    systemic contact dermatitis, 293–294
Hydrogen peroxide, 1053–1054
Hydrophobic bonds, 268
Hydroquinone, 88, 379, 1036–1037
Hyperirritable skin, 494–495
Hyperkeratosis, 244, 1033
Hyperostosis, 433
Hyperpigmentation
    cosmetics, 444–445

depigmenting, 377, 379
phototoxicity, 344
sulfur mustard, 403
transdermal drug delivery systems, 635, 639
Hyperplasticity, 244
Hypersensitivity, 171
    (*See also* Delayed type hypersensitivity)
Hypomelanosis, 377, 380
Hypopigmentation
    tert-butyl catechol, 379
    cosmetics, 444–445
    sulfur mustard, 403
    transdermal drug delivery systems, 635
Hyposensitization, 301–302

I

Iatrogenic agents, 362–365
ICAM-1 (intercellular adhesion molecule), 252, 1145
ICCVAM (*See* Interagency Coordinating Committee on the Validation of Alternative Methods)
ICD (*See* Irritant contact dermatitis)
Ichthyosis, 60, 202
ICU (*See* Immunologic contact urticaria)
IFN-gamma (gamma-interferon), 782–784
IL (*See* Interleukins)
Imidazolidinyl urea, 1044
Immediate contact reactions, 819–820
    diagnostic tests, 1017–1019
    (*See also* Contact urticaria syndrome)
Immersion tests
    animal models, 683
    human models, 688–689
    sodium lauryl sulfate, 486
Immune complex-mediated (Type II) reactions, 1012–1014
Immunity, carcinogenesis, 413
Immunoadjuvants
    complete Freund's adjuvant, 779–780
    contact allergen prospective testing, 775–792
    cyclophosphamide, 781
    cytokines, 782–787
    gamma-interferon, 782–784
    immunostimulatory DNA, 787

Interleukin-10, 786
Interleukin-12, 784–787
local anticancer drugs, 781–782
plasmids, 780, 786–787
Propionibacterium acnes, 780
Immunoglobin E (Ig E), 820, 826–828
Immunologic contact urticaria (ICU)
agents, 821–825
animal models, 999–1006
contact chemical allergy, 1003
cosmetics, 1032–1033
diagnostic tests, 833–835
IgE-mediated, 826–828
mechanisms, 1001–1002
protein allergy, 1003
respiratory chemical allergy,
1002–1003
Immunological adjuvants (See
Immunoadjuvants)
Immunological immediate contact
reactions, 1017–1018
Immunostimulatory DNA, 787
Immunotoxicology testing, 253–255
In vitro methods
alternatives to animal models, 851,
855–856, 861, 957–998
barrier creams, 1089–1090
diffusion receptor fluid absorption,
557, 558
epidermal constructs, 854–857, 859,
861–862
epidermal phototoxicity, 855–859
human epidermis, 849–869
iontophoresis, 157–158
irritation testing, 661–664, 684–686,
849–869
metabolism studies, 621–630
ocular phototoxicity, 459–463
percutaneous absorption, 519–529
phototoxicity testing, 849–869
sensitization testing, 666
skin metabolism, 621–630
tissue viability analysis, 859
transdermal drug delivery systems,
661–664, 666
In vitro-in vivo correlation, iontophoresis,
167–168
In vivo methods
alternative toxicity testing validation,
975–976
barrier creams, 1090–1095

iontophoresis, 158–159
irritation testing, 660–661, 663–664
isolated perfused porcine skin flaps,
575–576
ocular phototoxicity, 463–464
percutaneous absorption, 557, 558
sensitization testing, 664–668
transdermal drug delivery systems,
660–661, 663–668
Incomplete Freund's adjuvant, 778–779
Individual differences, 93–94
Induration, 635
INF (interferons), 782–784, 1143
Inflammation, cosmetics, 445
Ingredient patch testing, 1042–1043
Interagency Coordinating Committee
on the Validation of
Alternative Methods (ICC-
VAM), 800
Intercellular adhesion molecule-1
(ICAM-1), 252, 1144
Intercellular lamellae, 77–78
Intercellular lipids, 695–723
Intercorneocyte spaces, 533, 534
Interferons (INF), 782–784, 1143
Interlaboratory variability, 980–981
Interleukins (IL), 247–251, 1143–1145
Interleukin-1 alpha, 854–858,
860–861
Interleukin-8 alpha, 854–859,
860–861
Interleukin-10 (Il-10), 786
Interleukin-12 (Il-12), 784–787
Intradermal tests, 1010, 1013, 1017
Intraexperiment variability, 979
Intralaboratory variability, 979–980
Inverse Square Law (radiometry), 886
Invisible gloves (See Barrier creams)
'Invisible irritation', 949
Involucrin, 245
Ion transport pathways, 160–162
Ionic bonds, 268
Iontophoresis, 146, 151–180
advantages, 168
animal models, 160
competing ions, 163–164
concentration effects, 163
continuous versus pulsed current,
166
contraindications, 171
current density, 164–165

dermatological applications, 171–172
disadvantages, 169–171
electrode materials, 159–160
historical perspectives, 153–154
in vitro devices, 157–158
in vitro-in vivo correlation, 167–168
in vivo devices, 158–159
ion transport pathways, 160–162
molecular size, 163
pH effects, 162–163
sex differences, 165–166
site of application, 165–166
species differences, 165–166
theory, 154–157
IPPSF (*See* Isolated perfused porcine skin
        flaps)
Irradiance, 881, 883
Irritable skin, definition, 131–132
Irritant contact dermatitis (ICD), 679
    versus allergic contact dermatitis,
        237–263
    barrier creams, 509, 1087–1099
    clinical features, 188, 240–243
    cytokines, 246–252
    diagnostic tests, 1015–1017
    histology, 243–246
    immunohistochemical studies,
        243–246
    immunotoxicology testing, 253–255
    localization, 189
    transdermal drug delivery systems,
        143–144, 633–634
    water, 473, 475, 476
Irritation, 181–228
    acneiform irritant dermatitis, 187
    acute irritant dermatitis, 183–184
    age differences, 198–199
    airborne, 193–194
    anatomical differences, 195–196
    clinical aspects, 183–189
    cosmetics, 1024–1027
    cumulative irritant dermatitis, 186
    delayed, acute irritant contact
        dermatitis, 184
    environmental factors, 192–193
    exposure, 191–192
    exsiccation eszematoid, 187–188
    external factors, 190–194
    friction dermatitis, 188–189
    gender, 201
    histology, 206–208

histopathology, 206–208
in vitro epidermal analysis, 855–859
irritant reaction, 184–185
mechanism, 208–209
pathology, 206–208
population differences, 199–200
predictive irritancy testing, 203–206
predisposing factors, 194–203
pustular irritant dermatitis, 187
sensitive skin, 125
sensitization differentiation *in vitro*,
        860
skin diseases, 201–203
subclinical, 937–955
suberythematous irritation, 185
subjective/sensory irritation, 185,
        1019, 1026–1027
surfactant effects on stratum
        corneum intercellular lipids,
        697, 717
traumatic irritant dermatitis, 187
traumiterative irritant dermatitis, 187
treatment, 209–211
(*See also* Irritant contact dermatitis;
        Nonimmunologic)
Irritation testing, 677–694
    animal models, 679–684
    bioengineering methods, 690
    human models, 686–690
    in vitro assays, 684–686
    transdermal drug delivery systems,
        660–664
Isofenphos, 100–101
Isolated perfused porcine skin flaps
        (IPPSF), 563–588
    absorption studies, 572–574
    advantages, 565–566
    applications, 570–580
    cutaneous biotransformation,
        578–579
    dermal risk assessments, 581–582
    dermatopharmacokinetics, 575–578,
        581–582
    method overview, 567–570
    surgical preparation and perfusion,
        567–570
    vasoactive chemicals, 579–580

J

Japanese

cosmetics, 1035
irritation, 199–200
sensitive skin, 128, 129–131

K

Kaolin, 512
Kava, 303
Keratinization, 48–49
Keratinocytes, 232–233, 239
Keratohyalin granules, 474–475

L

Labeling of cosmetics, 1042–1043
Lacquer trees, 302
Lactate production, 571, 915, 923
Lactic acid test, 1019
  (*See also* Stingers)
Lactic dehydrogenase (LDH), 859,
  914–915, 923, 932
Lag time, percutaneous absorption,
  87–88
Lamellae (*See* Intercellular lamellae)
Lamellar granules, 74
Lamellated bodies, 46
Laminin, 397–400
Langerhans cells (LC), 45
  allergic contact dermatitis, 231,
    246–249
  irritant contact dermatitis, 246–249
  occlusion, 473
  skin sensitization, 795
Lanolin, 1047
Laser Doppler flowmetry (LDF), 19,
  488–489
Laser Doppler velocimetry (LDV), 19,
  20–21, 55–56, 88
Laser flash photolysis, 458–459
Latex rubber, 234, 827–828
Law of Conservation of Radiance, 886
LC (*See* Langerhans cells)
LDF (laser Doppler flowmetry), 19,
  488–489
LDH (lactic dehydrogenase), 859,
  914–915, 923, 932
LDV (laser Doppler velocimetry), 19,
  20–21, 55–56, 88
Lead acetate, 924–925
Lens damage, 463
Lesions, sulfur mustard, 397–405
Leukoderma, 377, 379–380, 1036

Lidocaine, 580, 581
Light microscopy, 571
Light transmission, eyes, 452–453
Light-induced dermal toxicity (*See*
  Phototoxicity)
Lipid envelope, 74–75
Lipids
  chemical structures, 75–77
  differentiation, 73, 74
  intercellular, surfactant effects,
    695–723
  intercellular lamellae, 77–78
  lamellar granules, 74
  percutaneous absorption, 71–81
  peroxidation hypothesis, 394
  regional differences, 52–53
  retinoids, 430–432
  stratum corneum, 533–534
    delipidization, 534–535, 539, 540
Lipoproteins, 430–432
LLNA (*See* Local lymph node assays)
LNC (lymph node cells), 795
  (*See also* Local lymph node assays)
Local anticancer drugs, 781–782
Local lymph node assays (LLNA)
  contact allergens, 793–816
  development, 796–798
  EC3 values, 803–805
  evaluation/validation, 798, 800–802
  international regulatory status, 802
  relative potency assessment, 802–805
  risk assessment, 805–806
  stimulation index, 797–798, 803
  transdermal drug delivery systems,
    656, 666–668
Localization, irritant contact dermatitis,
  189
Log P (octanol/water partition coefficient), 521
Luminescence, ocular phototoxicity,
  458–459
Lumped compartments, PB-PK models,
  595, 600–601
Lupus vulgaris, 171
Lymph node cells (LNC), 795
  (*See also* Local lymph node assays)

M

Macrolide antibiotics, 210–211
Maculo-papular rashes, 291

Magnetophoresis, 146
Malathion, 97–98
Management structure, validation
    testing, 967
Manicure (*See* Nails)
Marker compounds, 31–32, 570–572
Mass balance equations, 600–604
Mass spectrometry (MS), 460
Matrix-controlled devices, 140–141
Maturation (*See* Ageing skin)
Mazindol, 366
MBEH (monobenzyl ether of hydro-
    quinone), 377, 381–382
MDCM (mechanistically-defined
    chemical mixtures), 32, 35
MDT (modified Draize test), 737–739
MEA (multiple endpoint analysis),
    854–862
Mechanistically-defined chemical
    mixtures (MDCM), 32, 35
Melanin, 382, 383
Melanocytes, 45, 1130
Melanoma, 411
Membrane-controlled devices, 140–141
Mercury, 86–87, 300–301, 556–557, 558
Merkel cells, 45
Merthiolate, 305
Messenger RNA (mRNA), 1150
Metabolic constants, 605–606, 609
Metabolism
    allergic contact dermatitis, 275–277
    in vitro methods, 621–630
    PB-PK models, 600
    transdermal drug delivery systems,
        657
Metal salts, 801
Metals
    detection methods, 541–542
    percutaneous absorption, 556–557
    permeability, 321–340
    systemic contact dermatitis, 299–301
5-Methoxypsoralen (5-MOP), 344, 874,
    1133–1134
8-Methoxypsoralen (8-MOP), 344–345,
    347, 1129, 1133–1134
Methyl chloroform, 551–552
Methyl salicylate, 626–627
Mice (*See* Murine models)
Microbial growth, diffusion cells, 930
Microneedles, 642
Micropore tape, 536, 537, 538–539

Microscopy, 571
Minimal erythema doses (MEDs), 1112
Mitochondrial oxidation, 915
Mitomycin C, 294–295
Model irritants, 481
Models
    chemical partitioning, 105–121
    percutaneous absorption, 94–97
    pharmacokinetic, isolated perfused
        porcine skin flaps, 575–578
    physiologically-based pharmacoki-
        netic, 589–619
    QSARs, 116–118
    validation, 609–610
    (*See also* Animal models;
        Physiologically-based pharma-
        cokinetic models)
Modified Draize test (MDT), 737–739
Modified guinea pig maximization test,
    742–744
Moisturizers, 474–475, 509–510
    (*See also* Hydrating agents)
Molecular size, 163
Molecular volume, 325
Monobenzyl ether of hydroquinone
    (MBEH), 377, 381–382
Monosodium lauryl glutamate (SLG),
    706–711
5-MOP (5-methoxypsoralen), 344, 874,
    1133–1134
8-MOP (8-methoxypsoralen), 344–345,
    347, 1129, 1133–1134
Morphological endpoints, 571
Mouse ear sensitivity test (MEST), 656,
    666–668
    (*See also* Murine models)
Mouthwashes, 1064
mRNA (messenger RNA), 1152
MS (mass spectrometry), 460
MTT test, 854–855, 861–862
Mucocutaneous toxicity, 429–430
Multiple dosing
    Azone self-enhanced percutaneous
        absorption, 92–93
    bioavailability, 89–90
    percutaneous absorption, 89–93
Multiple endpoint analysis (MEA),
    854–862
Multiple simultaneous exposures,
    190–192
Murine models

cumulative irritation assays, 681
immunoadjuvants, 780–787
local lymph node assays, 796–807
mouse ear model, irritation testing,
    683–684
transdermal drug delivery systems,
    635, 656, 666–668
Musk xylol, 526–527
Mutagenicity tests, 916–933

N

Nails, cosmetics, 446, 1041, 1061–1064
Natural moisturizing factors (NMF),
    474–475
Natural rubber latex, 234, 827–828
NCE (new chemical entities), 656,
    659–660
Neomycin, 291
Nernst-Planck flux equation, 154–155,
    156–157
New chemical entities (NCE), 656,
    659–660
Nickel
    allergic responses in animal models,
        801
    barrier creams, 1090, 1091
    cosmetics, 1070
    systemic contact dermatitis, 287, 294,
        295–299
Nicorandil, 52
Nicotinates, 17
Nicotine, 637–638, 650–651
NICU (See Nonimmunologic contact
    urticaria)
(14C) 2 Nitro-p-phenylenediamine
    (2NPPD), 628–629
Nitrogen mustards, 391
Nitroglycerin
    explosion dangers, 637
    transdermal drug delivery systems,
        636–637, 650–651
Nitroxide molecules, 701–702
NMF (natural moisturizing factors),
    474–475
NMSC (non-melanoma skin cancer), 411
Non-eczematous atopic dry skin, 60
Nonimmunologic contact urticaria
    (NICU), 825–826, 829–832,
    833
    animal models, 999–1006

cosmetics, 1030–1032
    mechanisms, 1004
Nonimmunologic drug eruptions,
    1009–1010
Nonimmunologic immediate contact
    reactions, 1018–1019
Noninvasive bioengineering techniques,
    488–490
Non-linear processes, PB-PK models,
    591–592
Non-melanoma skin cancer (NMSC),
    411
Nonprescription drugs, 365–367
Nonpyrethroid subjective irritation,
    1026
Nonqualified data, 966
Non-sensitizing skin irritants, 801–802
Nonsteroidal anti-inflammatory drugs
    (NSAIDs), 345–346, 830
Norepinephrine, 580, 581
Normalization for photons absorbed,
    461–462
North American Contact Dermatitis
    Group, 767, 772
2NPPD ((14C) 2 nitro-p-phenylenedi-
    amine), 628–629
NSAID (non-steroidal anti-inflammatory
    drugs), 345–346, 830
Nucleophilic addition, 271
Nucleophilic substitution, 270–271
Nucleoside analysis, 919
Nummular eczema, 125

O

Objective irritation, 1024–1026
Occlusion, 13–28
    barrier function, 16–18
    hydration dermatitis, 17–18, 19
    quantification, 18–21
    sodium lauryl sulfate, 486
    subclinical barrier changes, 947–948
    transdermal drug delivery, 143
    water irritation, 473–475
Occupational agents
    chemically induced scleroderma,
        357–362
    contact dermititis, barrier creams,
        509, 510
    dermatitis, hairdressers, 184–185,
        1068–1070

Octanol/water partition coefficient (Log P), 521
Ocular phototoxicity
  biophysical studies, 458–459
  drug induced, 449–470
  eye structure/function, 451–453
  in vitro studies, 459–463
  in vivo studies, 463–464
  mechanism, 457–458
  protection measures, 464
  short screen prediction, 454–455
  tissue culture, 462–464
  xenobiotics, 453
Odland bodies, 46
OECD (*See* Organization for Economic Cooperation and Development)
OET (open epicutaneous test), 741–742
One-chambered diffusion cells, 521–523
Open applications
  animal irritant testing, 682–683
  sodium lauryl sulfate, 481, 482, 486
Open epicutaneous test (OET), 741–742
Open tests, contact urticaria, 1010, 1018
Optimization test, 734–736
Oral agents, phototoxicity, 344
Oral hygiene products, 1064
Order parameter S, 703–704, 707–717
Organic solvents, 359
Organization for Economic Cooperation and Development (OECD), 658, 660, 664, 667–668
Over-the-counter (OTC) products, 365–367, 511–512

P

p53 gene, 1138–1140, 1152–1153
PABA (p-aminobenzoic acid), 574, 625, 1056–1059
Parabens, 304
Parabens esters, 1044
Parathion, 35–36, 579
PARP (poly(ADP-ribose) polymerase), 393–395
Participating laboratories, validation testing, 967, 981–982
Partition coefficients, 604–605, 609
Partitioning, chemical, 105–121
Passive topical kinetic model, 576–578
Patch testing

ACD versus ICD, 243
contact dermatitis, 1015–1017
contact urticaria, 1010, 1013, 1014–1015
cosmetics, 1038–1041, 1042–1043
drug eruptions, 1009–1015
human irritation, 686–687
sodium lauryl sulfate, 481, 482
standard patch test series, 1016–1017
(*See also* Transdermal drug delivery systems)
PB-PK models (*See* Physiologically based pharmacokinetic models)
PCBs (polychlorinated biphenyls), 555, 558
PCT (photochemotherapy), 1132–1133
PDT (photodynamic therapy), 1137
Pearson correlation, 984–985
Penicillamine, 364
Penicillins, 291–292
Pentachloroethylene, 552
Pentachlorophenol, 553–555, 556, 558
Pentazocine, 363
Peptide immunization, 542
Peptide regulatory factors (PRF), 246
Percent of dose absorbed, 334
Perchloroethylene, 357–358
  metabolic constants, 606
  partition coefficients, 605
  percutaneous absorption, 552
Percutaneous absorption, 83–102
  Azone self-enhanced, 92–93
  chemicals in clothing, 97–98
  complex chemical mixtures, 29–41
  contaminated soil/water, 549–561
  diazinon, 98–99
  differentiation, 73, 74
  diffusion cell arrays, 901–935
  hair follicles, 53–54
  hazardous substances, 85–87
    from soil/water, 549–561
  human *in vivo*, 98–101
  in vitro and *in vivo* models, 94–97
  in vitro methods, 93–94, 519–529, 625–629
  individual differences, 93–94
  intercellular lamellae, 77–78
  isofenphos, 100–101
  isolated perfused porcine skin flaps, 572–574, 579–580
  lag time, 87–88

lamellar granules, 74
lipid envelope, 74–75
lipids, 71–81
multiple dosing, 89–93
piperonyl butoxide, 99–100
powdered human stratum corneum,
    111–112
pyrethrin, 99–100
regional differences, 51–52
short-term exposure, 85–87
skin permeability, 3–11
soil load, 557–558, 559
stratum corneum, 48, 71–81
versus tape stripping, 539–542
transdermal drug delivery, 139–140
vasoactive chemicals, 579–580
Performance measures, validation
    testing, 961–966
Perfusion (See Isolated perfused porcine
    skin flaps)
Periungual verrucae, 475
Permanent waves, 1049–1050
Permeability, 3–11
    age of skin, 328
    anatomical site, 328–329
    atrazine, 5–7
    borates, 7–8
    constants, in vitro methods, 527
    counter ions, 325
    depot formation, 327
    descriptors, 332–333
    dose, 324–325
    homeostatic controls, 329
    metal diffusion, 321–340
    molecular volume, 325
    pH effects, 327
    polarity, 325–326
    protein reactivity, 327
    risk assessment, 8–11
    solubility, 327
    strata, 329
    time factors, 327–328
    valence, 326–327
    vehicle, 325
    xenobiotics, 329–330
    (See also Percutaneous absorption)
Permeation coefficient, 332–333
Personal hygiene products, 1065
Pesticides, 361–362, 579
Petrolatum, 512, 1090, 1096
PG (prostaglandins), 1140–1142

PH effects
    iontophoresis, 162–163
    permeability, 327
    water irritation, 475
Pharmacokinetic models, 575–578,
    589–619
Phenanthrene, 627
Phenols, 378, 379
meta-Phenylenediamine, 360
Phenylenediamine (PPD), 1052–1053,
    1069–1070
Phonophoresis, 146
Photo tests, 1015
Photobiologically effective dose, 884
Photocarcinogenesis, 893
Photochemical waves, 146
Photochemotherapy (PCT), 1133–1134
Photodynamic therapy (PDT), 1138
Photoimmunology, 1147–1151
Photoirritation (See Phototoxicity)
Photometry, 882–883
Photon quantities, 884
Photopatch testing, 1014, 1038–1041
Photosensitivity, 444, 1037–1041
Photosensitized oxidations, 1135–1138
Photosensitizers, 454–457
Phototoxicity, 341–352, 1105–1178
    agents, 344–346
    cellular mediators, 1141–1147
    cellular targets, 1116
    DNA-protein cross-links, 1122–1125
    gene expression, 1151–1154
    in vitro epidermal analysis, 855–859
    investigative procedures, 348–349
    isolated perfused porcine skin flaps,
        572
    mechanisms, 347, 1116–1122
    mutations in cellular phenotype,
        1139–1141
    non-steroidal anti-inflammatory
        drugs, 345–346
    ocular, drug induced, 449–470
    photochemical mechanisms,
        1113–1118
    photoimmunology, 1147–1151
    photosensitized oxidations,
        1135–1138
    psoralens, 344–345, 347–349, 874,
        1116–1118, 1125–1134
    quantitative, 881–883
    tests, 346–347

in humans, 871–877
thymine photoproducts, 1117,
    1120–1122
transdermal drug delivery systems,
    658–659
ultraviolet characteristics, 1108–1113
Physiologically based pharmacokinetic
    (PB-PK) models, 589–619
    components, 594–606
    development, 606–613
    failure, 612
    future, 613
    nomenclature, 613–614
    percutaneous absorption, 551–553
    reason for use, 591–593
    situations of use, 594
    value, 612
Phytoalexins, 413
Phytosphingosines, 75–77
Pig ears, 566
Pig skin preparations
    chemical toxicity studies, 913–933
    lactate production, 915
    lactic dehydrogenase, 914–915
    mitochondrial oxidation, 915
    mutagenicity tests, 916–933
    nucleoside analysis, 919
    RNA terminal metabolites, 916–933
    statistical analysis, 907–908, 919–921
    test system, 903–904
    vehicle formulation, 904–913
    (See also Isolated perfused porcine
        skin flaps)
Pigmentation
    cosmetics, 444–445, 1035–1037, 1063
    depigmentation, 375–387,
        1036–1037
    hyperpigmentation, 344, 377, 379,
        403, 444–445, 635, 639
    hypopigmentation, 379, 403,
        444–445, 635
    occlusion, 19
    repigmentation, 381–382
    sodium lauryl sulfate, 492–493
    sulfur mustard, 403
    transdermal drug delivery systems,
        635, 639
Piperonyl butoxide, 99–100
Piroxicam, 56, 346
PKC (protein kinase C), 1132
Plant species, phototoxicity, 344

Plasmids, 780, 786–787
Poison ivy, 231, 276
Polarity, permeability, 325–326, 330
Poly(ADP-ribose) polymerase (PARP)
    hypothesis, 393–395
Polychlorinated biphenyls (PCBs),
    555–556, 558
Polymers/polymer extracts, 659–660
Population differences
    irritation, 199–200
    sensitive skin, 128, 129–131
    sodium lauryl sulfate, 492–493
Porphyrins, 454–457, 1118, 1135–1137
Powdered human stratum corneum
    (PHSC), 105–121
    barrier function, 112–113
    chemical decontamination, 114–115
    chemical partitioning, 109–111
    diseased skin, 113
    enhanced topical formulation,
        115–116
    environmental contaminants,
        113–114
    percutaneous absorption, 111–112
    physical properties, 108–109
    QSAR predictive modeling, 116–118
PPD (phenylenediamine), 1052–1053,
    1069–1070
Predictive methods
    irritation, 203–206
    skin sensitization potential, 766–767,
        768
    transdermal drug delivery systems,
        653–675
    validation, 963–969, 983
Preliminary irritation tests, 730
Preservatives, 1043–1046
Pretreatments, 636–637, 641
Prevesication, 396
Pre-work creams/gels (See Barrier creams)
PRF (peptide regulatory factors), 246
Prick tests, 1010, 1012
Prickle cell layer (See Stratum spinosum)
Primary irritation (See Acute irritant
        dermatitis)
Progesterone/estrogen, 640, 651
Prohaptens, 275–277
Pro-inflammatory mediators, 854–859,
        860–861
Prophylactics, 145
Propionibacterium acnes (P. acnes or C.

parvum), 780
Propylene glycol, 305
Prospective testing, 775–792
Prostaglandins (PG), 1141–1143
Protective clothing, 510
Protective creams/gels/ointments (*See* Barrier creams)
Protein allergy, 1003
Protein contact dermatitis, 819–820, 828–829
Protein kinase C (PKC), 1132
Protein reactivity, 327
Provocative testing, 481–482, 486
Provocative use tests, 1015
Pruritus, 473, 635
Psoralens, 344–345, 347–349, 874, 1116–1118, 1125–1134
Psoriasis
   allergic contact dermatitis, 244
   barrier function, 59–60
   irritation, 202
Pulse radiolysis, 458–459
Pustular irritant dermatitis, 187
Pyranocoumarins, 1128
Pyrethrin, 99–100
Pyrethroids, 1026–1027
Pyrimidine, 1124
Pyrimidine dimers, 1117, 1120–1122
Pyrocatechols, 1036–1037

Q

Q18B (quaternium-18 bentonite), 511, 1090, 1091, 1096–1097
QSAR (quantitative structure-activity relationship), 116–118, 656–657
Quantitative phototoxicity, 881–883
Quantitative structure-activity relationship (QSAR), 116–118, 656–657
Quantum quantities, 884
Quaternium-15, 1045
Quaternium-18 bentonite (Q18B), 511, 1090, 1091, 1096–1097
Quinoline antimalarials, 345

R

Rabbit models
   cumulative irritation assays, 682–683
   Draize tests, 660–661, 679–681

perfused skin systems, 566
transdermal drug delivery systems, 660–661
Race (*See* Population differences)
Radiance, 883
Radiant exposure, 881, 883
Radiant intensity, 884
Radioallergosorbent test (RAST), 1010–1011
Radiometry, 882, 883–884, 885–886
RAST (radioallergosorbent test), 1010–1011
Rat Skin Transcutaneous Electrical Resistance (TER) Assays, 685–686
Raynaud's phenomenon, 360, 362, 366
Receptor fluids, 524–525, 916–933
Receptor interactions, 428
Redness (*See* Erythema)
Reference set of test substances (RSTS), 968, 969–975, 977
Regional differences, 50–53
Relevance, validation, 960–961, 983–992
Reliability, validation, 960, 961–983
Repeat animal patch (RAP) test, 681
Repeat application patch testing, 682
Repetitive irritation test (RIT), 681–682
Repigmentation, 381–382
Reproducibility, validation, 963, 977–982
Reservoir-controlled devices, 140–141
Respiratory chemical allergy, 1002–1003
Respiratory depression, 641
Resveratrol, 413
Retinal damage, 463
13-cis-Retinoic acid, 422–423
Retinoids, 419–439
   ADME studies, 425–426
   adverse effects, 428–434
   anatomical site, 424–425
   binding, 423–424
   bone, 433–434
   central nervous system, 434
   classification, 421–423
   dyslipidemias, 430–42
   metabolism, 426–427
   mucocutaneous toxicity, 429–430
   pharmacokinetics, 426
   receptor interactions, 428
   species differences, 424–425
   teratogenicity, 432–433

triglycerides, 431
Retinyl palmitate, 627
Reverse iontophoresis, 171
Rhus
    allergies, 276
    barrier creams, 1092–1093
    dermatitis, 301–302
Risk assessment
    complex chemical mixtures, 31
    dermatopharmacokinetic templates,
        581–582
    error types, 9–11
    local lymph node assays, 805–806
    permeability, 8–11
    systemic contact dermatitis, 304–305
RNA terminal metabolites, 916–933
Rosacea, 125
RSTS (reference set of test substances),
        968, 969–975, 977
Rubber latex, 234, 827–828
'Rule of Ten' (radiometry), 886
Rutaceae, 344

S

Salicylates, 1059
Salicylic acid, 574, 904–913
SAR (structure-activity relationship), 656
Scaling, TDDS, 635
Scleroderma (*See* Chemically induced
        scleroderma)
Scopolamine, 144, 633–634, 650–651
Scratch tests, 1010, 1012
Scratch-chamber tests, 1010, 1018
Screening, ultraviolet, 873
Sculptured nails, 1063
Sebaceous glands, 53–55, 160–162
Seborrheic dermatitis, 495–496
Selenium, 414
Sensitive skin, 123–135
    cosmetics, 128, 129–131
    definition, 131–132
    population differences, 128, 129–131
    self reported, 126–128
    sodium lauryl sulfate, 493–494
    symptoms, 125–126
Sensitization
    animal models, 727–729
    classification, 731
    contact urticaria, 1002
    cosmetics, 1028

irritant contact dermatitis, 239
irritation differentiation *in vitro*, 860
mechanism, 795
occlusion, 19
relative potency assessment, 803
systemic contact dermatitis, 292
transdermal drug delivery systems,
        144, 145, 664–668
(*See also* Allergic contact dermatitis)
Sensitization potential
    diagnostic tests, 767, 772
    predictive tests, 766–767, 768
Sensory irritation (*See* Subjective
        irritation)
Sensory nerves, 830–831
Serum concentration-time profile,
        575–576
Sex (*See* Gender)
Shampoos, 1051–1052
Shark liver oil, 512
Short screen prediction, 454–455
Short-term exposure, 85–87
SIAT (single-injection adjuvant test),
        746–748
Silica, 360–361
Single continuous exposure, 90–92
Single-injection adjuvant test (SIAT),
        746–748
Skin cancer, 409–18
Skin color (*See* Pigmentation)
Skin compartments, PB-PK models,
        597–599, 601–602
Skin metabolism, 621–630, 657
Skin protective creams (SPCs) (*See* Barrier
        creams)
Skin sensitization potential
    diagnostic tests, 767, 772
    predictive tests, 766–767, 768
Skin structure, barrier function, 45–49
Skin viability assays, 624–625
SkinEthic®, 854
SLG (monosodium lauroyl glutamate),
        706–711
SLS (*See* Sodium lauryl sulfate)
Soap chamber techniques, 689
Sodium fluoride, 924–925
Sodium lauryl sulfate (SLS), 191–192,
        244, 479–506
    allergic contact dermatitis, 233
    application methods, 481–485
    barrier creams, 1090, 1091,

1092–1093
biologic endpoints, 485–491
ESCD guidelines on exposure tests, 485, 486
host-related factors, 491–496
local lymph node assays, 801–802
stratum corneum intercellular lipids, 705–715
subclinical barrier changes, 947–949
Soil, hazardous substances, 549–561
Soil load, 557–558, 559
Solubility, permeability, 327
Solvents
    chemically induced scleroderma, 358–359
    delipidization of stratum corneum, 534–535
    percutaneous absorption, 551–553
SOPs (standard operating procedures), 967–968
Sorbic acid, 304
SPCs (skin protective creams) (*See* Barrier creams)
Species differences
    barrier function, 50–53
    hair follicles, 54
    iontophoresis, 165–166
    PB-PK models, 592–593
    retinoids, 424–425
Species-specific physiological parameters, 608
Specificity, nonimmunologic contact urticaria, 832
Spectral bands, 884–885
Spectral quantities, 884
Spectroradiometers, 889, 892
Spin labeling, 698, 701–5, 717
Split adjuvant technique, 732–734
Spongiosis, 243–244
Squamometry, 944–949
Standard allergens, 770–771
Standard operating procedures (SOPs), 967–968
Standard patch test series, 1016–1017
Staphylococcus aureus, 16
Static diffusion cells, 521–522
Stearamidoethyl diethylamine phosphate, 1046–1047
Stevens test (*See* Ear/flank test)
Stimulation index, 797–798, 803
Stingers, 131–132, 1019, 1026

Stinging tests, 128, 129–131
Straighteners, hair, 1051
Stratum basale, 45–46
Stratum corneum (SC)
    barrier function, 47–49, 71
    cadaver, 704–712, 713, 714
    complex chemical mixtures, 32–33
    description, 533–534
    EPR spectroscopy, 698–705
    intercellular lamellae, 77–78
    lamellar granules, 74
    lipid envelope, 74–75
    lipid role in barrier function, 73
    lipid structures, 75–77
    metal permeability, 334–335
    occlusion, 15, 17, 19
    percutaneous absorption, 48, 71–81
    physical properties, 108–109
    removal methods, 534–536
    stripped human, 705, 712–715
    surfactant effects on intercellular lipids, 695–723
    tape stripping, 531–548
    thickness, tape stripping, 537–539
    transdermal drug delivery, 139–140, 146
    water role, 715–717
    (*See also* Barrier function; Powdered human stratum corneum)
Stratum granulosum, 46–47
Stratum lucidum, 47
Stratum spinosum, 46
Stray radiation, 896
Streptomycin, 292
Stripped human stratum corneum, 705, 712–715
Stripping (*See* Tape stripping)
Structure-activity relationship (SAR), 656
Styrene, 605, 606
Subacute reactions, 487
Subclinical changes, 940–949
Suberythematous irritation, 185
Subjective irritation, 185, 1019, 1026–1027
Sulfonamides, 292
Sulfur mustard, 389–408
    apoptosis, 401
    biochemical mechanism, 393–396
    clinical features, 401–403
    diagnosis, 404
    histopathology, 396–397

immunohistochemistry, 397–400
lesions, 397–405
long-term effects, 405
management of lesions, 404–405
toxicity, 392–393
ultrastructure, 396–397
Sunscreens, 344, 1056–1061
Surfactants
    animal immersion tests, 683
    cosmetics, 1046–1047
    human immersion tests, 688–689
    intercellular lipid effects, 695–723
    mutagenicity tests, 926–927
    subclinical barrier changes, 947–949
    (*See also* Sodium lauryl sulfate)
Surgical procedures, 567–570
Susceptibility evaluation, 481–482, 486
Sweat ducts, 160–162
Sweat glands, 53–55
Systemic challenge, 1010, 1011
Systemic contact dermatitis, 285–320
    antibiotics, 291–292
    antihistamines, 292
    chromium, 299–301
    clinical features, 289–291
    cobalt, 299–301
    corticosteroids, 293–294
    diagnosis, 305–306
    gold, 301
    immunology, 287–289
    mercury, 300–301
    nickel, 287, 294, 295–299
    para-amino compounds, 292–293
    plant species, 301–304
    risk assessment, 304–305
Systemic toxicity, 636, 641

T

T cells
    allergic contact dermatitis, 231, 239,
        245, 267
    immunoadjuvants, 777, 779,
        782–783, 784
    irritant contact dermatitis, 245
Tape stripping
    versus peptide immunization, 542
    versus percutaneous absorption/pen-
        etration, 539–542
    stratum corneum, 531–548
        removal methods, 534–536

versus stratum corneum thickness,
    537–539
stripping factors, 536–539
TDDS (*See* Transdermal drug delivery
    systems)
Tea tree oil, 303
Temperature
    sodium lauryl sulfate evaporation,
        483–484
    transdermal drug delivery systems,
        638, 641
TER (transcutaneous electrical resis-
    tance), 685–686
Teratogenicity, retinoids, 432–433
Testosterone, 640, 650–651
Tetracyclines, 345
TEWL (*See* Transepidermal water loss)
Theophylline, 574
Thermal injury, ultraviolet, 892
Thin layer chromatography (TLC), 461
Thioglycolic acid, 1050
Thiol depletion hypothesis, 394
Thymine, 1125–1126
Thymine photoproducts, 1118–1121
Tierexperimenteller nachweis test
    (TINA), 748–749
Tissue compartments, 595–597
Tissue culture, 462–464, 661–663,
    851–854
Tissue distribution profiles, 573–574
Tissue viability, 854–855, 856–857, 859,
    861–862
Titanium dioxide, 1061
TLC (thin layer chromatography), 461
TMA (trimellitic anhydride), 1002–1003
TMP (8-trimethylpsoralen), 1133–1134
TNCB (trinitrochlorobenzene), 253–254,
    1003
TNF (tumor necrosis factors), 247–249,
    782, 1143–1146
Tolazoline, 580, 581
Toluene, 605, 606
Toluene sulfonamide/formaldehyde
    resin (TSFR), 1062
Topical corticoids, 19, 22, 210
Topical drug delivery, 904
Topical skin protectants (*See* Barrier
    creams)
Toxic oil syndrome, 355–356
Toxicity, chemical, 913–933
Toxicity testing

alternative methods, 957–998
best performance, 984–989
data collection and analysis, 968–969
good laboratory practice, 969
in vivo toxicity data, 975–976
performance, 961–966, 989–990
prediction models, 963–969, 983
relevance, 960–961, 983–992
reliability, 960, 961–983
reproducibility, 963, 977–982
standard operating procedures, 967–968
supplemental data, 990–992
test substances, 968, 969–975, 977
transdermal drug delivery systems, 653
validation, 957–998
Toxicokinetic analysis-pharmacokinetic analysis, 658
Toxicology evaluation plan, 655–660
TPIS (Transdermal Periodic Iontophoretic System), 158, 166
Transcription factors, 1152
Transcutaneous electrical resistance (TER) assays, 685–686
Transdermal drug delivery systems (TDDS), 137–150, 631–651
active drug delivery, 641–642
advantages, 141–142
adverse reactions, 143–145
clonidine, 634–636
devices, 140–141
disadvantages, 142–143
estradiol, 638–639
estrogen, 640
fentanyl, 640–641
formulations, 141
irritation testing, 660–664
matrix systems, 639
nicotine, 637–638
nitroglycerin, 636–637
occlusion, 18, 19
percutaneous absorption, 139–140
predictive toxicology, 653–675
progesterone, 640
prophylactic measures against ACD, 145
reservoir systems, 639
scopolamine, 633–634
sensitization testing, 664–668

testosterone, 640
toxicology evaluation plan, 655–660
Transdermal Periodic Iontophoretic System (TPIS), 158, 166
Transdermal therapeutic systems (TTS) (*See* Transdermal drug delivery systems)
Transepidermal water loss (TEWL)
occlusion, 18, 20–21
sodium lauryl sulfate, 483, 484, 485, 488–490
subclinical barrier changes, 940–944
Transmission electron microscopy, 571
Transpore tape, 536, 537, 538–539
Traumatic irritant dermatitis, 187
Traumiterative irritant dermatitis, 187
Trichloroethylene, 357–358, 551–552
Triglycerides, 431
Trimellitic anhydride (TMA), 1002–1003
8-Trimethylpsoralen (TMP), 1133–1134
1,3,5-Trinitrobenzene, 925–926, 931
Trinitrochlorobenzene (TNCB), 253–254, 1003
Triple therapy (*See* Multiple dosing)
Tropical-immersion-foot, 473
L-Tryptophan, 365–366
TSFR (toluene sulfonamide/formaldehyde resin), 1062
TTS (transdermal therapeutic systems) (*See* Transdermal drug delivery systems)
Tubercle bacilli, 779
(*See also* Complete Freund's adjuvant)
Tumor necrosis factors (TNF), 247–924, 782, 1143–1146
Two-chambered diffusion cells, 523
Type IV collagen, 397–400
Tyrosine hydroxylase, 384

U

UK Health and Safety Executive, 802
Ulcerations, 188–189
Ultrasound, 489
Ultraviolet (UV)
action spectra, 894–897
carcinogenesis, 411–412
cellular mediators, 1141–1147
characteristics, 1108–1113
cosmetics, 444, 1037–1041
DNA-protein cross-links, 1122–1125

dosimetry, 881–883, 891–894
gene expression, 1151–1154
irritation, 211
isolated perfused porcine skin flaps,
    572
lamp sources, 875, 886–889
measuring and quantifying exposure,
    879–900
mutations in cellular phenotype,
    1139–1140
nonimmunologic contact urticaria,
    831
photobiology, 891
photoimmunology, 1147–1151
photosensitized oxidations,
    1135–1138
phototoxicity, 1105–1178
phototoxicity testing, 871–877
psoralens, 1125–1134
radiometry, 882, 883–884, 885–886
screening, 873
spectral bands, 884–885
sunscreens, 1056–1061
thymine photoproducts, 1117,
    1120–1122
transmission through eye, 452–453
(*See also* Phototoxicity)
Umbelliferae, 344
Urea, barrier creams, 1092–1093
Urea formaldehyde foam insulation, 356
Urocanic acid, 1111–1112, 1121,
    1150–1151
US Food and Drug Administration (FDA)
identified skin protectants, 511–512
transdermal drug delivery systems,
    655–656, 658, 667, 668

V

Valence, permeability, 326–327
Validation
    best performance, 984–989
    data collection and analysis, 968–639
    definition, 960–961
    flowchart, 962
    good laboratory practice, 969
    in vivo toxicity data, 975–976
    interlaboratory variability, 980–981
    intraexperiment variability, 979
    intralaboratory variability, 979–680
    management structure, 967

participating laboratories, 967,
    981–982
PB-PK models, 609–610
performance, 961–966
prediction models, 963–969, 983
relevance, 960–961, 983–992
reliability, 960, 961–983
reproducibility, 963, 977–982
standard operating procedures,
    967–968
test substances, 968, 969–975, 977
toxicity testing, 957–998
toxicological test methods, agencies,
    800–801
Vascular function, 570
Vasoactive chemicals, 579–580
Venous flux, 572–574
Vesicants, sulfur mustard, 389–408
Vesicular hand eczema, 290
Vesiculation, 635
Viability assays, 624–625
Viable epidermis, 33
Viable skin maintenance, 624
Vinyl chloride disease, 357
Viruses, carcinogenesis, 412–413
Visual scoring schemes, 485, 487
Vitamin A, 433
Vitamin D, 433
Volatile chemicals, 604–605

W

Water
    hazardous substances, 549–561
    irritation, 471–478
    solubility, percutaneous absorption,
        521
    stratum corneum surfactant effects,
        715–717
Weak allergen testing, 778
Wheal-and-flare reactions, 819, 833
White petrolatum, 512
Whole tissue culture, 462
Withdrawal
    nicotine patches, 638
    scopolamine patches, 634
Wound dressings, 16

X

Xanthotoxin (8-MOP), 344–345, 347,
    1129, 1133–1134

Xenobiotics
    ocular phototoxicity, 453
    permeability, 329–330
m-Xylene, 605, 606

Z

Zinc acetate, 512
Zinc carbonate, 512
Zinc oxide, 512